To my parents

MY MOTHER

Frances Mary

AND IN LOVING MEMORY OF MY FATHER

Arnold Lawrence

who taught me to always love, care, and be the best that I could be!

TO MY GRANDMOTHER

Beatrice Elizabeth Profiglio

my memories of her caring and love will remain in my heart forever.

SAUNDERS COMPREHENSIVE REVIEW for NCLEX-PN

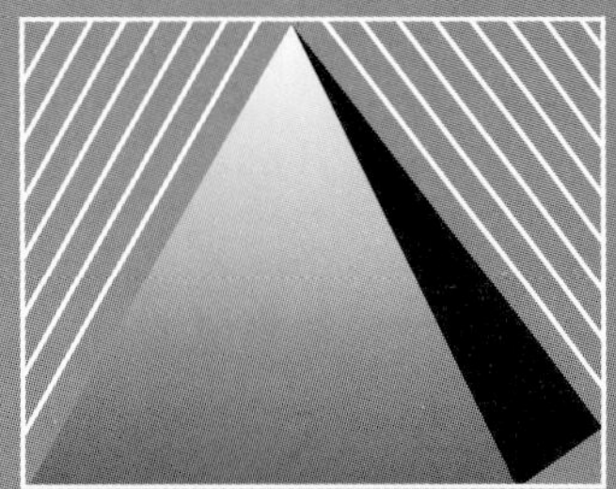

SAUNDERS COMPREHENSIVE REVIEW for NCLEX-PN

LINDA ANNE SILVESTRI, MSN, RN

Assistant Professor of Nursing,
Salve Regina University,
Newport, Rhode Island;
President, Nursing Reviews, Inc. and
Professional Nursing Seminars, Inc.
Charlestown, Rhode Island

SECOND EDITION

SAUNDERS
An Imprint of Elsevier

SAUNDERS
An Imprint of Elsevier

11830 Westline Industrial Drive
St. Louis, Missouri 63146

SAUNDERS COMPREHENSIVE REVIEW FOR NCLEX-PN ISBN 0-7216-9718-6

NOTICE

Nursing is an ever-changing field. Standard safety precautions must be followed, but as new research and clinical experience broaden our knowledge, changes in treatment and drug therapy may become necessary or appropriate. Readers are advised to check the most current product information provided by the manufacturer of each drug to be administered to verify the recommended dose, the method and duration of administration, and contraindications. It is the responsibility of the licensed prescriber, relying on experience and knowledge of the patient, to determine dosages and the best treatment for each individual patient. Neither the publisher nor the author assumes any liability for any injury and/or damage to persons or property arising from this publication.

Previous edition copyrighted 2000

International Standard Book Number 0-7216-9718-6

Vice President and Publishing Director, Nursing: Sally Schrefer
Executive Editor: Loren S. Wilson
Senior Developmental Editor: Michele D. Hayden
Publishing Services Manager: Patricia Tannian
Project Manager: Melissa Mraz Lastarria
Book Design Manager: Gail Morey Hudson
Cover Design: Jen Brockett

KI/MVB
Printed in United States of America

Last digit is the print number: 9 8 7 6 5

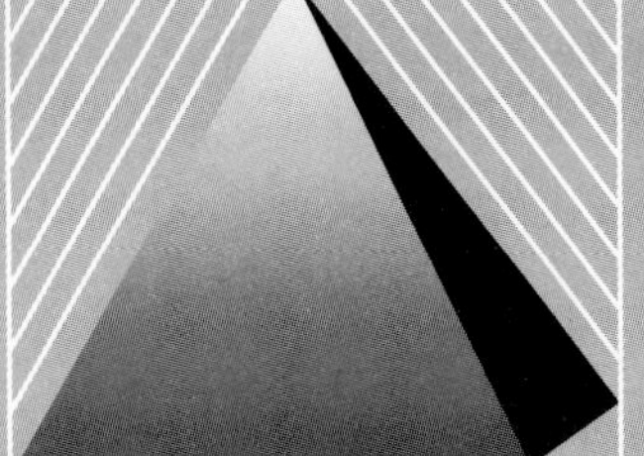

About the Author

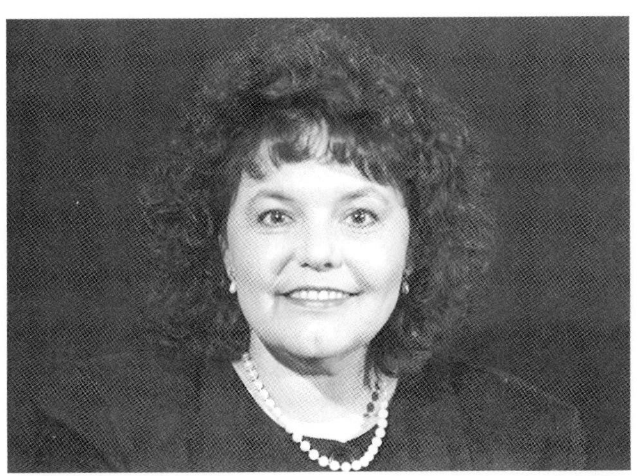

PHOTO BY LAURENT W. VALLIERE.

Linda Anne Silvestri received her diploma in nursing at Cooley Dickinson Hospital School of Nursing in Northampton, Massachusetts. Afterward, she worked at Baystate Medical Center in Springfield, Massachusetts. At Baystate Medical Center, she worked in acute medical-surgical units, the intensive care unit, the emergency department, pediatric units, and other acute care units. She later received an associate's degree from Holyoke Community College in Holyoke, Massachusetts, and then received her Bachelor of Science degree in nursing from American International College in Springfield, Massachusetts.

A native of Springfield, Massachusetts, Linda began her teaching career as an instructor of medical-surgical nursing and leadership-management nursing at Baystate Medical Center School of Nursing in 1981. In 1985 she earned her Master of Science degree in nursing from Anna Maria College, Paxton, Massachusetts, with a dual major in nursing management and patient education.

Linda relocated to Rhode Island in 1989 and began teaching advanced medical-surgical nursing and psychiatric nursing to RN and LPN students at the Community College of Rhode Island. While she was teaching at the Community College of Rhode Island, a group of students approached Linda, asking her to help them prepare for the NCLEX. On the basis of her experience as a nursing educator and as an NCLEX item writer, she developed a comprehensive review course to prepare nursing graduates for the NCLEX examination.

In 1994 Linda began teaching medical-surgical nursing at Salve Regina University in Newport, Rhode Island. She also prepares nursing students at Salve Regina University for the NCLEX examination. Currently, she is matriculated at the University of Rhode Island in the PhD in Nursing Program. Linda is also a member of Sigma Theta Tau.

In 1991 Linda established Professional Nursing Seminars, Inc., and in 2000 she established Nursing Reviews, Inc. Both companies are dedicated to conducting NCLEX-RN and NCLEX-PN review courses and to assisting nursing graduates to achieve their goals of becoming registered nurses or licensed practical or vocational nurses.

Today, Linda Silvestri's companies conduct NCLEX review courses throughout New England. She is the successful author of numerous NCLEX-RN and NCLEX-PN review products, including *Saunders Comprehensive Review for NCLEX-RN, Saunders Q&A Review for NCLEX-RN, Saunders Computerized Review for NCLEX-RN, Saunders Instructor's Resource Package for NCLEX-RN, Saunders Comprehensive Review for NCLEX-PN, Saunders Q&A Review for NCLEX-PN,* and *Saunders Instructor's Resource Package for NCLEX-PN.*

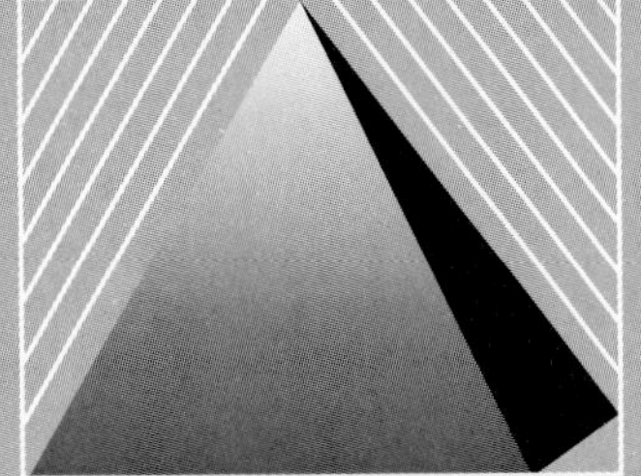

Contributors

Mary Ann Hogan, MSN, RN, CS
Clinical Assistant Professor
University of Massachusetts
Amherst, Massachusetts

Jo Ann Barnes Mullaney, PhD, APRN, BC
Professor of Nursing
Salve Regina University
Newport, Rhode Island

Laurent W. Valliere, BS
Vice President, Professional Nursing Seminars, Inc.
Charlestown, Rhode Island

Mary Wright, RN
Graduate, Department of Nursing
Rhode Island College
Providence, Rhode Island

The author and publisher would also like to acknowledge the following individuals for contributions to the first edition of this book.

Alicia M. Adams, MN, RN, CEN
Director, Practical Nursing and Allied Health
Uintah Basin Applied Technology Center
Roosevelt, Utah

Carole A. Baxter, EdD, RN
Assistant Dean of Nursing
Mount Wachusett Community College
Gardner, Massachusetts

Carol Boswell, EdD, RN
Associate Professor
Texas Tech University Health Sciences Center
Odessa, Texas

Sharen Brady, MSN, RN
Early Intervention Specialist and Associate Professor of Nursing in PN/ADN Program
Weber State University
Ogden, Utah

Brenda E. Caranicas, MS, RN
Former Director, Associate in Science of Practical Nursing Program
Fort Berthold Community College
New Town, North Dakota

Jean DeCoffe, MSN, RN
Assistant Professor of Nursing
Curry College
Milton, Massachusetts

Marcia M. Hamel, BSN, RN, M Ed
Meredith, New Hampshire

Lisa Ivers, BSN, RN
Instructor, Ivy Tech State College
Valparaiso, Indiana

Lula Johnson, MSN, RN
Director, JTPA School of Practical Nursing
Detroit, Michigan

Mary T. Kowalski, MSN, BA, RN
Director of Vocational Nursing and Health Career Programs
Cerro Coso Community College
Ridgecrest, California

Beverly McNeese, RN
Department Head, Practical Nursing Program
Louisiana Technical College
Baton Rouge Campus
Baton Rouge, Louisiana

Jan H. Mearkle, MSN, MS
Public Health Consultant
Summit, Mississippi

Joann E. Potts Peuterbaugh, MSN, RN
LPN Coordinator
F.W. Olin Vocational School of Practical Nursing
Alton, Illinois

Ann Leiphart Unholz, MS, RN
Director, Henrico County, St. Mary's Hospital School of Practical Nursing
Highland Springs, Virginia

Paula A. Viau, PhD, RN
Assistant Professor; Nursing
Director, Undergraduate Program College of Nursing
University of Rhode Island
Kingston, Rhode Island

Margaret Wafstet, MN, RN
Director, Practical Nursing Program
University of Montana-Missoula
College of Technology
Missoula, Montana

Mary Louise White, MSN, RN
Clinical Nurse Specialist
Delta College
University Center, Michigan

REVIEWERS

Marjorie L. (Gie) Archer, MS, RNC, WHCNP
Vocational Nursing Coordinator
Co-Chair, Department of Health Sciences and Human Services
North Central Texas College
Gainesville, Texas

Julie Barry, PhD, RN
Nursing Director, John Wood Community College
Quincy, Illinois

Dolores Cotton, MS, RN
Practical Nursing Coordinator
Meridian Technology Center
Stillwater, Oklahoma

Tammie Crook, BSN, RN
Nurse Manager, Med/Surg
Beckley Appalachian Regional Hospital
Beckley, West Virginia

Sally Flesch, PhD, RN
Professor, Allied Health Department
Black Hawk College
Moline, Iowa

Margaret M. Gingrich, MSN, RN
Associate Professor, Harrisburg Area Community College
Harrisburg, Pennsylvania

Rosemary Macy, MS, RN
Assistant Professor, Department of Nursing
Boise State University
Boise, Idaho

Cecilia Jane Maier, MS, RN, CCRN
Assistant Professor, Mount Carmel College of Nursing
Columbus, Ohio

Lorene Porter, MSN, RN
Professor of Nursing, Tomball College
Tomball, Texas

Pat Recek, MSN, RN
Coordinator, Vocational Nursing Program
Austin Community College
Austin, Texas

STUDENT REVIEWERS

Kristin Alberti
Salve Regina University
Newport, Rhode Island

Joanna Bort
Salve Regina University
Newport, Rhode Island

Sara Cabral
Salve Regina University
Newport, Rhode Island

April Oland Childs
Salve Regina University
Newport, Rhode Island

Danielle Darisse
Salve Regina University
Newport, Rhode Island

Jody DelliSante
Salve Regina University
Newport, Rhode Island

Danielle DeMelis
Salve Regina University
Newport, Rhode Island

Margaret Eldridge
Salve Regina University
Newport, Rhode Island

Kristen K. Foti
Salve Regina University
Newport, Rhode Island

Stephanie Hall
Salve Regina University
Newport, Rhode Island

Rebecca Hormanski
Salve Regina University
Newport, Rhode Island

Moira Houlihan
Salve Regina University
Newport, Rhode Island

Kristin Long
Salve Regina University
Newport, Rhode Island

Paul Lovely
Salve Regina University
Newport, Rhode Island

Nicole Mackin
Salve Regina University
Newport, Rhode Island

Lisa Mattson
Salve Regina University
Newport, Rhode Island

Kristin Roy
Salve Regina University
Newport, Rhode Island

Tonya Scharn
Salve Regina University
Newport, Rhode Island

Shandrea Silva
Salve Regina University
Newport, Rhode Island

Lindsay Stokes
Salve Regina University
Newport, Rhode Island

Kelly Sullivan
Salve Regina University
Newport, Rhode Island

Cristyna Vanasse
Salve Regina University
Newport, Rhode Island

To All Future Licensed Practical/Vocational Nurses:

Congratulations to you!

You should be very proud and pleased with yourself on your most recent accomplishment of completing your nursing program to become a licensed practical/vocational nurse. I know that you have worked very hard to become successful and you have proved to yourself that you can indeed achieve your goals.

In my opinion, you are about to enter the most wonderful and rewarding profession that exists. Your willingness, desire, and ability to assist those who need nursing care will bring great satisfaction to your life.

In the profession of nursing, your learning will be a lifelong process. This aspect of the profession makes it stimulating and dynamic. Your learning process will continue to expand and grow as the profession continues to evolve. Your next very important endeavor will be the learning process involved to achieve success in your examination to become a licensed practical/vocational nurse.

I am excited and pleased to be able to provide you with the *Saunders Pyramid to Success* products that will prepare you for your next important professional goal of becoming a licensed practical/vocational nurse. I want to thank all of my former nursing students that I have assisted in preparing for NCLEX-PN for their willingness to offer ideas regarding their needs in preparing for this examination. Student ideas have certainly added a special, unique aspect to all of the products available in the *Saunders Pyramid to Success*.

Saunders Pyramid to Success products provide you with everything that you need to prepare for NCLEX-PN. These products have been designed to include material that is required for all nursing students who are preparing to take the NCLEX-PN examination, regardless of the educational background, specific strengths, areas in need of improvement, or clinical experience during the nursing program.

So, let's get started and begin our journey through the *Saunders Pyramid to Success*, and welcome to the wonderful profession of nursing!

Sincerely,

Linda Anne Silvestri MSN, RN

Linda Anne Silvestri, MSN, RN

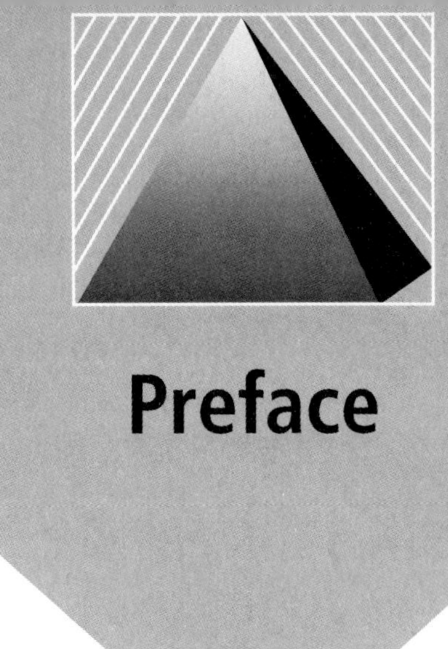

Preface

"To know that even one life has breathed easier because you have lived, this is to have succeeded."

RALPH WALDO EMERSON

Welcome to *Saunders Pyramid to Success*!

The *Saunders Comprehensive Review for NCLEX-PN* is one of a series of products designed to assist you in achieving your goal of becoming a licensed practical/vocational nurse. The *Saunders Comprehensive Review for NCLEX-PN* will provide you with a comprehensive review of all of the nursing content areas specifically related to the new 2002 CAT NCLEX-PN test plan implemented in April 2002 by the National Council of State Boards of Nursing.

ORGANIZATION

The *Saunders Comprehensive Review for NCLEX-PN* contains 21 units and 65 chapters. The chapters are designed to identify specific components of nursing content. Each chapter contains practice questions reflective of the content of the chapter and of the 2002 CAT NCLEX-PN test plan.

In the new test plan implemented in April 2002, the National Council of State Boards of Nursing has identified a test plan framework based on *Client Needs.* These Client Needs categories include Safe, Effective Care Environment; Health Promotion and Maintenance; Psychosocial Integrity; and Physiological Integrity. All of the chapters in this book address all components of the test plan framework. However, Units I through IV include content that specifically addresses the Client Needs category of Safe, Effective Care Environment; Units V through VII and Unit XX provide a focus on Health Promotion and Maintenance; Units VIII through XVIII emphasize Physiological Integrity; and Unit XIX focuses on Psychosocial Integrity.

UNIT I: NCLEX-PN PREPARATION

Chapter 1 addresses all of the information related to the 2002 CAT NCLEX-PN test plan and the testing procedures related to the examination. This chapter answers questions that you may have regarding the testing procedures.

Chapter 2 discusses the issue of NCLEX-PN preparation from a nonacademic view and provides an emphasis on a holistic approach for your individual test preparation. This chapter identifies the components of a structured study plan and pattern, anxiety reduction techniques, and personal focus issues.

Nursing students want to hear what other students have to say about their experiences with NCLEX-PN to learn what it is "really like" to take the examination. Chapter 3 is written by a nursing student who took the NCLEX-PN examination. This chapter addresses the issue of what the examination is all about and includes the student's "story of success."

Test-taking strategies are a key component of success in taking such an important examination. Chapter 4, *Test-Taking Strategies,* includes all of those important strategies that will teach you how to read a question, how not to read into a question, and how to use the process of elimination and various other strategies to select the correct response from the options presented.

UNIT II: ISSUES IN NURSING

Unit II addresses relevant nursing issues reflective of the components of the CAT NCLEX-PN test plan. Chapter 5, *Cultural Diversity,* identifies the specific common cultures and the related factors that promote maintenance of cultural identity when caring for culturally diverse clients. Chapter 6, *Ethical and Legal Issues,* provides a review of the ethical and legal considerations important to the practice of nursing and relevant to the components of the test plan. Chapter 7, *Leadership Issues and Priorities of Care,* identifies issues pertinent to the practice of nursing.

UNIT III: NURSING SCIENCES

The chapters in Unit III specifically address content that students have identified as areas requiring review. Chapter 8, *Fluids and Electrolytes,* and Chapter 9, *Acid-Base Balance,* highlight the key components of the physiology, then move toward the data collection and nursing interventions required to identify alterations that can occur in a client. Chapter 10, *Laboratory Values,* identifies the common laboratory studies, the normal values, and significant information related to the specific laboratory test. Chapter 11, *Nutritional Components of Care,* addresses the various food groups and important nutritional components of specific diet therapy. This chapter will assist you with your review of the selection of the correct food or the foods to avoid with certain physiological conditions, since these types of questions are certainly addressed in the CAT NCLEX-PN test plan. Chapter 12, *Intravenous Therapy and Blood Administration,* focuses on the nurses' role in monitoring these therapies and complications.

UNIT IV: FUNDAMENTAL SKILLS

Chapter 13, *Hygiene and Safety,* addresses nursing care specific to client safety and the measures that promote environmental safety. Chapter 14, *Medication and Intravenous Administration,* includes the important components related to conversion tables, calculation of medication dosages, and intravenous solutions and flow rates. Chapter 15, *Basic Life Support,* has been included to assist you in reviewing the steps in cardiopulmonary resuscitation and the Heimlich maneuver and to refresh your memory on the priorities to be addressed in emergency situations. Chapter 16, *Perioperative Nursing Care,* addresses the key components related to caring for the client requiring surgery. Chapter 17, *Positioning Clients,* identifies safe client positions specific to various surgical and diagnostic procedures. Chapter 18, *Care of a Client with a Tube,* addresses the various types of tubes, such as chest tubes, gastrointestinal tubes, or renal tubes, that have always been very confusing to students, particularly in terms of their purpose and nursing care involved.

UNITS V, VI, AND VII: GROWTH AND DEVELOPMENT ACROSS THE LIFE SPAN, AND MATERNITY AND PEDIATRIC NURSING

Units V, VI, and VII address many of the components of the Health Promotion and Maintenance category of Client Needs. Unit V, *Growth and Development Across the Life Span,* addresses the common theories of growth and development used in nursing. Unit VI, *Maternity Nursing,* includes chapters that address care of the pregnant client, care of the newborn, and maternity and newborn medications. Unit VII, *Pediatric Nursing,* focuses on the components of pediatric care and on the specifics related to administering medication to the child.

UNITS VIII THROUGH XVIII: ADULT HEALTH

Units VIII through XVIII address the components of Adult Health and are divided based on the specific body system, including the integumentary, endocrine, gastrointestinal, respiratory, cardiovascular, renal, eye and ear, neurological, musculoskeletal, and immune, and oncology nursing. These chapters incorporate all of the *Client Needs* components of the CAT NCLEX-PN test plan with a particular emphasis on Physiological Integrity. Each unit includes a pharmacology chapter that provides a comprehensive review of the medications specific to the body system.

UNIT XIX: MENTAL HEALTH NURSING

Unit XIX primarily addresses the *Psychosocial Integrity* of the Client Needs component of the test plan. Specific mental health disorders are addressed. A chapter that provides a comprehensive review of psychiatric medications is included.

UNIT XX: THE GERONTOLOGICAL CLIENT

Unit XX focuses on the variations related to caring for the gerontological client.

UNIT XXI: COMPREHENSIVE TEST

Unit XXI is a comprehensive test that includes practice questions related to all of the content areas addressed in this book. It consists of 85 questions representative of the percentages identified in the test plan for NCLEX-PN.

SPECIAL FEATURES OF THE BOOK

PYRAMID TERMS

Each content area begins with *Pyramid Terms,* the definitions of important related terms significant to the content contained in the chapter. In addition, these *Pyramid Terms* are in bold type throughout the content section.

PYRAMID TO SUCCESS

The *Pyramid to Success,* a unit or chapter introduction, provides you with an overview of the unit or chapter, guidance and direction regarding the focus of review in the particular content area, and its relative importance to the 2002 CAT NCLEX-PN test plan. Specific nursing content areas, as stipulated in the test plan, are identified. The *Pyramid to Success* reviews the Client Needs and the Integrated Concepts and Processes as they pertain to the content in that unit or chapter. These points are the specific components to keep in mind as you review the unit or chapter.

PYRAMID POINTS

Pyramid Points are the bullets that are placed next to specific content areas throughout the chapters. The *Pyramid Points* provide you with immediate recognition of content that is important in preparation for CAT NCLEX-PN. These bullets identify areas of content that typically appear on CAT NCLEX-PN.

PRACTICE QUESTIONS

While students are preparing for NCLEX-PN, it is crucial for them to practice questions. This book contains 1500 practice questions. The accompanying software includes all the questions from the book, plus an additional 1500 questions for a total of 3000 test questions. Each of the 65 chapters is followed by practice questions in NCLEX format. The answer section for the practice questions includes the correct answer and the rationale for the correct and incorrect answers. The structure of the answer section is unique and provides the following information for every question:

The Rationale. The rationale provides you with the significant information regarding both correct and incorrect options.

Test-Taking Strategy. The test-taking strategy provides you with the logical path in selecting the correct option and assists you in selecting an answer to a question should you need to guess. Specific suggestions for review are identified in the test-taking strategy.

Question Categories. Each question is identified on the basis of the categories used by the CAT NCLEX-PN test plan. Additional content categories are provided with each question to assist you in identifying areas in need of review. The categories identified with each question include Level of Cognitive Ability, Client Needs, Integrated Concept/Process, and the specific nursing Content Area. All categories are identified by their full names, so that you do not need to memorize codes or abbreviations.

Reference. A reference, including a page number, is provided so that you can easily find the information that you need to review in your nursing textbooks.

PHARMACOLOGY AND MEDICATION CALCULATIONS REVIEW

Students consistently say that pharmacology is an area in which they need assistance. This book includes 13 pharmacology chapters, a medication and intravenous administration chapter, and a pediatric medication calculation chapter. Each of these chapters is followed by a practice test using the same question format as described above. This book contains over 400 pharmacology questions.

BOXES, TABLES, AND FIGURES

Several boxes, tables, and figures have been included to provide you with the visualization of significant content areas represented in the CAT NCLEX-PN test plan.

NCLEX-PN REVIEW SOFTWARE

Packaged in this book you will find a CD-ROM containing NCLEX-PN review software. This software contains 3000 questions, 1500 from the book and 1500 additional questions. This Windows- and Macintosh-compatible program offers three testing modes for review.

Quiz—randomly chosen questions on a specific selected content area. The answer, rationale, test-taking strategy, question categories, reference, and results appear after you answer all questions.

Study—All questions on a specific selected content area. The answer, rationale, test-taking strategy, question categories, and reference, appear after you answer each question.

Examination—One hundred randomly chosen questions from the entire pool of 3000 questions. The answer, rationale, test-taking strategy, question categories, reference, and results appear after you answer all 100 questions.

The software allows you to customize your review and determine your areas of strength and weakness. It also provides you with a wealth of practice test questions while at the same time simulating the NCLEX-PN experience on computer.

HOW TO USE THIS BOOK

Saunders Comprehensive Review for NCLEX-PN is especially designed to help you with your successful journey to the peak of the *Saunders Pyramid to Success*, becoming a licensed practical/vocational nurse.

As you begin your journey through this book, you will be introduced to all of the important points regarding the CAT NCLEX-PN examination, the process of testing, and the unique and special tips regarding how to prepare yourself for this important examination.

You should begin your process through *Saunders Pyramid to Success* by reading all of Unit I and becoming familiar with the important points regarding the CAT NCLEX-PN examination, the process of testing, and the unique and special tips regarding how to prepare yourself for this examination. Read the chapter from the nursing graduate who passed NCLEX-PN and pay attention to what this graduate has to say about the examination. Read the chapter on test-taking strategies and practice these strategies as you proceed through your journey with this book. Continue on your journey by reading each of the chapters in the units that follow. Review the Pyramid Terms and the Pyramid to Success and identify the Client Needs and Integrated Concepts and Processes specific to the test plan in each area. Read each of the chapters, focusing on the Pyramid Points that identify those areas most likely to be tested on CAT NCLEX-PN.

As you read each chapter, identify your strengths and the areas that are in need of further review. Highlight these areas, and test your strengths and abilities by taking all of the practice tests provided at the end of the chapters. Be sure to read all of the rationales and the test-taking strategies. The rationale provides you with the significant information regarding both the correct and incorrect options. The test-taking strategy offers you the logical path to selecting the correct option. The strategy also identifies the content area that you need to review if you had difficulty with the question. Use the reference listed so that you can easily find the information that you need to review.

After reviewing all of the chapters in the book, turn to Unit XXI, the Comprehensive Test. Take this examination, and then review each question, answer, and rationale. Identify any areas requiring review; then take this time to review those areas again.

After using this book to review specific content areas, continue on your journey through *Saunders Pyramid to Success* with the companion book, *Saunders Q&A Review for NCLEX-PN,* for additional practice questions. This companion book and its accompanying software offer you 3000 practice questions in specific areas outlined by the 2002 CAT NCLEX-PN test plan. With practice questions uniquely focused on the Client Needs and the Integrated Concepts and Processes, you can assess your level of competence.

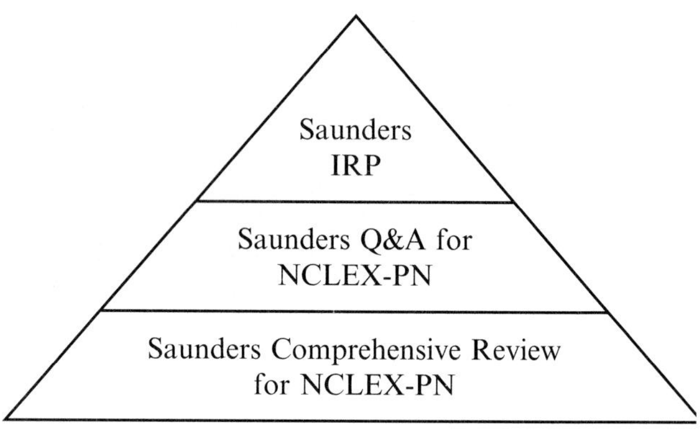

The final component of the *Saunders Pyramid to Success* is the *Saunders Instructor's Resource Package for NCLEX-PN.* This manual and CD-ROM accompany the Saunders program of NCLEX-PN review products. Be sure to ask your nursing program director and nursing faculty about the CD-ROM and its use for a review course or a self-paced review in your school's computer laboratory.

Good luck with your journey through the *Saunders Pyramid to Success.* I wish you continued success throughout your new career as a Licensed Practical/Vocational Nurse!

Linda Anne Silvestri, MSN, RN

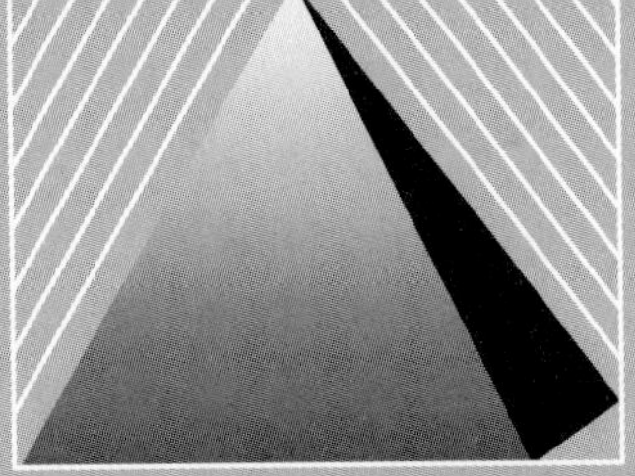

Acknowledgments

Sincere appreciation and warmest thanks are extended to the many individuals who in their own ways have contributed to the publication of this book.

First, I want to thank all of my nursing students at the Community College of Rhode Island in Warwick, who approached me in 1991 and persuaded me to assist them in preparing to take the NCLEX examination. Their enthusiasm and inspiration led to the commencement of my professional endeavors in conducting NCLEX review courses for nursing students. I also thank the numerous nursing students who have attended my review courses for their willingness to share their needs and ideas. Their input has certainly added a special uniqueness to this publication.

I wish to acknowledge all of the nursing faculty who taught in my NCLEX review courses. Their commitment, dedication, and expertise have certainly assisted nursing students in achieving success with the NCLEX examination. In addition, I want to acknowledge Laurent W. Valliere for his contribution to this publication, for teaching in my NCLEX review courses, and for his commitment and dedication in assisting my nursing students to prepare for NCLEX from a nonacademic point of view.

I sincerely acknowledge and thank two very important individuals from Elsevier Science. I thank Loren Wilson, Executive Editor, for all of her assistance throughout the preparation of this edition and for her continuous enthusiasm, support, and expert professional guidance. And, I thank Shelly Hayden, Senior Developmental Editor, for her continuous assistance and for keeping me on track. Her expert organizational skills maintained order for all of the work that I submitted for manuscript production.

A special thank you and acknowledgment go to another important individual, Sarah Miller, my assistant. She provided continuous support and dedication to my work both in the NCLEX review courses in and preparing the second edition of this book. I want to acknowledge all of the staff at Elsevier Science for their tremendous assistance throughout the preparation and production of this publication. A special thank you to all of them.

I thank all of the special people in the production department, Melissa Lastarria, Project Manager, whose consistent editing assisted in finalizing this publication, Trish Tannian, Publishing Services Manager, and Gail Morey Hudson, Book Design Manager. I sincerely thank Bob Boehringer, Marketing Manager, from the Nursing Marketing Department, whose support, hard work, and special creativity assisted with this publication.

I would also like to acknowledge Patricia Mieg, Educational Sales Representative, who encouraged me to submit my ideas and initial work for the first edition of this book to the W.B. Saunders Company and initiated my meeting with Maura Connor, my former Senior Acquisitions Editor. I want to thank Maura Connor for her professional direction that led me to success as I initially created *Saunders Pyramid to Success for NCLEX-PN.* I want to acknowledge my parents, who opened my door of opportunity in education. I thank my mother, Frances Mary, for all of her love, support, and assistance as I continuously worked to achieve my professional goals. I thank my father, Arnold Lawrence, who always provided insightful words of encouragement. My memories of his love and support will always remain in my heart. I also thank my sister, Dianne Elodia, my brother, Lawrence Peter, and my niece, Gina Marie, who were continuously supportive, giving, and helpful during my research and preparation of this publication. I want to acknowledge all of the contributors, who provided practice questions for this publication, and the many faculty and student reviewers for their thoughts and ideas. I sincerely thank Mary Ann Hogan, MSN, RN, from the

University of Massachusetts in Amherst, who has always encouraged and supported me through my professional endeavors. Her numerous contributions to this publication is a reflection of her dedication to the profession of nursing and to nursing students.

A special thank you to Dr. JoAnn Mullaney from Salve Regina University in Newport, Rhode Island, for her numerous and expert contributions to this publication, and to Mary Wright, for providing a chapter to this publication regarding her experiences with NCLEX.

I also need to thank Salve Regina University for the opportunity to educate nursing students in the baccalaureate nursing program and for its support during my research and writing of this publication. I would especially like to acknowledge Dr. Louise Murdock and Dr. Ellen McCarty, Co-Chairpersons of the Department of Nursing at Salve Regina University, for their continuous support, academic mentoring, and astute vision regarding the future of the profession of nursing.

I wish to acknowledge the University of Rhode Island, College of Nursing, for providing me with the opportunity for professional growth in my nursing education. I also wish to acknowledge the Community College of Rhode Island, which provided me the opportunity to educate nursing students in the Associate Degree of Nursing Program, and a special thank you to Patricia Miller, MSN, RN, and Michelina McClellan, MS, RN, from Baystate Medical Center, School of Nursing, in Springfield, Massachusetts, who were my first mentors in nursing education. Lastly, a very special thank you to all my nursing students, past, present, and future. Your love of and dedication to the profession of nursing and your commitment to provide health care will bring never-ending rewards!

Linda Anne Silvestri, MSN, RN

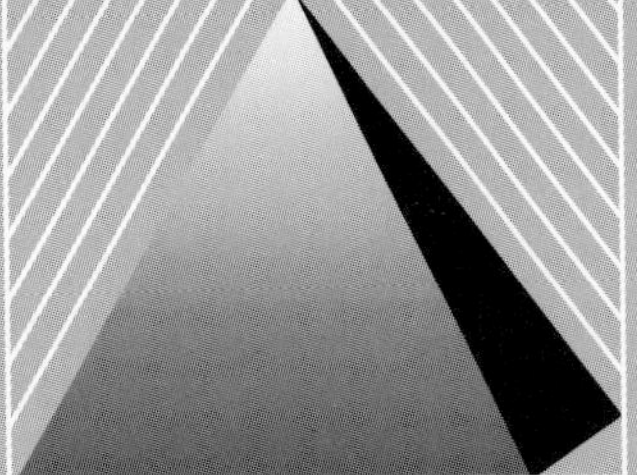

Contents

UNIT I

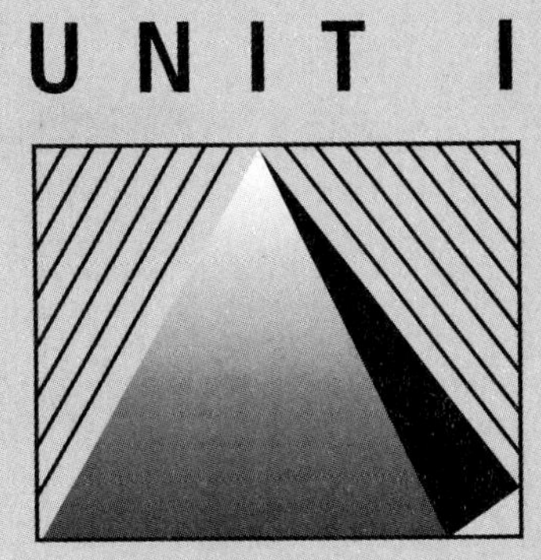

NCLEX-PN Preparation

NCLEX-PN Preparation

THE PYRAMID TO SUCCESS

Welcome to the Pyramid to Success!

Saunders Comprehensive Review for NCLEX-PN is specially designed to help you begin your successful journey to the peak of the Pyramid, becoming a Licensed Practical/Vocational Nurse!

As you begin your journey, you will be introduced to all of the important points regarding the NCLEX-PN examination and the process of testing, and the unique and special tips regarding how to prepare yourself for this very important examination. You will read what a nursing graduate who recently passed the examination has to say about the test. All those important Test-Taking Strategies are detailed. These details will guide you in selecting the correct option or assist you in selecting an answer to a question you must guess at.

Each of the content areas in this book begins with the Pyramid to Success. The Pyramid to Success addresses specific points related to NCLEX-PN, including the Pyramid Terms, the Client Needs, and the Integrated Concepts and Processes as identified in the test plan framework for the examination. Pyramid Terms are key words that are defined and are boldfaced throughout each chapter to direct your attention to those significant NCLEX-PN points. The Client Needs and the Integrated Concepts and Processes specific to the content of the chapter are identified.

Throughout each chapter, you will find Pyramid Point bullets that identify areas most likely to be tested on NCLEX-PN. Read each chapter, and identify your strengths and areas in need of further review. Test your strengths and abilities by taking all the practice tests provided in this book. Be sure to read all the rationales and the test-taking strategies. The rationale provides you with significant information regarding both the correct and incorrect options. The test-taking strategy provides you with the logical path to selecting the correct option. The test-taking strategy also identifies the content area to review, if required. The reference source and page number are provided so that you can easily find the information that you need to review. Each question is coded on the basis of the Level of Cognitive Ability, the Client Needs, the Integrated Concepts and Processes, and the nursing content area.

After completing your comprehensive review in this book, continue on your journey through the Pyramid to Success with the companion book, *Saunders Q&A Review for NCLEX-PN*, which provides you with 3000 practice questions based on the NCLEX-PN test plan.

Let's begin our journey through the Pyramid to Success!

THE EXAMINATION PROCESS

An important step in the Pyramid to Success is to become as familiar as possible with the examination process. A significant amount of anxiety can occur in candidates facing the challenge of this examination. Knowing what the examination is all about, and knowing what you will encounter during the process of testing will help alleviate fear and anxiety. The information contained in this chapter addresses the procedures related to the development of the NCLEX-PN Test Plan, the components of the Test Plan, and the answers to the questions most commonly asked by nursing students and graduates preparing to take the NCLEX-PN. The information related to the development of the NCLEX-PN Test Plan, the components of the Test Plan, and the testing procedures was adapted from *Test Plan for the National Council Licensure Examination for Practical/Vocational Nurses;* National Council of State Boards of Nursing, Chicago, 2001; and *The NCLEX Process: Serving as an Anchor for the NCLEX Examination,* National Council of State Boards of Nursing, Chicago, 2000.

DEVELOPMENT OF THE TEST PLAN

The initial step in developing the NCLEX-PN examination is the preparation of a test plan to guide the selection of content and behaviors to be tested. In the test development process, the National Council of State Boards of Nursing considers the legal scope of nursing practice as governed by state laws and regulations, including the Nurse Practice Act. The National Council uses these laws to define the areas on NCLEX-PN that will assess the competence of candidates for nurse licensure. The National Council of State Boards of Nursing also conducts a Practice Analysis study to determine the framework for the Test Plan for NCLEX-PN. Since nursing practice continues to change, this study is conducted every 3 years. Results of this study, most recently conducted in 2000, provided the structure for the new test plan implemented in April 2002.

PRACTICE ANALYSIS STUDY

Participants in this study include entry-level practical/vocational nurses. The participants are provided a list of nursing activities and are asked about the frequency of performing these specific activities, their impact on maintaining client safety, and the setting where the activities were performed. Analysis of the data obtained from this study guides the development of a framework for entry-level nurse performance that incorporates specific client needs and the concepts and processes fundamental to the practice of nursing. The NCLEX-PN Test Plan is derived from this framework.

THE TEST PLAN

The content of NCLEX-PN reflects the activities that an entry-level practical/vocational nurse must be able to perform to provide clients with safe and effective nursing care. The questions are written to address the Levels of Cognitive Ability, Client Needs, and Integrated Concepts and Processes as identified in the Test Plan.

Levels of Cognitive Ability

The NCLEX-PN examination consists of multiple-choice questions written at the cognitive levels of knowledge, comprehension, application, and analysis (Box 1-1).

BOX 1-1

Level of Cognitive Ability

A nurse is collecting data from a perinatal client with a history of left-sided heart failure. The nurse notes that the client is experiencing unusual episodes of a cough on minimal exertion. The nurse recognizes this finding as significant and associated with the first indicator of which of the following cardiac problems?

1. Orthopnea
2. Decreased blood volume
3. Right-sided heart failure
4. Pulmonary edema

Answer: 4

This question requires the test taker to analyze the data provided in order to recognize the client's problem. The test taker needs to know the complications of left-sided heart failure and the signs and symptoms of pulmonary edema. Analysis of the data provided in the question will direct the test taker to the correct option.

Level of Cognitive Ability: Analysis

Client Needs

In the new Test Plan implemented in April 2002, the National Council of State Boards of Nursing identifies a test plan framework based on *Client Needs.* This framework was selected based on the analysis of the findings in the Practice Analysis study. Additionally, Client Needs provides a structure for defining nursing actions and competencies across all settings for all clients and is congruent with state laws and statutes. The National Council of State Boards of Nursing identifies four major categories of Client Needs. These categories are further divided into subcategories, and the percentage of test questions in each subcategory is identified. (Table 1-1).

Safe, Effective Care Environment

The Safe, Effective Care Environment category includes two subcategories, Coordinated Care and Safety and Infection Control. Coordinated Care (6% to 12%) addresses content related to facilitating effective client care through collaboration with other health care team members. Safety and Infection Control (7% to 13%)

TABLE 1-1

Client Needs and the Percentage of Test Questions

Client Needs	Percentage
SAFE, EFFECTIVE CARE ENVIRONMENT	
Coordinated Care	6%-12%
Safety and Infection Control	7%-13%
HEALTH PROMOTION AND MAINTENANCE	
Growth and Development Through the Life Span	4%-10%
Prevention and Early Detection of Disease	4%-10%
PSYCHOSOCIAL INTEGRITY	
Coping and Adaptation	6%-12%
Psychosocial Adaptation	4%-10%
PHYSIOLOGICAL INTEGRITY	
Basic Care and Comfort	10%-16%
Pharmacological Therapies	5%-11%
Reduction of Risk Potential	11%-17%
Physiological Adaptation	13%-19%

addresses content that tests the knowledge, skills, and ability required to protect clients and health care personnel from environmental hazards (Box 1-2).

Health Promotion and Maintenance

The Health Promotion and Maintenance category includes two subcategories, Growth and Development Through the Life Span and the Prevention and Early Detection of Disease. Growth and Development Through the Life Span (4% to 10%) addresses content that tests the knowledge, skills, and ability required to assist the client and significant others during the normal expected stages of growth and development from conception through advanced old age. Prevention and Early Detection of Disease (4% to 10%) addresses content that tests the knowledge, skills, and ability required to provide client care related to prevention and early detection of health problems (Box 1-3).

BOX 1-2

Safe, Effective Care Environment

COORDINATED CARE

A nurse observes that a client becomes agitated and incoherent and suspects that the client is experiencing a reaction to medication. In planning a safe environment for this client, the most appropriate intervention is to:

1. Request that the physician order restraints and sedation
2. Ask the family to stay with the client
3. Ask a nursing assistant to stay with the client
4. Collaborate with the registered nurse to plan safe care

Answer: 4

This question addresses the subcategory, Coordinated Care, in the Client Needs category, Safe, Effective Care Environment. The nurse has the responsibility to facilitate safe and effective client care through collaboration with other health care team members.

SAFETY AND INFECTION CONTROL

A nurse is assigned to care for a client receiving an intravenous (IV) infusion. While caring for the client, the nurse implements which of the following nursing actions to decrease the risk for infection?

1. Takes the vital signs at 4-hour intervals
2. Changes the IV dressing every shift
3. Administers acetaminophen (Tylenol) every 4 hours
4. Uses aseptic technique when handling the intravenous solution and tubing

Answer: 4

This question addresses the subcategory, Safety and Infection Control, in the Client Needs category, Safe, Effective Care Environment. It addresses content related to surgical asepsis and protecting the client from infection.

Psychosocial Integrity

The Psychosocial Integrity category includes two subcategories, Coping and Adaptation and Psychosocial Adaptation. Coping and Adaptation (6% to 12%) addresses content that tests the knowledge, skills, and ability required to promote the client's and/or significant other's ability to cope, adapt, and/or problem solve situations related to illnesses, disabilities, or stressful events. Psychosocial Adaptation (4% to 10%) addresses content related to participating in recognizing and providing care for clients with maladaptive behavior and assisting with behavior management of the client with acute and/or chronic mental illness or a cognitive psychosocial disturbance (Box 1-4).

Physiological Integrity

The Physiological Integrity category includes four subcategories, Basic Care and Comfort, Pharmacological Therapies, Reduction of Risk Potential, and Physiological Adaptation. Basic Care and Comfort (10% to 16%) addresses content that tests the knowledge, skills, and ability required to provide comfort and assistance to the client in the performance of activities of daily living. Pharmacological Therapies (5% to 11%) addresses content that tests the knowledge, skills, and ability required to provide care related to the administration of medications, and monitoring clients receiving parenteral therapies. Reduction of Risk Potential (11% to 17%) addresses content that tests the knowledge, skills, and ability required to reduce the client's potential for developing complications or health problems related to existing conditions, treatments, or procedures. Physiological Adaptation (13% to 19%) addresses content related to participating in providing care to clients with acute, chronic, or life-threatening physical health conditions (Box 1-5).

Integrated Concepts and Processes

The National Council of State Boards of Nursing has identified six concepts and processes that are fundamental to the practice of nursing. These concepts and processes are a component of the Test Plan and are incorporated throughout the major categories of Client Needs (Box 1-6).

CAT NCLEX-PN

The term *NCLEX-PN* stands for National Council Licensure Examination for Practical/Vocational Nurses. CAT NCLEX-PN is a computer-administered examination that the nursing graduate must take and pass in order to practice as a practical/vocational nurse. This examination measures the test candidate's knowledge, skills, and abilities required to perform safely and

BOX 1-3

Health Promotion and Maintenance

GROWTH AND DEVELOPMENT THROUGH THE LIFE SPAN

A nurse is assisting in planning a health maintenance program for a group of older adults. Which of the following activities would best promote the maintenance of health among this group?

1. Gardening every day for an hour
2. Cycling three times a week for 20 minutes
3. Sculpting once a week for 40 minutes
4. Walking three to five times a week for 30 minutes

Answer: 4

This question addresses the subcategory, Growth and Development Through the Life Span, in the Client Needs category, Health Promotion and Maintenance. One of the best exercises for an older adult is walking, progressing to 30-minute sessions three to five times each week. Swimming and dancing are also beneficial. Exercise and activity are essential for health promotion and maintenance in the older adult and to achieve an optimal level of functioning.

PREVENTION AND EARLY DETECTION OF DISEASE

A nurse is reinforcing teaching points provided to a client by the registered nurse regarding measures that can be taken to prevent thrombophlebitis. Which of the following statements indicates that the client understands these measures?

1. "I need to sit with my legs elevated for most of the day."
2. "I need to avoid sitting or standing in one position for prolonged periods of time."
3. "I'm glad I don't need to wear those ugly stockings anymore."
4. "I have decreased my fluid consumption to one glass of water a day."

Answer: 2

This question addresses the subcategory, Prevention and Early Detection of Disease, in the Client Needs category, Health Promotion and Maintenance. The content addresses measures that will prevent thrombophlebitis. Avoidance of sitting or standing for a prolonged period of time is one of the measures for the prevention of venous stasis and thrombophlebitis.

BOX 1-4

Psychosocial Integrity

COPING AND ADAPTATION

A nurse is assigned to care for a client with ovarian cancer. While giving morning care, the client says, "If I can just live long enough to attend my daughter's graduation, I'll be ready to die." Which phase of coping is this client experiencing?

1. Isolation
2. Bargaining
3. Depression
4. Acceptance

Answer: 2

This question addresses the subcategory of Coping and Adaptation in the Client Needs category, Psychosocial Integrity. Bargaining is the phase of coping in which the dying person tries to negotiate, as in this case, making deals with their God or fate. The content addressed in this question is specific to coping mechanisms.

PSYCHOSOCIAL ADAPTATION

A nurse is collecting data regarding the lethality risk of a suicidal client. The best question for the nurse to ask the client is which of the following?

1. "Do you ever think about ending it all?"
2. "Have you ever thought of killing yourself?"
3. "Do you wish your life were over?"
4. "Do you have a death wish?"

Answer: 2

This question addresses the subcategory, Psychosocial Adaptation in the Client Needs category, Psychosocial Integrity. The question addresses mental illness concepts and crisis intervention. A lethality assessment requires direct communication between the client and the nurse concerning the client's intent. It is important to provide a question that is directly related to lethality.

effectively as a newly licensed, entry-level practical/vocational nurse.

COMPUTERIZED ADAPTIVE TESTING (CAT)

The word *CAT* stands for Computerized Adaptive Testing. CAT provides a uniqueness to the examination that the candidate will take; the examination adapts to each test taker's skill level. The CAT examination is assembled interactively as the candidate answers the questions. All of the test questions are stored in a large test bank and are categorized based on the test plan structure and the level of difficulty of the question. With the CAT method of testing, an examination is created and tailored to test the candidate's knowledge and skills while fulfilling Test Plan requirements. The candidate will not waste time answering questions that are far above or below his or her competency level.

BOX 1-5

Physiological Integrity

BASIC CARE AND COMFORT

A nurse notes that the client has slight weakness in the right leg. Based on this observation, the nurse recognizes that the client would benefit most from the use of a:

1. Walker
2. Wooden crutch
3. Lofstrand crutch
4. Straight leg cane

Answer: 4

This question addresses the subcategory of Basic Care and Comfort in the Client Needs category, Physiological Integrity. A straight leg cane is useful for the client with slight weakness in one leg. In this question, the nurse specifically assists the client in the performance of activities of daily living.

PHARMACOLOGICAL THERAPIES

A nurse is caring for a client with a diagnosis of chronic angina pectoris who is receiving sotalol (Betapace) 80 mg PO daily. Which of the following indicates to the nurse that the client is experiencing a side effect related to the medication?

1. Difficulty swallowing
2. Diaphoresis
3. Dry mouth
4. Bradycardia

Answer: 4

This question addresses the subcategory of Pharmacological Therapies in the Client Needs category, Physiological Integrity. Sotalol is a beta-adrenergic blocking agent. Side effects include bradycardia, palpitations, difficulty breathing, irregular heart beat, signs of congestive heart failure, and cold hands and feet. The content addressed in this question is specific to the side effects of a medication.

REDUCTION OF RISK POTENTIAL

A nurse is assigned to assist in caring for a client who has undergone cystoscopy. The nurse recognizes that which of the following is an abnormal sign if noted during the first few hours after the procedure?

1. Pink-tinged urine
2. Grossly bloody urine with clots
3. Clear yellow urine
4. Yellow-colored urine

Answer: 2

This question addresses the subcategory, Reduction of Risk Potential in the Client Needs category, Physiological Integrity. It involves a potential complication related to a procedure. Grossly bloody urine with clots is always an abnormal finding and should be reported immediately.

PHYSIOLOGICAL ADAPTATION

A nurse is assigned to care for a client with a diagnosis of pheochromocytoma. The nurse is told in report that the client's magnesium level is 7 mEq/L. Based on this laboratory result, the nurse recognizes which of the following signs as significant?

1. Drowsiness
2. Hypertension
3. Hyperpnea
4. Hyperactive reflexes

Answer: 1

This question addresses the subcategory, Physiological Adaptation in the Client Needs category, Physiological Integrity. It addresses an alteration in body systems. Neurological manifestations begin to occur at magnesium levels of 6 to 7 mEq/L and are noted as symptoms of neurological depression, such as drowsiness, sedation, lethargy, respiratory depression, muscle weakness, and areflexia.

BOX 1-6

Integrated Concepts and Processes

Caring
Clinical Problem Solving Process (Nursing Process)
Communication and Documentation
Cultural Awareness
Self-Care
Teaching/Learning

When you answer a question on CAT NCLEX-PN, the computer will calculate a competency skill estimate based on all earlier selected answers. An item determined to measure the candidate's ability most precisely in the appropriate test plan area is selected and presented on the computer screen. This process is repeated for each item and continues in this way until the test plan requirements are met and a reliable pass or fail decision is made.

THE PROCESS OF REGISTRATION

The initial step in the registration process is that a candidate apply to the state board of nursing in the state in which he or she intends to obtain licensure. (The addresses, telephone numbers, and web sites, if available, of boards of nursing in all states and territories of the United States are provided at the end of this chapter.) You need to obtain information from the board of nursing regarding the specific registration process, as the process may vary from state to state. It is very important that you follow the registration instructions and complete the registration forms precisely and accurately.

Registration forms not properly completed, or not accompanied by the proper fees in the required method of payment, will be returned to you and will delay testing. The initial fee for the application process may vary from state to state. Each board of nursing will set its initial license fee according to its own needs. The registration forms will identify the registration and testing service fees. When the board of nursing receives the completed registration form, based on the criteria established by the board, your eligibility is determined, and the board authorizes your admission to the examination.

Once your eligibility to test has been determined by the board of nursing in the jurisdiction in which licensure is requested, the valid NCLEX registration is processed and an Authorization to Test form will be sent to you. You cannot make an appointment until the board of nursing declares eligibility and you receive an Authorization to Test form. The Authorization to Test form will provide a candidate identification number and an authorization number, and these numbers will be needed to make an appointment with the testing center.

SPECIAL TESTING CIRCUMSTANCES

A candidate who is requesting special accommodations should contact the board of nursing before submitting a registration form. The board of nursing will provide you with the procedures for the request. The board of nursing must authorize special testing accommodations. Following board of nursing approval, the National Council of State Boards reviews the requested accommodations to ensure that the proposed modification does not affect the psychometric properties of NCLEX or cause a security risk. The National Council of State Boards must also approve the accommodations.

MAKING AN APPOINTMENT TO TEST

The CAT NCLEX-PN examination is administered year round. You will be provided with a list of testing centers and the telephone numbers. Note the expiration date on the Authorization to Test form. You must schedule and make an appointment before this expiration date. You may take the test at any approved testing center and do not have to test in the same jurisdiction in which you are seeking licensure. An eligible candidate taking NCLEX for the first time will be offered an appointment date within 30 days of the telephone call to the testing center. Repeat candidates will be offered an appointment date within 45 days of the telephone call to the testing center. A confirmation notice will not be sent to you; therefore it is important to note the date and time of the appointment. When you call the test center, it is also important to verify the address and the directions to the testing center.

CANCELING OR RESCHEDULING AN APPOINTMENT

If for any reason you need to cancel or reschedule your appointment to test, the scheduling change must be made before noon, two business days before the scheduled appointment. The original appointment must be canceled before a new appointment can be scheduled.

LATE ARRIVALS TO THE TEST CENTER

It is important that you arrive at the testing center 30 minutes before the test is scheduled. Candidates arriving late for the scheduled testing appointment may be required to forfeit the NCLEX appointment. If it is necessary for the appointment to be forfeited, candidates will need to re-register for the examination and pay an additional fee. The board of nursing will be notified that the candidate will not test.

A few days before your scheduled date of testing, take the time to drive to the testing center to determine its exact location, the length of time required to arrive to that destination, and any potential obstacles that might delay you, such as road construction, traffic, or parking sites.

THE TESTING CENTER

The test center is designed to ensure complete security of the testing process. Strict candidate identification requirements have been established. To be admitted to the testing center, it is imperative that you bring the Authorization to Test form, along with two forms of identification. You must sign both forms of identification, and one must contain your photograph. The name on the photograph identification must be the same as the name stated on the Authorization to Test form. Examples of acceptable forms of identification will be included in the information received with the Authorization to Test form. You will be required to sign in and out on the test center log form. Each candidate will be thumbprinted and photographed at the test center, and the photograph will accompany the NCLEX results to confirm the candidate's identity. Personal belongings are not allowed in the testing room. Secure storage will be provided for the candidate; however, storage space is limited, so you must plan accordingly. In addition, the testing center will not assume responsibility for your personal belongings. The testing waiting areas are generally small; therefore friends or family members who accompany you are not permitted to wait in the testing center while you are taking the NCLEX-PN.

Once you have completed the admission process and a brief orientation, the proctor will escort you to the assigned computer. You will be seated at an individual table area with an appropriate work space that includes computer equipment, appropriate lighting, scratch paper, and a pencil. Unauthorized scratch paper may not be brought into or removed from the testing room. Eating, drinking, and smoking are not allowed in the testing room. A video camera is located in the testing room, and full sound and motion videotaping of all test sessions occurs.

Keep your two forms of identification with you at all times. You cannot leave the testing room without the permission of the proctor. If you leave the testing room for any reason, you will be required to show two forms of identification to be readmitted. You must follow the directions given by the test center staff and must remain seated during the test, except when authorized to leave. If you feel that you have a problem with the computer, need more scratch paper, or need the proctor for any reason, you must raise your hand to notify the proctor.

THE COMPUTER

You do not need any computer experience to take the CAT NCLEX-PN examination. A keyboard tutorial is provided and administered to all test takers at the start of the examination. In addition, a proctor is present to assist in explaining the use of the computer to ensure your full understanding of how to proceed.

CAT NCLEX-PN TEST QUESTIONS

The examination is composed of individual (stand-alone) test questions. In other words, this examination does not present a case situation followed by several test questions that relate to that case situation. With an individual (stand-alone) test question, you can expect that the question will appear on the left-hand side of the screen with the four options on the right-hand side of the screen, or the question will appear across the top of the screen with the four options below (Box 1-7).

The test questions will be multiple choice (question and four options). You may be presented with a visual or image type of display and will be asked a question about the visual or image. For example, you may be presented with a visual that displays an adult client's thorax. In this visual, you may be asked to identify the area where the stethoscope would be placed to take an apical pulse rate.

When a test question is presented on the computer screen, it must be answered or the test will not move on. This means that you will not be able to skip questions, go back and review questions, or go back and change answers. Students preparing for CAT NCLEX-PN become anxious and frustrated because questions cannot be skipped and returned to at a later time during the examination process. Remember, in a CAT examination, once an answer is recorded, all subsequent questions administered depend, to an extent, on the answer selected for that question. Skipping and returning to earlier questions are not compatible with the logical methodology of a computerized adaptive test. In addition, it is important to recall the number of times you may have changed a correct answer to an incorrect one on a pencil and paper nursing examination during your nursing education. The inability to skip questions or go back to change previous answers will not be a disadvantage to you. Actually, you will not fall into that "trap" of changing a correct answer to an incorrect one with CAT. There is no penalty for guessing on CAT NCLEX-PN. Remember, the answer to the question will be right there in front of you. If you need to guess, use your nursing knowledge to its fullest extent, as well as all of the test-taking strategies provided to you in Chapter 4 of this book.

TESTING TIME

The maximum testing time is 5 hours, and this time period includes the tutorial, sample questions, and all rest breaks. There is no minimum amount of examination time. A mandatory 10-minute break will be taken after 2 testing hours, and an optional 10-minute break can be taken at the end of 3.5 hours of testing. The computer screen will notify you of the time for these breaks. You must leave the testing room during breaks. You may leave the room for additional, unscheduled breaks, but no additional testing time will be allowed.

BOX 1-7

Appearance of an Individual (Stand-Alone) Test Question on the Computer Screen

The most appropriate method for feeding the infant with a cleft lip or palate is:	1. With the head in an upright position 2. With the infant in a lying position 3. With the infant in a side-lying position 4. With the infant prone

A client is admitted to the hospital with a diagnosis of myasthenia gravis. Pyridostigmine (Mestinon) is prescribed for the client. An adverse effect of this medication is:

1. Muscle cramps
2. Mouth ulcers
3. Depression
4. Unexplained weight gain

LENGTH OF THE EXAMINATION

The minimum number of questions that you may need to answer in order to meet adequate testing in each area of the test plan is 85. Of these 85 questions, 70 will be real (scored) questions and 15 will be try-out (unscored) questions. The maximum number of questions in the test is 205. Fifteen of the total number of questions that you need to answer will be try-out (unscored) questions.

The try-out questions are questions that may be presented as scored questions on future NCLEX-PN examinations. These try-out questions are not identified as such. In other words, you do not know which questions are the try-out (unscored) questions.

COMPLETING THE EXAMINATION

Once the test is completed, you will complete a brief computer-delivered questionnaire about your testing experience. After this questionnaire is completed, the test proctor will collect all scratch paper, sign you out, and permit you to leave.

PROCESSING RESULTS

On completion of the examination, results are transmitted electronically to the data center for scoring. Your results are then transmitted to the board of nursing in the state in which you applied for licensure. The board of nursing will mail the results to the candidate.

INTERSTATE ENDORSEMENT

Since the CAT NCLEX-PN is a national examination, you can apply to take the examination in any state. Once licensure is received, the practical/vocational nurse can apply for Interstate Endorsement. The procedures and requirements for Interstate Endorsement may vary from state to state, and these procedures can be obtained from the state board of nursing in the state in which endorsement is sought.

ADDITIONAL INFORMATION REGARDING NCLEX-PN

Additional information regarding the NCLEX-PN examination can be obtained from the National Council of State Boards of Nursing, Inc, 676 St Clair Street, Suite 550, Chicago, IL 60611-2921. The telephone number for the National Council of State Boards of Nursing, Inc, is (312) 787-6555. The website is: http://www.ncsbn.org.

STATE BOARDS OF NURSING

Alabama Board of Nursing
770 Washington Avenue
RSA Plaza, Suite 250
Montgomery, AL 36130-3900
Phone: (334) 242-4060
FAX: (334) 242-4360
Web Site: http://www.abn.state.al.us/

Alaska Board of Nursing
Div. of Occupational Licensing
3601 C Street, Suite 722
Anchorage, AK 99503
Phone: (907) 269-8161
FAX: (907) 269-8196
Web Site: http://www.dced.state.ak.us/occ/pnur.htm

American Samoa Health Services
Regulatory Board
LBJ Tropical Medical Center
Pago Pago, AS 96799
Phone: (684) 633-1222
FAX: (684) 633-1869

Arizona State Board of Nursing
1651 E. Morten Avenue, Suite 210
Phoenix, AZ 85020
Phone: (602) 331-8111
FAX: (602) 906-9365
Web Site: http://www.azboardofnursing.org/

Arkansas State Board of Nursing
University Tower Building
1123 S. University, Suite 800
Little Rock, AR 72204-1619
Phone: (501) 686-2700
FAX: (501) 686-2714
Web Site: http://www.state.ar.us/nurse

California Board of Vocational Nursing
and Psychiatric Technician Examiners
2535 Capitol Oaks Drive, Suite 205
Sacramento, CA 95833
Phone: (916) 263-7800
FAX: (916) 263-7859
Web Site: http://www.bvnpt.ca.gov/

Colorado Board of Nursing
1560 Broadway, Suite 880
Denver, CO 80202
Phone: (303) 894-2430
FAX: (303) 894-2821
Web Site: http://www.dora.state.co.us/nursing/

Connecticut Board of Examiners for Nursing
Dept. of Public Health
410 Capitol Avenue, MS# 13PHO
PO Box 340308
Hartford, CT 06134-0328
Phone: (860) 509-7624
FAX: (860) 509-7553
Web Site: http://www.state.ct.us/dph/

Delaware Board of Nursing
861 Silver Lake Blvd
Cannon Building, Suite 203
Dover, DE 19904
Phone: (302) 739-4522
FAX: (302) 739-2711

District of Columbia Board of Nursing
Department of Health
825 N. Capitol Street, NE, 2nd Floor
Room 2224
Washington, DC 20002
Phone: (202) 442-4778
FAX: (202) 442-9431

Florida Board of Nursing
Capital Circle Officer Center
4052 Bald Cypress Way
Room 120
Tallahassee, FL 32399-3252
Phone: (850) 488-0595
Web Site: http://www.doh.state.fl.us/mqa/

Georgia State Board of Licensed
Practical Nurses
237 Coliseum Drive
Macon, GA 31217-3858
Phone: (478) 207-1300
FAX: (478) 207-1633
Web Site: http://www.sos.state.ga.us/ebd-lpn/

Guam Board of Nurse Examiners
PO Box 2816
1304 East Sunset Boulevard
Barrgada, GU 96913
Phone: (671) 475-0251
FAX: (671) 477-4733

Hawaii Board of Nursing
Professional & Vocational Licensing Division
PO Box 3469
Honolulu, HI 96801
Phone: (808) 586-3000
FAX: (808) 586-2689
Web Site: http://www.state.hi.us/dcca/pvl/areasnurse.html

Idaho Board of Nursing
280 N. 8th Street, Suite 210
PO Box 83720
Boise, ID 83720
Phone: (208) 334-3110
FAX: (208) 334-3262
Web Site: http://www.state.id.us/ibn/ibnhome.htm

Illinois Department of Professional Regulation
James R. Thompson Center
100 West Randolph, Suite 9-300
Chicago, IL 60601
Phone: (312) 814-2715
FAX: (312) 814-3145
Web Site: http://www.dpr.state.il.us/

Illinois Department of Professional Regulation
320 W. Washington St.
3rd Floor
Springfield, IL 62786
Phone: (217) 782-8556
FAX: (217) 782-7645

Indiana State Board of Nursing
Health Professions Bureau
402 W. Washington Street, Room W041
Indianapolis, IN 46204
Phone: (317) 232-2960
FAX: (317) 233-4236
Web Site: http://www.state.in.us/hpb/boards/isbn/

Iowa Board of Nursing
RiverPoint Business Park
400 S.W. 8th Street
Suite B
Des Moines, IA 50309-4685
Phone: (515) 281-3255
FAX: (515) 281-4825
Web Site: http://www.state.ia.us/government/nursing/

Kansas State Board of Nursing
Landon State Office Building
900 S.W. Jackson, Suite 551-S
Topeka, KS 66612
Phone: (785) 296-4929
FAX: (785) 296-3929
Web Site: http://www.ksbn.org

Kentucky Board of Nursing
312 Whittington Parkway, Suite 300
Louisville, KY 40222
Phone: (502) 329-7000
FAX: (502) 329-7011
Web Site: http://www.kbn.state.ky.us/

Louisiana State Board of Practical Nurse Examiners
3421 N. Causeway Boulevard, Suite 203
Metairie, LA 70002
Phone: (504) 838-5791
FAX: (504) 838-5279
Web Site: http://www.lsbpne.com/

Maine State Board of Nursing
158 State House Station
Augusta, ME 04333
Phone: (207) 287-1133
FAX: (207) 287-1149
Web Site: http://www.state.me.us/boardofnursing

Maryland Board of Nursing
4140 Patterson Avenue
Baltimore, MD 21215
Phone: (410) 585-1900
FAX: (410) 358-3530
Web Site: http://www.mbon.org

Massachusetts Board of Registration in Nursing
Commonwealth of Massachusetts
239 Causeway Street
Boston, MA 02114
Phone: (617) 727-9961
FAX: (617) 727-1630
Web Site: http://www.state.ma.us/reg/boards/rn/

Michigan CIS/Office of Health Services
Ottawa Towers North
611 W. Ottawa, 4th Floor
Lansing, MI 48933
Phone: (517) 373-9102
FAX: (517) 373-2179
Web Site: http://www.cis.state.mi.us/bhser/genover.htm

Minnesota Board of Nursing
2829 University Avenue SE
Suite 500
Minneapolis, MN 55414
Phone: (612) 617-2270
FAX: (612) 617-2190
Web Site: http://www.nursingboard.state.mn.us/

Mississippi Board of Nursing
1935 Lakeland Drive, Suite B
Jackson, MS 39216-5014
Phone: (601) 987-4188
FAX: (601) 364-2352
Web Site: http://www.msbn.state.ms.us/

Missouri State Board of Nursing
3605 Missouri Boulevard
PO Box 656
Jefferson City, MO 65102-0656
Phone: (573) 751-0681
FAX: (573) 751-0075
Web Site: http://www.ecodev.state.mo.us/pr/nursing/

Montana State Board of Nursing
301 South Park
PO Box 200513
Helena, MT 59620-0513
Phone: (406) 841-2340
FAX: (406) 841-2343
Web Site: http://www.discoveringmontana.com/dli/bsd/license/bsd_boards/nur_board/board_page.htm

Northern Mariana Islands
Commonwealth Board of Nurse Examiners
PO Box 501458
Saipan, MP 96950
Phone: (670) 664-4810
FAX: (670) 664-4813

Nebraska Health and Human Services System
Dept. of Regulation & Licensure, Nursing Section
301 Centennial Mall South
Lincoln, NE 68509-4986
Phone: (402) 471-4376
FAX: (402) 471-3577
Nursing and Nursing Support Web Site: http://www.hhs.state.ne.us/crl/nursing/nursingindex.htm

Nevada State Board of Nursing
License Certification and Education
4330 S. Valley View Boulevard
Suite 106
Las Vegas, NV 89103
Phone: (702) 486-5800
FAX: (702)) 486-5803
Web Site: http://www.nursingboard.state.nv.us

New Hampshire Board of Nursing
PO Box 3898
78 Regional Drive, BLDG B
Concord, NH 03302
Phone: (603) 271-2323
FAX: (603) 271-6605
Web Site: http://www.state.nh.us/nursing/

New Jersey Board of Nursing
PO Box 45010
124 Halsey Street, 6th Floor
Newark, NJ 07101
Phone: (973) 504-6586
FAX: (973) 648-3481
Web Site: http://www.state.nj.us/lps/ca/medical.htm

New Mexico Board of Nursing
4206 Louisiana Boulevard, NE
Suite A
Albuquerque, NM 87109
Phone: (505) 841-8340
FAX: (505) 841-8347
Web Site: http://www.state.nm.us/clients/nursing

New York State Board of Nursing
Education Bldg.
89 Washington Avenue
2nd Floor West Wing
Albany, NY 12234
Phone: (518) 474-3817 Ext. 120
FAX: (518) 474-3706
Web Site: http://www.nysed.gov/prof/nurse.htm

North Carolina Board of Nursing
3724 National Drive, Suite 201
Raleigh, NC 27612
Phone: (919) 782-3211
FAX: (919) 781-9461
Web Site: http://www.ncbon.com/

North Dakota Board of Nursing
919 South 7th Street, Suite 504
Bismarck, ND 58504
Phone: (701) 328-9777
FAX: (701) 328-9785
Web Site: http://www.ndbon.org/

Ohio Board of Nursing
17 South High Street, Suite 400
Columbus, OH 43215-3413
Phone: (614) 466-3947
FAX: (614) 466-0388
Web Site: http://www.state.oh.us/nur/

Oklahoma Board of Nursing
2915 N. Classen Boulevard, Suite 524
Oklahoma City, OK 73106
Phone: (405) 962-1800
FAX: (405) 962-1821
Web Site: http://www.youroklahoma.com/nursing

Oregon State Board of Nursing
800 NE Oregon Street, Box 25
Suite 465
Portland, OR 97232
Phone: (503) 731-4745
FAX: (503) 731-4755
Web Site: http://www.osbn.state.or.us/

Pennsylvania State Board of Nursing
124 Pine Street
Harrisburg, PA 17101
Phone: (717) 783-7142
FAX: (717) 783-0822
Web Site: http://www.dos.state.pa.us/bpoa/nurbd/mainpage.htm

Commonwealth of Puerto Rico
Board of Nurse Examiners
800 Roberto H. Todd Avenue
Room 202, Stop 18
Santurce, PR 00908
Phone: (787) 725-7506
FAX: (787) 725-7903

Rhode Island Board of Nurse
Registration and Nursing Education
105 Cannon Building
Three Capitol Hill
Providence, RI 02908
Phone: (401) 222-5700
FAX: (401) 222-3352
Web Site: http://www.health.state.ri.us

South Carolina State Board of Nursing
110 Centerview Drive
Suite 202
Columbia, SC 29210
Phone: (803) 896-4550
FAX: (803) 896-4525
Web Site: http://www.llr.state.sc.us/pol/nursing

South Dakota Board of Nursing
4300 South Louise Ave., Suite C-1
Sioux Falls, SD 57106-3124
Phone: (605) 362-2760
FAX: (605) 362-2768
Web Site: http://www.state.sd.us/dcr/nursing/

Tennessee State Board of Nursing
426 Fifth Avenue North
1st Floor - Cordell Hull Building
Nashville, TN 37247
Phone: (615) 532-5166
FAX: (615) 741-7899
Web Site: http://170.142.76.180/bmf-bin/BMFproflist. pl

Texas Board of Vocational Nurse Examiners
William P. Hobby Building, Tower 3
333 Guadalupe Street, Suite 3-400
Austin, TX 78701
Phone: (512) 305-8100
FAX: (512) 305-8101
Web Site: http://www.bvne.state.tx.us/

Utah State Board of Nursing
Heber M. Wells Bldg., 4th Floor
160 East 300 South
Salt Lake City, UT 84111
Phone: (801) 530-6628
FAX: (801) 530-6511
Web Site: http://www.commerce.state.ut.us/

Vermont State Board of Nursing
109 State Street
Montpelier, VT 05609-1106
Phone: (802) 828-2396
FAX: (802) 828-2484
Web Site: http://vtprofessionals.org/nurses/

Virgin Islands Board of Nurse Licensure
Veterans Drive Station
St. Thomas, VI 00803
Phone: (340) 776-7397
FAX: (340) 777-4003

Virginia Board of Nursing
6606 W. Broad Street, 4th Floor
Richmond, VA 23230
Phone: (804) 662-9909
FAX: (804) 662-9512
Web Site: http://www.dhp.state.va.us/

Washington State Nursing Care Quality
Assurance Commission
Department of Health
1300 Quince Street SE
Olympia, WA 98504-7864
Phone: (360) 236-4700
FAX: (360) 236-4738
Web Site: http://www.doh.wa.gov/nursing/

West Virginia Board of Examiners for Licensed Practical Nurses
101 Dee Drive
Charleston, WV 25311
Phone: (304) 558-3572
FAX: (304) 558-4367
Web Site: http://www.lpnboard.state.wv.us/

Wisconsin Department of Regulation and Licensing
1400 E. Washington Avenue
PO Box 8935
Madison, WI 53708
Phone: (608) 266-0145
FAX: (608) 261-7083
Web Site: http://www.drl.state.wi.us/

Wyoming State Board of Nursing
2020 Carey Avenue, Suite 110
Cheyenne, WY 82002
Phone: (307) 777-7601
FAX: (307) 777-3519
Web Site: http://nursing.state.wy.us/

REFERENCES

deWit S: *Fundamental concepts and skills for nursing,* Philadelphia, 2001, WB Saunders.

Hodgson B, Kizior R: *Saunders nursing drug handbook 2002,* Philadelphia, 2002, WB Saunders.

National Council of State Boards of Nursing, editors: *Test plan for the National Council Licensure Examination for Practical/Vocational Nurses,* Chicago, 2001, Author.

National Council of State Boards of Nursing, editors: *The NCLEX process: serving as an anchor for the NCLEX Examination,* Chicago, 2000, Author.

National Council of State Boards of Nursing. Web Site: http://www.ncsbn.org

Potter P, Perry A: *Fundamentals of nursing,* ed 5, St Louis, 2001, Mosby,

Riley J: *Communication in nursing,* ed 4, St Louis, 2000, Mosby.

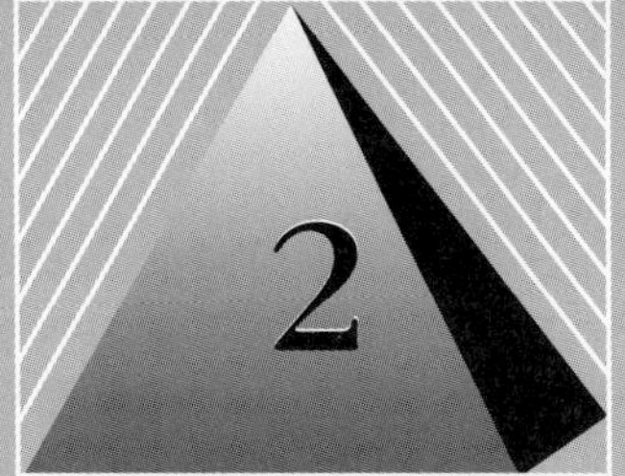

Pathways to Success

LAURENT W. VALLIERE

THE PYRAMID TO SUCCESS

Preparing to take the NCLEX-PN examination can produce a great deal of anxiety. You may be thinking that NCLEX-PN is the most important examination that you will ever have to take, and that it reflects the culmination of everything that you have worked so hard for. NCLEX-PN is an important examination because receiving that nursing license means that you can begin your career as a licensed practical/vocational nurse. Your success on NCLEX-PN involves expelling all thoughts that allow this examination to appear overwhelming and intimidating. Such thoughts will take complete control over your destiny. A positive attitude, a structured plan for preparation, and maintaining control in your pathway to success will ensure achievement in reaching the peak of the Pyramid to Success (Box 2-1).

THE FOUNDATION

The foundation of Pathways to Success begins with having a positive attitude and developing short- and long-term goals. Both will lead you toward achievement and success. Without these components, the Pathway to Success leads to nowhere and has no end point. You will expend energy and valuable time and will experience exhaustion without any accomplishment. Therefore, it is imperative that you take the time to develop that positive attitude and to establish your short- and long-term goals.

BOX 2-1

Pathways to Success

THE FOUNDATION
Maintaining a positive attitude
Thinking about short- and long-term realistic goals
Developing control

THE LIST
Documenting short- and long-term realistic goals
Maintaining control

THE PLAN
Developing a study plan and schedule
Deciding on the place to study
Balancing personal and work obligations with the study schedule
Sharing the study schedule and personal needs with others
Implementing the study plan

POSITIVE PAMPERING
Establishing healthy eating habits
Planning time for exercise and fun activities
Including activities in the schedule that provide positive mental stimulation

FINAL PREPARATION
Reviewing goals
Identifying goals achieved
Remaining focused to complete the plan of study
Writing down the date and time of the examination and posting it next to your name with the letters LPN/LVN following, and the word "YES!"
Planning a test drive to the testing center
Relaxing on the day before the examination

THE DAY OF THE EXAMINATION
Grooming yourself for success
Eating a healthy and nutritious breakfast
Maintaining a confident and positive attitude
Maintaining control
Meeting the challenges of the day
Reaching the peak of the Pyramid to Success

Where do you start? To begin this process, find a location that offers solitude. Sit or lie in a comfortable position, close your eyes, relax, inhale deeply, hold your breath to a count of 4, exhale slowly, and again, relax. Repeat this breathing exercise several times until you begin to feel relaxed and free from anxiety. Allow your mind to become void of all chatter. Now you are in control and your mind can see for miles. Your highway of life has a multitude of destinations to which you may travel. It is now time for you to plan the order of your journey to the Pyramid to Success.

THE LIST

It is time to create "The List." The List is your set of goals. At this time, you may or may not have a scheduled date for taking the NCLEX-PN examination. Begin by developing the goals you wish to accomplish today, tomorrow, and into the future. Allow yourself the opportunity to list all that is flowing from your uninhibited thought process. Write your goals on a piece of paper. When the List is complete, it is time to bank it away for 2 or 3 days. Then retrieve and review the List and begin the process of planning for preparing for the NCLEX-PN examination.

THE PLAN

Now that you have the List in order, look at your goals that relate to studying for the licensing examination. The first task is to decide what study pattern works best for you. Take the time to review what has worked most successfully for you in the past. There are questions that must be addressed in order to develop your plan for study (Box 2-2).

"The Plan" must include how you will manage your study needs and the demands of your family and friends. Take time to think about how you will balance your everyday commitments with your plan for study. Your family and friends are key players in your life and are going to become a part of your Pyramid to Success. After you have established your study needs, communicate your needs and the importance of your study plan in achieving your goal of becoming a licensed practical/vocational nurse to your family and friends.

A difficult part of the Plan may include how you will deal with those family and friends who choose not to participate in your Pyramid to Success. What if an individual or individuals choose not to be part of the Pyramid? Then you are faced with a decision. You must weight all of the factors carefully. You must keep your goals in mind and remember that your need for positive momentum is critical. Your decision may not be an easy one, but it must help you ensure that you achieve your goal of becoming a licensed practical/vocational nurse. Remember, a positive momentum and goal achievement need to be shared by all who support you.

The Plan must include a schedule. Establish a realistic schedule that includes your daily, weekly, and future goals, and adhere to it. This consistency will provide advantages to you and to those supporting you. A daily schedule allows you to plan more carefully your topic areas for study. Adherence to the Plan helps you develop a rhythm that can only enhance your retention and positive momentum. Those that are supporting you will share this rhythm and will be able to schedule their activities and life better because you are consistent with your study schedule. You are moving forward, and you are in control!

BOX 2-2

Developing a Plan for Study

Do I work better alone or in a group study environment? If I work best in a group, does the group consist of one, two, or more study partners?
Who are these study partners?
How long should my study sessions last?
Does the time of day that I study make a difference for me?
Do I retain more if I study in the morning?
How does my work schedule affect my study pattern?
How do I balance my family obligations with my need to study?
Do I have a comfortable study area at home, or do I need to find another environment that is conducive to my study needs?

POSITIVE PAMPERING

Positive momentum can be maintained only if you are properly balanced. This means that you must continue to care for yourself. Proper exercise, diet, and positive mental stimulation are critical to achieving your goal of becoming a licensed practical/vocational nurse.

Just as you have developed a schedule for study, you should have a schedule that includes some fun and form of physical activity. It is your choice—aerobics, running, weight lifting, bowling, or whatever makes you feel good about yourself. Time spent away from the hard study schedule and devoted to some form of fun and physical exercise pays its rewards 100-fold. You will feel alive and more energetic with a schedule that includes these activities.

Establish healthy eating habits. Stay away from fatty foods because they will slow you down. Eat lighter meals and eat more frequently. Include complex carbohydrates in your diet for energy, and be careful not to include too much caffeine in your daily diet.

Continue to feel good about yourself, because you are in control. Take the time to pamper yourself with activities that make you feel even better about who you are. Make dinner reservations at your favorite restaurant with someone who is special and is supporting your goal to become a licensed practical/vocational nurse. Take walks in a place that has a particular tranquility that enables you to reflect on the positive momentum that you have achieved and maintained. Whatever it is, wherever it takes you, allow yourself the time to do some positive pampering.

FINAL PREPARATION

You have established the foundation of your Pyramid. You have developed your list of goals and your study plan and have maintained your positive momentum. You are moving forward, and you are in control. When you receive your date and time for the NCLEX-PN examination, you may immediately think, "I am not ready!"

Stop! Reflect on all that you have achieved. Think about your goal achievement and the organization of the positive life momentum with which you have surrounded yourself. Think about all those individuals who love and support your effort to become a licensed practical/vocational nurse. Believe that the challenge that awaits you is one that you have successfully prepared for and will lead you to your goal, becoming a licensed practical/vocational nurse!

Take a deep breath and organize the remaining days so that they support your educational and personal needs. Support your positive momentum with a visual technique. Write your name in large letters and write the letters LPN/LVN after it. Post one or more of these visual reinforcements in areas that you frequent. This form of motivational technique works for many individuals preparing for this examination.

Through all that you have accomplished to this point, it is imperative that you not fall into the trap of expecting too much of yourself. The idea of perfection must not drive you to lose your positive momentum. You must believe in who you are, as you are, and stay focused on your goal. Allow yourself the opportunity to continue to carry out your plan in a manner that is most conducive to who you are, not someone else. The date and time are in hand. Write down the date and time and underneath write the word "YES." Post this next to your name plus LPN/LVN.

You must ensure that you have command over how to get to the testing center. A test run is a must. Time the drive, and allow for road construction or whatever may occur to slow the traffic. On the test run, when you arrive at the test facility, you may want to walk in. Become familiar with the lobby and the surroundings. This may help to alleviate some of the nervousness associated with entering an unknown building. Remember, you must do whatever it takes to keep yourself in control. If familiarizing yourself with the facility will help you to maintain positive momentum, by all means, be sure to do so! Who is in control? You are!

It is time to check your study plan and make the necessary adjustments now that a firm date and time are set. Adjust your review so that it flows to your needs and that your study plan ends 2 days before the examination. Remember that the mind is like a muscle. If it is overworked, it has no strength or stamina. Your strategy is to rest the body and the mind on the day before the examination. Your strategy is to stay in control and allow yourself the opportunity to be absolutely fresh and attentive the day of the examination. This will help you control the nervousness that is natural, achieve the clear thought processes required, and feel confident that you have done all that is necessary to prepare and conquer this challenge. The day before the examination is to be one of pleasure. Treat yourself to what you enjoy the most.

Relax! You have prepared yourself well for the challenge of tomorrow. Allow yourself a good night's sleep, and wake up the day of the examination knowing that you are absolutely ready to succeed. Look at your name with LPN/LVN after it and the word, "YES!"

THE DAY OF THE EXAMINATION

Wake up believing in yourself and that all you have accomplished is about to propel you to the level of licensed practical/vocational nurse. Allow yourself plenty of time, eat a nutritious breakfast, and groom yourself for success. You are ready to meet the challenges of the day and overcome any obstacle you may face. Today will soon be history, and tomorrow will bring you the envelope on which you read your name with the words, Licensed Practical/Vocational Nurse, after it.

Be proud and confident of your achievements. You have worked hard to reach your goal of becoming a licensed practical/vocational nurse. If you believe in yourself and your goals, no one person or obstacle can move you off the pathway that leads to success, to the peak of the Pyramid!

Congratulations and I wish you the very best in your career as a Licensed Practical/Vocational Nurse!

The NCLEX-PN Examination: From a Student's Perspective

MARY E. WRIGHT

When I graduated from nursing school, I was 32 years old. My three best friends graduated at the same time from the same nursing program, and all of us were the older students of the class. There were many commitments that all of us had to contend with during our education. We had many hats to wear, so to speak, and several roles and responsibilities: We were mothers, wives, friends, nursing students, and support systems to each other and everyone around us. Our path through the learning process in nursing school was not an easy one. There were many obstacles and many commitments to meet, but the perseverance and desire to become a nurse made all of the obstacles challenges—challenges that we all knew would lead to many rewards.

When we graduated from nursing school, we knew that we had one more major challenge to meet and that was to pass the NCLEX examination. My three friends and I lived quite a distance from the test site so we decided that we would pack up our bags, register at a luxurious hotel, and take the test together. We arrived at the hotel on the day before our scheduled and dreaded examination in a state of high anxiety. Were we ready to meet this last challenge? Yes, we were.

Suggestions about preparing for this examination were fortunately shared by the nursing graduates who took it the previous year, and by my nursing instructors. Whenever I became anxious, nervous, or felt as though I was losing confidence in my abilities to succeed, I thought about all of their suggestions, which helped get me back on track. I want to share with you some of the tips I received from others regarding the preparation for this important examination, as well as my own hints.

To begin, it is important to listen to what others have to say about preparing for this examination because their input will be very helpful. But remember that this test is all about you, and you must meet your own needs in preparing yourself.

You need to remember that balance in life can bring success. A study plan is important, but it needs to be structured and realistic to meet your needs and all of the commitments that you have in your life. An immediate instinct is to study every minute that you can right up to the time of the examination. My suggestion is that you spend two hours each day for intensive review. If you feel as though you can spend more than two hours, then do so; but I found that after the two hours, I became distracted and fatigued.

How do you proceed with your study? Practice questions—do as many as you possibly can. Read the rationales for the correct and incorrect answers and learn how to answer the question if you are unfamiliar with the content area. Make a list of the content that you will need to read, and refresh your memory on these areas from your nursing textbooks. But again, practice with as many questions as you can.

Do you study right up to the time of the examination? No. You need to relax and enjoy yourself the day before the examination. Remember, no cramming at the last minute. Be confident that you have what it takes to pass this test to become a licensed practical or vocational nurse. I needed to remember that I would not be taking this important examination if I didn't have what it takes.

In addition to your two hours' study time, make sure that you spend time having some fun. Each day, spend time doing what you like to do, whatever that may be. It is also very important that you save time for exercise and to prepare healthy meals for yourself. You need to be prepared physically and mentally.

On the night before the examination, don't study—have fun and get a good night's sleep. Again, remember that you are prepared. My nursing instructors told me that if I had difficulty sleeping, to try deep- and slow-breathing exercises because they would relax my body. That's what I did, and it helped. In fact, whenever I became distracted and nervous during the examination, I began to deep breathe and became relaxed so that I could proceed.

On the night before the examination, my friends and I went out for dinner and a relaxing evening; but as soon as we ordered our meals, my friends began asking questions about medications, medication calculations, and various other topics related to nursing. I could feel my stomach beginning to knot, and I finally told my friends that there would be no nursing conversations at this dinner table. I reminded them that we knew what we needed to know and that these last hours were not going to make a difference.

On the morning of the examination, we had a wake-up call in addition to four alarm clocks going off at the crack of dawn. You want to get up early enough to have time to prepare yourself physically and mentally. Eat a light, healthy breakfast and take something to eat for breaktime during the examination. It may be difficult to eat because your stomach may feel as though it is a big knot. But remember to feed your brain because your brain is what you will really need.

When you arrive at the testing center, you will need to complete all of the pretesting rituals. This will make you nervous because all you want to do is get on with the test and get it over with. Take those deep breaths and don't become frustrated because you will begin to block your thought process. You haven't started the test yet. Be patient. As you have probably been told, all of the questions are multiple choice. You will, just as I did, receive questions about nursing content that you do not know or have never heard of. When this happens, don't become nervous. Take a deep breath and remember this happens to everyone. Also, remember that the answer is right there in front of you, so read the question again, and make an educated guess just as you had to do with all of your practice questions.

When the examination was completed, I felt relieved, yet I kept experiencing ambivalent feelings. One minute I felt as though I did great, and then I would begin to feel nervous and anxious as though I had failed. You are likely to experience these same feelings. Remember, it is over with, you did the best that you could, now go on with your life.

The final component is the waiting game—waiting for the results. This is as difficult as any other part of the process. Keep yourself busy. I anxiously checked my mailbox every day awaiting the news. Finally, it came. It was a white, thin envelope. I could see my name through a clear opening in the envelope, but I could not see the letters LPN, so I feared opening it. But I remembered that I was told—a thin envelope is a good sign. So I carefully opened it and saw my name with LPN following it. I ran back into my house yelling "Yes!" all the way. I immediately called everyone that I knew to spread the great news. And then, I called my three friends. They passed, too. Now, we could begin the careers that we had dreamed of.

As a final thought, always remember that belief and a positive attitude will help guide you to your goal of becoming a Licensed Practical Nurse.

Congratulations to you and I wish you continued success in your new career as a Licensed Practical Nurse.

4 Test-Taking Strategies

I. PYRAMID TO SUCCESS (Box 4-1)

II. HOW TO AVOID READING INTO THE QUESTION

A. Pyramid points
   1. Identify the case situation from the stem of the question
   2. Identify what the question is asking
   3. Look for the key words
   4. Read every option
   5. Use the process of elimination
   6. As you read the question, avoid asking yourself "What if...?"

B. The case situation (Box 4-2)
   1. The case situation provides you with the information about a clinical health problem and the information that you need to consider in answering the question
   2. Read all of the information and every word in the case situation

C. The stem of the question (Box 4-2)
   1. The stem of the question follows the case situation and asks something specific about the case situation
   2. Read the stem carefully, and specifically identify exactly what is being asked

D. The options (Box 4-2)
   1. The options are all of the answers, and you must select one
   2. Read every option carefully and reread the stem of the question to be sure that you understand what is being asked
   3. Use the process of elimination
   4. Once you have eliminated two incorrect options, reread the stem of the question to identify specifically what the question is asking, before selecting the correct option

III. KEY WORDS (Box 4-3)

A. Key words focus your attention on critical ideas in the case situation, in the stem, and in the options

BOX 4-1

Pyramid to Success

Read the question and every option thoroughly and carefully!
Ask yourself, "What is the question specifically asking?"
Be alert to key words and true and false response stems!
Eliminate the incorrect options!
Use all of your nursing knowledge, your clinical experiences, and your test-taking skills and strategies to answer the question!

BOX 4-2

Case Situation, Stem, and Options

CASE SITUATION

A nurse is monitoring a child for bleeding after surgery for removal of a brain tumor. The nurse checks the head dressing for the presence of blood and notes a colorless drainage on the back of the dressing.

STEM

Which of the following would be the most appropriate nursing intervention?

Options

1. Circle the area of drainage and continue to monitor
2. Reinforce the dressing
3. Notify the registered nurse
4. Document the findings and continue to monitor

Answer: 3

BOX 4-3

Common Key Words

Early or late
Best
First
Initial
Immediately
Most likely or least likely
Most appropriate or least appropriate
On the day of
After several days

BOX 4-4

Key Words to Eliminate Incorrect Options

Which of the following is an EARLY sign of shock?
Which of the following is a LATE SIGN of shock?
ON THE DAY OF surgery, following a transurethral resection of the prostate (TURP), a nurse notes that the client's urine is bright red. Which of the following nursing actions is MOST APPROPRIATE?
AFTER SEVERAL DAYS, following a transurethral resection of the prostate (TURP), a nurse notes that the client's urine is bright red. Which of the following nursing actions is MOST APPROPRIATE?
Noting the key words in each of these situations will assist in directing you to select the correct option.
The EARLY signs of shock are quite different from the LATE signs of shock!
Bright red urine might be expected ON THE DAY OF surgery following a TURP, but would not be expected AFTER SEVERAL DAYS!

B. Key words are important to identify because they will assist in eliminating the incorrect options (Box 4-4)
C. Some of the key words may indicate that all of the options are correct, and that it will be necessary to prioritize in order to select the correct option

IV. THE CLIENT OF THE QUESTION

A. Identify the client of the question
B. The client is the person who is the focus of the question
C. It is important to remember that the client of the question may not necessarily be the person with the health problem; in the test question, the client may be a relative, friend, spouse, significant other, or another member of the health care team
D. After identifying the client of the question, select the option that relates to and most directly addresses that client

V. THE ISSUE OF THE QUESTION (Box 4-5)

A. Identify the issue of the question

BOX 4-5

The Issue of the Question

A nurse administers a dose of scopolamine to a preoperative client. The nurse monitors the client for which of the following *side effects*?
1. Excessive urination
2. Diaphoresis
3. Dry mouth
4. Pupillary constriction

Answer: 3

TEST-TAKING STRATEGY

Focus on the issue—the side effect of a medication. Use your nursing knowledge, clinical experiences, and test-taking skills and strategies to answer the question. Recalling that scopolamine is an anticholinergic medication that causes the frequent side effects of dry mouth, urinary retention, decreased sweating, and pupil dilation will direct you to the correct option.

B. The issue of the question is the specific subject content that the question is asking about
C. Identifying the issue of the question will assist in eliminating the incorrect options and direct you to selecting the correct option
D. The issue of the question can include
   1. A medication or intravenous (IV) therapy
   2. A side effect of a medication
   3. An adverse or toxic effect of a medication
   4. A treatment or procedure
   5. A complication of a health care problem, treatment, or procedure
   6. A specific nursing action

VI. TRUE OR FALSE RESPONSE STEMS

A. True response stem (Box 4-6)
   1. True response stems use key words that ask you to select an option that is true regarding the case situation in the question
   2. Common key words used in a true response stem
      a. Most or most appropriate
      b. Most likely
      c. Best
      d. Best judgment
      e. Initial
      f. First
      g. Chief
      h. Immediate
B. False response stem (Box 4-7)
   1. False response stems use key words that ask you to select an option that is NOT true regarding the case situation in the question
   2. Common key words used in a false response stem

BOX 4-6

True Response Stem

A nurse is reviewing the laboratory results of a client seen in the health care clinic. The nurse notes that the red blood cell count is decreased. The nurse determines that this finding *most likely* occurs in which of the following conditions?

1. Polycythemia vera
2. Dehydration
3. Severe diarrhea
4. Iron deficiency

Answer: 4

TEST-TAKING STRATEGY

This question identifies an example of a true response stem. Note the key words "most likely." Also, note the relationship between the words "decreased" in the case situation and "deficiency" in the correct option. These strategies will assist in directing you to the correct option.

BOX 4-7

False Response Stem

A nurse has reinforced discharge instructions to a client who underwent a right mastectomy with axillary lymph node dissection. Which statement by the client indicates a *need for further instruction* regarding home care measures?

1. "I need to be sure to wear thick mitt covers or use thick pot holders when I am cooking."
2. "I should inform all of my other health care providers that I have had this surgical procedure."
3. "It is alright to use a straight razor to shave under my arms?"
4. "I need to be sure that I do not have blood pressures measured or blood drawn from my right arm."

Answer: 3

TEST-TAKING STRATEGY

This question identifies an example of a false response stem. Note the key words "need for further instruction." These key words indicate that you need to select an option that identifies an incorrect client statement. Recalling that edema and infection are the concerns with this client and that the client needs to be instructed in the measures that will avoid trauma to the affected arm will direct you to the correct option.

a. Least likely
b. Need for further instructions or education
c. Lowest priority
d. Incorrect
e. Unsafe
f. Except, not, or avoid

VII. QUESTIONS THAT REQUIRE PRIORITIZING

A. Identify the key words in the question that indicate the need to prioritize

B. Common key words
   1. Initial
   2. Essential
   3. Vital
   4. Immediate
   5. Highest
   6. Best
   7. Most
   8. Priority

C. Use Maslow's Hierarchy of Needs theory as a guide to prioritize (Box 4-8)
   1. Physiological needs come FIRST; select an option that addresses a physiological need
   2. When a physiological need is not addressed in the question or noted in one of the options, safety needs receive priority; select an option that addresses safety

D. ABCs: airway, breathing, and circulation (Box 4-9)
   1. Use the ABCs when selecting an option
   2. Remember the order of priority: airway, breathing, and circulation

E. Clinical problem-solving process (Table 4-1)
   1. Guidelines
      a. Use the steps of the Clinical Problem-Solving Process (Nursing Process) to prioritize
      b. Remember that data collection is the first step in the process
      c. When you are asked to select your first and initial nursing action, follow the steps to select the correct option

BOX 4-8

Prioritizing: Maslow's Hierarchy of Needs Theory

A nurse is reviewing the plan of care for a pregnant client with a diagnosis of sickle cell anemia. Which nursing diagnosis, if stated on the plan of care, would the nurse select as receiving the *highest* priority?

1. Anxiety
2. Ineffective individual coping
3. Altered body image
4. Fluid volume deficit

Answer: 4

TEST-TAKING STRATEGY

Use Maslow's Hierarchy of Needs theory to prioritize, remembering that physiological needs come first. Using this guideline will direct you to option 4. Fluid volume deficit is a physiological need and is the priority nursing diagnosis.

TABLE 4-1

Steps of the Nursing Process

Data Collection	Follow the steps of the nursing process to select an option.
|	
Planning	The first step of the nursing process is data collection.
|	
Implementation	When the question asks you what the nurse's initial, first, or most appropriate action is, select the option that relates to data collection relative to the client.
|	
Evaluation	

BOX 4-9

Prioritizing: Use of the ABCs

A client with a diagnosis of cancer is receiving morphine sulfate, 10 mg subcutaneously every 3 to 4 hours for pain. When reviewing the plan of care for the client, the nurse understands that which of the following is the *priority* action?

1. Monitor the client's temperature
2. Monitor the urine output
3. Encourage the client to cough and deep breathe
4. Encourage increased fluids

Answer: 3

TEST-TAKING STRATEGY

Use the ABCs—airway, breathing, and circulation—as a guide to direct you to the correct option. Recall that morphine sulfate suppresses the cough reflex and the respiratory reflex. The correct option addresses airway.

BOX 4-10

Nursing Process: Data Collection

A nurse is reinforcing the prescribed dietary measures with a client with diabetes mellitus. The client expresses frustration in learning the dietary regimen. The nurse would initially:

1. *Identify* the cause of the frustration
2. Continue with the dietary instructions
3. Notify the registered nurse
4. Tell the client that the diet needs to be followed

Answer: 1

TEST-TAKING STRATEGY

Use the steps of the nursing process. Data collection is the first step. Of the four options presented, the only option that reflects the process of collecting data is option 1. Options 2, 3, and 4 identify the implementation step of the nursing process. The initial action is to identify the cause of the frustration.

   d. If an option contains the concept of data collection, select that option
2. Data collection (Box 4-10)
   a. Data collection questions address the process of gathering subjective and objective data relative to the client, communicating and documenting information gained in data collection, and contributing to the formulation of nursing diagnoses
   b. Remember that data collection is the first step in the nursing process
   c. When you are asked a question regarding your initial or first nursing action, select the option that addresses the process of data collection
   d. If a data collection action is not one of the options, follow the steps of the nursing process as your guide to select your initial or first action
   e. When answering questions that focus on data collection, look for key words in the options that reflect the collection of data relative to the client (Box 4-11)
3. Planning (Box 4-12)
   a. Planning questions will require providing input into plan development, assisting in the formulation of the goals of care, and assisting in the development of a plan of care
   b. Remember that this is a nursing examination and the answer to the question most likely involves something that is included in the nursing care plan, rather than the medical plan
4. Implementation (Box 4-13)
   a. This examination is about NURSING, so focus on the nursing action rather than on the medical action, unless the question is asking you what prescribed medical action is anticipated
   b. Implementation questions address the process of assisting with organizing and

BOX 4-11

Data Collection: Key Words

Check
Collect
Determine
Find out
Gather
Identify
Monitor
Observe
Obtain information
Recognize

BOX 4-12

Nursing Process: Planning

A nurse is preparing to assist with the care of a client after a gastroscopy procedure. The nurse suggests including which most appropriate nursing intervention in the *plan of care*?

1. Place the client in a supine position to provide comfort.
2. Monitor the client's vital signs every hour for 4 hours.
3. Provide saline gargles immediately on return to the nursing unit to aid in comfort.
4. Check the gag reflex by using a tongue depressor to stroke the back of client's throat.

Answer: 4

TEST-TAKING STRATEGY

Planning questions require providing input into plan development, assisting in the formulation of the goals of care, and assisting in the development of a plan of care. Use of the ABCs—airway, breathing, and circulation—will also assist in answering this question. Option 4 is the only option that addresses airway.

BOX 4-13

Nursing Process: Implementation

A nurse is assisting in caring for a client with preeclampsia who is at risk for eclampsia. The nurse understands that if the client progresses from preeclampsia to eclampsia, the *first action* is to:

1. Prepare for the administration of IV magnesium sulfate
2. Check the blood pressure and fetal heart tones
3. Clear and maintain an open airway
4. Administer oxygen by face mask

Answer: 3

TEST-TAKING STRATEGY

Implementation questions address the process of organizing and managing care. This question also requires that you prioritize for the nursing actions. Use the ABCs—airway, breathing, and circulation—to answer the question. The first action is to clear and maintain an open airway.

managing care, providing care to achieve established goals, and communicating and documenting nursing interventions thoroughly and accurately

c. On NCLEX-PN, the only client that you need to be concerned about is the client in the question that you are answering

d. When you are answering a question, remember that this client is your only assigned client

e. Answer the question as if the situation were textbook and ideal and the nurse had all the time and resources needed and readily available at the client's bedside

5. Evaluation (Box 4-14)
   a. Evaluation questions focus on comparing the actual outcomes of care with the expected outcomes, and communicating and documenting findings
   b. These questions focus on assisting in determining the client's response to care, and identifying factors that may interfere with implementation of the plan of care
   c. In an evaluation question, be alert to false response stems because they are frequently used in evaluation-type questions
   d. The question may ask for the client's statement that indicates INACCURATE information regarding the issue of the question

VIII. CLIENT NEEDS

A. Safe, effective care environment

1. These questions address the fact that the nurse provides nursing care, collaborates with other health care team members to facilitate effective client care, and protects clients, significant others, and health care personnel from environmental hazards
2. Be alert to safety needs addressed in a question, and remember the importance of hand-

BOX 4-14

Nursing Process: Evaluation

A nurse is interviewing the parents of a child with a seizure disorder to determine their adjustment to caring for their child. Which statement by one of the parents would indicate a *need for providing information* regarding the care of the child?

1. "Our child is involved in a swim program with neighbors and friends."
2. "Our child sleeps in our bedroom at night."
3. "Our babysitter just completed cardiopulmonary resuscitation (CPR) training."
4. "We worry about injuries when our child has a seizure."

Answer: 2

TEST-TAKING STRATEGY

This is an evaluation question and contains a false response stem as identified by the words "*need for providing information.*" Option 2 identifies a need to provide the parents with an alternate method to monitor for night seizures. Options 1 and 3 identify parental understanding of the disorder. Option 4 is a common concern.

washing, call bells, bed positioning, and the appropriate use of side rails

B. Physiological integrity
   1. These questions address the fact that the nurse provides comfort and assistance in the performance of activities of daily living, provides care related to the administration of medications, and monitors clients receiving parenteral therapies
   2. These questions also address the nurse's ability to reduce the client's potential for developing complications or health problems related to treatments, procedures, or existing conditions, and the nurse's role in participating in providing care to clients with acute, chronic, or life-threatening physical health conditions
   3. Use Maslow's Hierarchy of Needs theory and remember that physiological needs are a priority and are addressed first
   4. Use the ABCs, airway, breathing, and circulation and the steps of the nursing process when selecting an option addressing physiological integrity

C. Psychosocial integrity
   1. These questions address the fact that the nurse provides nursing care that promotes and supports the emotional, mental, and social well-being of the client and significant other(s)
   2. Content addressed in these questions relates to promoting the client or significant other's(s') ability to cope, adapt, or problem-solve in situations such as illnesses, disabilities, or stressful events
   3. Content also includes the nurse's role in recognizing and providing care for clients with maladaptive behavior, and assisting with behavior management of the client with an acute and/or chronic mental illness or a cognitive psychosocial disturbance
   4. Communication questions (Table 4-2)
      a. Identify the use of therapeutic communication tools
      b. Use of communication tools indicates a CORRECT option
      c. Use of communication blocks indicates an INCORRECT option
      d. Always focus on the client's feelings first; if an option reflects the client's feelings, select that option as the answer to the question (Box 4-15)

D. Health promotion and maintenance
   1. These questions address the fact that the nurse provides and assists in directing nursing care to promote and maintain health
   2. Content addressed in these questions relates to assisting the client and significant other(s)

BOX 4-15

Focusing on the Client's Feelings

A nurse in the mental health unit is having a conversation with a client diagnosed with posttraumatic stress disorder. The client is upset and is having difficulty with verbalizing realistic thoughts. The most appropriate nursing response to the client is which of the following?

1. "Don't worry so much."
2. "Everything is going to be all right."
3. "I can see that you are upset about this. Why don't we talk about it?"
4. "Why are you having so much trouble verbalizing realistic thoughts?"

Answer: 3

TEST-TAKING STRATEGY

Option 3 is the only option that addresses the client's feelings and concerns. Options 1 and 2 provide false reassurance and place the client's feelings on hold. Option 4 is a nontherapeutic communication technique.

TABLE 4-2

Communication Tools and Blocks

Tools	Blocks
Being silent	Giving advice
Offering self for assistance	Showing approval/disapproval
Showing empathy	Using cliches and false reassurance
Focusing	Requesting an explanation "Why?"
Restatement	Devaluing client feelings
Validation/clarification	Being defensive
Giving information	Focusing on inappropriate issues or persons
Dealing with the here and now	Placing the client's issues on "hold"

Always focus on the client's feelings FIRST!
If an option reflects the client's feelings, select that option!

during the normal expected stages of growth and development from conception through advanced old age, and providing client care related to the prevention and early detection of health problems

3. Use the Teaching/Learning theory if the question addresses client education, remembering that the nurse's role is to facilitate the acquisition of knowledge, skills, and attitudes that lead to a change in behavior
4. Be alert to false response stems with questions that address health promotion and maintenance

IX. PYRAMID POINTS (Box 4-16)

A. Unfamiliar content

1. Answer questions using your nursing knowledge, clinical experiences, and test-taking skills and strategies
2. If the content of the question is unfamiliar and you are unable to answer the question using your nursing knowledge, look for a global option, similar distracters, or similar words, behaviors, thoughts, or feelings in the question and in one of the options

B. Global option (Box 4-17)

1. When more than one option appears to be correct, look for a global option
2. A global option is one that is a general statement and may include the ideas of the other options within it

C. Similar distracters

1. If you don't know the answer, try looking for similar distracters
2. Remember that there is only ONE correct option
3. If two options say the same thing or include the same idea, then NEITHER OF THESE OPTIONS can be correct
4. The answer to the question is the option that is different

D. Similar words, behaviors, thoughts, or feelings

1. If you do not know the answer, look for a similar word, behavior, thought, or feeling used in the case situation or the stem of the question and in one of the options

BOX 4-16

Pyramid Points

If the question asks for an immediate action or response, all options may be correct; therefore, base your selection on priorities.

Reword a difficult question, but if you do so, be careful not to change the intent of the question.

Relate the situation to something that you are familiar with and try to visualize the client as you go through the case situation and the question.

If there are words in the case situation or stem of the question that are unfamiliar, try to figure out the meaning in terms of the context of the sentence or break down the word and use medical terminology skills.

If one option includes qualifiers such as GENERALLY, USUALLY, TENDS TO, POSSIBLY, or MAY, and other options do not, select that option.

Absolute terminology such as ALWAYS, NEVER, ALL, EVERY, NONE, MUST, and ONLY tend to make an option incorrect.

With medication calculations, talk yourself through each step and be sure the answer makes sense; recheck the calculation before selecting an option, particularly if the answer seems like an unusual dosage.

Remember, the only client you need to be concerned about is the one in the question you are answering, and answer the question as if the situation were ideal and the nurse had all the time and resources readily available at the client's bedside.

Pace yourself, concentrate, and focus on one item at a time; if you find yourself becoming distracted, take a few minutes to breathe deeply and then refocus.

SMILE!
BELIEF!
CONFIDENCE!
CONTROL!
SUCCESS!

BOX 4-17

Global Option

A nurse employed in an emergency room receives a telephone call from emergency medical services and is told that several victims who survived a plane crash will be transported to the hospital. The nurse is told that the victims are suffering from cold exposure because the plane plummeted and submerged into the local river. The initial nursing action of the nurse is which of the following?

1. Supply the triage rooms with bottles of sterile water and normal saline.
2. Call the laundry department and ask the department to send as many warm blankets as possible to the emergency room.
3. Call the nursing supervisor to activate the agency disaster plan.
4. Ask the intensive care unit to send nurses to the emergency room.

Answer: 3

TEST-TAKING STRATEGY

Option 3 is the global option. Activating the agency disaster plan will ensure that the interventions in options 1, 2, and 4 will occur.

2. If you find a word, behavior, thought, or feeling that is used in the case situation or the stem of the question and is repeated in one of the options, that option MAY be the correct one

E. Pharmacology questions
   1. If you are familiar with the medication, use nursing knowledge to answer the question
   2. Remember that the question will identify both the generic name and trade name of the medication
   3. If the case situation identifies a diagnosis, then you can make a relationship between the medication and the diagnosis; for example, you can determine that cyclophosphamide (Cytoxan) is an antineoplastic medication if the question refers to a client with breast cancer who is taking this particular medication
   4. Try to determine the classification of the medication being addressed to assist in answering the question; identifying the classification will assist in determining a medication action and/or side effects (Cardiazem is a cardiac medication)
   5. Use medical terminology, and break the name of the medication into parts; for example, Lopressor can be broken down into Lo and pressor, meaning lowering the blood pressure
   6. Look at the prefix and/or suffix of the medication name; "ase" indicates an enzyme, "sone" indicates a corticosteroid, "line" indicates a bronchodilator, and "lol" indicates a beta-blocker
   7. General principles to remember
      a. Clients are instructed to avoid alcohol with medications
      b. Capsules and sustained-released medications are not to be crushed
      c. The nurse never adjusts or changes the client's medication dosage and never discontinues a medication
      d. Medications are never administered if the order is difficult to read, is unclear, or identifies a medication dose that is not a normal one

REFERENCES

Hill S, Howlett H: *Success in practical/vocational nursing*, ed 4, Philadelphia, 2001, WB Saunders.

National Council of State Boards of Nursing, editors: *Test plan for the National Council Licensure Examination for Practical/Vocational Nurses.* Chicago, 2001, Author.

Potter P, Perry A: *Fundamentals of nursing*, ed 5, St Louis, 2001, Mosby,

Riley J: *Communication in nursing*, ed 4, St Louis, 2000, Mosby.

UNIT II

Issues in Nursing

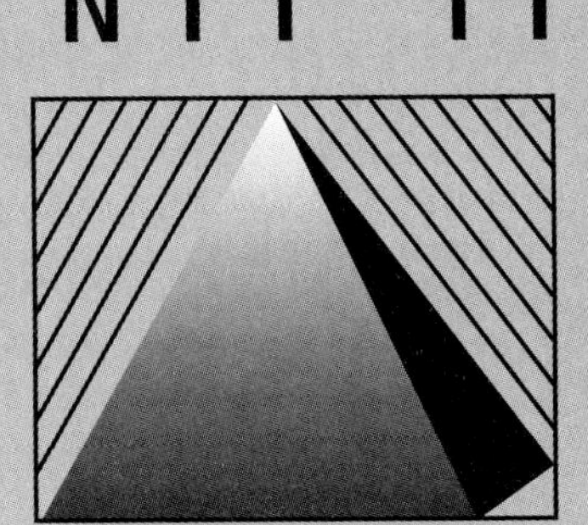

Cultural Diversity

PYRAMID TERMS

Acculturation Process of learning norms, beliefs, and behavioral expectations of a group.

Belief Something believed as true and accepted by an ethnocultural group.

Cultural Assimilation Occurs when individuals from a minority group are absorbed by the dominant culture and take on the characteristics of the dominant culture.

Cultural Competence Having the knowledge, understanding, and skills regarding a diverse culture that allow one to provide acceptable care.

Cultural Diversity The differences among people that result from ethnic, racial, and cultural variables.

Cultural Imposition The tendency to impose one's own beliefs, values, and patterns of behavior on individuals from another culture.

Culture The structures of knowledge, beliefs, behaviors, ideas, attitudes, values, habits, customs, languages, symbols, rituals, ceremonies, and practices that are unique to a particular group of people.

Dominant Culture The group whose values prevail within society.

Ethnic Relating to a group of people who have had different experiences from those of the dominant culture by status, background, residence, religion, education, or other factors that functionally unify the group.

Ethnicity A cultural group's perception of themselves, or the group identity. This self-perception influences how the group members are perceived by others.

Ethnocentrism An assumption of cultural superiority and an inability to accept another culture's ways.

Minority Group An ethnic, racial, or religious group that constitutes less than a numerical majority of the population.

Oppression Is based on cultural biases and stems from values, beliefs, traditions, and cultural expectations; occurs when the rules, modes, and ideals of one group are imposed on another group.

Race A grouping of people based on biological similarities. Members of a racial group have similar physical characteristics, such as blood group, facial features, and color of skin, hair, and eyes.

Racism Discrimination directed toward individuals who are misperceived to be inferior because of biological differences; a form of oppression.

Stereotyping An expectation that all people within the same racial, ethnic, or cultural group act alike and share the same beliefs and attitudes.

Subculture A group of people with characteristic patterns of behavior that distinguish the group from the larger culture or society.

Values Principles and standards that have meaning and worth to an individual, family, group, or community.

THE PYRAMID TO SUCCESS

Often, nurses are caring for clients who come from different ethnic, cultural, and religious backgrounds from their own. Awareness of and sensitivity to the unique health and illness beliefs and practices are essential for the delivery of safe and effective care. Acknowledgment and acceptance of cultural differences with a nonjudgmental attitude are essential in providing culturally sensitive care. The belief underlying the NCLEX-PN Test Plan is that people are unique individuals and define their own systems of daily living, which reflect their values, motives, and lifestyles. Cultural awareness is a concept and process that is fundamental to the practice of nursing. The primary Integrated Concepts and Processes addressed in this chapter are Cultural Awareness, Caring, Communication and Documentation.

CLIENT NEEDS

Safe, Effective Care Environment

Acting as a client advocate
Client rights
Confidentiality

Respecting client's control of personal environment/property
Establishing priorities
Ethical practice
Legal responsibilities
Communicating the need for referrals to members of the health care team

Health Promotion and Maintenance

Disease prevention
Family planning
Health screening and health promotion programs
Lifestyle choices

Psychosocial Integrity

Coping mechanisms
Religious and spiritual influences on health
Support systems
End-of-life issues
Therapeutic communication

Physiological Integrity

Basic care and comfort practices
Nutritional preferences (Box 5-1)

BOX 5-1

Dietary Preferences

AFRICAN-AMERICANS
Fried foods
Chicken, pork, greens, rice
Some pregnant African-Americans engage in pica

ASIAN-AMERICANS
Soy sauce
Raw fish
Rice

EUROPEAN (WHITE)-AMERICANS
Carbohydrates (potatoes)
Red meat

HISPANIC-AMERICANS
Beans
Fried foods
Spicy foods
Chili
Carbonated beverages

AMERICAN INDIANS, ALEUTS, ESKIMOS
Blue cornmeal
Fish
Game
Fruits and berries
Navajos prefer meat and blue cornmeal and tend to avoid consumption of milk.

Therapeutic procedures
Practices or restrictions related to procedures and treatments

I. AFRICAN-AMERICANS

A. Communication
1. Languages include English or Black English
2. Head nodding does not necessarily mean agreement
3. Direct eye contact is often viewed as being rude
4. Nonverbal communication is very important
5. It is considered to be intrusive to ask personal questions of someone on initial contact or meeting

B. Time orientation and space
1. Orientation is more to the present than the future
2. Close personal space is important
3. Touching another's hair is sometimes viewed as offensive

C. Social roles
1. Large extended-family networks are important
2. Many single-parent, female-headed households
3. Religion is usually Protestant (Baptist) (Box 5-2)
4. Strong church affiliation with community is important
5. Social organizations are strong within communities

D. Health and illness
1. Harmony with nature
2. No separation of body, mind, and spirit
3. Illness is a disharmonious state that may be caused by demons or spirits
4. Illness can be prevented by nutritious meals, rest, and cleanliness

E. Health risks
1. Sickle cell anemia
2. Hypertension
3. Coronary heart disease
4. Cancer (especially stomach and esophageal)
5. Lactose intolerance
6. Coccidioidomycosis

F. Implementation
1. Avoid **stereotyping**
2. Do not label Black English as an unacceptable form of language
3. Clarify meaning of client's verbal and nonverbal behavior
4. Be flexible and avoid rigidity in scheduling care
5. Encourage involvement with family

BOX 5-2

Religions and Dietary Practices

SEVENTH DAY ADVENTIST (CHURCH OF GOD)
Alcohol, coffee, and tea prohibited
Some groups prohibit meat

BAPTIST
Alcohol prohibited
Consumption of coffee and tea discouraged

BUDDHISM
Alcohol and drug use discouraged
Some sects are vegetarian

ROMAN CATHOLICISM
Avoid meat on Ash Wednesday and Good Friday
Optional fasting during Lent season
During Lent, discourage meat on Friday
Children and the ill are exempt from fasting

CHURCH OF JESUS CHRIST OF LATTER-DAY SAINTS (MORMON)
Alcohol, coffee, and tea prohibited
Limited consumption of meat
First Sunday of the month is time for fasting

HINDUISM
Beef and veal prohibited
Many individuals are vegetarians
Limited consumption of meat
Fasting occurs on specific days of the week according to which god the person worships
Children are not allowed to participate in fasting
Fasting rituals vary from complete abstinence to consumption of only one meal per day

ISLAM
Pork prohibited
Any meat product not ritually slaughtered is prohibited
Avoidance of alcohol or drugs
During Ramadan, fasting occurs during daytime

JEHOVAH'S WITNESS
Prohibition of any foods to which blood has been added
Can consume animal flesh that has been drained

JUDAISM
Dietary kosher laws must be adhered to by Orthodox believers
Meats allowed include animals that are vegetable eaters, cloven-hoofed animals, and animals that are ritually slaughtered
Fish that have scales and fins are allowed
Any combination of meat and milk is prohibited
During Yom Kippur, 24-hour fasting
Pregnant women and those who are seriously ill are exempt from fasting
During Passover week, only unleavened bread is eaten

PENTECOSTAL (ASSEMBLY OF GOD)
Alcohol is prohibited
Avoid consumption of anything to which blood has been added
Some individuals avoid pork

RUSSIAN ORTHODOX
Abstention from meat and dairy products on Wednesday, Friday, and during Lent
During Lent, all animal products, including dairy products, are forbidden
Fasting during Advent
Exceptions from fasting include illness and pregnancy

6. A folk healer or herbalist may be consulted before the individual seeks medical treatment

II. ASIAN-AMERICANS

A. Communication
   1. Languages include Chinese, Japanese, Korean, Vietnamese, and English
   2. Silence is valued
   3. Eye contact is considered rude
   4. Criticism or disagreement is not expressed verbally
   5. Head nodding does not necessarily mean agreement
   6. The word "no" is interpreted as disrespect for others

B. Time orientation and space
   1. Orientation is more to present
   2. Social distance is important
   3. Usually do not touch others during conversation 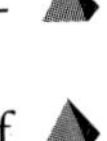
   4. Touching is unacceptable with members of opposite sex 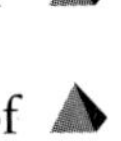
   5. The head is considered to be sacred; therefore touching someone on the head is disrespectful 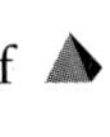

C. Social roles
   1. Devoted to tradition
   2. Large extended-family networks
   3. Loyalty to immediate and extended family and honor are valued
   4. Family unit is very structured and hierarchical

5. Men have the power and authority, and women are expected to be obedient
6. Education is viewed as important
7. Religions include Taoism (Buddhism), Islam, and Christianity (Box 5-2)
8. Social organizations are strong within the community

D. Health and illness
1. Health is a state of physical and spiritual harmony with nature and a balance between positive and negative energy forces (yin and yang)
2. A healthy body is viewed as a gift from ancestors
3. Illness is viewed as an imbalance between yin and yang
4. Yin foods are cold, and yang foods are hot; cold foods are eaten when one has a hot illness, and hot foods are eaten when one has a cold illness
5. Illness is contributed to by prolonged sitting or lying, or to overexertion

E. Health risks
1. Hypertension
2. Cancer (stomach and liver)
3. Lactose intolerance
4. Thalassemia
5. Coccidioidomycosis

F. Implementation
1. Avoid physical closeness and excessive touching; only touch a client's head when necessary, informing the client before doing so
2. Limit eye contact
3. Avoid gesturing with hands
4. Clarify responses to questions
5. Be flexible and avoid rigidity in scheduling care
6. Encourage involvement with family
7. A healer may be consulted before an individual seeks out traditional treatment

III. EUROPEAN (WHITE)-ORIGIN AMERICANS

A. Communication
1. Languages include national languages and English
2. Silence can be used to show respect or disrespect for another, depending on situation
3. Eye contact is viewed as indicating trustworthiness

B. Time orientation and space
1. Future oriented
2. Aloof and tend to avoid close physical contact
3. Handshakes are used for formal greetings

C. Social roles
1. The nuclear family is the basic unit; the extended family is also important
2. The man is the dominant figure
3. Religion includes Judeo-Christian (Box 5-2)
4. Community social organizations are important

D. Health and illness
1. Health is usually viewed as an absence of disease or illness
2. Have a tendency to be stoical when expressing physical concerns
3. Primarily rely on modern Western health care delivery system

E. Health risks
1. Breast cancer
2. Heart disease
3. Diabetes mellitus
4. Thalassemia

F. Implementation
1. Monitor and assess client's body language
2. Respect client's personal space

IV. HISPANIC-AMERICANS

A. Communication
1. Languages include Spanish or Portuguese, with various dialects
2. Tend to be verbally expressive, yet confidentiality is important
3. Eye behavior is significant; for example, the "evil eye" can be given to a child if a person looks at and admires a child without touching the child
4. Avoiding eye contact indicates respect and attentiveness
5. Direct confrontation is disrespectful, and the expression of negative feeling is impolite
6. Dramatic body language, such as gestures or facial expressions, is used to express emotion or pain

B. Time orientation and space
1. Oriented more to present
2. Comfortable with close proximity to others
3. Very tactile and use embraces and handshakes
4. Value the physical presence of others
5. Politeness and modesty are essential

C. Social roles
1. The nuclear family is the basic unit; there are also large extended family networks
2. The extended family is highly regarded
3. Needs of the family take precedence over individual family members' needs
4. Men are decision makers and bread winners, and women are the caretakers and homemakers
5. Religion includes Catholicism (Box 5-2)
6. Strong church affiliation
7. Social organizations strong within the community

D. Health and illness
   1. Health may be a reward from God or a result of good luck
   2. Health results from a state of balance between "hot and cold" forces and "wet and dry" forces
   3. Illness occurs as a result of God's punishment for sins
   4. Folk medicine traditions

E. Health risks
   1. Lactose intolerance
   2. Diabetes mellitus
   3. Parasites
   4. Coccidioidomycosis

F. Implementation
   1. Communicate with male head of family
   2. Protect privacy
   3. Offer to call priest or other clergy because of the significance of religious practices related to illnesses
   4. Always touch a child when examining him or her
   5. Be flexible and avoid rigidity in scheduling care

V. NATIVE-AMERICANS

A. Communication
   1. Languages include English, Navajo, and other tribal languages
   2. Silence indicates respect for the speaker
   3. Speak in a low tone of voice and expect others to be attentive
   4. Eye contact is avoided because it is a sign of disrespect
   5. Body language is important

B. Time orientation and space
   1. Orientation is more to present
   2. Personal space is very important
   3. Will lightly touch another person's hand during greetings
   4. Massage is used for the newborn infant to promote bonding between infant and mother
   5. Touching a dead body is prohibited in some tribes

C. Social roles
   1. Very family orientated
   2. Basic family unit is the extended family, which often includes people from several households
   3. In some tribes, grandparents are viewed as family leaders
   4. Elders are honored
   5. Children are taught to respect traditions
   6. The father does all the work outside the home, and the mother assumes responsibility for domestic duties
   7. Sacred myths and legends provide spiritual guidance
   8. Religion and healing practices are integrated
   9. Community social organizations are important

D. Health and illness
   1. Health is a state of harmony between the person, the family, and the environment
   2. Illness is caused by supernatural forces and disequilibrium between person and environment
   3. Traditional health and illness beliefs may continue to be observed; natural and magicoreligious folk medicine tradition
   4. Traditional healer: medicine man or woman

E. Health risks
   1. Alcohol abuse
   2. Accidents
   3. Heart disease
   4. Diabetes mellitus
   5. Tuberculosis
   6. Arthritis
   7. Lactose intolerance
   8. Gallbladder disease
   9. American Eskimos are susceptible to glaucoma

F. Implementation
   1. Clarify communication
   2. Understand that the client may be attentive even when eye contact is absent
   3. Be attentive to own use of body language
   4. Obtain input from extended family members
   5. Encourage client to personalize space in which health care is delivered; for example, encourage client to bring personal items or objects to the hospital
   6. In the home, assess for the availability of running water, and modify infection control and hygiene practices as necessary

VI. PROLONGATION OF LIFE

A. Christian Science religion is unlikely to use medical means to prolong life

B. Jewish faith generally opposes prolonging life after irreversible brain damage

VII. DEATH AND DYING PRACTICES

A. Autopsy may be prohibited, opposed, or discouraged by Eastern Orthodox religions, Muslims, Jehovah's Witnesses, and Orthodox Jews

B. Organ donation is prohibited by Jehovah's Witnesses and Muslims

C. Buddhists in America encourage organ donation and consider it an act of mercy

D. Cremation is discouraged, opposed, or prohibited by the Mormon, Eastern Orthodox, Islamic, and Jewish faiths
E. Hindus prefer cremation and cast the ashes in a holy river

PRACTICE QUESTIONS

1. A nurse is assisting in collecting data on an African-American client admitted to the ambulatory care unit who is scheduled for a hernia repair. Which of the following information about the client is of least priority during data collection?
   1. Cardiovascular
   2. Neurological
   3. Respiratory
   4. Psychosocial
2. A nursing instructor is providing a session on cultural beliefs related to health and illness. After the session, the instructor asks a nursing student to describe the beliefs of an African-American in regard to illness. Which of the following is the most appropriate response made by the student?
   1. "Illness is due to an imbalance between yin and yang."
   2. "Illness is a punishment for sins."
   3. "Illness is a disharmonious state that may be caused by demons and spirits."
   4. "Illness is due to lack of exercise."
3. A nurse is planning to reinforce instructions to the African-American client about nutrition. When developing the plan, the nurse is aware that a common dietary practice of African-Americans is to eat:
   1. Fried foods
   2. Rice as the basis for all meals
   3. Red meat
   4. Raw fish
4. A nurse is assigned to care for an Asian-American client. The nurse plans care knowing that which of the following most appropriately describes the Asian-American's view of illness?
   1. Illness is caused by supernatural forces
   2. Illness is a punishment for sins
   3. Illness is a disharmonious state that may be caused by demons and spirits
   4. Illness is due to an imbalance between yin and yang
5. A nursing student is discussing cultural diversity issues in a clinical conference. The nursing instructor asks a student to describe ethnocentrism. Which of the following if stated by the student would indicate a lack of understanding of the issue of ethnocentrism?
   1. "It is a tendency to view ones' own ways as best."
   2. "It is acting in a manner that is superior to other cultures."
   3. "It is believing that ones' own ways are the only acceptable way."
   4. "It is imposing one's beliefs on individuals from another culture."
6. A nurse consults with a nutritionist regarding the dietary preferences of an Asian-American client. Which of the following foods would the nurse most appropriately plan to include in the diet plan?
   1. Red meat
   2. Rice
   3. Fried foods
   4. Fruits
7. A nurse assists in developing a plan of care for a European-American client and considers the practices and preferences of the culture. Which of the following cultural practices or preferences are not a practice or preference of this cultural group?
   1. Community social organizations are important
   2. Health is often viewed as an absence of disease or illness
   3. Members appear stoic when expressing physical concerns
   4. The woman is the dominant figure
8. A Hispanic-American mother brings her child to the clinic for an examination. Which of the following is most important when gathering data about the child?
   1. Avoiding eye contact
   2. Touching the child during the examination
   3. Avoiding speaking to the child
   4. Using body language only
9. A nurse assists in developing a plan of care for the Native-American client considering the practices and preferences of the culture. Which of the following practices and preferences is not normally a characteristic of this ethnic group?
   1. Religion and healing practices
   2. Touching the body of a dead family member
   3. Avoiding eye contact
   4. Use of healing practices
10. A nurse caring for an Orthodox Jewish client plans a diet that adheres to the practices of Judaism. The nurse plans the diet knowing that which of the following concepts is not a practice of Judaism?
    1. Eating fish with scales and fins are allowed
    2. Meat is allowed if ritually slaughtered
    3. Only unleavened bread is eaten during Passover week
    4. Meat and milk can be eaten together

ANSWERS

1. *Answer:* 4
Rationale: The psychosocial data are the least priority during the initial admission data collection. In the African-American culture, it is considered to be intrusive to ask personal questions on the initial contact or meeting. Additionally, cardiovascular, neurological, and respiratory data include physiological assessments that would be the priority.
Test-Taking Strategy: Use the process of elimination. Note the key words "least priority." Use Maslow's Hierarchy of Needs theory to answer the question. Options 1, 2, and 3 address physiological needs. Review the characteristics of the African-American culture if you had difficulty with this question.
Level of Cognitive Ability: Comprehension
Client Needs: Physiological Integrity
Integrated Concept/Process: Cultural Awareness
Content Area: Fundamental Skills
Reference: Hill S, Howlett H: *Success in practical/vocational nursing*, ed 4, Philadelphia, 2002, WB Saunders, pp.138-139.

2. *Answer:* 3
Rationale: In the African-American culture, illness is viewed as a disharmonious state that may be caused by demons and spirits. The goal of treatment, from the traditional African perspective, is to remove the harmful spirit from the body of the ill person. Asian-Americans believe that illness is due to an imbalance between yin and yang and to prolonged sitting or lying, or to overexertion.
Test-Taking Strategy: Knowledge regarding the beliefs related to health and illness of the various cultures assists in answering the question. From this point, use the process of elimination to determine the correct option. Review the characteristics of the African-American culture if you had difficulty with this question.
Level of Cognitive Ability: Comprehension
Client Needs: Psychosocial Integrity
Integrated Concept/Process: Cultural Awareness
Content Area: Fundamental Skills
Reference: Potter P, Perry A: *Fundamentals of nursing*, ed 5, St Louis, 2001, Mosby, p. 123.

3. *Answer:* 1
Rationale: African-American food preferences include chicken, pork, greens, rice, and fried foods. Asian-Americans eat raw fish, rice, and soy sauce. Hispanic-Americans prefer beans, fried foods, spicy foods, chili, and carbonated beverages. European-Americans prefer carbohydrates and red meat.
Test-Taking Strategy: Knowledge regarding the food practices and preferences related to the various cultures is required to answer the question. Recalling that African-Americans are at risk for hypertension and coronary artery disease will assist in directing you to option 1. Review the food preferences of the African-American culture if you had difficulty with this question.
Level of Cognitive Ability: Comprehension
Client Needs: Physiological Integrity
Integrated Concept/Process: Cultural Awareness
Content Area: Fundamental Skills
Reference: Grodner M, Anderson S, DeYoung S: *Foundations and clinical applications of nutrition: a nursing approach*, St Louis, 2000, Mosby, p. 790.

4. *Answer:* 4
Rationale: Asian-Americans believe that illness is due to an imbalance between yin and yang, and to prolonged sitting or lying, or to overexertion. In the African-American culture, illness is viewed as a disharmonious state that may be caused by demons and spirits. Native Americans believe that illness is caused by supernatural forces.
Test-Taking Strategy: Knowledge regarding the beliefs related to health and illness of the various cultures assists in answering the question. From this point, use the process of elimination to determine the correct option. Review the characteristics of the Asian-American culture if you had difficulty with this question.
Level of Cognitive Ability: Comprehension
Client Needs: Psychosocial Integrity
Integrated Concept/Process: Cultural Awareness
Content Area: Fundamental Skills
Reference: Potter P, Perry A: *Fundamentals of nursing*, St Louis, 2001, Mosby, p. 123.

5. *Answer:* 4
Rationale: Ethnocentrism is a tendency to view one's own ways of life as the most desirable, acceptable, or best, and to act in a superior manner toward another culture. Cultural imposition is the tendency to impose one's own beliefs, values, and patterns of behavior on individuals from another culture.
Test-Taking Strategy: Use the process of elimination and note the key words "indicate a lack of understanding" in the stem of the question. Also, note the similarity between options 1, 2, and 3. If you had difficulty with this question, review culturally related concepts.
Level of Cognitive Ability: Comprehension
Client Needs: Psychosocial Integrity
Integrated Concept/Process: Cultural Awareness
Content Area: Fundamental Skills
Reference: Harkreader H: *Fundamentals of nursing: caring and clinical judgment*, Philadelphia, 2000, WB Saunders, p. 60.

6. *Answer:* 2
Rationale: Asian-Americans' food preferences include raw fish, rice, and soy sauce. African-American food preferences include chicken, pork, greens, rice, and fried foods. Hispanic-Americans prefer beans, fried foods, spicy foods, chili and carbonated beverages. European-Americans prefer carbohydrates and red meat.
Test-Taking Strategy: Knowledge regarding the food practices and preferences related to the various cultures is required to answer the question. Correlate rice with Asian-Americans. This may assist when answering other questions similar to this one. Review the food preferences associated with the Asian-American culture if you had difficulty with this question.
Level of Cognitive Ability: Comprehension
Client Needs: Physiological Integrity
Integrated Concept/Process: Cultural Awareness
Content Area: Fundamental Skills
Reference: Grodner M., Anderson S, DeYoung S: *Foundations and clinical applications of nutrition: a nursing approach*, St Louis, 2000, Mosby, p. 790.

7. *Answer:* 4
Rationale: In the European-American culture, the man is the dominant figure. Community social organizations are important in this culture. European-Americans tend to be aloof and avoid physical contact and appear stoic when expressing physical concerns.
Test-Taking Strategy: Use knowledge regarding the practices and preferences associated with the European-American culture to answer the question. Review these practices and preferences if you had difficulty with this question.
Level of Cognitive Ability: Comprehension
Client Needs: Psychosocial Integrity
Integrated Concept/Process: Cultural Awareness
Content Area: Fundamental Skills
Reference: Potter P, Perry A: *Fundamentals of nursing*, ed 5, St Louis, 2001, Mosby, p. 118.

8. *Answer:* 2
Rationale: In the Hispanic-American culture, eye behavior is significant. The "bad (evil) eye" can be given to a child if a person looks at and admires a child without touching the child. Therefore, touching the child during the examination is very important. Although avoiding eye contact indicates respect and attentiveness, this is not the most important intervention. Avoiding speaking to the child and using body language only are not therapeutic interventions.
Test-Taking Strategy: Use the process of elimination. Eliminate options 3 and 4 first because they are similar. From the remaining options, select the intervention that is most therapeutic, that is, touch. Review the characteristics of the Hispanic-American culture if you had difficulty with this question.
Level of Cognitive Ability: Application
Client Needs: Psychosocial Integrity
Integrated Concept/Process: Cultural Awareness
Content Area: Fundamental Skills
Reference: Potter P, Perry A: *Fundamentals of nursing*, ed 5, St. Louis, 2001, Mosby, p. 126.

9. *Answer:* 2
Rationale: In the Native-American culture, touching a dead body is normally prohibited. The use of religion and healing practices is integrated into health care and illness practices. Eye contact is avoided because it is a sign of disrespect.
Test-Taking Strategy: Use the process of elimination and note the key word "not." Eliminate options 1 and 4 first because they are similar. From the remaining options, remembering that eye contact is a sign of disrespect will direct you to option 2. Review the practices and preferences of this culture if you had difficulty with this question.
Level of Cognitive Ability: Comprehension
Client Needs: Psychosocial Integrity
Integrated Concept/Process: Cultural Awareness
Content Area: Fundamental Skills
Reference: Potter P, Perry A: *Fundamentals of nursing*, ed 5, St Louis, 2001, Mosby, p. 126.

10. *Answer:* 4
Rationale: Dietary kosher laws must be adhered to by Orthodox believers. Meats allowed include animals that are vegetable eaters, cloven-hoofed animals, and animals that are ritually slaughtered. Fish that have scales and fins are allowed; however any combination of meat and milk is prohibited. During Passover week, only unleavened bread is eaten.
Test-Taking Strategy: Use the process of elimination and note the key word "not" in the stem of the question. Knowledge regarding the dietary practices in Judaism is required to answer the question. Review these practices if you had difficulty with this question.
Level of Cognitive Ability: Comprehension
Client Needs: Psychosocial Integrity
Integrated Concept/Process: Cultural Awareness
Content Area: Fundamental Skills
Reference: Potter P, Perry A: *Fundamentals of nursing*, ed 5, St Louis, 2001, Mosby, p. 120

REFERENCES

Grodner M, Anderson S, DeYoung S: *Foundations and clinical applications of nutrition: a nursing approach*, St Louis, 2000, Mosby.

Harkreader H: *Fundamentals of nursing: caring and clinical judgment*, Philadelphia, 2000, WB Saunders.

Hill S, Howlett H: *Success in practical/vocational nursing*, ed 4, Philadelphia, 2001, WB Saunders.

National Council of State Boards of Nursing, editors: *Test plan for the National Council Licensure Examination for Practical/Vocational Nurses*, Chicago, 2001, Author.

Potter P, Perry A: *Fundamentals of nursing*, ed 5, St Louis, 2001, Mosby.

Riley J: *Communication in nursing*, ed 4, St Louis, 2000, Mosby.

Ethical and Legal Issues

PYRAMID TERMS

Advance Directive Written document, recognized by state law, that provides directions concerning the provision of care when a person is unable to make his or her own treatment choices.

Advocacy Acting on the behalf of the clients, protecting the clients' rights to make their own decisions.

Consent Voluntary act by which a person agrees to allow someone else to do something.

Ethics Deals with the rules of conduct and what the nurse should do in a particular situation.

Informed Consent The client understands the reason for the purposed intervention, with its benefits and risks, and agrees to the treatment by signing a consent form.

Law In nursing, the rules and regulations that control the practice of nursing.

Malpractice Failure to meet the standards of acceptable care, which results in harm to another person.

Negligence Failure to provide care that a reasonable person would ordinarily use in a similar circumstance.

Nurse Practice Act Legal guideline in nursing.

Patient's Bill of Rights Includes the rights and responsibilities of clients receiving care.

Values Beliefs and attitudes that may influence behavior and the process of decision making

THE PYRAMID TO SUCCESS

Across all settings in the practice of nursing, nurses are frequently confronted with ethical and legal issues related to client care. It is the responsibility of the nurse to be aware of the ethical principles, laws, and guidelines related to providing safe and quality care to clients. In the Pyramid to Success, focus on ethical practices; the Nurse Practice Act, client rights, particularly confidentiality and informed consent; and advocacy, documentation, advance directives, death and dying, and organ donation. The primary Integrated Concepts and Processes addressed in this chapter are the Clinical Problem-Solving Process (Nursing Process), Caring, and Communication and Documentation.

CLIENT NEEDS

Safe, Effective Care Environment

Acting as an advocate
Advance directives
Client rights
Confidentiality
Continuous quality improvement
Establishing priorities
Ethical practice
Incident/irregular occurrence reports
Informed consent
Legal responsibilities
Organ donation
Resource management

Health Promotion and Maintenance

Developmental stages and transitions
Family interaction patterns
Lifestyle choices

Psychosocial Integrity

Abuse and neglect
Chemical dependency
Coping mechanisms
End-of-life issues
Grief and loss
Support systems

Physiological Integrity

Basic care and comfort
Potential for alterations in body systems
Palliative care
Potential complications of tests and procedures

I. ETHICS AND VALUES

A. **Ethics**: The branch of philosophy that concerns the distinction between right and wrong on the basis of a body of knowledge, not just on the basis of opinions

B. **Morality**: Behavior in accordance with customs or tradition, usually reflecting personal or religious beliefs

C. **Ethical Principles**: Codes that direct or govern our actions (Box 6-1)

D. **Values**: Beliefs and attitudes that may influence behavior and the process of decision making

E. **Values Clarification**: Process of analyzing one's own **values** to better understand what is truly important

F. **Ethical Codes**
1. Provide broad principles for determining and evaluating client care
2. Are not legally binding, but in most states, the Board of Nursing has authority to reprimand nurses for unprofessional conduct that results from violation of the ethical codes
3. Specific ethical codes
   a. National Federation of Licensed Practical Nurses (NFLPN) Code for Licensed Practical/Vocational Nurses
   b. NFLPN Nursing Practice Standards
   c. NFLPN Specialized Nursing Practice Standards
   d. National Association of Practical Nurse Education and Service (NAPNES) code of ethics
   e. NAPNES Standards of Practice for Practical/Vocational Nurses

G. **Ethical Dilemma**
1. Occurs when there is a conflict between two or more ethical principles
2. There is no correct decision
3. The nurse must make a choice between two alternatives that are equally unsatisfactory
4. Ethical reasoning is the process of thinking through what one ought to do in an orderly and systematic manner to provide justification for actions based on principles

H. **Advocate**
1. A person who speaks up for or acts on the behalf of the client, protects the client's right to make his or her own decisions, and upholds the principle of fidelity
2. Represents the client's viewpoint to others
3. Avoids letting personal **values** influence **advocacy** for the client
4. Supports the client's decision even when it conflicts with his or her own preferences or choices

I. **Ethics Committees**
1. Multidisciplinary approach to facilitate dialogue regarding ethical dilemmas
2. Develop and establish policies and procedures for the prevention and resolution of dilemmas

BOX 6-1

Ethical Principles

Autonomy	Respect for an individual's right to maintain control over health care decisions
Nonmaleficence	The obligation to do or cause no harm to another
Beneficence	The obligation of doing good with nursing actions and preventing and removing harm. Paternalism is an undesirable outcome of beneficence, in which the health care provider decides what is best for the client and attempts to encourage the client to act against his or her own choices
Justice	Providing fair and equitable treatment to clients
Veracity	The obligation to tell the truth
Fidelity	The duty to do what one has promised

II. REGULATION OF NURSING PRACTICE

A. Nurse Practice Act
1. On a state level, defines the duties and functions that the nurse can perform
2. Defines what nursing is, what it is not, and under what circumstances nursing can be practiced for compensation
3. Additional issues covered by the **Nurse Practice Act** include licensure requirements for protection of the public, grounds for disciplinary action, rights of the nurse licensee if a disciplinary action is taken, and related topics
4. All nurses are responsible for knowing the provisions of the act of the state or province in which they work
5. No physician, registered professional nurse, or agency can give the licensed practical/vocational nurse the right to do more than can be performed legally

B. Standards of care

1. Guidelines by which the nurse should practice
2. Guidelines for determining whether nurses performed duties in an appropriate manner
3. If nurses do not perform duties within accepted standards of care, they place themselves in jeopardy of legal action
4. If a nurse is named as defendant in a **malpractice** lawsuit and it is shown that neither the accepted standards of care outlined by the state or province nursing practice act nor the policies of the employing institution were followed, the nurse's legal liability is clear

C. Employee guidelines
1. Respondent superior: Employer will be held liable for any negligent acts of an employee if the alleged negligent act occurred during the employment relationship and was within the scope of the employee's responsibilities
2. Contracts
   a. Nurses are responsible for carrying out the terms of contractual agreement with the employee agency and the client
   b. The nurse employee relationship is governed by established employee handbooks and client care policies and procedures that create obligations, rights, and duties between those parties
3. Institutional policies
   a. Written policies and procedures of the employing institution that detail how nurses are to perform their duties
   b. Policies and procedures are usually quite specific and are located in manuals in most health care facilities
   c. Although policies are not **laws**, courts generally rule against nurses who violate policies
   d. If the nurse practices nursing in accordance with the client care policies and procedures established by the employer, functions within the job responsibility, and provides care consistent with the care in a nonnegligent manner, the potential for liability is minimized

D. Hospital staffing
1. Nurses should not walk out when staffing is inadequate because charges of abandonment can be made
2. Nurses in short staffing situations are obligated to notify the nursing supervisor

E. Floating
1. An acceptable legal practice used by hospitals to solve their understaffing problems
2. Legally, a nurse cannot refuse to float unless a union contract guarantees that nurses can work only in a specified area or the nurse can prove lack of knowledge for the performance of assigned tasks
3. Nurses in a floating situation must not assume responsibility beyond their level of experience or qualification
4. Nurses who float should inform the supervisor of any lack of experience in caring for the type of clients on the new nursing unit
5. The nurse should request and be given orientation to the new unit

F. Disciplinary action
1. Boards of nursing may deny, revoke, or suspend any license to practice as a practical/vocational nurse in accordance with their statutory authority
2. Causes for disciplinary action
   a. Unprofessional conduct
   b. Conduct that could adversely affect the health and welfare of the public
   c. Breach in client confidentiality
   d. Failure to use sufficient knowledge, skills, or nursing judgment
   e. Physically or verbally abusing a client
   f. Assuming duties without sufficient preparation
   g. Knowingly delegating nursing care to unlicensed personnel that places the client at risk for injury
   h. Failure to accurately maintain a record for each client
   i. Falsifying a client's record
   j. Leaving a nursing assignment without properly notifying appropriate personnel

III. LEGAL LIABILITY

A. **Laws**
1. Nurses are governed by civil and criminal **law** in roles as providers of services, employees of institutions, and private citizens
2. A nurse has a personal and legal obligation to provide a standard of client care expected of a reasonably competent nurse
3. Nurses are held responsible (liable) for harm resulting from their negligent acts, or omissions to act

B. Types of **laws** (Box 6-2)

C. **Negligence** and **Malpractice**
1. Conduct that falls below the standard of care
2. Can include an act of commission (was not done correctly) as well as an act of omission (was not done)
3. If a nurse gives care that does not meet appropriate standards, he or she may be held liable for **negligence**
4. **Malpractice** is **negligence** on the part of a nurse

BOX 6-2

Types of Laws

Contract law	Concerned with enforcement of agreements among private individuals
Civil law	Concerned with relationships among people and the protection of a person's rights Violation may cause harm to an individual or property, but no grave threat to society exists
Criminal law	Concerned with relationships between individuals and governments and with acts that threaten society and its order A crime is an offense against society that violates a law and is defined as a misdemeanor (less serious nature) or felony (serious nature)
Tort law	Civil wrong, other than a breach in contract, in which the law allows an injured person to seek damage from a person who caused the injury

5. **Malpractice** is determined if the nurse owed a duty to the client and did not carry out the duty, and the client was injured because the nurse failed to perform the duty
6. Proof of liability
   a. Duty: The nurse's responsibility to provide care in an acceptable way
   b. Breach of duty: The nurse did not adhere to the nursing standard of practice
   c. Causation: The breach of the duty was the legal cause of injury to the client
   d. Injury: The client experienced injury or damages or both and can be compensated by **law**

D. Professional liability insurance
1. Nurses need their own liability insurance for protection against **malpractice** lawsuits
2. Having one's own insurance provides the nurse protection as an individual and, in a lawsuit, allows the nurse to have present an attorney who has only the nurse's interests in mind

E. Good Samaritan **laws**
1. Passed by a state legislature
2. Encourage health care professionals to assist in emergency situations without fear of being sued for the care provided
3. These **laws** limit liability and offer legal immunity for people helping at the scene of an accident, providing they give reasonable care
4. Immunity from suit applies only when all conditions of the state **law** are met; for example, the health care provider receives no compensation for the care provided and the care given is not intentionally negligent

F. Controlled substances
1. The nurse must adhere to facility policies and procedures concerning administration of controlled substances, which is governed by federal and state **laws**
2. Controlled substances must be kept securely locked, and only authorized personnel should have access to them

IV. COLLECTIVE BARGAINING

A. Formalized decision-making process between representatives of management and representatives of labor to negotiate wages and conditions of employment

B. When collective bargaining breaks down because an agreement cannot be reached, the employees usually call a strike

C. Striking presents a moral dilemma to many nurses because nursing practice is a service to people

V. LEGAL RISK AREAS

A. Assault
1. Occurs when a person puts another person in fear of a harmful or an offensive contact
2. The victim fears and believes that harm will occur as a result of the threat

B. Battery: An intentional touching of another's body without the other's **consent**

C. Invasion of privacy: Includes violating confidentiality, intruding on private client or family matters, and sharing client information with unauthorized persons

D. False imprisonment
1. Occurs when a client is not allowed to leave a health care facility when there is no legal justification to detain the client
2. Occurs when restraining devices are used without an appropriate clinical need
3. A client can sign an "Against Medical Advice" form when the client is competent to make decisions, refuses care, and is requesting to leave the health care facility
4. Document circumstances in the medical record to avoid allegations by the client that cannot be defended

E. Defamation: Occurs when information that causes damage to someone's reputation is communicated to a third party either in writing (libel) or verbally (slander)

F. Fraud: Results from a deliberate deception intended to produce unlawful gains

VI. CLIENT RIGHTS

A. Patient's Bill of Rights
   1. Increase health care providers' awareness of the need to treat clients in an ethical and legal manner and encourages protection of rights
   2. Key elements of a client's rights with which nurses should be familiar include **informed consent** and confidentiality

B. Confidentiality
   1. A special relationship exists between two people in which information discussed will not be shared with a third party who is not directly involved in the client's care
   2. Nurses are bound to protect client confidentiality by most **nurse practice acts**, by ethical principles and standards, and by institutional and agency policies and procedures
   3. Treatment records cannot be released to any third party without the client's written **consent** and only after agency policies and procedures are followed
   4. Information release may be mandatory when ordered by a court, or when state statutes require reporting abuse, communicable diseases, or other associated incidents

C. Privileged communication
   1. Information given to a professional person who is forbidden by law from disclosing the information in a court without the consent of the person who provided it
   2. The nurse should seek legal counsel in regard to a privileged communication and should become familiar with the rights and privileges of the client and the nurse

D. **Informed consent**
   1. **Consent** is the client's approval to have his or her body touched by a specific individual
   2. Legally, the client must be mentally competent to give **consent** for procedures
   3. Before granting a **consent**, the client must be fully informed regarding treatment, tests, surgery, and so on, and must understand both the intended outcome and the potentially harmful results
   4. **Consent** must be obtained by the physician, surgeon, or other medical practitioner performing the treatment or procedure
   5. In most states, when a nurse is involved in the **informed consent** process, the nurse is only witnessing the signature of the client on the **informed consent** form
   6. If a client is determined by a court to be unable to make decisions and is declared incompetent or under a legal disability, a personal guardian is appointed by the court to make decisions
   7. An **informed consent** can be waived for urgent medical and surgical intervention as long as institutional policy so indicates
   8. Parental or guardian **consent** should be obtained before treatment is initiated on a minor except in an emergency, in situations where the **consent** of the minor is sufficient such as treatment of a sexually transmitted disease, or if a court order or other legal authorization has been obtained
   9. Minors who are married or emancipated from parents and those seeking treatment for sexually transmitted diseases can sign an informed **consent** form
   10. A client has the right to refuse information and waive the **informed consent** and undergo treatment, but this decision must be documented in the medical record

VII. LEGAL SAFEGUARDS

A. Risk management
   1. A planned method to identify, analyze, and evaluate risks followed by a plan for reducing the frequency of accidents and injuries
   2. Programs are based on a systematic reporting of incidents or unusual occurrences.

B. Incident reports
   1. A tool used as a means of identifying and improving client care
   2. Written as soon as possible after the occurrence by the person who witnessed the incident
   3. Follow specific documentation guidelines
   4. The report should be legible, factual, accurate, and objective
   5. The report form should not be copied or placed in the client's record
   6. No reference should be made to the report form in client's record, although the incident itself is recorded in the client's chart

C. Physician's orders
   1. The nurse is obligated to carry out a physician's orders except when the nurse believes the order is inappropriate
   2. A nurse carrying out an inaccurate order may be legally responsible for any harm suffered by the client
   3. A nurse must clarify an unclear or inappropriate order with the physician

4. If no resolution occurs regarding the order in question, the nursing supervisor needs to be contacted
5. See Box 6-3 concerning telephone orders

D. Documentation
1. Legally required by accrediting agencies, state licensing **laws**, and state nurse and medical practice acts
2. Follow agency guidelines and procedures (Box 6-4)

BOX 6-3

Telephone Orders

Date and time the entry.
Repeat the order to the physician and record the order given.
Sign the order beginning with t.o. (telephone order), write the physician's name, and sign the order.
If another nurse witnessed the order, that signature follows.
The physician needs to countersign the order within a time frame according to agency policy.

BOX 6-4

Documentation Guidelines

NARRATIVE
Use a black pen with permanent ink.
Date and time entries.
Provide objective, factual, accurate, and complete documentation.
Document entries in chronological order.
Document care, medications, treatments, and procedures as soon as possible after completion.
Document client responses to interventions.
Document consent for or refusal of treatments.
Document calls made to other health care providers.
Use quotes as appropriate for subjective data.
Use correct spelling, grammar, and punctuation.
Sign and title each entry.
Do not document for others or change documentation for other individuals.
Avoid unacceptable abbreviations.
Avoid judgmental or evaluative statements, such as "uncooperative client."
Do not leave blank spaces on documentation forms.
Follow agency policies when an error is made (draw one line through the error, initial, and date).
Follow agency guidelines regarding late entries.

COMPUTERIZED
Use the user identification (ID) code, name, or password.
Never lend access ID to another person.
Maintain privacy and confidentiality of documented information printed from the computer.

E. Client/family teaching
1. Client and family teaching is the responsibility of the registered nurse (RN), and the practical nurse reinforces teaching once the instruction and education have been started by the RN
2. The practical nurse initiates client teaching in the area of basic health care
3. Provide complete instructions in a language the client can understand
4. Document client and family teaching, what was taught, evaluation of understanding, and who was present during the teaching
5. Inform the client of what would happen if information shared during teaching is not followed

VIII. LEGAL DOCUMENTS FOR DECISION MAKING

A. Wills
1. Some agencies have specific policies that prohibit the nurse from signing as witness to this legal document for a client
2. If a nurse witnesses a legal document, the nurse must document the event and the factual circumstances surrounding the signing in the medical record
3. Documentation should include who was present, any significant comments by the client, and the nurse's observations of the client's conduct during this process

B. **Advance directives**
1. Written document recognized by state **law** that provides directions concerning the provision of care when a person is unable to make his or her own treatment choices
2. It must be made part of the medical record
3. A physician must be notified of its presence so that orders can be written consistent with the client's wishes

C. Living will: Document prepared by a competent adult that provides direction regarding medical care in the event of a person's incapacitation or otherwise becoming unable to make decisions personally

D. Durable power of attorney
1. Also called health care proxy
2. An authorization that enables any competent individual to name someone to exercise decision-making authority under specific circumstances on the individual's behalf

IX. DEATH AND DYING

A. Right of informed refusal: A competent adult has the right to refuse treatment, even life-sustaining treatment

B. Do not resuscitate (DNR) orders
   1. A written order must be present and must be reviewed on a regular basis
   2. Specific agency guidelines must be followed regarding when and under what circumstances an oral DNR order is acceptable
   3. The client or legal representative must provide **informed consent** for the DNR status
   4. Both DNR and cardiopulmonary resuscitation (CPR) must be clearly defined so that other treatment not refused by the client will be continued

C. Death certificate: The physician is responsible for signing a death certificate

D. Care of the body
   1. The nurse is responsible for preparing the body for the morgue or mortuary
   2. Follow agency guidelines and the wishes of the family of the deceased
   3. Treat the body with dignity

E. Organ transplant: The option to accept an organ transplant can be refused

F. Organ donation
   1. Any person 18 years or older may become an organ donor by written **consent**
   2. Informed choice to donate an organ can take place with the use of a written document signed by the client before death, a will, donor card, or **advance directive**
   3. A family member or legal guardian may authorize donation of the decedent's organs in the absence of appropriate documentation
   4. All 50 states have adopted the Uniform Anatomical Gift Act for cadaveric organ donation

G. Autopsy
   1. Medical examination of the body after death for the purpose of determining the cause of death
   2. Required by state **law** in certain circumstances, such as a sudden death or a death that occurs under suspicious circumstances
   3. If no oral or written instructions were given by the decedent, state **law** determines who has the authority to **consent** to any autopsy requested on a voluntary basis
   4. Documentation regarding **consent** must be present before the body can be released for autopsy

H. Assisted suicide
   1. Legal support exists for a client to refuse life-sustaining procedures and for health care providers to honor the client's voluntary and informed decision by withdrawing or withholding treatment
   2. Taking an active role in assisting a client to die is a criminal offense in most states

X. REPORTING RESPONSIBILITIES

A. Requirements: Nurses are required to report certain communicable diseases or criminal activities such as abuse, gunshot or stab wounds, assaults, homicides, and suicides to the appropriate authorities

B. The impaired nurse
   1. If a nurse suspects that a co-worker is abusing chemicals, the nurse must report the individual to nursing administration in a confidential manner with the goal of treatment for the individual being the issue
   2. Nursing administration then notifies the board of nursing regarding the nurse's behavior

C. Occupational Safety and Health Act (OSHA)
   1. Requires that an employer provide a safe workplace for employees according to regulations
   2. Employees can confidentially report working conditions that violate regulations
   3. An employee who does not report unsafe working conditions can be retaliated against by the employer

D. Sexual harassment
   1. Prohibited by state and federal **laws**
   2. Includes unwelcome conduct of a sexual nature
   3. Follow agency policies and procedures to handle reporting a concern or complaint

PRACTICE QUESTIONS

1. A nurse enters a client's room and finds the client lying on the floor. The nurse checks the client and then calls the nursing supervisor and the physician to inform them of the occurrence. The nursing supervisor instructs the nurse to complete an incident report. The nurse completes the incident report, understanding that it allows the analysis of adverse client events through:
   1. A method of promoting quality care and risk management
   2. Determining the effectiveness of interventions in relation to outcomes
   3. The appropriate method of reporting to local, state, and federal agencies
   4. Providing clients with necessary stabilizing treatments

2. A nurse observes that a client received pain medication 1 hour ago from another nurse, but that the client still has severe pain. The nurse has previously observed this same occurrence. Based on the Nurse Practice Act, the observing nurse plans to do which of the following?

1. Talk with the nurse who gave the medication
2. Report the information to a nursing supervisor
3. Call the Impaired Nurse Organization
4. Report the information to the police

3. A client has died and a family member is asked about the funeral arrangements. The family member refuses to discuss the issue. The nurse's most appropriate action is to:
   1. Provide information needed for decision making
   2. Suggest a referral to a mental health professional
   3. Show acceptance of liability of feelings
   4. Remain with the family member without discussing funeral arrangements
4. A client arrives in the emergency room and is staggering, confused, and verbally abusive. The client complains of a headache from drinking alcohol and is asking for medication. The nurse explains to the client that the physician will need to perform an assessment before the administration of medication. When the client becomes verbally abusive, the nurse threatens to place the client in restraints. Which of the following can the client legally charge the nurse as a result of the nursing action?
   1. Assault
   2. Battery
   3. Negligence
   4. Invasion of privacy
5. A nurse lawyer provides an education session to the nursing staff regarding client rights. A nurse asks the lawyer to describe an example that might relate to invasion of client privacy. A nursing action that indicates a violation of this right is:
   1. Taking photographs of the client without consent
   2. Telling the client that they cannot leave the hospital
   3. Threatening to place a client in restraints
   4. Performing a surgical procedure without consent
6. A nurse calls a physician of a client scheduled for a cardiac catheterization because the client has numerous questions regarding the procedure and has requested to speak to the physician. The physician is very upset and arrives at the unit to visit the client after prompting by the nurse. The nurse is outside of the client's room and hears the physician tell the client in a derogatory manner that the nurse "doesn't know anything." The nurse plans to address the physician's remark understanding that the physician has violated which legal tort?
   1. Libel
   2. Slander
   3. Assault
   4. Negligence
7. A nurse employed in a long-term care facility calls the physician regarding a new medication order because the dose prescribed is higher than the recommended dosage. The nurse is unable to locate the physician and the medication is due to be administered. Which of the following actions does the nurse take?
   1. Hold the medication until the physician can be contacted
   2. Administer the dose prescribed
   3. Administer the recommended dose until the physician can be located
   4. Contact the nursing supervisor
8. A nurse enters a client's room and finds the client sitting on the floor. The nurse checks the client thoroughly and then assists the client back to bed. The nurse completes an incident report and notifies the nursing supervisor and the physician of the incident. Which of the following is the next appropriate nursing action regarding the incident?
   1. Make a copy of the incident report for the physician
   2. Place the incident report in the client's chart
   3. Document a complete entry in the client's record concerning the incident
   4. Document in the client's record that an incident report has been completed
9. A nursing graduate who recently passed NCLEX-PN is employed as a licensed practical nurse (LPN) in a local hospital. During orientation, the nurse educator asks the LPN about his or her understanding of the need to obtain professional liability insurance. The most appropriate response by the LPN is:
   1. "The hospital's liability insurance will cover my actions."
   2. "It is very expensive and not necessary."
   3. "Nurses are encouraged to have their own malpractice insurance."
   4. "The majority of suits are filed against physicians and the hospital."
10. A nurse witnesses an automobile accident and provides care to an open wound at the scene of the accident to a young child. The family is extremely grateful and insists that the nurse accept monetary compensation for the care provided to the child. Because of the family insistence, the nurse accepts the compensation to avoid offending the family. The child develops an infection and sepsis, and is hospitalized. The family files suit against the nurse who provided care to the child at the scene of the accident. The nurse understands that which of the following is accurate regarding immunity from this suit?
    1. The Good Samaritan Law will protect the nurse
    2. The Good Samaritan Law will protect the nurse if the care given at the scene was not negligent
    3. The Good Samaritan Law will not provide immunity from suit if the nurse accepted compensation for the care provided
    4. The Good Samaritan Law protects laypersons and not professional health care providers

11. A client is brought to the emergency room after a serious accident, is unconscious, and is bleeding profusely. Surgery is required immediately to save the client's life. In regard to informed consent for the surgical procedure, which of the following is the best action?
    1. Try calling the client's spouse to obtain telephone consent before the surgical procedure
    2. Transport the client to the operating room immediately as required by the physician without obtaining an informed consent
    3. Ask the friend that accompanied the client to the emergency room to sign the consent form
    4. Call the nursing supervisor to initiate a court order for the surgical procedure
12. A nurse arrives at work and is told to report (float) to the pediatric unit for the day because the unit is understaffed and needs additional nurses to care for the children. The nurse has never worked in the pediatric unit. Which of the following is the most appropriate nursing action?
    1. Refuse to float to the pediatric unit
    2. Call the hospital lawyer
    3. Call the nursing supervisor
    4. Report to the pediatric unit and identify tasks that can be safely performed
13. A nurse enters a client's room and notes that the client's lawyer is present, and that the client is preparing a living will. The living will requires that the client's signature is witnessed and the client asks the nurse to witness the signature. Which of the following is the most appropriate nursing action?
    1. Sign the living will as a witness to signature only
    2. Sign the will clearly identifying credentials and employment agency
    3. Decline from signing the will
    4. Call the hospital lawyer before signing the will
14. An elderly woman is brought to the emergency room. When caring for the client, the nurse notes old and new ecchymotic areas on both arms and buttocks. The nurse asks the client how the bruises were sustained. The client, although reluctant, tells the nurse in confidence that the daughter frequently hits her if she gets in the way. Which of the following is the most appropriate nursing response?
    1. "I promise I will not tell anyone but let's see what we can do about this."
    2. "I have a legal obligation to report this type of abuse."
    3. "Let's talk about ways that will prevent your daughter from hitting you."
    4. "This should not be happening, and if it happens again you must call the emergency room."
15. A client tells the nurse of his/her decision to refuse external cardiac massage. Which of the following would be the most appropriate initial nursing action?
    1. Notify the physician of the client's request
    2. Document the client's request in the client's record
    3. Conduct a client conference to share the client's request
    4. Discuss the client's request with the family

ANSWERS

1. *Answer:* 1

Rationale: Proper documentation of unusual occurrences, incidents, and accidents, and the nursing actions taken as a result of the occurrence are internal to the institution or agency. Documentation on the incident report allows the nurse and administration to review the quality of care and determine any potential risks present. Options 2, 3, and 4 are incorrect.

Test-Taking Strategy: Use the process of elimination. Eliminate options 2 and 4 because incident reports are not routinely filled out for interventions or treatment measures. Eliminate option 3 because incident reports are not used to report occurrences to other agencies. Medical records are used for this purpose. Review the purpose of incident reports if you had difficulty with this question.

Level of Cognitive Ability: Application

Client Needs: Safe, Effective Care Environment

Integrated Concept/Process: Nursing Process/Implementation

Content Area: Fundamental Skills

Reference: Hill S, Howlett H: *Success in practical/vocational nursing: from student to leader,* ed 4, Philadelphia, 2001, WB Saunders, p. 307.

2. *Answer:* 2

Rationale: Nurse practice acts require reporting the suspicion of impaired nurses. The Board of Nursing has jurisdiction over the practice of nursing and may develop plans for treatment and supervision. This suspicion needs to be reported to the nursing supervisor who will then report to the Board of Nursing. Option 1 may cause a conflict. Options 3 and 4 are inappropriate.

Test-Taking Strategy: Use the principles of prioritizing when answering this question. By reporting the information, the nurse alerts the institution to the potential problem and sets the stage for further investigation and appropriate action. Review the actions to take regarding reporting the suspicion of an impaired nurse if you had difficulty with this question.

Level of Cognitive Ability: Application

Client Needs: Safe, Effective Care Environment

Integrated Concept/Process: Nursing Process/Planning

Content Area: Fundamental Skills

Reference: Hill S, Howlett H: (2001). *Success in practical/vocational nursing: from student to leader,* ed 4, Philadelphia, 2001, WB Saunders, pp. 181-182.

3. *Answer:* 4
Rationale: The family member is exhibiting the first stage of grief—denial. Option 1 may be an appropriate intervention for the bargaining stage. Option 2 may be an appropriate intervention for depression. Option 3 is an appropriate intervention for the acceptance or reorganization and restitution stage.
Test-Taking Strategy: Note the key words "most appropriate." Use therapeutic communication techniques to direct you to option 4. Remember to address client and family feelings first. Review the grieving process and therapeutic communication techniques if you had difficulty with this question.
Level of Cognitive Ability: Application
Client Needs: Psychosocial Integrity
Integrated Concept/Process: Caring
Content Area: Fundamental Skills
Reference: Potter P, Perry A: *Fundamentals of nursing,* ed 5, St Louis, 2001, Mosby, p. 614.

4. *Answer:* 1
Rationale: An assault occurs when a person puts another person in fear of a harmful or offensive contact. For this intentional tort to be actionable, the victim must be aware of the threat of harmful or offensive contact. Battery is the actual contact with one's body. Negligence involves actions below the standards of care. Invasion of privacy occurs when the individual's private affairs are unreasonably intruded into.
Test-Taking Strategy: Use the process of elimination. Note the key word "threatens" in the question. This will easily direct you to option 1. Review the descriptions associated with each term in the options if you had difficulty with this question.
Level of Cognitive Ability: Comprehension
Client Needs: Safe, Effective Care Environment
Integrated Concept/Process: Nursing Process/Implementation
Content Area: Fundamental Skills
Reference: Potter P, Perry A: *Fundamentals of nursing,* ed 5, St Louis, 2001, Mosby, p. 425.

5. *Answer:* 1
Rationale: Invasion of privacy takes place when an individual's private affairs are unreasonably intruded upon. Not allowing a client to leave the hospital constitutes false imprisonment. Threatening to place a client in restraints constitutes assault. Performing a surgical procedure without consent is an example of battery.
Test-Taking Strategy: Use the process of elimination. Note the key words "invasion of client privacy." These words should direct you to option 1. Review those situations that include invasion of client privacy if you had difficulty with this question.
Level of Cognitive Ability: Comprehension
Client Needs: Safe, Effective Care Environment
Integrated Concept/Process: Nursing Process/Implementation
Content Area: Fundamental Skills
Reference: Potter P, Perry A: *Fundamentals of nursing,* ed 5, St Louis, 2001, Mosby, p. 425.

6. *Answer:* 2
Rationale: Defamation takes place when something untrue is said (slander) or written (libel) about a person resulting in injury to that person's good name and reputation. An assault occurs when a person puts another person in fear of a harmful or an offensive contact. Negligence involves the actions of professionals that fall below the standard of care for a specific professional group.
Test-Taking Strategy: Use the process of elimination and focus on the information in the question. You can easily eliminate options 3 and 4 first recalling the definition of these terms. From the remaining options, recalling that slander constitutes verbal defamation will direct you to option 2. Review the torts identified in the options if you had difficulty with this question.
Level of Cognitive Ability: Application
Client Needs: Safe, Effective Care Environment
Integrated Concept/Process: Nursing Process/Planning
Content Area: Fundamental Skills
Reference: Potter P, Perry A: *Fundamentals of nursing,* ed 5, St Louis, 2001, Mosby, p. 426.

7. *Answer:* 4
Rationale: If the physician writes an order that requires clarification, it is the nurse's responsibility to contact the physician for clarification. If there is no resolution regarding the order, because the physician cannot be located, or because the order remains as it was written after talking with the physician, the nurse should then contact the nurse manager or supervisor for further clarification as to what the next step should be. Under no circumstances should the nurse proceed to carry out the order until clarification is obtained.
Test-Taking Strategy: Use the process of elimination. Eliminate options 2 and 3 first because they are similar and unsafe actions. Holding the medication can result in client injury. The nurse needs to take action. Option 4 clearly identifies the required action in this situation. Review nursing responsibilities related to physician's orders if you had difficulty with this question.
Level of Cognitive Ability: Application
Client Needs: Safe, Effective Care Environment
Integrated Concept/Process: Nursing Process/Implementation
Content Area: Fundamental Skills
Reference: Potter P, Perry A: *Fundamentals of nursing,* ed 5, St Louis, 2001, Mosby, p. 508.

8. *Answer:* 3
Rationale: The incident report is confidential and privileged information and should not be copied, placed in the chart, or referred to in the client's record. The incident report is not a substitute for a complete entry in the client's record concerning the incident.
Test-Taking Strategy: Use the process of elimination. Eliminate options 2 and 4 first because they are similar. Recalling that incident reports should not be copied will direct you to option 3. Review nursing responsibilities related to incident reports if you had difficulty with this question.
Level of Cognitive Ability: Application
Client Needs: Safe, Effective Care Environment
Integrated Concept/Process: Nursing Process/Implementation
Content Area: Fundamental Skills
Reference: Potter P, Perry A: *Fundamentals of nursing,* ed 5, St Louis, 2001, Mosby, p. 440.

9. *Answer:* 3
Rationale: Nurses need their own liability insurance for protection against malpractice lawsuits. Nurses erroneously assume that they are protected by an agency's professional liability policies. Usually when a nurse is sued, the employer is also sued for the nurse's actions or inactions. Even though this is the norm, nurses are encouraged to have their own malpractice insurance.
Test-Taking Strategy: Note that the issue of the question relates to "professional liability insurance." Focusing on this issue should easily direct you to option 3. Review liability related to malpractice insurance if you had difficulty with this question.
Level of Cognitive Ability: Comprehension
Client Needs: Safe, Effective Care Environment
Integrated Concept/Process: Nursing Process/Implementation
Content Area: Fundamental Skills
Reference: Potter P, Perry A: *Fundamentals of nursing,* ed 5, St Louis, 2001, Mosby, p. 427.

10. *Answer:* 3
Rationale: A Good Samaritan Law is passed by a state legislator to encourage nurses and other health care providers to provide care to a person when an accident, emergency, or injury occurs, without fear of being sued for the care provided. Called immunity from suit, this protection usually applies only if all of the conditions of the law are met, for example, the heath care provider receives no compensation for the care provided, and the care given is not willfully and wantonly negligent.
Test-Taking Strategy: Read the question carefully and note the key words "accept monetary compensation." This will easily direct you to option 3. Additionally, options 1, 2, and 4 are similar. Review the Good Samaritan Law if you had difficulty with this question.
Level of Cognitive Ability: Comprehension
Client Needs: Safe, Effective Care Environment
Integrated Concept/Process: Nursing Process/Implementation
Content Area: Fundamental Skills
Reference: Potter P, Perry A: *Fundamentals of nursing,* ed 5, St Louis, 2001, Mosby, p. 429.

11. *Answer:* 2
Rationale: Generally there are only two instances in which the informed consent of an adult client is not needed. One instance is when an emergency is present and delaying treatment for the purpose of obtaining informed consent would result in injury or death to the client. The second instance is when the client waives the right to give informed consent. Options 1, 3, and 4 are inappropriate.
Test-Taking Strategy: Use the process of elimination. Option 3 can be easily eliminated first. Note the key words "surgery is required immediately." Options 1 and 4 would delay treatment and should be eliminated. Review the issues surrounding informed consent if you had difficulty with this question.
Level of Cognitive Ability: Application
Client Needs: Safe, Effective Care Environment
Integrated Concept/Process: Nursing Process/Implementation
Content Area: Fundamental Skills
Reference: Potter P, Perry A: *Fundamentals of nursing,* ed 5, St Louis, 2001, Mosby, p. 432.

12. *Answer:* 4
Rationale: Floating is an acceptable legal practice used by hospitals to solve their understaffing problems. Legally, a nurse cannot refuse to float unless a union contract guarantees that nurses can only work in a specified area, or the nurse can prove the lack of knowledge for the performance of assigned tasks. When encountered with this situation, the nurse should identify potential areas of harm to the client.
Test-Taking Strategy: Use the process of elimination. Note the key words "most appropriate." Options 1 and 2 can be eliminated first because they are inappropriate. From the remaining options, eliminate option 3 because it is premature to call the nursing supervisor. Review nursing responsibilities related to "floating" if you had difficulty with this question.
Level of Cognitive Ability: Application
Client Needs: Safe, Effective Care Environment
Integrated Concept/Process: Nursing Process/Implementation
Content Area: Fundamental Skills
Reference: Hill S, Howlett H: *Success in practical/vocational nursing: from student to leader,* ed 4, Philadelphia, 2001, WB Saunders, pp. 317-318.

13. *Answer:* 3
Rationale: Living wills are required to be in writing and signed by the client. The client's signature must be either witnessed by specified individuals or notarized. Many states prohibit any employee, including a nurse of a facility where the declarer is receiving care, from being a witness.
Test-Taking Strategy: Use the process of elimination. Note the key words "most appropriate." Options 1 and 2 are similar and should be eliminated first. From the remaining options, option 3 is most appropriate. Review legal implications associated with wills if you had difficulty with this question.
Level of Cognitive Ability: Application
Client Needs: Safe, Effective Care Environment
Integrated Concept/Process: Nursing Process/Implementation
Content Area: Fundamental Skills
Reference: Hill S, Howlett H: *Success in practical/vocational nursing: from student to leader,* ed 4, Philadelphia, 2001, WB Saunders, pp. 301, 318.

14. *Answer:* 2
Rationale: Confidential issues are not to be discussed with nonmedical personnel or the person's family or friends without the person's permission. Clients should be assured that information is kept confidential, unless it places the nurse under a legal obligation. The nurse must report situations related to child or elderly abuse, gunshot wounds, stabbings, and certain infectious diseases.
Test-Taking Strategy: Use the process of elimination. Option 4 can be eliminated first because this action does not protect the client from injury. Options 1 and 3 are similar and should be eliminated next. Review the nursing responsibilities related to reporting obligations if you had difficulty with this question.
Level of Cognitive Ability: Application
Client Needs: Psychosocial Integrity
Integrated Concept/Process: Communication and Documentation
Content Area: Fundamental Skills
Reference: Potter P, Perry A: *Fundamentals of nursing,* ed 5, St Louis, 2001, Mosby, p. 503.

15. ***Answer:*** 1

Rationale: External cardiac massage is one type of treatment that a client can refuse. The most appropriate initial action is to notify the physician because a written Do Not Resuscitate (DNR) order from the physician must be present. The DNR order must be reviewed or renewed on a regular basis per agency policy.

Test-Taking Strategy: Use the process of elimination. The key words "most appropriate initial" may indicate that more than one option may be correct. Although options 2, 3, and 4 may be appropriate, remember that first a written physician's order is necessary. Review DNR procedures if you had difficulty with this question.

Level of Cognitive Ability: Application

Client Needs: Safe, Effective Care Environment

Integrated Concept/Process: Nursing Process/Implementation

Content Area: Fundamental Skills

Reference: Potter P, Perry A: *Fundamentals of nursing,* ed 5, St Louis, 2001, Mosby, p. 434.

REFERENCES

DeWit S: *Fundamental concepts and skills for nursing,* Philadelphia, 2001, WB Saunders.

Hill S, Howlett H: *Success in practical/vocational nursing: from student to leader,* ed 4, Philadelphia, 2001, WB Saunders.

National Council of State Boards of Nursing, editors: *Test plan for the National Council Licensure Examination for Practical/Vocational Nurses,* Chicago, 2001, Author.

Potter P, Perry A: *Fundamentals of nursing,* ed 5, St Louis, 2001, Mosby.

Riley J: *Communication in nursing,* ed 4, St Louis, 2000, Mosby.

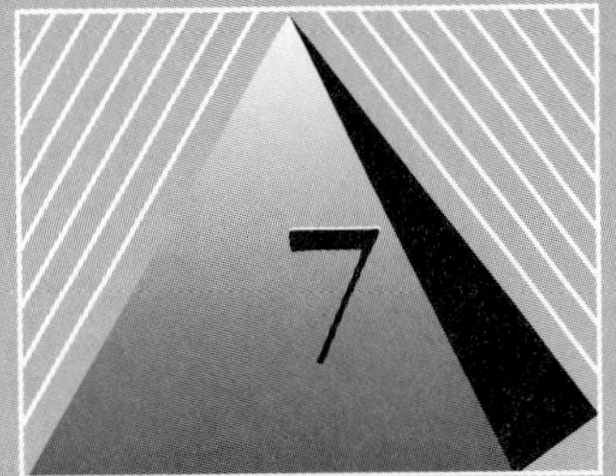

Leadership Issues and Priorities of Care

PYRAMID TERMS

Accountability A moral concept that involves acceptance by the nurse of the consequences of a decision or action.

Case Management An interdisciplinary health care delivery system designed to promote appropriate use of hospital personnel and material resources to maximize hospital revenues while providing for optimal outcome of care.

Critical Paths Provide effective clinical management systems for monitoring care and for reducing or controlling the length of hospital stay.

Delegation Process of transferring a selected nursing task in a situation to an individual who is competent to perform that specific task.

Empowerment An interpersonal process of enabling others to do for themselves.

Leadership An interpersonal process that involves motivating and guiding others to achieve goals.

Management The accomplishment of tasks either by oneself or by directing others.

Prioritizing Deciding which needs or problems require immediate action and which ones could be delayed until a later time because they are not urgent.

Responsibility The duty to act.

Variances Actual deviations or detours from the critical paths.

PYRAMID TO SUCCESS

The nurse is both a leader and a manager. As described in the NCLEX-PN Test Plan, the nurse needs to collaborate with other health care team members to facilitate effective care. Pyramid points focus on concepts of management and supervision, leadership responsibilities, resource management, making client care assignments, establishing priorities among a group of clients, and the principles of time management. The primary Integrated Concepts and Processes addressed in this chapter include the Clinical Problem-Solving Process (Nursing Process), Communication and Documentation, and Self-Care.

CLIENT NEEDS

Safe, Effective Care Environment

Client care assignments
Concepts of management and supervision
Consultation with members of the health care team
Continuous quality improvement
Establishing priorities
Identifying practice limitations
Resource management
Variance reports

Health Promotion and Maintenance

Client's ability to perform self-care
Disease prevention
Health screening
Health promotion programs

Psychosocial Integrity

Religious, cultural, and spiritual influences on health
Support systems
Therapeutic environment

Physiological Integrity

Basic care and comfort
Prioritizing client care

I. HEALTH CARE DELIVERY SYSTEMS
   A. Managed care
      1. Designed to control the cost of health services and promote a continuum of care through the development and use of integrated services
      2. Emphasizes the promotion of health, client education and responsible self-care, early

identification of disease, and the use of health care resources
3. The practice of prospectively paying predetermined amounts of money to selected providers to maintain the health of a defined population
4. To control health care costs, employers limit employee choices to less costly managed programs or encourage employees to elect managed care options
5. Managed care organizations, through contractual agreements, enter into a variety of relationships with providers to meet the needs of members
6. Less costly to provide this type of care than that associated with acute care and hospitalization
7. Physicians receive a specific monetary amount per member per month to provide care irrespective of services rendered, which provides the incentive to keep the client healthy
8. Requires that physicians authorize specialty care and limit use of hospital-based services to promote efficient, cost-effective care and appropriate use of resources

B. Health maintenance organization (HMO)
1. Offers comprehensive coverage for hospital and physician services in exchange for a fixed, prepaid fee
2. Both an insurance company and a health care delivery system

C. **Case management**
1. Represents an interdisciplinary health care delivery system designed to promote appropriate use of hospital personnel and material resources to maximize hospital revenues while providing the optimal amount of care
2. Provides a care process that assists hospitals and health care providers to standardize the appropriate use of resources
3. Manages client care by managing the client care environment

D. **Critical paths**
1. Developed on the basis of appropriate standards of care
2. Provide effective clinical **management** systems for monitoring care and for reducing or controlling the length of hospital stay
3. Developed through the collaborative efforts of physicians, nurses, pharmacists, and other interdisciplinary caregivers, with the goal of improving the quality and outcomes of care
4. The goal of **critical paths** is to anticipate and recognize negative **variance** early so that appropriate action can be taken and better client outcomes can result
5. **Variances**
   a. Actual deviations or detours from the **critical paths**
   b. Positive **variance** occurs when the client achieves maximum benefit and is discharged earlier than anticipated on his or her **critical path**
   c. Negative **variance** occurs when untoward events prevent a timely discharge, and the length of hospital stay is longer than planned for a client on a specific **critical path**
   d. **Variance** analysis occurs continually as the case manager and other caregivers monitor client outcomes against the **critical path**
   e. Accurate monitoring of **critical paths** with **variance** analysis can estimate the financial impact of client care
   f. If the **variance** is predictable, negotiation with insurers for an additional length of hospital stay can maximize client care revenues

E. Levels of prevention
1. Primary prevention: Relates to heath promotion activities and specific protection for disease or illness
2. Secondary prevention: Focuses on the early diagnosis and prompt treatment of disease
3. Tertiary prevention: Represented by rehabilitative services

F. Health care settings
1. Hospital care
2. Home care
3. Hospice care
4. Long-term care
5. Surgical centers
6. Ambulatory care
7. Public health departments

II. FORMAL ORGANIZATIONS

A. Mission statement: Communicates in broad terms an organization's reason for existence, the geographical area the organization serves, and attitudes and beliefs within which the organization functions

B. Goals and objectives: Measurable activities specific to the development of designated services and programs of an organization

C. Organizational chart: Depicts and communicates how activities are arranged, how authority relationships are defined, and how communication channels are established

D. Procedures and protocols
1. Guides in defining appropriate courses of actions

2. Procedure defines a task
3. Protocol signifies the definition of a clinical process

E. Centralization: When decisions are made by a limited number of individuals at the top of the organization, or by managers of a department or unit, and thereafter communicated to the employees

F. Decentralization: Authority is distributed throughout the organization to allow for increased **responsibility** and **delegation** in decision making

III. NURSING DELIVERY SYSTEMS

A. Functional Nursing: involves a task approach to client care, with major tasks being delegated by the charge nurse to individual members of the team

B. Team Nursing: the team is generally led by a charge nurse and each staff member works fully within the realm of his or her educational and clinical expertise

C. Primary Nursing: focuses on the client outcomes as opposed to nursing tasks and is concerned with keeping the nurse at the bedside and actively involved in individualized client care

IV. PROFESSIONAL RESPONSIBILITIES

A. **Accountability**
1. The process that mandates that individuals are answerable for their actions and have an obligation (or duty) to act
2. Assuming only the responsibilities that are within one's scope of practice
3. Not assuming **responsibility** for activities in which competence has not been achieved
4. Involves admitting mistakes rather than blaming others, and evaluating the outcomes of one's own actions
5. Includes a **responsibility** to the client to be competent, to render nursing services in accordance with standards of nursing practice, and to adhere to professional ethics

B. **Leadership**
1. The interpersonal process that involves motivating and guiding others to achieve goals
2. A method of modeling accountable behavior to others

C. **Leadership** Styles
1. Autocratic: leader maintains strong control, makes the decisions, and solves all problems
2. Democratic: also called participative **leadership,** based on the belief that every group member should have input into development of goals and problem solving
3. Laissez-Faire: leader assumes a passive, nondirective, and inactive approach and all decision making is left to the group, with the leader giving little if any guidance, support, or feedback
4. Situational: utilizing a combination of styles based on current circumstances and events

D. **Leadership** Qualities (Box 7-1)

E. **Management**: The accomplishment of tasks either by oneself or by directing others

V. EMPOWERMENT

A. An interpersonal process of enabling others to do for themselves

B. Occurs when individuals are better able to influence what happens to them

C. Involves open communication, mutual goal setting, and decision making

D. Nurses can **empower** clients through advocacy

VI. ASSIGNMENTS AND DELEGATION

A. Process of transferring a selected nursing task in a situation to an individual who is competent to perform that specific task

B. Delegation is a tool for nurse leaders that encourages team members to develop skills

C. Licensed practical nurses may be responsible, depending on the state Nurse Practice Act, to assign and delegate tasks to nursing assistants and other unlicensed assistive personnel (UAP)

D. Even though a task may be delegated to someone, the nurse who delegates maintains **accountability** for the overall nursing care of the client

E. Only the task, not the ultimate **accountability,** may be delegated to another

F. Guidelines for client care assignments
1. Always ensure client safety
2. Be aware of individual variations in work abilities
3. Determine which tasks can be delegated and to whom

BOX 7-1

Leadership Qualities

Communication
Credibility
Critical thinking
Initiating action
Risk taking

4. Match the task to the delegate on the basis of the Nurse Practice Act and appropriate position descriptions
5. Provide directions that are clear, concise, accurate, and complete
6. Validate the person's understanding of the directions
7. Communicate a feeling of confidence to the delegate, and provide feedback promptly after the task is performed
8. Maintain continuity of care as much as possible when assigning client care

VII. PRIORITIES OF CARE

A. **Prioritizing**: Deciding which needs or problems require immediate action and which ones could be delayed until a later time because they are not urgent

B. Guidelines for **prioritizing**

1. The nurse and client mutually rank the client's needs in order of importance based on the client's desires, needs, and safety
2. Priorities are classified as high, intermediate, or low
   a. Client needs that are life-threatening or that could result in harm to the client if they are left untreated are high priorities
   b. Non-emergency and non-life-threatening client needs are intermediate priorities
   c. Client needs that are not directly related to the client's illness or prognosis are low priorities
3. When providing care, the nurse needs to decide which needs or problems require immediate action and which ones could be delayed until a later time because they are not urgent
4. Client problems that involve actual or life-threatening concerns are considered before potential health-threatening concerns
5. When **prioritizing** care, the nurse must consider time constraints and available resources
6. Problems identified as important by the client must be given high priority
7. Priority setting may be guided by principles, models, and/or theories, such as Maslow's Hierarchy of Needs
8. Maslow's Hierarchy of Needs theory identifies the levels of physiological needs, safety, love and belonging, self-esteem, and self-actualization; basic needs are met before moving to other needs in the hierarchy
9. Use the ABCs: airway, breathing, and circulation; client needs related to maintaining a patent airway are always the priority

VIII. TIME MANAGEMENT

A. Description

1. A technique designed to assist in completing tasks within a definite time period
2. Involves efficiency in completing tasks as quickly as possible, and effectiveness in deciding on the most important task to do, and doing it correctly

B. Guidelines

1. Identify tasks, obligations, and activities, and write them down
2. Organize the workday; identify which tasks must be completed in specified time frames
3. Prioritize client needs according to importance
4. Anticipate the needs of the day, and provide time for unexpected and unplanned tasks that may arise
5. Focus on beginning the daily tasks working on the most important first, while keeping goals in mind; look at the final goal for the day, which will help to break down tasks into manageable parts
6. Begin client rounds at the beginning of the shift, collecting data on each assigned client
7. Delegate tasks when appropriate
8. Keep a daily hour-by-hour log to assist in providing structure to the tasks that must be accomplished, and cross tasks off the list as they are accomplished
9. Use agency resources wisely, anticipating resource needs and gathering the necessary supplies before beginning the task
10. Organize paperwork and continuously document task completion and necessary client data throughout the day
11. At the end of the day, evaluate the effectiveness of time management

PRACTICE QUESTIONS

1. A nurse is assigned to care for four clients. In planning client rounds, which client would the nurse collect data on first?
   1. A client receiving oxygen via nasal cannula who had difficulty breathing during the previous shift
   2. A postoperative client preparing for discharge
   3. A client scheduled for a chest x-ray study
   4. A client requiring daily dressing changes
2. A nurse is assisting in reviewing the critical paths of the clients on the nursing unit. In performing a variance analysis, which of the following indicates the need for further action?

1. A client's family attending a diabetic teaching session
2. Canceling physical therapy sessions on the weekend
3. Normal vital signs and the absence of wound infection in a postoperative client
4. A client demonstrating accurate medication administration following teaching

3. A licensed practical nurse (LPN) is attending an agency orientation regarding the nursing model of practice implemented in the facility. The nurse is told that the nursing model is a team nursing approach. The nurse understands that which of the following is a characteristic of this type of nursing model of practice?
   1. A task approach method is used to provide care to clients
   2. A single registered nurse (RN) is responsible for providing nursing care to a group of clients
   3. Managed care concepts and tools are used in providing client care
   4. Nursing personnel are led by an RN leader in providing care to a group of clients

4. A nurse is assigned to assist with working with food services in a rural, poor school setting. A goal for the school dietary program is to avoid nutritional deficiencies and enhance children's nutritional status through healthy dietary practices. In implementing interventions by levels of prevention, which of the following would be a primary prevention intervention that the nurse could suggest?
   1. Case finding in the school to identify dietary practices
   2. School screening programs for early detection of children with poor eating habits
   3. Providing educational programs, literature, and posters to promote awareness of healthy eating
   4. Conducting a community-wide dietary screening activity to detect community dietary trends

5. A nurse is assisting with working with disaster relief after a tornado. The nurse's goal with the overall community is to prevent as much injury and death as possible from the uncontrollable event. Finding safe housing for survivors, providing support to families, organizing counseling, and securing physical care when needed are all examples of which type of prevention?
   1. The primary level of prevention
   2. The secondary level of prevention
   3. The tertiary level of prevention
   4. Aggregate care prevention

6. A nurse is planning the client assignments. Which of the following is the least appropriate assignment for the nursing assistant?
   1. Assist a 12-year-old boy with Down syndrome, who is profoundly developmentally disabled, to eat lunch
   2. Obtain frequent oral temperatures on a client
   3. Accompany a 51-year-old man, being discharged to home after a bowel resection 8 days ago, to his transportation
   4. Collect a urine specimen from a 70-year-old woman admitted 3 days ago

7. A nurse is asked by another nurse about the definition of case management. Which of the following would not be a component of the response?
   1. Case management represents a primary health prevention focus managed by a single case manager
   2. Case management manages client care by managing the client care environment
   3. Case management is designed to promote appropriate use of hospital personnel and material resources
   4. Case management maximizes hospital revenues while providing for optimal outcome of client care

8. A nurse employed in a long-term care facility is planning the client assignments for the shift. Which of the following clients would the nurse most appropriately assign to the nursing assistant?
   1. A client requiring BID dressing changes
   2. A client requiring frequent ambulation
   3. A client on a bowel management program requiring rectal suppositories and a daily enema
   4. A diabetic client requiring daily insulin and reinforcement of dietary measures

9. A nurse has received the client assignment for the day and is organizing the required tasks. Which of the following will not be a component of the plan for time management?
   1. Prioritizing client needs and daily tasks
   2. Providing time for unexpected tasks
   3. Gathering supplies before beginning a task
   4. Documenting task completion at the end of the day

10. A nurse is giving a bed bath to a client. A nursing assistant enters the client's room and tells the nurse that another client is in pain and needs pain medication. The most appropriate action is which of the following?
    1. Finish the bed bath and then administer the pain medication to the other client
    2. Cover the client, raise the side rails, tell the client that you will return shortly, and administer the pain medication to the other client
    3. Ask the nursing assistant to tell the client in pain that medication will be administered as soon as the bed bath is complete
    4. Ask the nursing assistant to find out when the last pain medication was given to the client

ANSWERS

1. *Answer:* 1
Rationale: Airway is always a high priority and the nurse would attend to the client who has been experiencing an airway problem first. The clients described in options 2, 3, and 4 would be an intermediate priority.
Test-Taking Strategy: Use Maslow's Hierarchy of Needs theory and the ABCs—airway, breathing, and circulation—to answer the question. Remember that airway is always the first priority. Review these prioritizing principles if you had difficulty with this question.
Level of Cognitive Ability: Application
Client Needs: Safe, Effective Care Environment
Integrated Concept/Process: Nursing Process/Planning
Content Area: Fundamental Skills
Reference: DeWit S: *Fundamental concepts and skills for nursing*, Philadelphia, 2001, WB Saunders, p. 53.

2. *Answer:* 2
Rationale: Variances are actual deviations or detours from the critical paths. Variances can be either positive or negative, avoidable or unavoidable, and can be caused by a variety of things. Positive variance occurs when the client achieves maximum benefit and is discharged earlier than anticipated. Negative variance occurs when untoward events prevent a timely discharge. Variance analysis occurs continually to anticipate and recognize negative variance early so that appropriate action can be taken.
Test-Taking Strategy: Note the key words "need for further action." Use the process of elimination to identify the negative variance. Options 1, 3, and 4 identify positive outcomes. Option 2 identifies a negative outcome. Review the purpose of variance analysis if you had difficulty with this question.
Level of Cognitive Ability: Comprehension
Client Needs: Safe, Effective Care Environment
Integrated Concept/Process: Nursing Process/Evaluation
Content Area: Fundamental Skills
Reference: DeWit S: *Fundamental concepts and skills for nursing*, Philadelphia, 2001, WB Saunders, p. 111.

3. *Answer:* 4
Rationale: In team nursing, nursing personnel are led by an RN leader in providing care to a group of clients. Option 1 identifies functional nursing. Option 2 identifies primary nursing. Option 3 identifies a component of case management.
Test-Taking Strategy: Note that the issue of the question relates to team nursing. Keep this issue in mind and use the process of elimination. Option 4 is the only option that identifies the concept of a team approach. Review the various types of nursing delivery systems if you had difficulty with this question.
Level of Cognitive Ability: Comprehension
Client Needs: Safe, Effective Care Environment
Integrated Concept/Process: Nursing Process/Implementation
Content Area: Fundamental Skills
Reference: DeWit S: *Fundamental concepts and skills for nursing*, Philadelphia, 2001, WB Saunders, p. 9.

4. *Answer:* 3
Rationale: Primary prevention interventions are those measures that keep illness, injury, or potential problems from occurring. Option 1 is a tertiary prevention measure; options 2 and 4 are secondary prevention measures that seek to detect existing health problems or trends.
Test-Taking Strategy: Note the issue of the question "primary prevention intervention." Recalling that primary prevention interventions are those measures that keep illness from occurring will direct you to option 3. Review the levels of prevention if you had difficulty with this question.
Level of Cognitive Ability: Comprehension
Client Needs: Health Promotion and Maintenance
Integrated Concept/Process: Nursing Process/Planning
Content Area: Fundamental Skills
Reference: DeWit S: *Fundamental concepts and skills for nursing*, Philadelphia, 2001, WB Saunders, p. 27.

5. *Answer:* 3
Rationale: Tertiary prevention involves the reduction of the amount and degree of disability, injury, and damage after a crisis. Primary prevention means keeping the crisis from ever occurring and secondary prevention focuses on reducing the intensity and duration of the crisis during the crisis itself. There is no known aggregate care prevention level.
Test-Taking Strategy: Identify the scenario in the question. Focus on this scenario and use knowledge regarding the various levels of prevention to answer the question. Review these levels if you had difficulty with this question.
Level of Cognitive Ability: Application
Client Needs: Safe, Effective Care Environment
Integrated Concept/Process: Nursing Process/Implementation
Content Area: Fundamental Skills
Reference: DeWit S: *Fundamental concepts and skills for nursing*, Philadelphia, 2001, WB Saunders, p. 27.

6. *Answer:* 1
Rationale: The nurse must determine the most appropriate assignment based on the skills of the staff member and the needs of the client. In this case, the least appropriate assignment for the nursing assistant would be assisting with feeding a profoundly developmentally disabled child. The child is likely to have difficulty eating and, therefore, has a higher potential for complications such as choking and aspiration. The remaining options do not include data that indicate that these tasks carry any unforeseen risk.
Test-Taking Strategy: Note the key words "least appropriate." Use the ABCs—airway, breathing, and circulation—and recall the principles of delegation and supervision of the work of others in answering the question. Remember work that is delegated to others must be done consistent with the individual's level of expertise and licensure or lack of licensure. Review the principles related to assignments and delegation if you had difficulty with this question.
Level of Cognitive Ability: Application
Client Needs: Safe, Effective Care Environment
Integrated Concept/Process: Nursing Process/Implementation
Content Area: Fundamental Skills
Reference: DeWit S: *Fundamental concepts and skills for nursing*, Philadelphia, 2001, WB Saunders, p. 34.

7. *Answer:* 1
Rationale: Case management represents an interdisciplinary health care delivery system to promote appropriate use of

hospital personnel and material resources to maximize hospital revenues while providing for optimal outcome of care. Options 2, 3, and 4 identify the components of managed care.
Test-Taking Strategy: Note the key word "not." Use the process of elimination and knowledge regarding the characteristics of case management to answer this question. Also, note the key word "single" in the correct option. Review the characteristics of case management if you had difficulty with this question.
Level of Cognitive Ability: Comprehension
Client Needs: Safe, Effective Care Environment
Integrated Concept/Process: Nursing Process/Planning
Content Area: Fundamental Skills
Reference: DeWit S: *Fundamental concepts and skills for nursing,* Philadelphia, 2001, WB Saunders, p. 111.

8. ***Answer:*** 2
Rationale: Assignment of tasks needs to be implemented based on the job description of the individual, the level of clinical competence, and state law. Options 1, 3, and 4 involve care that requires the skill of a licensed nurse.
Test-Taking Strategy: Use the process of elimination and knowledge regarding tasks that can be safely delegated to the nursing assistant. Eliminate options 1, 3, and 4 because these clients require care that needs to be provided by a licensed nurse. Review the principles related to assignments and delegation if you had difficulty with this question.
Level of Cognitive Ability: Application
Client Needs: Safe, Effective Care Environment
Integrated Concept/Process: Nursing Process/Planning
Content Area: Fundamental Skills
Reference: DeWit S: *Fundamental concepts and skills for nursing,* Philadelphia, 2001, WB Saunders, p. 34.

9. ***Answer:*** 4
Rationale: The nurse should document task completion continuously throughout the day. Options 1, 2, and 3 identify accurate components of time management.
Test-Taking Strategy: Note the key word "not." Use the process of elimination and knowledge regarding the guidelines for time management to answer the question. Review these guidelines if you had difficulty with this question.
Level of Cognitive Ability: Application
Client Needs: Safe, Effective Care Environment
Integrated Concept/Process: Nursing Process/Planning
Content Area: Fundamental Skills
Reference: DeWit S: *Fundamental concepts and skills for nursing,* Philadelphia, 2001, WB Saunders, p. 102.

10. ***Answer:*** 2
Rationale: The most appropriate action is to provide safety to the client who is receiving the bed bath and prepare to administer the pain medication. Options 1 and 3 delay the administration of medication to the client in pain. Option 4 is not a responsibility of the nursing assistant.
Test-Taking Strategy: Use the process of elimination and principles related to priorities of care. Options 1 and 3 delay the administration of pain medication, and option 4 is not a responsibility of the nursing assistant. The most appropriate action is to plan to administer the medication. Review the principles related to priorities of care if you had difficulty with this question.
Level of Cognitive Ability: Application
Client Needs: Safe, Effective Care Environment
Integrated Concept/Process: Nursing Process/Implementation
Content Area: Fundamental Skills
Reference: DeWit S: *Fundamental concepts and skills for nursing,* Philadelphia, 2001, WB Saunders, p. 53.

REFERENCES

DeWit S: *Fundamental concepts and skills for nursing,* Philadelphia, 2001, WB Saunders.

Hill S, Howlett H: *Success in practical/vocational nursing: from student to leader,* ed 4, Philadelphia, 2001, WB Saunders.

National Council of State Boards of Nursing, editors: *Test plan for the National Council Licensure Examination for Practical/Vocational Nurses,* Chicago, 2001, Author.

Potter P, Perry A: *Fundamentals of nursing,* ed 5, St Louis, 2001, Mosby.

UNIT III

Nursing Sciences

Fluids and Electrolytes

PYRAMID TERMS

Fluid Volume Deficit Dehydration in which water and electrolytes are lost in the same proportion. The goal of treatment is to restore fluid volume, replace electrolytes as needed, and eliminate the cause of the fluid volume deficit.

Fluid Volume Excess An actual excess of total body fluid or a relative fluid excess in one or more fluid compartments. Also called overhydration or fluid overload. The goal of treatment is to restore fluid balance, correct electrolyte balances if present, and eliminate or control the underlying cause of the overload.

Homeostasis The tendency of biological systems to maintain relatively constant conditions in the internal environment while continuously interacting with and adjusting to changes originating within or outside the system.

Hypercalcemia A serum calcium level that exceeds 10 mg/dL.

Hypocalcemia A serum calcium level below 8.6 mg/dL.

Hyperkalemia A serum potassium level that exceeds 5.1 mEq/L.

Hypokalemia A serum potassium level below 3.5 mEq/L.

Hypermagnesemia A serum magnesium level that exceeds 2.6 mg/dL.

Hypomagnesemia A serum magnesium level below 1.6 mg/dL.

Hypernatremia A serum sodium level that exceeds 145 mEq/L.

Hyponatremia A serum sodium level below 135 mEq/L.

Hyperphosphatemia A serum phosphorus level that exceeds 4.5 mg/dL.

Hypophosphatemia A serum phosphorus level below 2.7 mg/dL.

Third Space Losses A fluid shift from the intravascular space into another part of the body where the fluid is not functional.

PYRAMID TO SUCCESS

Pyramid points focus primarily on data collection related to a fluid and electrolyte imbalance, implementation, and evaluating the expected outcomes. Fluid and electrolytes constitute a content area that is complex and sometimes difficult to understand. It is important to understand cell functions and properties and the concepts related to body fluids as outlined in this chapter. Review this content. Pyramid points focus on the common fluid and electrolyte disturbances. Focus on the pyramid points related to the causes, data collection, and related treatments. The primary Integrated Concepts and Processes addressed in this chapter are the Clinical Problem-Solving Process (Nursing Process), Communication and Documentation, Self-Care, and Teaching/Learning.

CLIENT NEEDS

Safe, Effective Care Environment

Accident prevention
Asepsis
Establishing priorities
Standard (universal) precautions
Handling hazardous and infectious materials

Health Promotion and Maintenance

Health screening and potential risk for a fluid and electrolyte imbalance
Instructions related to medication and diet management
Instructions related to the signs and symptoms of an imbalance
Measures to prevent an imbalance

Psychosocial Integrity

Reassure the client experiencing symptoms related to a fluid and electrolyte imbalance
Provide support and continuously inform the client of the purpose for prescribed interventions

Physiological Integrity

Identify clients at risk for a fluid or electrolyte imbalance
Monitor laboratory values
Monitor for complications related to the imbalance
Assist in managing emergencies
Identify the expected and unexpected responses to treatment and document accordingly

I. CELL PROPERTIES (Box 8-1)

II. CONCEPTS OF FLUID AND ELECTROLYTE BALANCE

A. Electrolytes
1. Description: When a substance is dissolved in solution and some of its molecules split or dissociate into electrically charged atoms or ions
2. Measurement
a. To measure volume of fluids, the metric system is used and measures liters (L) or milliliters (mL)
b. The unit of measure that expresses the combining activity of an electrolyte is the milliequivalent (mEq)

B. Body fluid compartments (Box 8-2)
1. Fluid in each of the body compartments contain electrolytes
2. Each compartment has a particular composition of electrolytes, which differs from that of other compartments
3. To function normally, body cells must have fluids and electrolytes
4. The electrolytes must be in the right compartments in the right amounts
5. A specific kind and amount of certain electrolytes must be available for normal cell function
6. Whenever an electrolyte moves out of a cell, another electrolyte moves in to take its place
7. The number of cations and anions must be the same for **homeostasis** to exist
8. Compartments are separated by semipermeable membranes

C. Third-Spacing
1. The accumulation and sequestration of trapped extracellular fluid in an actual or potential body space as a result of disease or injury
2. The trapped fluid represents a volume loss and is unavailable for normal physiological processes
3. Fluid may be trapped in body spaces such as the pericardial, pleural, peritoneal, or joint cavities; the bowel; or the abdomen; or within soft tissues after trauma or burns
4. Assessing the intravascular fluid loss is difficult; it may not be reflected in weight changes or intake and output (I&O) records, and may

BOX 8-1

Cell Properties

Atom - The smallest part of an element that still has the properties of the element.
Composed of particles known as the proton (positive charge), neutron (neutral), and electron (negative charge).
Protons and neutrons are in the nucleus of the atom; therefore, the nucleus is positively charged.
Electrons carry a negative charge and revolve around the nucleus. As long as the number of electrons is the same as the number of protons, there is no net charge on the atom; that is, it is neither positive nor negative. Atoms may gain, lose, or share electrons and then no longer are neutral.
Molecule - When two or more atoms combine to form a substance.
Ion - When an atom carries an electrical charge because it has either gained or lost electrons. Some ions carry a negative electrical charge, and some carry a positive charge.
Cation - When an ion carries a positive charge and it has given away or lost electrons.
The result is fewer electrons than protons and a positive charge.
Anion - An ion that has gained electrons and therefore carries a negative charge.
When an ion has gained or taken on electrons, it assumes a negative charge and the result is a negatively charged ion.

BOX 8-2

Body Fluid Compartments

Intracellular Compartment - Refers to all fluid inside the cells. Most of the body fluids are inside the cells
Extracellular Compartment - Refers to all fluid outside the cells
Intravascular Compartment - Fluid that is within blood vessels
Interstitial Fluids - Fluid between the cells and blood vessels

not become apparent until after organ malfunction occurs

D. Edema
   1. An excess accumulation of fluid in the interstitial spaces
   2. Localized edema occurs as a result of traumatic injury from accidents or surgery, local inflammatory processes, and burns
   3. Generalized edema, also called anasarca, is an excessive accumulation of fluid in the interstitial space throughout the body as a result of a condition such as cardiac, renal, or liver failure

E. Body fluid
   1. Description
      a. Provides transportation of nutrients to the cells and carries waste products from the cells
      b. Total body fluid amounts to about 60% of body weight
      c. A loss of 10% of body fluid in the adult is serious
      d. A loss of 20% of the body fluid in the adult is fatal
   2. Constituents of body fluids
      a. Body fluids consist of water and dissolved substances
      b. The largest single fluid constituent of the body is water

F. Body fluid transport
   1. Diffusion
      a. The movement of particles in all directions through a solution
      b. Occurs within fluid compartments and from one compartment to another if the barrier between the compartments is permeable to the diffusing substances
      c. Diffusion of a solute (substance that is dissolved) will spread the molecules from an area of high concentration to an area of lower concentration
      d. A permeable membrane will allow substances to pass through it without restriction
      e. A selectively permeable membrane will allow some solutes to pass through without restriction but will prevent other solutes from passing freely
   2. Osmosis
      a. Osmotic pressure is the force that draws the water from a less concentrated solution through a selectively permeable membrane into a more concentrated solution
      b. If a membrane is permeable to water but not to all the solutes present, it is a selective or semipermeable membrane
      c. When the solvent (solution in which the solute is dissolved) or water moves across this membrane, it is called osmosis
   3. Filtration
      a. Filtration is the movement of solutes and solvents by hydrostatic pressure
      b. Hydrostatic pressure is the force exerted by the weight of a solution
      c. The movement is from an area of greater pressure to an area of lesser pressure
   4. Osmolality
      a. Refers to the number of osmotically active particles per kilogram of water
      b. In the body, osmotic pressure is measured in milliosmols
      c. The normal osmolality of plasma is 280 to 294 mOsm/kg
   5. Hydrostatic pressure
      a. The force of the fluid pressing outward against some surface
      b. When there is a difference in the hydrostatic pressure on two sides of a membrane, water and diffusible solutes move out of the solution that has the higher hydrostatic pressure by the process of filtration
      c. At the arterial end of the capillary, the hydrostatic pressure is greater than the osmotic pressure; therefore, fluids and diffusible solutes move out of the capillary
      d. At the venous end, the osmotic pressure or pull is greater than the hydrostatic pressure, and fluids and some solutes move into the capillary
      e. The excess fluid and solutes remaining in the interstitial spaces are returned to the intravascular compartment by the lymph channels

G. Movement of body fluid
   1. Description
      a. Cell membranes separate the interstitial fluid from the intravascular fluid
      b. These barriers are selectively permeable; that is, the cell membrane and the capillary wall will allow water and some solutes free passage through them
      c. Several forces affect the movement of water and solutes through the walls of cells and capillaries
      d. The greater the number of particles in the concentrated solution, the more pull there will be to move the water through the membrane
      e. Fluids and electrolytes must be kept in balance for health; when they remain out of balance, death can occur

f. If the body loses more electrolytes than fluids, as can happen in diarrhea, then the extracellular fluid will contain fewer electrolytes or solutes than the intracellular fluid

2. Isotonic solutions (Table 8-1)
   a. When the solutions on both sides of a selectively permeable membrane have established equilibrium or are equal in concentration, they are then isotonic
   b. An isotonic solution is isotonic to human cells and thus there will be very little osmosis
3. Hypotonic solutions (Table 8-1)
   a. When a solution contains a lower concentration of salt than other solutions, it is hypotonic
   b. A hypotonic solution has less salt or more water than an isotonic solution
4. Hypertonic solutions: A solution that has a higher concentration of solutes than another solution (Table 8-1)
5. Osmotic pressure
   a. The force that draws the solvent from a solution with more solvent activity through a selectively permeable membrane to a solution with less solvent activity
   b. When the solutions on each side of a selectively permeable membrane are equal in concentration, they are isotonic
   c. A hypotonic solution has less solute than an isotonic solution, whereas a hypertonic solution contains more solute
6. Active transport
   a. If an ion is to move through a membrane from an area of low concentration to an area of high concentration, an active transport system is necessary
   b. An active transport system moves molecules or ions uphill against concentration and osmotic pressure
   c. The energy for active transport is supplied by metabolic processes in the cell
   d. Substances that are actively transported through the cell membrane include ions of sodium, potassium, calcium, iron, hydrogen, some of the sugars, and the amino acids

H. Body fluid excretion (Box 8-3)
1. Description
   a. Fluids leave the body by several routes including the skin, lungs, gastrointestinal tract (GI) tract, and kidneys
   b. The kidneys excrete the largest quantity of fluid
   c. As long as all organs are functioning normally, the body is able to maintain balance in its fluid content
2. Skin
   a. Water is lost through the skin by diffusion in the amounts of 300 to 400 mL/day
   b. Water is also lost through the skin by perspiration
   c. The amount of water lost by perspiration will vary depending on the temperature of the environment and of the body
   d. Average amount of water lost by perspiration is 100 mL/day
3. Lungs
   a. Water is lost from the lungs through expired air that is saturated with water vapor
   b. The amount of water lost from the lungs will vary with the rate and the depth of respiration
   c. The average amount of water lost from the lungs is 300 to 400 mL/day
   d. Water lost from the lungs and the skin by diffusion is called insensible loss because the individual is unaware of losing that water
4. GI tract
   a. Large quantities of water are secreted into the GI tract, but almost all of this fluid is reabsorbed
   b. The average amount of water lost in the feces is 200 mL/day, equal to the amount of

TABLE 8-1

Tonicity of IV Fluids

Solution	Tonicity
0.45% normal saline (1/2 NS)	Hypotonic
0.9% normal saline (NS)	Isotonic
5% dextrose in water (5% D/W)	Isotonic
5% dextrose in 0.225% saline (5% D/1/4 NS)	Isotonic
Lactated Ringer's solution	Isotonic
5% dextrose in lactated Ringer's solution	Hypertonic
5% dextrose in 0.45% saline (5% D/1/2 NS)	Hypertonic
5% dextrose in 0.9% saline (5% D/NS)	Hypertonic
10% dextrose in water (10% D/W)	Hypertonic

BOX 8-3

Daily Body Fluid Excretion

Skin by diffusion = 350 mL
Skin by perspiration =100 mL
Lungs = 350 mL
Feces = 200 mL
Kidneys = 1400 mL

water gained through the oxidation of foods

c. Severe diarrhea will result in the loss of large quantities of fluids and electrolytes

5. Kidneys
   a. Play a major role in regulating fluid and electrolyte balance
   b. Normal kidneys can adjust the amount of water and electrolytes leaving the body
   c. The usual quantity of urine output is approximately 1400 mL/day; however, this will vary greatly depending on fluid intake, amount of perspiration, and other factors

I. Body fluid replacement
1. Description: Water enters the body through three sources: oral liquids, water in foods, and water formed by oxidation of foods
2. Amounts
   a. The average total amount of water taken into the body by all three sources is 2400 mL/day
   b. About 10 mL of water is released by the metabolism of each 100 calories of fat, carbohydrates, or proteins
3. Electrolytes
   a. Electrolytes are present in both foods and liquids
   b. With a normal diet, an excess of essential electrolytes is taken in and the unused electrolytes are excreted

J. Maintaining fluid and electrolyte balance
1. Description
   a. Homeostasis is a term that indicates the relative stability of the internal environment
   b. Concentration and composition of body fluids must be nearly constant
   c. In the client, when one of the substances, either fluids or electrolytes, is deficient, it must be replaced either normally by the intake of food and water or by therapy such as IVs, and/or medications
   d. When the client has an excess of fluid or electrolytes, therapy is directed toward assisting the body to eliminate the excess
2. Kidneys: Play a major role in controlling all types of balance in fluid and electrolytes
3. Adrenal glands: Through the secretion of aldosterone, the adrenal glands also aid in controlling extracellular fluid volume by regulating the amount of sodium reabsorbed by the kidneys
4. Antidiuretic hormone (ADH): ADH from the pituitary gland regulates the osmotic pressure of extracellular fluid by regulating the amount of water reabsorbed by the kidney

III. FLUID VOLUME DEFICIT

A. Description
1. Dehydration in which water and electrolytes are lost in the same proportion
2. The goal of treatment is to restore fluid volume, replace electrolytes as needed, and eliminate the cause

B. Causes
1. Vomiting and/or diarrhea
2. Continuous GI irrigation
3. GI suctioning
4. Ileostomy or colostomy drainage
5. Draining wounds, burns, or fistulas
6. Increased urine output from the use of diuretics

C. Data collection
1. Thirst
2. Poor skin turgor and dry mucous membranes
3. Increased heart rate, thready pulse, postural hypotension
4. Rapid weight loss
5. Flat neck or hand veins
6. Dizziness or weakness
7. Decrease in urine volume and dark, concentrated urine
8. Increased specific gravity of the urine
9. Confusion
10. Increased hematocrit

D. Implementation
1. Monitor vital signs
2. Check mucous membranes and skin turgor
3. Monitor weight daily
4. Monitor I&O (intake and output)
5. Test urine for specific gravity
6. Monitor hematocrit and electrolyte values
7. Replace fluids by PO, NG, or IV (lactated Ringer's solution, 0.9% normal saline) as prescribed

IV. FLUID VOLUME EXCESS

A. Description
1. An actual excess of total body fluid or a relative fluid excess in one or more fluid compartments
2. Also called overhydration or fluid overload
3. The goal of treatment is to restore fluid balance, correct electrolyte imbalances if present, and eliminate or control the underlying cause of the overload

B. Causes
1. Excessive administration of oral or IV fluids 
2. Excessive irrigation of body cavities such as tap-water enemas
3. Decreased kidney function

4. Conditions such as congestive heart failure (CHF), syndrome of inappropriate antidiuretic hormone (SIADH), cirrhosis, and Cushing's syndrome

C. Data collection
1. Cough and dyspnea
2. Lung crackles
3. Increased respirations and heart rate
4. Increased blood pressure and bounding pulse
5. Pitting edema
6. Weight gain
7. Neck and hand vein distention
8. Decreased hematocrit
9. Confusion

D. Implementation
1. Monitor vital signs
2. Position client in semi-Fowler's
3. Check for edema
4. Monitor I&O
5. Monitor weight
6. Administer diuretics as prescribed
7. Monitor hematocrit and electrolyte values
8. Restrict fluids as prescribed
9. Provide a low-sodium diet as prescribed

V. HYPOKALEMIA (Table 8-2)

A. Description (Box 8-4)
1. A serum potassium level below 3.5 mEq/L
2. Potassium deficit is the most common electrolyte imbalance and is potentially life threatening

B. Implementation
1. Monitor vital signs
2. Monitor neuromuscular activity
3. Monitor I&O
4. Check renal function before administering potassium
5. Administer potassium supplements as prescribed (orally or monitor by IV)
6. Oral potassium chloride has an unpleasant taste and should be taken with juice or other desired liquid
7. Oral potassium preparations can cause GI irritation and should not be taken on an empty stomach
8. If the client complains of abdominal pain, distention, nausea, vomiting, diarrhea, or GI bleeding, the oral potassium may need to be discontinued

TABLE 8-2

Potassium Imbalances

Hypokalemia	Hyperkalemia
CAUSES	**CAUSES**
Use of non-potassium-sparing diuretics	Renal failure
Diarrhea	Intestinal obstruction
Vomiting	Cell damage
Inadequate intake of potassium	Excessive oral or parenteral administration of potassium
Excessive gastric suction	Metabolic acidosis
Excessive fistula drainage	Addison's disease
Cushing's syndrome	Excessive use of potassium-based salt substitutes
Chronic use of corticosteroids	Transfusion of stored blood with red blood cell (RBC) release of potassium
Renal disease	
Total parenteral nutrition	
Uncontrolled diabetes	
Alkalosis	
SIGNS AND SYMPTOMS	**SIGNS AND SYMPTOMS**
Leg and abdominal cramps	Muscle weakness
Lethargy and weakness	Paresthesias
Shallow respirations and thready pulse	Hypotension
Confusion	Diarrhea
Decreased or absent reflexes	Hyperactive bowel sounds
Hypoactive bowel sounds and ileus	Wide, flat P waves, widened QRS complex, prolonged PR interval, depressed ST segment, and narrow, peaked T waves
Postural hypotension	
Peaked P waves, flat T waves, depressed ST segment and U waves	

BOX 8-4

Potassium (K)

NORMAL VALUE
3.5 mEq/L to 5.1 mEq/L

COMMON FOOD SOURCES
Apricots
Avocado
Bananas
Beef
Cantaloupes
Carrots
Chocolate
Figs
Peaches
Pork
Potato
Prunes
Raisins
Spinach
Tomatoes
Veal

9. When potassium is added to an IV solution, shake the bag and invert it to ensure that the potassium is evenly distributed
10. An IV bolus injection of potassium is never administered; it is always diluted
11. A client receiving more than 10 mEq/hr should be placed on a cardiac monitor, and the infusion should be controlled by an infusion device
12. Monitor for cardiac changes during the administration of potassium
13. Monitor electrolyte values
14. Monitor IV site; if phlebitis or infiltration occurs, the IV should be stopped immediately and restarted at another site
15. Instruct the client not to use salt substitutes containing potassium unless prescribed by the physician

VI. **HYPERKALEMIA** (Table 8-2)
   A. Description: A serum potassium level that exceeds 5.1 mEq/L (Box 8-4)
   B. Implementation
      1. Monitor vital signs
      2. Monitor for cardiac changes
      3. Decrease potassium intake
      4. Administer potassium excreting diuretics as prescribed
      5. Monitor I&O
      6. Monitor laboratory values
      7. Emergency treatment includes rapid IV administration of dextrose with regular insulin to move excess potassium into the cells
      8. Administer sodium polystyrene sulfonate (Kayexalate) orally or by enema as prescribed, which absorbs the potassium into the GI tract
      9. Monitor for calcium and magnesium loss when using sodium polystyrene sulfonate
      10. Monitor renal function
      11. Prepare for peritoneal or hemodialysis as prescribed
      12. When blood transfusions are prescribed for a client with a potassium imbalance, the client should receive fresh blood if possible because transfusions of stored blood may elevate the potassium level as the breakdown of older blood cells releases potassium
      13. Instruct the client to avoid foods high in potassium
      14. Instruct the client to avoid the use of salt substitutes or other potassium-containing substances

VII. **HYPONATREMIA** (Table 8-3)
   A. Description: A serum sodium level below 135 mEq/L (Box 8-5)
   B. Implementation
      1. Monitor vital signs
      2. Monitor I&O
      3. Monitor weight
      4. Assess skin turgor and mucous membranes
      5. Restrict water intake and avoid tap water enemas 

BOX 8-5

Sodium

NORMAL VALUE
135 to 145 mEq/L

COMMON FOOD SOURCES
Table salt
Soy sauce
Cured pork
Cottage cheese
American cheese
Milk
Butter
White and whole-wheat bread
Ketchup
Mustard
Bacon
Frankfurters
Lunch meat
Canned food
Processed food
Snack food

TABLE 8-3

Sodium Imbalances

Hyponatremia	Hypernatremia
CAUSES	**CAUSES**
Inadequate sodium intake (NPO, low sodium diet)	Decreased water intake or excessive loss of water
Gastrointestinal suction	Fever
Excessive intake of water	Excessive perspiration
Irrigation of GI tubes with plain water	Dehydration
Potent diuretics	Hyperventilation
Increased perspiration	Watery diarrhea
Draining skin lesions	Enteral nutrition and total parenteral nutrition deplete the cells of water
Burns	Diabetes insipidus
Nausea and vomiting	Cushing's syndrome
Diabetic ketoacidosis (DKA)	Impaired renal function
Syndrome of inappropriate artidiuretic hormone secretion (SIADH)	Use of corticosteroids
Retention of fluid such as with kidney or heart failure	Excessive administration of sodium bicarbonate
SIGNS AND SYMPTOMS	**SIGNS AND SYMPTOMS**
Rapid, thready pulse	Dry mucous membranes
Postural blood pressure changes	Loss of skin turgor
Weakness	Thirst
Abdominal cramping	Flushed skin
Poor skin turgor	Elevated temperature
Muscle twitching and seizures	Oliguria
Mental confusion	Muscle twitching
Apprehension	Fatigue
	Confusion
	Seizures

6. Use normal saline rather than sterile water for irrigation
7. Administer sodium replacement as prescribed and monitor electrolyte values
8. Encourage foods high in sodium
9. If the client is taking lithium carbonate, monitor the lithium level, as **hyponatremia** can cause diminished lithium excretion, resulting in toxicity

VIII. HYPERNATREMIA (Table 8-3)

A. Description: A serum sodium level that exceeds 145 mEq/L (Box 8-5)

B. Implementation
1. Monitor vital signs
2. Monitor I&O
3. Monitor electrolyte values
4. Increase water intake orally
5. Encourage the client to drink 8 to 10 glasses of water daily
6. Provide water between meals or tube feedings

IX. HYPOCALCEMIA (Table 8-4)

A. Description: A serum calcium level below 8.6 mg/dL (Box 8-6)

BOX 8-6

Calcium

NORMAL VALUE
8.6 to 10.0 mg/dL

COMMON FOOD SOURCES
Yogurt, low-fat
Milk
Rhubarb
Collard greens
Cheese
Tofu
Spinach
Broccoli
Green beans
Carrots

TABLE 8-4

Calcium Imbalances

Hypocalcemia	Hypercalcemia
CAUSES	**CAUSES**
Inadequate dietary intake of calcium	Excessive intake of calcium supplements, milk, and antacids products containing calcium
Increased absorption of calcium from intestinal tract	Excessive intake of vitamin D
Inadequate vitamin D consumption	Increased bone reabsorption or destruction from conditions such as bone tumors, fractures, osteoporosis, immobility
Diarrhea	Decreased excretion of calcium
Long-term immobilization and bone demineralization	Renal failure
Excessive GI losses from diarrhea or wound draining	Use of thiazide diuretics
End-stage renal disease	Hyperparathyroidism
Calcium-excreting medications such as diuretics, caffeine, anticonvulsants, heparin, laxatives, nicotine	Use of lithium
Decreased secretion of parathyroid hormone	Use of glucocorticoids
Acute pancreatitis	Adrenal insufficiency
Crohn's disease	
Excessive administration of blood	
SIGNS AND SYMPTOMS	**SIGNS AND SYMPTOMS**
Tachycardia	Increased heart rate and blood pressure
Hypotension	Bounding pulse
Paresthesias	Bradycardia (late stage)
Twitching	Shortened QT interval and widened T wave
Cramps	Muscle weakness (hypotonicity)
Tetany	Diminished deep tendon reflexes
Positive Chvostek's or Trousseau's sign	Nausea and vomiting
Diarrhea	Constipation
Hyperactive bowel sounds	Abdominal distention
Prolongation of QT interval	Confusion, lethargy, coma

B. Implementation
1. Monitor vital signs
2. Monitor for the presence of Chvostek's and Trousseau's signs
3. Provide a quiet environment and avoid overstimulation
4. Initiate seizure precautions
5. Administer calcium orally or monitor IV as prescribed
6. Administer vitamin D as prescribed to aid in the absorption of calcium from the intestinal tract
7. Administer calcium supplements 1 to 2 hours after meals to maximize intestinal absorption
8. Keep 10% calcium gluconate available for acute calcium deficit
9. Monitor calcium levels closely after thyroid surgery
10. Instruct the client taking calcium-excreting medications to have serum calcium levels checked periodically
11. Teach proper use of antacids or laxatives
12. Instruct the client to consume foods high in calcium

X. HYPERCALCEMIA (Table 8-4)

A. Description: A serum calcium level that exceeds 10 mg/dL (Box 8-6)

B. Implementation
1. Monitor vital signs
2. Monitor for dysrhythmias
3. Restrict calcium intake
4. Increase mobility
5. Assist with passive range of motion exercises when ambulation is not possible
6. Move clients carefully
7. Monitor for the development of pathological fractures
8. Strain urine to check for urinary stones
9. Monitor for severe flank or abdominal pain
10. Monitor level of consciousness
11. Monitor for confusion and neurological changes
12. Avoid large doses of vitamin D supplements
13. Avoid the use of thiazide diuretics
14. Prepare for the administration of phosphate as prescribed

15. Prepare for the administration of calcitonin (Calcimar) as prescribed to inhibit calcium resorption from the bone

XI. HYPOMAGNESEMIA (Table 8-5)

A. Description: A serum magnesium level below 1.6 mg/dL (Box 8-7)

B. Implementation
1. Monitor vital signs
2. Monitor for dysrhythmias
3. Monitor for neuromuscular changes
4. Monitor I&O
5. Initiate seizure precautions
6. Administer magnesium supplements and monitor laboratory values
7. Monitor serum magnesium levels every 12 to 24 hours when client is receiving magnesium by IV

BOX 8-7

Magnesium

NORMAL VALUE

1.6 to 2.6 mg/dL

COMMON FOOD SOURCES

Green leafy vegetables such as spinach and broccoli
Avocado
Canned white tuna fish
Low fat yogurt
Cooked rolled oats
Milk
Peas
Potatoes
Pork, beef, chicken
Raisins
Peanut butter
Cauliflower

TABLE 8-5

Magnesium Imbalances

Hypomagnesemia	Hypermagnesemia
CAUSES	**CAUSES**
Malnutrition	Overuse of antacids or laxatives containing magnesium
Diarrhea	Renal insufficiency and renal failure
Celiac disease	Treatment of toxemia of pregnancy with magnesium
Crohn's disease	
Alcoholism	**SIGNS AND SYMPTOMS**
Prolonged gastric suctioning	Hypotension
Ileostomy or colostomy, intestinal fistulas	Bradycardia
Acute pancreatitis	Weak pulse
Diabetic ketoacidosis	Sweating and flushing
Eclampsia	Respiratory depression
Chemotherapy	Loss of deep tendon reflexes
Sepsis	Peaked T waves, prolonged PR and QT intervals, widened QRS complexes
SIGNS AND SYMPTOMS	
Twitching	
Paresthesias	
Hyperactive reflexes	
Irritability	
Confusion	
Positive Chvostek's or Trousseau's signs	
Shallow respirations	
Tetany	
Seizures	
Tachycardia	
Broadening of T waves, shortening of ST segment, prolonged QT interval, and widened QRS	
In severe deficiency, inverted T waves and prominent U waves	

8. Monitor for reduced deep tendon reflexes suggesting hypermagnesemia during the administration of magnesium
9. Instruct the client to eat food high in magnesium

XII. HYPERMAGNESEMIA (Table 8-5)

A. Description: A serum magnesium level that exceeds 2.6 mg/dL (Box 8-7)

B. Implementation

1. Monitor vital signs
2. Monitor for respiratory depression
3. Monitor for hypotension, bradycardia, and dysrhythmias
4. Monitor neurological and muscular activity
5. Monitor level of consciousness
6. Remove the source of the excess magnesium
7. Monitor laboratory values
8. Increase renal excretion by encouraging fluids or administering loop diuretics as prescribed
9. Prepare for the administration of 10% calcium gluconate if serum levels are more than 7 mEq/L
10. Instruct the client regarding avoiding the use of laxatives and antacids containing magnesium

XIII. HYPOPHOSPHATEMIA (Table 8-6)

A. Description: A serum phosphorus level below 2.7 mg/dL (Box 8-8)

B. Implementation

1. Monitor vital signs
2. Monitor respiratory status
3. Move the client carefully
4. Administer phosphate as prescribed
5. Check the renal system before administering phosphate
6. Monitor calcium, phosphorus, sodium, and chloride levels

BOX 8-8

Phosphorus

NORMAL VALUE

2.7 to 4.5 mg/dL

COMMON FOOD SOURCES

Fish
Pork, beef, chicken
Organ meats
Nuts
Whole-grain breads and cereals

TABLE 8-6

Phosphorus Imbalances

Hypophosphatemia	Hyperphosphatemia
CAUSES	**CAUSES**
Decreased nutritional intake and malnutrition	Excessive dietary intake of phosphorus
Use of magnesium-based or aluminum hydroxide-based antacids	Overuse of phosphate-containing laxatives or enemas
Renal failure	Vitamin D intoxication
Hyperparathyroidism	Hypoparathyroidism
Malignancy	Renal insufficiency
Hypercalcemia	Chemotherapy
Alcohol withdrawal	
Diabetic ketoacidosis	
Respiratory alkalosis	
SIGNS AND SYMPTOMS	**SIGNS AND SYMPTOMS**
Confusion	Neuromuscular irritability
Seizures	Muscle weakness
Weakness	Hyperactive reflexes
Decreased deep tendon reflexes	Tetany
Shallow respirations	Positive Chvostek's or Trousseau's sign
Increased bleeding tendency	
Immunosuppression	
Bone pain	

7. Administer vitamin D
8. Monitor for decreased neuromuscular activity
9. Monitor for calcium excess and kidney stones
10. Monitor for hematologic changes
11. Decrease intake of calcium-rich foods and increase intake of meats and whole grains that contain phosphorus
12. Instruct the client regarding the use of antacids

XIV. HYPERPHOSPHATEMIA (Table 8-6)

A. Description: A serum phosphorus level that exceeds 4.5 mg/dL (Box 8-8)

B. Implementation
1. Increase fecal excretion of phosphorus by binding phosphorus from food in the GI tract (aluminum hydroxide gel)
2. Monitor laboratory values
3. Prepare for dialysis if prescribed
4. Monitor for signs of **hypocalcemia**
5. Administer calcium as prescribed if **hypocalcemia** exists
6. Monitor for neuromuscular irritability
7. Monitor for hyperreflexia, tetany, and seizures
8. Monitor for Chvostek's and Trousseau's signs
9. Instruct the client to avoid phosphate-containing medications, including laxatives and enemas
10. Instruct the client to decrease the intake of foods high in phosphorus
11. Instruct the client how to take phosphate-binding medications, emphasizing that these should be taken with meals or immediately after meals

PRACTICE QUESTIONS

1. The registered nurse (RN) tells the licensed practical nurse (LPN) that the physician has prescribed a hypotonic IV solution for the client. Which of the following IV solutions would the LPN obtain for administration to the client?
   1. 0.45% saline (1/2 NS)
   2. 5% dextrose in water (5% D/W)
   3. 10% dextrose in water (10% D/W)
   4. 5% dextrose in 0.9% saline (5% D/NS)
2. Intravenous (IV) lactated Ringer's solution is prescribed for a postoperative client. A nursing student is caring for the client and the nursing instructor asks the student about the tonicity of the prescribed IV solution. The student responds by telling the instructor that the solution is:
   1. Isotonic
   2. Normotonic
   3. Hypotonic
   4. Hypertonic
3. A nurse is reading the physician's progress notes in the client's record and reads that the physician has documented "insensible fluid loss of approximately 800 mL daily." The nurse understands that this type of fluid loss can occur through:
   1. The gastrointestinal (GI) tract
   2. Urinary output
   3. Wound drainage
   4. The skin
4. A nurse is reviewing the health records of assigned clients. The nurse plans care knowing that which of the following clients is least likely at risk for the development of third spacing?
   1. The client with cirrhosis
   2. The client with diabetes mellitus
   3. The client with sepsis
   4. The client with renal failure
5. A nurse is reviewing the health records of assigned clients. The nurse plans care knowing that which client is at risk for fluid volume deficit?
   1. A client with a colostomy
   2. A client with cirrhosis
   3. A client with congestive heart failure (CHF)
   4. A client with decreased kidney function
6. A nurse is caring for a client who has been taking diuretics on a long-term basis. A fluid volume deficit is suspected. Which of the following findings would be noted in the client with this condition?
   1. Rales
   2. Increased blood pressure
   3. Decreased hematocrit
   4. Increased specific gravity of the urine
7. A nurse is caring for a client with cirrhosis. The nurse notes that the client is dyspneic and crackles are heard on auscultation. The nurse suspects fluid volume excess. What additional signs would the nurse expect to note in this client if a fluid volume excess is present?
   1. Flat hand and neck veins
   2. A weak and thready pulse
   3. An increase in blood pressure
   4. An increased urine output
8. The nurse is reviewing the health records of assigned clients. The nurse plans care knowing that which of the following clients are at risk for a potassium deficit?
   1. The client on nasogastric (NG) suction
   2. The client with renal disease
   3. The client with Addison's disease
   4. The client with metabolic acidosis
9. A nurse is instructing a client how to decrease the intake of magnesium in the diet. The nurse tells the client that which of the following food items would contain the least amount of magnesium?
   1. Processed drinking water
   2. Peanut butter

3. Spinach
4. Broccoli

10. A nurse instructs a client at risk for hypokalemia about the foods high in potassium that should be included in the daily diet. The nurse tells the client that which of the following foods provide the least amount of potassium?
    1. Spinach
    2. Carrots
    3. Apricots
    4. Apple
11. A nurse reviews a client's electrolyte results and notes a potassium level of 5.5 mEq/L. The nurse understands that a potassium value at this level would most likely be noted in which condition?
    1. The client who sustained a traumatic burn
    2. The client with Cushing's syndrome
    3. The client with colitis
    4. The client who has been overusing laxatives
12. A nurse reviews a client's electrolyte results and notes that the potassium level is 5.4 mEq/L. Which of the following would the nurse note on the cardiac monitor as a result of the laboratory value?
    1. Narrow peaked T waves
    2. Prominent U wave
    3. ST elevation
    4. Peaked P wave
13. A nurse prepares to administer sodium polystyrene sulfonate (Kayexalate) to the client. Before administering the medication, the nurse reviews the action of the medication and understands that it:
    1. Releases bicarbonate in exchange for primarily sodium ions
    2. Releases sodium ions in exchange for primarily bicarbonate ions
    3. Releases sodium ions in exchange for primarily potassium ions
    4. Releases potassium ions in exchange for primarily sodium ions
14. A nurse reviews electrolyte values and notes a sodium level of 130 mEq/L. The nurse understands that which of the following clients are at risk for the development of a sodium value at this level?
    1. The client with syndrome of SIADH
    2. The client with an inadequate daily water intake
    3. The client with watery diarrhea
    4. The client with diabetes insipidus
15. A nurse is caring for a client with leukemia. When caring for the client, the nurse notes that the client has poor skin turgor and has flat neck and hand veins. The nurse suspects hyponatremia. What additional signs would the nurse expect to note in this client if hyponatremia is present?
    1. Dry mucous membranes
    2. Postural blood pressure changes
    3. Intense thirst
    4. Slow bounding pulse
16. A nurse is caring for a client with a nasogastric (NG) tube. NG tube irrigations are prescribed to be performed once every shift. The client's serum electrolyte results indicate a potassium level of 4.5 mEq/L and a sodium level of 132 mEq/L. Based on these laboratory findings, which solution is the most appropriate to use for the NG irrigation?
    1. Tap water
    2. Distilled water
    3. Sterile water
    4. Normal saline
17. A nurse reviews a client's serum sodium level and notes that the level is 150 mEq/L. The physician prescribes dietary instructions for the client based on the sodium level. Which of the following foods will the nurse instruct the client to avoid?
    1. Spinach
    2. Squash
    3. Processed oat cereals
    4. Molasses
18. A nurse reviews the serum calcium level and notes that the client's level is 4.0 mEq/L. The nurse understands that which of the following conditions most likely caused this serum calcium level?
    1. Prolonged bed rest
    2. Excessive administration of vitamin D
    3. Renal disease
    4. Multiple myeloma
19. A nurse is caring for a client with a suspected diagnosis of hypocalcemia. Which of the following signs would not be an indication of this diagnosis?
    1. Hypotonicity of the muscles
    2. Twitching
    3. Hyperactive bowel sounds
    4. Positive Trousseau's sign
20. A nurse is instructing a client how to decrease the intake of calcium in the diet. The nurse tells the client that which of the following food items would contain the least amount of calcium?
    1. Butter
    2. Milk
    3. Spinach
    4. Broccoli
21. A nurse is caring for a client with hyperparathyroidism and notes that the client's serum calcium level is 13 mg/dL. Which of the following medications would the nurse prepare to administer as prescribed to the client?
    1. Calcium gluconate
    2. Calcium chloride
    3. Calcitonin (Calcimar)
    4. Large doses of vitamin D
22. A nurse is instructing a client how to decrease the intake of potassium in the diet. The nurse tells the

client that which of the following foods contains the least amount of potassium?

1. Potatoes
2. Apricots
3. Avocado
4. Lettuce

23. The nurse is caring for a client with renal failure. The laboratory results reveal a magnesium level of 3.6 mg/dL. Which of the following signs would the nurse most likely expect to note in the client based on this magnesium level?
    1. Twitching
    2. Hyperactive reflexes
    3. Irritability
    4. Loss of deep tendon reflexes
24. The nurse reviews the serum phosphorus level and notes that the client's level is 2.0 mg/dL. The nurse understands that which of the following conditions most likely caused this serum phosphorus level?
    1. Alcoholism
    2. Hypoparathyroidism
    3. Chemotherapy
    4. Vitamin D intoxication
25. A nurse is instructing a client how to decrease the intake of phosphorus in the diet. The nurse tells the client that which of the following foods would contain the least amount of phosphorus?
    1. Oranges
    2. Fish
    3. Whole grain bread
    4. Almonds

ANSWERS

1. *Answer:* 1

Rationale: 5% dextrose in water is an isotonic solution. 10% dextrose in water and 5% dextrose in 0.9% saline are hypertonic solutions. 0.45% saline is hypotonic and is probably the only hypotonic solution used in clinical situations. Distilled water is another example of a hypotonic solution. Hypotonic solutions contain a lower concentration of salt or more water than an isotonic solution.
Test-Taking Strategy: Use the process of elimination. Note the similarities in options 2, 3, and 4. All of these solutions contain dextrose. Option 1 is different from the others. Review the tonicity of IV solutions if you had difficulty with this question.
Level of Cognitive Ability: Application
Client Needs: Physiological Integrity
Integrated Concept/Process: Nursing Process/Implementation
Content Area: Fundamental Skills
Reference: DeWit S: *Fundamental concepts and skills for nursing,* Philadelphia, 2001, WB Saunders, p. 715.

2. *Answer:* 1

Rationale: Lactated Ringer's solution is an isotonic solution. Other isotonic solutions include 5% dextrose in water, 0.9% saline, and 5% dextrose in 0.225% saline. 0.45% saline is hypotonic. 10% dextrose in water, 5% dextrose in 0.9% saline, and 5% dextrose in 0.45% saline are hypertonic solutions.
Test-Taking Strategy: Knowledge regarding the tonicity of the various IV solutions is required to answer the question. Review this information if you had difficulty with this question.
Level of Cognitive Ability: Comprehension
Client Needs: Physiological Integrity
Integrated Concept/Process: Nursing Process/Implementation
Content Area: Fundamental Skills
Reference: DeWit S: *Fundamental concepts and skills for nursing,* Philadelphia, 2001, WB Saunders, p. 715.

3. *Answer:* 4

Rationale: Sensible losses are those the person is aware of, such as through wound drainage, GI tract losses, and urination. Insensible losses may occur without the person's awareness. Insensible losses occur daily through the skin and lungs.
Test-Taking Strategy: Note that the issue of the question is fluid loss. Use the process of elimination, noting the similarity between options 1, 2, and 3. These types of losses can be measured for accurate output. Fluid loss through the skin cannot be accurately measured, only approximated. If you had difficulty with this question, review the difference between sensible and insensible fluid loss.
Level of Cognitive Ability: Comprehension
Client Needs: Physiological Integrity
Integrated Concept/Process: Nursing Process/Data Collection
Content Area: Fundamental Skills
Reference: DeWit S: *Fundamental concepts and skills for nursing,* Philadelphia, 2001, WB Saunders, p. 336.

4. *Answer:* 2

Rationale: Fluid that shifts into the interstitial spaces and remains there is referred to as third space fluid. Common sites for third spacing include the abdomen, pleural cavity, peritoneal cavity, and the pericardial sac. Third space fluid is physiologically useless because it does not circulate to provide nutrients for the cells. Risk factors include clients with liver or kidney disease, major trauma, burns, sepsis, wound healing or major surgery, malignancy, malabsorption syndrome, malnutrition, and alcoholic or elderly clients.
Test-Taking Strategy: Use the process of elimination. Note the key words "least likely." Eliminate options 1 and 4 first, because it is likely that fluid balance disturbances will occur with these conditions. From the remaining options, sepsis is the option that is most acute and therefore is most similar to options 1 and 4. Review the risk factors associated with third spacing if you had difficulty with this question.
Level of Cognitive Ability: Application

Client Needs: Physiological Integrity
Integrated Concept/Process: Nursing Process/Planning
Content Area: Fundamental Skills
Reference: DeWit S: *Fundamental concepts and skills for nursing,* Philadelphia, 2001, WB Saunders, p. 445.

5. *Answer:* 1
Rationale: Causes of a fluid volume deficit include vomiting, diarrhea, conditions that cause increased respirations or increased urinary output, insufficient IV fluid replacement, draining fistulas, or an ileostomy or colostomy. A client with cirrhosis, CHF, or decreased kidney function is at risk for fluid volume excess.
Test-Taking Strategy: Use the process of elimination. Read the question carefully noting that it asks for the client at risk for a deficit. Read each option and think about the fluid imbalance that can occur in each. The clients presented in options 2, 3, and 4 retain fluid. The only condition that can cause a fluid volume deficit is the condition noted in option 1. If you had difficulty with this question review the causes of fluid volume deficit.
Level of Cognitive Ability: Comprehension
Client Needs: Physiological Integrity
Integrated Concept/Process: Nursing Process/Planning
Content Area: Fundamental Skills
Reference: DeWit S: *Fundamental concepts and skills for nursing,* Philadelphia, 2001, WB Saunders, p. 445.

6. *Answer:* 4
Rationale: Findings in a client with a fluid volume deficit include increased respirations and heart rate, decreased central venous pressure (CVP), weight loss, poor skin turgor, dry mucous membranes, decreased urine volume, increased specific gravity of the urine, dark-colored and odorous urine, an increased hematocrit, and altered level of consciousness. The signs in options 1, 2, and 3 are seen in a client with fluid volume excess.
Test-Taking Strategy: Use the process of elimination. Eliminate option 1 and 2 first. Rales are noted in fluid volume excess as is an increased blood pressure. Remember that the specific gravity of the urine would be increased in a client with a fluid volume deficit. If you had difficulty with this question review the findings noted in fluid volume deficit.
Level of Cognitive Ability: Comprehension
Client Needs: Physiological Integrity
Integrated Concept/Process: Nursing Process/Data Collection
Content Area: Fundamental Skills
Reference: DeWit S: *Fundamental concepts and skills for nursing,* Philadelphia, 2001, WB Saunders, p. 445.

7. *Answer:* 3
Rationale: Findings associated with fluid volume excess include cough, dyspnea, crackles, tachypnea, tachycardia, an elevated blood pressure and a bounding pulse, an elevated central venous pressure, weight gain, edema, neck and hand vein distension, altered level of consciousness, and a decreased hematocrit.
Test-Taking Strategy: Use the process of elimination. Note the similarities in options 1, 2, and 4. Each of these signs relates to a decrease in fluid volume. Option 3 reflects an increase. If you had difficulty with this question review the assessment signs noted in fluid volume excess.
Level of Cognitive Ability: Comprehension
Client Needs: Physiological Integrity
Integrated Concept/Process: Nursing Process/Data Collection
Content Area: Fundamental Skills
Reference: DeWit S: *Fundamental concepts and skills for nursing,* Philadelphia, 2001, WB Saunders, p. 446.

8. *Answer:* 1
Rationale: Potassium-rich gastrointestinal (GI) fluids are lost through GI suction, placing the client at risk for hypokalemia. The client with renal disease, Addison's disease, and/or metabolic acidosis is at risk for hyperkalemia.
Test-Taking Strategy: Read the question carefully noting that it asks for the client at risk for hypokalemia. Read each option and think about the electrolyte loss that can occur in each. Option 1 clearly identifies a loss of body fluid. If you had difficulty with this question review the causes of hypokalemia.
Level of Cognitive Ability: Application
Client Needs: Physiological Integrity
Integrated Concept/Process: Nursing Process/Planning
Content Area: Fundamental Skills
Reference: DeWit S: *Fundamental concepts and skills for nursing,* Philadelphia, 2001, WB Saunders, p. 447.

9. *Answer:* 1
Rationale: Drinking water that has not been processed through a water softener is high in magnesium. Peanut butter, spinach, and broccoli are magnesium-containing foods and should be avoided by the client on a magnesium-restricted diet.
Test-Taking Strategy: Use the process of elimination and note the key words "least amount." Eliminate options 3 and 4 first because they are similar. Recalling that unprocessed water is high in magnesium will easily direct you to option 1. Review the foods that are high in magnesium if you had difficulty with this question.
Level of Cognitive Ability: Application
Client Needs: Health Promotion and Maintenance
Integrated Concept/Process: Teaching/Learning
Content Area: Fundamental Skills
Reference: Williams S: *Basic nutrition & diet therapy,* ed 11, St Louis, 2001, Mosby, p. 122.

10. *Answer:* 4
Rationale: An apple provides approximately 3 mEq of potassium per serving. Spinach and carrots (1/2 cup cooked) and 4 apricots provide approximately 7 mEq of potassium per serving.
Test-Taking Strategy: Use the process of elimination and note the key words "least amount." Recalling the potassium content of the foods identified will direct you to option 4. Review the foods high in potassium if you had difficulty with this question.
Level of Cognitive Ability: Application
Client Needs: Health Promotion and Maintenance
Integrated Concept/Process: Teaching/Learning
Content Area: Fundamental Skills
Reference: Williams S: *Basic nutrition & diet therapy,* ed 11, St Louis, 2001, Mosby, p. 122.

11. *Answer:* 1
Rationale: A serum potassium level greater than 5.1 mEq/L is indicative of hyperkalemia. Clients who experience cellular shifting of potassium as in the early stages of massive cell destruction, such as in trauma, burns, sepsis, or with metabolic or respiratory acidosis, are at risk for hyperkalemia. The client with Cushing's syndrome or colitis, and the client who has been overusing laxatives is at risk for hypokalemia.
Test-Taking Strategy: Use the process of elimination to eliminate options 3 and 4 first because they are similar and reflect a gastrointestinal loss. From the remaining options, remembering that cell destruction causes potassium shifts will assist in directing you to the correct option. Remember that Cushing's syndrome presents a risk for hypokalemia and Addison's disease presents a risk for hyperkalemia. Review the causes of hyperkalemia if you had difficulty with this question.
Level of Cognitive Ability: Analysis
Client Needs: Physiological Integrity
Integrated Concept/Process: Nursing Process/Data Collection
Content Area: Fundamental Skills
Reference: DeWit S: *Fundamental concepts and skills for nursing,* Philadelphia, 2001, WB Saunders, p. 447.

12. *Answer:* 1
Rationale: A serum potassium level of 5.4 mEq/L is indicative of hyperkalemia. Cardiac changes include a wide flat P wave, prolonged PR interval, widened QRS complex, narrow peaked T waves, and a depressed ST segment.
Test-Taking Strategy: From the information in the question, you need to determine that this condition is a hyperkalemic one. From this point, it is necessary to know the cardiac changes that are expected when hyperkalemia exists. Review these cardiac changes if you had difficulty with this question.
Level of Cognitive Ability: Analysis
Client Needs: Physiological Integrity
Integrated Concept/Process: Nursing Process/Data Collection
Content Area: Fundamental Skills
Reference: DeWit S: *Fundamental concepts and skills for nursing,* Philadelphia, 2001, WB Saunders, p. 447.

13. *Answer:* 3
Rationale: Sodium polystyrene sulfonate (Kayexalate) is a cation exchange resin used in the treatment of hyperkalemia. The resin either passes through the intestine or is retained in the colon. It releases sodium ions in exchange for primarily potassium ions. The therapeutic effect occurs 2 to 12 hours after oral administration and longer after rectal administration.
Test-Taking Strategy: Use the process of elimination. Looking at the name of the medication (Kayexalate) closely will assist in recalling the action of the medication. If you had difficulty with this question, review the action of this medication.
Level of Cognitive Ability: Comprehension
Client Needs: Physiological Integrity
Integrated Concept/Process: Nursing Process/Planning
Content Area: Pharmacology
Reference: Hodgson B, Kizior R: *Saunders nursing drug handbook 2002,* Philadelphia, 2002, WB Saunders, p. 1016.

14. *Answer:* 1
Rationale: Hyponatremia is a serum sodium level below 135 mEq/L. Hyponatremia can result secondary to SIADH. The client with an inadequate daily water intake, watery diarrhea, or with diabetes insipidus is at risk for hypernatremia.
Test-Taking Strategy: Knowledge regarding the normal sodium level and the causes of hyponatremia is required to answer the question. Review these causes if you had difficulty with this question.
Level of Cognitive Ability: Analysis
Client Needs: Physiological Integrity
Integrated Concept/Process: Nursing Process/Data Collection
Content Area: Fundamental Skills
Reference: DeWit S: *Fundamental concepts and skills for nursing,* Philadelphia, 2001, WB Saunders, p. 447.

15. *Answer:* 2
Rationale: Postural blood pressure changes occur in the client with hyponatremia. Dry mucous membranes and intense thirst are seen in clients with hypernatremia. A slow, bounding pulse is not indicative of hyponatremia. In hyponatremia, a rapid, thready pulse would be noted.
Test-Taking Strategy: Use the process of elimination and note the information provided in the question. Eliminate options 1 and 3 first because they are similar. A client with dry mucous membranes is likely to have intense thirst. From the remaining options, it is necessary to recall the signs of hyponatremia. If you have difficulty with this question review the signs associated with hyponatremia.
Level of Cognitive Ability: Comprehension
Client Needs: Physiological Integrity
Integrated Concept/Process: Nursing Process/Data Collection
Content Area: Fundamental Skills
Reference: DeWit S: *Fundamental concepts and skills for nursing,* Philadelphia, 2001, WB Saunders, p. 447.

16. *Answer:* 4
Rationale: A potassium level of 4.5 mEq/L is within normal range. A sodium level of 132 mEq/L is low, indicating hyponatremia. In clients with hyponatremia, normal (isotonic) saline should be used rather than water for GI irrigations.
Test-Taking Strategy: Use the process of elimination. Note that sterile water, distilled water, and tap water are similar. The only option that is different is option 4. If you had difficulty with this question review the care to the client experiencing hyponatremia.
Level of Cognitive Ability: Application
Client Needs: Physiological Integrity
Integrated Concept/Process: Nursing Process/Implementation
Content Area: Fundamental Skills
Reference: DeWit S: *Fundamental concepts and skills for nursing,* Philadelphia, 2001, WB Saunders, p. 447.

17. *Answer:* 3
Rationale: The normal serum sodium level is 135 to 145 mEq/L. A serum sodium level of 150 mEq/L is indicative of hypernatremia. Based on this finding, the nurse would instruct the client to avoid foods high in sodium. Spinach and molasses are good food sources of calcium. Squash is high in phosphorus.

Test-Taking Strategy: Note the key word "avoid." Recall the normal serum sodium level. After determining that the client has hypernatremia, determining the food to avoid is the issue. Eliminate options 1 and 2 first because these are basically very healthy foods. From the remaining options, note the word "processed" in option 3. Processed foods tend to be higher in sodium content. This is the food to avoid. Review foods high in sodium content if you had difficulty with this question.
Level of Cognitive Ability: Application
Client Needs: Health Promotion and Maintenance
Integrated Concept/Process: Teaching/Learning
Content Area: Fundamental Skills
Reference: Williams S: *Basic nutrition & diet therapy*, ed 11, St Louis, 2001, Mosby, p. 120.

18. *Answer:* 1
Rationale: The normal serum calcium level is 8.6 to 10.0 mg/dL. A client with a serum calcium level of 4.0 mEq/L is experiencing hypocalcemia. The excessive administration of vitamin D, renal disease, and multiple myeloma are causative factors associated with hypercalcemia. Although immobilization can initially cause hypercalcemia, the long-term effect of prolonged bed rest is hypocalcemia.
Test-Taking Strategy: Knowledge regarding the normal serum calcium level will assist in determining that the client is experiencing hypocalcemia. This should assist in eliminating option 2. Recalling the causative factors associated with hypocalcemia is necessary to select the correct option from those remaining. If you had difficulty with this question review the causative factors associated with hypocalcemia.
Level of Cognitive Ability: Analysis
Client Needs: Physiological Integrity
Integrated Concept/Process: Nursing Process/Data Collection
Content Area: Fundamental Skills
Reference: DeWit S: *Fundamental concepts and skills for nursing*, Philadelphia, 2001, WB Saunders, p. 448.

19. *Answer:* 1
Rationale: Hypotonicity of the muscles is seen in hypercalcemia. Options 2, 3, and 4 identify signs of hypocalcemia.
Test-Taking Strategy: Note the key word "not." Use the process of elimination, noting that options 2, 3, and 4 are similar in that they all reflect a hyperactivity of body systems. The option that is different is option 1. Review the signs noted in hypocalcemia if you had difficulty with this question.
Level of Cognitive Ability: Analysis
Client Needs: Physiological Integrity
Integrated Concept/Process: Nursing Process/Data Collection
Content Area: Fundamental Skills
Reference: DeWit S: *Fundamental concepts and skills for nursing*, Philadelphia, 2001, WB Saunders, p. 448.

20. *Answer:* 1
Rationale: Butter comes from milk fat and does not contain significant amounts of calcium. Milk, spinach, and broccoli are calcium-containing foods and should be avoided by the client on a calcium-restricted diet.
Test-Taking Strategy: Use the process of elimination. Note the key words "least amount." Option 2 can be easily eliminated first. Eliminate options 3 and 4 next because they are similar. Review the foods high in calcium if you had difficulty with this question.
Level of Cognitive Ability: Application
Client Needs: Health Promotion and Maintenance
Integrated Concept/Process: Teaching/Learning
Content Area: Fundamental Skills
Reference: Williams S: *Basic nutrition & diet therapy*, ed 11, St Louis, 2001, Mosby, p. 115.

21. *Answer:* 3
Rationale: The normal serum calcium level is 8.6 to 10.0 mg/dL. This client is experiencing hypercalcemia. Calcium gluconate and calcium chloride are medications used in the treatment of tetany that occurs from acute hypocalcemia. In hypercalcemia, large doses of vitamin D need to be avoided. Calcitonin, a thyroid hormone, decreases the plasma calcium level by inhibiting bone resorption and lowering the serum calcium concentration.
Test-Taking Strategy: Recalling the normal serum calcium level will assist in determining that the client is experiencing hypercalcemia. With this knowledge, you can easily eliminate options 1 and 2 because you would not administer medication that would add calcium to the body. Remembering that excessive vitamin D is a causative factor of hypercalcemia will assist in eliminating option 4. If you had difficulty with this question, review the treatment for hypercalcemia.
Level of Cognitive Ability: Application
Client Needs: Physiological Integrity
Integrated Concept/Process: Nursing Process/Implementation
Content Area: Pharmacology
Reference: DeWit S: *Fundamental concepts and skills for nursing*, Philadelphia, 2001, WB Saunders, p. 448.

22. *Answer:* 4
Rationale: Lettuce contains less than 100 mg of potassium. Potatoes, apricots, and avocado are potassium-containing foods and should be avoided by the client on a potassium-restricted diet.
Test-Taking Strategy: Note the key words "least amount." The question asks for the food that contains the least amount of potassium. Recalling the foods high in potassium will direct you to option 4. If you had difficulty with the question review these foods.
Level of Cognitive Ability: Application
Client Needs: Health Promotion and Maintenance
Integrated Concept/Process: Teaching/Learning
Content Area: Fundamental Skills
Reference: Williams S: *Basic nutrition & diet therapy*, ed 11, St Louis, 2001, Mosby, p. 122.

23. *Answer:* 4
Rationale: The normal magnesium level is 1.6 to 2.6 mg/dL. A client with a magnesium level of 3.6 mg/dL is experiencing hypermagnesemia. Options 1, 2, and 3 would be noted in a client with hypomagnesemia.
Test-Taking Strategy: Knowledge regarding the normal magnesium level and the associated signs related to an imbalance is helpful in answering the question. Use the process of elimination, noting that options 1, 2, and 3 are similar, in that they

reflect neurological excitability. If you had difficulty with this question review the signs noted in magnesium imbalances.
Level of Cognitive Ability: Analysis
Client Needs: Physiological Integrity
Integrated Concept/Process: Nursing Process/Data Collection
Content Area: Fundamental Skills
Reference: DeWit S: *Fundamental concepts and skills for nursing,* Philadelphia, 2001, WB Saunders, p. 448.

24. ***Answer:*** **1**
Rationale: The normal serum phosphorus level is 2.7 to 4.5 mg/dL. The client in this question is experiencing hypophosphatemia. Causative factors relate to decreased nutritional intake and malnutrition. A poor nutritional state is associated with alcoholism. Hypoparathyroidism, chemotherapy, and vitamin D intoxication are causative factors of hyperphosphatemia.
Test-Taking Strategy: Knowledge regarding the normal phosphorus level is required to determine the condition this client is experiencing. From this point, it is necessary to know the causes of hypophosphatemia. If you had difficulty with this question review the causative factors associated with hypophosphatemia.
Level of Cognitive Ability: Analysis
Client Needs: Physiological Integrity
Integrated Concept/Process: Nursing Process/Data Collection
Content Area: Fundamental Skills
Reference: DeWit S: *Fundamental concepts and skills for nursing,* Philadelphia, 2001, WB Saunders, p. 448.

25. ***Answer:*** 1
Rationale: An orange contains the least amount of phosphorus. Foods high in phosphorus include fish, pork, beef, chicken, organ meats, nuts, whole-grain breads, and cereals.
Test-Taking Strategy: Note the key words "least amount." The question asks for the food that contains the least amount of phosphorus. Recalling the foods that are high and low in phosphorus will direct you to option 1. Review these foods if you had difficulty with this question.
Level of Cognitive Ability: Application
Client Needs: Health Promotion and Maintenance
Integrated Concept/Process: Teaching/Learning
Content Area: Fundamental Skills
Reference: Williams S: *Basic nutrition & diet therapy,* ed 11, St Louis, 2001, Mosby, p. 117.

REFERENCES

DeWit S: *Fundamental concepts and skills for nursing,* Philadelphia, 2001, WB Saunders.

Hodgson B, Kizior R: *Saunders nursing drug handbook 2002,* Philadelphia, 2002, WB Saunders.

National Council of State Boards of Nursing, editors: *Test plan for the National Council Licensure Examination for Practical/Vocational Nurses.* Chicago, 2001, Author.

Potter P, Perry A: *Fundamentals of nursing,* ed 5, St Louis, 2001, Mosby.

Williams S: *Basic nutrition & diet therapy,* ed 11, St Louis, 2001, Mosby.

Acid Base Balance

PYRAMID TERMS

Allen Test Testing for collateral circulation to the hand by evaluating the patency of the radial and ulnar arteries.

Respiratory Acidosis The total concentration of buffer base is lower than normal, with a relative increasing hydrogen ion (H^+) concentration; thus a greater number of H^+ are circulating in the blood than can be absorbed by the buffer system. Caused by primary defects in the function of the lungs or by changes in normal respiratory patterns as a result of secondary problems. Any condition that causes an obstruction of the airway or depresses respiratory status can cause respiratory acidosis.

Respiratory Alkalosis A deficit of carbonic acid (H_2CO_3) or a decease in H^+ concentration. Results from the accumulation of base or from a loss of acid without a comparable loss of base in the body fluids. Caused by conditions that cause overstimulation of the respiratory status.

Metabolic Acidosis The total concentration of buffer base is lower than normal, with a relative increase in the H^+ concentration. It occurs as a result of losing buffer bases or retaining too many acids without sufficient bases. It occurs in conditions such as renal failure, diabetic ketoacidosis, from the production of lactic acid, and from the ingestion of toxins, such as aspirin.

Metabolic Alkalosis A deficit of or loss of H^+ or acids or an excess of base (bicarbonate). Results from the accumulation of base or from a loss of acid without a comparable loss of base in the body fluids. Caused by conditions resulting in hypovolemia, the loss of gastric fluid, excessive bicarbonate intake, the massive transfusion of whole blood, and hyperaldosteronism.

PYRAMID TO SUCCESS

Acid base imbalance is a content area that is sometimes viewed as complex to understand. It is important to understand the description of each imbalance and then review the causes of each disorder, correlating the pathophysiology to each cause. From this point, note the signs and symptoms related to each disorder and the treatment associated with the clinical manifestations. The primary Integrated Concepts and Processes addressed in this chapter are Clinical Problem-Solving Process (Nursing Process), Communication and Documentation, Self-Care, and Teaching/Learning.

CLIENT NEEDS

Safe, Effective Care Environment

Invasive procedures, such as arterial blood gas specimens or treatments, related to the various acid base imbalances
Asepsis, standard (universal) precautions
Providing safety to the client when implementing various treatments for the acid base disorder

Health Promotion and Maintenance

Identify those clients at risk for an acid base disturbance
Reinforce instructions to the client and family about the prevention, early detection, and treatment measures for health disorders

Psychosocial Integrity

Provide emotional support to the client and to the family
Support systems

Physiological Integrity

Identify clients at risk for an acid-base disturbance
Reduce the likelihood that an alteration will occur
Monitor for changes in status and complications
Administer and monitor medications, IV fluids, and other prescribed therapies
Document the expected and unexpected responses to the therapy

Assist with obtaining arterial blood gases
Provide wound care when blood is obtained for a blood gas determination
Assist with determining the results from an arterial blood gas study

I. HYDROGEN IONS, ACIDS, AND BASES

A. Hydrogen ions (H^+)
1. Vital to life
2. Expressed as pH
3. pH of body fluid is normally alkaline (between 7.35 and 7.45)

B. Acids
1. Produced as end products of metabolism
2. Contain hydrogen ions
3. Hydrogen ion donors, which means that acids give up H^+ to neutralize or decrease the strength of an acid or to form a weaker base
4. The number of hydrogen ions in body fluid determines its acidity, alkalinity, or if it is neutral

C. Bases
1. Contain no H^+
2. Hydrogen ion acceptors
3. Accept H^+ from acids to neutralize or decrease the strength of a base or to form a weaker acid

II. REGULATORY SYSTEMS FOR H^+ CONCENTRATION IN THE BLOOD

A. Buffers
1. The fastest-acting regulatory system
2. Provide immediate protection against changes in H^+ concentration in the extracellular fluid
3. Serve as a transport mechanism that carries excess H^+ to the lungs
4. Once the primary buffer systems react, they are consumed, and this leaves the body less able to withstand further stress until they are replaced

B. Primary buffer systems in extracellular fluid
1. Hemoglobin (Hgb) system
   a. In the red blood cells (RBCs)
   b. Maintains acid base balance by a process called chloride shift
   c. Chloride shifts in and out of the cells in response to the level of oxygen (O_2) in the blood
2. Plasma proteins system
   a. Functions in conjunction with the liver to vary the amount of H^+ in the chemical structure of protein
   b. Plasma proteins have the ability to attract or release H^+
3. Carbonic acid/bicarbonate system
   a. Maintains a pH of 7.4 with a ratio of 20 parts bicarbonate to 1 part carbonic acid (20:1)
   b. This ratio (20:1) determines H^+ concentration of body fluid
   c. Carbonic acid concentration is controlled by the excretion of CO_2 by the lungs; the rate and depth of respiration changes in response to changes in CO_2
   d. Bicarbonate concentration is controlled by the kidneys, which selectively retain or secrete bicarbonates in response to the body needs
4. Phosphate buffer system
   a. Present in the cells and body fluids
   b. Especially active in the kidneys
   c. Acts like bicarbonate and clears spare H^+

C. Lungs
1. Body's second defense that interacts with the buffer system to maintain acid base balance
2. In acidosis, the pH goes down and the respiratory rate and depth go up in an attempt to blow off acids; the carbonic acid created by the neutralizing action of bicarbonate can be carried to the lungs, where it is reduced to CO_2 and water and exhaled, thus H^+ are inactivated and excreted
3. In alkalosis, the pH goes up and the respiratory rate and depth go down; the CO_2 is retained, and the carbonic acid builds to neutralize and decrease the strength of excess bicarbonate
4. The action of the lungs is reversible in controlling an excess or deficit
5. The lungs can hold H^+ until the deficit is corrected or can inactivate H^+, changing them to water molecules to be exhaled as CO_2, thus correcting the excess
6. The lungs are capable of inactivating only H^+ carried by carbonic acid (H_2CO_3); excess H^+ created by other problems must be excreted by the kidneys

D. Kidneys
1. The ultimate correction of acid base disturbances is dependent on the kidneys, even though the renal excretion of acids and alkali occurs more slowly
2. Compensation requires a few hours to several days; however, it is more thorough and selective than that of other regulators
3. In acidosis, the pH goes down, and excess H^+ are secreted into the tubules and combine with buffers for excretion in the urine
4. In alkalosis, the pH goes up, and bicarbonate ions move into the tubules, combine with sodium, and are excreted in the urine

5. Selective regulation of bicarbonate in the kidneys
   a. The kidneys restore bicarbonate by the release of H^+ and holding bicarbonate ions
   b. Extra H^+ are excreted in the urine in the form of phosphoric acid
   c. The alteration of certain amino acids in the renal tubules results in a diffusion of ammonia into the kidneys, and the ammonia combines with extra H^+ and is excreted in the urine

E. Potassium
1. Plays an exchange role in maintaining acid base balance
2. The body changes the potassium (K) level by drawing H^+ into the cell or by pushing them out of the cell
3. In acidosis, the body protects itself from the acid state by moving H^+ into the cell; therefore K moves out to make room for H^+; the K level goes up
4. In alkalosis, the cells release H^+ into the blood in an attempt to increase the acidity of the blood and combat alkalinity; the K moves into the cells and the K level goes down

III. RESPIRATORY ACIDOSIS

A. Description: The total concentration of buffer base is lower than normal, with a relative increasing hydrogen ion (H^+) concentration; thus a greater number of H^+ are circulating in the blood than can be absorbed by the buffer system

B. Causes
1. Due to primary defects in the function of the lungs or by changes in normal respiratory patterns from secondary problems
2. Remember that any condition that causes an obstruction of the airway or depresses respiratory status can cause **respiratory acidosis**
3. Hypoventilation
4. Chronic obstructive pulmonary disease (COPD)
5. Pulmonary edema
6. Pneumonia
7. Atelectasis
8. Asthma
9. Bronchitis or bronchiectasis
10. Infection
11. Medications such as sedatives, narcotics, or anesthetics
12. Brain trauma

C. Data collection
1. In an attempt to compensate, the respiratory rate and depth increase
2. pH less than 7.35 and PCO_2 greater than 45 mm Hg
3. Mental status changes such as confusion
4. Drowsiness
5. Restlessness
6. Weakness
7. Dizziness
8. Dyspnea
9. Hyperkalemia

D. Implementation
1. Maintain patent airway
2. Monitor for signs of respiratory distress
3. Administer oxygen as prescribed
4. Place client in semi-Fowler's position unless contraindicated
5. Encourage and assist the client to turn, cough, and deep breathe
6. Prepare to administer chest physiotherapy and postural drainage as prescribed
7. Encourage hydration to thin secretions unless excess fluid intake is contraindicated
8. Suction the client as necessary
9. Monitor electrolyte values
10. Avoid the use of tranquilizers, narcotics, and hypnotics because they further depress respirations
11. Administer antibiotics for infection as prescribed

IV. RESPIRATORY ALKALOSIS

A. Description: A deficit of carbonic acid (H_2CO_3) or a decease in H^+ concentration; results from the accumulation of base or from a loss of acid without a comparable loss of base in the body fluids

B. Causes
1. Due to conditions that cause overstimulation of the respiratory status
2. Hyperventilation
3. Hypoxemia
4. Fever
5. Early stages of salicylate poisoning
6. Reactions to certain medications
7. Pain
8. Anxiety
9. Hysteria

C. Data collection
1. Initially, the hyperventilation and respiratory stimulation will cause abnormal rapid and deep respirations (tachypnea); in an attempt to compensate, respiratory rate and depth then go down
2. pH is greater than 7.45 and PCO_2 is less than 35 mm Hg

3. Mental status changes
4. Pallor around the mouth
5. Tingling of the fingers
6. Dizziness
7. Spasms of the muscles of the hands
8. Hypokalemia

D. Implementation
1. Maintain a patent airway
2. Provide emotional support and reassurance to the client
3. Encourage appropriate breathing patterns
4. Provide cautious care with ventilator clients so that the client is not forced to take breaths too deeply or rapidly
5. Monitor electrolyte values
6. Administer sedatives as prescribed

V. METABOLIC ACIDOSIS

A. Description: The total concentration of buffer base is lower than normal, with a relative increase in the H^+ concentration; occurs as a result of losing buffer bases or retaining too many acids without sufficient bases

B. Causes
1. Excessive burning of fats such as occurs in the client with diabetes mellitus or in the client who is on a low carbohydrate, high protein diet to lose weight
2. Abnormal carbohydrate metabolism in which, in the absence of oxygen, lactic acid accumulates in the blood
3. Failure of the kidneys to reabsorb bicarbonate
4. Severe diarrhea: Intestinal and pancreatic secretions are normally alkaline; therefore, excessive loss of base leads to acidosis
5. Malnutrition

C. Data collection
1. In an attempt to blow off the extra CO_2 and compensate for the acidosis, hyperpnea with Kussmaul's respirations occurs
2. pH less than 7.35 and a HCO_3 less than 22 mEq/L
3. Headache
4. Weakness
5. Malaise
6. Fruity-smelling breath
7. Hyperkalemia
8. Stupor, unconsciousness, coma, and death, if acidosis is not resolved

D. Implementation
1. Based on the cause of the acidosis
2. Maintain a patent airway
3. Prepare for the administration of IV bicarbonate or lactate
4. Monitor electrolyte values
5. Initiate safety precautions
6. Frequent mouth care using an alkaline mouthwash such as baking soda
7. Monitor the potassium level very closely; when acidosis is being treated, potassium will move back into the cell and the blood level will drop

E. Implementation in diabetes mellitus/diabetic ketoacidosis: Insulin is given to hasten the movement of serum glucose into the cell, thereby decreasing the concurrent ketosis

F. Implementation in renal failure: Dialysis may be used to remove protein and waste products, thereby lessening the acidotic state

VI. METABOLIC ALKALOSIS

A. Description: A deficit of or loss of H^+ or acids or an excess of base (bicarbonate); results from the accumulation of base or from a loss of acid without a comparable loss of base in the body fluids

B. Causes
1. Hypokalemia
2. Vomiting
3. Gastric suction
4. Intestinal fistulas
5. Diuretics
6. Corticosteroid therapy

C. Data collection
1. In an attempt to compensate, respiratory rate and depth go down to conserve carbon dioxide (CO_2)
2. Slow, shallow respirations
3. Decreased chest movements
4. Cyanosis
5. Irritability
6. Disorientation
7. Lethargy
8. Convulsions
9. Hypokalemia
10. Hypocalcemia

D. Implementation
1. Maintain a patent airway
2. Monitor vital signs
3. Monitor I&O
4. Monitor electrolyte values
5. Institute safety precautions
6. Prepare to replace potassium and calcium as prescribed
7. Prepare to administer medications as prescribed to promote the kidney's excretion of bicarbonate
8. Prepare to administer acidifying solutions as prescribed

VII. ARTERIAL BLOOD GASES (Box 9-1)

A. Description: Reflect the ability of the lungs to exchange oxygen and carbon dioxide, the effectiveness of the kidneys in balancing retention and elimination of bicarbonate, and the effectiveness of the heart as a pump

B. Obtaining an arterial blood gas specimen
1. Obtain vital signs
2. Perform **Allen's test** to determine the presence of collateral circulation (Box 9-2)
3. Identify factors that may affect the accuracy of the results, such as changes in the O_2 settings on respiratory assistive devices, suctioning within the last 20 minutes, and client activities
4. Assist with the specimen draw by preparing a heparinized syringe
5. Provide emotional support to the client
6. Apply pressure immediately to the puncture site for 5 minutes, and for 10 minutes if the client is taking anticoagulants
7. Appropriately label the specimen and transport on ice to the laboratory
8. Record the client's temperature and the type of supplemental oxygen that the client is receiving on the laboratory form

C. Respiratory imbalances (Box 9-3)
1. Remember, the respiratory function indicator is the PCO_2
2. In a respiratory imbalance, you will find an opposite response between the pH and the PCO_2; in other words, the pH will be up with a PCO_2 down, or the pH will be down with an elevated PCO_2
3. Remember the pH is down in an acidotic condition and is elevated in an alkalotic condition
4. Look at the pH and the PCO_2 to determine if the condition is a respiratory problem
5. **Respiratory acidosis**
   a. The pH is down
   b. The PCO_2 is up
6. **Respiratory alkalosis**
   a. The pH is up
   b. The PCO_2 is down

D. Metabolic imbalances (Box 9-3)
1. Remember, the metabolic function indicator is the bicarbonate (HCO_3)
2. In a metabolic imbalance, you will find a corresponding response between the pH and the HCO_3
3. In other words, the pH will be up and the HCO_3 will be up, or the pH will be down and the HCO_3 will be down
4. Remember, the pH is down in an acidotic condition and is elevated in an alkalotic condition
5. Look at the pH and the HCO_3 to determine if the condition is a metabolic problem
6. **Metabolic acidosis**
   a. The pH is down

BOX 9-1

Normal Blood Gas Values

pH 7.35-7.45
PCO_2 35-45 mm Hg
HCO_3 22-27 mEq/L
PO_2 80-100 mm Hg

BOX 9-2

Performing Allen's Test

Apply direct pressure over the client's ulnar and radial arteries simultaneously.
While pressure is applied, ask the client to open and close the hand repeatedly; the hand should blanch.
Release pressure from the ulnar artery while compressing the radial artery and assess the color of the extremity distal to the pressure point.
If pinkness fails to return within 6 seconds, the ulnar artery is insufficient, indicating that the radial artery should not be used for obtaining a blood specimen.

BOX 9-3

Analyzing Arterial Blood Gas Results

If you can remember the following pyramid points and steps, you will be able to analyze any blood gas report.

PYRAMID POINTS
In acidosis, the pH is down
In alkalosis, the pH is up
The respiratory function indicator is the PCO_2
The metabolic function indicator is the HCO_3

PYRAMID STEPS
Look at the blood gas report
Pyramid Step 1
Look at the pH. Is it up or down? If it is up, it reflects alkalosis. If it is down, it reflects acidosis.
Pyramid Step 2
Look at the PCO_2. Is it up or down? If it reflects an opposite response as the pH, then you know that the condition is a respiratory imbalance. If it does not reflect an opposite response as the pH, then move on to Pyramid Step 3.
Pyramid Step 3
Look at the HCO_3. Does the HCO_3 reflect a corresponding response with the pH? If it does, then the condition is a metabolic imbalance.

b. The HCO_3 is down

7. **Metabolic alkalosis**

a. The pH is up

b. The HCO_3 is up

E. Analyzing arterial blood gas results (Box 9-3)

PRACTICE QUESTIONS

1. A nurse is caring for a client with a diagnosis of chronic obstructive pulmonary disease (COPD). The nurse monitors the client for which acid base imbalance that most likely occurs in this condition?
   1. Respiratory acidosis
   2. Respiratory alkalosis
   3. Metabolic acidosis
   4. Metabolic alkalosis
2. A licensed practical nurse (LPN) is assigned to care for a client with Guillain-Barré syndrome. The registered nurse (RN) reviews the results of the arterial blood gases with the LPN and tells the LPN that the client is experiencing respiratory acidosis. The LPN would expect to note which of the following?
   1. pH 7.40, PCO_2 52 mm Hg
   2. pH 7.35, PCO_2 40 mm Hg
   3. pH 7.25, PCO_2 50 mm Hg
   4. pH 7.50, PCO_2 30 mm Hg
3. A nurse is caring for a client with respiratory insufficiency. Arterial blood gas results indicate a pH of 7.50 and a PCO_2 of 30 mm Hg and the nurse is told that the client is experiencing respiratory alkalosis. Which of the following additional laboratory values would the nurse expect to note?
   1. Sodium level, 145 mEq/L
   2. Potassium level, 3.2 mEq/L
   3. Magnesium level, 2.4 mg/dL
   4. Phosphorus level, 4.0 mg/dL
4. The nurse is caring for a client with pneumonia. The nurse is told that the blood gas results indicate a pH of 7.50 and a PCO_2 of 30 mm Hg. The nurse determines that these results indicate:
   1. Metabolic acidosis
   2. Metabolic alkalosis
   3. Respiratory alkalosis
   4. Respiratory acidosis
5. A client is scheduled for blood to be drawn from the radial artery for an arterial blood gas (ABG) determination. A nurse assists in performing an Allen's test before drawing the blood gas to determine the adequacy of the:
   1. Brachial circulation
   2. Ulnar circulation
   3. Femoral circulation
   4. Carotid circulation
6. A nurse is caring for a client with a nasogastric tube that is attached to low suction. The nurse monitors the client closely for which of the following acid base disorders that is most likely to occur in this client?
   1. Respiratory acidosis
   2. Respiratory alkalosis
   3. Metabolic acidosis
   4. Metabolic alkalosis
7. A nurse is caring for a client with an ileostomy. The nurse monitors the client closely, understanding that this client is at risk for developing which of the following acid base disorders?
   1. Respiratory acidosis
   2. Respiratory alkalosis
   3. Metabolic acidosis
   4. Metabolic alkalosis
8. A nurse is caring for a client with diabetic ketoacidosis and documents that the client is experiencing Kussmaul's respirations. Based on this documentation, which of the following did the nurse most likely observe?
   1. Respirations that are abnormally deep, regular, and increased in rate
   2. Respirations that are regular but abnormally slow
   3. Respirations that are labored and increased in depth and rate
   4. Respirations that cease for several seconds
9. A nurse is collecting data from a client with a suspected diagnosis of gastric ulcer. The client tells the nurse that oral antacids are taken frequently throughout the day. The nurse continues to collect data from the client, understanding that the client is at risk for which of the following acid base disturbances?
   1. Respiratory alkalosis
   2. Respiratory acidosis
   3. Metabolic acidosis
   4. Metabolic alkalosis
10. A nurse is caring for a client with renal failure. The nurse is told that the blood gas results indicate a pH of 7.30 and a HCO_3 20 mEq/L and that the client is experiencing metabolic acidosis. The nurse reviews the laboratory results and expects to note which of the following?
    1. Sodium level, 145 mEq/L
    2. Magnesium level, 2.6 mg/dL
    3. Potassium level, 5.2 mEq/L
    4. Phosphorus level, 4.5 mg/dL

ANSWERS

1. *Answer:* 1
Rationale: Respiratory acidosis most often occurs as a result of primary defects in the function of the lungs or changes in normal respiratory patterns from secondary problems. Chronic respiratory acidosis is most commonly caused by COPD. Acute respiratory acidosis also occurs in these clients when superimposed respiratory infection or concurrent respiratory disease increases the work of breathing. Options 2, 3, and 4 are not likely to occur unless other conditions complicate the COPD.
Test-Taking Strategy: Use the process of elimination. Remembering that primary defects in the function of the lungs results in respiratory acidosis will direct you to the correct option. Review the causes of respiratory acidosis if you had difficulty with this question.
Level of Cognitive Ability: Comprehension
Client Needs: Physiological Integrity
Integrated Concept/Process: Nursing Process/Data Collection
Content Area: Fundamental Skills
Reference: DeWit S: *Fundamental concepts and skills for nursing,* Philadelphia, 2001, WB Saunders, p. 451.

2. *Answer:* 3
Rationale: The normal pH is 7.35 to 7.45. The normal PCO_2 is 35 to 45 mm Hg. In respiratory acidosis the pH is down and the PCO_2 is up.
Test-Taking Strategy: Remember that in a respiratory imbalance you will find an opposite response between the pH and the PCO_2. Also remember that the pH is down in an acidotic condition. Options 1 and 4 reflect an elevated pH, which indicates an alkalotic condition. Option 2 reflects a normal blood gas result. Option 3 is the only option that reflects an acidotic condition. Review the interpretation of arterial blood gas results if you had difficulty with this question.
Level of Cognitive Ability: Analysis
Client Needs: Physiological Integrity
Integrated Concept/Process: Nursing Process/Data Collection
Content Area: Adult Health/Neurological
Reference: DeWit S: *Fundamental concepts and skills for nursing,* Philadelphia, 2001, WB Saunders, p. 451.

3. *Answer:* 2
Rationale: Clinical manifestations of respiratory alkalosis include tachypnea, mental status changes, dizziness, pallor around the mouth, spasms of the muscles of the hands, and hypokalemia. Options 1, 3, and 4 identify normal laboratory results.
Test-Taking Strategy: Recalling the clinical manifestations of respiratory alkalosis and the normal laboratory values will assist in answering the question. By the process of elimination, you can then determine that the only abnormal laboratory value is the potassium level. Review the clinical manifestations of respiratory alkalosis if you had difficulty with this question.
Level of Cognitive Ability: Analysis
Client Needs: Physiological Integrity
Integrated Concept/Process: Nursing Process/Data Collection
Content Area: Adult Health/Respiratory
Reference: DeWit S: *Fundamental concepts and skills for nursing.* Philadelphia, 2001, WB Saunders, p. 452.

4. *Answer:* 3
Rationale: The normal pH is 7.35 to 7.45. In a respiratory condition, an opposite effect will be seen between the pH and the PCO_2. In an alkalotic condition, the pH is up. Clients with pneumonia are at risk for respiratory alkalosis as a result of hypoxemia.
Test-Taking Strategy: Remember that in a respiratory condition you will find an opposite response between the pH and the PCO_2. Therefore options 1 and 2 can be eliminated. Also, remember that the pH is up in an alkalotic condition. Review the steps related to reading blood gas values if you had difficulty with this question.
Level of Cognitive Ability: Analysis
Client Needs: Physiological Integrity
Integrated Concept/Process: Nursing Process/Data Collection
Content Area: Adult Health/Respiratory
Reference: DeWit, S: *Fundamental concepts and skills for nursing,* Philadelphia, 2001, WB Saunders, p. 452.

5. *Answer:* 2
Rationale: Before radial puncture for obtaining an arterial specimen for ABGs, an Allen's test should be performed to determine adequate ulnar circulation. Failure to assess collateral circulation could result in severe ischemic injury to the hand, if damage to the radial artery occurs with arterial puncture.
Test-Taking Strategy: Knowledge regarding the purpose and procedure for the Allen's test is required to answer this question. Review this test if you had difficulty with this question.
Level of Cognitive Ability: Analysis
Client Needs: Physiological Integrity
Integrated Concept/Process: Nursing Process/Evaluation
Content Area: Adult Health/Cardiovascular
Reference: Potter P, Perry A: *Fundamentals of nursing,* ed 5, St Louis, 2001, Mosby, p. 790.

6. *Answer:* 4
Rationale: Loss of gastric fluid via nasogastric suction or vomiting causes metabolic alkalosis due to the loss of hydrochloric acid. This results in an alkalotic condition.
Test-Taking Strategy: Remember that hydrochloric acid is lost when the client is on nasogastric suction. This will direct you to the options identifying an alkalotic condition. Since the question addresses a situation other than a respiratory one, the acid-base disorder would be a metabolic condition. If you had difficulty with this question review the causes of metabolic alkalosis.
Level of Cognitive Ability: Analysis
Client Needs: Physiological Integrity
Integrated Concept/Process: Nursing Process/Data Collection
Content Area: Adult Health/Gastrointestinal
Reference: DeWit S: *Fundamental concepts and skills for nursing,* Philadelphia, 2001, WB Saunders, p. 529.

7. *Answer:* 3
Rationale: Intestinal secretions high in bicarbonate may be lost through enteric drainage tubes, an ileostomy, or with

diarrhea. The decreased bicarbonate level creates the actual base deficit of metabolic acidosis.
Test-Taking Strategy: Note that the client condition described in the question is a client with a gastrointestinal disorder. This will direct you to think about a metabolic disorder. Remembering that intestinal fluids are primarily alkaline will assist in selecting the correct option. When excess bicarbonate is lost, acidosis will result. Review the causes of metabolic acidosis if you had difficulty with this question.
Level of Cognitive Ability: Analysis
Client Needs: Physiological Integrity
Integrated Concept/Process: Nursing Process/Data Collection
Content Area: Adult Health/Gastrointestinal
Reference: DeWit S: *Fundamental concepts and skills for nursing,* Philadelphia, 2001, WB Saunders, p. 452.

8. ***Answer:*** 1
Rationale: Kussmaul's respirations are abnormally deep, regular, and increased in rate. In bradypnea, respirations are regular but abnormally slow. In hyperpnea, respirations are labored and increased in depth and rate. Apnea is described as respirations that cease for several seconds.
Test-Taking Strategy: Knowledge regarding the descriptions for alterations in breathing pattern is required to answer the question. Remember, Kussmaul's respirations occur in diabetic ketoacidosis. Review the characteristics of these types of respirations if you had difficulty with this question.
Level of Cognitive Ability: Comprehension
Client Needs: Physiological Integrity
Integrated Concept/Process: Nursing Process/Data Collection
Content Area: Fundamental Skills
Reference: DeWit S: *Fundamental concepts and skills for nursing,* Philadelphia, 2001, WB Saunders, p. 358.

9. ***Answer:*** 4
Rationale: Increases in base components occur as a result of oral or parenteral ingestion of bicarbonates, carbonates, acetates, citrates, and lactates. Excessive use of oral antacids containing sodium or calcium bicarbonate can cause a metabolic alkalosis.
Test-Taking Strategy: Remembering that antacids contain bicarbonate and that an excess oral intake will increase bicarbonate will assist in directing you to the correct option. Review the causes of metabolic alkalosis if you had difficulty with the question.
Level of Cognitive Ability: Analysis
Client Needs: Physiological Integrity
Integrated Concept/Process: Nursing Process/Data Collection
Content Area: Adult Health/Gastrointestinal
Reference: DeWit S: *Fundamental concepts and skills for nursing,* Philadelphia, 2001, WB Saunders, p. 452.

10. ***Answer:*** 3
Rationale: Clinical manifestations of metabolic acidosis include weakness, malaise, and headache. Hyperkalemia will occur. The pH will be less than 7.35 and the HCO_3 lower than 22 mEq/L.
Test-Taking Strategy: Knowledge regarding the clinical manifestations of metabolic acidosis along with normal laboratory values will assist you in answering the question. By the process of elimination, you can then determine that the only abnormal laboratory value is the potassium level. Review the manifestations of metabolic acidosis if you had difficulty with this question.
Level of Cognitive Ability: Analysis
Client Needs: Physiological Integrity
Integrated Concept/Process: Nursing Process/Data Collection
Content Area: Adult Health/Renal
Reference: DeWit S: *Fundamental concepts and skills for nursing,* Philadelphia, 2001, WB Saunders, p. 452.

REFERENCES

DeWit S: *Fundamental concepts and skills for nursing,* Philadelphia, 2001, WB Saunders.

Hodgson B, Kizior R: *Saunders nursing drug handbook 2002,* Philadelphia, 2002, WB Saunders.

National Council of State Boards of Nursing, editors: *Test plan for the National Council Licensure Examination for Practical/Vocational Nurses,* Chicago, 2001, Author.

Potter P, Perry A: *Fundamentals of nursing,* ed 5, St Louis, 2001, Mosby.

10 Laboratory Values

PYRAMID TERMS

Capillary Puncture Preferred for a peripheral blood smear.

Plasma The fluid ground substance; what remains after the cells have been removed from a sample of whole blood.

Serum Blood plasma from which clotting agents have been removed.

Venipuncture Puncture into a vein to obtain a blood specimen for testing; the antecubital veins are the veins of choice because of ease of access.

PYRAMID TO SUCCESS

This chapter identifies the normal adult values of the most common laboratory tests. If you are familiar with the normal values, you will be able to determine if an abnormality exists. It is unlikely that a question on NCLEX-PN will simply ask you what a normal value may be. The questions on NCLEX-PN related to laboratory values will require you to identify whether the laboratory value is normal or abnormal, and then you will be required to think about the effects of the laboratory value in terms of the client. Pyramid points focus on awareness of the normal values of the most common laboratory tests, therapeutic levels in the serum of commonly prescribed medications, and interventions based on the findings. When a question is presented on NCLEX-PN regarding a specific laboratory value, note the disorder presented in the question and the associated body organ that is affected as a result of the disorder. This process will assist you in determining the correct answer. For example, if the question is asking you about the immune status of a client receiving chemotherapy, monitoring laboratory values will focus on the white blood cell count and the neutrophils because this client may be at risk for infection. In the client receiving chemotherapy who has a low white blood cell count, the plan of care focuses on the immune system and protecting the client from infection. Implementation focuses on preventive interventions related to infection, such as protective isolation measures. Evaluation may focus on maintenance of a normal temperature in the client. The primary Integrated Concepts and Processes addressed in this chapter are Clinical Problem-Solving Process (Nursing Process), Communication and Documentation, Self-Care, and Teaching/Learning. Box 10-1 lists abbreviations found in laboratory values.

CLIENT NEEDS

Safe, Effective Care Environment

Informed consent for specific procedures
Handling infectious materials
Asepsis
Standard (universal) and other precautions

BOX 10-1

Pyramid Abbreviations

g/dL - grams per deciliter
µg/dL - micrograms per deciliter
mg/dL - milligrams per deciliter
mEq/L - milliequivalents per liter
U/L - units per liter
mm/hr - millimeters per hour
IU/L - International Units per liter
µg/mL - micrograms per milliliter
ng/mL - nanograms per milliliter
µU/mL - microunits per milliliter
mL/kg - milliliters per kilogram

Health Promotion and Maintenance

Client preparation for laboratory test
Post-test procedures
Importance of follow-up laboratory studies
Community resources available for follow-up studies

Psychosocial Integrity

Communicate purpose of test to client
Provide psychosocial comfort during testing
Identify support systems
Describe specific interventions required based on the results

Physiological Integrity

Comfort interventions
Normal values of the most common laboratory tests
Significant laboratory results
Therapeutic serum medication levels of commonly prescribed medications
Monitoring for clinical manifestations associated with the abnormal laboratory value
Monitoring for potential complications related to the test
Signs and symptoms that need to be reported

I. ELECTROLYTES (Table 10-1)
   A. **Serum** sodium (Na)
      1. Description
         a. A major cation of extracellular fluid
         b. Maintains osmotic pressures and acid-base balance and assists in transmission of nerve impulses
         c. Absorbed from the small intestine and excreted in the urine in amounts dependent on dietary intake
         d. Minimum daily requirement of Na is 15 mEq
      2. Nursing consideration: Drawing blood samples proximal to IV infusion of sodium chloride will falsely elevate results
   B. **Serum** potassium (K)
      1. Description
         a. A major intracellular cation; regulates cellular water balance, electrical conduction in muscle cells, and acid-base balance

TABLE 10-1

Normal Adult Electrolyte Values

Sodium	135-145 mEq/L
Potassium	3.5-5.1 mEq/L
Chloride	98-107 mEq/L
Bicarbonate (venous)	22-29 mEq/L

         b. The body obtains K through dietary ingestion, and the kidneys either preserve or excrete K depending on cellular need
         c. K levels are used to evaluate cardiac function, renal function, gastrointestinal (GI) function, and the need for IV replacement therapy
      2. Nursing considerations
         a. Use of a tourniquet and pumping the hand before venous sampling can increase the value
         b. Do not draw blood from a site where an IV infusion exists
         c. If the client is receiving K, note on the laboratory form
         d. Clients with elevated white blood cell (WBC) counts and platelet counts may have falsely elevated K levels
   C. **Serum** chloride
      1. Description
         a. A hydrochloric acid salt that is the most abundant body anion in the extracellular fluid
         b. Functions in counterbalancing cations, such as sodium, and acts as a buffer during oxygen and carbon dioxide exchange in red blood cells
         c. Aids in digestion and maintaining osmotic pressure and water balance
      2. Nursing considerations
         a. Draw blood from an extremity that does not have saline infusing into it
         b. Do not allow the client to clench/unclench the hand before the blood draw
         c. Any condition accompanied by prolonged vomiting, diarrhea, or both will alter levels

II. COAGULATION STUDIES
   A. Activated partial thromboplastin time (aPTT)
      1. Description
         a. Evaluates how well the coagulation sequence is functioning by measuring the amount of time it takes for recalcified, citrated **plasma** to clot after partial thromboplastin is added to it
         b. Screens for deficiencies and inhibitors of all factors except VII and XIII
         c. Most commonly used to monitor heparin therapy and screen for coagulation disorders
      2. Value: 20 to 36 seconds, depending on the type of activator used
      3. Nursing considerations
         a. If the client is on intermittent heparin therapy, draw sample 1 hour before next scheduled dose

b. Do not draw samples from an arm into which heparin is infusing
c. Transport specimen to laboratory immediately
d. The aPTT should be between 1.5 and 2.5 times normal when the client is receiving heparin therapy; if the value is prolonged, initiate bleeding precautions

B. Prothrombin time (PT) and international normalized ratio (INR)
1. Description
a. Prothrombin is a vitamin K-dependent glycoprotein produced by the liver that is necessary for firm fibrin clot formation
b. Each laboratory establishes a normal value or control based on the method used to perform the test (PT)
c. The PT measures the amount of time it takes for clot formation and is used to monitor response to warfarin sodium (Coumadin) therapy or to screen for dysfunction of the extrinsic system resulting from liver disease, vitamin K deficiency, or disseminated intravascular coagulation (DIC)
d. A PT value within 2 seconds (plus or minus) of the control is considered normal
e. The INR standardizes the PT ratio and is calculated in the laboratory setting by raising the observed PT ratio to the power of the International Sensitivity Index specific to the thromboplastin reagent used
2. Values
a. PT: 9.6 to 11.8 seconds (adult male) and 9.5 to 11.3 seconds (adult female)
b. INR: 2.0 to 3.0 for standard warfarin sodium (Coumadin) therapy
c. INR: 3.0 to 4.5 for high-dose warfarin sodium (Coumadin) therapy
3. Nursing considerations
a. Baseline PT should be drawn before starting anticoagulation therapy
b. Note time of collection on laboratory form
c. Provide direct pressure to the site for 3 to 5 minutes if a coagulation defect is present
d. Concurrent warfarin sodium (Coumadin) therapy with heparin therapy can lengthen the PT for up to 5 hours after dosing
e. Diets high in green leafy vegetables can increase the absorption of vitamin K, which shortens the PT
f. A PT greater than 30 seconds places the client at risk for hemorrhage
g. Oral anticoagulation therapy usually maintains the PT at 1.5 to 2 times the laboratory control value

C. Clotting time
1. Description: Measures the time required for the interaction of all factors involved in the clotting process
2. Value: 8 to 15 minutes
3. Nursing considerations
a. The client should not receive heparin therapy for 3 hours before specimen collection
b. The test result is prolonged by any anticoagulant therapy, test tube agitation, or high temperature changes that may affect the specimen

D. Platelet count
1. Description
a. Platelets function in hemostatic plug formation, clot retraction, and coagulation factor activation
b. Platelets are produced by the bone marrow to function in hemostasis
2. Value: 150,000 to 400,000 cells/μL
3. Nursing considerations
a. Monitor the site for bleeding in clients with known thrombocytopenia
b. High altitudes, chronic cold weather, and exercise increase platelet counts
c. Bleeding precautions should be instituted in clients with a low platelet count

III. SERUM GASTROINTESTINAL STUDIES

A. Albumin
1. Description
a. A main **plasma** protein of blood
b. Maintains oncotic pressure and transports bilirubin, fatty acids, medications, hormones, and other substances that are insoluble in water
2. Value: 3.4 to 5 g/dL
3. Nursing considerations
a. Draw from an extremity the does not have an IV infusing into it
b. Instruct the client to consume a low-fat diet on the day of the test

B. Alkaline phosphatase
1. Description
a. An enzyme normally found in bone, liver, intestine, and placenta
b. The level rises during periods of bone growth, liver disease, and bile duct obstruction
2. Value: 4.5 to 13 King-Armstrong units/dL
3. Nursing considerations
a. The client may be requested to fast 10 to 12 hours before the test
b. Administration of hepatotoxic medications within 12 hours before specimen collection invalidates the test

c. Transport specimen to laboratory immediately

C. Ammonia

1. Description

a. A waste product from nitrogen breakdown during protein metabolism

b. Metabolized by the liver and excreted by the kidneys as urea

c. Elevated levels resulting from hepatic dysfunction may lead to encephalopathy

d. Not a reliable indicator of hepatic coma

2. Value: 35 to 65 μg/dL

3. Nursing considerations

a. Instruct the client to fast, except for water, and to refrain from smoking for 8 to 10 hours before the test

b. Place the specimen in an ice water bath

c. Transport to the laboratory immediately

D. Amylase

1. Description

a. An enzyme produced by the pancreas and salivary glands that aids in the digestion of complex carbohydrates and is excreted by the kidneys

b. In acute pancreatitis, the amylase level is greatly increased; the level starts rising in 3 to 6 hours after the onset of pain, peaks at about 24 hours, and returns to normal in 2 to 3 days after the onset of pain

2. Value: 25 to 151 IV/L

3. Nursing considerations

a. On the laboratory form, list medications that the client has taken 24 hours before the test

b. Note that many medications may cause false-positive or false-negative results

c. Results are invalidated if the specimen was obtained less than 72 hours after cholecystography with radiopaque dyes

E. Bilirubin

1. Description

a. Produced by the liver, spleen, and bone marrow and is also a by-product of hemoglobin breakdown

b. Total bilirubin levels can be broken down into direct bilirubin, which is primarily excreted via the intestinal tract, and indirect bilirubin, which circulates primarily in the bloodstream

c. Total bilirubin levels rise with any type of jaundice, whereas direct and indirect levels rise depending on the etiology of the jaundice

2. Values

a. Bilirubin, direct: 0 to 0.3 mg/dL

b. Bilirubin, indirect: 0.1 to 1.0 mg/dL

c. Bilirubin, total: less than 1.5 mg/dL

3. Nursing considerations

a. Instruct the client to eat a diet low in yellow foods, such as carrots, yams, yellow beans, and pumpkins, for 3 to 4 days before sampling

b. Instruct the client to fast for 4 hours before sampling

c. Note that results will be elevated with the use of alcohol, morphine sulfate, theophylline, ascorbic acid, and aspirin

d. Note that results are invalidated if the client received a radioactive scan within 24 hours before the test

F. Lipase

1. Description

a. A pancreatic enzyme that changes fats and triglycerides into fatty acids and glycerol

b. Elevated lipase levels occur in pancreatic disorders; elevations may not occur until 24 to 36 hours after the onset of illness and may remain elevated for up to 14 days

2. Value: 10 to 140 U/L

3. Nursing considerations

a. Endoscopic retrograde cholangiopancreatography (ERCP) may increase lipase activity

b. Traumatic **venipuncture** can inhibit lipase activity

G. Lipids

1. Description

a. Blood lipids consist primarily of cholesterol, triglycerides, and phospholipids

b. Lipid assessment includes total cholesterol, high-density lipoprotein (HDL), low-density lipoprotein (LDL), and triglycerides

c. Cholesterol is present is all body tissues and is a major component of LDL, brain and nerve cells, cell membranes, and some gallstones

d. Triglycerides constitute a major part of very-low-density lipoproteins (VLDL) and a small part of LDL

e. Triglycerides are synthesized in the liver from fatty acids, protein, and glucose, and are obtained from the diet

2. Values:

a. Cholesterol: 140 to 199 mg/dL

b. LDL: less than 130 mg/dL

c. HDL: 30 to 70 mg/dL

d. Triglycerides: less than 200 mg/dL

3. Nursing considerations

a. Oral contraceptives may increase the levels of lipids in the **serum**

b. Instruct the client to abstain from foods and fluid, except for water, for 12 to 14 hours and from alcohol for 24 hours before the test

c. Instruct the client that the evening meal before the test should be free of high-cholesterol foods

d. Cholesterol levels tend to decrease temporarily with major illness or surgery

H. Protein

1. Description

a. Reflects the total amount of albumin and globulins in the **serum**

b. Regulates osmotic pressure and is comprised of coagulation factors for hemostasis, enzymes, hormones, tissue growth and repair, and pH buffers

2. Value: 6.0 to 8.0 g/dL

3. Nursing considerations

a. Do not draw in an extremity with an IV infusion

b. Instruct the client to avoid a high-fat diet for 8 hours before the test

I. Uric acid

1. Description

a. Formed as the purines, adenine and guanine, and is continuously metabolized during the formation and degradation of DNA and RNA, and from the metabolism of dietary purines

b. Elevated amounts deposit in joints and soft tissue and cause gout

c. Conditions of fast cell turnover, as well as slowed renal excretion of uric acid, may cause uricemia

d. Elevated amounts of urinary uric acid precipitate into urate stones in the kidneys

2. Values

a. Male: 4.5 to 8 mg/dL

b. Female: 2.5 to 6.2 mg/dL

3. Nursing considerations

a. Instruct the client to fast for 8 hours before test

b. Aminophylline, caffeine, and vitamin C may cause falsely elevated results

IV. GLUCOSE STUDIES

A. Fasting blood glucose (FBS)

1. Description

a. Glucose is a monosaccharide found in fruits and is formed from the digestion of carbohydrates and the conversion of glycogen by the liver

b. Glucose is the body's main source of cellular energy and is essential for brain and erythrocyte function

c. FBS levels are used to help diagnose diabetes mellitus and hypoglycemia (Table 10-2)

2. Nursing considerations

a. Instruct the client to fast for 8 to12 hours before test

b. Instruct a client with diabetes mellitus to withhold morning insulin or oral hypoglycemic medication until after the blood is drawn

B. Glucose tolerance test (GTT) (Table 10-2)

1. Description

a. Aids in the diagnosis of diabetes mellitus

b. If the glucose levels peak at higher than normal at 1 and 2 hours after injection or ingestion of glucose and are slower than normal to return to fasting levels, then diabetes mellitus is confirmed

2. Nursing considerations

a. Instruct the client to eat a high-carbohydrate (200 to 300 g) diet for 3 days before the test

b. Instruct the client to avoid alcohol, coffee, and smoking for 36 hours before testing

c. Instruct the client to fast for 10 to 16 hours before the test

d. Instruct the client to avoid strenuous exercise for 8 hours before and after the test

e. Instruct the client with diabetes mellitus to withhold morning insulin or oral hypoglycemic medication

f. Instruct the client that the test will take 3 to 5 hours, requires intravenous or oral administration of glucose, and multiple blood samples

C. Glycosylated hemoglobin

1. Description

a. Glycosylated hemoglobin is blood glucose bound to hemoglobin

b. HbA_{1c} (glycosylated hemoglobin A) is a reflection of how well blood glucose levels have been controlled for up to the prior 4 months

TABLE 10-2

Normal Adult Glucose Values

Test	Value
Glucose, fasting	70-110 mg/dL
Glucose monitoring (capillary blood)	60-110 mg/dL
Glucose tolerance test, oral	
Baseline fasting	70-110 mg/dL
30 minute fasting	110-170 mg/dL
60 minute fasting	120-170 mg/dL
90 minute fasting	100-140 mg/dL
120 minute fasting	70-120 mg/dL
Glucose, 2 hour postprandial	< 140 mg/dL

c. Hyperglycemia in diabetics is usually a cause of an increase in HbA_{1c}

2. Values
   a. Values are expressed as a percentage of total hemoglobin
   b. Diabetic with good control: 7.5% or less
   c. Diabetic with fair control: 7.6% to 8.9%
   d. Diabetic with poor control: 9% or greater
3. Nursing consideration: Fasting is not required before the test

V. RENAL FUNCTION STUDIES

A. **Serum** creatinine

1. Description
   a. A very specific indicator of renal function, revealing the balance between creatinine formation and excretion
   b. Increased levels indicate a slowing of the glomerular filtration rate
2. Value: 0.6 to 1.3 mg/dL
3. Nursing considerations: Instruct the client to avoid excessive exercise for 8 hours and avoid excessive red meat intake for 24 hours before the test

B. Blood urea nitrogen (BUN)

1. Description
   a. Urea nitrogen is the nitrogen portion of urea, a substance formed in the liver through an enzymatic protein breakdown process
   b. Urea is normally freely filtered through the renal glomeruli, with a small amount reabsorbed in the tubules and the remainder excreted in the urine
   c. Elevated values may be a result of prerenal, renal, or postrenal causes
2. Value: 8 to 25 mg/dL
3. Nursing considerations: Both creatinine levels and urea nitrogen levels should be analyzed when evaluating renal function

VI. SERUM ENZYMES/CARDIAC MARKERS

A. Creatine kinase (CK)

1. Description
   a. An enzyme found in muscle and brain tissue; reflects tissue catabolism resulting from cell trauma
   b. The test is performed to detect myocardial or skeletal muscle damage or central nervous system damage; normal CK is 26 to 174 U/L
   c. Isoenzymes include CK-MB (cardiac), CK-BB (brain), and CK-MM (muscle)
   d. CK-MB is found mainly in cardiac muscle, CK-BB is found mainly in brain tissue, and CK-MM is found mainly is skeletal muscle
2. Values
   a. CK-MB: 0% to 5% of total
   b. CK-MM: 95% to 100% of total
   c. CK-BB: 0%
3. Nursing considerations
   a. If the test is to evaluate skeletal muscle, instruct the client to avoid strenuous physical activity for 24 hours before the test
   b. Instruct the client to avoid ingestion of alcohol for 24 hours before the test
   c. Invasive procedures and IM injections may falsely elevate CK levels

B. Lactate dehydrogenase (LD or LDH)

1. Description
   a. The isoenzymes that are particularly affected with acute myocardial infarction are the LDH_1 and LDH_2
   b. This enzyme begins to elevate approximately 24 hours after myocardial infarction and peaks in 48 to 72 hours; thereafter it returns to normal, usually within 7 to 14 days (Table 10-3)
   c. The presence of an LD flip (when LD_1 is higher than LD_2), is helpful in diagnosing a myocardial infarction
2. Nursing considerations
   a. LDH isoenzymes should be interpreted in view of the clinical findings
   b. Testing should be repeated on 3 consecutive days

C. Troponins

1. Description
   a. Troponin is a regulatory protein found in striated muscle
   b. The troponins function together in the contractile apparatus for striated muscle in skeletal muscle and in the myocardium
   c. Increased amounts of troponins are released into the bloodstream when an infarction causes damage to the myocardium

TABLE 10-3

Normal Adult Lactate Dehydrogenase

Lactate dehydrogenase (LDH)	140-280 U/L
Lactate dehydrogenase isoenzymes	
LDH_1	14%-26%
LDH_2	29%-39%
LDH_3	20%-26%
LDH_4	8%-16%
LDH_5	6%-16%

d. Serial measurements are important to compare with a baseline test
2. Values:
   a. Troponin I: less than 0.6 ng/mL; greater than 1.5 ng/mL is consistent with a myocardial infarction
   b. Troponin T: greater than 0.1 to 0.2 ng/mL is consistent with a myocardial infarction
3. Nursing consideration: Client does not need to be fasting

VII. ERYTHROCYTE STUDIES

A. Erythrocyte sedimentation rate
1. Description
   a. The rate at which erythrocytes settle out of anticoagulated blood in 1 hour
   b. Not diagnostic of any particular disease but indicates that a disease process is ongoing
2. Value: 0 to 30 mm/hr, depending on age of client
3. Nursing consideration: Fasting is not necessary, but a fatty meal may cause **plasma** alterations

B. Hemoglobin and hematocrit
1. Description
   a. Hemoglobin is the main component of erythrocytes and serves as the vehicle for the transportation of oxygen and carbon dioxide
   b. Hemoglobin determinations are important in determining anemia
   c. Hematocrit represents red blood cell mass and is an important measurement in the identification of anemia or polycythemia (Table 10-4)
2. Nursing consideration: Fasting is not required

C. **Serum** iron
1. Description
   a. Iron is mostly found in hemoglobin
   b. Iron acts as a carrier of oxygen from the lungs to the tissues and indirectly aids in the return of carbon dioxide to the lungs

TABLE 10-4

Normal Adult Hemoglobin and Hematocrit Levels

Hemoglobin	
Male	14-16.5 g/dL
Female	12-15 g/dL
Hematocrit	
Male	42%-52%
Female	35%-47%

   c. Aids in diagnosing anemias and hemolytic disorders
2. Values
   a. Male: 65-175 μg/dL
   b. Female: 50-170 μg/dL
3. Nursing consideration: Level will be increased if the client has ingested iron before test

D. Red blood cell (RBC) count
1. Description
   a. RBCs function in hemoglobin transport, which results in delivery of oxygen to the body tissues
   b. RBCs are formed by red bone marrow, have a life span of 120 days, and are removed from the blood by the liver, spleen, and bone marrow
   c. Aids in diagnosing anemias and blood dyscrasias
   d. Evaluates the body's ability to produce red blood cells in sufficient numbers
2. Values
   a. Female: 4 to 5.5 million/μL
   b. Male: 4.5 to 6.2 million/μL
3. Nursing consideration: Fasting is not required

VIII. ELEMENTS

A. Calcium
1. Description
   a. A cation that is absorbed into the bloodstream from dietary sources and functions in bone formation, nerve impulse transmission, and contraction of myocardial and skeletal muscles
   b. Aids in blood clotting by converting prothrombin to thrombin
2. Value: 8.6 to 10.0 mg/dL
3. Nursing considerations
   a. Instruct the client to eat a diet with normal calcium levels (800 mg/day) for 3 days before test
   b. Instruct the client that fasting may be required for 8 hours before the test

B. Magnesium
1. Description
   a. Used as an index to determine metabolic activity and renal function
   b. Magnesium is needed in the blood-clotting mechanism, regulates neuromuscular activity, acts as a cofactor that modifies the activity of many enzymes, and has an effect on the metabolism of calcium
2. Value: 1.6 to 2.6 mg/dL
3. Nursing considerations
   a. Prolonged use of magnesium products will cause increased levels

b. Long-term total parenteral nutrition therapy or excessive loss of body fluids may cause decreased levels

C. Phosphorus
1. Description
a. Important in bone formation, energy storage and release, urinary acid-base buffering, and carbohydrate metabolism
b. Absorbed from food and excreted by the kidneys
c. High concentrations of phosphorus are stored in bone and skeletal muscle
2. Value: 2.7 to 4.5 mg/dL
3. Nursing considerations: Instruct the client to fast before the test

IX. THYROID STUDIES

A. Description
1. Performed if a thyroid disorder is suspected
2. Helpful to differentiate primary thyroid disease from secondary causes and from abnormalities in thyroxine-binding globulin levels

B. Values
1. Thyroid-stimulating hormone (thyrotropin; TSH): 0.2 to 5.4 μU/mL
2. Thyroxine (T_4): 5.0 to 12.0 μg/dL
3. Thyroxine, free (FT_4): 0.8 to 2.4 ng/dL
4. Triiodothyronine (T_3): 80 to 230 ng/dL

C. Nursing consideration: Test results are invalid if client had undergone a radionuclide scan within 7 days before the test

X. WHITE BLOOD CELL (WBC) COUNT

A. Description
1. WBCs function in the body's immune defense system
2. The WBC count assesses each leukocyte distribution

B. Value: 4500 to 11,000/μL (Table 10-5)

C. Nursing considerations
1. A "shift to the left" means that there is an increased number of immature neutrophils in the peripheral blood
2. A low total WBC count with a left shift indicates a recovery from bone marrow depression or an infection of such intensity that the demand for neutrophils in the tissue is greater than the capacity of the bone marrow to release them into the circulation
3. A high total WBC count with a left shift indicates an increased release of neutrophils by the bone marrow in response to an overwhelming infection or inflammation
4. A "shift to the right" means that cells have more than the usual number of nuclear segments; found in liver disease, Down syndrome, or megaloblastic and pernicious anemia

TABLE 10-5

Normal Adult White Blood Cell Differential

Neutrophils	56% or 1800-7800/μL
Bands	3% or 0-700/μL
Eosinophils	2.7% or 0-450/μL
Basophils	0.3% or 0-200/μL
Lymphocytes	34% or 1000-4800/μL
Monocytes	4% or 0-800/μL

XI. HEPATITIS TESTS

A. Description
1. Tests include radioimmune assay (RIA), enzyme-linked immunosorbent assay (ELISA), and microparticle enzyme immunoassay (MEIA)
2. Serologic tests for specific hepatitis virus markers assist in defining the specific type of hepatitis

B. Values
1. The presence of IgM antibody to hepatitis A virus (IgM anti-HAV) and the total antibody to hepatitis A virus (total anti-HAV) identify the disease
2. Detection of core antigen (HBcAg), envelope antigen (HBeAg), and surface antigen (HBsAg), or their corresponding antibodies, constitutes hepatitis B assessment
3. Hepatitis C is confirmed by the presence of antibodies to hepatitis C (anti-HCV)
4. Serological hepatitis delta virus (HDV) determination is made by detection of the hepatitis D antigen (HDAg) early in the course of the infection and by detection of anti-HDV antibody in the later disease stages
5. Specific serologic tests for hepatitis E virus (HEV) include detection of IgM and IgG antibodies to hepatitis E (anti-HEV)
6. Hepatitis G (HGV) has been found in some blood donors, IV drug users, hemodialysis clients, and clients with hemophilia; however, HGV does not appear to cause significant liver disease

C. Nursing consideration: If the RIA technique is being used, the injection of radionuclides within 1 week before the test may falsely elevate results

XII. HUMAN IMMUNODEFICIENCY VIRUS (HIV) AND ACQUIRED IMMUNODEFICIENCY SYNDROME (AIDS) TESTING

A. Description
1. Detects HIV types 1 and 2 (HIV-1/2), which causes AIDS
2. Tests used to determine the presence of antibodies to HIV-1 include ELISA, Western blot (WB), and indirect fluorescent antibody (IFA)
3. A single reactive ELISA test by itself cannot be used to diagnose AIDS and should be repeated in duplicate with the same blood sample; if repeatedly reactive, follow-up tests using WB or IFA should be done
4. A positive WB or IFA is considered confirmatory for HIV
5. A positive ELISA that fails to be confirmed by WB or IFA should not be considered negative, and repeat testing should take place in 3 to 6 months

B. Nursing considerations
1. Maintain issues of confidentiality surrounding HIV and AIDS testing
2. Follow prescribed state regulations and protocols related to reporting positive test results

XIII. URINE TESTS (Table 10-6)

XIV. THERAPEUTIC SERUM MEDICATION LEVELS (Table 10-7)

PRACTICE QUESTIONS

1. A nurse is reviewing the laboratory results of an adult client with Addison's disease. The nurse identifies that the magnesium level is normal if which of the following are noted?
   1. 2.0 mg/dL
   2. 3.0 mg/dL

TABLE 10-6

Normal Adult Values: Urine Tests

Name of Test	Value
Chloride	110-250 mEq/24 hr
Magnesium	7.3-12.2 mg/dL/day
Potassium	25-125 mEq/24 hr
Protein	40-150 mg/24 hr
Sodium	40-220 mEq/24 hr
Uric acid	250-750 mg/24 hr
pH	4.5-7.8
Specific gravity	1.016 to 1.022

TABLE 10-7

Therapeutic Serum Medication Levels

Medication	Therapeutic Range
Acetaminophen (Tylenol)	10-20 μg/mL
Carbamazepine (Tegretol)	5-12 μg/mL
Digoxin (Lanoxin)	0.5-2.0 ng/mL
Gentamicin (Garamycin)	5-10 μg/mL
Lithium (Lithobid)	0.5-1.3 mEq/L
Magnesium sulfate	4-7 mg/dL
Phenytoin (Dilantin)	10-20 μg/mL
Salicylate	100-250 μg/mL
Theophylline (Aminophylline, Theo-Dur)	10-20 μg/mL
Tobramycin (Nebcin)	5-10 μg/mL
Valproic acid (Depakene)	50-100 μg/mL

   3. 4.0 mg/dL
   4. 5.0 mg/dL
2. A client is suspected of having a myocardial infarction. The nurse would expect elevations in which of the following isoenzyme values reported with the creatine kinase (CK) level?
   1. MM
   2. MB
   3. BB
   4. MK
3. An adult male client has had laboratory work done as part of a routine physical examination. The nurse reviews the client's record and identifies that the client may have a mild degree of renal insufficiency if which of the following serum creatinine levels is found?
   1. 0.6 mg/dL
   2. 1.1 mg/dL
   3. 1.9 mg/dL
   4. 3.5 mg/dL
4. A client with a seizure disorder is taking phenytoin (Dilantin). A serum dilantin level is drawn and the nurse evaluates that the medication therapy is effective if the laboratory result is:
   1. 3 μg/mL
   2. 8 μg/mL
   3. 16 μg/mL
   4. 24 μg/mL
5. A client who takes theophylline for chronic obstructive pulmonary disease (COPD) is seen in the urgent care center for respiratory distress. Just before initiating therapy, a baseline theophylline level is drawn. The nurse determines that the client may not be compliant with medication therapy if the result is:
   1. 6 μg/mL
   2. 11 μg/mL
   3. 15 μg/mL
   4. 18 μg/mL

6. A nurse is told that the laboratory result for a serum digoxin level is 2.4 ng/mL. The nurse plans to do which of the following?
   1. Record the normal value on the client's flow-sheet
   2. Administer the next dose of the medication as scheduled
   3. Check the client's last pulse rate
   4. Hold the medication
7. A client with atrial fibrillation who is receiving maintenance therapy of warfarin sodium (Coumadin) has a prothrombin time (PT) of 30 seconds. The nurse anticipates that which of the following will be prescribed?
   1. Holding the next dose of warfarin sodium
   2. Administering the next dose of warfarin sodium
   3. Increasing the next dose of warfarin sodium
   4. Adding a dose of heparin
8. An adult client who has had preadmission testing before surgery has had blood drawn for determination of serum electrolytes. The nurse identifies which of the following as an abnormal value?
   1. Sodium of 148 mEq/L
   2. Potassium of 3.8 mEq/L
   3. Chloride of 101 mEq/L
   4. Bicarbonate of 26 mEq/L
9. An adult client with a critically high potassium level has received sodium polystyrene sulfonate (Kayexalate). The nurse evaluates that the medication was most effective if the client's repeat serum potassium level is:
   1. 6.2 mEq/L
   2. 5.8 mEq/L
   3. 5.4 mEq/L
   4. 4.9 mEq/L
10. The client with a history of cardiac disease is due for a morning dose of furosemide (Lasix). The nurse reviews the client's record and would report which of the following serum potassium levels before administering the dose of furosemide?
    1. 3.8 mEq/L
    2. 3.2 mEq/L
    3. 4.8 mEq/L
    4. 4.2 mEq/L
11. A client with diabetes mellitus has a fasting blood glucose drawn. The nurse identifies which of the following results as a critical value?
    1. 150 mg/dL
    2. 200 mg/dL
    3. 220 mg/dL
    4. 340 mg/dL
12. An adult client with a history of gastrointestinal bleeding has a platelet count of 300,000 cells/μL. Which of the following actions by the nurse is most appropriate on reading this report?
    1. Report the abnormally low count
    2. Report the abnormally high count
    3. Place the client on bleeding precautions
    4. Place the normal report in the client's medical record
13. An adult client with hepatic cirrhosis has been taking a diet with optimal amounts of protein, since neither excess nor deficiency of protein has been helpful. The nurse evaluates the client's status as most satisfactory if the total protein level is which of the following values in the normal range?
    1. 0.4 g/dL
    2. 3.7 g/dL
    3. 6.4 g/dL
    4. 9.8 g/dL
14. A client is seen in the urgent care center for complaints of chest pain 3 days ago. Since that time, the client has not been feeling well and fatigues easily. The nurse reviews the results of the laboratory tests and would suspect myocardial infarction at the time of chest pain if which of the following isoenzymes for lactic dehydrogenase (LDH) came back positive?
    1. LDH_1
    2. LDH_3
    3. LDH_4
    4. LDH_5
15. An adult client was diagnosed with acute pancreatitis 9 days ago. The nurse interprets that the client is recovering from this episode if the serum lipase level drops to which of the following values, which is just beneath the upper limit of normal?
    1. 20 U/L
    2. 80 U/L
    3. 135 U/L
    4. 250 U/L
16. A nurse has an order to test the stool of a client with Hemoccult slides. The nurse reviews the client's record knowing that which of the following medications can cause false-negative results?
    1. Ascorbic acid
    2. Colchicine
    3. Iodine
    4. Acetylsalicylic acid (aspirin)
17. An adult female client has a hemoglobin level of 10.8 g/dL. The nurse interprets that this result is most likely due to which of the following factors in the client's history?
    1. Chronic obstructive pulmonary disease (COPD)
    2. Heart failure
    3. Dehydration
    4. Iron deficiency anemia
18. An adult male client admitted with dehydration has received fluid volume replacement. The nurse evaluates that the client has had adequate fluid resuscitation if the client's repeat hematocrit level has

decreased to which of the following values in the normal range?

1. 56%
2. 48%
3. 39%
4. 34%

19. A client with diabetes mellitus has a glycosylated hemoglobin HbA_{1c} level of 8%. Based on this test result, the nurse plans to reinforce teaching measures with the client about the need to:
    1. Avoid infection
    2. Take in adequate fluids
    3. Prevent hyperglycemia
    4. Prevent hypoglycemia
20. A client has been diagnosed as having syndrome of inappropriate antidiuretic hormone secretion (SIADH) following cranial surgery. The nurse interprets that this complication is not resolving if which of the following urine specific gravity measurements is obtained?
    1. 1.002
    2. 1.016
    3. 1.020
    4. 1.030
21. A nurse is caring for a client with a diagnosis of cancer who is immunosuppressed. The nurse knows that neutropenic precautions will be implemented if the client's white blood cell (WBC) count is:
    1. 2000/μL
    2. 5800/μL
    3. 8400/μL
    4. 11,500/μL
22. A nurse volunteering at the health screening clinic teaches a 22-year-old client that diet and exercise should be used as tools to keep the total cholesterol level under:
    1. 150 mg/dL
    2. 200 mg/dL
    3. 250 mg/dL
    4. 300 mg/dL
23. A client has been admitted for urinary tract infection and dehydration. The nurse evaluates that the client has received adequate volume replacement if the blood urea nitrogen (BUN) level drops to:
    1. 35 mg/dL
    2. 29 mg/dL
    3. 15 mg/dL
    4. 6 mg/dL
24. A nurse is reviewing the laboratory results of a female adult client suspected of having iron deficiency anemia. The nurse reviews the results knowing that the normal hemoglobin level for this client is:
    1. 10 g/dL
    2. 14 g/dL
    3. 17 g/dL
    4. 19 g/dL
25. A nurse is assigned to a 40-year-old client admitted with chronic pancreatitis. The nurse reviews the client's record and expects to note a serum amylase level that is most similar to which of the following values?
    1. 25 IV/L
    2. 100 IV/L
    3. 300 IV/L
    4. 500 IV/L

ANSWERS

1. *Answer:* 1

Rationale: The normal magnesium level in an adult client is 1.6 to 2.6 mg/dL. Options 2, 3, and 4 indicate elevated values.
Test-Taking Strategy: Use the process of elimination. Knowledge regarding the normal magnesium level in an adult client is required to answer this question. Review this level if you had difficulty with this question.
Level of Cognitive Ability: Comprehension
Client Needs: Physiological Integrity
Integrated Concept/Process: Nursing Process/Data Collection
Content Area: Fundamental Skills
Reference: Chernecky C, Berger B: *Laboratory tests and diagnostic procedures*, ed 3, Philadelphia, 2001, WB Saunders, p. 709.

2. *Answer:* 2

Rationale: CK is a cellular enzyme that can be fractionated into three isoenzymes. The MM band reflects CK from skeletal muscle. The MB band reflects CK from cardiac muscle. This is the level that elevates with myocardial infarction. The BB band reflects CK from the brain. There is no MK band.
Test-Taking Strategy: To answer this question correctly, it is necessary to have specific knowledge of the isoenzymes that are produced with elevations in this enzyme. Review this information if you had difficulty with this question.
Level of Cognitive Ability: Comprehension
Client Needs: Physiological Integrity
Integrated Concept/Process: Nursing Process/Data Collection
Content Area: Fundamental Skills
Reference: Chernecky C, Berger B: *Laboratory tests and diagnostic procedures*, ed 3, Philadelphia, 2001, WB Saunders, p. 305.

3. *Answer:* 3

Rationale: The normal serum creatinine level is 0.6 to 1.3 mg/dL. The client with a mild degree of renal insufficiency would have a slightly elevated level, which would be the value of 1.9 mg/dL. Creatinine levels of 3.5 mg/dL may be associated with acute or chronic renal failure.
Test-Taking Strategy: Note that the key word "mild." This tells you that the correct option will be an abnormal value, but perhaps not the most abnormal of all the options. Use your knowledge of this common laboratory test to direct you to

option 3. Review the normal value of this laboratory test if you had difficulty with this question.
Level of Cognitive Ability: Analysis
Client Needs: Physiological Integrity
Integrated Concept/Process: Nursing Process/Data Collection
Content Area: Fundamental Skills
Reference: Chernecky C, Berger B: *Laboratory tests and diagnostic procedures*, ed 3, Philadelphia, 2001, WB Saunders, p. 399.

4. *Answer:* 3
Rationale: The therapeutic range for serum phenytoin (Dilantin) level is 10 to 20 μg/mL. If the level is below the therapeutic range, the client may continue to experience seizure activity. If the level is too high, the client could experience phenytoin toxicity.
Test-Taking Strategy: To answer this question accurately, specific knowledge is needed about the normal range of results for this laboratory test. Review this normal range if you had difficulty with this question.
Level of Cognitive Ability: Comprehension
Client Needs: Physiological Integrity
Integrated Concept/Process: Nursing Process/Evaluation
Content Area: Fundamental Skills
Reference: Chernecky C, Berger B: *Laboratory tests and diagnostic procedures*, ed 3, Philadelphia, 2001, WB Saunders, p. 817.

5. *Answer:* 1
Rationale: The therapeutic range for the serum theophylline level is 10 to 20 μg/mL. If the level is below the therapeutic range, the client may experience frequent exacerbations of the disorder. If the level is within the therapeutic range, the client is most likely compliant with medication therapy.
Test-Taking Strategy: Note the key words "may not be compliant." Recalling the therapeutic level of theophylline will direct you to option 1. Review this therapeutic range if you had difficulty with this question.
Level of Cognitive Ability: Analysis
Client Needs: Physiological Integrity
Integrated Concept/Process: Nursing Process/Evaluation
Content Area: Fundamental Skills
Reference: Hodgson B, Kizior R: *Saunders nursing drug handbook 2002*, Philadelphia, 2002, WB Saunders, p. 47.

6. *Answer:* 4
Rationale: The normal therapeutic range for digoxin is 0.5 to 2.0 ng/mL. A value of 2.4 exceeds the therapeutic range and could be toxic to the client. The most important action is to hold further doses of digoxin. Option 1 is incorrect because the value is not normal. The next dose should not be administered automatically. Checking the client's pulse is not incorrect but may have limited value. Depending on the time that has elapsed since the last pulse check, it may be more useful to do a current assessment of the client's status.
Test-Taking Strategy: Knowledge regarding the therapeutic range for this medication will assist in answering this question. Noting that the value is high will direct you to option 4. Review this therapeutic level if you had difficulty with this question.
Level of Cognitive Ability: Application
Client Needs: Physiological Integrity
Integrated Concept/Process: Nursing Process/Implementation
Content Area: Fundamental Skills
Reference: Hodgson B, Kizior R: *Saunders nursing drug handbook 2002*, Philadelphia, 2002, WB Saunders, p. 344.

7. *Answer:* 1
Rationale: The normal PT is 9.6 to 11.8 seconds (adult male) and 9.5 to 11.3 seconds (adult female). Since the value stated is extremely high (and perhaps near the critical range), the nurse should anticipate that the client would not receive further doses at this time. If the level were too high, then the antidote (vitamin K) may be prescribed.
Test-Taking Strategy: To answer this question accurately, it is necessary to be familiar with the normal PT level. Review this level if you had difficulty with this question.
Level of Cognitive Ability: Comprehension
Client Needs: Physiological Integrity
Integrated Concept/Process: Nursing Process/Planning
Content Area: Fundamental Skills
Reference: Chernecky C, Berger B: *Laboratory tests and diagnostic procedures*, ed 3, Philadelphia, 2001, WB Saunders, p. 865.

8. *Answer:* 1
Rationale: The normal serum electrolyte ranges for adults is as follows: sodium, 135 to 145 mEq/L; potassium, 3.5 to 5.1 mEq/L; chloride 98 to107 mEq/L; bicarbonate (venous) 22 to 29 mEq/L. The only abnormal value identified is the serum sodium level.
Test-Taking Strategy: Focus on the issue, an abnormal value. Recalling the normal serum electrolyte values will direct you to option 1. Review the normal electrolyte values if you had difficulty with this question.
Level of Cognitive Ability: Comprehension
Client Needs: Physiological Integrity
Integrated Concept/Process: Nursing Process/Data Collection
Content Area: Fundamental Skills
Reference: Chernecky C, Berger B: *Laboratory tests and diagnostic procedures*, ed 3, Philadelphia, 2001, WB Saunders, p. 460.

9. *Answer:* 4
Rationale: The normal serum potassium level in the adult is 3.5 to 5.1 mEq/L. Option 4 is the only option reflecting a value that has dropped down into the normal range.
Test-Taking Strategy: Note the key words "critically high." You would expect that this medication is administered to lower the potassium level. Recalling the normal serum potassium level will direct you to option 4. Review this normal level if you had difficulty with this question.
Level of Cognitive Ability: Analysis
Client Needs: Physiological Integrity
Integrated Concept/Process: Nursing Process/Evaluation
Content Area: Fundamental Skills
Reference: Chernecky, C, Berger, B: *Laboratory tests and diagnostic procedures*, ed 3, Philadelphia, 2001, WB Saunders, p. 549.

10. *Answer:* 2
Rationale: The normal serum potassium level in the adult is 3.5 to 5.1 mEq/L. Option 2 is the only value that falls below the therapeutic range. Administering furosemide to a client

with a low potassium level and a cardiac history could precipitate ventricular dysrhythmias in the client.
Test-Taking Strategy: Use the process of elimination. Familiarity with the normal serum potassium level is needed to answer this question. This will assist you in identifying the value that is not within normal range. Review this normal value if you had difficulty with this question.
Level of Cognitive Ability: Application
Client Needs: Physiological Integrity
Integrated Concept/Process: Nursing Process/Implementation
Content Area: Fundamental Skills
Reference: Chernecky C, Berger B: *Laboratory tests and diagnostic procedures*, ed 3, Philadelphia, 2001, WB Saunders, p. 459.

11. ***Answer:*** 4
Rationale: The normal fasting blood glucose is 70 to110 mg/dL in the adult client. A critical level is considered to be one that exceeds 300 mg/dL. This makes option 4 the correct option.
Test-Taking Strategy: Use the process of elimination and knowledge of the normal fasting blood glucose level to answer the question. Noting the key words "critical value" will direct you to option 4. Review this laboratory test if you had difficulty with this question.
Level of Cognitive Ability: Comprehension
Client Needs: Physiological Integrity
Integrated Concept/Process: Nursing Process/Data Collection
Content Area: Fundamental Skills
Reference: Chernecky C, Berger B: *Laboratory tests and diagnostic procedures*, ed 3, Philadelphia, 2001, WB Saunders, p. 560.

12. ***Answer:*** 4
Rationale: A normal platelet count ranges from 150,000 to 400,000 cells/μL. The nurse should place the report containing the normal laboratory value in the client's medical record.
Test-Taking Strategy: Use the process of elimination. Remember that options that are similar are not likely to be correct. With this in mind, eliminate options 1 and 3 first. From the remaining options, recalling the normal range for this laboratory test will direct you to option 4. Review this normal value if you had difficulty with this question.
Level of Cognitive Ability: Application
Client Needs: Physiological Integrity
Integrated Concept/Process: Nursing Process/Implementation
Content Area: Fundamental Skills
Reference: Chernecky C, Berger B: *Laboratory tests and diagnostic procedures*, ed 3, Philadelphia, 2001, WB Saunders, p. 827.

13. ***Answer:*** 3
Rationale: The normal range for the protein level in the adult client is 6.0 to 8.0 g/dL, making option 3 the correct option. Options 1 and 2 indicate low levels. Option 4 indicates an elevated level.
Test-Taking Strategy: Note the key words "most satisfactory." Recalling the normal protein level will direct you to option 3. Review this normal level if you had difficulty with this question.
Level of Cognitive Ability: Analysis
Client Needs: Physiological Integrity
Integrated Concept/Process: Nursing Process/Evaluation
Content Area: Fundamental Skills
Reference: Chernecky C, Berger B: *Laboratory tests and diagnostic procedures*, ed 3, Philadelphia, 2001, WB Saunders, p. 334.

14. ***Answer:*** 1
Rationale: The isoenzymes that are particularly affected with acute myocardial infarction are LDH_1 and LDH_2. LDH begins to elevate approximately 24 hours after myocardial infarction and peaks in 48 to 72 hours. Thereafter, it returns to normal, usually within 7 to 14 days.
Test-Taking Strategy: Familiarity with the cardiac isoenzymes for LDH is needed to answer this question. Review these enzymes if you had difficulty with this question.
Level of Cognitive Ability: Comprehension
Client Needs: Physiological Integrity
Integrated Concept/Process: Nursing Process/Data Collection
Content Area: Fundamental Skills
Reference: Chernecky C, Berger B: *Laboratory tests and diagnostic procedures*, ed 3, Philadelphia, 2001, WB Saunders, p. 305.

15. ***Answer:*** 3
Rationale: The normal serum lipase level is 10 to 140 U/L. The client who is recovering from acute pancreatitis usually has elevated lipase levels for approximately 10 days after onset of symptoms. This makes lipase a valuable test in monitoring the client's pancreatic function. Option 3 is the only option that contains a value just beneath the upper limit of normal.
Test-Taking Strategy: Note the key words "just beneath the upper limit of normal." Recalling the normal lipase level will direct you to option 3. Review this normal level if you had difficulty with this question.
Level of Cognitive Ability: Comprehension
Client Needs: Physiological Integrity
Integrated Concept/Process: Nursing Process/Evaluation
Content Area: Fundamental Skills
Reference: Chernecky C, Berger B: *Laboratory tests and diagnostic procedures*, ed 3, Philadelphia, 2001, WB Saunders, p. 679.

16. ***Answer:*** 1
Rationale: Ascorbic acid can interfere with the result of occult blood testing, causing false negative results. Colchicine and iodine can cause false-positive results. Acetylsalicylic acid would either have no effect on results or could cause a positive result, since this medication is irritating to the stomach lining.
Test-Taking Strategy: Specific knowledge of interfering factors with occult blood testing is needed to answer this question accurately. Focusing on the issue, a false-negative result, will assist in directing you to option 1. Review the medications that can affect this test if you had difficulty with this question.
Level of Cognitive Ability: Comprehension
Client Needs: Physiological Integrity
Integrated Concept/Process: Nursing Process/Data Collection
Content Area: Fundamental Skills
Reference: Chernecky C, Berger B: *Laboratory tests and diagnostic procedures*, ed 3, Philadelphia, 2001, WB Saunders, p. 239.

17. ***Answer:*** 4
Rationale: The normal hemoglobin level for an adult female client is 12 to 15 g/dL. Iron deficiency anemia can result in

lower hemoglobin levels. Heart failure and COPD may increase the hemoglobin level due to the need by the body for more oxygen carrying capacity. Dehydration may increase the hemoglobin level by hemoconcentration.
Test-Taking Strategy: Use the process of elimination. Evaluate each of the conditions in the options in terms of whether it is likely to raise or lower the hemoglobin level. Review the normal hemoglobin level and the causes of a low level if you had difficulty with this question.
Level of Cognitive Ability: Analysis
Client Needs: Physiological Integrity
Integrated Concept/Process: Nursing Process/Data Collection
Content Area: Fundamental Skills
Reference: Chernecky C, Berger B: *Laboratory tests and diagnostic procedures,* ed 3, Philadelphia, 2001, WB Saunders, p. 594.

18. *Answer:* 2
Rationale: The normal hematocrit level for an adult male is 42% to 52%. The client who is dehydrated has an elevated level owing to hemoconcentration. The client's level may be expected to drift back down to within the normal range once fluid volume has been adequately restored. Thus, option 2 is the only correct choice. Option 1 is too high, while options 3 and 4 are low.
Test-Taking Strategy: Use the process of elimination and note the key words "normal range." Recalling the normal hematocrit level for an adult male will direct you to option 2. Review this normal value if you had difficulty with this question.
Level of Cognitive Ability: Comprehension
Client Needs: Physiological Integrity
Integrated Concept/Process: Nursing Process/Data Collection
Content Area: Fundamental Skills
Reference: Chernecky C, Berger B: *Laboratory tests and diagnostic procedures,* ed 3, Philadelphia, 2001, WB Saunders, p. 592.

19. *Answer:* 3
Rationale: The glycosylated hemoglobin measures the amount of glucose that has become permanently bound to the red blood cells from circulating glucose. Elevations in blood glucose will cause elevations in the amount of glycosylation. Thus the test is useful in detecting clients who have periods of hyperglycemia that are undetected in other ways. Values are expressed as a percentage of total hemoglobin and include diabetic with good control of 7.5% or less; diabetic with fair control of 7.6% to 8.9%; diabetic with poor control of 9% or greater. Elevations indicate continued need for teaching related to prevention of hyperglycemic episodes.
Test-Taking Strategy: Use the process of elimination and focus on the level identified in the question. Recalling the expected values related to this test and their significance will assist in answering correctly. Review this test if you had difficulty with this question.
Level of Cognitive Ability: Application
Client Needs: Health Promotion and Maintenance
Integrated Concept/Process: Teaching/Learning
Content Area: Fundamental Skills
Reference: Chernecky C, Berger B: *Laboratory tests and diagnostic procedures,* ed 3, Philadelphia, 2001, WB Saunders, p. 573.

20. *Answer:* 4
Rationale: The normal range for urine specific gravity is between 1.016 and 1.022. Elevations may occur with SIADH, because the kidneys are stimulated to reabsorb water, thus causing unusual concentration of the urine. Option 1 represents a low value, which may be seen in the client with diabetes insipidus. Options 2 and 3 reflect normal values.
Test-Taking Strategy: Use the process of elimination and note the key words "not resolving." Recalling the normal values for this test will assist in eliminating options 2 and 3. From the remaining options, recalling the pathophysiology associated with SIADH will direct you to option 4. Review this test if you had difficulty with this question.
Level of Cognitive Ability: Analysis
Client Needs: Physiological Integrity
Integrated Concept/Process: Nursing Process/Evaluation
Content Area: Fundamental Skills
Reference: Chernecky C, Berger B: *Laboratory tests and diagnostic procedures,* ed 3, Philadelphia, 201, WB Saunders, p. 410.

21. *Answer:* 1
Rationale: The normal WBC count ranges from 4500 to 11,000/μL. The client who is immunosuppressed has a decrease in the number of circulating WBCs. The nurse implements neutropenic precautions when the client's values fall sufficiently below the low-normal level.
Test-Taking Strategy: Knowledge regarding the normal WBC count and the purpose of neutropenic precautions will direct you to option 1. Review this laboratory test if you had difficulty with this question.
Level of Cognitive Ability: Comprehension
Client Needs: Safe, Effective Care Environment
Integrated Concept/Process: Nursing Process/Implementation
Content Area: Fundamental Skills
Reference: Chernecky C, Berger B: *Laboratory tests and diagnostic procedures,* ed 3, Philadelphia, 2001, WB Saunders, p. 374.

22. *Answer:* 2
Rationale: The normal cholesterol level is 140 to 199 mg/dL. The client should be counseled to keep the total cholesterol level under 200 mg/dL. This will aid in prevention of atherosclerosis, which can lead to a number of cardiovascular disorders later in life.
Test-Taking Strategy: Recalling the normal cholesterol level will direct you to option 2. Review this normal level if you had difficulty with this question.
Level of Cognitive Ability: Application
Client Needs: Health Promotion and Maintenance
Integrated Concept/Process: Teaching/Learning
Content Area: Fundamental Skills
Reference: Chernecky C, Berger B: *Laboratory tests and diagnostic procedures,* ed 3, Philadelphia, 2001, WB Saunders, p. 680.

23. *Answer:* 3
Rationale: The normal BUN for the adult is 8 to 25 mg/dL. Thus option 3 is correct. Values such as those in options 1 and 2 reflect continued dehydration. Option 4 reflects a lower than normal value, which may occur with fluid overload, among other conditions.

Test-Taking Strategy: Use the process of elimination and note the key words "adequate volume replacement." Recalling the normal BUN level will direct you to option 3. Review this level if you had difficulty with this question.
Level of Cognitive Ability: Comprehension
Client Needs: Physiological Integrity
Integrated Concept/Process: Nursing Process/Evaluation
Content Area: Fundamental Skills
Reference: Chernecky C, Berger B: *Laboratory tests and diagnostic procedures*, ed 3, Philadelphia, 2001, WB Saunders, p. 237.

24. *Answer:* 2
Rationale: The normal hemoglobin level for an adult female is 12 to 15 g/dL. Option 1 is a low value and would indicate an anemia. Options 3 and 4 are elevated values.
Test-Taking Strategy: Knowledge regarding the normal hemoglobin level will direct you to option 2. If you are unfamiliar with this laboratory value, review its normal value.
Level of Cognitive Ability: Comprehension
Client Needs: Physiological Integrity
Integrated Concept/Process: Nursing Process/Data Collection
Content Area: Fundamental Skills
Reference: Chernecky C, Berger B: *Laboratory tests and diagnostic procedures*, ed 3, Philadelphia, 2001, WB Saunders, p. 594.

25. *Answer:* 3
Rationale: The normal serum amylase level is 25 to 151 IV/L. With chronic cases of pancreatitis, the rise in serum amylase levels usually does not exceed three times the normal value. In acute pancreatitis, the value may exceed five times the normal value.
Test-Taking Strategy: Familiarity with the normal serum amylase level is needed to answer this question. Note the key word "chronic." It is also necessary to understand the effects of chronic pancreatitis on this laboratory value. Review these effects if you had difficulty with this question.
Level of Cognitive Ability: Analysis
Client Needs: Physiological Integrity
Integrated Concept/Process: Nursing Process/Data Collection
Content Area: Fundamental Skills
Reference: Chernecky C, Berger B: *Laboratory tests and diagnostic procedures*, ed 3, Philadelphia, 2001, WB Saunders, p. 158.

REFERENCES

Chernecky C, Berger B: *Laboratory tests and diagnostic procedures*, ed 3, Philadelphia, 2001, WB Saunders.

DeWit S: *Fundamental concepts and skills for nursing*, Philadelphia, 2001, WB Saunders.

Hodgson B, Kizior R: *Saunders nursing drug handbook 2002*, Philadelphia, 2002, WB Saunders.

National Council of State Boards of Nursing, editors: *Test plan for the National Council Licensure Examination for Practical/Vocational Nurses.* Chicago, 2001, Author.

Potter P, Perry A: *Fundamentals of nursing*, ed 5, St Louis, 2001, Mosby.

Nutritional Components of Care

PYRAMID TERMS

Absorption Passage of digested nutrients through the wall of the stomach or small intestine into the blood or lymph system.

Anorexia A lack of appetite with no desire to eat.

Central Parenteral Nutrition (CPN) Parenteral nutrition, administered through the subclavian or internal jugular vein, that is used when feeding must last longer than 7 days; known as total parenteral nutrition (TPN).

Digestion The breakdown of carbohydrates, fats, and proteins into monosaccharides, fatty acids, and amino acids.

Enteral Nutrition Administering nutrition with liquefied foods into the gastrointestinal (GI) tract via a tube.

Malnutrition Deficiency of the nutrients required for development and maintenance of the human body.

Metabolism Ongoing chemical process within the body that converts digested nutrients into energy for the functioning of body cells.

Nutrients Includes carbohydrates, fats/lipids, proteins, vitamins, minerals, and water. Must be supplied in adequate amounts to provide energy, growth, development, and maintenance of the human body.

PYRAMID TO SUCCESS

Nutrition is a basic need that must be met for all clients. Nurses must have the knowledge required to educate and care for healthy clients, as well as clients with nutritional needs or disorders requiring alterations in dietary measures. NCLEX-PN will address the dietary measures required for basic needs and for particular body system alterations. When presented with a question related to nutrition, consider the client's diagnosis and the particular requirement or restriction necessary for treatment of the disorder. Pyramid points focus on the common types of therapeutic diets, nutrients contained in food items, and enteral feedings. The Integrated Concepts and Processes addressed in this chapter include Clinical Problem-Solving Process (Nursing Process), Caring, Communication and Documentation, Cultural Awareness, Self-Care, and Teaching/Learning.

CLIENT NEEDS

Safe, Effective Care Environment

Standard (universal) and other precautions
Asepsis
Informed consent
Dietary consultation
Home care referral

Health Promotion and Maintenance

Lifestyle choices
Disease prevention
Health promotion programs
Collecting physical data
Client and family dietary teaching

Psychosocial Integrity

Religious and cultural influences on health
Role changes
Promoting self-care
Support systems

Physiological Integrity

Nutrition and oral hydration
Assistance with care
Elimination
Enteral feedings
Laboratory values
Alteration in body systems

Monitoring for potential complications of enteral feedings
Monitoring for expected effects of treatment
Documentation

I. NUTRIENTS

A. Carbohydrates (Table 11-1)
1. The preferred source of energy
2. Include sugars, starches, and cellulose, and provides 4 cal/g
3. Promote normal fat **metabolism**, spare protein, and enhance lower GI function
4. Major food sources include milk, grains, fruits, and vegetables
5. Inadequate carbohydrate intake affects **metabolism**

B. Fats (Table 11-2)
1. Provide a concentrated source and a stored form of energy
2. Protect internal organs and maintain body temperature
3. Enhance **absorption** of the fat-soluble vitamins
4. Provide 9 cal/g
5. Inadequate fat intake leads to clinical manifestations of sensitivity to cold, skin lesions, increased risk of infection, and amenorrhea in women
6. Diets high in fat can lead to obesity and increase the risk of cardiac disease and some cancers

C. Proteins (Box 11-1)
1. Made from amino acids, critical to all aspects of growth and development of body tissues, and provides 4 cal/g
2. Build and repair body tissues, regulate fluid balance, maintain acid-base balance, produce antibodies, provide energy, and produce enzymes and hormones
3. Essential amino acids (EAAs) are required in the diet because the body cannot manufacture them
4. High-quality proteins or complete proteins such as eggs, dairy products, meat, fish, and poultry contain adequate amounts of EAAs
5. Foods that do not contain the EAAs in sufficient amounts are lower-quality or incomplete proteins
6. Inadequate protein can cause protein-energy **malnutrition** and severe wasting of fat and muscle tissue

D. Vitamins (Box 11-2)
1. Facilitate **metabolism** of proteins, fats, and carbohydrates; act as catalysts for metabolic functions; promote life and growth processes; and maintain and regulate body functions
2.  Fat-soluble vitamins A, D, E, and K can be stored in the body, so an excess can cause toxicity
3. The B vitamins and vitamin C are water soluble, are not stored in the body, and can be excreted in the urine
4.  Vitamin K acts as a catalyst for facilitating blood-clotting factors, especially prothrombin

TABLE 11-1

Carbohydrate Food Sources

Glucose	Fructose	Cellulose	Lactose
Grapes	Honey	Bran	Milk
Oranges	Fruits	Apples	
Dates		Beans	
Corn		Cabbage	
Carrots			
Sucrose		**Starch**	
Granulated table sugar		Wheat	
Molasses		Corn	
Apricots		Oats	
Peaches		Rye	
Plums		Barley	
Honeydew and cantaloupe		Potatoes and pasta	
Peas and corn		Beets, carrots, and peas	

TABLE 11-2

Fat Food Sources

Saturated Fats	Cholesterol
Beef	Animal products
Lunch meats	Egg yolks
Hard yellow cheeses	Liver and organ meats
Butter	
Polyunsaturated Fats	**Monounsaturated Fats**
Safflower oil	Duck and goose
Corn oil	Eggs
Sunflower oil	Olive and peanut oils

BOX 11-1

Protein Food Sources

Meats
Dairy products
Cereal products
Dried beans

BOX 11-2

Food Sources of Vitamins

WATER SOLUBLE

Vitamin C (ascorbic acid): Citrus fruits, tomatoes, broccoli, cabbage

Vitamin B_1 (thiamine): Pork and nuts, whole grain cereals, and legumes

Vitamin B_2 (riboflavin): Milk, lean meats, fish, grains

Niacin: Meats, poultry, fish, beans, peanuts, grains

Vitamin B_6 (pryidoxine): Yeast, corn, meat, poultry, fish

Vitamin B_{12} (cobalamin): Meat, liver

Folic acid: Green, leafy vegetables; liver, beef, and fish; legumes; grapefruit, and oranges

FAT SOLUBLE

Vitamin A: Liver, egg yolk, whole milk, green or orange vegetables, fruits

Vitamin D: Fortified milk, fish oils, cereals

Vitamin E: Vegetable oils; green, leafy vegetables; cereals; apricots, apples, and peaches

Vitamin K: Green, leafy vegetables; cauliflower, and cabbage

5. Vitamin C produces collagen, a vital component in wound healing
6. Vitamin A maintains eyesight and epithelial linings

E. Minerals (Box 11-3)
1. Components of hormones, cells, tissues, and bones
2. Act as catalysts for chemical reactions and enhancers of cell function
3. Almost all foods contain some form of minerals
4. A deficiency of minerals can occur in chronically ill or hospitalized clients

II. FOOD GUIDE PYRAMID (Figure 11-1)

A. Groups six broad families of foods with similar kinds of **nutrients** together

B. Levels of the pyramid
1. Level one (base of the pyramid)
   a. Bread, cereal, rice, and pasta group
   b. Daily recommendation is 6 to 11 servings
2. Level two
   a. Vegetables and fruit group
   b. Daily recommendation is 3 to 5 servings of vegetables and 2 to 4 servings of fruit
3. Level three
   a. Includes the milk, yogurt, and cheese group and the meats, poultry, fish, dry beans and peas, eggs, and nuts group
   b. Daily recommendation is 2 to 3 servings for each group
   c. The recommendation for the milk group depends on the various life stage of the individual
4. Peak of the pyramid
   a. Includes fats, oils, and sweets group
   b. Foods are high in fats, sugar, or alcohol and are to be eaten sparingly because they are kilocalorie-dense, nutrient-sparse foods

III. THERAPEUTIC DIETS

A. Clear liquid diet
1. Indications
   a. Serves a primary function of providing fluids and electrolytes to prevent dehydration
   b. Initial feeding after complete bowel rest
   c. Used initially to feed a malnourished person or a person who has not had any oral intake for some time
   d. Bowel preparation for surgery or tests
   e. Postsurgical diet
   f. Diarrhea
2. Nursing considerations
   a. Clear liquid is deficient in energy and most **nutrients**
   b. The body digests and absorbs clear liquids easily
   c. Contributes to little or no residue in the GI tract
   d. Can be unappetizing and boring
   e. Client should not stay on a clear liquid diet for more than a day or two
   f. Consists of foods that are relatively transparent to light, and are clear and liquid at room and body temperature
   g. Foods include such items as water, bouillon, clear broth, carbonated beverages, gelatin, hard candy, lemonade, Popsicles, and either regular or decaffeinated coffee or tea
   h. The nurse should limit the amount of caffeine consumed by the client because caffeine can cause an upset stomach and sleeplessness
   i. Client may have salt or sugar
   j. Dairy products are not allowed

B. Full liquid diet
1. Indication: May be used as a second diet after clear liquids after surgery, or for the client who is unable to chew or swallow
2. Nursing considerations
   a. Nutritionally deficient in energy and most **nutrients**
   b. Includes both clear and opaque liquid foods and those that liquefy at body temperature 

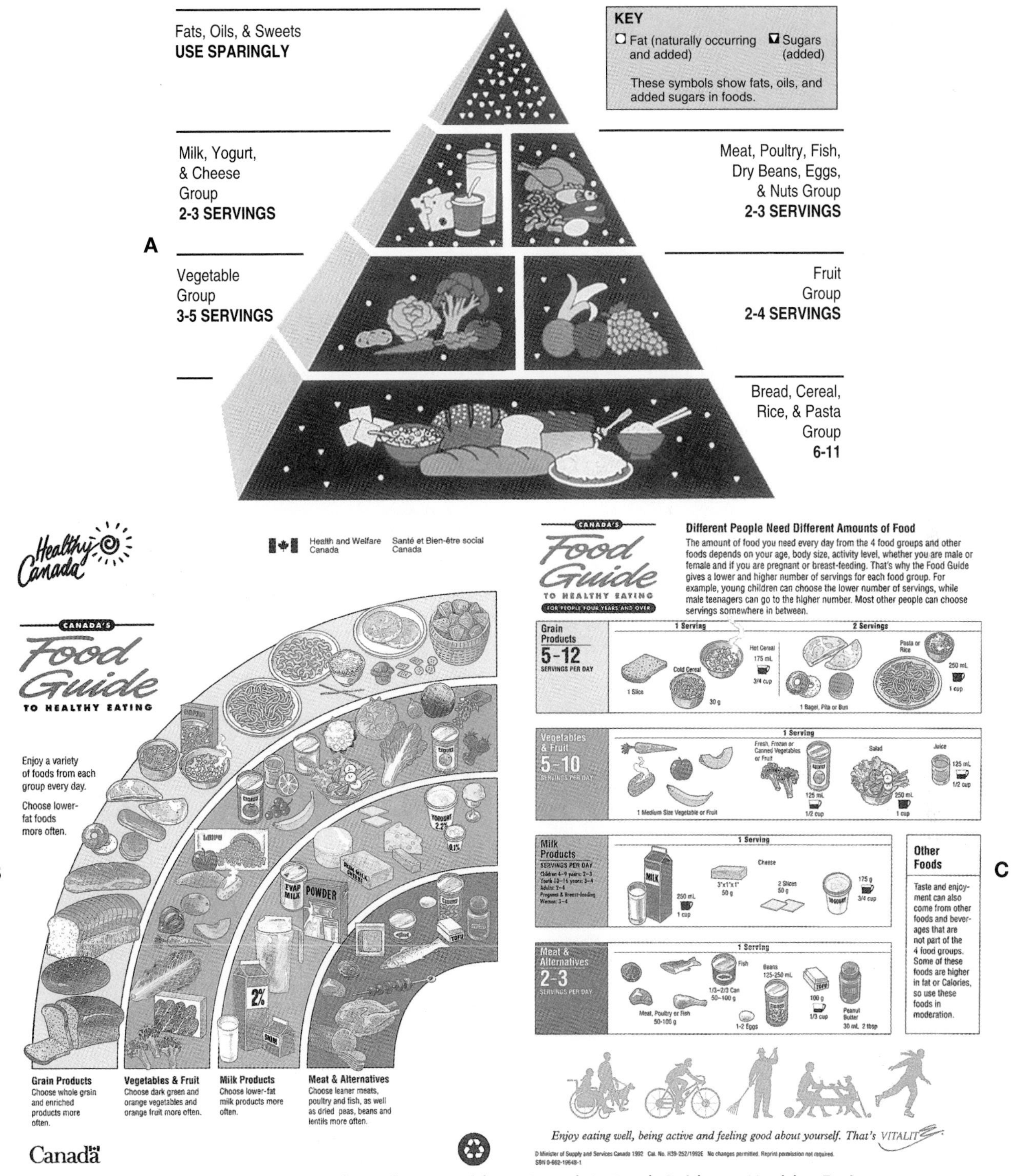

FIG. 11-1 A, U.S. Food Guide Pyramid. B, Canada's Food Guide to Healthy Eating. (From U.S. Department of Agriculture: *USDA's food guide pyramid*, USDA Human Nutrition Information Service Pub No. 249, Washington DC, 1996, U.S. Government Printing Office; and Ottawa, 1992, Health and Welfare Canada, Minister of Supply and Services Canada: Catalogue H-39-252/1992.)

c. Foods include all clear liquids, and such items as plain ice cream, sherbet, breakfast drinks, milk, pudding and custard, soups that are strained, and strained vegetable juices

C. Soft diet
   1. Indications
      a. Used in clients with dental problems, clients with poor-fitting dentures, and clients who have difficulty chewing or swallowing

BOX 11-3

Food Sources of Minerals

CALCIUM
Yogurt, low-fat
Milk
Rhubarb
Collard greens
Cheese
Tofu
Spinach
Broccoli
Green beans
Carrots

CHLORIDE
Salt

MAGNESIUM
Green leafy vegetables
Avocado
Canned white tuna fish
Low-fat yogurt
Cooked rolled oats
Milk
Peas
Potatoes
Pork, beef, chicken
Raisins
Peanut butter
Cauliflower

PHOSPHORUS
Fish
Pork, beef, chicken
Organ meats
Nuts
Whole-grain breads and cereals

ZINC
Meats, eggs, leafy vegetables, protein-rich foods

POTASSIUM
Avocado
Raisins
Pork, beef, veal
Cantaloupe
Spinach
Bananas
Fish
Oranges
Strawberries
Mushrooms
Carrots
Potatoes
Tomatoes

SODIUM
Table salt
Soy sauce
Cured pork
Cottage cheese
American cheese
Milk
Butter
White and whole-wheat bread
Ketchup
Mustard
Bacon
Frankfurters
Lunch meat
Canned food
Processed food
Snack food

IRON
Liver, meats, egg yolk, dark-green vegetables, breads and cereals

b. Used for ulcerations of the mouth or gums, oral surgery, broken jaw, plastic surgery of the head or neck, dysphasia, or for the stroke client
c. Therapeutic for clients with impaired **digestion** and/or **absorption** as a result of conditions such as ulcerative colitis and Crohn's disease

2. Nursing considerations

a. Clients with mouth sores should be served foods at cooler temperatures

b. Clients who have difficulty chewing and swallowing because of a reduced flow of saliva can increase salivary flow by sucking on sour candy
c. Encourage the client to eat a variety of foods
d. Provide plenty of fluids with meals to ease chewing and swallowing of foods
e. Sucking fluids through a straw may be easier than drinking them from a cup or glass
f. All foods and seasonings are permitted; however, liquid, chopped, or puréed foods, or regular foods with a soft consistency are best tolerated
g. Avoid foods than contain nuts or seeds, which can become easily trapped in the mouth and cause discomfort
h. Raw fruits and vegetables, fried foods, and whole grains are avoided

D. Bland diet
  1. Indication: May be used for the client with gastritis, ulcers, reflux esophagitis, congestive heart failure (CHF), or myocardial infarction (MI)
  2. Nursing considerations
    a. Bland foods are less likely to form gas than regular diets
    b. Eliminate foods that stimulate gastric acid secretions
    c. Eliminate foods that are irritating to the gastric mucosa
    d. Foods to be avoided include alcohol; caffeine and caffeine-containing beverages such as cola, cocoa, coffee, and tea; fried foods; pepper and spicy foods

E. Low-residue/low-fiber diet
  1. Indications
    a. Supplies foods that are least likely to form an obstruction when the intestinal tract is narrowed by inflammation or scarring, or when GI motility is slowed
    b. Used for inflammatory bowel disease, ileostomy, colostomy, partial obstructions of the intestinal tract, enteritis, or diarrhea
  2. Nursing considerations
    a. Foods high in carbohydrate are usually low in residue and include white bread, cereals, and pasta
    b. Foods to be avoided are raw fruits (except bananas), vegetables, seeds, plant fiber, and whole grains
    c. Dairy products are limited to two servings a day

F. High-fiber diet
  1. Indications
    a. Used in constipation
    b. Used in irritable bowel syndrome when the primary symptom is alternating constipation and diarrhea
    c. Helps regulate blood glucose in clients with diabetes mellitus
    d. Helps control blood cholesterol in clients with heart disease
  2. Nursing considerations
    a. Provides 20 to 25 g of dietary fiber daily
    b. Adds volume and weight to the stool and speeds the movement of undigested materials through the intestine
    c. Consists of fruits and vegetables

G. Fat-controlled diet (Table 11-2)
  1. Indications
    a. Indicated for atherosclerosis, diabetes mellitus, hyperlipidemia, hypertension, MI, nephrotic syndrome, and renal failure
    b. Reduces the risk of heart disease
  2. Nursing consideration: Limit both the total amount of fats and amounts of polyunsaturated, monounsaturated, and saturated fats and cholesterol

H. High-calorie diet
  1. Indications: Severe stress, burns, cancer, human immunodeficiency virus (HIV) infections, acquired immunodeficiency syndrome (AIDS), chronic obstructive pulmonary disease (COPD), respiratory failure, or any other type of debilitating disease
  2. Nursing considerations
    a. The high-calorie diet should also be high in protein because the purpose of the diet is to build or maintain lean body mass
    b. Add fats to foods whenever possible
    c. Add nuts and dried fruits such as raisins to desserts or cereals if the client can tolerate and eat these foods
    d. Add sugar to food, and provide high-calorie desserts
    e. Encourage snacks between meals, such as milkshakes and instant breakfasts

I. Sodium restriction diet
  1. Indications: Hypertension, CHF, kidney diseases, cardiac diseases, and cirrhosis of the liver
  2. Nursing considerations (Box 11-4)
    a. The amount of sodium allowed varies from 250 mg to about 4 g of sodium daily
    b. A no-added-salt diet includes no salt at the table and lightly salting foods during cooking
    c. Cereals allowed on a sodium-restricted diet include dried or instant cereals, puffed wheat, puffed rice, and shredded wheat

J. Protein-restriction diet
  1. Indications: Acute renal failure, chronic renal disease, cirrhosis of the liver, and hepatic coma
  2. Nursing considerations
    a. Provide enough protein to maintain nutritional status but not an amount that will allow the build-up of waste products from protein **metabolism** (40 to 60 g of protein daily)
    b. The smaller the amount of protein allowed, the more important it becomes that all protein included in the diet be of high quality
    c. An adequate total energy intake from foods is critical for clients on protein-restricted diets (protein will be used for energy, rather than for protein synthesis)
    d. Special low-protein products, such as pastas, bread, cookies, wafers, and gelatin made with wheat starch, can improve energy intake and add variety to the diet

BOX 11-4

Sodium-Free Spices and Flavorings

Allspice
Almond extract
Bay leaves
Caraway seeds
Cinnamon
Curry powder
Garlic powder or garlic
Ginger
Lemon extract
Maple extract
Marjoram
Mustard powder
Nutmeg

e. Carbohydrates in powdered or liquid forms can also provide additional energy
f. Vegetables and fruits contain some protein, and for very low-protein diets, these foods must be calculated into the diet
g. Foods are limited from the milk, meat, bread, and starch exchange

K. High-protein diet
1. Indications: Tissue building, burns, liver disease, and maternity clients
2. Nursing considerations
a. High-protein diets correct protein loss or assist with tissue repair by increasing the intake of protein food sources
b. Increase foods such as meat, fish, fowl, and dairy products
c. The client may need protein supplements

L. Low-calcium diet
1. Indication: To prevent renal calculi (Table 11-3)
2. Nursing considerations: Decrease the total intake of calcium to prevent further stone formation; avoid whole grains, milk and dairy products, and green, leafy vegetables

M. High-calcium diet
1. Indications: Calcium is needed during bone growth and in adulthood to prevent osteoporosis
2. Nursing considerations
a. Primary dietary sources of calcium are dairy products (refer to Chapter 8, Box 8-6, for food items high in calcium)
b. Clients experiencing lactose intolerance need to regularly incorporate sources of calcium other than dairy products into their dietary patterns

N. Low-purine diet
1. Indication: Used to treat gout
2. Nursing considerations

TABLE 11-3

Diets for Renal Calculi

ALKALINE ASH DIET
Purpose: **To increase pH**
Foods:
Milk
Fruits except cranberries, blueberries, plums, and prunes
Rhubarb
Vegetables
Small amounts of beef, halibut, veal, trout, and salami allowed

ACID ASH DIET
Purpose: To decrease pH
Foods:
Eggs
Meat
Cranberries, blueberries, plums, prunes
Fish
Poultry
Oysters

a. Purine is a precursor for uric acid that forms stones and crystals
b. The client needs to avoid consuming fish such as anchovies, herring, mackerel, sardines, and scallops
c. The client needs to avoid consuming glandular meats, gravies, meat extracts, wild game, goose, and sweetbreads

O. High-iron diet
1. Indication: Used in anemia
2. Nursing considerations
a. Replaces iron deficit from inadequate intake or loss
b. Includes organ meats, meat, egg yolks, whole wheat products, leafy vegetables, dried fruit, legumes

P. Diet for diverticular disease
1. Symptomatic diverticulitis: fiber is avoided because fiber is irritating to the bowel
2. Asymptomatic diverticular disease: a high-fiber diet is consumed to prevent constipation
3. The client should maintain a liberal fluid intake of 2500 to 3000 mL/day, unless contraindicated
4. Seeds and nuts should be avoided because they get trapped in the diverticula and cause irritation
5. Gas-forming foods need to be avoided (Box 11-5)

Q. Fluid restriction (Box 11-6)
1. Indications: Acute renal failure–oliguric phase, chronic renal disease, cirrhosis of the liver, CHF, hepatic coma, and MI

BOX 11-5

Gas-Forming Foods

Apples
Artichokes
Barley
Beans
Bran
Broccoli
Brussels sprouts
Cabbage
Celery
Cherries
Coconuts
Eggplant
Figs
Honey
Melons
Milk
Molasses
Nuts
Onions
Radishes
Soybeans
Wheat
Yeast

BOX 11-6

Measures to Relieve Thirst

Chew gum or suck hard candy
Freeze fluids so they take longer to consume
Add lemon juice to water to make it more refreshing
Gargle with refrigerated mouthwash

2. Nursing considerations: Usually this diet restricts those foods that are composed largely of water such as carbonated beverage, coffee, juices, milk, tea, water, frozen yogurt, gelatin, ice-cream, ice milk, Popsicles, sherbet, soup, cream, liquid medications

R. Carbohydrate-controlled diet
1. Indications
a. Helps maintain normal glucose levels in clients with disorders that cause blood glucose levels to rise or fall abnormally
b. Used for diabetes mellitus, hypoglycemia, lactose intolerance, galactosemia, dumping syndrome, and obesity
2. Nursing considerations
a. Adjust energy intake from foods so as to provide specific amounts and types of carbohydrates
b. The exchange list system is used most frequently to plan carbohydrate-controlled diets

S. Miscellaneous diets: Refer to Chapter 8 Boxes 8-4; 8-5; 8-7; 8-8 for foods high in potassium, sodium, magnesium, and phosphorus, respectively

IV. THE EXCHANGE SYSTEM

A. Starches and breads
1. One bread is equal to 15 g of carbohydrate, 3 g of protein, trace of fat, and 80 calories
2. One bread is equal to 3/4 cup ready-to-eat cereal, 1/3 cup cooked beans, 1/2 cup corn

B. Meats
1. One lean meat is equal to 7 g of protein, 3 g of fat, and 55 calories
2. One meat exchange is equal to 1 ounce
3. One ounce of lean meat is equal to 1 ounce of chicken meat without skin, 1 ounce of any fish, 1/4 cup canned tuna, 1 ounce low-fat cheese
4. Medium-fat meats
a. One medium-fat meat is equal to 7 g of protein, 5 g of fat, and about 75 calories
b. One ounce medium-fat meat is equal to 1 ounce lean meat in protein content but has 5 g of fat
c. Equal to 1 ounce pork loin, 1 egg, 1/4 cup creamed cottage cheese
5. High-fat meats
a. One high-fat meat is equal to 7 g of protein, 8 g of fat, and 100 calories
b. A hotdog counts as 1 high-fat meat exchange plus 1 fat exchange
c. One ounce high-fat meat is equal to 1 ounce lean meat in protein content but includes an extra 1 fat
d. Equal to 1 ounce ham, 1 ounce cheddar cheese, 1 small hotdog
e. Peanut butter is like a meat in terms of its protein content
f. One tablespoon peanut butter is equal to 1 high-fat meat
g. One tablespoon peanut butter is equal to 7 g of protein, 8 g of fat, and 100 calories

C. Vegetables
1. One vegetable is equal to 5 g of carbohydrate, 2 g of protein, and 25 calories
2. A half cup of carrots is equal to 1/2 cup of greens, 1/2 cup of brussels sprouts, 1/2 cup of beets

D. Fruits
1. One fruit is equal to 15 g of carbohydrate and 60 calories
2. One-half banana is equal to one small apple, 1/2 grapefruit, 1/2 cup orange juice

E. Milks

1. One milk is equal to 12 g of carbohydrate, 8 g of protein, trace of fat, and 90 calories
2. One cup nonfat milk is equal to 1 cup of nonfat plain yogurt, 1 cup of nonfat butter milk, 1/2 cup evaporated nonfat milk

F. Fats
1. One fat is equal to 5 g of fat and 45 calories
2. One teaspoon (tsp) of butter is equal to 1 tsp margarine, 1 tsp any oil, 1 tablespoon salad dressing, 1 strip of bacon, 5 large olives, 10 whole peanuts

G. Legumes
1. Similar to meats, are rich in protein and iron, and are lower in fat than meat
2. Contain starch
3. One cup of legumes is equal to 1 lean meat plus 2 starches
4. One cup of legumes is equal to 30 g of carbohydrates, 13 g of protein, 3 g of fat, and 215 calories

V. ENTERAL NUTRITION

A. Description: Provides liquefied foods into the GI tract via a tube

B. Indications
1. When the GI tract is functional but oral intake is not feasible
2. Used for clients with swallowing problems, burns, major trauma, liver failure, or severe **malnutrition**

C. Nursing considerations
1. Clients with lactose intolerance need to be placed on lactose-free formulas
2. Refer to Chapter 18 for information regarding administering GI tube feedings

VI. TOTAL PARENTERAL NUTRITION (TPN)

A. Description
1. Supplies necessary nutrients via veins
2. Supplies carbohydrates in the form of dextrose, fats in a special emulsified form, proteins in the form of amino acids, vitamins, and minerals
3. Prevents subcutaneous fat and muscle protein from being catabolized by the body for energy

B. Indications
1. When the GI tract is severely dysfunctional or nonfunctional
2. Clients who can take some oral nutrition, but not enough to meet the body's needs
3. Clients with multiple GI surgeries, GI trauma, severe intolerance to enteral feedings, intestinal obstructions, or when the bowel needs to rest for healing
4. Clients with acquired immunodeficiency syndrome (AIDS), cancer, or malnutrition

C. Intravenous sites
1. Peripheral Parenteral Nutrition (PPN)
   a. Administered through a peripheral vein
   b. Used for short periods (5 to 7 days) and when the client needs only small concentrations of carbohydrates, fats, and proteins
2. **Central Parenteral Nutrition (CPN)**
   a. Administered through the subclavian or internal jugular veins
   b. Used when feeding must last longer than 7 days

D. Complications (Box 11-7)

E. Precautions
1. Assist with insertion of catheter; position the client in Trendelenburg position with a towel under the scapula
2. Ask the client to perform the Valsalva maneuver during insertion to prevent air emboli
3. When the central line is inserted, placement is confirmed by chest x-ray study
4. TPN catheter is not used for blood draws or the administration of other medications or fluids
5. TPN is always delivered via an electronic infusion device
6. Solutions should be stored under refrigeration
7. TPN solution is changed every 24 hours

F. Nursing interventions
1. Maintain aseptic technique
2. Monitor vital signs
3. Monitor weight and I&O daily
4. Monitor site for redness, swelling, tenderness, or drainage
5. Monitor urine for glucose and acetone four times a day
6. Electrolytes, glucose, and blood urea nitrogen (BUN) are monitored as prescribed
7. Monitor infusion rate hourly
8. If sepsis is suspected, a blood culture will be drawn, and the tip of the catheter will be cultured for bacteria
9. Monitor for signs of fluid overload such as a bounding pulse, jugular vein distention, headache, increased blood pressure, and lung crackles

BOX 11-7

Complications of TPN

Infection
Hyperglycemia
Fluid overload
Air embolism

10. If the IV tubing disconnects, instruct the client to perform the Valsalva maneuver
11. Monitor for signs of an air embolus such as confusion, pallor, light-headedness, tachycardia, tachypnea, hypotension, anxiety, and unresponsiveness
12. Place the client in the left side-lying position with head lower than feet if air embolism is suspected, and contact the physician

G. Fat emulsion
1. Assess for allergy to eggs, a contraindication for lipid infusion
2. Administer slowly for the first 15 to 30 minutes and monitor the client for adverse reactions such as dyspnea, cyanosis, and allergic responses
3. Monitor for signs and symptoms of fat overload, which include fever, leukocytosis, hyperlipidemia, pruritic urticaria, and possibly focal seizures

PRACTICE QUESTIONS

1. A low-sodium diet has been prescribed for a client with hypertension. After diet teaching, which of the following foods, if selected from the menu by the client, would best indicate an understanding of this diet?
   1. Tomato soup
   2. Baked turkey
   3. Chicken gumbo soup
   4. Boiled shrimp
2. A nurse is providing dietary instructions to a client with gout. Which of the following foods would the nurse instruct the client to avoid?
   1. Macaroni products
   2. Corn bread
   3. Scallops
   4. Chocolate
3. A clear liquid diet has been prescribed for a client with gastroenteritis. Which of the following items would be most appropriate to offer to the client?
   1. Orange juice
   2. Strained soup
   3. Fat-free broth
   4. Soft custard
4. A client with diabetes mellitus has been instructed in the dietary exchange system. The client asks the nurse if bacon is allowed in the diet. Which of the following responses is most appropriate?
   1. "Bacon is much too high in fat."
   2. "Bacon is not allowed."
   3. "One strip of bacon may be eaten if you eliminate one teaspoon of butter."
   4. "Bacon may be eaten if you eliminate one meat item from your diet."
5. A client has been diagnosed with enteritis. Which of the following diets would the nurse anticipate to be prescribed for the client?
   1. High residue
   2. Low residue
   3. High carbohydrate
   4. Low fat
6. A client with heart disease is instructed regarding a low-fat diet. The nurse evaluates that the client understands the diet if the client states a food item to avoid is:
   1. Apples
   2. Oranges
   3. Avocado
   4. Cherries
7. A nurse instructs a client to increase the content of riboflavin in the diet. The nurse instructs the client to select which of the following food items that is high in riboflavin?
   1. Milk
   2. Tomatoes
   3. Citrus fruits
   4. Green, leafy vegetables
8. A nurse instructs a client to increase the content of thiamine in the diet. The nurse instructs the client to select which of the following food items that is especially high in thiamine?
   1. Chicken
   2. Broccoli
   3. Pork
   4. Milk
9. A nurse caring for a client with a neurological disorder is assisting in planning care to maintain nutritional status. The nurse is concerned about the client's swallowing ability. The nurse avoids including which of the following food items in this client's diet?
   1. Cheese casserole
   2. Scrambled eggs
   3. Mashed potatoes
   4. Spinach
10. A burned client is transferred to the nursing unit and a regular diet has been prescribed. The nurse encourages the client to eat which dietary items to promote wound healing?
   1. Veal, potatoes, Jell-O, orange juice
   2. Peanut butter and jelly sandwich, cantaloupe, tea
   3. Chicken breast, broccoli, strawberries, milk
   4. Spaghetti with tomato sauce, garlic bread, ginger ale
11. A nurse is assisting a client who has had a cerebrovascular accident (CVA) to eat. The nurse implements which of the following that will best promote independence?

1. Offer only pureed foods
2. Sit the client in high Fowler's position
3. Place the food tray on the unaffected side
4. Encourage the client to eat with other clients who have had CVAs

12. A nurse has completed diet teaching for a client on a low-sodium diet to treat hypertension. The nurse evaluates that further teaching is necessary when the client makes which of these statements?
    1. "This diet will help to lower my blood pressure."
    2. "The reason I need lower salt intake is to reduce fluid retention."
    3. "This diet is not a replacement for my antihypertensive medications."
    4. "Frozen foods are lowest in sodium."
13. A client is on a diet designed to avoid concentrated sugars. The nurse evaluates that the client understands the diet plan if which of these diets is selected by the client?
    1. Strawberry yogurt, lettuce salad, coffee
    2. Chicken salad, tomato, Jell-O, instant iced tea
    3. Peanut butter and jelly sandwich, sherbet, cola
    4. Tuna sandwich, lettuce salad, watermelon, herbal tea
14. A nurse is assigned to care for a client receiving enteral feedings. The nurse plans care knowing that which of the following is of highest priority for this client?
    1. Altered nutrition
    2. Risk for aspiration
    3. Risk for fluid volume deficit
    4. Risk for diarrhea
15. A client receiving total parenteral nutrition (TPN) may begin to take small amounts of clear liquids today. The nurse's priority is to collect data regarding which of the following before giving the client anything by mouth?
    1. Client's appetite
    2. Client's weight today
    3. Presence of swallow reflex
    4. Adequate pulse and blood pressure
16. A nurse is preparing to administer a feeding to the client receiving enteral nutrition through a nasogastric tube. The nurse performs which of the following as the priority nursing action?
    1. Measuring intake and output
    2. Weighing the client
    3. Adding blue food coloring to the formula
    4. Determining tube placement
17. A nurse has reinforced discharge teaching with the family of a client who is to have enteral feedings at home. The nurse uses which method of evaluation to best determine the family's competence in performing the feeding procedure?
    1. Return demonstration of the feeding procedure
    2. Selection of appropriate equipment for the feeding procedure
    3. Written testing on the steps of the feeding procedure
    4. Verbal description of the feeding procedure by each member of the family
18. A nurse is asked to assist in preparing a client who will be receiving total parenteral nutrition (TPN) solution via the central line. The nurse plans to obtain which of the following most essential pieces of equipment for this procedure?
    1. Electronic infusion pump
    2. Blood glucose meter
    3. Urine test strips
    4. Noninvasive blood pressure monitor
19. A client is receiving nutrition by means of total parenteral nutrition (TPN). The nurse monitors the client for which of the following signs of hyperglycemia, a complication of this therapy?
    1. Nausea, vomiting, and oliguria
    2. Sweating, chills, and abdominal pain
    3. Pallor, weak pulse, and thirst
    4. Nausea, thirst, and increased urine output
20. A client receiving total parenteral nutrition (TPN) complains of a headache. The nurse notes that the client has an increased blood pressure and a bounding pulse. The nurse reports the findings knowing that these signs are indicative of which complication of TPN therapy?
    1. Hyperglycemia
    2. Air embolism
    3. Sepsis
    4. Fluid overload

ANSWERS

1. *Answer:* 2

Rationale: Regular soup (1 cup) contains 900 mg of sodium. Fresh shellfish (1 oz) contains 50 mg sodium. Poultry (1 oz) contains 25 mg sodium.

Test-Taking Strategy: Use the process of elimination. Eliminate options 1 and 3 first because they are similar. Also, recall that canned foods are high in sodium. From the remaining options, select option 2 over option 4 remembering that shellfish is also high in sodium. Review foods high in sodium if you had difficulty with this question.

Level of Cognitive Ability: Analysis

Client Needs: Health Promotion and Maintenance

Integrated Concept/Process: Self-Care

Content Area: Fundamental Skills

Reference: Williams S: *Basic nutrition and diet therapy,* ed 11, St Louis, 2001, Mosby, p. 120.

2. *Answer:* 3
Rationale: Scallops should be omitted from the diet of a client who has gout because of the high purine content. The food items identified in options 1, 2, and 4 contain a negligible purine content and may be consumed daily by the client with gout.
Test-Taking Strategy: Use the process of elimination. Recalling the food items that are high in purine will direct you to option 3. Review foods high in purine if you had difficulty with this question.
Level of Cognitive Ability: Application
Client Needs: Health Promotion and Maintenance
Integrated Concept/Process: Teaching/Learning
Content Area: Fundamental Skills
Reference: Williams S: *Basic nutrition and diet therapy*, ed 11, St Louis, 2001, Mosby, p. 412.

3. *Answer:* 3
Rationale: A clear liquid diet consists of foods that are relatively transparent. The food items in options 1, 2, and 4 would be included in a full liquid diet.
Test-Taking Strategy: Remember that a clear liquid diet consists of foods that are relatively transparent. By the process of elimination you should easily select option 3 because this is the only food item that is transparent. Review food items allowed on a clear liquid and full liquid diet if you had difficulty with this question.
Level of Cognitive Ability: Application
Client Needs: Physiological Integrity
Integrated Concept/Process: Nursing Process/Implementation
Content Area: Fundamental Skills
Reference: Williams S: *Basic nutrition and diet therapy*, ed 11, St Louis, 2001, Mosby, p. 328.

4. *Answer:* 3
Rationale: Bacon is a component of the fat group in the exchange system. One teaspoon of butter is equal to 1 tsp margarine, 1 tsp of any oil, 1 tablespoon of salad dressing, one strip of bacon, five large olives, or 10 whole peanuts.
Test-Taking Strategy: Note the key words "most appropriate" in the stem of the question. Eliminate options 1 and 2 because they are similar. Select option 3 over option 4 knowing that bacon is an item of the fat group. Review foods in the exchange system if you had difficulty with this question.
Level of Cognitive Ability: Application
Client Needs: Health Promotion and Maintenance
Integrated Concept/Process: Teaching/Learning
Content Area: Fundamental Skills
Reference: Williams S: *Basic nutrition and diet therapy*, ed 11, St Louis, 2001, Mosby, p. 219.

5. *Answer:* 2
Rationale: A low-residue (low-fiber) diet places less strain on the intestines because this type of diet is easier to digest. This diet is prescribed for clients with inflammatory bowel disease, ileostomy, colostomy, partial obstructions of the intestinal tract, enteritis, or diarrhea.
Test-Taking Strategy: Note that the diagnosis in the question refers to an inflammation in the colon. With this in mind, you should easily be directed to option 2, the diet that would place the least strain on the intestinal tract. Review the indications for a low-residue diet if you had difficulty with this question.
Level of Cognitive Ability: Comprehension
Client Needs: Physiological Integrity
Integrated Concept/Process: Nursing Process/Planning
Content Area: Fundamental Skills
Reference: DeWit S: *Fundamental concepts and skills for nursing*, Philadelphia, 2001, WB Saunders, p. 494.

6. *Answer:* 3
Rationale: Fruits and vegetables, except avocado, olives, and coconut, contain minimal amounts of fat.
Test-Taking Strategy: Use the process of elimination and knowledge regarding the fat content of fruits to eliminate options 1 and 2. Recalling that avocado is high in fat content will direct you to option 3 from the remaining options. Review the fruits high in fat if you had difficulty with this question.
Level of Cognitive Ability: Analysis
Client Needs: Health Promotion and Maintenance
Integrated Concept/Process: Self-Care
Content Area: Fundamental Skills
Reference: Williams S: *Basic nutrition and diet therapy*, ed 11, St Louis, 2001, Mosby, p. 469.

7. *Answer:* 1
Rationale: Food sources of riboflavin include milk, lean meats, fish, and grains. Tomatoes and citrus fruits are high in vitamin C. Green, leafy vegetables are high in folic acid.
Test-Taking Strategy: Knowledge regarding food items high in riboflavin is required to answer this question. Review these foods if you had difficulty with this question.
Level of Cognitive Ability: Application
Client Needs: Health Promotion and Maintenance
Integrated Concept/Process: Teaching/Learning
Content Area: Fundamental Skills
Reference: Williams S: *Basic nutrition and diet therapy*, ed 11, St Louis, 2001, Mosby, p. 469.

8. *Answer:* 3
Rationale: Thiamine is present in a variety of foods of plant and animal origin. Pork products are especially rich in the vitamin. Other good sources include nuts, whole grain cereals, and legumes. Poultry is high in pyridoxine. Broccoli is high in vitamin C. Milk is high in riboflavin.
Test-Taking Strategy: Knowledge regarding food items high in thiamine is required to answer this question. Review these foods if you had difficulty with this question.
Level of Cognitive Ability: Application
Client Needs: Health Promotion and Maintenance
Integrated Concept/Process: Teaching/Learning
Content Area: Fundamental Skills
Reference: Williams S: *Basic nutrition and diet therapy*, ed 11, St Louis, 2001, Mosby, p. 87.

9. *Answer:* 4
Rationale: Moist pastas, casseroles, egg dishes, and potatoes are usually well tolerated by the client who has difficulty swallowing. Raw vegetables, chunky vegetables such as diced beets, and stringy vegetables such as spinach, corn and peas, are

foods commonly excluded from the diet of a client who has difficulty swallowing.
Test-Taking Strategy: Note the key words "swallowing ability" and "avoids." Use the process of elimination to select option 4 as the food that would be most difficult to swallow. Review the foods to avoid in a client who has difficulty swallowing if you had difficulty with this question.
Level of Cognitive Ability: Application
Client Needs: Physiological Integrity
Integrated Concept/Process: Nursing Process/Planning
Content Area: Fundamental Skills
Reference: Williams S: *Basic nutrition and diet therapy*, ed 11, St Louis, 2001, Mosby, p. 321.

10. *Answer:* 3
Rationale: Protein and vitamin C are necessary for wound healing. Poultry and milk are good sources of protein. Broccoli and strawberries are good sources of vitamin C. Peanut butter is a source of niacin. Jell-O and jelly have no nutrient value. Spaghetti is a complex carbohydrate.
Test-Taking Strategy: Use the process of elimination. Eliminate options 1 and 2 first because jelly and Jell-O have no nutrient value related to healing. Recall that protein and vitamin C are necessary for wound healing. From the remaining options, select option 3 over option 4 because of the greater nutrient value in these food items. Review foods high in protein and vitamin C if you had difficulty with this question.
Level of Cognitive Ability: Application
Client Needs: Physiological Integrity
Integrated Concept/Process: Nursing Process/Implementation
Content Area: Fundamental Skills
Reference: Williams S: *Basic nutrition and diet therapy*, ed 11, St Louis, 2001, Mosby, p. 84.

11. *Answer:* 3
Rationale: Independence is promoted by allowing the client to have control in a given situation. Placing the client's tray on the unaffected side will facilitate the client's ability to perform the activity of eating. Options 1, 2, and 4 do not offer the client control.
Test-Taking Strategy: Note the key words "promote independence." With this issue in mind, by the process of elimination, you should easily be directed to option 3. Review measures that will promote independence in the client with a CVA if you had difficulty with this question.
Level of Cognitive Ability: Application
Client Needs: Psychosocial Integrity
Integrated Concept/Process: Nursing Process/Implementation
Content Area: Fundamental Skills
Reference: Black J, Hawks J, Keene A: *Medical-surgical nursing: clinical management for positive outcomes*, ed 6, Philadelphia, 2001, WB Saunders, p. 1968.

12. *Answer:* 4
Rationale: A low-sodium diet is used as an adjunct to antihypertensive medications for the treatment of hypertension. Sodium retains fluid that leads to hypertension secondary to increased fluid volume. Frozen foods use salt as a preservative and should not be encouraged as part of a low-sodium diet.
Test-Taking Strategy: Use the process of elimination noting the key words "further teaching is necessary." Eliminate options 1, 2, and 3 because these are accurate statements related to hypertension. Review the purpose of a low-sodium diet if you had difficulty with this question.
Level of Cognitive Ability: Analysis
Client Needs: Health Promotion and Maintenance
Integrated Concept/Process: Self-Care
Content Area: Fundamental Skills
Reference: Williams S: *Basic nutrition and diet therapy*, ed 11, St Louis, 2001, Mosby, p. 120.

13. *Answer:* 4
Rationale: Concentrated sugars are found in fruit yogurt, gelatin desserts, prepared drink mixes, jelly, and sherbet.
Test-Taking Strategy: Use the process of elimination. Note that option 4 is the only option that does not identify a prepackaged food item. Review foods containing concentrated sugar if you had difficulty with this question.
Level of Cognitive Ability: Analysis
Client Needs: Health Promotion and Maintenance
Integrated Concept/Process: Nursing Process/Evaluation
Content Area: Fundamental Skills
Reference: Williams S: *Basic nutrition and diet therapy*, ed 11, St Louis, 2001, Mosby, p. 26.

14. *Answer:* 2
Rationale: Any condition in which gastrointestinal motility is slowed or esophageal reflux is possible places a client at risk for aspiration. Options 1 and 4 may be appropriate nursing diagnoses, but are not of highest priority. Option 3 is not likely to occur in this client.
Test-Taking Strategy: Note the key words "highest priority." Use the ABCs, airway, breathing, and circulation. Option 2 addresses airway management. Options 1, 3, and 4 are possible problems, but not as high a priority as airway maintenance. Review care to the client receiving enteral feedings if you had difficulty with this question.
Level of Cognitive Ability: Application
Client Needs: Physiological Integrity
Integrated Concept/Process: Nursing Process/Planning
Content Area: Fundamental Skills
Reference: DeWit, S: *Fundamental concepts and skills for nursing*, Philadelphia, 2001, WB Saunders, p. 463.

15. *Answer:* 3
Rationale: The nurse ensures that the client has intact gag and swallow reflexes. The nurse would also check for the presence of bowel sounds. Pulse, blood pressure, and weight require ongoing monitoring, but are not the most important, given the wording of the question. The client may be expected to have a poor appetite after being without oral intake for a period of time.
Test-Taking Strategy: Focus on the issue of the question noting the key word "priority." Option 3 is most closely associated with the issue of the question, feeding the client, and addresses prevention of aspiration. Review nursing care measures for the client resuming an oral intake if you had difficulty with this question.
Level of Cognitive Ability: Application

Client Needs: Physiological Integrity
Integrated Concept/Process: Nursing Process/Data Collection
Content Area: Fundamental Skills
Reference: DeWit S: *Fundamental concepts and skills for nursing,* Philadelphia, 2001, WB Saunders, p. 489.

16. *Answer:* 4
Rationale: Initiating a tube feeding before checking tube placement can lead to serious complications such as aspiration. Options 1 and 2 are part of the total plan of care for a client on enteral feedings. Option 3 is instituted for a client who has been identified as a high risk for aspiration. Option 4 is the priority nursing action.
Test-Taking Strategy: Use the ABCs—airway, breathing, and circulation—and the nursing process to answer the question. Option 4 relates to the risk of aspiration. If you had difficulty with this question, review nursing interventions when initiating a tube feeding.
Level of Cognitive Ability: Application
Client Needs: Physiological Integrity
Integrated Concept/Process: Nursing Process/Implementation
Content Area: Fundamental Skills
Reference: DeWit S: *Fundamental concepts and skills for nursing,* Philadelphia, 2001, WB Saunders, p. 495.

17. *Answer:* 1
Rationale: Return demonstration is the most reliable evaluation of procedure performance. Selection of equipment is included in a return demonstration. Written testing is not useful for performance testing of procedures. Verbal description does not allow the nurse to observe the psychomotor skill needed to perform the procedure.
Test-Taking Strategy: Note the similar words in the question and option. "Performing" in the question and "demonstration" in the option indicate action. Review basic teaching/learning principles if you had difficulty with this question.
Level of Cognitive Ability: Application
Client Needs: Health Promotion and Maintenance
Integrated Concept/Process: Teaching/Learning
Content Area: Fundamental Skills
Reference: DeWit S: *Fundamental concepts and skills for nursing,* Philadelphia, 2001, WB Saunders, p. 122.

18. *Answer:* 1
Rationale: The nurse obtains an electronic infusion pump in preparation for this procedure. It is necessary to use an infusion pump to ensure that the solution does not infuse too rapidly or fall too far behind. Because the client's blood glucose is monitored every 6 to 8 hours during administration of TPN, a blood glucose meter will also be needed, but it is not the most essential item needed. Urine test strips may be needed to measure glucose. A noninvasive blood pressure cuff is unnecessary for this procedure.
Test-Taking Strategy: Note that the question contains the key words "most essential." Use knowledge of principles of TPN administration to eliminate each of the incorrect options easily. Review these principles if you had difficulty with this question.
Level of Cognitive Ability: Application
Client Needs: Physiological Integrity
Integrated Concept/Process: Nursing Process/Planning
Content Area: Fundamental Skills
Reference: DeWit S: *Fundamental concepts and skills for nursing,* Philadelphia, 2001, WB Saunders, p. 506.

19. *Answer:* 4
Rationale: The high glucose concentration in TPN places the client at risk for hyperglycemia. Signs of hyperglycemia include polyuria, polydipsia (thirst), blurred vision, nausea and vomiting, and abdominal pain.
Test-Taking Strategy: Use the process of elimination. Remember that in order for an option to be correct, all of the parts of that option must be correct. Recalling the signs of hyperglycemia will easily direct to option 4. Review the signs of hyperglycemia if you had difficulty with this question.
Level of Cognitive Ability: Application
Client Needs: Physiological Integrity
Integrated Concept/Process: Nursing Process/Data Collection
Content Area: Fundamental Skills
Reference: DeWit S: *Fundamental concepts and skills for nursing,* Philadelphia, 2001, WB Saunders, p. 506.

20. *Answer:* 4
Rationale: The client's signs and symptoms are consistent with fluid overload. The increased intravascular volume increases the blood pressure, while the pulse rate increases as the heart tries to pump the extra fluid volume. A fever would be present in sepsis. Signs and symptoms of an air embolus include confusion, pallor, light-headedness, tachycardia, tachypnea, hypotension, anxiety, and unresponsiveness. Polyuria, polydipsia, and polyphagia are manifestations of hyperglycemia.
Test-Taking Strategy: Use the process of elimination. Focus on the data in the question and recall the complications of TPN and their manifestations. Review these complications and manifestations if you had difficulty with this question.
Level of Cognitive Ability: Analysis
Client Needs: Physiological Integrity
Integrated Concept/Process: Nursing Process/Implementation
Content Area: Fundamental Skills
Reference: DeWit S: *Fundamental concepts and skills for nursing,* Philadelphia, 2001, WB Saunders, p. 506.

REFERENCES

Black J, Hawks J, Keene A: *Medical-surgical nursing: clinical management for positive outcomes,* ed 6, Philadelphia, 2001, WB Saunders.

DeWit S: *Fundamental concepts and skills for nursing,* Philadelphia, 2001, WB Saunders.

National Council of State Boards of Nursing, editors: *Test plan for the National Council Licensure Examination for Practical/Vocational Nurses,* Chicago, 2001, Author.

Potter P, Perry A: *Fundamentals of nursing,* ed 5, St Louis, 2001, Mosby.

Williams S: *Basic nutrition and diet therapy,* ed 11, St Louis, 2001, Mosby.

Intravenous Therapy and Blood Administration

PYRAMID TERMS

ABO ABO represents a type of antigen system. The ABO type of the donor should be compatible with the recipient's. Type A can match with types A or O; type B can match with types B or O; type O can match only with type O; type AB can match with A, B, or O.

Air Embolism A bolus of air enters the vein through an inadequately primed intravenous (IV) line, from a loose connection, or during tubing change or removal of the IV.

Circulatory Overload A complication resulting from the infusion of blood at a rate too rapid for body size, cardiac status, or clinical condition of the recipient.

Compatibility Determined by two different types of antigen systems, the ABO system antigens and the RH antigen, present on the membrane surface of the red blood cells (RBCs).

Crossmatching The testing of the donor's blood and the recipient's blood for compatibility.

Infiltration See page of the intravenous fluid out of the vein into the surrounding tissue.

Phlebitis An inflammation of the vein that can occur from either mechanical or chemical (medication) trauma or a local infection.

Rh Represents a type of antigen system. Rh-negative blood can be given to an Rh-negative or Rh-positive recipient.

Septicemia The presence of infective agents or their toxins in the bloodstream. A serious infection that must be treated promptly; otherwise, the infection leads to circulatory collapse, profound shock, and death.

Transfusion Reaction A hemolytic transfusion reaction is caused by blood type or Rh incompatibility. An allergic transfusion reaction is most often seen in clients with a history of allergy. A febrile transfusion reaction most commonly occurs in clients with antibodies directed against the transfused white blood cells (WBCs). A bacterial transfusion reaction is seen after transfusion of contaminated blood products.

PYRAMID TO SUCCESS

The nurse is responsible for monitoring clients receiving parenteral therapies. Pyramid points focus on the safety related to monitoring an infusion rate, and monitoring for complications related to the IV. Focus on the signs and symptoms of infiltration, phlebitis, circulatory overload, and air embolism and the treatment measures associated with each. Pyramid points also focus on safety related to monitoring a client receiving a blood transfusion, and monitoring for complications related to the transfusion. Focus on the signs and symptoms of a transfusion reaction and the immediate interventions if a transfusion reaction occurs. Documentation of expected and unexpected effects of the therapy is also a pyramid point. The primary Integrated Concepts and Processes addressed in this chapter are Caring, Communication and Documentation, Cultural Awareness, Clinical Problem-Solving Process (Nursing Process), and Teaching/Learning.

CLIENT NEEDS

Safe, Effective Care Environment

Informed consent for therapy
Continuity of care
Close supervision during IV infusion
Error prevention in monitoring IVs
Handling hazardous or infectious materials
Asepsis
Standard (universal) precautions

Health Promotion and Maintenance

Lifestyle choices related to the transfusion
Techniques of collecting physical data

Psychosocial Integrity

Identifying coping mechanisms
Support systems for the client
Communication regarding the procedure for IV infusion and blood administration
Religious and cultural considerations related to blood administration

Physiological Integrity

Safe administration of IV and blood transfusion
Monitoring infusion rates
Monitoring for expected effects
Monitoring for complications
Documentation

I. INTRAVENOUS THERAPY (Table 12-1)

A. Used to sustain clients who are unable to take substances orally
B. Replaces water, electrolytes, and nutrients more rapidly than oral administration
C. Provides immediate access to the vascular system for the rapid delivery of specific solutions without the time required for gastrointestinal (GI) tract absorption
D. Provides a vascular route for the administration of medication or blood components

II. INTRAVENOUS DEVICES

A. IV cannulas
1. Steel needles or butterfly set

TABLE 12-1

Types of Intravenous Solutions

Type	Description
Isotonic	Solutions with the same osmolality as body fluids
Hypotonic	Solutions that are more dilute or have a lower osmolality than body fluids
Hypertonic	Solutions that are more concentrated or have a higher osmolality than body fluids

Solution	Tonicity
0.45% normal saline (1/2 NS)	Hypotonic
0.9% normal saline (NS)	Isotonic
5% dextrose in water (5% D/W)	Isotonic
5% dextrose in 0.225% saline (5% D/1/4 NS)	Isotonic
Lactated Ringer's solution	Isotonic
5% dextrose in lactated Ringer's solution	Hypertonic
5% dextrose in 0.45% saline (5% D/1/2 NS)	Hypertonic
5% dextrose in 0.9% saline (5% D/NS)	Hypertonic
10% dextrose in water (10% D/W)	Hypertonic

a. Used when the infusion time will be short
b. **Infiltration** is more common with these devices
c. The butterfly infusion set may commonly be used in children and elderly clients, whose veins are likely to be small or fragile

2. Plastic cannulas
a. Used when a longer infusion time is expected
b. Can cause catheter embolism if the tip of the cannula breaks

B. IV gauges
1. The smaller the gauge number, the larger the outside diameter of the cannula
2. The size used depends on the solution to be administered and the diameter of the available vein
3. For rapid emergency fluid administration, blood products, or anesthetics, a large needle such as 14, 16, 18, or 19 gauge is used
4. For standard IV fluid, a 22 or 24 gauge is used
5. If the client has very small veins, a 24 to 25 gauge is used

C. IV containers (Figure 12-1)
1. Container may be glass or plastic
2. Squeeze the plastic bag or check the glass bottle to ensure intactness and check for any small punctures or cracks

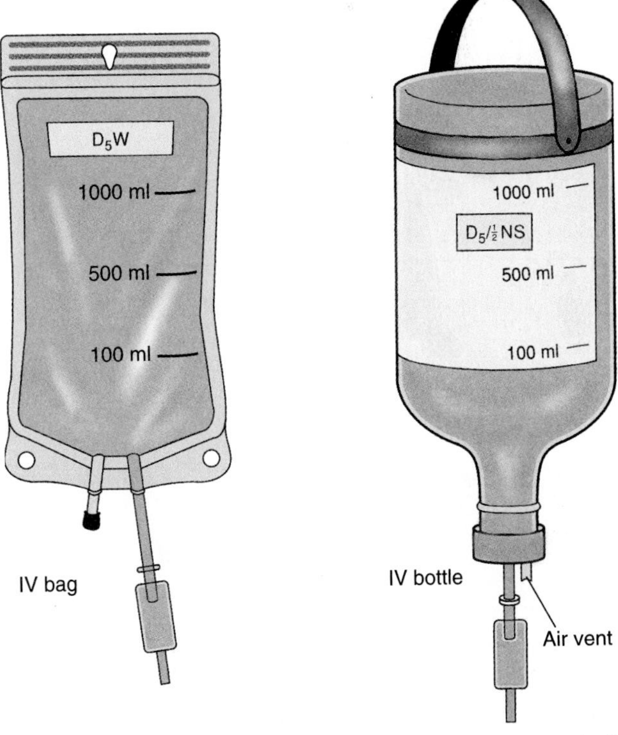

FIG. 12-1 Intravenous containers. (From Kee J, Marshall S: *Clinical calculations*, ed 4, Philadelphia, 2000, WB Saunders.)

3. Do not write on the plastic IV bag with a marking pen because it may be absorbed into the solution
4. Use a label and a ballpoint pen for marking the bag, placing the label onto the bag

D. Intravenous tubing (Figure 12-2)
1. Contains a spike end for the bag or bottle, a drop chamber, a roller clamp, a Y-site, and an adapter end for attachment to the needle
2. Some tubing contains a vent that allows air to enter the IV container as the fluid leaves
3. Vented tubing is used for glass or rigid plastic containers to allow air to enter and displace the fluid as it leaves; fluid will not flow from a rigid IV container unless it is vented
4. Nonvented tubing may be used for flexible plastic containers
5. Extension tubing may be attached to the IV tubing for children, clients who are restless, or clients who have special mobility needs

E. Drip chambers (Figure 12-3)
1. Microdrip chamber
a. Normally this has a short vertical metal piece where the drop forms
b. Delivers 60 drops per millimeter
c. Read the tubing package to determine how many drops per millimeter are delivered (drop factor)

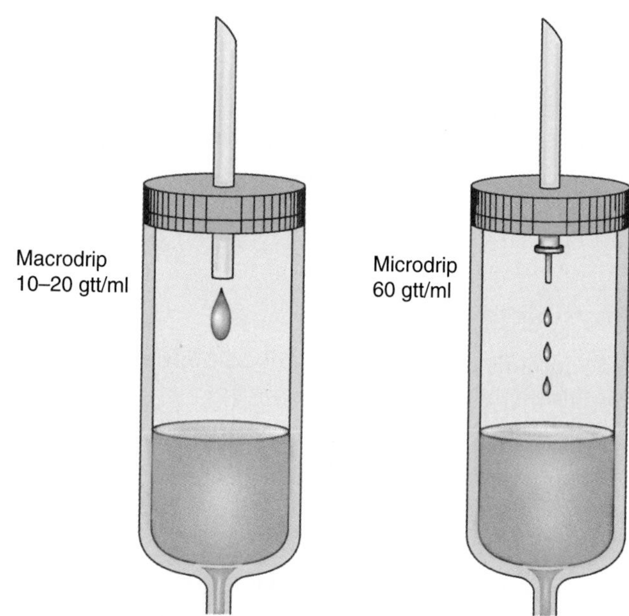

FIG. 12-3 Macrodrip and microdrip sizes. (From Kee J, Marshall S: *Clinical calculations*, ed 4, Philadelphia, 2000, WB Saunders.)

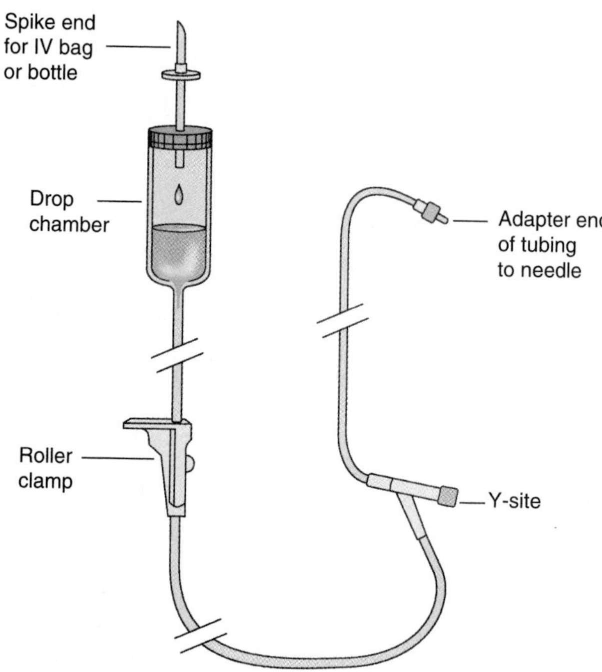

FIG. 12-2 Intravenous tubing. (From Kee J, Marshall S: *Clinical calculations*, ed 4, Philadelphia, 2000, WB Saunders.)

d. Used if fluid will be infused at a slow rate (less than 50 mL per hour), if the solution contains medication, and in the pediatric client
2. Macrodrip chamber
a. Drop factor varies from 8 to 20 drops per millimeter
b. Used if the solution is thick or is to infuse rapidly
c. Read the tubing package to determine how many drops per millimeter are delivered (drop factor)

F. Filters: may be used in IV lines to trap small particles and provide protection by preventing particles from entering the client's veins

G. Needleless systems: includes recessed needles, plastic cannulas, or one-way valves that decrease the exposure to contaminated needles

H. Intermittent infusion sets: used when intravascular accessibility is desired for intermittent administration of medications or solutions

III. PERIPHERAL IV SITES

A. The most frequently used sites are the veins of the forearm because the bones of the forearm act as a natural support and splint

B. Veins in the lower extremities are not suitable because of the risk of thrombus formation and possible pooling in areas of decreased venous return

C. Veins in the scalp and feet may be suitable sites for infants
D. Bending the elbow on the arm with an IV may easily obstruct the flow of solution, causing **infiltration** that could lead to thrombophlebitis
E. Avoid checking the blood pressure on the arm receiving the IV infusion
F. Do not place restraints over the venipuncture site
G. An arm board may be prescribed when the venipuncture site is located in an area of flexion

IV. ADMINISTERING IV SOLUTIONS

A. The IV solution should be checked against the physician's orders for the type, amount, percent of solution, and rate of flow
B. Wash hands thoroughly and use sterile technique when working with an IV
C. When preparing a new solution for administration, clamp the tubing, attach the spike end of the tubing to the IV bag, and then prime the tubing to remove air from the tubing and IV system
D. Change the IV tubing every 24 to 72 hours depending on agency policy
E. Do not let an IV bag or bottle hang for more than 24 hours
F. Do not allow the IV tubing to touch the floor
G. Change the IV dressing every 72 hours, when the dressing is wet or contaminated, or as specified by the agency policy
H. Label the tubing, dressing, and solution bags clearly, including the date and time when changed

V. IV PRECAUTIONS

A. Can cause initial pain and discomfort for the client
B. Provides a route of entry for microorganisms into the body
C. Fluid overload or electrolyte imbalances can occur from an excessive or too rapid infusion of fluids; an IV infusion should be checked at least once per hour in an adult client
D. Incompatibilities between certain solutions can occur
E. Clients with cardiac, respiratory, renal, or liver diseases, and the elderly and very young persons cannot tolerate an excessive fluid volume, and the risk of fluid overload exists with these clients
F. A client with congestive heart failure is usually not given a saline solution because this type of fluid encourages the retention of water and therefore exacerbates heart failure by increasing the fluid overload
G. A client with diabetes mellitus does not typically receive dextrose (glucose) solutions

VI. COMPLICATIONS (Table 12-2)

A. Infection
  1. Description
    a. The entry of microorganisms into the body through the venipuncture site
    b. Venipuncture interrupts the integrity of the skin, the first line of defense against infection
    c. The longer the therapy continues, the greater the risk of infection
  2. At-risk clients
    a. Immunocompromised client from diseases such as cancer or acquired immunodeficiency syndrome (AIDS)
    b. Clients receiving treatments such as chemotherapy that have an altered or lowered WBC count
    c. Elderly clients, because aging alters the effectiveness of the immune system
  3. Prevention and implementation
    a. Maintain strict asepsis when caring for the IV site
    b. Monitor vital signs, particularly temperature

TABLE 12-2

Signs of Complications of Intravenous Therapy

Complication	Signs
Phlebitis	Heat, redness, tenderness at site Not swollen or hard IV infusion sluggish
Thrombophlebitis	Hard and cordlike vein Heat, redness, tenderness at site IV infusion sluggish
Infiltration	Edema, pain, and coolness at site May or may not have a blood return
Catheter embolism	Decrease in blood pressure (BP) Pain along vein Weak, rapid pulse Cyanosis of nail beds Loss of consciousness
Fluid overload	Increased BP Rapid breathing Dyspnea Moist cough and crackles
Air embolus	Tachycardia Dyspnea Cyanosis Hypotension Decreased level of consciousness

c. Monitor for local inflammation at the IV site
d. Check fluid containers for cracks, leaks, or cloudiness or other evidence of contamination
e. Change the tubing and site dressing every 24 to 72 hours according to agency policy
f. Antimicrobial ointment is used at the IV site
g. Ensure that the IV solution is not hanging for more than 24 hours
h. Monitor for systemic infection, which will include malaise, headache, chills, fever, nausea, vomiting, backache, tachycardia
i. If infection occurs, the IV is discontinued and the physician is notified; blood cultures may be prescribed

B. **Phlebitis** and thrombophlebitis
1. Description
a. An inflammation of the vein that can occur from either mechanical or chemical (medication) trauma, or a local infection
b. Phlebitis can cause the development of a clot (thrombophlebitis)
2. Prevention and implementation
a. An IV cannula smaller than the vein is used, and very small veins or veins over an area of flexion are avoided
b. Anchor the cannula and a loop of tubing securely with tape
c. Use an armboard or a splint as prescribed if the client is restless or active
d. If **phlebitis** occurs, the IV device is removed immediately
e. The physician is notified if **phlebitis** is suspected, and warm, moist compresses are applied as prescribed

C. **Infiltration**
1. Description
a. A form of tissue damage that is also called extravasation
b. Seepage of the intravenous fluid out of the vein into the surrounding tissues occurs
c. Occurs when an IV device has become dislodged or perforates the wall of the vein
2. Prevention and implementation
a. IV sites over an area of flexion are avoided
b. Anchor the cannula and a loop of tubing securely with tape
c. Use an armboard or a splint as prescribed if the client is restless or active
d. Monitor the IV site for pain, edema, or coolness, comparing it with the opposite extremity
e. Monitor the IV rate for a decrease or a halt in flow
f. If **infiltration** has occurred, the IV device is removed immediately
g. Do not rub an infiltrated area because this can cause the development of a hematoma
h. If **infiltration** has occurred, the extremity is elevated and compresses are applied (warm or cool, depending on the physician's preference or agency policy) over the affected area

D. Catheter embolism
1. Description: the tip of the catheter breaks off during IV insertion or removal resulting in the possibility of an embolus
2. Prevention and implementation
a. Remove the IV catheter carefully and inspect the catheter when removed
b. If the catheter tip has broken off, the physician is notified; a tourniquet is placed high on the limb of IV site as prescribed and an x-ray study is obtained
c. The client may require surgery to remove the catheter pieces

E. Fluid (circulatory) overload
1. Description: results from the administration of fluids too rapidly or in a client at risk for fluid overload
2. Prevention and implementation
a. Identify clients at risk for fluid overload
b. Calculate and monitor the drip rate frequently
c. An infusion controller device may be used for clients at risk for overload
d. If fluid overload occurs, the physician is notified

F. **Air embolism**
1. Description: A bolus of air enters the vein through an inadequately primed IV line, from a loose connection, or during tubing change or removal of the IV
2. Prevention and implementation
a. Prime the tubing with fluid before use and monitor for any air bubbles in tubing
b. Secure all connections
c. Replace IV fluid before the bag or bottle is dry
d. If an air embolus is suspected, the tubing is clamped, the client is turned on the left side with the head of the bed lowered to trap the air in the right atrium, and the physician is notified

VII. CENTRAL VENOUS CATHETERS (Figure 12-4)
A. Description
1. Used to deliver hyperosmolar solutions, to measure central venous pressure, to infuse

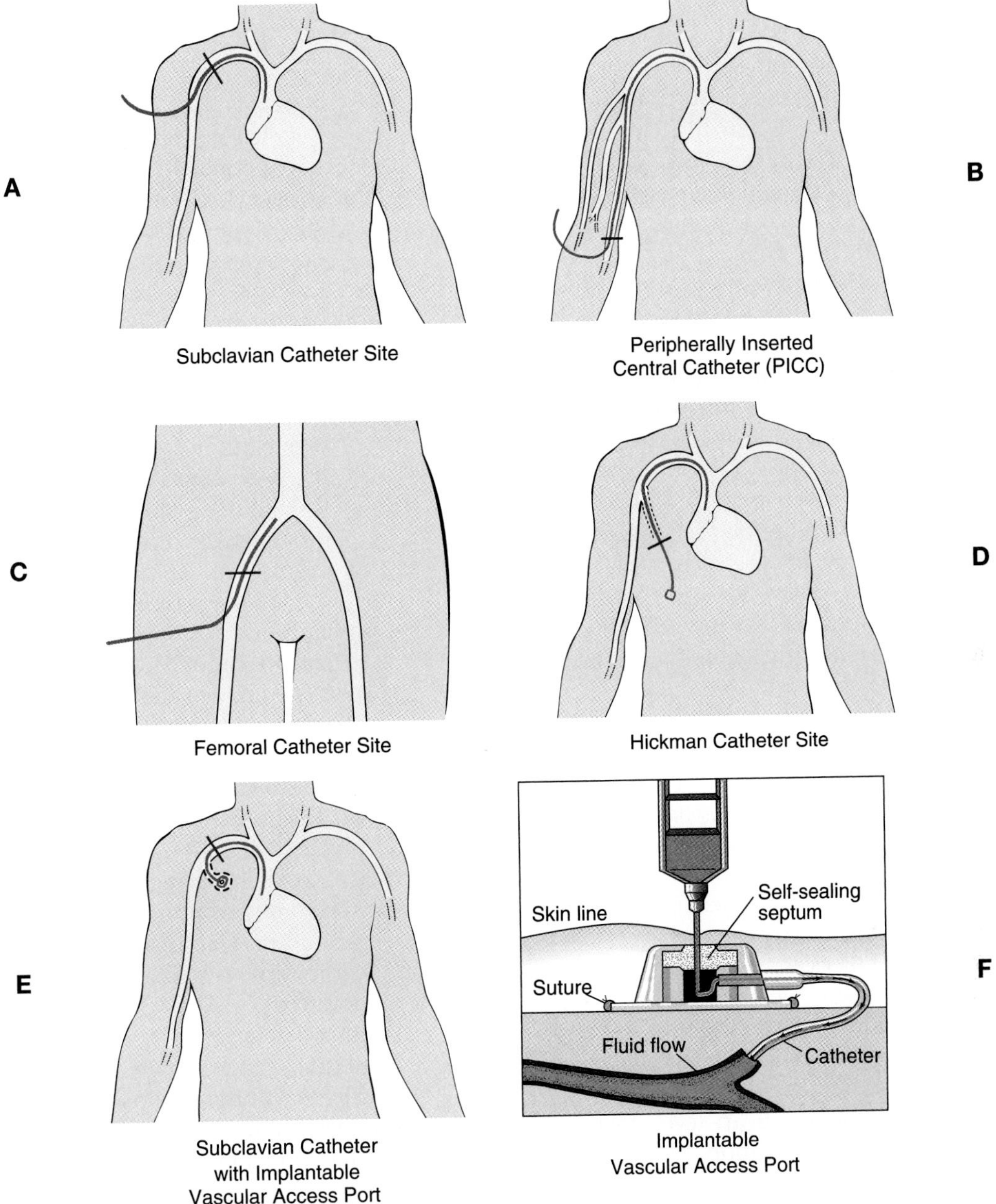

FIG. 12-4 Central venous access sites. (From Kee J, Marshall S: *Clinical calculations*, ed 4, Philadelphia, 2000, WB Saunders. Redrawn from Winters B: *Oncol Nurs Forum* 11(6): 25, 1984.)

total parenteral nutrition (TPN), or multiple IV infusions or medications

2. Catheter position is determined by x-ray study after insertion
3. May have a single, double, or triple lumen
4. May be inserted peripherally and threaded through the basilic or cephalic vein into the superior vena cava, inserted centrally through the internal jugular or subclavian veins, or surgically tunneled through subcutaneous tissue into the cephalic vein
5. With multilumen catheters, more than one medication can be administered at the same time without incompatibility problems, and there is only one insertion site for care
6. For central line insertion, tubing change, and line removal, place the client in Trendelenburg position if not contraindicated, or supine position, and instruct the client to perform the Valsalva maneuver to increase pressure in the central veins when the IV system is open

B. Tunneled central venous catheters
   1. A more permanent type of catheter, such as the Hickman, Broviac, or Groshong catheter, that is used for long-term IV therapy

2. May be single or multilumen
3. Inserted in the operating room, and the catheter is threaded into the lower part of the vena cava at the entrance of the right atrium
4. The catheter will be fitted with an intermittent infusion device to allow access as needed and to keep the system closed and intact
5. Patency is maintained by flushing with a diluted heparin solution as per agency policy
6. Groshong catheters require only normal saline flush to maintain patency

C. Vascular access ports (implantable port)
1. Surgically implanted under the skin, such as a Port-a-Cath, Mediport, or Infusaport; used for long-term administration of repeated IV therapy
2. For access, requires palpation and injection through the skin into the self-sealing port with a noncoring needle such as a Huber-point needle
3. Patency is maintained by periodic flushing with a diluted heparin solution per agency policy

D. Peripherally inserted central catheter (PICC) line
1. Used for long-term IV therapy, frequently in the home
2. The basilic vein is usually used, but the median cubital and cephalic veins in the antecubital area can also be used
3. Threaded so that the catheter tip may terminate in either the axillary or subclavian vein or the superior vena cava
4. A small amount of bleeding may occur at the time of insertion and continue for 24 hours, but bleeding thereafter is not expected
5. **Phlebitis** is a common complication
6. Insertion is below the heart level; therefore, **air embolism** is not common

VIII. BLOOD ADMINISTRATION

A. Types of blood components
1. Red blood cells (RBCs)
   a. Used to replace erythrocytes
   b. Evaluation of an effective response is based on the resolution of the symptoms of anemia and an increase of the erythrocyte count
2. Whole blood
   a. Rarely used because treatment with a specific blood component is usually prescribed
   b. Used to resolve hypovolemic shock resulting from hemorrhage
   c. Contains RBCs, plasma, and plasma proteins
   d. Evaluation of an effective response is based on the resolution of the symptoms of hypovolemia
3. Platelets
   a. Platelets are used to treat thrombocytopenia and platelet dysfunctions
   b. **Crossmatching** is not required but is usually done (platelet concentrates contain few RBCs)
   c. Evaluation of an effective response is based on improvement in the platelet count
4. Fresh-frozen plasma
   a. Fresh-frozen plasma may be used to provide clotting factors or volume expansion; it contains no platelets
   b. **Rh** and **ABO** compatibility are required for the transfusion of plasma products
   c. Evaluation of an effective response is assessed by monitoring coagulation studies

B. Compatibility
1. To ensure proper identity, client blood samples are drawn and labeled at the bedside; client is asked to state his or her name and this is compared to the identification bracelet
2. The recipient's **ABO** and **Rh** type are identified
3. An antibody screen is done to determine the presence of antibodies
4. **Crossmatch** testing is done in which donor RBCs are combined with the recipient's serum and Coombs' serum; a **crossmatch** is compatible if no RBC agglutination has occurred
5. In an emergency, O-negative RBCs and AB plasma can be safely administered to most clients without serological testing

C. Implementation
1. The temperature is checked before beginning a transfusion; a fever may be a cause for delaying the transfusion; in addition, a fever will mask a possible symptom of an acute transfusion reaction
2. During the transfusion, the client is monitored for signs and symptoms of a **transfusion reaction**; the first 10 to 15 minutes of the transfusion are the most critical and the nurse must stay with client; if a major **ABO** incompatibility exists or a severe allergic reaction occurs, it is usually evident within the first 50 mL of the transfusion
3. The client is instructed to immediately report anything unusual
4. If a reaction occurs, the transfusion is stopped and the physician is notified; the blood bag and tubing are returned to the blood bank

5. If a reaction occurs, the client is monitored for any life-threatening symptoms and the appropriate blood and urine samples are obtained as prescribed
6. Document the client's tolerance to the administration of the blood product

D. **Transfusion Reactions**
1. Immediate **transfusion reaction**
   a. Chills and diaphoresis
   b. Rapid, thready pulse
   c. Pallor and cyanosis
   d. Muscle aches, back pain, or chest pain
   e. Headache
   f. Apprehension
   g. Tingling and numbness
   h. Dyspnea, cough, or wheezing
   i. Nausea, vomiting, abdominal cramping, and diarrhea
   j. Rashes, hives, itching, and swelling
2. Delayed **transfusion reaction**
   a. Reactions can occur days to years after a transfusion
   b. Signs include fever, mild jaundice, and a decreased hematocrit level

PRACTICE QUESTIONS

1. A client has an order to receive 1000 mL 5% dextrose in 0.45% sodium chloride. After gathering the appropriate equipment, the nurse takes which of the following actions first before spiking the IV bag with the tubing?
   1. Uncaps the spike portion of the tubing
   2. Uncaps the distal end of the tubing
   3. Closes the roller clamp on the IV tubing
   4. Opens the roller clamp on the IV tubing
2. A nurse is checking the IV dressing of a client with a peripheral intravenous solution infusing. The date on the dressing is 2/9 (February 9). The nurse calculates that the dressing should be changed on which of the following dates?
   1. 2/10
   2. 2/12
   3. 2/14
   4. 2/16
3. A nurse is doing a routine assessment of a client's peripheral IV site. The nurse notes that the site is cool, pale, and swollen and that the IV has stopped running. The nurse interprets that which of the following has probably occurred?
   1. Infiltration
   2. Phlebitis
   3. Thrombosis
   4. Infection
4. A nurse is assigned to care for a client with a peripheral IV infusion. The nurse is providing hygiene care to the client and would avoid which of the following while changing the client's hospital gown?
   1. Use a hospital gown with snaps at the sleeves
   2. Put the bag and tubing through the sleeve, followed by the client's arm
   3. Disconnect the IV tubing from the catheter in the vein
   4. Check the IV flow rate immediately after changing the hospital gown
5. A nurse is making a worksheet and is listing the tasks that need to be done during the shift on assigned clients. The nurse writes on the plan to check the IV of an assigned client receiving fluid replacement therapy every:
   1. 4 hours
   2. 3 hours
   3. 2 hours
   4. 1 hour
6. A nurse is checking the insertion site of a peripheral intravenous catheter. The nurse notes the site to be reddened, warm, painful, and slightly edematous in the area of the vein that is proximal to the IV catheter. The nurse interprets that this is most likely due to:
   1. Infiltration of the IV line
   2. Phlebitis of the vein
   3. Hypersensitivity to the IV solution
   4. Allergic reaction to the IV catheter material
7. A nurse has been instructed to discontinue an intravenous line. The nurse removes the catheter by withdrawing the catheter while applying pressure to the site with a(n):
   1. Alcohol swab
   2. Betadine swab
   3. Band-Aid
   4. Sterile 2 × 2 gauze
8. A nurse is preparing an IV solution and tubing for a client requiring IV fluids. While preparing to prime the tubing, the tubing drops and hits the top of the medication cart. The nurse should plan to do which of the following?
   1. Scrub the tubing before attaching it to the IV bag
   2. Change the IV tubing
   3. Wipe the tubing with Betadine
   4. Scrub the tubing with an alcohol swab
9. A nurse is completing a time tape for a 1000 mL IV bag that is scheduled to infuse over 8 hours. The nurse has just placed the 11:00 marking at the 500 mL level. The nurse would place the mark for 12:00 at which of the following levels on the time tape?
   1. 425 mL
   2. 400 mL
   3. 375 mL
   4. 350 mL
10. A nurse is assisting in caring for a client receiving a unit of packed red blood cells. The nurse tells the

client that it is most important to report which of the following signs immediately?
1. Mild discomfort at the catheter site
2. Chills, itching, or rash
3. Unusual sleepiness or fatigue
4. Headache, nausea, or vomiting

11. A nurse is assisting in caring for a client who will receive a unit of blood. Just before the infusion, it is most important for the nurse to assess the client's:
1. Skin color
2. Oxygen saturation
3. Vital signs
4. Latest hematocrit

12. A client receiving a blood transfusion rings the call bell for the nurse. Upon entering the room, the nurse notes that the client is flushed, dyspneic, and is complaining of generalized itching. The nurse interprets that the client is experiencing:
1. Fluid overload
2. Bacteremia
3. Hypovolemic shock
4. Transfusion reaction

13. A client who was receiving a blood transfusion has experienced a transfusion reaction. The nurse sends the blood bag used for the client to which of the following areas?
1. Risk management department
2. Laboratory
3. Pharmacy
4. Blood bank

14. A nurse takes a client's temperature before giving a blood transfusion. The temperature is 100° F orally. The nurse reports the finding to the registered nurse and anticipates that which of the following actions will take place?
1. The transfusion will begin as prescribed
2. The blood will be held and the physician will be notified
3. The transfusion will begin after administering an antihistamine
4. The transfusion will begin after administering 600 mg of acetaminophen (Tylenol)

15. A nurse is assisting in caring for a client who has received a transfusion of platelets. The nurse evaluates that the client is benefiting most from this therapy if the client exhibits which of the following?
1. Decline of temperature to normal
2. Decrease in oozing from puncture sites and gums
3. Increased hemoglobin level
4. Increased hematocrit level

ANSWERS

1. *Answer:* 3

Rationale: The nurse should first clamp the tubing to prevent the solution from running freely through the tubing once it is attached to the IV bag. The nurse should next uncap the proximal (spike) portion of the tubing and attach it to the IV bag. Then, the roller clamp is opened slowly and the fluid is allowed to flow through the tubing in a controlled fashion to prevent air from remaining in parts of the tubing.

Test-Taking Strategy: Use the process of elimination and note the key word "first." This question tests a specific procedure related to intravenous therapy. Attempt to visualize this process to answer the question correctly. Review this procedure if you had difficulty with this question.

Level of Cognitive Ability: Application

Client Needs: Physiological Integrity

Integrated Concept/Process: Nursing Process/Implementation

Content Area: Fundamental Skills

Reference: Potter P, Perry A: *Fundamentals of nursing,* ed 5, St Louis, 2001, Mosby, p. 1220.

2. *Answer:* 2

Rationale: The IV site dressing should be changed every 48 to 72 hours, which is every 2 to 3 days. With an insertion date of 2/9, the due date for change depending on agency policy would be either 2/11 or 2/12. Changing the dressing every 5 to 7 days (options 3 and 4) would place the client at risk of infection. Changing the dressing on a daily basis is not necessary, unless the dressing becomes wet.

Test-Taking Strategy: Use the process of elimination. Recalling that the IV site dressing should be changed every 48 to 72 hours will direct you to option 2. Review the standard accepted guidelines for intravenous site maintenance if you had difficulty with this question.

Level of Cognitive Ability: Application

Client Needs: Physiological Integrity

Integrated Concept/Process: Nursing Process/Planning

Content Area: Fundamental Skills

Reference: Potter P, Perry A: *Fundamentals of nursing,* ed 5, St Louis, 2001, Mosby, p. 1239.

3. *Answer:* 1

Rationale: An infiltrated IV is one that has dislodged from the vein and is lying in subcutaneous tissue. The pallor, coolness, and swelling are the result of IV fluid being deposited in the subcutaneous tissue. When the pressure in the tissues exceeds the pressure in the tubing, the flow of the IV solution will stop. The other three options identify complications that are likely to be accompanied by warmth at the site, not coolness.

Test-Taking Strategy: Focus on the data in the question and note the key word "cool." Recalling that coolness occurs at the site of IV infiltration will direct you to option 1. Review the signs of infiltration if you had difficulty with this question.

Level of Cognitive Ability: Analysis

Client Needs: Physiological Integrity

Integrated Concept/Process: Nursing Process/Data Collection

Content Area: Fundamental Skills
Reference: Potter P, Perry A: *Fundamentals of nursing,* ed 5, St Louis, 2001, Mosby, p. 1235.

4. *Answer:* 3
Rationale: The tubing should not be removed from the IV catheter. With each break in the system, there is an increased chance of introducing bacteria into the system, leading to infection. This is poor aseptic technique. Options 1 and 2 are appropriate. The flow rate should be checked immediately after changing the hospital gown because the position of the roller clamp may have been affected during the change.
Test-Taking Strategy: Use the process of elimination and note the key word "avoid." Visualize this procedure and use knowledge of the basic principles related to intravenous therapy and asepsis to direct you to option 3. Review these principles if you had difficulty with this question.
Level of Cognitive Ability: Application
Client Needs: Safe, Effective Care Environment
Integrated Concept/Process: Nursing Process/Implementation
Content Area: Fundamental Skills
Reference: Potter P, Perry A: *Fundamentals of nursing,* ed 5, St Louis, 2001, Mosby, p. 1237.

5. *Answer:* 4
Rationale: Safe nursing practice includes monitoring an IV infusion at least once per hour in an adult client. Options 1, 2, and 3 do not provide time frames that are safe or acceptable.
Test-Taking Strategy: Use the process of elimination. To answer this question accurately, it is necessary to be familiar with the specific time frames indicated in this nursing procedure. In questions similar to this one, it is best to select the most frequent time frame. Review the precautions related to administering IV fluid if you had difficulty with this question.
Level of Cognitive Ability: Application
Client Needs: Physiological Integrity
Integrated Concept/Process: Communication and Documentation
Content Area: Fundamental Skills
Reference: Potter P, Perry A: *Fundamentals of nursing,* ed 5, St Louis, 2001, Mosby, pp. 1234-1235.

6. *Answer:* 2
Rationale: Phlebitis at an IV site can be distinguished by client discomfort at the site, as well as by redness, warmth, and swelling proximal to the IV catheter. The IV catheter should be removed, and a new IV should be inserted at a different site. The remaining options are incorrect.
Test-Taking Strategy: Use the process of elimination. Remember that options that are similar are not likely to be correct. In this case, options 3 and 4 are similar and are therefore eliminated. Recalling that warmth occurs at the site of phlebitis will direct you to option 2 from the remaining options. Review the signs of phlebitis if you had difficulty with this question.
Level of Cognitive Ability: Analysis
Client Needs: Physiological Integrity
Integrated Concept/Process: Nursing Process/Data Collection
Content Area: Fundamental Skills
Reference: Potter P, Perry A: *Fundamentals of nursing,* ed 5, St Louis, 2001, Mosby, p. 1235.

7. *Answer:* 4
Rationale: A dry sterile dressing such as a sterile 2 × 2 gauze is used to apply pressure to the site while the catheter is discontinued and removed. This material is absorbent, sterile, and nonirritating to the site. A Betadine swab or alcohol swab would irritate the opened puncture site and would not stop the blood flow. A Band-Aid may be used to cover the site once hemostasis has occurred.
Test-Taking Strategy: Use the process of elimination. Visualize this procedure and think about each of the items identified in the options to answer the question. Familiarity with this basic nursing procedure is needed to answer this question correctly. Noting the word "sterile" in option 4 will assist in directing you to this option. Review this procedure if you had difficulty with this question.
Level of Cognitive Ability: Application
Client Needs: Safe, Effective Care Environment
Integrated Concept/Process: Nursing Process/Implementation
Content Area: Fundamental Skills
Reference: Potter P, Perry A: *Fundamentals of nursing,* ed 5, St Louis, 2001, Mosby, pp. 1239-1240.

8. *Answer:* 2
Rationale: The nurse should change the IV tubing. The tubing has become contaminated and could result in systemic infection to the client if used. Wiping or scrubbing the tubing is insufficient to prevent systemic infection.
Test-Taking Strategy: Use knowledge of basic infection control measures and intravenous therapy concepts to answer this question. Note the similarity between options 1, 3, and 4 and eliminate these options. Review aseptic technique and IV therapy if you had difficulty with this question.
Level of Cognitive Ability: Application
Client Needs: Safe, Effective Care Environment
Integrated Concept/Process: Nursing Process/Implementation
Content Area: Fundamental Skills
Reference: Potter P, Perry A: *Fundamentals of nursing,* ed 5, St Louis, 2001, Mosby, p. 1240.

9. *Answer:* 3
Rationale: If the IV is scheduled to run over 8 hours, then the hourly rate is 125 mL per hour. Using 500 mL as the reference point for 11:00, the next hourly marking (12:00) would be at 375 mL, which is 125 mL less than 500.
Test-Taking Strategy: Use basic principles related to pharmacology calculations and IV administration to answer this question. Review the procedure for time taping an IV bag if you had difficulty with this question.
Level of Cognitive Ability: Application
Client Needs: Physiological Integrity
Integrated Concept/Process: Nursing Process/Implementation
Content Area: Fundamental Skills
Reference: DeWit S: *Fundamental concepts and skills for nursing,* Philadelphia, 2001, WB Saunders, p. 723.

10. *Answer:* 2
Rationale: The client is told to report chills, itching, or rash immediately. These could possibly be signs of a transfusion reaction. Mild discomfort at the catheter site may be indicative of a problem, or could result from the size of the IV catheter

required to infuse the blood product. Sleepiness, fatigue, headache, nausea, and vomiting are unrelated to a transfusion reaction.
Test-Taking Strategy: Note the key words "most important" and "immediately." This tells you that more than one or all of the options may be partially or totally correct. Knowing that a transfusion reaction is of most concern to the nurse, you must prioritize your answer to select the option that characterizes this problem. Review the signs of a transfusion reaction if you had difficulty with this question.
Level of Cognitive Ability: Application
Client Needs: Physiological Integrity
Integrated Concept/Process: Nursing Process/Implementation
Content Area: Fundamental Skills
Reference: Potter P, Perry A: *Fundamentals of nursing,* ed 5, St Louis, 2001, Mosby, p. 1243.

11. *Answer:* 3
Rationale: A change in vital signs may indicate that a transfusion reaction is occurring. The nurse assesses the client's vital signs before the procedure to obtain a baseline, every 15 minutes for the first half hour after beginning the transfusion, and every half hour thereafter.
Test-Taking Strategy: Note the key words "just before" and "most important." This tells you that more than one of the options may be partially or totally correct. Recalling the signs of a blood transfusion reaction will direct you to option 3. Additionally, vital signs is the most global option. Review these signs if you had difficulty with this question.
Level of Cognitive Ability: Application
Client Needs: Physiological Integrity
Integrated Concept/Process: Nursing Process/Data Collection
Content Area: Fundamental Skills
Reference: Potter P, Perry A: *Fundamentals of nursing,* ed 5, St Louis, 2001, Mosby, p. 1243.

12. *Answer:* 4
Rationale: The signs and symptoms exhibited by the client are consistent with a transfusion reaction. With fluid overload, the client would have crackles in addition to dyspnea. With bacteremia, the client would have a fever, which is not part of the clinical picture presented. There is no correlation between the signs mentioned in the question and hypovolemic shock. The signs identified in the question are indicative of an allergic reaction, which is one type of blood transfusion reaction.
Test-Taking Strategy: Use the process of elimination and focus on the data in the question. Recalling the signs of a transfusion reaction will direct you to option 4. Review the complications of blood administration and the signs of a transfusion reaction if you had difficulty with this question.
Level of Cognitive Ability: Analysis
Client Needs: Physiological Integrity
Integrated Concept/Process: Nursing Process/Data Collection
Content Area: Fundamental Skills
Reference: Potter P, Perry A: *Fundamentals of nursing,* ed 5, St Louis, 2001, Mosby, p. 1244.

13. *Answer:* 4
Rationale: The nurse prepares to return the blood transfusion bag containing any remaining blood to the blood bank. This allows the blood bank to complete any follow-up testing procedures needed once a transfusion reaction has been documented.
Test-Taking Strategy: Use the process of elimination. Recalling that blood is issued from the blood bank will help you to eliminate each of the incorrect options. Review the procedures to follow when a blood transfusion reaction occurs if you had difficulty with this question.
Level of Cognitive Ability: Application
Client Needs: Physiological Integrity
Integrated Concept/Process: Nursing Process/Implementation
Content Area: Fundamental Skills
Reference: Potter P, Perry A: *Fundamentals of nursing,* ed 5, St Louis, 2001, Mosby, p. 1245.

14. *Answer:* 2
Rationale: If the client has a temperature equal to or greater than 100° F, the unit of blood should be held until the physician is notified and has the opportunity to give further orders. The other options are incorrect.
Test-Taking Strategy: Use the process of elimination. Eliminate options 1, 3, and 4 because they are similar. Remember that the physician needs to be notified before initiating a blood transfusion, if the temperature is elevated. Review the procedures related to administering a blood transfusion if you had difficulty with this question.
Level of Cognitive Ability: Application
Client Needs: Physiological Integrity
Integrated Concept/Process: Nursing Process/Planning
Content Area: Fundamental Skills
Reference: Potter P, Perry A: *Fundamentals of nursing,* ed 5, St Louis, 2001, Mosby, p. 1243.

15. *Answer:* 2
Rationale: Platelets are necessary for proper blood clotting. The client with insufficient platelets may exhibit frank bleeding, or oozing of blood from puncture sites, wounds, and mucous membranes. A temperature would decline to normal after infusion of granulocytes if those transfused cells were then instrumental in fighting infection in the body. Increased hemoglobin and hematocrit levels would be seen when the client has received a transfusion of red blood cells.
Test-Taking Strategy: Use the process of elimination. Recalling that bleeding is a concern when the platelets are low will easily direct you to option 2. Review the action of platelets if you had difficulty with this question.
Level of Cognitive Ability: Analysis
Client Needs: Physiological Integrity
Integrated Concept/Process: Nursing Process/Evaluation
Content Area: Fundamental Skills
Reference: Potter P, Perry A: *Fundamentals of nursing,* ed 5, St Louis, 2001, Mosby, p. 1273.

REFERENCES

DeWit S: *Fundamental concepts and skills for nursing,* Philadelphia, 2001, WB Saunders.

Kee J, Marshall S: *Clinical calculations,* ed 4, Philadelphia, 2000, WB Saunders.

National Council of State Boards of Nursing, editors: *Test plan for the National Council Licensure Examination for Practical/Vocational Nurses.* Chicago, 2001, Author.

Potter P, Perry A: *Fundamentals of nursing,* ed 5, St Louis, 2001, Mosby.

UNIT IV

Fundamental Skills

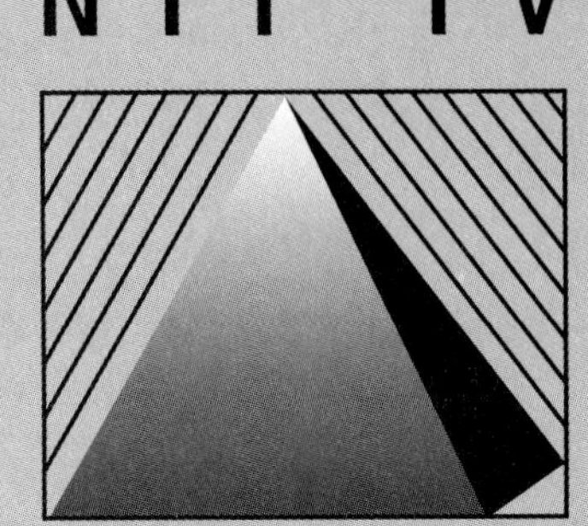

13 Hygiene and Safety

PYRAMID TERMS

Chemical Restraints Medications given to inhibit a specific behavior or movement.

Nosocomial Infections Infections acquired in the hospital or other health care facility that were not present or incubating at the time of the client's admission; also referred to as hospital-acquired infections.

Physical Restraints Devices that are applied to restrict movement.

Poison Any substance that impairs health and destroys life when ingested, inhaled, or otherwise absorbed by the body.

Standard (Universal) Precautions Guidelines used by all health care providers with all clients to reduce the risk of infection for clients and caregivers.

Transmission-Based Precautions Guidelines that are used in addition to standard precautions; used for specific syndromes that are highly suggestive of infections until a diagnosis is confirmed.

PYRAMID TO SUCCESS

Safety and Infection Control is a subcategory of the Client Needs component, Safe, Effective Care Environment, of the test plan for NCLEX-PN. Pyramid points focus on maintaining environmental safety, preventing accidents, the use of restraints, and priority nursing actions in the event of an emergency or a disaster. Pyramid points also focus on standard (universal) and transmission-based precautions and the measures required to handle hazardous and infectious materials. The primary Integrated Concepts and Processes addressed in this chapter include the Clinical Problem-Solving Process (Nursing Process), Communication and Documentation, Self-Care, and Teaching/Learning.

CLIENT NEEDS

Safe, Effective Care Environment

Disaster planning
Establishing priorities
Guidelines regarding the use of restraints
Handling hazardous and infectious materials
Maintaining precautions to prevent accidents
Standard and transmission-based precautions

Health Promotion and Maintenance

Assisting clients and families to identify environmental hazards in the home
Client and family education regarding accident prevention
Client and family education to prevent the spread of infection
Client and family education regarding measures to be implemented in an emergency
Disease prevention
Home safety measures

Psychosocial Integrity

Cultural and religious lifestyles
Sensory/perceptual alterations
Support systems

Physiological Integrity

Assisting the client with activities of daily living (ADLs)
Managing and providing care to clients with infectious diseases
Priority nursing actions in an emergency
Providing comfort and assistance to the client
Use of assistive devices to prevent injury

I. HYGIENE

A. Description
1. The activity of providing care or promoting self-care, which includes bathing and grooming
2. Includes care of the skin, hair, nails, mouth, teeth, eyes, ears, nasal cavities, and perineal and genital areas
3. Personal hygiene is the activity of self-care, including bathing and grooming

B. General principles
1. Wash hands and wear gloves
2. Ensure privacy
3. Explain procedures to the client
4. Determine the client's health status and readiness for hygiene procedures
5. Determine the client's routine hygiene practices
6. Use proper body mechanics during bathing and hygiene activities
7. Use time spent with client as an opportunity for communication and teaching
8. Maintain and encourage independence as much as possible

II. ENVIRONMENTAL SAFETY

A. Fire safety (Box 13-1)
1. Keep open spaces free of clutter
2. Clearly mark fire exits
3. Know the location of all fire alarms, exits, and extinguishers (Table 13-1; Box 13-2)
4. Know the telephone number for reporting fires
5. Know the agency's fire drill and evacuation plan
6. Never use the elevator in the event of a fire
7. Turn off oxygen and appliances in the vicinity of the fire
8. In the event of a fire, if the client is on life support, maintain the client's respiratory status manually with an Ambu-bag until the client is moved away from the threat of the fire
9. In the event of a fire, ambulatory clients can be directed to walk by themselves to a safe area, and in some cases may be able to assist in moving clients in wheelchairs
10. Bedridden clients are generally moved from the scene of a fire by a stretcher, their beds, or a wheelchair
11. If a client must be carried from the area of a fire, appropriate transfer techniques need to be used
12. If the fire department personnel are at the scene of the fire, they can help evacuate clients

B. Electrical safety
1. Electrical equipment must be maintained in good working order and should be grounded
2. Use a three-pronged electrical cord 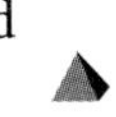
3. In a three-pronged electrical cord, the third, longer prong of the cord is the ground; the other two prongs carry the power to the piece of electrical equipment
4. Any electrical equipment that the client brings into the health care facility must be inspected for safety before use 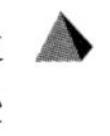
5. Check electrical cords and outlets for exposed, frayed, or damaged wires
6. Avoid overloading any circuit
7. Read warning labels on all equipment; never operate unfamiliar equipment
8. Use safety extension cords only when absolutely necessary, and tape them to the floor with electrical tape
9. Never run electrical wiring under carpets

BOX 13-1

Priority Actions in the Event of a Fire

Remember the mnemonic **RACE** to set priorities in the event of a fire:
R-Rescue: Remove all clients from the vicinity of a fire
A-Alarm: Activate the fire alarm; report a fire before attempting to extinguish it
C-Confine: Close doors and windows when a fire is detected
E-Extinguish: Extinguish the fire, using the appropriate fire extinguisher

BOX 13-2

Using a Fire Extinguisher

Remember the mnemonic **PASS** to use a fire extinguisher:
P-Pull the pin
A-Aim at the base of the fire
S-Squeeze the handles
S-Sweep the fire from side to side

TABLE 13-1

Fire Extinguishers

Type of Extinguishers	Class of Fires
Type A: Water	Wood, draperies, upholstery, paper, and rubbish
Types B or C: Carbon dioxide or dry chemical	Flammable liquids or gases, grease, and electrical
Types A, B, or C: Multipurpose, dry chemical	Any fire

10. Never pull a plug using the cord; always grasp the plug itself
11. Never use electrical appliances near sinks, bathtubs, or other water sources
12. Always disconnect a plug from the outlet before cleaning equipment or appliances
13. If a client receives an electrical shock, turn off the electricity before touching the client

C. Radiation safety
1. Know the health care agency protocols and guidelines
2. Label potentially radioactive material
3. To reduce exposure to radiation:
    a. The time spent near the source should be limited
    b. The distance from the source should be as great as possible
    c. A shielding device such as a lead apron should be used
4. Monitor radiation exposure with a film badge
5. Place the client who has a radiation implant in a private room
6. Never touch dislodged implants
7. Wear gloves when handling body discharges

D. Disposal of infectious wastes
1. Handle all infectious materials as a hazard
2. Dispose of waste in designated areas only, using proper containers for disposal
3. Ensure that infectious material is properly labeled
4. Needles should not be recapped, bent, or broken
5. Dispose of all sharps immediately after use in closed, puncture-resistant disposal containers that are leak proof and labeled or color-coded

E. Falls (See Box 13-3 for measures to prevent falls)

BOX 13-3

Measures to Prevent Falls

Assess the client's risk for falling
Assign the clients at risk for falling to rooms near the nurses' station
Alert all personnel to the client's risk for falling
Orient the client to physical surroundings
Instruct the client to seek assistance when getting up
Explain the use of the call bell system to the client
Keep the bed in the low position with side rails up if required
Lock all beds, wheelchairs, and stretchers
Keep personal items within reach
Eliminate clutter and obstacles in client's room
Provide adequate lighting
Reduce bathroom hazards
Maintain the client's toileting schedule throughout the day

F. Restraints
1. Protective devices used to limit the physical activity of a client or to immobilize a client or an extremity
2. **Physical Restraints**: Restrict client movement through the application of a device
3. **Chemical Restraints**: Medications given to inhibit a specific behavior or movement
4. Implementation
    a. When **restraints** are necessary, the physician's orders should state the type of restraint, identify specific client behaviors for which restraints are to be used, and identify a limited time frame for use
    b. Physicians' orders for **restraints** should be renewed within a specific time frame according to the agency's policy
    c. **Restraints** are not to be ordered PRN
    d. The reason for the **restraints** should be given to the client and the family, and their permission should be sought
    e. **Restraints** should not interfere with any treatments or affect the client's health problem
    f. Use a clove hitch knot so that the restraint can be changed and released easily
    g. Ensure that there is enough slack on the straps to allow some movement of the body part
    h. Secure restraint to bed frame, not to the side rails
    i. Assess skin integrity and neurovascular and circulatory status every 30 minutes; release the **restraint** at least every 1 to 2 hours or as designated by agency policy to permit muscle exercise and promote circulation
    j. Continually assess the need for **restraints** (Box 13-4)
5. Alternatives to **restraints**
    a. Orient client and family to surroundings
    b. Explain all procedures and treatments to the client and family

BOX 13-4

Documentation Points with the Use of a Restraint

Reason for restraint
Method of restraint
Date and time of application of restraint
Duration of use of the restraint and client's response
Release from restraint with periodic exercise and circulatory, neurovascular, and skin assessment
Assessment of continued need for restraint
Evaluation of the client's response

c. Encourage family and friends to stay with client, and utilize sitters for clients who need supervision
d. Assign confused and disoriented clients to rooms near the nurses' station
e. Provide appropriate visual and auditory stimuli to the client, such as clocks, calendars, television, and a radio
f. Place familiar items, such as family pictures, near the client's bedside
g. Maintain toileting routines
h. Eliminate bothersome treatments, such as tube feedings, as soon as possible
i. Evaluate all medications that the client is receiving
j. Use relaxation techniques with the client
k. Institute exercise and ambulation schedules as the client's condition allows

G. **Poisons**
1. Any substance that impairs health and destroys life when ingested, inhaled, or otherwise absorbed by the body
2. Specific antidotes or treatments are available for only some types of **poisons**
3. The capacity of body tissue to recover from a **poison** determines the reversibility of the effect
4. **Poison** can impair the respiratory, circulatory, central nervous, hepatic, gastrointestinal (GI), and renal systems of the body
5. The toddler, the preschooler, and the young school-aged child must be protected from accidental poisoning
6. In older adults, diminished eyesight and impaired memory may result in accidental ingestion of poisonous substances or an overdose of prescribed medications
7. The **Poison** Control Center phone number should be visible on the telephone itself in homes with small children; in all cases of suspected poisoning, the number should be called immediately
8. Implementation
a. Remove any obvious materials from the mouth, eyes, or body area immediately
b. Identify the type and amount of substance ingested
c. Call the **Poison** Control Center before attempting an intervention
d. If the victim vomits or vomiting is induced, save the vomitus if requested to do so, and deliver it to the **Poison** Control Center
e. If instructed by the **Poison** Control Center to take the person to the emergency department, call an ambulance
f. Vomiting is never induced after ingestion of lye, household cleaners, grease, or petroleum products
g. Vomiting is never induced in an unconscious victim

III. DISASTERS
A. Know the agency's disaster plan
B. Internal disasters are those in which the agency is in danger
C. External disasters occur in the community, and victims will be brought to the health care facility for care
D. When the health care agency is notified of a disaster, plans specified in the agency policy must be carried out

IV. NOSOCOMIAL INFECTIONS (Box 13-5)
A. Also referred to as hospital-acquired infections
B. Infections acquired in the hospital or other health care facility that were not present or incubating at the time of the client's admission
C. Illness impairs the body's normal defense mechanisms
D. The hospital environment provides exposure to a variety of virulent organisms that the client has not been exposed to in the past; therefore, the client has not developed resistance to these organisms
E. Infections can be transmitted by health care personnel who fail to practice proper hand washing procedures or fail to change gloves between client contacts

V. STANDARD (UNIVERSAL) PRECAUTIONS
A. Description
1. Must be practiced with all clients in any setting regardless of the diagnosis or presumed infectiousness
2. Promotes hand washing and the use of gloves, masks, eye protection, and gowns, when appropriate, for client contact
3. These precautions apply to blood; all body fluids, secretions, and excretions regardless of

BOX 13-5

Common Drug-Resistant Nosocomial Infections

Vancomycin-resistant enterococci (VRE)
Methicillin-resistant *Staphylococcus aureus* (MRSA)
Multidrug-resistant (MDR) tuberculosis

whether they contain blood; nonintact skin; and mucous membranes

B. Implementation
   1. Handle all blood and body fluids from all clients as if they were contaminated
   2. Hands are washed between client contacts; after contact with blood, body fluids, secretions, and excretions, and after contact with equipment or articles contaminated by them; and immediately after gloves are removed
   3. Gloves are worn when touching blood, body fluids, secretions, excretions, nonintact skin, mucous membranes, or contaminated items; gloves should be removed and hands washed between client care
   4. Masks, eye protection, or face shields are worn if client care activities may generate splashes or sprays of blood or body fluid
   5. Gowns are worn if soiling of clothing is likely from blood or body fluid; wash hands after removing a gown
   6. Client care equipment is properly cleaned and reprocessed, and single-use items are discarded
   7. Contaminated linen is placed in leak-proof bags and handled to prevent skin and mucous membrane exposure
   8. All sharp instruments and needles are discarded in a puncture-resistant container; needles are disposed of uncapped, or a mechanical device for recapping is used if necessary
   9. Spills of blood or body fluids are cleaned with a solution of bleach and water (diluted 1:10) or agency approved disinfectant

VI. TRANSMISSION-BASED PRECAUTIONS

A. Airborne precautions
   1. Diseases
      a. Measles
      b. Chickenpox (varicella)
      c. Disseminated varicella zoster
      d. Pulmonary or laryngeal tuberculosis (TB)
   2. Barrier protection for airborne precautions
      a. Single room maintained under negative pressure; door is kept closed except when someone is entering or exiting the room
      b. Negative air-flow pressure in the room with a minimum of 6 to 12 air exchanges per hour depending on the health care agency
      c. Mask or respiratory protection device
   3. Barrier protection for TB
      a. Includes airborne precautions and the additional following precautions
         1. Use of ultraviolet germicide irradiation or HEPA filter, which may reduce the number of droplet nuclei
         2. Use of personal respiratory protective devices (masks), capable of filtration of 95% efficiency, when personnel enter the isolation room; ability to fit-test masks to obtain a face-seal leakage of less than or equal to 10%
         3. Place a mask on the client when the client is out of the room; the client leaves the room only if necessary

B. Droplet precautions
   1. Diseases
      a. Diphtheria (pharyngeal)
      b. Rubella
      c. Streptococcal pharyngitis
      d. Mycoplasma pneumonia or menigococcal pneumonia or sepsis
      e. Scarlet fever in infants and younger children
      f. Pertussis
      g. Mumps
      h. Pneumonic plague
   2. Barrier protection
      a. Private room or cohort client
      b. Use of a mask
      c. Place a mask on the client when out of the room; the client leaves the room only if necessary

C. Contact precautions
   1. Diseases
      a. Respiratory syncytial virus (RSV)
      b. Shigella and other enteric pathogens
      c. Major wound infections
      d. Herpes simplex
      e. Scabies
      f. Varicella zoster (disseminated)
      g. Colonization or infection with multidrug-resistant organism (Box 13-5)
   2. Barrier protection
      a. Private room or cohort client
      b. Use of gloves and a gown when in contact with the client

PRACTICE QUESTIONS

1. A nurse enters a client's room and finds that the wastebasket is on fire. The nurse immediately assists the client out of the room. The next nursing action would be to:
   1. Confine the fire by closing the room door
   2. Activate the fire alarm
   3. Call for help
   4. Extinguish the fire

2. A nurse enters the nursing lounge and discovers that a chair is on fire. The nurse activates the alarm, closes the lounge door, and obtains the fire extinguisher to extinguish the fire. The nurse pulls the pin on the fire extinguisher. The next appropriate action would be to:
   1. Squeeze the handle on the extinguisher
   2. Aim at the base of the fire
   3. Sweep the fire from side to side with the extinguisher
   4. Sweep the fire from top to bottom with the extinguisher
3. A nurse conducts a home safety assessment with a client preparing for discharge and the client tells the nurse that a space heater is used to heat the apartment. Which of the following instructions would the nurse provide to the client regarding the use of the space heater?
   1. A space heater should not be used in an apartment
   2. The space heater needs to be placed at least 3 feet from anything that can burn
   3. The space heater should be placed in the hallway at nighttime
   4. The space heater should be kept at low setting at all times
4. A nurse is preparing to initiate a tube feeding to a client and the physician has prescribed the use of an electronic food pump. The nurse brings the pump to the bedside to plug the pump cord into the wall and discovers that there is no available plug in the wall socket. Which of the following would be the most appropriate nursing action?
   1. Use an extension cord from the nurse's lounge for the pump plug
   2. Initiate the feeding without the use of a pump
   3. Plug in the pump cord in the available plug above the room sink
   4. Contact the electrical maintenance department for assistance
5. A nurse obtains an order from the physician to restrain a client using a jacket restraint. The nurse instructs the nursing assistant to apply the restraint to the client. Which of the following observations, if made by the nurse, would indicate inappropriate application of the restraint?
   1. A clove hitch knot in the restraint strap
   2. Restraint straps are safely secured to the side rails
   3. The jacket restraint is secure and two fingers can easily slide between the restraint and the client's skin
   4. The jacket restraint strap does not tighten when force is applied against it
6. A nurse is providing directions to the nursing assistant who will be caring for a client with hand restraints. The nurse instructs the nursing assistant to remove the restraints to permit muscle exercise and promote circulation at least:
   1. Every 2 hours
   2. Every 3 hours
   3. Every 4 hours
   4. Once during the shift
7. A nurse is planning care for a client with an internal radiation implant. Which of the following is not an appropriate component for the nurse to include in the plan of care?
   1. Placing the client in a semiprivate room at the end of the hallway
   2. Wearing gloves when emptying the client's bedpan
   3. Keeping all linens in the room until the implant is removed
   4. Wearing a lead apron when providing direct care to the client
8. A mother calls a neighborhood nurse and tells the nurse that her 3-year-old child has just ingested liquid furniture polish. The nurse would direct the mother to immediately:
   1. Administer Ipecac to induce vomiting
   2. Bring the child to the emergency room
   3. Call an ambulance
   4. Call the Poison Control Center
9. An emergency room nurse receives a telephone call and is informed that a tornado hit a local residential area and numerous casualties have occurred. The victims will be brought to the emergency room. The initial nursing action would be which of the following?
   1. Prepare the triage rooms
   2. Obtain additional supplies from the central supply department
   3. Activate the agency disaster plan
   4. Obtain additional nursing staff to assist in treating the casualties
10. A nurse is caring for a client with a nosocomial infection caused by methicillin-resistant *Staphylococcus aureus* (MRSA) who is on contact precautions. The nurse prepares to provide colostomy care to the client. Which of the following protective items will be required to perform this procedure?
    1. Gloves, gown, and goggles
    2. Gloves and goggles
    3. Gloves, gown, and shoe protectors
    4. Gloves and a gown

ANSWERS

1. *Answer:* 2
Rationale: The order of priority in the event of a fire is to rescue the clients in immediate danger. The next step is to activate the fire alarm. The fire is then confined by closing all doors and lastly, the fire is extinguished.
Test-Taking Strategy: Remember the mnemonic RACE to prioritize in the event of a fire. R = Rescue clients in immediate danger; A = Alarm, sound the alarm; C = Confine the fire by closing all doors; E = Extinguish or evacuate. Review fire safety procedures if you had difficulty with this question.
Level of Cognitive Ability: Application
Client Needs: Safe, Effective Care Environment
Integrated Concept/Process: Nursing Process/Implementation
Content Area: Fundamental Skills
Reference: DeWit S: *Fundamental concepts and skills for nursing,* Philadelphia, 2001, WB Saunders, p. 326.

2. *Answer:* 2
Rationale: A fire can be extinguished by smothering it with a blanket or by the use of a fire extinguisher. To use the extinguisher, the pin is pulled first. The extinguisher should then be aimed at the base of the fire. The handle of the extinguisher is then squeezed and the fire is extinguished by sweeping from side to side to coat the area evenly.
Test-Taking Strategy: Note the key word "next." Remember the mnemonic PASS to prioritize in the use of a fire extinguisher. PASS = Pull the pin; A = Aim at the base of the fire; S = Squeeze the handle; S = Sweep from side to side to coat the area evenly. Review the procedures related to the use of a fire extinguisher if you had difficulty with this question.
Level of Cognitive Ability: Application
Client Needs: Safe, Effective Care Environment
Integrated Concept/Process: Nursing Process/Implementation
Content Area: Fundamental Skills
Reference: DeWit S: *Fundamental concepts and skills for nursing,* Philadelphia, 2001, WB Saunders, p. 325.

3. *Answer:* 2
Rationale: Space heaters need to be used appropriately because they present a great risk of fire. A space heater needs to be placed at least 3 feet from anything that can burn. Placing a heater in a hallway does not guarantee that it will be 3 feet from anything that can burn. A low setting does not reduce the risk of fire. A space heater can be used in an apartment if there is ample space and safety precautions are followed.
Test-Taking Strategy: Use the process of elimination keeping in mind the issue related to fire safety. Note that option 2 is the only option that specifically defines a safety measure related to the use of a space heater. Review fire safety prevention measures in the home if you had difficulty with this question.
Level of Cognitive Ability: Application
Client Needs: Safe, Effective Care Environment
Integrated Concept/Process: Teaching/Learning
Content Area: Fundamental Skills
Reference: DeWit S: *Fundamental concepts and skills for nursing,* Philadelphia, 2001, WB Saunders, p. 326.

4. *Answer:* 4
Rationale: The nurse needs to use hospital resources for assistance. A regular extension cord should not be used because it poses the risk of fire. The use of electrical appliances near a sink also presents a hazard. If the use of a pump is prescribed, the nurse must provide the safe means for its use.
Test-Taking Strategy: Use the process of elimination. Eliminate option 2 because the physician has ordered the use of an electronic pump. Recalling safety issues related to electrical hazards will assist in eliminating options 1 and 3. Review electrical safety if you had difficulty with this question.
Level of Cognitive Ability: Application
Client Needs: Safe, Effective Care Environment
Integrated Concept/Process: Nursing Process/Implementation
Content Area: Fundamental Skills
Reference: Potter P, Perry A: *Fundamentals of nursing,* ed 5, St Louis, 2001, Mosby, p. 1046.

5. *Answer:* 2
Rationale: A clove hitch knot should be used for applying a restraint because it does not tighten when force is applied against it and allows quick and easy removal of the restraint in the case of an emergency. The restraint strap is secured to the bed frame and never to the side rail to avoid accidental injury in the event that the side rail is released. The jacket restraint should be secure and one to two fingers should slide easily between the restraint and the client's skin.
Test-Taking Strategy: Note the key word "inappropriate." This indicates that you are looking for an option that identifies an inaccurate measure related to the application of restraints. The words "secured to the side rails" in option 2 should direct you to this option as an inappropriate action. Review guidelines related to the application of restraints if you had difficulty with this question.
Level of Cognitive Ability: Comprehension
Client Needs: Safe, Effective Care Environment
Integrated Concept/Process: Teaching/Learning
Content Area: Fundamental Skills
Reference: DeWit S: *Fundamental concepts and skills for nursing,* Philadelphia, 2001, WB Saunders, p. 331.

6. *Answer:* 1
Rationale: The nurse should instruct the nursing assistant to release the restraints at least every 2 hours to permit muscle exercise and promote circulation. Agency guidelines regarding the use of restraints should always be followed.
Test-Taking Strategy: Use the process of elimination. In this situation, it is best to select the option that identifies the most frequent time frame. Review guidelines related to the use of restraints if you had difficulty with this question.
Level of Cognitive Ability: Application
Client Needs: Physiological Integrity
Integrated Concept/Process: Teaching/Learning
Content Area: Fundamental Skills
Reference: DeWit S: *Fundamental concepts and skills for nursing,* Philadelphia, 2001, WB Saunders, p. 327.

7. *Answer:* 1
Rationale: A private room with a private bath is essential if a client has an internal radiation implant. This is necessary to prevent accidental exposure of radiation to other clients. Options 2, 3, and 4 are accurate interventions for a client with a radiation implant.

Test-Taking Strategy: Use the process of elimination. Note the key words "not an appropriate." Option 2 can be eliminated first because this is a component of standard precautions for all clients. Options 3 and 4 can be eliminated next because they directly relate to radiation safety. Review radiation safety principles if you had difficulty with this question.
Level of Cognitive Ability: Application
Client Needs: Safe, Effective Care Environment
Integrated Concept/Process: Nursing Process/Planning
Content Area: Fundamental Skills
Reference: DeWit S: *Fundamental concepts and skills for nursing,* Philadelphia, 2001, WB Saunders, p. 739.

8. *Answer:* 4
Rationale: If a poisoning occurs, the Poison Control Center should be contacted immediately. Vomiting should not be induced if the victim is unconscious or if the substance ingested was a strong corrosive or petroleum product. Bringing the child to the emergency room and calling an ambulance would not be the initial actions, as these would delay treatment. The Poison Control Center may advise the mother to bring the child to the emergency room, and if this is the case, the mother should call an ambulance.
Test-Taking Strategy: Use the process of elimination. Note the key word "immediately." Eliminate options 2 and 3 because these options will delay treatment. Recalling that vomiting should not be induced if a corrosive substance was ingested will assist in eliminating option 1. Review poison control measures if you had difficulty with this question.
Level of Cognitive Ability: Application
Client Needs: Physiological Integrity
Integrated Concept/Process: Nursing Process/Implementation
Content Area: Child Health
Reference: DeWit S: *Fundamental concepts and skills for nursing,* Philadelphia, 2001, WB Saunders, p. 326.

9. *Answer:* 3
Rationale: In an external disaster, many people will be brought to the emergency room for treatment. Although options 1, 2, and 4 may be a component of preparing for the casualties, the initial nursing action must be to activate the disaster plan.
Test-Taking Strategy: Note the key word "initial." Use the process of elimination in determining the priority action. Note that option 3 is the global option. Review procedures related to management of a disaster if you had difficulty with this question.
Level of Cognitive Ability: Application
Client Needs: Safe, Effective Care Environment
Integrated Concept/Process: Nursing Process/Implementation
Content Area: Fundamental Skills
Reference: DeWit S: *Fundamental concepts and skills for nursing,* Philadelphia, 2001, WB Saunders, p. 53.

10. *Answer:* 1
Rationale: Goggles are worn to protect the mucous membranes of the eye during interventions that may produce splashes of blood, body fluids, secretions, and excretions. In addition, contact precautions require the use of gloves, and a gown should be worn if direct client contact is anticipated. Shoe protectors are not necessary.
Test-Taking Strategy: Note the key words "contact precautions" and "colostomy." Use the process of elimination in determining the necessary items required caring for this client. Review this type of precautions if you had difficulty with this question.
Level of Cognitive Ability: Application
Client Needs: Safe, Effective Care Environment
Integrated Concept/Process: Nursing Process/Implementation
Content Area: Fundamental Skills
Reference: DeWit S: *Fundamental concepts and skills for nursing,* Philadelphia, 2001, WB Saunders, p. 230.

REFERENCES

DeWit S: *Fundamental concepts and skills for nursing,* Philadelphia, 2001, WB Saunders.

Kee J, Marshall S: *Clinical calculations,* ed 4, Philadelphia, 2000, WB Saunders.

National Council of State Boards of Nursing, editors: *Test plan for the National Council Licensure Examination for Practical/Vocational Nurses,* Chicago, 2001, Author.

Potter P, Perry A: *Fundamentals of nursing,* ed 5, St Louis, 2001, Mosby.

Medication and Intravenous Administration

PYRAMID TERMS

Conversion The first step in the calculation of a medication problem.

Generic Name The common or chemical name of a medication; printed on the label in smaller letters, usually under the trade name.

Milliequivalent Milliequivalent, abbreviated mEq, is an expression of the number of grams of a medication contained in 1 mL of a normal solution.

Parenteral Parenteral always means injection route. Injections are administered by intravenous (IV), intramuscular (IM), and subcutaneous (SQ, SC) routes.

Percentage Solutions Percentage solutions express the number of grams of the medication per 100 mL of solution.

Reconstitution Powders must be dissolved with a sterile diluent before use, and usually sterile water or normal saline is used. The dissolving procedure is called reconstitution.

Ratio Solutions Ratio solutions express the number of grams of the medication per total milliliters of solution.

Trade Name Also called the brand name; printed on the label in large bold letters.

Unit Unit, abbreviated as U or u, is measurement of a medication in terms of its action, not its physical weight.

PYRAMID TO SUCCESS

When a medication or intravenous calculation question is presented, a nurse should always use the appropriate formula to solve the problem. Short cuts should not be used in making these calculations. The problem and answer should be expressed in the correct units of measurement. Be careful with decimal points. It is important to place the decimal points in the correct places, or the answer will be incorrect. When solving a medication calculation problem, the nurse determines whether the answer is within reason and makes sense. In the clinical setting, the nurse should always seek assistance if he or she is unsure of the accuracy of a calculation.

On CAT NCLEX-PN, you will be provided with an optional drop-down calculator for calculating dosages. Even if you use the calculator to calculate dosages, it is important to check the calculation before selecting the answer to the question. REMEMBER, on CAT NCLEX-PN, the correct answer will be on the screen. Following the formula, placing the decimal points in the correct places, and checking the accuracy of the calculation will ensure selection of the correct answer. Remember, practice makes perfect!

The Integrated Concepts and Processes addressed in this chapter are Caring, the Clinical Problem-Solving Process (Nursing Process), Communication and Documentation, Cultural Awareness, Self-Care, and Teaching/Learning.

CLIENT NEEDS

Safe, Effective Care Environment

Asepsis
Client rights
Error prevention
Establishing priorities
Handling hazardous and infectious materials
Intravenous fluid and medication calculations
Standard precautions

Health Promotion and Maintenance

Collecting physical data
Disease prevention
Reinforcing teaching regarding prescribed medication(s) or IV therapy

Psychosocial Integrity

Caring and providing emotional comfort

Communication
Cultural awareness
Use of coping mechanisms
Use of support systems

Physiological Integrity

Actions, side effects, and untoward effects of medications and IV therapy
Administration of medications and monitoring IV therapy
Alterations in body systems
Expected effects of pharmacological therapy
Fluid and electrolyte imbalances
Laboratory values
Unexpected responses to therapy

I. DRUG MEASUREMENT SYSTEMS

A. Metric System
1. The basic units of metric measures are meter, liter, and gram (Table 14-1)
2. Meter measures length
3. Liter measures volume
4. Gram measures weight

B. Apothecary and household systems (Table 14-2)
1. The apothecary and household systems are the oldest of the medication measurement systems
2. The four apothecary measures sometimes used are the grain, minim, dram, and ounce
3. Grain measures weight
4. Minim, dram, and ounce measure volume
5. The three household measures commonly used are tablespoon, teaspoon, and drop

C. Additional common medication measures
1. **Milliequivalent**
a. Abbreviated mEq
b. Is an expression of the number of grams of a medication contained in 1 mL of a normal solution
c. Example: potassium

TABLE 14-1

Metric System

Abbreviations	Equivalents
meter - m	1 L = 1000 mL
liter - L	1 mL = 0.001 L or 1 cc
gram - g, gm, Gm	1 mL = 1 cc or 0.001 L
milligram - mg, mgm	1 g = 1000 mg
microgram - μg, mcg	1 mg = 1000 mcg or 0.001 g
kilogram - kg, Kg	1 mcg = 0.000001 g
milliliter - mL	1 kg = 1000 g
cubic centimeter - cc	1 kg = 2.2 lb

TABLE 14-2

Apothecary and Household Systems

Abbreviations	Equivalents
grain - gr	gr 1 = 60 mg
dram - dr	gr 5 = 300 mg
ounce - oz	gr 15 = 1000 mg or 1 gm
minim - min, M or m	gr 1/150 = 0.4 mg
quart - qt1	1 oz = 30 mL
pint - pt	1 dr = 4 mL
drop - gtt1	1 T = 15 mL or 3 tsp
teaspoon - t or tsp	1 t or tsp = 5 mL
tablespoon - T or tbs	1 min = 1 gtt
pound - lb	15 min = 1 mL
	60 min = 1 dr
	8 dr = 1 oz
	1 qt = 2 pt or 32 oz
	1 qt = 1000 mL or 1 L
	1 pt = 16 oz
	16 oz = 1 lb
	2.2 lbs = 1 kg

2. **Unit**
a. Abbreviated as U or u; measures a medication in terms of its action, not its physical weight
b. Examples: penicillin, heparin, insulin

II. CONVERSIONS

A. Conversion between metric units (Box 14-1)
1. The metric system is a decimal system; therefore, conversions between the units in this system can be done by either dividing or multiplying by 1000 or by moving the decimal point three places to the right or three places to the left

BOX 14-1

Conversion Between Metric Units

1. Problem:
Convert 2 grams to milligrams.
Solution
Change a larger unit to a smaller unit.
2.000 grams = 2000 mg (moving the decimal three places to the right)
2. Problem:
Convert 250 mL to liters
Solution
Change a smaller unit to a larger unit
250 mL = 0.250 L or 0.25 L (moving the decimal three places to the left)

2. In the metric system, to convert larger to smaller, multiply by 1000 or move the decimal three places to the right
3. In the metric system, to convert smaller to larger, divide by 1000 or move the decimal three places to the left

B. Conversion between apothecary, household, and metric systems
1. Conversions between the metric, apothecary, and household measures are equivalent, not equal, measures
2. Conversion to equivalent measures between systems is necessary when a medication order is written in one system but the medication label is stated in another
3. Medications are not always ordered and prepared in the same system of measurement; therefore it is necessary to convert units from one system to another
4. Conversion is the first step in the calculation of dosages
5. Calculating equivalents between two systems may be done using the method of ratio and proportion (Box 14-2)

III. CELSIUS AND FAHRENHEIT TEMPERATURE (Table 14-3)

A. To convert Fahrenheit to Celsius, subtract 32 and divide the result by 1.8

B. To convert Celsius to Fahrenheit, multiply by 1.8 and add 32

IV. MEDICATION LABELS

A. A medication label will contain both the **generic** and **trade name** of the medication

B. The **generic name** is the common or chemical name of a medication; the **generic name** is not capitalized

BOX 14-2

Calculating Equivalents Between Two Systems

Calculating equivalents between two systems may be done using the method of ratio and proportion

PROBLEM

The physician orders nitroglycerin, gr 1/150. The medication label reads 0.4 mg per tablet. How many tablets will you administer to the client?

gr 1 : 60 mg = gr 1/150 : X mg

$60 \times 1/150 = x$

x = 0.4 mg (1 tablet)

TABLE 14-3

Celsius and Fahrenheit Temperature

FAHRENHEIT TO CELSIUS

To convert Fahrenheit to Celsius, subtract 32 and divide the result by 1.8

Formula: C = (F - 32) divided by 1.8

CELSIUS TO FAHRENHEIT

To convert Celsius to Fahrenheit, multiply by 1.8 and add 32

Formula: F = 1.8 C + 32

C. The **trade name,** also called brand name, is printed on the medication label in large bold letters

D. Each medication has only one official name but may have several trade names, each for the exclusive use of the company that manufactures the medication

E. Always check expiration dates on the medication labels

V. MEDICATION ORDERS (Box 14-3)

A. In a medication order, the name of the medication is written first, followed by the dosage, route, and frequency

B. If there are any questions or inconsistencies with the written order, the person who wrote the order must be contacted immediately, and the order must be verified

VI. ORAL MEDICATIONS

A. Scored tablets contain an indented marking to make breakage for partial dosages possible; when necessary, scored tablets (those marked for division) can be divided in halves or quarters

B. Enteric-coated tablets and sustained-released capsules delay absorption until the medication reaches the small intestine; these medications should not be crushed

C. Capsules contain a powered or oily medication in a gelatin cover

BOX 14-3

Medication Orders

Name of client
Date and time when order was written
Name of medication to be given
Dosage of medication
Route
Time and frequency of administration
Signature of person writing the order

D. Oral liquids are supplied in solution form and contain a specific amount of medication in a given amount of solution, as stated on the label
E. The Medicine Cup (Figure 14-1)
   1. Has a capacity of 30 mL or 1 ounce
   2. Is used for oral liquids
   3. Is calibrated to measure teaspoons, tablespoons, and drams
   4. To pour accurately, hold the medication cup at eye level, then line up the measure that is needed and pour
F. Volumes of less than 5 mL are measured using a syringe with the needle removed
G. A calibrated dropper is used when giving medicine to children and when adding small amounts of liquid to water or juice; calibrations are in milliliters, cubic centimeters, drops, or minims

VII. PARENTERAL MEDICATIONS

A. **Parenteral** always means injection route, and **parenteral** medications are administered by intravenous (IV), intramuscular (IM), or by subcutaneous (SC) routes
B. **Parenteral** medications are packaged in single-use ampules, single and multiple-use rubber stoppered vials, and in premeasured syringes and cartridges

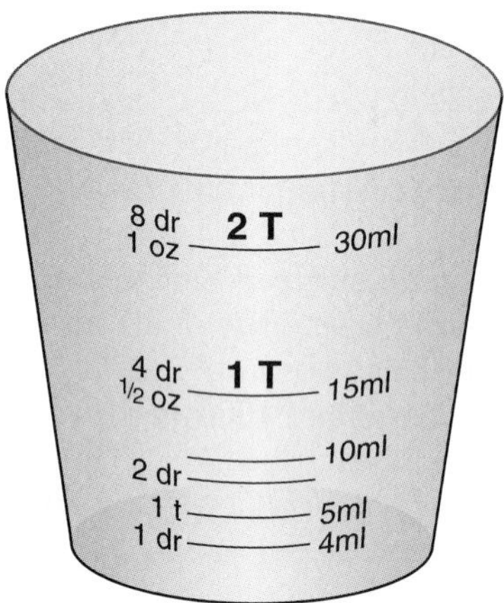

FIG. 14-1 Medicine cup. (From Kee J, Marshall S: *Clinical calculations*, ed 4, Philadelphia, 2000, WB Saunders.)

C. The nurse should not administer more than 3 mL per IM or SC injection site because volumes larger than 3 mL are difficult for a single injection site to absorb
D. Always question excessively large or small volumes of medication
E. The standard 3-mL (cubic centimeter [cc]) syringe is used to measure most injectable medications; it is calibrated in tenths (0.1) of a mL (Figure 14-2)
F. The calibrations on a syringe are read from the top black ring on the syringe, not the raised middle section and not the bottom ring
G. Prefilled medication cartridge and cartridge holder/syringe (Figure 14-3)
   1. Tubex and Carpuject are trade names of two widely used, reusable, metal or plastic cartridge holders
   2. The medication cartridge slips into the cartridge holder, which provides a plunger for injection of the medication
   3. The medication cartridge is prefilled with medication and is labeled with the medication name and dosage
   4. The medication cartridge is routinely overfilled with 0.1 to 0.2 mL of medication to allow for manipulation of the holder to expel air from the needle before injection
   5. The medication cartridge is designed to provide sufficient capacity to allow for the addition of a second medication when combined dosages are prescribed
   6. The prefilled medication cartridge is to be used once and discarded; if the nurse is to give less than a full single dose provided, the nurse needs to discard the extra amount before giving the client the injection, following agency policies and procedures
H. Standard medication doses for adults are to be rounded to the nearest tenth (0.1) of a mL or cc and measured on the mL scale; for example, 1.25 mL is rounded to 1.3 mL
I. When volumes larger than 3 mL are required, a 5-, 6-, 10-, or 12- mL syringe may be used; these syringes are calibrated in fifths (Figure 14-4)

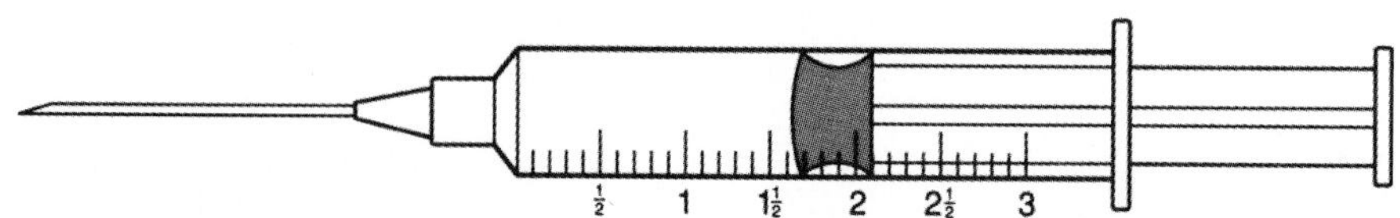

FIG. 14-2 A 3-mL syringe. (From Kee J, Marshall S: *Clinical calculations*, ed 4, Philadelphia, 2000, WB Saunders.)

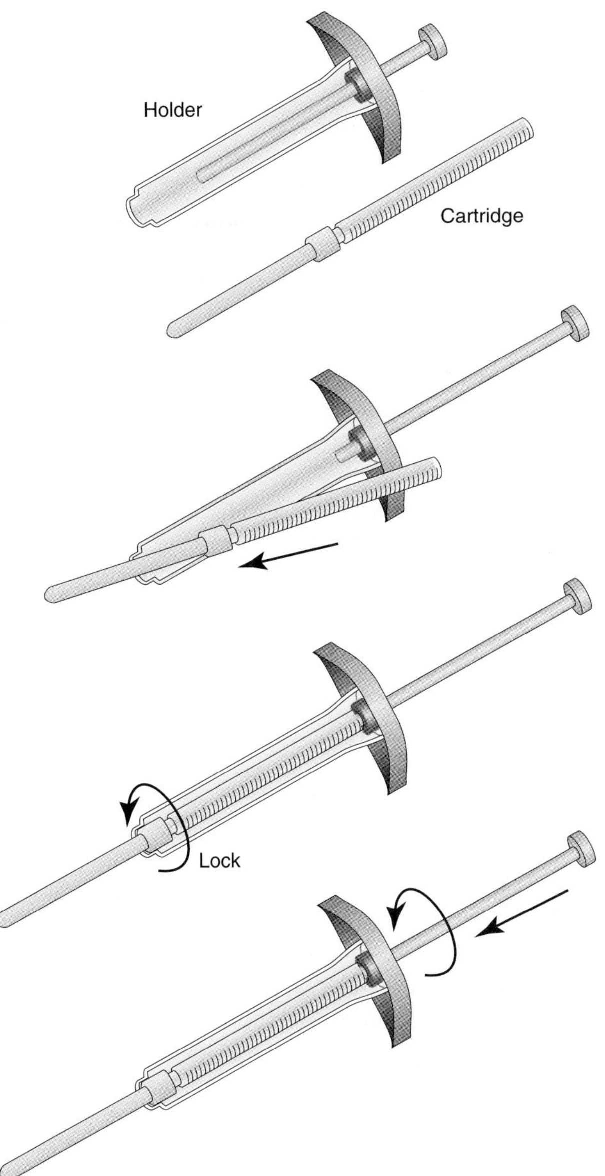

FIG. 14-3 Cartridge-type syringes. (From Leahy J, Kizilay P: *Foundations of nursing practice*, Philadelphia, 1998, WB Saunders.)

J. Syringes larger than 12 mL are calibrated in full mL measures
K. Tuberculin syringe (Figure 14-5)
   1. Holds a total capacity of 1 mL or cc and is used to measure small or critical amounts of medications such as allergen extract, vaccine, or a child's medication
   2. It is calibrated in hundredths (0.01) of a mL, with each one tenth (0.1) marked on the metric scale
L. Insulin syringe (Figure 14-6)
   1. The standard U-100 insulin syringe is used to measure U-100 insulin only; it is calibrated for a total of 100 units, or 1 mL (cc)
   2. Insulin should not be measured in any other type of syringe
   3. When the insulin order states to combine Regular and NPH insulin, remember to draw the Regular insulin first, and then draw the NPH insulin

VIII. INJECTABLE MEDICATIONS IN POWDER FORM

A. Some medications become unstable when stored in solution form and are therefore packaged in powder form
B. Powders must be dissolved with a sterile diluent before use, and usually sterile water or normal saline is used. The dissolving procedure is called **reconstitution** (Box 14-4)

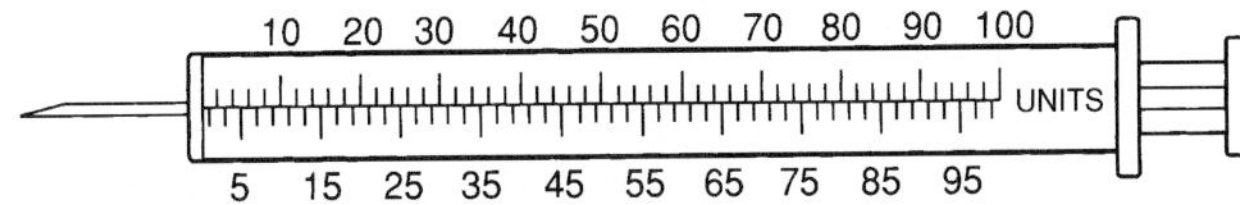

FIG. 14-6 Insulin syringe. (From Kee J, Marshall S: *Clinical calculations*, ed 4, Philadelphia, 2000, WB Saunders.)

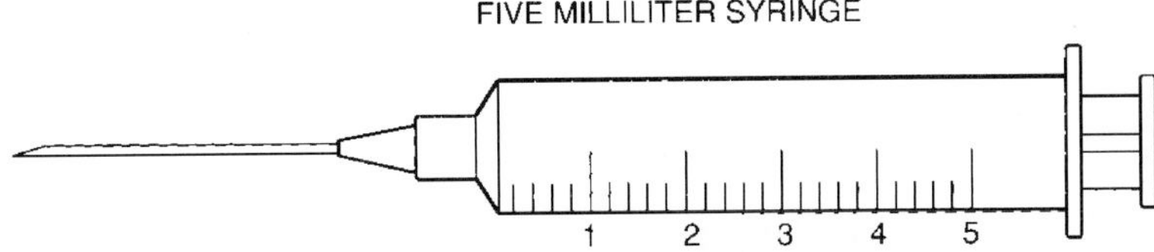

FIG. 14-4 A 5-mL syringe. (From Kee J, Marshall S: *Clinical calculations*, ed 4, Philadelphia, 2000, WB Saunders.)

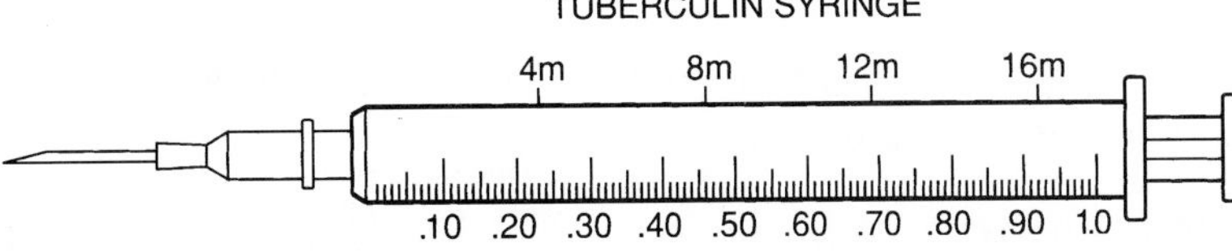

FIG. 14-5 Tuberculin syringe. (From Kee J, Marshall S: *Clinical calculations*, ed 4, Philadelphia, 2000, WB Saunders.)

BOX 14-4

Reconstitution

In reconstituting the medication, locate the instructions on the label or in the vial package insert and read and follow the directions carefully.

Instructions will state the volume of diluent to be used and the resulting volume of the reconstituted medication.

Often the powdered medication adds volume to the solution in addition to the amount of diluent added.

When you reconstitute a multiple dose vial, label the medication vial with the date and time of preparation, your initials, and the date of expiration.

It is also important to label the strength per volume.

The total volume of the prepared solution will always exceed the volume of the diluent that you add.

IX. CALCULATING THE CORRECT DOSAGE (Table 14-4)

A. When calculating oral medications, check the calculation and question an order if the amount is for more than three tablets

B. When calculating parenteral medications, check the calculation and question an order if the amount to be given is too large a dose

C. Regardless of the source of the error, if the nurse gives an incorrect dose, the nurse is legally responsible for the action

D. Be sure that all measures are in the same system, and all units are in the same size, converting when necessary; carefully consider what is the reasonable amount of the medication that should be administered

E. Round standard injection doses to tenths and measure in a 3-mL syringe

F. Round small, critical, or children's doses to hundredths and measure in the 1-mL tuberculin syringe

X. CALCULATING DOSAGES EXPRESSED AS RATIO OR PERCENT

A. **Percentage solutions**

1. Express the number of grams of the medication per 100 mL of solution
2. Example: calcium gluconate 10% = 10 g of pure medication per 100 mL of solution

B. **Ratio solutions**

1. Express the number of grams of the medication per total milliliters of solution
2. Example: epinephrine 1:1000 = 1 g pure medication per 1000 mL solution

XI. INTRAVENOUS FLOW RATES (Table 14-5)

A. Monitor IVs every 30 minutes to 1 hour for adults and every 15 minutes for children as specified by agency policy

B. If the IV is running behind schedule, collaborate with the registered nurse and/or the physician to determine the client's ability to tolerate an increased flow rate, particularly those clients with cardiac, pulmonary, renal, and neurological conditions

C. The nurse should never arbitrarily speed up an IV to catch up if the IV is running behind schedule

D. Whenever an IV rate is increased, the nurse should monitor the client for increased heart rate, increased respirations, or increased lung congestion, which could indicate fluid overload

E. IV fluids are most frequently ordered on the basis of mL per hour to be administered

F. The volume ordered is administered by adjusting the rate at which the IV infuses, which is counted in drops (gtt) per minute

G. Most flow rate calculations involve changing mL per hour into gtt per minute

H. IV Tubing

1. Calibrated in gtt per milliliter, and this calibration is needed for calculating flow rates
2. A standard or macrodrip set is used for routine adult IV administrations; depending on

TABLE 14-4

Formula for Calculating Medication Dosage

$$\frac{\text{D (Desired)}}{\text{A (Available)}} \times \text{Q (Quantity)} = \text{X}$$

D (Desired) = The dosage that the physician ordered

A (Available) = The dosage strength as stated on the medication label

Q (Quantity) = The volume that the dosage strength is available in, such as tablets, capsules, or mL

TABLE 14-5

Formulas for IV Calculations

FLOW RATES

$$\frac{\text{Total volume} \times \text{gtt factor}}{\text{Time in minutes}} = \text{gtt per min}$$

INFUSION TIME

$$\frac{\text{Total volume to infuse}}{\text{mL per hour being infused}} = \text{Infusion time}$$

the manufacturer and type of tubing, it will require 10, 15, or 20 gtt to equal 1 mL
3. A minidrip or microdrip set is used when more exact measurements are needed, and in pediatric units
4. In a minidrip or microdrip set, 60 gtt is equal to 1 mL
5. The calibration, in gtt per mL is written on the IV tubing package

XII. ELECTRONIC IV FLOW RATE REGULATORS

A. Controller
1. Works on the same principle of gravity as a regular IV drip, with the rate of flow being maintained by rapid compression and decompression of the IV tubing by the machine
2. The desired flow rate is set on the controller in milliliters per hour
3. Because controllers work by gravity, the height of the solution bag is critical and must be maintained at a minimum of 36 inches above the controller
4. The nurse should continue to monitor the amount of IV solution in the IV container and monitor the controller to ensure proper functioning of the machine

B. Pump
1. A pump is different from a controller in that it physically pumps fluids against resistance
2. Gravity is not a factor in the use of a pump, and the height of the IV solution bag is not a critical factor
3. The flow rate on a pump is set in milliliters per hour
4. The nurse should continue to monitor the amount of IV solution in the IV container and monitor the pump to ensure proper functioning of the machine

PRACTICE QUESTIONS

1. A physician orders 1000 mL of 0.9% NS to run over 12 hours. The drop factor is 15 drops per 1 mL. The nurse plans to adjust the flow rate at how many drops per minute?
   1. 15 drops per minute
   2. 17 drops per minute
   3. 21 drops per minute
   4. 23 drops per minute
2. A physician orders an IM dose of 400,000 units of penicillin G benzathine (Bicillin). The label on the 10 mL ampule sent from the pharmacy reads penicillin G benzathine (Bicillin) 300,000 units per mL. The nurse prepares to administer how many mL to administer the correct dose?
   1. 1.3 mL
   2. 13 mL
   3. 1.5 mL
   4. 10 mL
3. A physician orders 3000 mL of 5% dextrose to run over a 24-hour period. The drop factor is 10 drops per 1 mL. The nurse plans to adjust the flow rate at how many drops per minute?
   1. 15 drops per minute
   2. 17 drops per minute
   3. 21 drops per minute
   4. 24 drops per minute
4. A physician's order reads phenytoin (Dilantin) 0.2 g PO BID. The medication label states 100-mg capsules. How many capsule(s) will the nurse prepare to administer one dose?
   1. 1 capsule
   2. 2 capsules
   3. 3 capsules
   4. 4 capsules
5. A physician orders 1000 mL of 1/2% NS to run over 8 hours. The drop factor is 15 drops per 1 mL. The nurse plans to adjust the flow rate at how many drops per minute?
   1. 20 drops per minute
   2. 22 drops per minute
   3. 28 drops per minute
   4. 31 drops per minute
6. A physician orders 2000 mL of D_5 1/2% NS to run over 24 hours. The drop factor is 15 drops per 1 mL. The nurse plans to adjust the flow rate at how many drops per minute?
   1. 15 drops per minute
   2. 17 drops per minute
   3. 21 drops per minute
   4. 28 drops per minute
7. A physician's order reads cyanocobalamin (vitamin B_{12}) 100 mcg IM. The medication label reads cyanocobalamin (vitamin B_{12}), 0.5 mg per mL. The nurse administers how many mL to the client?
   1. 0.2 mL
   2. 0.5 mL
   3. 1 mL
   4. 2 mL
8. A physician orders 3000 mL of 5% dextrose to be administered over a 24-hour period. The nurse prepares to set the infusion rate knowing that how many mL per hour are to be administered?
   1. 50 mL per hour
   2. 75 mL per hour
   3. 100 mL per hour
   4. 125 mL per hour
9. A physician's order reads levothyroxine (Synthroid), 150 mcg PO daily. The medication label reads levothyroxine 0.1 mg per tablet. The

nurse prepares to administer how many tablet(s) to the client?
1. 1 tablet
2. 1.5 tablets
3. 2 tablets
4. 2.5 tablets

10. A physician orders 1000 mL 5% dextrose to run at 125 mL per hour. The nurse calculates the infusion rate knowing that it will take how many hours for 1 liter to infuse?
1. 8 hours
2. 10 hours
3. 12 hours
4. 15 hours

11. A physician orders one unit of packed red blood cells to run over 4 hours. The unit of blood contains 250 mL. The drop factor is 10 drops per 1 mL. The registered nurse (RN) asks the licensed practical nurse (LPN) to assist in monitoring the flow rate during the infusion. The LPN monitors the flow rate knowing that how many drops per minute should infuse?
1. 10 drops
2. 15 drops
3. 17 drops
4. 20 drops

12. A physician's order reads triazolam (Halcion), 125 mcg PO at HS daily. The medication bottle is labeled triazolam (Halcion), 0.125-mg tablets. The nurse prepares how many tablet(s) to administer one dose?
1. 1 tablet
2. 1.5 tablets
3. 2 tablets
4. 2.5 tablets

13. A physician's order reads atenolol (Tenormin), 0.025 g PO QD. The medication bottle reads atenolol (Tenormin) 50 mg-tablets. The nurse prepares how many tablet(s) to administer the dose?
1. 0.5 tablet
2. 1 tablet
3. 2 tablets
4. 3 tablets

14. A physician's order reads hydromorphone hydrochloride (Dilaudid), 3 mg IM q4h PRN. The medication label reads hydromorphone hydrochloride (Dilaudid), 4 mg per 1 mL. The nurse prepares to administer which of the following to the client?
1. 1.3 mg
2. 1.5 mL
3. 0.8 mL
4. 4 mg

15. A physician's order reads digoxin (Lanoxin), 0.25 mg PO daily. The medication label reads digoxin (Lanoxin), 0.125 mg per tablet. The nurse prepares how many tablet(s) to administer the dose?
1. 0.5 tablet
2. 1 tablet
3. 1.5 tablets
4. 2 tablets

16. A physician's order reads meperidine hydrochloride (Demerol), 80 mg IM PRN. The medication label reads meperidine hydrochloride (Demerol), 100 mg per mL. The nurse prepares to administer how many mL to the client?
1. 100 mL
2. 1.25 mL
3. 1 mL
4. 0.8 mL

17. A physician orders heparin sodium (Liquaemin), 650 units SC q12h. The medication vial reads heparin sodium (Liquaemin), 1000 units per mL. The nurse prepares how many mL to administer one dose?
1. 0.7 mL
2. 1.0 mL
3. 1.3 mL
4. 1.5 mL

18. A physician orders trimethobenzamide hydrochloride (Tigan), 250 mg IM PRN. The medication label reads trimethobenzamide hydrochloride (Tigan) 200 mg per 2 mL. The nurse plans to prepare how much medication to administer the dose?
1. 0.4 mL
2. 1.0 mL
3. 1.25 mL
4. 2.5 mL

19. A physician orders meperidine hydrochloride (Demerol), 35 mg IM stat. The medication label states meperidine hydrochloride (Demerol), 50 mg per mL. The nurse plans to prepare how much medication to administer the dose?
1. 0.5 mL
2. 0.6 mL
3. 0.7 mL
4. 1.0 mL

20. A physician orders prochlorperazine (Compazine), 20 mg q4h IM PRN. The medication label states prochlorperazine (Compazine), 10 mg per mL. The nurse prepares how much medication to administer the dose?
1. 0.5 mL
2. 2.0 mL
3. 2.5 mL
4. 2.9 mL

21. A physician orders atropine sulfate, 0.4 mg IM stat. The medication label states atropine sulfate, 0.3 mg per 0.5 mL. The nurse prepares how much medication to administer the dose?
1. 0.1 mL
2. 0.4 mL
3. 0.5 mL
4. 0.7 mL

22. A physician orders levodopa (Dopar), 1 g PO BID. The medication label states 500-mg tablets. The nurse prepares to administer how many tablets at the evening dose?
    1. 2 tablets
    2. 3 tablets
    3. 4 tablets
    4. 5 tablets
23. A physician orders zidovudine (AZT), 0.2 g PO q4h. The medication label states zidovudine (AZT), 100-mg tablets. The nurse prepares to administer how many tablets for one dose?
    1. 0.5 tablet
    2. 1 tablet
    3. 1.5 tablets
    4. 2 tablets
24. A physician orders atropine sulfate, gr 1/300 to be administered. The medication label states atropine sulfate, 0.5 mg per 0.5 mL. How many mL will the nurse prepare to administer to the client?
    1. 0.1 mL
    2. 0.2 mL
    3. 1 mL
    4. 2 mL
25. A physician's order states to administer aspirin (acetylsalicylic acid), 650 mg PO for a temperature above 38° C. The medication bottle states aspirin (acetylsalicylic acid), gr 5 per tablet. The nurse takes the client's temperature and notes that it is 101° F. The nurse plans to take which of the following actions?
    1. Not administer the aspirin at this time
    2. Check the client's temperature in 30 minutes
    3. Administer 2 aspirin tablets
    4. Administer 3 aspirin tablets

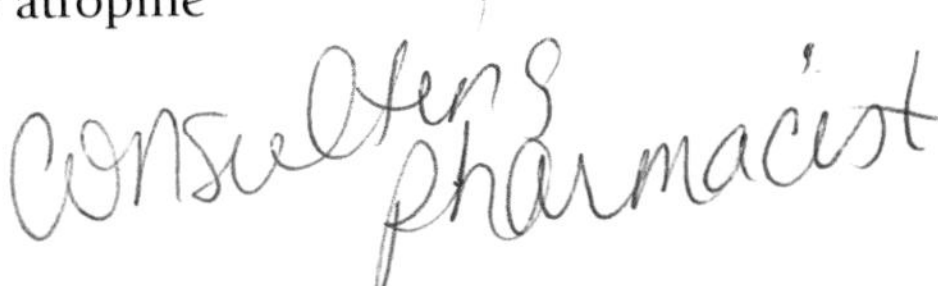

ANSWERS

1. *Answer:* 3

Rationale: The prescribed 1000 mL is to be infused over 12 hours. Follow the formula and multiply 1000 mL by 15 (gtt factor). Then, divide the result by 720 minutes (12 hours × 60 minutes). The infusion is to run at 20.8 or 21 drops per minute.

Formula:

$$\frac{\text{Total volume in mL} \times \text{drop factor}}{\text{Time in minutes}} = \text{Flow Rate in drops per minute}$$

$$\frac{1000 \text{ mL} \times 15 \text{ drops}}{720 \text{ minutes}} = \frac{15{,}000}{720} = 20.8 \text{ or } 21 \text{ drops per minute}$$

Test-Taking Strategy: Follow the formula for calculating the infusion rate for an IV. Label the problem and the answer. Make sure that the answer makes sense. Be sure to change 12 hours to minutes. Review the formula for calculating infusion rates if you had difficulty with this question.
Level of Cognitive Ability: Application
Client Needs: Physiological Integrity
Integrated Concept/Process: Nursing Process/Planning
Content Area: Fundamental Skills
Reference: DeWit S: *Fundamental concepts and skills for nursing,* Philadelphia, 2001, WB Saunders, p. 723.

2. *Answer:* 1

Rationale: Follow the formula for dosage calculation.

$$\frac{\text{Desired}}{\text{Available}} \times \text{mL} = \text{mL per dose} \quad \frac{400{,}000 \text{ units}}{300{,}000 \text{ units}} \times 1 \text{ mL} = 1.3 \text{ mL per dose}$$

Test-Taking Strategy: Follow the formula for the calculation of the correct dose. Label each figure including the answer. Focus on the key information: 300,000 units per mL. Recheck your work and make sure that the answer makes sense. Review medication calculation problems if you had difficulty with this question.
Level of Cognitive Ability: Application
Client Needs: Physiological Integrity
Integrated Concept/Process: Nursing Process/Planning
Content Area: Fundamental Skills
Reference: DeWit S: *Fundamental concepts and skills for nursing,* Philadelphia, 2001, WB Saunders, p. 642.

3. *Answer:* 3

Rationale: The prescribed 3000 mL is to be infused over 24 hours. Follow the formula and multiply 3000 mL by 10 (gtt factor). Then, divide the result by 1440 minutes (24 hours × 60 minutes). The infusion is to run at 20.8 or 21 drops per minute.

Formula:

$$\frac{\text{Total volume in mL} \times \text{drop factor}}{\text{Time in minutes}} = \text{Flow rate in drops per minute}$$

$$\frac{3000 \text{ mL} \times 10 \text{ drops}}{1440 \text{ minutes}} = \frac{30{,}000}{1440} = 20.8 \text{ or } 21 \text{ drops per minute}$$

Test-Taking Strategy: Follow the formula for calculating the infusion rate for an IV. Label the problem and the answer. Make sure that the answer makes sense. Be sure to change 24 hours to minutes. Review the formula for calculating infusion rates if you had difficulty with this question.
Level of Cognitive Ability: Application
Client Needs: Physiological Integrity
Integrated Concept/Process: Nursing Process/Planning
Content Area: Fundamental Skills
Reference: DeWit S: *Fundamental concepts and skills for nursing,* Philadelphia, 2001, WB Saunders, p. 723.

4. *Answer:* 2

Rationale: Convert 0.2 g to mg. In the metric system, to convert larger to smaller multiply by 1000 or move the decimal 3 places to the right. Therefore, 0.2 g = 200 mg.

Formula:

$$\frac{\text{Desired}}{\text{Available}} \times \text{Capsules} = \text{Capsules per dose}$$

$$\frac{200 \text{ mg}}{100 \text{ mg}} \times 1 \text{ capsule} = 2 \text{ capsules}$$

Test-Taking Strategy: In this medication calculation problem, it is necessary to first convert grams to milligrams. Follow the formula for conversion and read the question carefully. Recheck your work and make sure that the answer makes sense. Review medication calculations and conversions if you had difficulty with this question.
Level of Cognitive Ability: Application
Client Needs: Physiological Integrity
Integrated Concept/Process: Nursing Process/Implementation
Content Area: Fundamental Skills
Reference: DeWit S: *Fundamental concepts and skills for nursing,* Philadelphia, 2001, WB Saunders, p. 642.

5. ***Answer:*** 4
Rationale: The prescribed 1000 mL is to be infused over 8 hours. Follow the formula and multiply 1000 mL by 15 (gtt factor). Then, divide the result by 480 minutes (8 hours × 60 minutes). The infusion is to run at 31.2 or 31 drops per minute.
Formula:

$$\frac{\text{Total volumes in mL x drop factor}}{\text{Time in minutes}} = \text{Flow rate in drops per minute}$$

$$\frac{1000 \text{ mL} \times 15 \text{ drops}}{480 \text{ minutes}} = \frac{15{,}000}{480} = 31.2 \text{ or } 31 \text{ drops per minute}$$

Test-Taking Strategy: Follow the formula for calculating the infusion rate for an IV. Label the problem and the answer. Make sure that the answer makes sense. Be sure to change 8 hours to minutes. Review the formula for calculating infusion rates if you had difficulty with this question.
Level of Cognitive Ability: Application
Client Needs: Physiological Integrity
Integrated Concept/Process: Nursing Process/Planning
Content Area: Fundamental Skills
Reference: DeWit S: *Fundamental concepts and skills for nursing,* Philadelphia, 2001, WB Saunders, p. 723.

6. ***Answer:*** 3
Rationale: The prescribed 2000 mL is to be infused over 24 hours. Follow the formula and multiply 2000 mL by 15 (gtt factor). Then, divide the result by 1440 minutes (24 hours × 60 minutes). The infusion is to run at 20.8 or 21 drops per minute.
Formula:

$$\frac{\text{Total volumes in mL x drop factor}}{\text{Time in minutes}} = \text{Flow rate in drops per minute}$$

$$\frac{2000 \text{ mL} \times 15 \text{ drops}}{1440 \text{ minutes}} = \frac{30{,}000}{1440} = 20.8 \text{ or } 21 \text{ drops per minute}$$

Test-Taking Strategy: Follow the formula for calculating the infusion rate for an IV. Label the problem and the answer. Make sure that the answer makes sense. Be sure to change 24 hours to minutes. Review the formula for calculating infusion rates if you had difficulty with this question.
Level of Cognitive Ability: Application
Client Needs: Physiological Integrity
Integrated Concept/Process: Nursing Process/Planning
Content Area: Fundamental Skills
Reference: DeWit S: *Fundamental concepts and skills for nursing,* Philadelphia, 2001, WB Saunders, p. 723.

7. ***Answer:*** 1
Rationale: Convert 100 mcg to mg. In the metric system, to convert smaller to larger divide by 1000 or move the decimal 3 places to the left. Therefore, 100 mcg = 0.1 mg.
Formula:

$$\frac{\text{Desired}}{\text{Available}} \times \text{mL} = \text{mL per dose}$$

$$\frac{0.1 \text{ mg}}{0.5 \text{ mg}} \times 1 \text{ mL} = \frac{0.1}{0.5} = 0.2 \text{ mL}$$

Test-Taking Strategy: In this medication calculation problem, it is necessary to first convert mcg to mg. Follow the formula for conversion and read the question carefully. Focus on the key information, 0.5 mg per mL. Recheck your work and make sure that the answer makes sense. Review medication calculations and conversions if you had difficulty with this question.
Level of Cognitive Ability: Application
Client Needs: Physiological Integrity
Integrated Concept/Process: Nursing Process/Implementation
Content Area: Fundamental Skills
Reference: DeWit S: *Fundamental concepts and skills for nursing,* Philadelphia, 2001, WB Saunders, p. 642.

8. ***Answer:*** 4
Rationale: To determine how many mL per hour are to be administered, simply divide the total prescribed amount of IV solution by the prescribed time period for infusion.
Formula:

$$\frac{\text{Total volume in mL}}{\text{Number of hours}} = \text{Amount of mL per hour}$$

$$\frac{3000 \text{ mL}}{24 \text{ hours}} = 125 \text{ mL per hour}$$

Test-Taking Strategy: Focus on the issue of the question, mL per hour. Follow the formula and simply dividing will direct you to the correct option. Review the formula for determining the amount of mL to infuse per hour if you had difficulty with this question.
Level of Cognitive Ability: Application
Client Needs: Physiological Integrity
Integrated Concept/Process: Nursing Process/Planning
Content Area: Fundamental Skills
Reference: DeWit S: *Fundamental concepts and skills for nursing,* Philadelphia, 2001, WB Saunders, p. 723.

9. ***Answer:*** 2
Rationale: Convert 150 mcg to mg. In the metric system, to convert smaller to larger divide by 1000 or move the decimal 3 places to the left. Therefore, 150 mcg = 0.15 mg.
Formula:

$$\frac{\text{Desired}}{\text{Available}} \times \text{Tablet(s)} = \text{Tablet(s) per dose}$$

$$\frac{0.15 \text{ mg}}{0.1 \text{ mg}} \times 1 \text{ tablet} = 1.5 \text{ tablets}$$

Test-Taking Strategy: In this medication calculation problem, it is necessary to first convert mcg to mg. Follow the formula for conversion and read the question carefully. Recheck your work and make sure that the answer makes sense. Review medication calculations and conversions if you had difficulty with this question.
Level of Cognitive Ability: Application
Client Needs: Physiological Integrity
Integrated Concept/Process: Nursing Process/Planning
Content Area: Fundamental Skills
Reference: DeWit S: *Fundamental concepts and skills for nursing,* Philadelphia, 2001, WB Saunders, p. 642.

10. *Answer:* 1
Rationale: To determine how many hours it will take for 1 liter to infuse, first recall that 1 liter is equal to 1000 mL. Next, divide the 1000 mL by the amount being delivered in one hour.
Formula:

$$\frac{\text{Total volume in mL}}{\text{mL per hour}} = \text{Infusion time in hours} \quad \frac{1000\text{ mL}}{125\text{ mL}} = 8\text{ hours}$$

Test-Taking Strategy: Focus on the issue of the question, how many hours for 1 liter to infuse. Follow the formula and simply dividing will direct you to the correct option. Review the formula for determining the infusion time if you had difficulty with this question.
Level of Cognitive Ability: Application
Client Needs: Physiological Integrity
Integrated Concept/Process: Nursing Process/Implementation
Content Area: Fundamental Skills
Reference: DeWit S: *Fundamental concepts and skills for nursing,* Philadelphia, 2001, WB Saunders, p. 723.

11. *Answer:* 1
Rationale: The prescribed 250 mL is to be infused over 4 hours. Follow the formula and multiply 250 mL by 10 (gtt factor). Then, divide the result by 240 minutes (4 hours × 60 minutes). The infusion is to run at 10.4 or 10 drops per minute.
Formula:

$$\frac{\text{Total volume in mL} \times \text{drop factor}}{\text{Time in minutes}} = \text{Flow rate in drops per minute}$$

$$\frac{250\text{ mL} \times 10\text{ drops}}{240\text{ minutes}} = \frac{2500}{240} = 10.4\text{ or }10\text{ drops per minute}$$

Test-Taking Strategy: Follow the formula for calculating the infusion rate for an IV. Label the problem and the answer. Make sure that the answer makes sense. Be sure to change 4 hours to minutes. Review the formula for calculating infusion rates if you had difficulty with this question.
Level of Cognitive Ability: Application
Client Needs: Physiological Integrity
Integrated Concept/Process: Nursing Process/Implementation
Content Area: Fundamental Skills
Reference: DeWit S: *Fundamental concepts and skills for nursing,* Philadelphia, 2001, WB Saunders, p. 723.

12. *Answer:* 1
Rationale: Convert 125 mcg to mg. In the metric system, to convert smaller to larger divide by 1000 or move the decimal 3 places to the left. Therefore, 125 mcg = 0.125 mg. One tablet is administered.
Test-Taking Strategy: In this medication calculation problem, it is necessary to first convert mcg to mg. Follow the formula for conversion and read the question carefully. Recheck your work and make sure that the answer makes sense. Review medication calculations and conversions if you had difficulty with this question.
Level of Cognitive Ability: Application
Client Needs: Physiological Integrity
Integrated Concept/Process: Nursing Process/Planning
Content Area: Fundamental Skills
Reference: DeWit S: *Fundamental concepts and skills for nursing,* Philadelphia, 2001, WB Saunders, p. 642.

13. *Answer:* 1
Rationale: Convert 0.025 g to mg. In the metric system, to convert larger to smaller multiply by 1000 or move the decimal 3 places to the right. Therefore, 0.025 g = 25.0 mg.
Formula:

$$\frac{\text{Desired}}{\text{Available}} \times \text{Tablet} = \text{Number of tablets per dose}$$

$$\frac{25.0\text{ mg}}{50\text{ mg}} = 1\text{ Tablet} = 0.5\text{ tablet}$$

Test-Taking Strategy: In this medication calculation problem, it is necessary to first convert grams to milligrams. Follow the formula for conversion and read the question carefully. Recheck your work and make sure that the answer makes sense. Review medication calculations and conversions if you had difficulty with this question.
Level of Cognitive Ability: Application
Client Needs: Physiological Integrity
Integrated Concept/Process: Nursing Process/Planning
Content Area: Fundamental Skills
Reference: DeWit S: *Fundamental concepts and skills for nursing,* Philadelphia, 2001, WB Saunders, p. 642.

14. *Answer:* 3
Rationale: Follow the formula for dosage calculation.
Formula:

$$\frac{\text{Desired}}{\text{Available}} \times \text{mL} = \text{mL per dose} \quad \frac{3\text{ mg}}{4\text{ mg}} = 1\text{ mL} = 0.75\text{ or }0.8\text{ mL}$$

Test-Taking Strategy: Follow the formula for the calculation of the correct dose. Label each figure including the answer. Focus on the key information: 4 mg per 1 mL. Recheck your work and make sure that the answer makes sense. Review medication calculations if you had difficulty with this question.
Level of Cognitive Ability: Application
Client Needs: Physiological Integrity
Integrated Concept/Process: Nursing Process/Planning
Content Area: Fundamental Skills
Reference: DeWit S: *Fundamental concepts and skills for nursing,* Philadelphia, 2001, WB Saunders, p. 642.

15. *Answer:* 4
Rationale: Follow the formula for dosage calculation.
Formula:

$$\frac{\text{Desired}}{\text{Available}} \times \text{Tablets} = \text{Number of tablets per dose}$$

$$\frac{0.25\text{ mg}}{0.125\text{ mg}} \times 1\text{ tablet} = 2\text{ tablets}$$

Test-Taking Strategy: Follow the formula for the calculation of the correct dose. Label each figure including the answer. Focus on the key information: 0.125 mg per tablet. Recheck your work and make sure that the answer makes sense. Review medication calculations if you had difficulty with this question.
Level of Cognitive Ability: Application
Client Needs: Physiological Integrity
Integrated Concept/Process: Nursing Process/Planning
Content Area: Fundamental Skills
Reference: DeWit S: *Fundamental concepts and skills for nursing,* Philadelphia, 2001, WB Saunders, p. 642.

16. ***Answer:*** 4
Rationale: Follow the formula for dosage calculation.
Formula:

$$\frac{\text{Desired}}{\text{Available}} \times \text{mL} = \text{mL per dose} \quad \frac{80\text{ mg}}{100\text{ mg}} \times 1\text{ mL} = 0.8\text{ mL}$$

Test-Taking Strategy: Follow the formula for the calculation of the correct dose. Label each figure including the answer. Focus on the key information: 100 mg per mL. Recheck your work and make sure that the answer makes sense. Review medication calculations if you had difficulty with this question.
Level of Cognitive Ability: Application
Client Needs: Physiological Integrity
Integrated Concept/Process: Nursing Process/Planning
Content Area: Fundamental Skills
Reference: DeWit S: *Fundamental concepts and skills for nursing,* Philadelphia, 2001, WB Saunders, p. 642.

17. ***Answer:*** 1
Rationale: Follow the formula for dosage calculation.
Formula:

$$\frac{\text{Desired}}{\text{Available}} \times \text{mL} = \text{mL per dose}$$

$$\frac{650\text{ mg}}{1000\text{ mg}} \times 1\text{ mL} = 0.65\text{ mL or } 0.7\text{ mL}$$

Test-Taking Strategy: Follow the formula for the calculation of the correct dose. Label each figure including the answer. Focus on the key information: 1000 Units per mL. Recheck your work and make sure that the answer makes sense. Review medication calculations if you had difficulty with this question.
Level of Cognitive Ability: Application
Client Needs: Physiological Integrity
Integrated Concept/Process: Nursing Process/Planning
Content Area: Fundamental Skills
Reference: DeWit S: *Fundamental concepts and skills for nursing,* Philadelphia, 2001, WB Saunders, p. 642.

18. ***Answer:*** 4
Rationale: Follow the formula for dosage calculation.
Formula:

$$\frac{\text{Desired}}{\text{Available}} \times \text{mL} = \text{mL per dose}$$

$$\frac{250\text{ mg}}{200\text{ mg}} \times 2\text{ mL} = 2.5\text{ mL}$$

Test-Taking Strategy: Follow the formula for the calculation of the correct dose. Label each figure including the answer. Focus on the key information: 200 mg per 2 mL. Recheck your work and make sure that the answer makes sense. Review medication calculations if you had difficulty with this question.
Level of Cognitive Ability: Application
Client Needs: Physiological Integrity
Integrated Concept/Process: Nursing Process/Planning
Content Area: Fundamental Skills
Reference: DeWit S: *Fundamental concepts and skills for nursing,* Philadelphia, 2001, WB Saunders, p. 642.

19. ***Answer:*** 3
Rationale: Follow the formula for dosage calculations.
Formula:

$$\frac{\text{Desired}}{\text{Available}} \times \text{mL} = \text{mL per dose}$$

$$\frac{35\text{ mg}}{50\text{ mg}} \times 1\text{ mL} = 0.7\text{ mL}$$

Test-Taking Strategy: Follow the formula for the calculation of the correct dose. Label each figure including the answer. Focus on the key information: 50 mg per mL. Recheck your work and make sure that the answer makes sense. Review medication calculations if you had difficulty with this question.
Level of Cognitive Ability: Application
Client Needs: Physiological Integrity
Integrated Concept/Process: Nursing Process/Planning
Content Area: Fundamental Skills
Reference: DeWit S: *Fundamental concepts and skills for nursing,* Philadelphia, 2001, WB Saunders, p. 642.

20. ***Answer:*** 2
Rationale: Follow the formula for dosage calculation.
Formula:

$$\frac{\text{Desired}}{\text{Available}} \times \text{mL} = \text{mL per dose}$$

$$\frac{20\text{ mg}}{10\text{ mg}} \times 1\text{ mL} = 2.0\text{ mL}$$

Test-Taking Strategy: Follow the formula for the calculation of the correct dose. Label each figure including the answer. Focus on the key information: 10 mg per mL. Recheck your work and make sure that the answer makes sense. Review medication calculations if you had difficulty with this question.
Level of Cognitive Ability: Application
Client Needs: Physiological Integrity
Integrated Concept/Process: Nursing Process/Planning
Content Area: Fundamental Skills
Reference: DeWit S: *Fundamental concepts and skills for nursing,* Philadelphia, 2001, WB Saunders, p. 642.

21. ***Answer:*** 4
Rationale: Follow the formula for dosage calculation.
Formula:

$$\frac{\text{Desired}}{\text{Available}} \times \text{mL} = \text{mL per dose}$$

$$\frac{0.4\text{ mg}}{0.3\text{ mg}} \times 0.5\text{ mL} = 0.66 \text{ or } 0.7\text{ mL}$$

Test-Taking Strategy: Follow the formula for the calculation of the correct dose. Label each figure including the answer. Focus on the key information: 0.3 mg per 0.5 mL. Recheck your work and make sure that the answer makes sense. Review medication calculations if you had difficulty with this question.
Level of Cognitive Ability: Application
Client Needs: Physiological Integrity
Integrated Concept/Process: Nursing Process/Planning
Content Area: Fundamental Skills
Reference: DeWit S: *Fundamental concepts and skills for nursing,* Philadelphia, 2001, WB Saunders, p. 642.

22. ***Answer:*** 1
Rationale: Convert 1 g to mg. In the metric system, to convert larger to smaller multiply by 1000 or move the decimal 3 places to the right. Therefore, 1 g = 1000 mg.
Formula:

$$\frac{\text{Desired}}{\text{Available}} \times \text{Tablet} = \text{Number of tablets per dose}$$

$$\frac{1000\text{ mg}}{500\text{ mg}} \times 1\text{ tablet} = 2\text{ tablets}$$

Test-Taking Strategy: In this medication calculation problem, it is necessary to first convert grams to milligrams. Follow the formula for conversion and read the question carefully. Recheck your work and make sure that the answer makes sense. Review medication calculations and conversions if you had difficulty with this question.
Level of Cognitive Ability: Application
Client Needs: Physiological Integrity
Integrated Concept/Process: Nursing Process/Planning
Content Area: Fundamental Skills
Reference: DeWit S: *Fundamental concepts and skills for nursing,* Philadelphia, 2001, WB Saunders, p. 642.

23. ***Answer:*** 4
Rationale: Convert 0.2 g to mg. In the metric system, to convert larger to smaller multiply by 1000 or move the decimal 3 places to the right. Therefore, 0.2 g = 200 mg.
Formula:

$$\frac{\text{Desired}}{\text{Available}} \times \text{Tablet} = \text{Number of tablets per dose}$$

$$\frac{200\text{ mg}}{100\text{ mg}} \times 1\text{ tablet} = 2\text{ tablets}$$

Test-Taking Strategy: In this medication calculation problem, it is necessary to first convert grams to milligrams. Follow the formula for conversion and read the question carefully. Recheck your work and make sure that the answer makes sense. Review medication calculations and conversions if you had difficulty with this question.
Level of Cognitive Ability: Application
Client Needs: Physiological Integrity
Integrated Concept/Process: Nursing Process/Planning
Content Area: Fundamental Skills
Reference: DeWit S: *Fundamental concepts and skills for nursing,* Philadelphia, 2001, WB Saunders, p. 642.

24. ***Answer:*** 2
Rationale: Convert gr 1/300 to mg using ratio and proportion. Then, use the dosage calculation formula.

$$\text{gr } 1{:}\ 60\text{ mg} = \text{gr } 1/300{:}\ X\text{mg}$$
$$60 \times 1/300 = X$$
$$X = 0.2\text{ mg}$$

$$\frac{\text{Desired}}{\text{Available}} \times \text{mL} = \text{mL per dose}$$

$$\frac{0.2\text{ mg}}{0.5\text{ mg}} \times 0.5\text{ mL} = 0.2\text{ mL}$$

Test-Taking Strategy: In this medication calculation problem, it is necessary to first convert grains to milligrams. Follow the formula for conversion and read the question carefully. Focus on the issue: 0.5 mg per 0.5 mL. Recheck your work and make sure that the answer makes sense. Review medication calculations and conversions if you had difficulty with this question.
Level of Cognitive Ability: Application
Client Needs: Physiological Integrity
Integrated Concept/Process: Nursing Process/Planning
Content Area: Fundamental Skills
Reference: DeWit S: *Fundamental concepts and skills for nursing,* Philadelphia, 2001, WB Saunders, p. 642.

25. ***Answer:*** 3
Rationale: Calculation of this problem requires more than one step. Convert Fahrenheit to Celsius, convert mg to gr, and then calculate the dose to be administered.
Step 1: Convert Fahrenheit to Celsius
Formula: To convert Fahrenheit to Celsius, subtract 32 and divide the result by 1.8.
C = (101-32) divided by 1.8; C = (69) divided by 1.8; C = 38.3
Step 2: Convert mg to gr
gr 1 : 60 mg :: x gr : 650 mg
60 x = 650
x = gr 10.8
Step 3: Dosage calculation

$$\frac{\text{Desired}}{\text{Available}} \times \text{Tablet} = \text{Number of tablets per dose}$$

$$\frac{\text{gr } 10.8}{\text{gr } 5} \times 1\text{ tablet} = 2.16 \text{ or } 2\text{ tablets}$$

Test-Taking Strategy: Focus on what the question is asking you to determine. In this medication calculation problem, it is necessary to first convert Fahrenheit to Celsius, then you need to convert mg to gr. Follow the formula for conversion and read the question carefully. Recheck your work and make sure that the answer makes sense. Review these formulas if you had difficulty with this question.
Level of Cognitive Ability: Application

Client Needs: Physiological Integrity
Integrated Concept/Process: Nursing Process/Planning
Content Area: Fundamental Skills

Reference: DeWit S: *Fundamental concepts and skills for nursing,* Philadelphia, 2001, WB Saunders, p. 642.

REFERENCES

DeWit S: *Fundamental concepts and skills for nursing,* Philadelphia, 2001, WB Saunders.

Hodgson B, Kizior R: *Saunders nursing drug handbook 2002,* Philadelphia, 2002, WB Saunders.

Kee J, Marshall S: *Clinical calculations,* ed 4, Philadelphia, 2000, WB Saunders.

National Council of State Boards of Nursing, editors: *Test plan for the National Council Licensure Examination for Practical/Vocational Nurses,* Chicago, 2001, Author.

Potter P, Perry A: *Fundamentals of nursing,* ed 5, St Louis, 2001, Mosby.

Basic Life Support

PYRAMID TERMS

Automated External Defibrillator (AED) Converts ventricular fibrillation into a perfusing rhythm and allows for early defibrillation by first responders.

Basic Life Support (BLS) Providing oxygen to the brain, heart, and other vital organs until help arrives.

Cardiopulmonary Resuscitation (CPR) An interchangeable term for Basic Life Support.

Head Tilt-Chin Lift Preferred method to open a victim's airway.

Heimlich Maneuver Method of rescue to remove foreign objects from a choking victim.

Jaw Thrust Maneuver Method used to open a victim's airway if a neck injury is suspected.

PYRAMID TO SUCCESS

The Pyramid to Success focuses on the emergency measures related to performing Basic Life Support. Focus on the points related to the breaths and compression ratio with adult CPR and CPR in the infant and child. Pyramid points focus on airway management in CPR and in performing the Heimlich maneuver. Focus on the correct hand placements for cardiac compressions and the differences between the adult, child, and infant. Remember, before initiating CPR, determining unresponsiveness is the initial action. Remember the ABCs—airway, breathing, and circulation—when performing CPR. The primary Integrated Concepts and Processes addressed in this chapter include Caring, the Clinical Problem-Solving Process (Nursing Process), Communication and Documentation, Cultural Awareness, and Teaching/Learning.

CLIENT NEEDS

Safe, Effective Care Environment

Advanced directives regarding the client's documented requests
Advocacy regarding the client's wishes
Client rights
Establishing priorities
Ethical and legal responsibilities
Standard (universal) and other precautions

Health Promotion and Maintenance

Health promotion programs
Teaching the significant other to perform BLS
Techniques of data collection

Psychosocial Integrity

Potential end-of-life issues
Emotional support to significant other
Religious and spiritual influences
Therapeutic communication

Physiological Integrity

Administration of emergency medications and intravenous lines
Alterations in the cardiopulmonary system
Handling medical emergencies
Use of special equipment
Documentation of response to BLS

I. BASIC LIFE SUPPORT (BLS) (Box 15-1)

A. Providing oxygen to the brain, heart, and other vital organs until help arrives
B. Also known as **cardiopulmonary resuscitation (CPR)**

II. ADULT BLS

A. Description: An adult can be defined as a person who is 8 years of age or older
B. Airway
  1. Remember that data collection is the first step of the nursing process; assessing a victim of sudden illness or accident for unconsciousness is the initial action; assess for 5 to 10 seconds
  2. Gently shake the victim's shoulders and ask "Are you OK?"; be alert to the potential for a head or neck injury
  3. Activate the emergency medical system (EMS): "phone first," children 8 years of age and older and adults; "phone last," children less than 8 years old
  4. Place the victim in a supine position on a firm, flat surface (logroll the victim, using spine precautions)
    a. One-person rescue: The rescuer is positioned on his or her knees, parallel to victim's sternum and facing the victim
    b. Two-person rescue: One rescuer faces the victim, kneeling parallel to the victim's head; the second rescuer moves to the opposite side and faces the victim, kneeling parallel to the victim's sternum
    c. The rescuers apply gloves and a face shield, if available
  5. Open the airway
  6. The **head-tilt-chin-lift** is the preferred method for opening the airway; if there is a neck injury, the **jaw thrust maneuver** is used to open the airway
  7. Look for any foreign material, liquids, or solids in the victim's mouth; wipe out any foreign material with a hooked index or middle finger

BOX 15-1

The ABCs of Basic Life Support (BLS)

A - Airway
B - Breathing
C - Circulation
Each step of the ABCs of BLS begins with data collection!

C. Breathing
  1. Assess breathing, maintaining an open airway
  2. The rescuer places his or her ear over the victim's nose and mouth and looks for the chest to rise and fall, listens for air moving in and out of the lungs, and feels for the flow of air
  3. Breathing victim
    a. Place the victim on his or her side if no cervical trauma is suspected; logroll the victim onto his or her side as a unit (without twisting) to help maintain an open airway
    b. If trauma or injury is suspected, the victim should not be moved
  4. Nonbreathing victim
    a. Maintain the **head-tilt-chin-lift**; pinch the nostrils closed, give two, slow full ventilations (breaths) of 2 seconds per breath (use resuscitation bag or face shield if available, ensuring an adequate air seal); allow victim to exhale between breaths
    b. Give 10 to 12 ventilations per minute
    c. If unsuccessful at giving the breath or ventilation, reposition the victim's head and try again (improper chin and head position is the most common cause of difficulty in ventilating the victim)

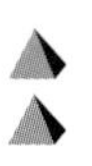

    d. If still unsuccessful, check the victim's mouth for a foreign body or for loose dentures (remove dentures only if they interfere with the mouth seal), clear the airway, and try to ventilate again
    e. Be alert to gastric distention when giving ventilations
  5. Mouth to nose: Recommended when it is impossible to ventilate through the victim's mouth, the mouth cannot be opened, the mouth is seriously injured, or a tight mouth-to-mouth seal is difficult to achieve
  6. Mouth to stoma: Used for the victim who has had a laryngectomy or has a temporary tracheostomy; to be effective, an adequate seal over the victim's mouth and nose is necessary
D. Circulation
  1. Assess circulation; always check for the absence of a pulse before beginning chest compressions on the victim
  2. Maintain an open airway and palpate for a carotid pulse for 5 to 10 seconds
  3. If there is a pulse, continue to give 10 to 12 ventilations per minute

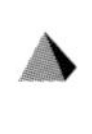

  4. Recheck the pulse after 1 minute; if there is no pulse, start chest compressions
E. Chest compressions
  1. Hand placement
    a. Correct hand placement for chest compressions is crucial

b. Hand placement is on the lower half of the sternum
c. With the hand closest to the victim's feet, locate the lower margin of the rib cage
d. Move the fingertips along the margin to the notch where the ribs meet the sternum
e. Place the middle finger on the notch and the index finger next to middle finger
f. Place the heel of the opposite hand next to the index finger, and place the other hand on top

2. Complications of chest compressions
   a. Laceration of internal organs
   b. Punctured lungs
   c. Fractured ribs or sternum

III. ADULT ONE-MAN BLS

A. The ratio is 15:2; that is, 15 chest compressions to 2 ventilations
B. The rate of compressions is 100 a minute at a depth of 1.5 to 2 inches
C. Perform four complete cycles, then reassess the victim
D. Check the carotid pulse after the first four cycles of **CPR** and every few minutes thereafter; if no pulse is felt, continue **CPR**

IV. ADULT TWO-MAN BLS

A. One person is at the victim's side performing chest compressions; one person is at the victim's head, maintaining an open airway, monitoring the carotid pulse, and doing the rescue breathing
B. The adult ratio for two-man **BLS** is 15:2; that is 15 compressions at a rate of 100 per minute, and 2 ventilations at 2 seconds per breath
C. When the second rescuer arrives at the scene, he or she must identify himself or herself and tell the first rescuer that he or she knows two-man **CPR**
D. That second rescuer then activates EMS, if this has not been done, and then returns to the scene to help
E. The second rescuer can perform one-man **CPR** if the first rescuer is fatigued; or, the first rescuer finishes 15 compressions, gives 2 ventilations, moves to the head, opens the airway, and checks the carotid pulse
F. If there is no pulse, the first rescuer announces "No pulse, continue **CPR**"
G. The second rescuer locates the landmark for chest compressions
H. The two rescuers begin **CPR** at a ratio of 15 compressions to 2 ventilations
I. At the end of 1 minute, the ventilator checks for a pulse and checks for breathing; if there is none, the ventilator says, "No pulse, continue **CPR**"
J. When the compressor becomes tired, the compressor should change positions with minimal interruption of chest compressions
K. The rescuer ventilating the victim assumes responsibility for monitoring for signs of circulation and breathing

V. PEDIATRIC DIFFERENCES

A. Description
   1. A child can be defined as a person between 1 and 8 years old
   2. An infant can be defined as a person less than 1 year old

B. Airway: Assess unresponsiveness

C. Breathing
   1. Breathing victim: Keep the airway open
   2. Nonbreathing victim
      a. Give two ventilations at 1 to 1.5 seconds per breath
      b. With the infant, provide ventilations by mouth-to-mouth and nose
      c. With the larger child, provide ventilations by mouth-to-mouth
      d. With the infant or the child, give 20 ventilations per minute; activate EMS as soon as possible

D. Circulation
   1. Assess circulation
   2. If the victim is older than 1 year, assess circulation via the carotid pulse
   3. If the victim is younger than 1 year, assess circulation via the brachial pulse
   4. The ratio is 5 compressions to 1 ventilation
   5. Reassess every few minutes
   6. Infant chest compressions
      a. The imaginary line between the nipples is located over the breastbone (sternum)
      b. The index finger of the hand farthest from the infant's head is placed just under the intermammary line where it intersects the sternum
      c. The area of compression is one finger width below this intersection, at the location of the middle and ring fingers
      d. With the use of 2 to 3 fingers, the breast bone is compressed 0.5 to 1 inch at 100 times a minute
      e. Two-thumb encircling hands technique is the preferred two-rescuer technique
   7. Chest compressions for a child
      a. The location for hand placement is the same as for an adult

b. Depress the chest 1 to 1.5 inches at 100 times a minute with the heel of one hand

VI. THE CHOKING VICTIM AND HEIMLICH MANEUVER

A. Conscious adult
   1. Ask the victim, "Are you choking?" (the victim will not be able to speak or cough if he or she is choking)
   2. If the victim's airway is partially obstructed, a crowing sound is heard; encourage the victim to cough
   3. Relieve the obstruction by the **Heimlich maneuver** (Box 15-2)
   4. Perform the **Heimlich maneuver** until the object is dislodged or the victim becomes unconscious

B. Unconscious adult
   1. Assess unconsciousness
   2. Call for help; activate EMS as soon as possible
   3. Open the airway
   4. Assess breathing
   5. Attempt ventilation
   6. Reposition the head if unsuccessful; reattempt ventilation
   7. Relieve the obstruction by the **Heimlich maneuver** with five thrusts; then finger sweep the mouth
   8. To perform the **Heimlich maneuver**, straddle the victim's thighs, place the heel of one hand on top of the other between the umbilicus and xiphoid process, and give five thrusts in and up with the heel of the bottom hand
   9. Reattempt ventilation
   10. Repeat the sequence of tongue-jaw lift, finger sweep, breaths, and **Heimlich maneuver** until successful
   11. Be sure to assess the victim's pulse and respirations
   12. Perform **CPR** if required

C. Choking child or infant
   1. Choking is suspected in infants and children experiencing acute respiratory distress associated with coughing, gagging, or stridor (high-pitched noisy breathing)
   2. Allow the victim to continue to cough if the cough is forceful
   3. If the cough is ineffective or the victim develops increased respiratory difficulty accompanied by a high-pitched noise while inhaling, help is needed
   4. Conscious child
      a. Assess for obstruction by asking the child, "Are you choking?"
      b. Relieve the obstruction by the **Heimlich maneuver** until the obstruction is dislodged or the child becomes unconscious
   5. Unconscious child
      a. Assess unconsciousness
      b. Open the airway by the tongue-jaw lift
      c. Check for breathing and look for a foreign object
      d. Attempt ventilation
      e. If unsuccessful, reposition the head; reattempt ventilation
      f. Relieve the obstruction using the **Heimlich maneuver,** giving five abdominal thrusts, and finger sweep the mouth only if the object is seen
      g. Assess airway for foreign object and reattempt ventilation
      h. Repeat the sequence
      i. Assess pulse and respirations and perform **CPR** if required
   6. Conscious infant
      a. Assess for obstruction and note breathing problems
      b. Relieve the obstruction by five back blows and five chest thrusts 
      c. Straddle the infant over the arm, place the infant's head lower than the trunk, and support the head firmly, holding the jaw
      d. Give five back blows with the heel of the hand between the shoulder blades
      e. Turn the infant; place the head lower than the trunk
      f. Give five chest thrusts at the same location as for chest compressions
      g. Check for the object and remove if seen 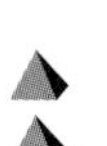
      h. Blind finger sweeps are avoided in infants and small children, since the object may be pushed back farther into the airway, causing further obstruction
      i. Continue until the object is removed or the infant becomes unconscious
   7. Unconscious infant
      a. Assess unconsciousness by gentle taps
      b. Open the airway by the tongue-jaw lift

BOX 15-2

Heimlich Maneuver

Stand behind the victim
Place arms around the victim's waist
Make a fist
Place the thumb side of the fist just above the umbilicus and well below the xiphoid process
Perform five quick in and up thrusts (between the umbilicus and xiphoid process)
Use chest thrusts for the obese or pregnant victim

c. Check for breathing and look for a foreign object
d. Attempt ventilation
e. Reposition the head if unsuccessful; reattempt ventilation
f. Relieve the obstruction by five back blows and five chest thrusts
g. Finger sweep the mouth only if the object is seen
h. Reattempt ventilation and repeat the sequence
i. Activate EMS after 1 minute of unresponsiveness
j. Perform **CPR** if required

VII. PREGNANT OR OBESE VICTIM

A. **Heimlich Maneuver**
1. Place arms under the victim's axilla and across the chest
2. Place the thumb side of a clenched fist against the middle of the sternum, and place the other hand over the fist
3. Perform backward chest thrusts until the foreign object is expelled or until the victim becomes unconscious
4. If unable to ventilate, position the hands as for chest compressions and deliver chest thrusts firmly to remove the obstruction
5. If the pregnant victim becomes unconscious, place her on her back; a wedge, such as a pillow or rolled blanket, should be placed under the right abdominal flank and hip to displace the uterus to the left side of the abdomen

B. Defibrillation in the pregnant victim: If defibrillation is needed, place the paddles one rib interspace higher than usual because the heart is displaced slightly by the enlarged uterus

VIII. AUTOMATED EXTERNAL DEFIBRILLATOR (AED)

A. Description
1. Used to convert ventricular fibrillation into a perfusing rhythm
2. Differentiates nonventricular fibrillation rhythms and allows for early defibrillation by first responders

B. Implementation
1. Attach **AED** leads to the victim
2. Turn on the **AED** and push the button to activate the analyzer
3. Follow instructions given for the **AED**, usually to "assess," "stand back," "shock," and "reassess"

BOX 15-3

Pyramid Points

Do not interrupt CPR for more than 5 seconds!

STOP CPR ONLY IF:
Pulse and respiration return
Emergency Medical System arrives
To administer automated external defibrillator (AED)
A physician declares the victim deceased

4. Evaluate for return of the pulse, and if the victim is pulseless, repeat defibrillation as directed up to three times; if defibrillation is still ineffective, perform **CPR** for 1 minute, and then deliver another series of three shocks (Box 15-3)

PRACTICE QUESTIONS

1. A nurse on the day shift walks into a client's room and finds the client unresponsive. The client is not breathing and does not have a pulse. The nurse immediately calls out for help. The next nursing action is which of the following?
   1. Ventilate with a mouth-to-mask device
   2. Start chest compressions
   3. Give the client oxygen
   4. Open the airway
2. A nurse is performing cardiopulmonary resuscitation (CPR) on an adult client. When performing chest compressions, the nurse understands that correct hand placement is located over the:
   1. Lower third of the sternum
   2. Upper half of the sternum
   3. Upper third of the sternum
   4. Lower half of the sternum
3. A nurse witnesses a neighbor's husband sustain a fall from the roof of the house. The nurse rushes to the victim and determines the need to open the airway. The nurse opens the airway in this victim using which most appropriate method?
   1. Head tilt-chin lift
   2. Flexed position
   3. Modified head tilt-chin lift
   4. Jaw thrust maneuver
4. A nurse is preparing to do the Heimlich maneuver on a 3-year-old conscious child. The nurse performs this maneuver by placing the hands between the:
   1. Umbilicus and the groin
   2. Groin and the abdomen
   3. Umbilicus and xiphoid process
   4. Lower abdomen and chest

5. A nurse is performing basic life support (BLS) on a 7-year-old child. The nurse delivers how many breaths per minute to the child?
   1. 12
   2. 16
   3. 18
   4. 20
6. A nurse is performing cardiopulmonary resuscitation (CPR) on an infant. When performing chest compressions, the nurse understands that the compression rate is:
   1. 60 times per minute
   2. 80 times per minute
   3. 100 times per minute
   4. 160 times per minute
7. A nursing instructor teaches a group of students about basic life support (BLS). The instructor asks a student to identify the most appropriate location to assess the pulse of an infant less than 1 year old. Which of the following, if stated by the student, would indicate that the student understands the appropriate procedure?
   1. Brachial
   2. Carotid
   3. Popliteal
   4. Radial
8. A nurse is teaching cardiopulmonary resuscitation (CPR) to a group of community members. The nurse asks a member of the group to describe the reason that blind finger sweeps are avoided in infants. The nurse determines that the member understands this reason if the member makes which statement?
   1. "The object may be forced back farther into the throat."
   2. "The mouth is too small to see the object."
   3. "The object may have been swallowed."
   4. "The infant may bite down on the finger"
9. A nurse is performing cardiopulmonary resuscitation (CPR) on an adult client. The nurse understands that when performing chest compressions, the sternum should be depressed:
   1. ½ to ¾ inch
   2. ¾ to 1 inch
   3. 1 ½ to 2 inches
   4. 2 ½ to 3 inches
10. A nursing instructor asks a nursing student to describe the procedure of performing the Heimlich maneuver on an unconscious pregnant woman at 8 months' gestation. The student describes the procedure correctly if the student states to:
   1. Perform abdominal thrusts until the object is dislodged
   2. Place the hands in the pelvis to perform the thrusts
   3. Place a rolled blanket under the right abdominal flank and hip area
   4. Perform left lateral abdominal thrusts until the object is dislodged

ANSWERS

1. *Answer:* 4
Rationale: The next nursing action would be to open the airway. Ventilation cannot be initiated unless the airway is opened. Chest compressions are started after the airway is opened and ventilation is initiated. Oxygen may be helpful at some point, but the airway is opened first.
Test-Taking Strategy: Visualize the steps of basic life support to answer the question. Recalling the ABCs, airway, breathing, and circulation will assist in directing you to option 4. Review the steps of BLS if you had difficulty with this question.
Level of Cognitive Ability: Application
Client Needs: Physiological Integrity
Integrated Concept/Process: Nursing Process/Implementation
Content Area: Fundamental Skills
Reference: Perry A, Potter P: *Clinical nursing skills and techniques*, ed 5, St Louis, 2002, Mosby, p. 429.

2. *Answer:* 4
Rationale: If a pulse is not present, chest compressions will need to be initiated. Proper hand placement for chest compressions is determined by locating the notch where the rib margin meets the sternum, and placing the middle finger on this notch and the index finger next to it. Then, the heel of the opposite hand is placed on the lower half of the sternum close to the index finger. The first hand is removed and placed on top of the hand on the sternum and chest compressions are begun. This location is the lower half of the sternum.
Test-Taking Strategy: Use the process of elimination. Eliminate options 2 and 3 first because this location would be ineffective. Visualize the procedure and consider the anatomical location of the heart to select from the remaining options. Review the procedure for chest compressions if you had difficulty with this question.
Level of Cognitive Ability: Comprehension
Client Needs: Physiological Integrity
Integrated Concept/Process: Nursing Process/Implementation
Content Area: Fundamental Skills
Reference: Perry A, Potter P: *Clinical nursing skills and techniques*, ed 5, St Louis, 2002, Mosby, p. 431.

3. *Answer:* 4
Rationale: If a neck injury is suspected, the jaw thrust maneuver is used to open the airway. The head tilt/chin lift produces

hyperextension of the neck and could cause complications if a neck injury is present. A flexed position is an inappropriate position for opening the airway
Test-Taking Strategy: Use the process of elimination. Eliminate options 1 and 3 first because they are similar. Next, eliminate option 2 since this position would not open the airway. Review the procedures for BLS if you had difficulty with this question.
Level of Cognitive Ability: Application
Client Needs: Physiological Integrity
Integrated Concept/Process: Nursing Process/Implementation
Content Area: Fundamental Skills
Reference: Perry A, Potter P: *Clinical nursing skills and techniques*, ed 5, St Louis, 2002, Mosby, p. 429.

4. ***Answer:*** 3
Rationale: To perform the Heimlich maneuver in a child, the rescuer stands behind the victim and places the arms directly under the victim's axillae and around the victim. The thumb side of one fist is placed against the victim's abdomen in the midline slightly above the umbilicus and well below the tip of the xiphoid process. The fist is grasped with the other hand and up to five thrusts are delivered. Care must be taken not to touch the xiphoid process or the lower margins of the rib cage because force applied to these structures may damage internal organs.
Test-Taking Strategy: Use the process of elimination noting the age of the child. Eliminate options 1 and 2 first because they are similar. From the remaining options, consider the anatomical location and the effect of the maneuver in dislodging an obstruction. Review the Heimlich maneuver if you had difficulty with this question.
Level of Cognitive Ability: Application
Client Needs: Physiological Integrity
Integrated Concept/Process: Nursing Process/Implementation
Content Area: Fundamental Skills
Reference: Schulte E, Price D, Gwin J: *Thompson's pediatric nursing*, ed 8, Philadelphia, 2001, WB Saunders, p. 176.

5. ***Answer:*** 4
Rationale: In a pediatric victim, 20 breaths per minute are delivered. Initially, the nurse would give the child two breaths at 1 to 1.5 seconds per breath. Options 1, 2, and 3 are incorrect.
Test-Taking Strategy: Use the process of elimination. Recalling the normal respiratory rate in a child at this age will assist in directing you to option 4. Review BLS in a pediatric victim if you had difficulty with this question.
Level of Cognitive Ability: Application
Client Needs: Physiological Integrity
Integrated Concept/Process: Nursing Process/Implementation
Content Area: Fundamental Skills
Reference: Perry A, Potter P: *Clinical nursing skills and techniques*, ed 5, St Louis, 2002, Mosby, p. 432.

6. ***Answer:*** 3
Rationale: In an infant, the rate of chest compressions is 100 times per minute. Options 1 and 2 identify rates that are too low and option 4 identifies a rate that is too high.
Test-Taking Strategy: Use the process of elimination considering the normal heart rate of an infant. Eliminate options 1 and 2 because of the low rates identified in the options. Eliminate option 4 because this rate would be much too rapid for an infant. Review BLS for an infant if you had difficulty with this question.
Level of Cognitive Ability: Application
Client Needs: Physiological Integrity
Integrated Concept/Process: Nursing Process/Implementation
Content Area: Fundamental Skills
Reference: Perry A, Potter P: *Clinical nursing skills and techniques*, ed 5, St Louis, 2002, Mosby, p. 432.

7. ***Answer:*** 1
Rationale: When assessing a pulse in an infant (under 1 year of age), the pulse should be checked at the brachial artery. The infant's relatively short, fat neck makes palpation of the carotid artery difficult. The popliteal and radial pulses are also difficult to palpate in an infant.
Test-Taking Strategy: Use the process of elimination and knowledge regarding circulatory assessment in an infant. Options 3 and 4 can be easily eliminated. Consider the body structure of an infant to assist in directing you to option 1. Review cardiac assessment and BLS in an infant if you had difficulty with this question.
Level of Cognitive Ability: Comprehension
Client Needs: Physiological Integrity
Integrated Concept/Process: Teaching/Learning
Content Area: Fundamental Skills
Reference: Perry A, Potter P: *Clinical nursing skills and techniques*, ed 5, St Louis, 2002, Mosby, p. 430.

8. ***Answer:*** 1
Rationale: Blind finger sweeps are not recommended for infants and children because of the risk of forcing the object farther down into the airway. Options 2, 3, and 4 are not directly related to the issue of the question.
Test-Taking Strategy: Use the ABCs—airway, breathing, and circulation—to answer this question. Option 1 addresses the concern of airway patency. Review obstructed airway management for an infant or child if you had difficulty with this question.
Level of Cognitive Ability: Comprehension
Client Needs: Health Promotion and Maintenance
Integrated Concept/Process: Teaching/Learning
Content Area: Fundamental Skills
Reference: Perry A, Potter P: *Clinical nursing skills and techniques*, ed 5, St Louis, 2002, Mosby, p. 416.

9. ***Answer:*** 3
Rationale: When performing CPR on an adult client, the sternum should be depressed 1.5 to 2 inches. Options 1 and 2 identify compression depths that would be ineffective in an adult. Option 4 identifies a depth that could cause injury to the client.
Test-Taking Strategy: Use the process of elimination. Note the key word "adult" in the question. Consider the normal body structure of an adult to assist in answering the question. Review adult BLS if you had difficulty with this question.
Level of Cognitive Ability: Application

Client Needs: Physiological Integrity
Integrated Concept/Process: Nursing Process/Implementation
Content Area: Fundamental Skills
Reference: Perry A, Potter P: *Clinical nursing skills and techniques*, ed 5, St Louis, 2002, Mosby, p. 432.

10. *Answer:* 3
Rationale: To perform the Heimlich maneuver in an advanced pregnant woman, the woman is placed on her back. A wedge, such as a pillow or rolled blanket, should be placed under the right abdominal flank and hip to displace the uterus to the left side of the abdomen. Options 1, 2, and 4 are incorrect and can cause harm to the woman and the fetus.
Test-Taking Strategy: Use the process of elimination and note that the client is an unconscious pregnant woman at 8 months' gestation. Recall the concepts associated with hypotension and vena cava syndrome to assist in directing you to option 3. Review the principles associated with performing the Heimlich maneuver on a pregnant woman if you had difficulty with this question.
Level of Cognitive Ability: Comprehension
Client Needs: Physiological Integrity
Integrated Concept/Process: Teaching/Learning
Content Area: Fundamental Skills
Reference: Perry A, Potter P: *Clinical nursing skills and techniques*, ed 5, St Louis, 2002, Mosby, p. 413.

REFERENCES

American Heart Association and International Liaison Committee on Resuscitation: *Guidelines 2000 for cardiopulmonary resuscitation and emergency cardiovascular care*, Dallas, 2000, Author.

Lowdermilk D, Perry S, Bobak I: *Maternity and women's health care*, ed 7, St Louis, 2000, Mosby.

Potter P, Perry A: *Fundamentals of nursing*, ed 5, St Louis, 2001, Mosby.

Wong D: *Whaley and Wong's nursing care of infants and children*, ed 6, St Louis, 1999, Mosby.

Perioperative Nursing Care

PYRAMID TERMS

Atelectasis A collapsed or airless state of the lung that may be the result of airway obstruction because of accumulated secretions or failure of the client to deep breathe. It is the most common postoperative complication and usually occurs 1 to 2 days after surgery.

Extended Postoperative Stage The period of at least 1 to 4 days after surgery.

Immediate Postoperative Stage The period of 1 to 4 hours after surgery.

Intermediate Postoperative Stage The period of 4 to 24 hours after surgery.

Wound Dehiscence An opening of the wound edges.

Wound Evisceration Protrusion of internal organs through an opening in wound edges.

PYRAMID TO SUCCESS

Pyramid points focus on reinforcing instructions to the client and family or significant other in the preoperative stage, preparing the client for the operative procedure, ensuring that prescribed preoperative procedures have been performed, and that the results of the procedures are within expected range and are documented. In the postoperative stage, pyramid points focus on monitoring for surgical complications and on the implementation of initial nursing measures if a complication arises. Pyramid points also focus on preparing the client for discharge, reinforcing instructions related to the prescribed treatments, and identifying the need for home care support services. The primary Integrated Concepts and Processes addressed in this chapter include Caring, Communication and Documentation, Cultural Awareness, the Clinical Problem-Solving Process (Nursing Process), Self-Care, and Teaching/Learning.

CLIENT NEEDS

Safe, Effective Care Environment

Advance directives
Client rights
Establishing priorities
Informed consent for the surgical procedure
Informing the client of the surgical process
Providing safety to the medicated client
Surgical asepsis
Standard (universal) precautions

Health Promotion and Maintenance

Expected body image changes
Reinforcing instructions related to the prescribed discharge plan
Preventing complications
Promoting lifestyle choices
Suggesting appropriate support services

Psychosocial Integrity

Assisting the client to develop coping methods
Promoting an environment that will allow the client to express concerns
Support systems
Unexpected body image changes

Physiological Integrity

Initiating nursing interventions when surgical complications arise
Monitoring for surgical complications
Monitoring for unexpected responses to treatments and procedures

Providing respiratory care
Providing basic care and comfort
Safe administration of preoperative and postoperative medications

I. PREOPERATIVE CARE

A. Obtaining informed consent
   1. The surgeon is responsible for obtaining the consent for surgery
   2. No sedation should be administered to the client before signing the consent
   3. Minors may need a parent or legal guardian to sign the consent form
   4. Older clients may need a legal guardian to sign the consent form
   5. The nurse may witness the client signing the preoperative consent, but the nurse must be sure that the client has understood the surgeon's explanation of the surgery
   6. The nurse needs to document the witnessing of the signing of the operative consent after the client acknowledges understanding the procedure

B. Nutrition
   1. Check the physician's orders regarding the NPO status before surgery
   2. Solid foods and liquids are generally withheld for 6 to 8 hours before general anesthesia and for 3 hours before surgery with local anesthesia, to avoid aspiration
   3. Monitor IV fluids if prescribed
   4. Note that total parenteral nutrition (TPN) may be prescribed for clients who are malnourished, have protein or metabolic deficiencies, or cannot ingest foods

C. Elimination
   1. If the client is to have intestinal or abdominal surgery, an enema or laxative or both may be prescribed the night before surgery
   2. The client should void immediately before surgery
   3. Prepare to insert a Foley catheter if prescribed
   4. If there is a Foley catheter in place, it should be emptied immediately before surgery and the amount and quality of urine output documented

D. Surgical site
   1. Prepare to clean the surgical site with a mild antiseptic soap the night before surgery, as prescribed
   2. Prepare to shave the operative site as prescribed
   3. Hair should be shaved only if it will interfere with the surgical procedure and only if prescribed
   4. Shaving of hair, if prescribed, should be done in the direction of hair growth with a sharp razor, and caution should be used to prevent cuts or epidermal damage

E. Reinforcing preoperative instructions
   1. Inform the client about what to expect after surgery
   2. Inform the client to notify the nurse if they experience any postoperative pain and that pain medication will be prescribed to be given as the client requests
   3. Instruct the client to use the noninvasive pain relief techniques before the pain occurs and as soon as the pain is noticed
   4. Reinforce instructions about the use of a client-controlled analgesia pump if its use is prescribed
   5. Inform the client that requesting a narcotic after surgery will not make the client a drug addict
   6. The client should be instructed not to smoke for at least 12 hours before surgery
   7. Instruct the client in deep breathing and coughing techniques, the use of incentive spirometry, and the importance of performing the techniques after surgery to prevent the development of pneumonia and **atelectasis** (Box 16-1 and Figure 16-1)
   8. Instruct the client in leg and foot exercises to prevent venous stasis of blood and facilitate venous blood return (Box 16-1 and Figure 16-2)

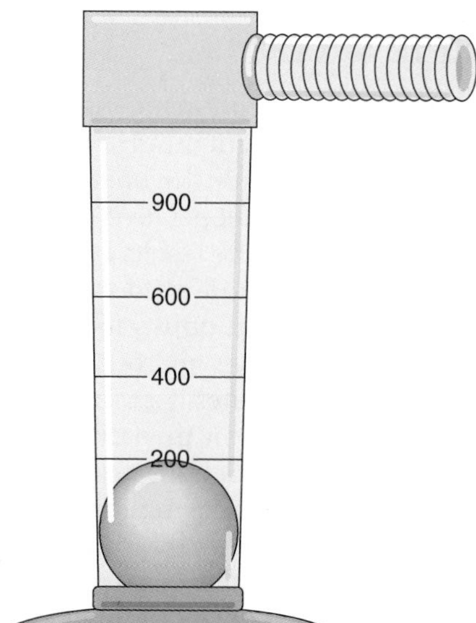

FIG. 16-1 Incentive spirometer. (From Phipps W, Sands J, Marek J: *Medical-surgical nursing: concepts and clinical practice*, ed 6, St Louis, 1999, Mosby. Courtesy University Hospitals of Cleveland, Cleveland, Ohio.)

BOX 16-1

Preoperative Instructions

DEEP BREATHING AND COUGHING EXERCISES

Instruct the client that a sitting position gives the best lung expansion for coughing and deep breathing exercises.
Instruct the client to breathe deeply three times, inhaling through the nostrils and exhaling slowly through pursed lips.
Instruct the client that the third breath should be held for 3 seconds; then the client should cough deeply three times.
The client should perform this exercise every 2 hours.

INCENTIVE SPIROMETRY

Instruct the client to assume a sitting position.
Instruct the client to place the mouth tightly around the mouthpiece.
Instruct the client to inhale slowly to raise and maintain the flow rate indicator between the 600 and 900 marks.
Instruct the client to hold the breath for 5 seconds, and then to exhale through pursed lips.
Instruct the client to repeat this process 10 times every hour.

LEG AND FOOT EXERCISES

Gastrocnemius (calf) pumping: Instruct the client to move both ankles by pointing the toes up and then down.
Quadriceps (thigh) setting: Instruct the client to press the back of the knees against the bed, and then to relax the knees; this contracts and relaxes the thigh and calf muscles to prevent thrombus formation.
Foot circles: Instruct the client to rotate each foot in a circle.
Hip and knee movements: Instruct the client to flex the knee and thigh and to straighten the leg and hold the position for 5 seconds before lowering (not performed if the client is having abdominal surgery or if the client has a back problem).

SPLINTING THE INCISION

If the surgical incision is abdominal or thoracic, instruct the client to place a pillow, or one hand with the other hand on top, over the incisional area.
During deep breathing and coughing, the client presses gently against the incisional area to splint or support it.

9. Instruct the client how to splint an incision and to turn and reposition (Box 16-1 and Figure 16-3)
10. Inform the client of any invasive devices that may be needed after surgery
11. Inform the client not to pull on any of the invasive devices, as they will be removed as soon as possible

F. Psychosocial preparation
1. Be alert to the client's anxiety level
2. Ask the client about questions or concerns the client may have regarding surgery
3. Allow time for privacy for the client to prepare psychologically for surgery
4. Provide support and assistance as needed

G. Preoperative checklist
1. Ensure that the client has an identification bracelet on
2. Check for client allergies (refer to Chapter 58 for information on latex allergy)
3. Review the preoperative check list to be sure that each item is addressed before the client is transported to surgery
4. Ensure that consent forms were signed for the operative procedure, for anesthesia, for any blood transfusions, for disposal of a limb, or for surgical sterilization procedures
5. Ensure that a history and physical examination was completed and documented in the client's record
6. Ensure that consultations prescribed were completed and documented in the client's record
7. Ensure that the prescribed laboratory results are documented in the client's record
8. Ensure that ECG and chest radiograph reports are noted in the client's record
9. Ensure that blood type and screen or type and crossmatch is noted in the client's record
10. Document that the client has voided before surgery
11. Remove jewelry, makeup, dentures, hairpins, nail polish, glasses, and any prosthesis
12. Document that valuables were given to the client's family members or locked in the hospital safe
13. Document that the prescribed preoperative medication was given (Box 16-2)
14. Monitor and document the client's vital signs
15. Document the last time the client ate or drank

H. Preoperative medications
1. Prepare to administer preoperative medications as prescribed, or on call to the operating room immediately before the surgery

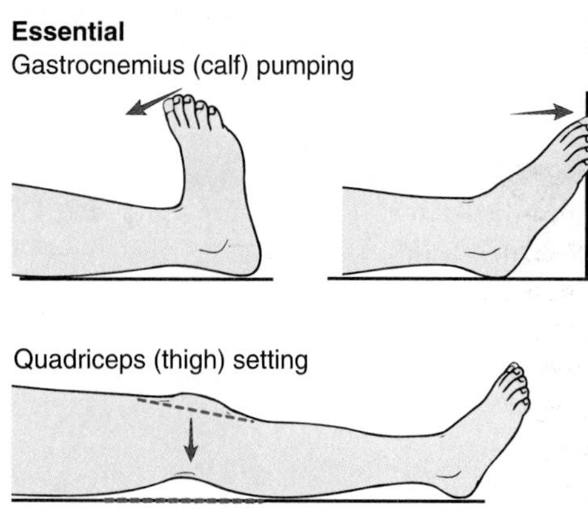

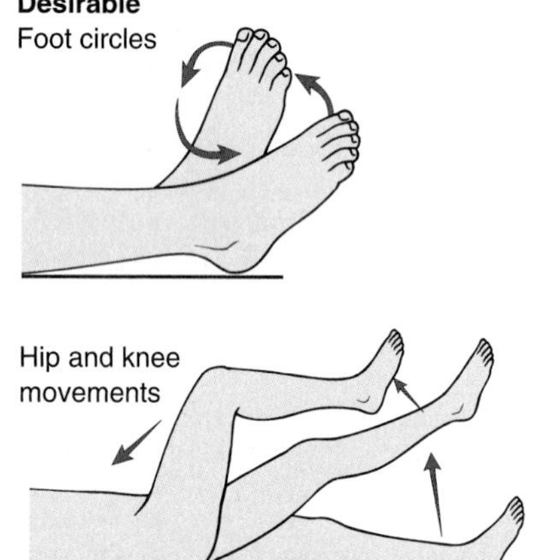

FIG. 16-2 Postoperative leg exercises. (From Lewis S, Heitkemper M, Dirksen S: *Medical-surgical nursing: assessment and management of clinical problems*, St Louis, 2000, Mosby.)

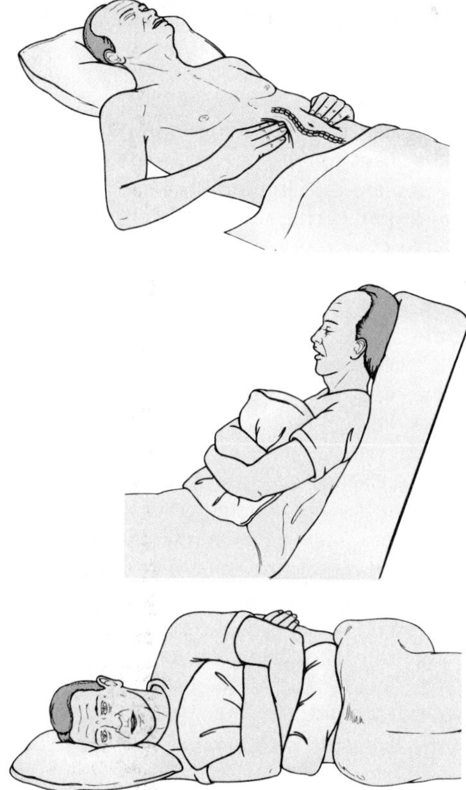

FIG. 16-3 Techniques for splinting wound when coughing. (From Lewis S, Heitkemper M, Dirksen S: *Medical-surgical nursing: assessment and management of clinical problems*, St Louis, 2000, Mosby.)

2. Instruct the client that he or she will feel drowsy after the medications are given
3. After administering the preoperative medications, keep the client in bed with the side rails up
4. Place the call bell next to the client, instruct the client not to get out of bed and to call for assistance if needed

I. Arrival at the operating room
1. When the client arrives to the operating room, the operating room nurse will verify the identification bracelet with the client's verbal response and will review the client's chart
2. The operating room nurse will confirm the operative procedure and site to be operated on
3. The client's chart will be checked for completeness
4. The client's chart will be reviewed for consent forms, history and physical examination, and allergic reaction information
5. The physician's orders will be reviewed and their completion verified
6. The IV line may be initiated at this time if prescribed
7. The anesthesia team will administer the prescribed anesthesia

II. POSTOPERATIVE CARE

A. Immediate stage
1. Description: the period of 1 to 4 hours after surgery
2. Respiratory system
   a. Monitor vital signs
   b. Monitor airway patency and adequate ventilation, since prolonged mechanical ventilation during anesthesia may affect postoperative lung function
   c. Remember that extubated clients who are lethargic may not be able to maintain an airway

BOX 16-2

Medications That Can Affect the Surgical Client

ANTIBIOTICS

Potentiate the action of anesthetic agents.

If taken for 2 weeks before surgery, aminoglycosides such as gentamycin (Garamycin), tobramycin (Nebcin), and neomycin (Mycifradin) may cause mild respiratory depression as a result of depressed neuromuscular transmission.

ANTIDYSRHYTHMICS

Reduce cardiac contractility and impair cardiac conduction during anesthesia.

ANTICOAGULANTS

Alter normal clotting factors and increase the risk of hemorrhaging.

Acetylsalicylic acid (aspirin, ASA) and ibuprofen (Motrin, Advil) are commonly used medications that can alter clotting mechanisms.

These medications should be discontinued at least 48 hours before surgery.

ANTICONVULSANTS

Long-term use of certain anticonvulsants can alter the metabolism of anesthetic agents.

ANTIHYPERTENSIVES

Can interact with anesthetic agents and cause bradycardia, hypotension, and impaired circulation.

CORTICOSTEROIDS

Cause adrenal atrophy and reduce the body's ability to withstand stress.

Before and during surgery, dosages may be temporarily increased.

INSULIN

The need for insulin after surgery in a client with diabetes mellitus either may be reduced because the client's nutritional intake is decreased or may be increased because of the stress response and IV administration of glucose solutions.

DIURETICS

Potentiate electrolyte imbalances after surgery.

ANTIDEPRESSANTS

May lower the blood pressure during anesthesia.

ANTICHOLINERGICS

Medications with anticholinergic effects increase the potential for confusion.

d. Monitor for secretions and remove by suctioning if the client is unable to clear the airway by coughing
e. Observe chest movement for symmetry and the use of accessory muscles
f. Monitor oxygen administration if prescribed
g. Monitor pulse oximetry as prescribed
h. Encourage coughing and deep-breathing exercises as soon as possible
i. Note the rate, depth, and quality of respirations: the respiratory rate should be greater than 10 and less than 30
j. Monitor the client for signs of **atelectasis**, pneumonia, and pulmonary embolism

3. Cardiovascular system
   a. Check the client's color
   b. Observe capillary refill, mucous membranes, and sclera
   c. Check peripheral pulses and for peripheral edema
   d. Monitor for bleeding
   e. Check pulse for rate and rhythm; a bounding pulse may indicate hypertension, fluid overload, or anxiety
   f. Monitor for signs of hypertension and hypotension
   g. Monitor for cardiac irregularities
   h. Check for Homan's sign, particularly in clients in the lithotomy position during surgery, as these clients may be predisposed to developing deep vein thrombosis
4. Musculoskeletal system
   a. Check the client for moving extremities

b. Check the physician's orders regarding client positioning or restrictions
c. Unless contraindicated, place the client in a low Fowler's position after surgery to increase the size of the thorax
d. Avoid positioning the client in a supine position until pharyngeal reflexes have returned
e. If the client is comatose or semicomatose, position on the side unless contraindicated

5. Neurological system
   a. Check level of consciousness
   b. Closely monitor the client who may be drowsy or unconscious
   c. Periodic frequent attempts to awaken the client should continue until the client awakens
   d. Orient the client to the environment
   e. Speak in a soft tone and filter out extraneous noises in the environment
   f. Maintain body temperature and prevent heat loss by providing the client with warm blankets and raising the room temperature as necessary
6. Temperature control
   a. Monitor temperature
   b. Monitor for signs of hypothermia that may result from anesthesia, a cool operating room, and exposure of the skin and internal organs during surgery
   c. Apply warm blankets and continue oxygen as prescribed if the client is shivering
7. Integumentary system
   a. Check surgical site, drains, and wound dressings
   b. Monitor for and document any drainage or bleeding from the surgical site
   c. Check skin for redness, abrasions, or breakdown that may have resulted from surgical positioning
8. Fluid and electrolyte balance
   a. Monitor IV administration as prescribed
   b. Accurately record I&O
9. Gastrointestinal system
   a. Monitor for nausea and vomiting
   b. Maintain patency of nasogastric tube, if present, as prescribed
   c. Monitor for abdominal distention
   d. Monitor for return of bowel sounds
10. Renal system
    a. Check bladder for distention
    b. Monitor color, quantity, and quality of urine output if a Foley catheter is present
    c. Expect the client to void 6 to 8 hours after the surgical procedure, depending on the type of anesthesia administered
11. Pain management
    a. Check for pain
    b. Note the type of anesthetic used and preoperative medication that the client received, and note if the client received any pain medications in the postanesthesia period
    c. Ask the client to rate the degree of pain on a scale of 1 to 10, with 10 being the most severe
    d. Monitor such objective data as facial expressions, body gestures, pulse rate, blood pressure, and respirations
    e. Inquire about the effectiveness of the last pain medication
    f. If a narcotic has been prescribed, during the initial administration check the client every 30 minutes for respiratory rate and pain relief
    g. Use noninvasive measures to relieve postoperative pain including distraction, comfort measures, positioning, backrubs, and providing a quiet and restful environment
    h. Document effectiveness of pain medication

B. Intermediate stage
1. Description
   a. The period of 4 to 24 hours after surgery
   b. Nursing care implemented during the immediate stage is continued
2. Respiratory system: Encourage coughing and deep breathing
3. Cardiovascular system: Encourage the use of antiembolism stockings if prescribed to promote venous return, strengthen muscle tone, and prevent pooling of secretions in the lungs
4. Musculoskeletal system
   a. Before ambulation, instruct the client to sit at the edge of the bed with the feet supported
   b. If client is unable to walk, turn the client every 1 to 2 hours
5. Neurological system: Check level of consciousness
6. Integumentary system
   a. Monitor wound for signs of infection
   b. Maintain a dry and intact dressing
   c. Reinforce with a sterile dressing if necessary and notify the primary health care provider if bleeding occurs from the site
   d. Change dressings as prescribed, noting the amount of bleeding or drainage, odor, and intactness of sutures or staples
   e. Use an abdominal binder for obese and debilitated individuals to prevent rupture of the incision (Figure 16-4)

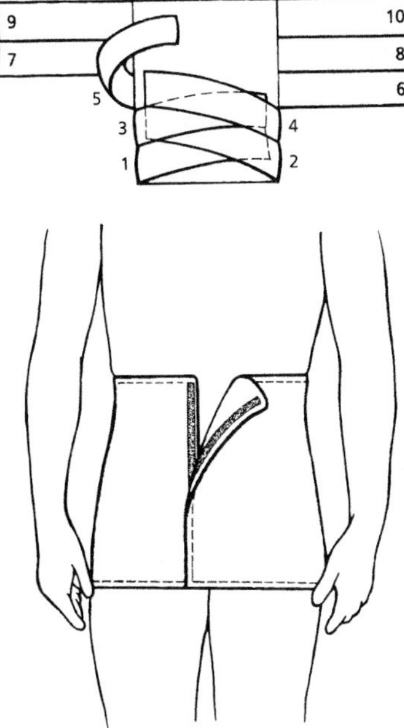

FIG. 16-4 Abdominal binders. (From Perry P, Potter A: *Clinical nursing skills and techniques*, ed 5, St Louis, 2002, Mosby.)

f. Drains should be patent and there should be minimal bleeding or drainage
g. Prepare to assist with the removal of drains as prescribed by the physician when the drainage amount becomes insignificant

7. Gastrointestinal system
   a. Turn the unconscious client to a side-lying position if vomiting occurs, and have suctioning equipment available and ready to use
   b. Administer frequent mouth care
   c. Maintain the NPO status until the gag reflex and peristalsis return
   d. Assess for bowel sounds in all four quadrants
   e. When oral fluids are permitted, start with ice chips and water
   f. Monitor the client for gas pains and encourage ambulation, positioning, and a rectal tube as prescribed
8. Renal system
   a. Monitor urinary output (should be greater than 30 mL per hour)
   b. If the client does not have a Foley catheter, client is expected to void within 6 to 8 hours after the surgical procedure and ensure that the amount is at least 200 mL
9. Pain management
   a. Use noninvasive measures to relieve postoperative pain
   b. Administer pain medication as prescribed
   c. Document effectiveness of pain medication

C. Extended stage
1. Description: The period of at least 1 to 4 days after the surgical procedure
2. Implementation
   a. Continue to check and observe the client's body systems during this stage
   b. Monitor for signs of infection such as redness, swelling, and tenderness at the surgical site, fever, and leukocytosis
   c. Encourage active range of motion every 2 hours
   d. Continue to encourage ambulation that will promote peristalsis and the passage of fluid and flatus
   e. Increase ambulation every day to increase muscle strength
   f. Encourage the client to perform as many activities of daily living as possible
   g. Instruct the client to eat foods that are high in protein and vitamin C content to promote wound healing

III. PNEUMONIA AND ATELECTASIS (Box 16-3 and Figure 16-5)

A. Description
1. Pneumonia, an inflammation of the alveoli caused by infectious process, may develop 3 to 5 days after the surgical procedure because of infection, aspiration, or immobility

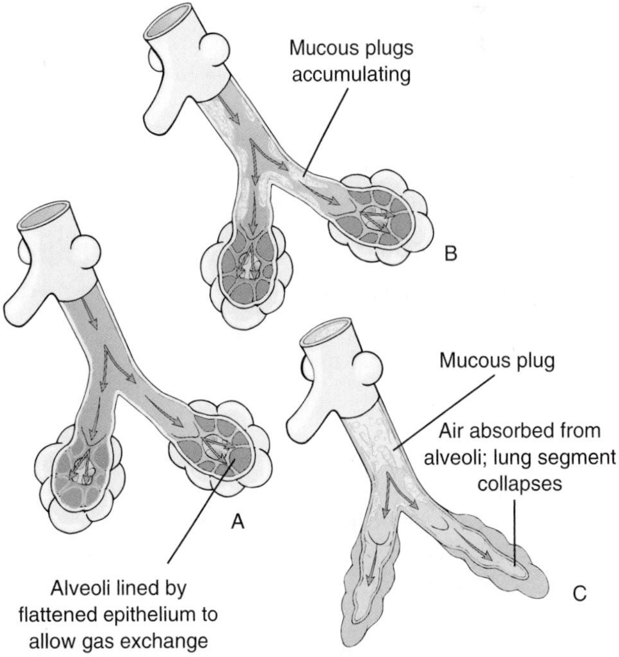

FIG. 16-5 Postoperative atelectasis. (From Lewis S, Heitkemper M, Dirksen S: *Medical-surgical nursing: assessment and management of clinical problems*, St Louis, 2000, Mosby.)

BOX 16-3

Postoperative Complications*

Pneumonia and atelectasis
Hypoxia
Pulmonary embolism
Hemorrhage
Shock
Thrombophlebitis
Urinary retention
Constipation
Paralytic ileus
Wound infection
Wound dehiscence
Wound evisceration

*The nurse always notifies the RN and/or physician if signs of complications are noted.

2. **Atelectasis**, a collapse of the alveoli with retained mucous secretions, is the most common postoperative complication and usually occurs 1 to 2 days after the surgical procedure

B. Data collection
   1. Dyspnea
   2. Increased respiratory rate
   3. Elevated temperature
   4. Productive cough
   5. Chest pain
   6. Crackles over involved lung area

C. Implementation
   1. Monitor temperature
   2. Encourage ambulation
   3. Reposition the client every 1 to 2 hours
   4. Encourage the client to use incentive spirometer, and to cough and deep breathe
   5. Suction to clear secretions if the client is unable to cough
   6. Encourage fluid intake

IV. HYPOXIA (Box 16-3)

A. Description: An inadequate concentration of oxygen in arterial blood

B. Data collection
   1. Restlessness
   2. Dyspnea
   3. Diaphoresis
   4. Increased heart rate and blood pressure
   5. Cyanosis

C. Implementation
   1. Eliminate cause of hypoxia
   2. Encourage coughing and deep breathing and use of incentive spirometry
   3. Turn and reposition client frequently
   4. Monitor pulse oximetry
   5. Administer oxygen as prescribed

V. PULMONARY EMBOLISM (Box 16-3)

A. Description: An embolus blocking the pulmonary artery and disrupting blood flow to one or more lobes of the lung

B. Data collection
   1. Dyspnea
   2. Sudden sharp chest or upper abdominal pain
   3. Increased heart rate and a decrease in blood pressure
   4. Cyanosis

C. Implementation
   1. Notify the registered nurse and/or physician immediately
   2. Monitor vital signs

VI. HEMORRHAGE (Box 16-3)

A. Description: The loss of a large amount of blood externally or internally in a short period of time

B. Data collection
   1. Restlessness
   2. Weak, rapid pulse and hypotension
   3. Cool, clammy skin
   4. Rapid breathing
   5. Reduced urine output

C. Implementation
   1. Provide pressure to the site of bleeding
   2. Notify the registered nurse and/or physician immediately

VII. SHOCK (Box 16-3)

A. Description: loss of circulatory fluid volume that is usually caused by hemorrhage

B. Data collection
   1. Restlessness
   2. Weak, rapid pulse and hypotension
   3. Cool clammy skin
   4. Rapid breathing
   5. Reduced urine output
   6. Disorientation

C. Implementation
   1. If shock develops, elevate the legs
   2. If the client had spinal anesthesia, do not elevate the legs any higher than placing them on the pillow; otherwise diaphragm muscles could be impaired
   3. Notify the registered nurse and/or physician immediately

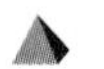

VIII. THROMBOPHLEBITIS (Box 16-3)

A. Description
   1. Inflammation of a vein, often accompanied by clot formation

2. Veins in the legs are most commonly affected

B. Data collection
1. Aching or cramping leg pain
2. Vein feels hard and cordlike and is tender to touch
3. Elevated temperature
4. Positive Homan's sign

C. Implementation
1. Monitor legs for swelling, inflammation, cyanosis, pain, tenderness, and venous distention
2. Elevate the extremity 30 degrees without allowing any pressure on the popliteal area
3. Encourage coughing and deep breathing
4. Encourage the use of antiembolism stockings as prescribed, removing them twice a day to wash and inspect the legs
5. Use intermittent pulsatile compression device as prescribed (Figure 16-6)
6. Perform passive range of motion every 2 hours if the client is on bed rest
7. Do not allow the client to dangle
8. Instruct the client not to sit in one position for an extended period of time
9. Heparin or warfarin (Coumadin) may be prescribed

IX. URINARY RETENTION (Box 16-3)

A. Description
1. Involuntary accumulation of urine in the bladder from loss of muscle tone
2. Occurs as a result of the effects of anesthetics and narcotic analgesics
3. Appears 6 to 8 hours after surgery

B. Data collection
1. Restlessness
2. Inability to void and a distended bladder
3. Lower abdominal pain

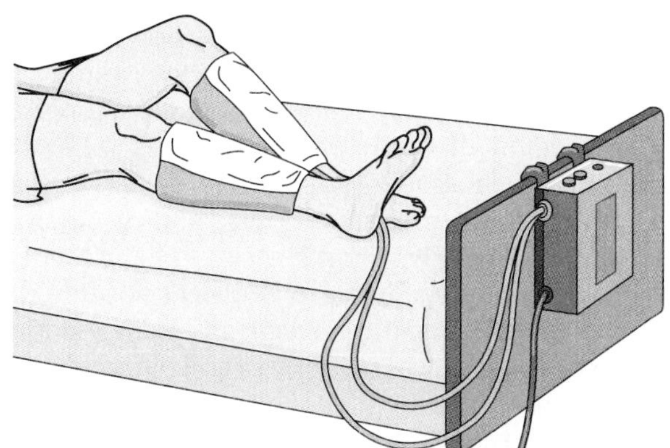

FIG. 16-6 Intermittent pulsatile compression device. (From Phipps W, Sands J, Marek J: *Medical-surgical nursing: Concepts and clinical practice*, ed 6, St Louis, 1999, Mosby. Courtesy University Hospitals of Cleveland, Cleveland, Ohio.)

4. Elevated blood pressure
5. Diaphoresis
6. On percussion, the bladder sounds like a drum

C. Implementation
1. Check for distended bladder
2. Encourage ambulation when prescribed
3. Encourage fluid intake unless contraindicated
4. Provide privacy when attempting to void
5. Assist the client to void by helping to stand
6. Pour warm water over the perineum
7. Allow the client to hear running water
8. Catheterize the client as prescribed after all noninvasive techniques have been attempted

X. CONSTIPATION (Box 16-3)

A. Description
1. Infrequent passage of stool
2. When the client resumes a solid diet after surgery, failure to pass stool within 48 hours is a cause for concern

B. Data collection
1. Abdominal distention
2. Absence of bowel movements

C. Implementation
1. Check bowel sounds
2. Encourage fluid intake up to 3000 mL per day unless contraindicated
3. Encourage early ambulation
4. Encourage consumption of fiber and roughage
5. Administer stool softeners and laxatives as prescribed
6. Provide privacy and adequate time for bowel elimination

XI. ILEUS (Box 16-3)

A. Description
1. Failure of appropriate forward movement of bowel contents
2. May occur as a result of anesthetic medications or manipulation of the bowel during the surgical procedure

B. Data collection
1. Postoperative nausea and vomiting
2. Abdominal distention
3. Absence of bowel sounds, bowel movement, or flatus

C. Implementation
1. Maintain NPO status until bowel sounds return
2. Maintain patency of nasogastric (NG) tube
3. Encourage ambulation
4. Monitor IV fluids as prescribed

5. Administer medications as prescribed to increase gastrointestinal (GI) motility and secretions

XII. WOUND INFECTION (Box 16-3)

A. Description
   1. Caused by poor aseptic technique or a contaminated wound before surgical exploration
   2. Usually occurs 3 to 6 days after surgery
   3. Purulent material may exit from the drains or separated wound edges
B. Data collection
   1. Fever and chills
   2. Warm, tender, painful, and inflamed incision site
   3. Edematous skin at incision and tight skin sutures
   4. Elevated white blood cell count
C. Implementation
   1. Monitor temperature
   2. Monitor incision site for approximation of suture line, edema or bleeding, and signs of infection
   3. Maintain patency of drains and keep drain and tubes away from incision line
   4. Monitor drains and assess drainage amount, color, and consistency
   5. Change dressing as prescribed
   6. Administer antibiotics as prescribed

XIII. WOUND DEHISCENCE (Box 16-3 and Figure 16-7)

A. Description
   1. Separation of the wound edges at the suture line
   2. Usually occurs 6 to 8 days after surgery
B. Data collection
   1. Increased drainage
   2. Opened wound edges
   3. Appearance of underlying tissues through the wound
C. Implementation
   1. Notify the registered nurse and/or physician immediately
   2. Place the client in low Fowler's position with knees bent to prevent abdominal tension on abdominal wounds
   3. Cover the wound with a sterile normal saline dressing
   4. Prevent wound infection
   5. Administer antiemetics as prescribed to prevent vomiting and further strain on the incision
   6. Instruct the client to splint the incision when coughing

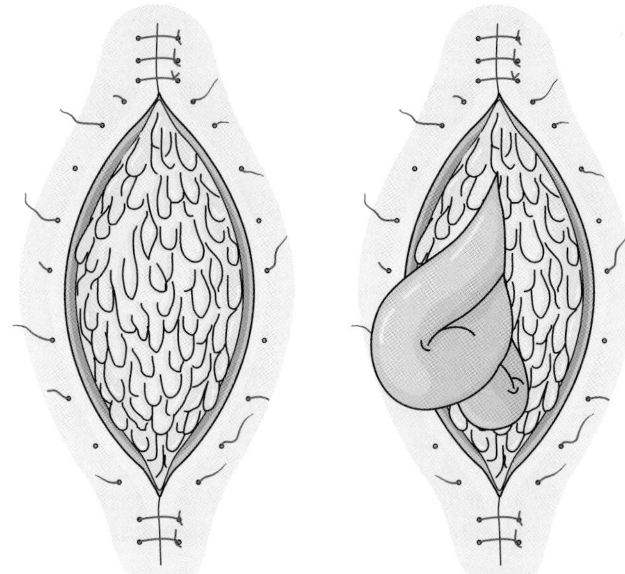

FIG. 16-7 Wound dehiscence and wound evisceration. (From Phipps W, Sands J, Marek J: *Medical-surgical nursing: concepts and clinical practice*, ed 6, St Louis, 1999, Mosby.)

XIV. WOUND EVISCERATION (Box 16-3 and Figure 16-7)

A. Description
   1. Protrusion of the internal organs and tissues through an opening in the wound edges
   2. Most common among obese clients, clients who have had abdominal surgery, or those who have poor wound-healing ability
   3. Usually occurs 6 to 8 days after surgery
   4. Wound evisceration is an emergency
B. Data collection
   1. Discharge of serosanguineous fluid from a previously dry wound
   2. The appearance of loops of bowel or other abdominal contents through the wound
   3. The client may report feeling a popping sensation after coughing or turning
C. Implementation
   1. Notify the registered nurse and/or physician immediately
   2. Place the client in a low Fowler's position with the knees bent to prevent abdominal tension
   3. Cover the wound with a sterile normal saline dressing
   4. Prevent wound infection
   5. Administer antiemetics as prescribed to prevent vomiting and further strain on the incision
   6. Instruct the client to splint the incision when coughing

XV. AMBULATORY SURGERY

A. Criteria for client discharge
   1. Is alert and oriented
   2. Has voided
   3. Has no respiratory distress
   4. Is able to ambulate, swallow, and cough
   5. Has minimal pain
   6. Is not vomiting
   7. Has minimal, if any, bleeding from incision site
   8. A responsible adult is available to drive the client home
   9. The surgeon has signed a release form

B. Reinforcing discharge instructions (Box 16-4)
   1. Should be performed before the date of the scheduled procedure
   2. Provide written instructions to the client and family regarding the specifics of care
   3. Instruct the client and family about postoperative complications that can occur
   4. Suggest appropriate resources for home care support
   5. Instruct the client not to drive for 24 hours if he or she had a general anesthetic
   6. Inform the client to call the surgeon, ambulatory center, or emergency department if postoperative problems occur
   7. Instruct the client to keep follow-up appointments with the surgeon

PRACTICE QUESTIONS

1. A nurse is reviewing the laboratory results of a client scheduled for surgery. Which of these laboratory results would indicate to the nurse that the surgery may be postponed?
   1. Sodium 140 mEq/L
   2. Hemoglobin 9.2 g/dL
   3. Platelets 200,000/mm^3
   4. Serum creatinine 0.9 mg/dL
2. A nurse is preparing a client for surgery. The nurse would plan to implement which of the following on the day of surgery?
   1. Remove colored nail polish
   2. Immediately report an increase in blood pressure of 120/72 mmHg to 128/84 mmHg
   3. Verify that the client has not eaten for the last 24 hours
   4. Avoid oral hygiene and rinsing with mouthwash
3. Emergency surgery is scheduled for a client with a bowel obstruction. The licensed practical nurse (LPN) tells the registered nurse (RN) that he or she is unable to obtain informed consent from the client because the client has received narcotic analgesics and is very sedated. The LPN understands that the most appropriate action is which of the following?
   1. Performing the surgery without an informed consent
   2. Calling the family and telling them that they must come to the hospital immediately to sign the informed consent
   3. Obtaining a telephone consent from the family member ensuring that the oral consent is witnessed by two persons
   4. Having the client sign the consent form because this is an emergency situation
4. A nurse is caring for a client scheduled for surgery. The client is concerned about the surgical procedure. To alleviate the client's fears and misconceptions about surgery, the nurse should first:

BOX 16-4
Reinforcing Discharge Instructions

Demonstrate care to the incision and how to change the dressing.
Instruct the client to cover the incision with plastic if showering is allowed.
Be sure the client is provided with a 48-hour supply of dressings for home use.
Instruct the client on the importance of returning to the physician's office for follow-up care.
Instruct the client that sutures are usually removed in the physician's office 7 to 10 days after surgery.
Inform the client that staples are usually removed 7 to 14 days after surgery and that they may become slightly reddened when they are ready to be removed.
Steri-strips may be applied to provide extra support after the sutures are removed.
Instruct the client on the use of medications, as well as their purpose, doses, administration, and side effects.
Instruct the client on diet.
Instruct the client to drink 6 to 8 glasses of liquid a day unless contraindicated.
Instruct the client on activity levels.
The client should be instructed to resume normal activities gradually.
Instruct the client to avoid lifting for 6 weeks if a major surgical procedure was performed.
Instruct the client with abdominal incisions not to lift anything weighing 10 pounds or more and not to engage in any activities that involve pushing or pulling.
The client can usually return to work in 6 to 8 weeks as prescribed by the physician.
Instruct the client on the signs and symptoms of complications and when to call the physician.

1. Provide explanations about the procedures involved in the planned surgery
2. Explain all nursing care and possible discomfort that may result
3. Tell the client that preoperative fear is normal
4. Ask the client to discuss information known about the planned surgery

5. A nurse is reinforcing instructions to a client regarding the use of the incentive spirometer. Which of the following client statements would indicate that the client does not clearly understand the procedure?
   1. "My lips should cover the mouthpiece completely."
   2. "I should inhale slowly to maintain a constant flow through the unit."
   3. "After maximum inspiration, I should hold my breath for 2 to 3 seconds then exhale slowly."
   4. "I can use the incentive spirometer in any position to achieve optimal lung expansion."

6. A nurse is collecting data from a client who is scheduled for surgery in 1 week in the ambulatory care surgical center. The nurse notes that the client has a history of arthritis and has been taking acetylsalicylic acid (aspirin, ASA). The nurse reports the information to the physician and anticipates that the physician will prescribe which of the following?
   1. Continue to take the aspirin as prescribed
   2. Decrease the dose of the aspirin to half of what is normally taken
   3. Discontinue the aspirin immediately
   4. Discontinue the aspirin 48 hours before the scheduled surgery

7. A nurse preparing a client for surgery reviews the client's medication record. The client is to be NPO after midnight. Which of the following medications, if noted on the client's record, would the nurse question?
   1. Cyclobenzaprine (Flexeril)
   2. Fentanyl (Duragesic)
   3. Allopurinol (Zyloprim)
   4. Prednisone (Deltasone)

8. A nurse obtains the vital signs on a postoperative client. The client's blood pressure (BP) is 100/60 mm Hg, pulse is 90 beats per minute, and respiration rate is 20 breaths per minute. Based on these findings, which of the following nursing actions should be performed?
   1. Cover the client with a warm blanket
   2. Shake gently to arouse
   3. Continue to monitor the vital signs
   4. Call the surgeon immediately

9. A client arrives to the surgical nursing unit after surgery. The initial nursing action is to check the:
   1. Dressing for bleeding
   2. Tubes or drains for patency
   3. Patency of the airway
   4. Vital signs to compare with preoperative measurements

10. A nurse is monitoring an adult client for postoperative complications. Which of the following would be most indicative of a potential postoperative complication that requires further observation?
    1. Urinary output of 20 mL per hour
    2. Temperature of 37.6° C (99.6° F)
    3. Serous drainage on the surgical dressing
    4. Blood pressure of 100/70 mm Hg

11. A nurse monitors the postoperative client frequently for the presence of secretions in the lungs knowing that accumulated secretions can lead to:
    1. Pulmonary edema
    2. Pneumonia
    3. Fluid imbalance
    4. Carbon dioxide retention

12. A nurse is caring for a postoperative client who has a drain inserted in the surgical wound. Which of the following nursing actions would be inappropriate in the care of the drain?
    1. Maintain aseptic technique when emptying
    2. Observe for bright red bloody drainage
    3. Check the drain for patency
    4. Secure the drain by curling or folding it and taping it firmly to body

13. A nurse checks the client's surgical incision for signs of infection. Which of the following would not be indicative of a potential infection?
    1. The presence of serous drainage
    2. Warm, red, tender skin around the incision
    3. Chills and fever
    4. The presence of purulent drainage

14. A nurse is checking a client's surgical incision and notes an increase in the amount of drainage, a separation of the incision line, and the appearance of underlying tissue. Which of the following is the most appropriate initial action?
    1. Clean the wound using aseptic technique and apply a sterile dry dressing
    2. Apply a sterile dressing soaked with normal saline to the wound
    3. Leave the incision open to the air to assist in drying the drainage
    4. Cover the wound with a Betadine soaked dressing

15. A nurse monitors a postoperative client for signs of complications. Which of the following would the nurse determine to be indicative of a sign of a potential complication?
    1. Faint bowel sounds heard in all four quadrants
    2. A negative Homan's sign
    3. A blood pressure of 120/70 mm Hg with a pulse of 90 beats per minute
    4. Increasing restlessness

ANSWERS

1. *Answer:* 2
Rationale: Routine screening tests include a complete blood cell count, serum electrolyte analysis, coagulation studies, and serum creatinine tests. The complete blood count includes the hemoglobin analysis. All of these values are within normal range except the hemoglobin. If a client has a low hemoglobin level, the surgery may be postponed.
Test-Taking Strategy: Use the process of elimination. Recalling the normal values for serum sodium, hemoglobin, platelets, and creatinine will direct you to option 2. This is the only abnormal value. Review these normal laboratory values if you had difficulty with this question.
Level of Cognitive Ability: Analysis
Client Needs: Physiological Integrity
Integrated Concept/Process: Nursing Process/Data Collection
Content Area: Fundamental Skills
Reference: Potter P, Perry A: *Fundamentals of nursing,* ed 5, St Louis, 2001, Mosby, p. 1665.

2. *Answer:* 1
Rationale: Nail polish should be removed from at least one nail for the pulse oximeter to check oxygen saturation. Some increase in blood pressure is common because of anxiety. The client usually has a restriction of food and fluids for 8 hours before surgery, not 24 hours. Oral hygiene is allowed, but the client should not swallow any water.
Test-Taking Strategy: Use the principles associated with prioritization when answering this question. Use the ABCs—airway, breathing, and circulation. Monitoring the oxygen saturation level through the nails would assess airway, breathing, and circulation. Review general preoperative care if you had difficulty with this question.
Level of Cognitive Ability: Application
Client Needs: Physiological Integrity
Integrated Concept/Process: Nursing Process/Implementation
Content Area: Fundamental Skills
Reference: Potter P, Perry A: *Fundamentals of nursing,* ed 5, St Louis, 2001, Mosby, p. 704.

3. *Answer:* 3
Rationale: Every effort must be made to obtain permission from a responsible family member to perform surgery if the client is unable to sign the consent form. A telephone consent must be witnessed by two persons who hear the family member's oral consent. The two witnesses then sign the consent and document the name of the family member, noting that an oral consent was obtained. In emergencies, the client may be unable to sign and family members may not be available. In this type of a situation, the physician is legally permitted to perform surgery without consent. Consent is not informed if it is obtained from the client that is confused, unconscious, mentally incompetent, or under the influence of sedatives.
Test-Taking Strategy: Use the process of elimination. Note the key words "most appropriate." Eliminate options 1 and 4 first because they are inappropriate. From the remaining options, select option 3 because it is legally acceptable to obtain telephone permission from a family member if two persons witness it. Review the issues related to informed consent if you had difficulty with this question.
Level of Cognitive Ability: Comprehension
Client Needs: Safe, Effective Care Environment
Integrated Concept/Process: Nursing Process/Implementation
Content Area: Fundamental Skills
Reference: Potter P, Perry A: *Fundamentals of nursing,* ed 5, St. Louis, 2001, Mosby, p. 432.

4. *Answer:* 4
Rationale: Explanations should begin with the information that the client knows. Option 3 is a block to communication. Options 1 and 2 may produce additional anxiety in the client.
Test-Taking Strategy: Use the process of elimination. Note the key word "first." Remember to always focus on the client's feelings first. This will direct you to option 4. Additionally, option 4 is the only option that addresses data collection, the first step of the nursing process. Review the psychosocial aspects related to the preoperative client if you had difficulty with this question.
Level of Cognitive Ability: Application
Client Needs: Psychosocial Integrity
Integrated Concept/Process: Caring
Content Area: Fundamental Skills
Reference: DeWit S: *Fundamental concepts and skills for nursing,* Philadelphia, 2001, WB Saunders, p. 88.

5. *Answer:* 4
Rationale: For optimal lung expansion with incentive spirometer, the client should assume the semi-Fowler's or high Fowler's position. The mouthpiece should be covered completely while the client inhales slowly with a constant flow through the unit. The breath should be held for 2 to 3 seconds before exhaling slowly.
Test-Taking Strategy: Use the process of elimination and note the key words "does not clearly understand." Remember that for optimal lung expansion, the head should be elevated to decrease the pressure of the internal organs on the diaphragm and to increase the expansion of the diaphragm. If you had difficulty with this question, review the correct procedure related to the use of an incentive spirometer.
Level of Cognitive Ability: Analysis
Client Needs: Physiological Integrity
Integrated Concept/Process: Nursing Process/Evaluation
Content Area: Fundamental Skills
Reference: DeWit S: *Fundamental concepts and skills for nursing,* Philadelphia, 2001, WB Saunders, p. 535.

6. *Answer:* 4
Rationale: Anticoagulants alter normal clotting factors and increase the risk of hemorrhage. Aspirin has properties that can alter the clotting mechanism and should be discontinued at least 48 hours before surgery.
Test-Taking Strategy: Use the process of elimination. Remembering that aspirin has properties that can alter normal clotting factors and that it should be discontinued at least 48 hours before surgery will assist in directing you to option 4. Review the medications that affect the preoperative client if you had difficulty with this question.
Level of Cognitive Ability: Application
Client Needs: Physiological Integrity
Integrated Concept/Process: Nursing Process/Planning
Content Area: Fundamental Skills

Reference: DeWit S: *Fundamental concepts and skills for nursing,* Philadelphia, 2001, WB Saunders, p. 756.

7. *Answer:* 4
Rationale: Prednisone is a corticosteroid that can cause adrenal atrophy, which reduces the body's ability to withstand stress. Before and during surgery, dosages may be temporarily increased. Cyclobenzaprine is a skeletal muscle relaxant. Fentanyl is an opioid analgesic. Allopurinol is an antigout medication.
Test-Taking Strategy: Use the process of elimination and knowledge regarding the medications that may have special implications for the surgical client to answer this question. Review these medications if you had difficulty with this question.
Level of Cognitive Ability: Application
Client Needs: Physiological Integrity
Integrated Concept/Process: Nursing Process/Implementation
Content Area: Fundamental Skills
References: Lehne R: *Pharmacology for nursing care,* ed 4, Philadelphia, 2001, WB Saunders, p. 659.

8. *Answer:* 3
Rationale: A slightly lower than normal BP and an increased pulse rate are common after surgery. Warm blankets are applied to maintain the client's body temperature. Level of consciousness can be determined by checking the client's response to light touch and verbal stimuli, rather than by shaking the client. There is no reason to contact the surgeon.
Test-Taking Strategy: Focus on the data in the question. Noting that the vital signs are within normal limits will direct you to option 3. Review expected postoperative findings if you had difficulty with this question.
Level of Cognitive Ability: Application
Client Needs: Physiological Integrity
Integrated Concept/Process: Nursing Process/Implementation
Content Area: Fundamental Skills
Reference: DeWit S: *Fundamental concepts and skills for nursing,* Philadelphia, 2001, WB Saunders, p. 767.

9. *Answer:* 3
Rationale: If the airway is not patent, immediate measures must be taken for the survival of the client. After checking the client's airway, the nurse would next check the client's vital signs, and then check the dressing and tubes and drains.
Test-Taking Strategy: Use the ABCs—airway, breathing, and circulation. Airway patency is the first action to be taken. Options 1, 2, and 4 are all nursing actions that should be performed after a patent airway has been established. Review care to the postoperative client if you had difficulty with this question.
Level of Cognitive Ability: Application
Client Needs: Physiological Integrity
Integrated Concept/Process: Nursing Process/Implementation
Content Area: Fundamental Skills
Reference: DeWit S: *Fundamental concepts and skills for nursing,* Philadelphia, 2001, WB Saunders, p. 767.

10. *Answer:* 1
Rationale: Urine output is maintained at a minimum of at least 30 mL per hour for an adult. An output of less than 30 mL for each of two consecutive hours should be reported to the physician. A temperature above 37.7° C (100° F) or below 36.1° C (97° F) and a falling systolic blood pressure under 90 mm Hg are to be reported. The client's preoperative or baseline blood pressure is used to make informed postoperative comparisons. Moderate or light serous drainage from the surgical site is considered normal.
Test-Taking Strategy: Knowledge of the normal ranges for temperature, blood pressure, urinary output, and wound drainage is necessary to determine the correct option. Through the process of elimination, you can determine that the urinary output is the only observation that is not within the normal range. Review expected postoperative findings if you had difficulty with this question.
Level of Cognitive Ability: Analysis
Client Needs: Physiological Integrity
Integrated Concept/Process: Nursing Process/Data Collection
Content Area: Fundamental Skills
Reference: DeWit S: *Fundamental concepts and skills for nursing,* Philadelphia, 2001, WB Saunders, p. 7.

11. *Answer:* 2
Rationale: The most common postoperative respiratory problems are atelectasis, pneumonia, and pulmonary emboli. Pneumonia is the inflammation of lung tissue that causes productive cough, dyspnea, and crackles. Pulmonary edema usually results from left-sided heart failure and can be caused by medications, fluid overload, and smoke inhalation. Carbon dioxide retention results from the inability to exhale carbon dioxide in conditions such as chronic obstructive pulmonary disease. Fluid imbalance can be a deficit or excess related to fluid loss or overload.
Test-Taking Strategy: Use the process of elimination and note the key words "presence of secretions in the lungs." Focusing on the issue of the question, the postoperative client, will direct you to option 2. Options 1, 3, and 4 most commonly occur with other conditions. Review postoperative complications if you had difficulty with this question.
Level of Cognitive Ability: Application
Client Needs: Physiological Integrity
Integrated Concept/Process: Nursing Process/Data Collection
Content Area: Fundamental Skills
Reference: DeWit S: *Fundamental concepts and skills for nursing,* Philadelphia, 2001, WB Saunders, p. 723.

12. *Answer:* 4
Rationale: Aseptic technique must be used when emptying the drainage container or changing the dressing to avoid contamination of the wound. Usually the drainage from the wound is pale, red, and watery. Active bleeding will be bright red in color. The drain should be checked for patency to provide an exit for the fluid or blood to promote healing. The nurse needs to ensure that drainage flows freely and that there are no kinks in the drains. Curling or folding the drain prevents the flow of the drainage.
Test-Taking Strategy: Use the process of elimination and note the key word "inappropriate." Remember that the nurse needs to ensure that drainage flows freely from a drain. Review care to the surgical client with a drain if you had difficulty with this question.

Level of Cognitive Ability: Application
Client Needs: Physiological Integrity
Integrated Concept/Process: Nursing Process/Implementation
Content Area: Fundamental Skills
Reference: DeWit S: *Fundamental concepts and skills for nursing,* Philadelphia, 2001, WB Saunders, p. 768.

13. *Answer:* 1
Rationale: Signs and symptoms of a wound infection include warm, red, and tender skin around the incision. The client may have fever and chills. Purulent material may exit from drains or from separated wound edges. It may be caused by poor aseptic technique and a contaminated wound before surgical exploration. It appears 3 to 6 days after surgery. Serous drainage is not indicative of a wound infection.
Test-Taking Strategy: Note the key word "not." Options 2, 3, and 4 indicate signs of infection. Serous drainage is sometimes normally noted at a surgical incision. Remember however, that an increased flow of serosanguineous drainage from a surgical incision may be a sign of dehiscence. Review the signs of a wound infection if you had difficulty with this question.
Level of Cognitive Ability: Comprehension
Client Needs: Physiological Integrity
Integrated Concept/Process: Nursing Process/Data Collection
Content Area: Fundamental Skills
Reference: DeWit S: *Fundamental concepts and skills for nursing,* Philadelphia, 2001, WB Saunders, p. 782.

14. *Answer:* 2
Rationale: Wound dehiscence is the separation of wound edges at the suture line. Signs and symptoms include increased drainage and the appearance of underlying tissues. It usually occurs 6 to 8 days after surgery. The client should be instructed to remain quiet and to avoid coughing or straining. The client should be positioned to prevent further stress on the wound. Sterile dressings soaked with sterile normal saline should be used to cover the wound. The physician needs to be notified.
Test-Taking Strategy: Use the process of elimination. Eliminate option 3 first because this action would expose the open wound and underlying tissues to infection. Eliminate options 1 and 4 next. A dry dressing and a dressing soaked with Betadine will irritate the exposed body tissues. Review emergency care when dehiscence or evisceration occurs if you had difficulty with this question.
Level of Cognitive Ability: Application
Client Needs: Physiological Integrity
Integrated Concept/Process: Nursing Process/Implementation
Content Area: Fundamental Skills
Reference: DeWit S: *Fundamental concepts and skills for nursing,* Philadelphia, 2001, WB Saunders, p. 773.

15. *Answer:* 4
Rationale: Increasing restlessness noted in a client is a sign that requires continuous and close monitoring, because it could be indicative of a potential indication of a complication such as hemorrhage or shock. Faint bowel sounds heard in all four quadrants is a normal occurrence. A negative Homan's sign is also normal. A positive Homan's sign, however, may be indicative of thrombophlebitis. A blood pressure of 120/70 mm Hg with a pulse of 90 is a relatively normal sign.
Test-Taking Strategy: Use the process of elimination. Eliminate options 1, 2, and 3 because these are normal expected findings. Review the normal expected postoperative findings if you had difficulty with this question.
Level of Cognitive Ability: Analysis
Client Needs: Physiological Integrity
Integrated Concept/Process: Nursing Process/Data Collection
Content Area: Fundamental Skills
Reference: DeWit S: *Fundamental concepts and skills for nursing,* Philadelphia, 2001, WB Saunders, p. 773.

REFERENCES

DeWit S: *Fundamental concepts and skills for nursing,* Philadelphia, 2001, WB Saunders.

Hodgson B, Kizior R: *Saunders nursing drug handbook 2002,* Philadelphia, 2002, WB Saunders.

National Council of State Boards of Nursing, editors: *Test plan for the National Council Licensure Examination for Practical/Vocational Nurses,* Chicago, 2001, Author.

O'Neill P: *Caring for the older adult,* Philadelphia, 2002, WB Saunders.

Potter P, Perry A: *Fundamentals of nursing,* ed 5, St Louis, 2001, Mosby.

17 Positioning Clients

PYRAMID TERMS

Fowler's Position The client is supine and the head of the bed is elevated to 45 degrees.

Low Fowler's Position (Semi-Fowler's) The client is supine and the head of the bed is elevated to 30 degrees.

High Fowler's Position The client is supine and the head of the bed is elevated to 90 degrees.

Lateral (Side-Lying) Position The client is lying on the side and the head and shoulders are aligned with the hips and the spine and are parallel to the edge of the mattress. The head, neck, and upper arm are supported by a pillow. The lower shoulder is pulled forward slightly and, along with the elbow, flexed at 90 degrees. The legs are flexed or extended. A pillow is placed to support the back.

Lithotomy Position The client is lying on the back with the hips and knees flexed at right angles and the feet in stirrups.

Prone Position The client is lying on the abdomen with head turned to the side. The shoulders are abducted and rotated 90 degrees, with arms flexed at the elbows and palms facing downward along the side of the head. The legs are extended and slightly separated. The feet should extend over the bottom of the mattress with the ankles at a 90-degree angle, or be supported at a 90-degree angle with sandbags.

Supine (Dorsal Recumbent) Position The client is lying on the back. The head and shoulders are usually slightly elevated with a small pillow. The arms and legs are extended, and the legs are slightly abducted.

Sims' Position (Semiprone) The client is lying on the side with the body turned prone at 45 degrees. The spine is parallel with the mattress, and shoulders and hips are aligned. The face is supported by a small pillow. The lower arm is behind the body, with the shoulder retracted and hyperextended, and the elbow is slightly flexed. The lower leg is extended, with the upper leg flexed at the hip and knee to a 45- to 90-degree angle. The ankles are supported at 90 degrees.

PYRAMID TO SUCCESS

Nursing responsibility includes positioning clients in a safe and appropriate manner to provide safety and comfort. Knowledge regarding the client position required for a certain procedure or condition is important (Figure 17-1). It is the nurse's responsibility to assist in preventing the development of complications related to an existing condition, prescribed treatment, or medical and surgical procedure. The nurse must review the physician's orders after treatments and procedures regarding client positioning and mobility. The primary Integrated Concepts and Processes addressed in this chapter include Caring, Communication and Documentation, the Clinical Problem-Solving Process (Nursing Process), and Teaching/Learning.

CLIENT NEEDS

Safe, Effective Care Environment

Appropriate positioning
Environmental and personal safety
Establishing priorities
Informed consent
Medical and surgical asepsis
Protective measures

Health Promotion and Maintenance

Instructions regarding the need for prescribed therapies
Techniques of collecting physical data

Psychosocial Integrity

Assisting the client to use coping mechanisms
Keeping the family informed of client progress
Providing comfort and support to the client

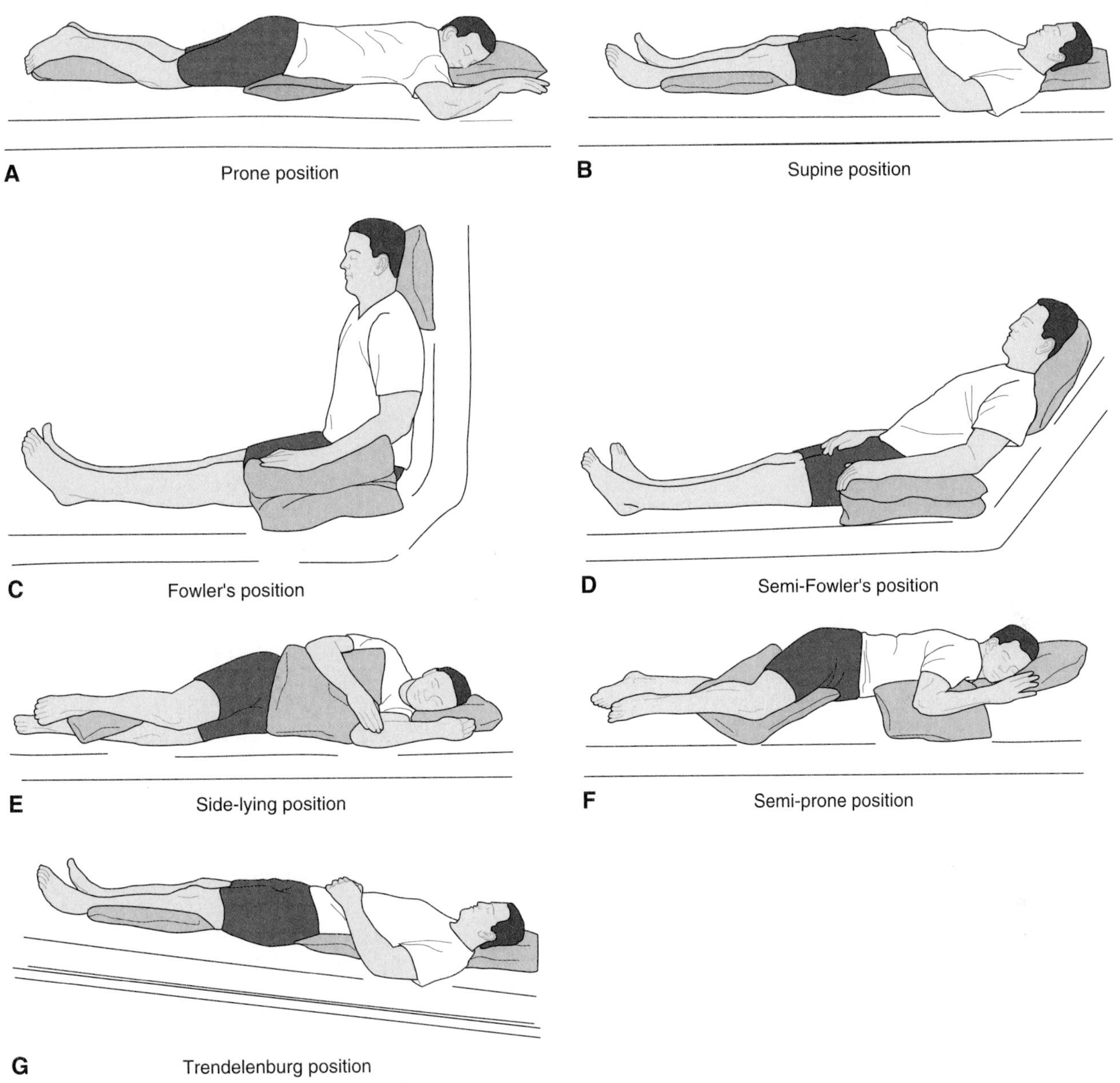

A Prone position

B Supine position

C Fowler's position

D Semi-Fowler's position

E Side-lying position

F Semi-prone position

G Trendelenburg position

FIG. 17-1 Basic positions for patients in bed. (From Lindeman C, McAthie M: *Fundamentals of contemporary nursing practice*, Philadelphia, 1999, WB Saunders.)

Physiological Integrity

Comfort measures for rest and sleep
Immobility
Preventing complications
Providing nutrition and oral intake
Providing personal hygiene as needed
Use of assistive devices

I. INTEGUMENTARY SYSTEM
   A. Autograft: After surgery, site is immobilized for 3 to 7 days to provide the time needed for the graft to adhere and attach to the wound bed

   B. Burns of the face and head: Elevate the head of the bed to prevent or reduce facial and tracheal edema
   C. Circumferential burns of the extremities: Elevate the extremities above the level of the heart to prevent or reduce dependent edema
   D. Skin graft: Elevate and immobilize the graft site to prevent movement and shearing of the graft and disruption of tissue

II. REPRODUCTIVE SYSTEM
   A. Mastectomy
      1. Position the client with the head of the bed elevated at least 30 degrees **(semi-Fowler's)**, with the affected arm elevated on a pillow to promote lymphatic fluid return after removal of axillary lymph nodes

2. Turn the client only to the back and unaffected side

B. Perineal and vaginal procedures: Place the client in **lithotomy position**

III. ENDOCRINE SYSTEM

A. Hypophysectomy: Elevate the head of the bed to prevent increased intracranial pressure

B. Thyroidectomy

1. Place in **semi-Fowler's position** to reduce swelling and edema in the neck area
2. Sandbags or pillows may be used to support the client's head or neck

IV. GASTROINTESTINAL SYSTEM

A. Hemorrhoidectomy: Assist the client to a **lateral (side-lying) position** to prevent pain and bleeding

B. Liver biopsy

1. During the procedure: To provide for maximal exposure of the right intercostal space, position the client **supine** with the right side of upper abdomen exposed; the client's right arm is raised and extended over the left shoulder behind the head
2. After the procedure: Assist the client into a right **(lateral) side-lying position**; place a small pillow or folded towel under the puncture site for at least 3 hours

C. Intestinal tubes (Miller-Abbott, Cantor, and Harris tubes): After insertion, place the client on right side to facilitate passage of the tube into the duodenum

D. Nasogastric tube irrigations and tube feedings: Elevate the head of the bed 30 degrees **(semi-Fowler's)** to prevent aspiration; maintain head elevation for continuous feedings and for 1 hour after an intermittent feeding

E. Rectal enemas/irrigations: Place the client in left **Sims' position** to allow the solution to flow by gravity in the natural direction of the colon

V. RESPIRATORY SYSTEM

A. Chronic obstructive pulmonary disease: In advanced disease, positioning in a sitting position, leaning forward, with the client's arms over several pillows or an overbed table will assist the client to breathe easier

B. Laryngectomy (radical neck dissection): Position the client in **semi-Fowler's** or **Fowler's position** to maintain a patent airway and minimize edema

C. Bronchoscopy postprocedure: Place the client in a **semi-Fowler's position** to prevent choking or aspiration caused by impaired ability to swallow

D. Postural drainage: The lung segment to be drained should be in the uppermost position

E. Thoracentesis: During the procedure, to facilitate removal of fluid from the chest wall, position the client sitting on the edge of bed leaning over the bedside table, with the feet supported on a stool, or lying in bed on the unaffected side with the head of the bed elevated 45 degrees **(Fowler's)**

VI. CARDIOVASCULAR SYSTEM

A. Abdominal aneurysm resection: After surgery, limit elevation of head of bed to 45 degrees **(Fowler's)** to avoid flexion of the graft

B. Amputation of the Lower Extremity

1. During the first 24 hours after amputation, elevate the foot of bed (but not the stump itself) to reduce edema, then keep the bed flat to prevent hip flexion contractures
2. Consult with the physician, and then position the client **prone** every 3 to 4 hours for 20 to 30 minutes to stretch muscles and prevent flexion contractures of the hip
3. When the client is in the **prone position**, keep the client's legs close together to prevent abduction
4. Teach the client to contract the gluteal muscles of the buttocks

C. Arterial vascular grafting of an extremity: To promote graft patency after the procedure, bed rest is maintained for at least 24 hours and the affected extremity is kept straight; limit movement and avoid flexion of the hip and knee

D. Cardiac catheterization

1. After cardiac catheterization, the extremity in which the catheter was inserted is kept straight for 4 to 6 hours
2. If the femoral artery was used, strict bed rest is enforced for 6 to 12 hours; the client may turn from side to side
3. The affected leg is kept straight and the head elevated no greater than 30 degrees until hemostasis is adequately achieved

E. Congestive heart failure and pulmonary edema: Position the client upright, preferably with the legs dangling over the side of the bed, to decrease venous return and lung congestion

F. Peripheral arterial disease

1. Obtain the physician's order for positioning
2. Because swelling can prevent arterial blood flow, clients may be advised to elevate their feet at rest, but they should not raise their legs above the level of the heart because extreme elevation slows arterial blood flow

G. Thrombophlebitis
   1. Place the client on bed rest, with an elevation of the affected extremity
   2. No knee gatch or pillow is placed under the knees

H. Vein ligation and stripping: Elevate the feet above the level of heart and instruct the client to avoid leg dangling and chair sitting

VII. SENSORY SYSTEM

A. Cataract surgery
   1. Postoperatively, elevate the head of the bed 30 to 45 degrees **(semi-Fowler's to Fowler's)**
   2. Turn the client to back or the nonoperative side to prevent development of edema at the operative site

B. Retinal reattachment
   1. Obtain physician's order regarding positioning
   2. If gas is used as a tamponade to flatten the retina, the client may have to be specially positioned to make the gas bubble float into the best position
   3. Some clients must lie face down or on the side for a time period as prescribed by the physician

VIII. NEUROLOGICAL SYSTEM

A. Autonomic dysreflexia: Elevate the head of the bed to a **high Fowler's position** to assist with adequate ventilation and to help prevent hypertensive stroke

B. Cerebral aneurysm: Complete bed rest with the head of the bed elevated 30 to 45 degrees **(semi-Fowler's to Fowler's)** to prevent pressure on the aneurysm site

C. Cerebral angiography: Maintain bed rest as prescribed and keep extremity into which the contrast medium was injected straight and immobilized for approximately the length of the bed rest

D. Cerebrovascular accident (CVA)
   1. In clients with hemorrhagic strokes, the head of the bed is elevated to 30 degrees to reduce intracranial pressure (ICP) and to facilitate venous drainage
   2. For clients with ischemic strokes, the head of the bed is kept flat
   3. Maintain the head in a midline, neutral position to facilitate venous drainage from the head
   4. Avoid extreme hip and neck flexion; extreme hip flexion may increase intrathoracic pressure, whereas extreme neck flexion prohibits venous drainage from the brain

E. Craniotomy
   1. The client should NOT be positioned on the site that was operated on, especially if the bone flap has been removed, because the brain has no bony covering on the affected site
   2. Elevate the head of bed 30 to 45 degrees **(semi-Fowler's** to **Fowler's)** and maintain the head in a midline, neutral position to facilitate venous drainage from the head
   3. Avoid extreme hip and neck flexion; extreme hip flexion may increase intrathoracic pressure, whereas extreme neck flexion prohibits venous drainage from the brain

F. Laminectomy
   1. Logroll the client, by turning the client all at once, to keep the back as straight as possible
   2. When the client is out of bed, the client's back is kept straight and the client is placed in a straight-backed chair, with the feet resting comfortably on the floor

G. Intracranial pressure
   1. Elevate head of bed 30 to 45 degrees **(semi-Fowler's** to **Fowler's)** and maintain the head in a midline, neutral position to facilitate venous drainage from the head
   2. Avoid extreme hip and neck flexion; extreme hip flexion may increase intrathoracic pressure, whereas extreme neck flexion prohibits venous drainage from the brain

H. Lumbar puncture
   1. During procedure: Assist the client to the **lateral (side-lying) position** with the back bowed at the edge of the examining table, the knees flexed up to the abdomen, and the head bent so that the chin is resting on the chest
   2. After procedure: Place the client in the **dorsal recumbent** (supine) **position** for 4 to 12 hours

I. Myelogram postprocedure
   1. If water-soluble dye is used, the head of the bed should be elevated for at least 8 hours to keep the dye from irritating the cerebral meninges
   2. If an oil-based dye is used, position the client flat in bed 6 to 8 hours after the dye is removed, to prevent leakage of cerebrospinal fluid

J. Spinal cord injury
   1. Immobilize the client on a spinal backboard, with the head in a neutral position, to prevent incomplete injury from becoming complete
   2. Prevent head flexion, rotation, or extension; the head is immobilized with a firm, padded cervical collar

3. Maintain traction and alignment of head by placing the hand on either side of the head by the client's ears
4. Logroll the client; no part of the body should be twisted or turned nor should client be allowed to assume a sitting position

IX. MUSCULOSKELETAL SYSTEM

A. Hip surgery
1. Avoid extreme positions and acute flexion of the operative hip, and keep affected leg abducted
2. Place a pillow between the client's legs to maintain abduction; instruct the client not to cross the legs
3. Prevent external rotation of the operative leg by placing a trochanter roll beside the external aspect of the thigh, and elevate the heels
4. Check the physician's orders regarding elevation of the head of the bed
5. Turn the client only after checking the physician's orders, as many clients are permitted to turn to the nonoperated side and to the back only

PRACTICE QUESTIONS

1. A client returns to the nursing unit after an above-the-knee amputation of the right leg. The nurse positions the client:
   1. With the stump flat on the bed
   2. With the foot of the bed elevated
   3. In reverse Trendelenburg
   4. Prone
2. A nurse is assigned to assist in caring for a client who had an autograft placed on the lower extremity. The nurse plans to:
   1. Maintain the surgical extremity in a flat position
   2. Keep the surgical extremity covered with a blanket
   3. Maintain the client in a prone position
   4. Elevate and immobilize the surgical extremity
3. A nurse is assigned to assist in caring for a client after cardiac catheterization. The nurse plans to maintain bed rest with:
   1. Head elevation at 45 degrees
   2. Head elevation no greater than 30 degrees
   3. Bathroom privileges only
   4. In high-Fowler's position
4. A nurse is reinforcing home care instructions to a client and family regarding care after right eye cataract removal. Which of the following statements, if made by the client, would indicate an understanding of the instructions?
   1. "I will not sleep on my right side."
   2. "I will not sleep on my left side."
   3. "I will take aspirin if I have any pain."
   4. "I will not wear my glasses until my physician says it is OK."
5. After a liver biopsy, the nurse places the client in which of the following positions?
   1. Supine
   2. Prone
   3. A left side-lying position with a small pillow or folded towel under the puncture site
   4. A right side-lying position with a small pillow or folded towel under the puncture site
6. A nurse is administering a cleansing enema to a client with a fecal impaction. Before administering the enema, the nurse assists the client to which of the following positions?
   1. On the left side of the body, with the head of the bed elevated 45 degrees
   2. On the right side of the body, with the head of the bed elevated 45 degrees
   3. Left Sims' position
   4. Right Sims' position
7. A client is being prepared for a thoracentesis. The nurse assigned to care for the client assists the client to which of the following positions for the procedure?
   1. Lying in bed on the affected side, with the head of the bed elevated 45 degrees
   2. Lying in bed on the unaffected side, with the head of the bed elevated 45 degrees
   3. Prone, with the head turned to the side supported by a pillow
   4. Sims' position, with the head of the bed flat
8. A nurse assists the physician with the insertion of a Miller-Abbott tube in a client with a bowel obstruction. After insertion of the tube, the nurse assigned to care for the client assists the client to which of the following positions?
   1. Prone
   2. Supine
   3. Right side
   4. Left side
9. A client is diagnosed with thrombophlebitis. The nurse tells the client that which of the following is necessary?
   1. Bed rest, with the affected extremity in a dependent position
   2. Bed rest, with bathroom privileges only
   3. Bed rest, keeping the affected extremity flat
   4. Bed rest, with elevation of the affected extremity
10. A nurse is assisting in caring for a client after a craniotomy. The nurse plans to position the client:
   1. Prone
   2. Supine
   3. Semi-Fowler's position
   4. Dorsal recumbent

ANSWERS

1. *Answer:* 2
Rationale: During the first 24 hours after amputation, the nurse elevates the foot of bed (but not the stump itself) to reduce edema. After the first 24 hours, the bed is kept flat to prevent hip flexion contractures. The physician's postoperative orders regarding positioning are always followed.
Test-Taking Strategy: Note the key words "returns to the nursing unit after." Recalling that edema is a concern after surgery will direct you to option 2. Review postoperative positioning after amputation if you had difficulty with this question.
Level of Cognitive Ability: Application
Client Needs: Physiological Integrity
Integrated Concept/Process: Nursing Process/Implementation
Content Area: Fundamental Skills
Reference: Black J, Hawks J, Keene A: *Medical-surgical nursing: clinical management for positive outcomes*, ed 6, Philadelphia, 2001, WB Saunders, p. 1412.

2. *Answer:* 4
Rationale: Autografts placed over joints or on lower extremities are often elevated and immobilized after surgery for 3 to 7 days. This period of immobilization allows the autograft time to adhere and attach to the wound bed.
Test-Taking Strategy: Use the process of elimination. Options 2 and 3 can be eliminated first because both a blanket and a prone position can easily disrupt a graft. From the remaining options, note that option 4 specifically addresses immobilization of the extremity. Review care after an autograft if you had difficulty with this question.
Level of Cognitive Ability: Application
Client Needs: Physiological Integrity
Integrated Concept/Process: Nursing Process/Planning
Content Area: Fundamental Skills
Reference: Black J, Hawks J, Keene A: *Medical-surgical nursing: clinical management for positive outcomes*, ed 6, Philadelphia, 2001, WB Saunders, p. 1321.

3. *Answer:* 2
Rationale: After cardiac catheterization, the extremity in which the catheter was inserted is kept straight for the time period as prescribed. The client may turn from side to side. The head of the bed is not elevated higher than 30 degrees to keep the affected leg straight at the groin and prevent arterial occlusion. Bathroom privileges are not allowed in the immediate post catheterization period. In high-Fowler's position the head of the bed is elevated 90 degrees.
Test-Taking Strategy: Use the process of elimination. Recalling that a concern after this procedure is bleeding and arterial occlusion will direct you to option 2. Review care to the client after cardiac catheterization if you had difficulty with this question.
Level of Cognitive Ability: Application
Client Needs: Physiological Integrity
Integrated Concept/Process: Nursing Process/Planning
Content Area: Fundamental Skills
Reference: DeWit S: *Fundamental concepts and skills for nursing*, Philadelphia, 2001, WB Saunders, p. 409.

4. *Answer:* 1
Rationale: After cataract surgery, the client should not sleep on the side of the body that was operated on. Clients should be instructed not to take aspirin or medications containing aspirin. Acetaminophen (Tylenol) can be taken as needed for pain. Clients may wear their glasses.
Test-Taking Strategy: Use the process of elimination. If you can remember to instruct clients to stay off the operative side, this will assist you with answering questions related to cataract surgery. Review care after this type of surgery if you had difficulty with this question.
Level of Cognitive Ability: Comprehension
Client Needs: Health Promotion and Maintenance
Integrated Concept/Process: Teaching/Learning
Content Area: Fundamental Skills
Reference: DeWit S: *Fundamental concepts and skills for nursing*, Philadelphia, 2001, WB Saunders, p. 841.

5. *Answer:* 4
Rationale: After a liver biopsy, the client is assisted to assume a right side-lying position with a small pillow or folded towel under the puncture site for at least 3 hours. Options 1, 2, and 3 are incorrect positions.
Test-Taking Strategy: Knowledge regarding the anatomy of the body will assist in answering this question. Remember that the liver is on the right side of the body, and that the application of pressure on the right side will minimize the escape of blood or bile through the puncture site. Review care after a liver biopsy if you had difficulty with this question.
Level of Cognitive Ability: Application
Client Needs: Physiological Integrity
Integrated Concept/Process: Nursing Process/Implementation
Content Area: Fundamental Skills
Reference: DeWit S: *Fundamental concepts and skills for nursing*, Philadelphia, 2001, WB Saunders, p. 432.

6. *Answer:* 3
Rationale: When administering an enema, the client is placed in a left Sims' position so that the enema solution can flow by gravity in the natural direction of the colon. The head of the bed is not elevated.
Test-Taking Strategy: Recalling the anatomy of the bowel will assist in eliminating options 2 and 4. Option 1 can be eliminated next because the head of the bed should be flat during enema administration. Review the procedure for enema administration if you had difficulty with this question.
Level of Cognitive Ability: Application
Client Needs: Physiological Integrity
Integrated Concept/Process: Nursing Process/Implementation
Content Area: Fundamental Skills
Reference: DeWit S: *Fundamental concepts and skills for nursing*, Philadelphia, 2001, WB Saunders, p. 591.

7. *Answer:* 2
Rationale: To facilitate removal of fluid from the chest wall, the client is positioned sitting on the edge of bed leaning over the bedside table with the feet supported on a stool, or lying in bed on the unaffected side with the head of the bed elevated 45 degrees (Fowler's).

Test-Taking Strategy: Attempt to visualize this procedure. Option 1 can be eliminated because if the client was lying on the affected side it would be very difficult to perform the procedure. Option 4 can be eliminated because the Sims' position is primarily used for rectal enemas or irrigations. In the prone position, the client is lying on the abdomen, which is not an appropriate position for this procedure. Review this procedure if you had difficulty with this question.
Level of Cognitive Ability: Application
Client Needs: Physiological Integrity
Integrated Concept/Process: Nursing Process/Implementation
Content Area: Fundamental Skills
Reference: DeWit S: *Fundamental concepts and skills for nursing,* Philadelphia, 2001, WB Saunders, p. 409.

8. *Answer:* 3
Rationale: The Miller-Abbott tube is a mercury-weighted intestinal tube. The weight of the mercury tube carries the tube by gravity. When the tube is inserted, it is sometimes difficult to get this intestinal tube to pass through the pylorus. To accomplish this, the client is instructed to lie on the right side.
Test-Taking Strategy: Recalling the anatomy of the gastrointestinal tract and that the Miller-Abbott tube is an intestinal tube will assist in answering this question. Review care to the client with this type of tube if you had difficulty with this question.
Level of Cognitive Ability: Application
Client Needs: Physiological Integrity
Integrated Concept/Process: Nursing Process/Implementation
Content Area: Fundamental Skills
Reference: DeWit S: *Fundamental concepts and skills for nursing,* Philadelphia, 2001, WB Saunders, p. 495.

9. *Answer:* 4
Rationale: Elevation of the affected leg facilitates blood flow by the force of gravity and also decreases venous pressure that in turn relieves edema and pain. The foot of the bed is elevated and bed rest is indicated to prevent emboli and to prevent pressure fluctuations in the venous system that occurs with walking.
Test-Taking Strategy: Use the process of elimination. Recalling the pathophysiology related to the venous system will assist in directing you to option 4. Review care to the client with thrombophlebitis if you had difficulty with this question.
Level of Cognitive Ability: Application
Client Needs: Physiological Integrity
Integrated Concept/Process: Nursing Process/Implementation
Content Area: Fundamental Skills
Reference: DeWit S: *Fundamental concepts and skills for nursing,* Philadelphia, 2001, WB Saunders, p. 722.

10. *Answer:* 3
Rationale: After craniotomy, the head of the bed is elevated 30 to 45 degrees (semi-Fowler's to Fowler's) and the client's head is maintained in a midline, neutral position to facilitate venous drainage. Options 1, 2, and 4 are incorrect positions.
Test-Taking Strategy: Focus on the surgical procedure. Recalling that a goal of care after this surgery is to facilitate venous drainage will direct you to option 3. Review care to the client after craniotomy if you had difficulty with this question.
Level of Cognitive Ability: Application
Client Needs: Physiological Integrity
Integrated Concept/Process: Nursing Process/Planning
Content Area: Fundamental Skills
Reference: Black J, Hawks J, Keene A: *Medical-surgical nursing: clinical management for positive outcomes,* ed 6, Philadelphia, 2001, WB Saunders, p. 1938.

REFERENCES

Black J, Hawks J, Keene A: *Medical-surgical nursing: clinical management for positive outcomes,* ed 6, Philadelphia, 2001, WB Saunders.

DeWit S: *Fundamental concepts and skills for nursing,* Philadelphia, 2001, WB Saunders.

Hodgson B, Kizior R: *Saunders nursing drug handbook 2002,* Philadelphia, 2002, WB Saunders.

National Council of State Boards of Nursing, editors: *Test plan for the National Council Licensure Examination for Practical/Vocational Nurses,* Chicago, 2001, Author.

O'Neill P: *Caring for the older adult,* Philadelphia, 2002, WB Saunders.

Potter P, Perry A: *Fundamentals of nursing,* ed 5, St Louis, 2001, Mosby.

Care of a Client with a Tube

PYRAMID TERMS

Chest Tube Returns negative pressure to the intrapleural space; used to remove abnormal accumulations of air and fluids from the plural space.

Gastrointestinal (GI) Intubation Refers to the insertion of a tube into the stomach or intestine.

Endotracheal Tube Used to maintain a patent airway and is indicated when the client needs mechanical ventilation.

Intestinal Tubes Passed nasally and designed to enter the small intestine through the pyloric sphincter because of the weight of a small bag of mercury at the end of the tube; used to decompress the bowel or to remove intestinal contents.

Miller-Abbott Tube A double lumen tube passed nasally into the small intestine that is used to decompress the bowel or to remove intestinal contents.

Sengstaken-Blakemore Tube Triple lumen gastric tube with an inflatable esophageal balloon, an inflatable gastric balloon, and a gastric aspiration lumen; used as a treatment modality for the client with esophageal varices.

Tracheostomy Artificial opening created into the trachea to establish an airway.

PYRAMID TO SUCCESS

The Pyramid to Success focuses on the common types of tubes used in the clinical setting. NCLEX-PN is likely to address content areas related to the appropriate care of certain tubes and the immediate interventions required if a complication arises. Focus on the specific data collection points related to the specific type of tube. Review procedures for verifying correct placement of a tube and procedures for administering medications or feedings through a tube, if appropriate. Pyramid points also focus on interventions associated with complications or emergencies that may occur. The primary Integrated Concepts and Processes addressed in this chapter include Caring, Clinical Problem-Solving Process (Nursing Process), Communication and Documentation, and Teaching/Learning.

CLIENT NEEDS

Safe, Effective Care Environment

Advance directives
Advocacy related to client's concerns
Asepsis in administering care
Client rights
Consultations and referrals as prescribed
Establishing priorities
Handling infectious materials
Informed consent for invasive procedure
Standard (universal) precautions

Health Promotion and Maintenance

Client/family instructions regarding care at home
Disease prevention
Lifestyle choices
Techniques of collecting physical data

Psychosocial Integrity

Situational role changes
Support systems
Unexpected body image changes

Physiological Integrity

Administering medications through a GI tube
Assisting with emergency interventions for complications
Diagnostic tests to confirm accurate placement of tube
Laboratory values
Measures to ensure basic care and comfort
Nutrition and hydration
Potential complications associated with the tube

I. NASOGASTRIC (NG) TUBES (Figure 18-1)

A. Description
   1. Short tubes used to intubate the stomach
   2. Inserted from the nose to the stomach

B. Types of tubes
   1. Levine
      a. Single-lumen nasogastric tube
      b. Used to remove gastric contents via intermittent suction, or to provide tube feedings
   2. Salem sump
      a. Double-lumen nasogastric tube with an air vent
      b. Used for decompression with continuous suction
      c. Air vent is not to be clamped and is to be kept above the level of the stomach
      d. If leakage occurs through the air vent, instill 30 mL of air into the air vent and irrigate the main lumen with normal saline (NS)

C. Determining Placement
   1. Note that the most reliable method to determine placement is by x-ray study, which should be performed after initial placement
   2. Determine tube placement every 4 hours and before administering feedings or medications
   3. Determine tube placement by aspirating gastric contents and measuring the pH, which should be 4 or less (pH values greater than 6 indicate intestinal placement)
   4. Inserting 5 to 10 mL of air into the NG tube and listening for the rush of air over the stomach with a stethoscope is an alternative method for determining placement, but is not as reliable as an x-ray study or checking gastric pH

D. Checking residual

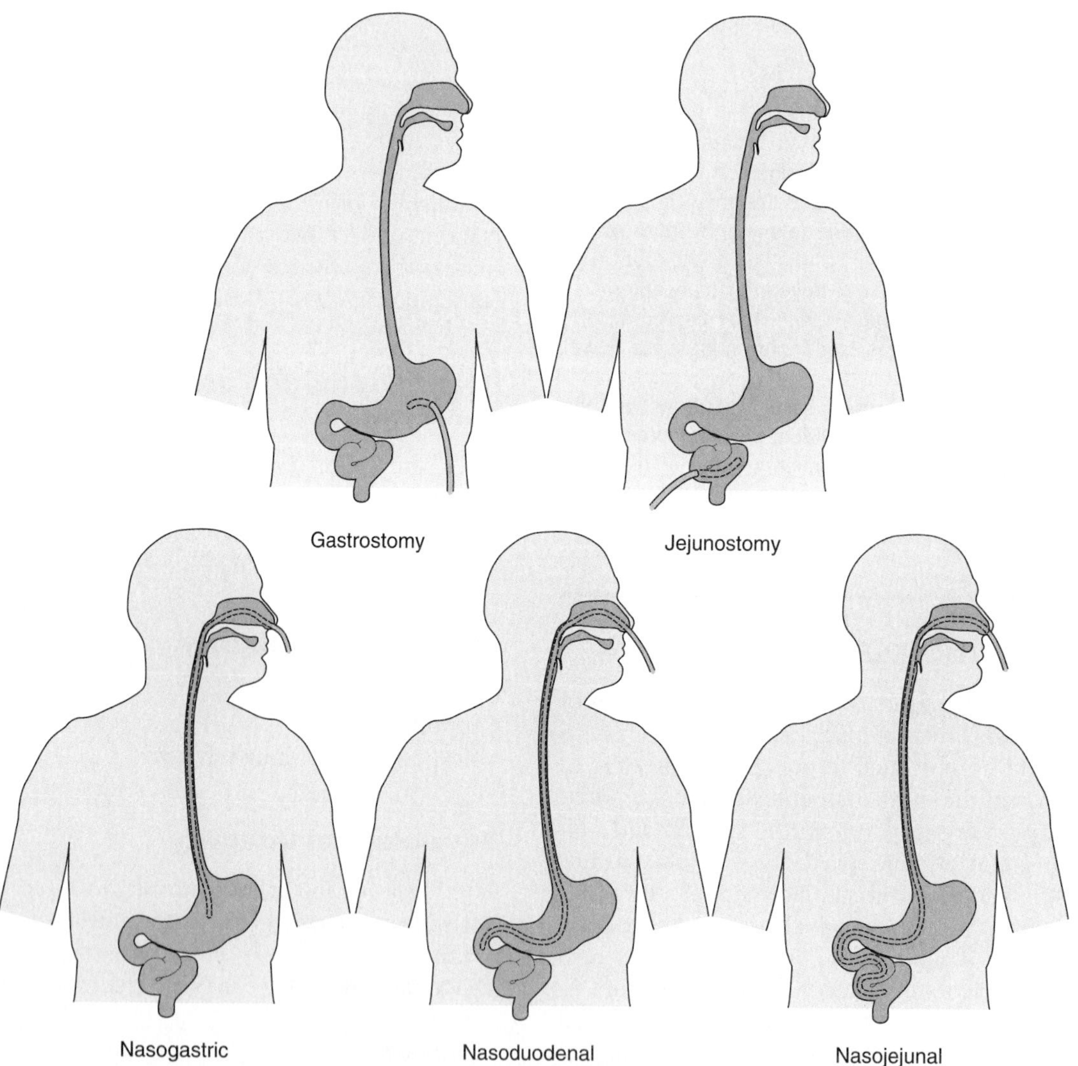

FIG. 18-1 Positioning of feeding tubes. (From Lindeman C, McAthie m: *Fundamentals of contemporary nursing practice*, Philadelphia, 1999, WB Saunders.)

1. Check residual volumes every 4 hours, before each feeding, or before giving medications
2. Aspirate all stomach contents (residual) and measure amount
3. Reinstill residual feeding to prevent excessive fluid and electrolyte losses unless the residual volume appears abnormal
4. Usually if the residual is less than 100 to 150 mL, feeding, if prescribed, is administered; if greater than 150 mL, hold the feeding

E. Irrigating
1. Check patency of tube every 4 hours
2. Check placement before irrigating
3. Gently instill 30 to 50 mL water or normal saline (depending on agency policy) with an irrigation syringe
4. Pull back on the syringe plunger to withdraw the fluid to check patency; repeat if the tube remains sluggish

F. Removal of an NG tube: Ask the client to take a deep breath and hold; remove the tube slowly and evenly over the course of 3 to 6 seconds (coil the tube around the hand as it is being removed)

II. GI TUBE FEEDINGS

A. Tubes
1. Nasogastric: nose to stomach
2. Gastrostomy: stomach
3. Jejunostomy: jejunum

B. Types of administration
1. Intermittent (bolus)
   a. Resembles normal meal feeding patterns
   b. Approximately 300 to 400 mL of formula is administered over a 30- to 60-minute period every 3 to 6 hours
2. Continuous
   a. Administered continuously for 24 hours
   b. An infusion pump regulates the flow
3. Cyclical
   a. Administered either in the daytime or nighttime for 8 to 16 hours
   b. An infusion pump regulates the flow
   c. Feedings at night allow for more freedom during the day

C. Administering feedings
1. If feedings are prescribed, x-ray confirmation should be done before initiating feedings after insertion of the tube
2. Position the client in high Fowler's and on the right side if comatose
3. Warm feeding to room temperature to prevent diarrhea and cramps
4. Aspirate all stomach contents (residual), measure amount, and return contents to stomach to prevent electrolyte imbalances (unless residual appears abnormal)
5. Usually if residual is less than 100 to 150 mL, feeding is administered; if greater than 150 mL, hold the feeding
6. Check tube placement by aspirating gastric contents and measuring the pH (should be 4 or less)
7. Check bowel sounds; feeding is held and the physician is notified if bowel sounds are absent
8. Use a feeding pump for continuous or cyclic feedings
9. For an intermittent (bolus) feeding, leave the client in a high Fowler's position for 30 minutes after feeding
10. For a continuous feeding, keep the client in a semi-Fowler's position at all times

D. Precautions
1. Change feeding container and tubing every 24 hours
2. Do not hang more solution than will be required for a 4-hour period to prevent bacterial growth
3. Check the expiration date on the formula before administering
4. Shake the formula well before inserting it into the container
5. Always check placement of the tube before feeding
6. Always check bowel sounds, and do not administer any feedings if bowel sounds are absent
7. If an obstruction occurs, try flushing with water, saline, cranberry juice, ginger ale, or cola, if not contraindicated, after checking placement
8. Add a drop of methyline blue to the feeding, particularly with clients who have **endotracheal** or tracheal tubes; suspect tracheoesophageal fistula when blue gastric contents appear in tracheal excretion; if this is noted, notify the physician immediately
9. Administer the feeding at the prescribed rate, or via gravity flow (intermittent, bolus feedings) with a 60 mL syringe with the plunger removed (Figure 18-2)
10. Gently flush with 30 to 50 mL water or normal saline (depending on agency policy) with an irrigation syringe after feeding

III. MEDICATIONS VIA NG OR GASTROSTOMY TUBE

A. Crush medications or use elixir forms of medications

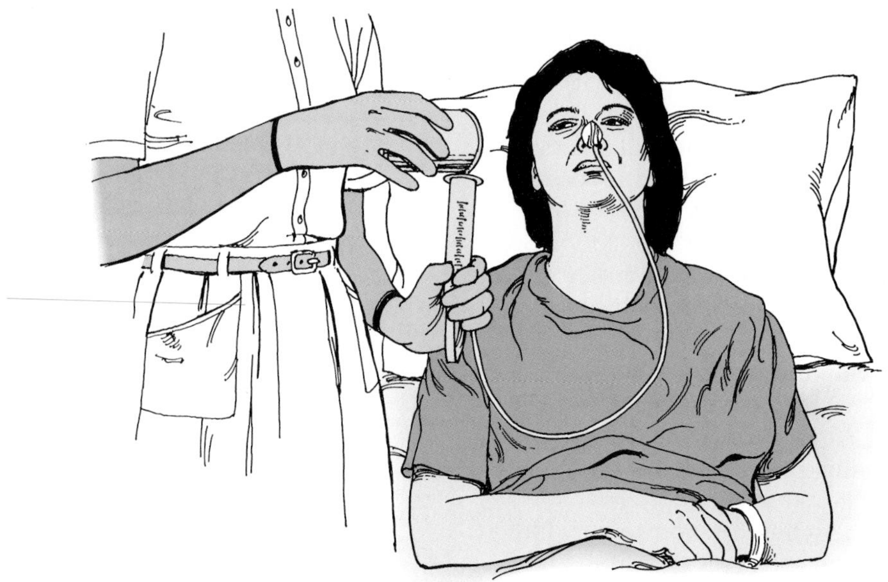

FIG. 18-2 Intermittent feeding. (From Perry A, Potter P: *Clinical nursing skills and nursing techniques*, St Louis, 2002, Mosby, p. 674.)

B. Ensure that the medication ordered can be crushed or that the capsule can be opened
C. Dissolve in 5 to 10 mL of water
D. Check placement and residual before instilling medications
E. Draw up the medication into a catheter tip syringe, clear excess air, and insert the medication into the tube
F. Flush with 30 mL of water (depending on agency policy)
G. Clamp the tube for 30 to 60 minutes (depending on the medication and agency policy)

IV. INTESTINAL TUBES

A. Description
  1. Passed nasally into the small intestine
  2. Used to decompress the bowel or to remove intestinal contents
  3. Designed to enter the small intestine through the pyloric sphincter because of the weight of a small bag of mercury at the end
B. Types of tubes
  1. Cantor and Harris tubes
    a. Single-lumen tubes with a reservoir for 5 to 10 mL of mercury located at its tip, below the level of the drainage holes
    b. Mercury is inserted before the tube is passed through the nose, making the procedure uncomfortable
    c. The Harris tube is also used for lavage and suction
  2. **Miller-Abbott Tube** (Figure 18-3)
    a. Double-lumen tube

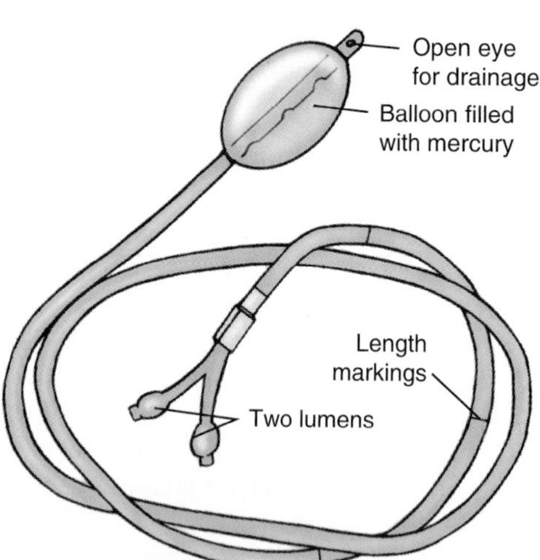

Miller-Abbott tube
A long double-lumen tube used to drain and decompress the small intestine. One lumen leads to a balloon that is filled with mercury once it is in the stomach; the second is for irrigation and drainage.

FIG. 18-3 The Miller-Abbott tube. (From Monahan F, Neighbors M: *Medical-surgical nursing*, ed 2, Philadelphia, 1998, WB Saunders.)

b. One lumen is for the instillation of mercury once the tube is in the stomach, and the other is for irrigation or drainage

C. Implementation

1. Position the client on the right side to facilitate passage of the mercury weights within the tube through the pylorus of the stomach and into the small intestine
2. Do not secure the tube to the client's face with tape until it has reached final placement (may take several hours) in the intestines
3. Allow tube to advance over several hours
4. An x-ray study is performed to verify desired placement
5. Monitor drainage from the tube
6. If the tube becomes blocked, the physician is notified; a small amount of air injected into the lumen may be prescribed to clear the tube
7. Check the abdomen and measure abdominal girth
8. When the tube is removed, dispose of the mercury in the appropriate manner as per agency policy

V. ESOPHAGEAL AND GASTRIC TUBES

A. Description

1. Used to apply pressure against esophageal veins to control bleeding
2. Not used if the client has ulceration or necrosis of the esophagus or had previous esophageal surgery

B. **Sengstaken-Blakemore Tube** (Figure 18-4)

1. Triple lumen gastric tube with an inflatable esophageal balloon, an inflatable gastric balloon, and a gastric aspiration lumen
2. The gastric balloon applies pressure at the cardioesophageal junction to decrease blood flow to esophageal varices, and directly compresses gastric varices; traction is applied to maintain the gastric balloon in place
3. The esophageal balloon directly compresses esophageal varices
4. An x-ray study of the upper abdomen and chest confirms placement
5. Gastric contents are aspirated by gastric lavage or intermittent suction via the gastric aspiration port
6. With the **Sengstaken-Blakemore tube**, a nasogastric tube is also inserted in the opposite nares to collect secretions that accumulate above the esophageal balloon

C. Implementation

1. The patency and integrity of all balloons are checked before insertion, and each lumen is labeled

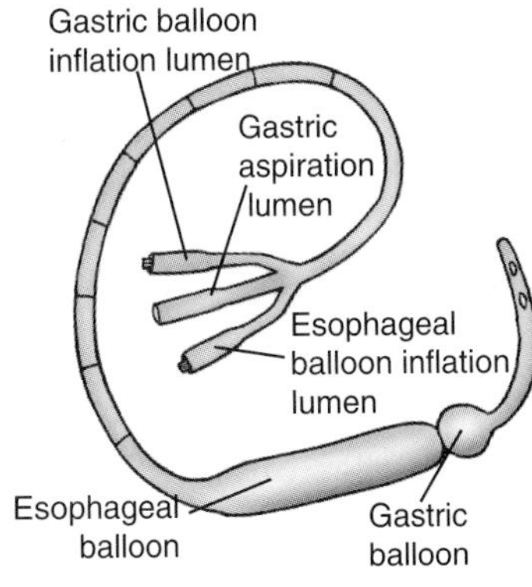

Sengstaken-Blakemore tube
A three-lumen tube. Two ports inflate an esophageal and a gastric balloon for tamponade, and the third is used for nasogastric suction. This tube does not provide esophageal suction, but a nasogastric tube may be inserted in the opposite naris or the mouth and allowed to rest on top of the esophageal balloon. Esophageal suction is then possible, reducing the risk of aspiration.

FIG. 18-4 The Sengstaken-Blakemore tube. (From Monahan F, Neighbors M: *Medical-surgical nursing*, ed 2, Philadelphia, 1998, WB Saunders.)

2. The client is placed in the left lateral or semi-Fowler's position for insertion
3. Prepare the client for an x-ray study immediately after insertion to verify placement
4. Maintain head elevation once the tube is in place
5. The balloon ports are double clamped to prevent air leaks
6. Scissors are kept at the bedside at all times
7. The client is monitored for respiratory distress; if it occurs, notify the registered nurse immediately; the tubes will be cut to deflate the balloons
8. Monitor for increased bloody drainage that may indicate persistent bleeding
9. Monitor for signs of esophageal rupture that include a drop in blood pressure, increased heart rate, back and upper abdominal pain (esophageal rupture is an emergency and must be reported immediately)

VI. URINARY AND RENAL TUBES

A. Routine urinary catheter care

1. Use gloves and wash the perineal area with warm soapy water
2. With the nondominant hand, pull back the labia or foreskin to expose the meatus (return the foreskin to its normal position)
3. Cleanse along the catheter with soap and water
4. Anchor the catheter to the thigh
5. Maintain the catheter bag below the level of the bladder

B. Ureteral and nephrostomy tubes

1. Never clamp
2. Maintain patency
3. Monitor output closely

4. Urine output of less than 30 mL per hour or a lack of output for more than 15 minutes should be reported immediately

VII. RESPIRATORY SYSTEM TUBES

A. **Endotracheal tubes**
   1. Description
      a. Used to maintain a patent airway
      b. Indicated when the client needs mechanical ventilation
   2. Orotracheal
      a. Allows use of a larger-diameter tube and reduces the work of breathing
      b. Indicated when the client has a nasal obstruction or a predisposition to epistaxis
      c. Uncomfortable and can be manipulated by the tongue, causing airway obstruction
   3. Nasotracheal
      a. Smaller-sized tube that increases resistance and increases the client's work of breathing
      b. Discouraged in clients with bleeding disorders
      c. More comfortable for the client and client is unable to manipulate with tongue
   4. Implementation
      a. Placement is confirmed by chest x-ray study (correct placement is 1 to 2 cm above the carina) and by auscultating both sides of chest while manually ventilating with a resuscitation bag
      b. The tube is secured immediately after intubation with adhesive tape
      c. Monitor the position of tube at the lip or nose
      d. Monitor skin and mucous membranes
      e. Suction only when needed
      f. Keep a resuscitation (Ambu) bag at bedside at all times
      g. Cuff inflation is maintained to create a seal and allow for complete mechanical control of respiration

B. **Tracheostomy**
   1. Description: artificial opening created in the trachea to establish an airway
   2. Single cannula tube: Has an outer but no inner cannula and is used for clients with a thick neck or on the client when a standard tube would not enter the trachea
   3. Cuffed tube: has an outer and inner cannula, obturator, and a cuff
   4. Cuffless tube
      a. Has an outer cannula, an open and a plugged inner cannula, and an obturator
      b. Used for long term, for evaluating the client's ability to breathe through the upper airway, and for the client no longer at risk for aspiration
   5. Fenestrated tube (Figure 18-5)
      a. Has an opening along the posterior wall of the outer cannula
      b. When the tube is capped, the client can breathe through the upper airway and can speak
      c. The cuff is always deflated before capping the tube
   6. Foam cuffed tube
      a. Cuff is larger than the standard cuffed tube
      b. Is filled with foam, which may apply less pressure to the tracheal mucosa
   7. Metal tube
      a. Has an outer and inner cannula and can be reused after sterilization
      b. Does not have a cuff and is most often used after a permanent **tracheostomy** or laryngectomy
   8. Implementation
      a. Monitor respirations
      b. Monitor pulse oximetry
      c. Encourage coughing and deep breathing
      d. Maintain a semi- to high-Fowler's position
      e. Monitor for bleeding, difficulty breathing, and crepitus, which are indications of hemorrhage, pneumothorax, and subcutaneous emphysema
      f. Provide respiratory treatments as prescribed
      g. Suction as needed; hyperoxygenate the client before suction
      h. If the client is allowed to eat, sit the client up for meals and for 30 minutes after meals and ensure that the cuff is inflated (if

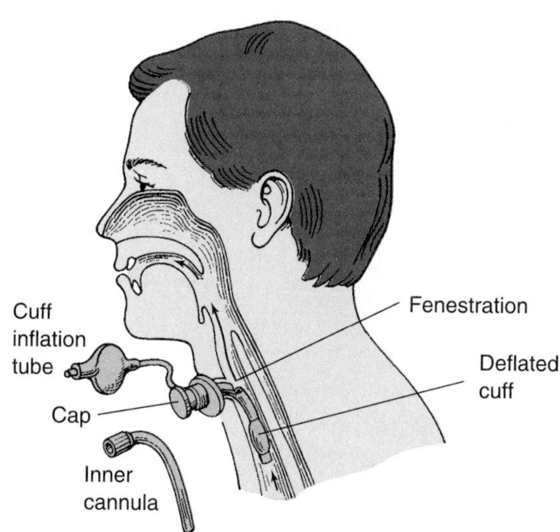

FIG. 18-5 Tracheostomy tube (fenestrated). (From Perry A, Potter P: *Clinical nursing skills and nursing techniques*, St Louis, 2002, Mosby.)

the tube is not capped) for meals and for 1 hour after meals

i. Assess the stoma and secretions for blood or purulent drainage

j. Follow the physician's orders and agency policy for cleaning the **tracheostomy** site and inner cannula; usually half-strength hydrogen peroxide is used

k. Administer humidified oxygen as prescribed because the normal humidification process is bypassed in a client with a **tracheostomy**

l. Obtain assistance in changing tracheostomy ties; after placing the new ties, cut and remove the old ties holding the tracheostomy tube in place (Figure 18-6)

m. Keep a resuscitation (Ambu) bag, obturator, clamps, and tracheotomy set at the bedside

VIII. CHEST TUBE DRAINAGE SYSTEM (Figures 18-7 and 18-8)

A. Description
   1. Returns negative pressure to the intrapleural space
   2. Used to remove abnormal accumulations of air and fluids from the plural space

B. Collection chamber
   1. Where the **chest tube** from the client connects to the system
   2. Drainage from the tube drains into and collects in a series of calibrated columns in this chamber

C. Water seal chamber
   1. The tip of the tube is underwater, allowing fluid and air to drain from the pleural space and preventing air from entering the pleural space
   2. Water oscillates (moves up as the client inhales and moves down as the client exhales)
   3. Bubbling indicates an air leak in the **chest tube** system

D. Suction control chamber
   1. Provides the suction, which can be controlled to provide negative pressure to the chest

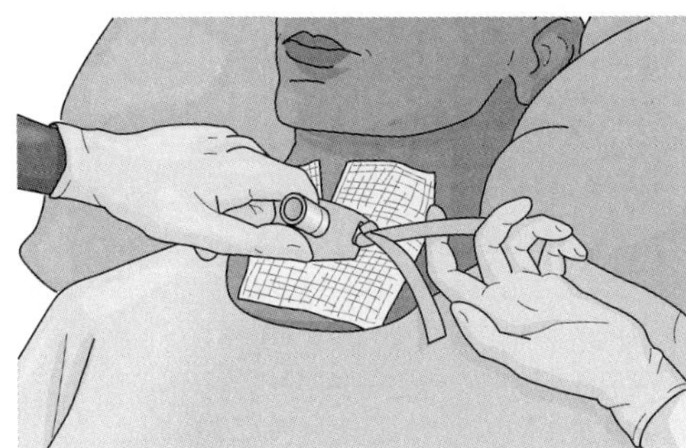

FIG. 18-6 Tracheostomy ties properly placed. (From Perry A, Potter P: *Clinical nursing skills and nursing techniques*, St Louis, 2002, Mosby.)

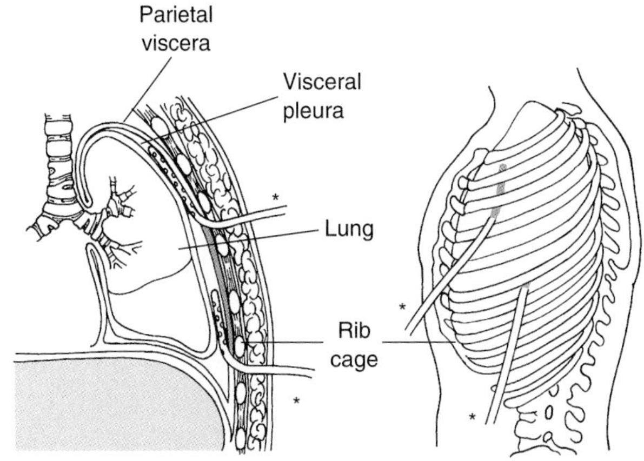

FIG. 18-7 Diagram of sites for chest tube placement (sites indicated by *). (From Perry A, Potter P: *Clinical nursing skills and nursing techniques*, St Louis, 2002, Mosby.)

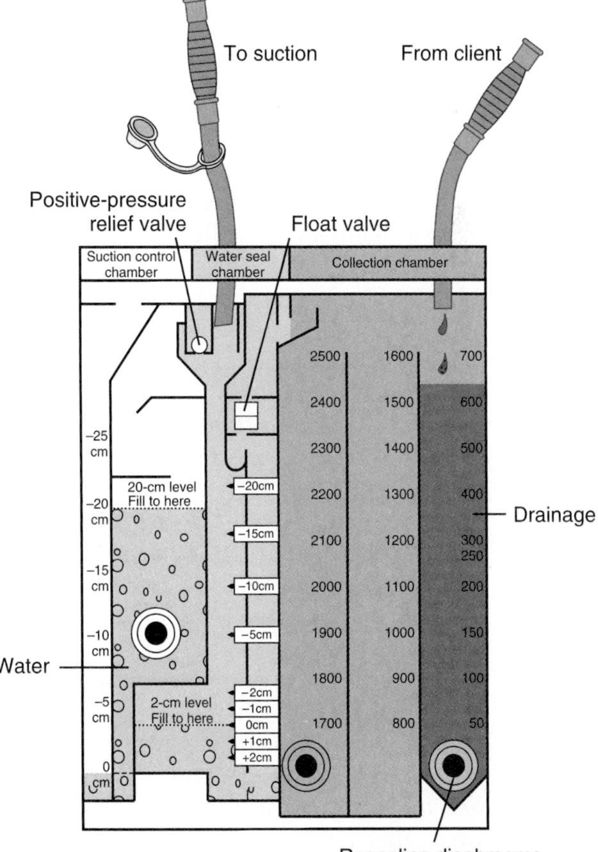

FIG. 18-8 A commonly used disposable chest drainage system combines the three bottles into a single device. (From Black J, Hawks J, Keene A: *Medical-surgical nursing*, ed 6, Philadelphia, 2001, WB Saunders. Courtesy of Deknatel, Fall River, MA.)

2. This chamber is filled with various levels of water to achieve the desired level of suction; without this control, lung tissue could be sucked into the **chest tube**
3. Gentle bubbling in this chamber indicates that there is suction, and it does not indicate that air is escaping from the pleural space

E. Dry suction system
1. Because this is a dry suction system, absence of bubbling is noted in the suction control chamber
2. A knob on the collection device is used to set the prescribed amount of suction; then the wall suction source dial is turned until a small orange floater valve appears in the window on the device (when the orange floater valve is in the window, the correct amount of suction is applied)

F. Implementation
1. An occlusive sterile dressing is maintained at the insertion site
2. A chest x-ray study determines the position of the tube and whether the lung has reexpanded
3. The apparatus and all connections must remain airtight at all times, and all connections must be taped
4. Keep the drainage system below the level of the chest, free of kinks, dependent loops, or other obstructions
5. Never pin the tubing to the bed clothes
6. Do not empty the drainage containers
7. Keep a clamp and a sterile occlusive dressing at the bedside at all times
8. Monitor the respiratory status
9. Monitor for client ease in breathing, pain, level of consciousness and orientation, and anxiety and restlessness
10. Monitor the entry site for unusual drainage and the presence of subcutaneous emphysema (crepitus)
11. Encourage coughing and deep breathing
12. Change the client's position frequently to promote drainage and ventilation
13. A **chest tube** is never clamped without a written order from the physician; also, agency policy for clamping **chest tubes** is followed
14. If the drainage system cracks or breaks, the tube is inserted into a bottle of sterile water and the registered nurse is immediately notified; the cracked or broken system is removed and replaced with a new system
15. If the **chest tube** is accidentally pulled out of the chest, pinch the skin opening together, apply an occlusive sterile dressing, cover the dressing with overlapping pieces of 2-inch tape, and immediately notify the registered nurse

G. Conditions requiring immediate attention
1. Respiratory distress
2. Persistent bubbling in the water seal chamber
3. Fluid drainage accumulating at a rate of more than 100 mL per hour
4. The presence of crepitus
5. Leakage of air around the junctions in the chest tube and drainage tube and disposable drainage device
6. Accidental removal or disconnection of the tube

H. **Chest tube** removal
1. When the **chest tube** is removed, the client is asked to take a deep breath and hold it, and the tube is removed; a dry sterile dressing, petroleum gauze dressing, or Telfa dressing (depending on physician's preference) is taped in place after removal of the **chest tube**
2. Depending on physician's preference, when the **chest tube** is removed, the client may be asked to take a deep breath, exhale, and bear down (Valsalva maneuver)
3. Medicate client 30 to 60 minutes before chest tube removal

PRACTICE QUESTIONS

1. A registered nurse is preparing to insert a nasogastric (NG) tube in a client and asks the licensed practical nurse (LPN) to obtain supplies needed for the procedure. Which of the following supplies if obtained by the LPN indicates a need for education regarding this procedure?
   1. One-half inch tape
   2. Oil-soluble lubricant
   3. A straw
   4. 50-mL catheter tip syringe
2. A nurse is checking for correct placement of a nasogastric (NG) tube. The nurse aspirates the stomach contents and checks the contents for pH. Which of the following pH values indicates correct placement of the tube?
   1. pH of 7.5
   2. pH of 7.35
   3. pH of 7.0
   4. pH of 4.0
3. A licensed practical nurse (LPN) is preparing to assist the registered nurse (RN) in removing a nasogastric (NG) tube from the client. The LPN would plan to instruct the client to do which of the following?
   1. To perform a Valsalva maneuver
   2. To take and hold a deep breath
   3. To exhale
   4. To inhale and exhale quickly

4. A nurse is preparing to administer medication through a nasogastric (NG) tube that is connected to suction. Which of the following indicates the accurate procedure related to the medication administration?
   1. Aspirate the NG tube after medication administration to maintain patency
   2. Position the client supine to assist in medication absorption
   3. Clamp the NG tube for 30 minutes after administration of the medication
   4. Change the suction setting to low intermittent suction for 30 minutes after medication administration
5. A nurse assists a physician with the insertion of a Miller-Abbott tube. After insertion of the tube, the nurse would assist the client to which of the following positions?
   1. On the right side
   2. On the left side
   3. Prone
   4. Left lateral Sims'
6. A nurse is assigned to assist in caring for a client with esophageal varices who has a Sengstaken-Blakemore tube inserted. The nurse checks the client's room to ensure that which of the following priority items is at the bedside?
   1. An irrigation set
   2. A pair of scissors
   3. A Kelly clamp
   4. An obturator
7. A nurse is inserting an indwelling urinary catheter into the urethra of a male client. As the nurse inflates the balloon, the client complains of discomfort. The most appropriate nursing action is to:
   1. Remove the syringe from the balloon; discomfort is normal and temporary
   2. Aspirate the fluid, advance the catheter farther, reinflate the balloon
   3. Aspirate the fluid, withdraw the catheter slightly, reinflate the balloon
   4. Aspirate the fluid, remove the catheter, and reinsert a new catheter
8. A nurse is inserting an indwelling urinary catheter into a male client. As the catheter is inserted into the urethra, urine begins to flow into the tubing. At this point, the nurse:
   1. Immediately inflates the balloon
   2. Withdraws the catheter approximately 1 inch and inflates the balloon
   3. Inserts the catheter until resistance is met and inflates the balloon
   4. Inserts the catheter 2.5 to 5 cm and inflates the balloon
9. A nurse is assigned to assist in caring for a client who has a chest tube. The nurse notes fluctuation of the fluid level in the water seal chamber. Based on this observation, which of the following actions would be most appropriate?
   1. Empty the drainage
   2. Encourage the client to deep breathe
   3. Continue to monitor as this is an expected finding
   4. Encourage the client to periodically hold the breath
10. A nurse is assigned to assist the physician with the removal of a chest tube. The nurse prepares to tell the client to do which of the following during removal of the chest tube?
    1. Stay very still
    2. Inhale and exhale quickly
    3. Inhale as the tube is pulled out
    4. Perform the Valsalva maneuver
11. A nurse is preparing to change the neck ties on a tracheostomy tube. To perform this procedure, the nurse would most appropriately plan to:
    1. Remove the old ties, clean the site, and then apply the new ties
    2. Obtain a second health care team member to assist
    3. Call the physician for assistance in changing the ties
    4. Call the respiratory therapy department for assistance in changing the ties
12. A nurse is preparing to begin a continuous tube feeding on a client with a nasogastric tube. The nurse positions the client:
    1. Supine
    2. Supine on the right side
    3. With the head elevated 15 degrees
    4. With the head elevated 45 degrees
13. A nurse is preparing to administer an intermittent tube feeding to a client with a nasogastric tube. The nurse checks the residual and obtains an amount of 200 mL. The nurse would:
    1. Administer the feeding
    2. Flush the tubing with 30 mL of water
    3. Hold the feeding
    4. Elevate the head of the bed to 90 degrees and administer the feeding
14. A nurse is preparing to administer a continuous tube feeding to a client with a nasogastric tube. The physician has prescribed an amount of 100 mL per hour. The nurse plans to fill the feeding bag with:
    1. 400 mL of formula
    2. 600 mL of formula
    3. 800 mL of formula
    4. Enough formula to last for 8 hours
15. A nurse is preparing to suction a client through a tracheostomy tube. The nurse avoids which of the following when performing this procedure?

1. Moistening the catheter tip in sterile saline solution before suctioning
2. Preoxygenating the client before suctioning
3. Introducing the catheter into the tracheostomy tube using a sterile gloved hand
4. Placing suction on the catheter while introducing the catheter into the tracheostomy tube

16. A nurse is suctioning a client through a tracheostomy tube. The nurse plans to apply suction during the withdrawal of the catheter for a period of time no greater than:
    1. 10 seconds
    2. 20 seconds
    3. 25 seconds
    4. 30 seconds
17. A nurse is told that an assigned client will have a fenestrated tracheostomy tube inserted. The nurse prepares the client for the procedure knowing that this type of tube:
    1. Is necessary for mechanical ventilation
    2. Enables the client to speak
    3. Prevents air from being inhaled through the tracheostomy opening
    4. Prevents the client from speaking
18. A nurse is told that an assigned client will have the chest tubes removed. In preparation for the procedure, the nurse plans to:
    1. Clamp the chest tubes
    2. Disconnect the drainage system
    3. Empty the drainage system
    4. Administer pain medication 30 minutes before the procedure
19. A nurse is assisting in caring for a client with a chest tube. The nurse understands that which of the following is an incorrect action in the care of the client?
    1. Be sure all connections remain airtight
    2. Be sure all connections are taped
    3. Pin the tubing to the bed clothes
    4. Do not allow the tubing to become kinked or obstructed by the weight of the client
20. A nurse is assigned to care for a client who has a chest tube. The nurse is told to monitor the client for subcutaneous emphysema. The nurse monitors the client for this complication by:
    1. Monitoring respirations hourly
    2. Palpating for leakage of air into the subcutaneous tissues
    3. Monitoring for pain
    4. Checking the blood pressure every 2 hours

ANSWERS

1. Answer: 2

Rationale: Water-soluble lubricant is used to lubricate 3 inches of the tube at the insertion end. An oil lubricant is not used because if the tube accidentally goes into the bronchus, pneumonia can develop. One-half inch tape is used to secure the tube after correct placement is verified. A 50-mL catheter tip syringe is used to aspirate gastric contents to confirm placement. The client will be asked to take a sip of water through a straw to help with the passage of the tube.
Test-Taking Strategy: Note the key words "indicates a need for education" in the stem of the question. Remember that water-soluble lubricant must be used to lubricate the tube. Review this procedure if you had difficulty with this question.
Level of Cognitive Ability: Comprehension
Client Needs: Physiological Integrity
Integrated Concept/Process: Teaching/Learning
Content Area: Fundamental Skills
Reference: DeWit S: *Fundamental concepts and skills for nursing*, Philadelphia, 2001, WB Saunders, p. 496.

2. *Answer:* 4

Rationale: If the NG tube is in the stomach, the pH of the contents will be acidic. Option 1 indicates an alkaline pH. Option 2 indicates a neutral pH. Option 3 indicates a slightly acidic pH.
Test-Taking Strategy: Use the process of elimination. Recalling that gastric contents are acidic will easily direct you to option 4. Review the procedure for checking NG tube placement if you had difficulty with this question.
Level of Cognitive Ability: Comprehension
Client Needs: Physiological Integrity
Integrated Concept/Process: Nursing Process/Evaluation
Content Area: Fundamental Skills
Reference: DeWit S: *Fundamental concepts and skills for nursing*, Philadelphia, 2001, WB Saunders, p. 497.

3. *Answer:* 2

Rationale: When the nurse removes an NG tube, the client is instructed to take and hold a deep breath. This will close the epiglottis and the airway will be temporarily obstructed during the tube removal. This allows for easy withdrawal through the esophagus into the nose. The nurse removes the tube with one very smooth continuous pull.
Test-Taking Strategy: Use the process of elimination and focus on the issue, removing an NG tube. Visualize the procedure as a guide considering what each client action identified in the options would produce. Review the procedure for removing an NG tube if you had difficulty with this question.
Level of Cognitive Ability: Application
Client Needs: Physiological Integrity
Integrated Concept/Process: Nursing Process/Implementation

Content Area: Fundamental Skills
Reference: DeWit S: *Fundamental concepts and skills for nursing,* Philadelphia, 2001, WB Saunders, p. 499.

4. *Answer:* 3
Rationale: If a client has an NG tube connected to suction, the nurse should wait up to 30 minutes before reconnecting the tube to the suction apparatus to allow adequate time for medication absorption. Aspirating the NG tube will remove the medication just administered. Low intermittent suction will also remove the medication just administered. The client should not be placed in the supine position because of the risk for aspiration.
Test-Taking Strategy: Use the process of elimination. Eliminate options 1 and 4 first because these actions are similar and will produce the same effect. Recalling that the client should not be placed in a supine position will assist in eliminating option 2. Review the procedure for administering medications through an NG tube if you had difficulty with this question.
Level of Cognitive Ability: Application
Client Needs: Physiological Integrity
Integrated Concept/Process: Nursing Process/Implementation
Content Area: Fundamental Skills
Reference: DeWit S: *Fundamental concepts and skills for nursing,* Philadelphia, 2001, WB Saunders, p. 499.

5. *Answer:* 1
Rationale: A Miller-Abbott tube is an intestinal tube that has a double lumen, one for a mercury balloon, and the other for suction or drainage. After insertion of the tube, the tube is allowed to advance over several hours. The client is positioned on the right side to facilitate passage through the pylorus of the stomach and into the small intestine.
Test-Taking Strategy: Use the process of elimination. Eliminate options 2 and 4 because they are similar. From the remaining options, recalling the purpose of this tube and the anatomy of the body will assist in directing you to option 1. Review care to the client with a Miller-Abbott tube if you had difficulty with this question.
Level of Cognitive Ability: Application
Client Needs: Physiological Integrity
Integrated Concept/Process: Nursing Process/Implementation
Content Area: Fundamental Skills
Reference: Black J, Hawks J, Keene A: *Medical-surgical nursing: clinical management for positive outcomes,* ed 6, Philadelphia, 2001, WB Saunders, p. 706.

6. *Answer:* 2
Rationale: When the client has a Sengstaken-Blakemore tube, a pair of scissors must be kept at the client's bedside at all times. The client needs to be observed for sudden respiratory distress that occurs if the gastric balloon ruptures and the entire tube moves upward. If this occurs, the registered nurse (RN) is notified immediately and the balloon lumens will be cut. An obturator and a Kelly clamp are kept at the bedside of a client with a tracheostomy. An irrigation set may be kept at the bedside, but it is not the priority item.
Test-Taking Strategy: Use knowledge regarding the structure, function, and placement of a Sengstaken-Blakemore tube to answer this question. Note the key word "priority" in the stem of the question. This should assist in eliminating options 1, 3, and 4. Review care of a client with a Sengstaken-Blakemore tube if you had difficulty with this question.
Level of Cognitive Ability: Application
Client Needs: Safe, Effective Care Environment
Integrated Concept/Process: Nursing Process/Implementation
Content Area: Fundamental Skills
Reference: Black J, Hawks J, Keene A: *Medical-surgical nursing: clinical management for positive outcomes,* ed 6, Philadelphia, 2001, WB Saunders, p. 1243.

7. *Answer:* 2
Rationale: If the balloon is malpositioned in the urethra, inflating the balloon could produce trauma and pain will occur. If pain occurs, the fluid should be aspirated and the catheter inserted a little farther to provide sufficient space to inflate the balloon. The catheter's balloon is behind the opening at the insertion tip. Inserting the catheter the extra distance will ensure that the balloon is inflated inside the bladder and not in the urethra. There is no need to remove the catheter and reinsert a new one. Pain when the balloon is inflated is not normal or temporary.
Test-Taking Strategy: Visualize the procedure to answer the question. Option 1 can be eliminated since discomfort is neither normal nor temporary when caused by the balloon being inflated. It is not necessary to withdraw the catheter and reinsert a new catheter. Option 3 will not properly position the balloon in the bladder for safe balloon inflation. Review the procedure for inserting a urinary catheter if you had difficulty with this question.
Level of Cognitive Ability: Application
Client Needs: Physiological Integrity
Integrated Concept/Process: Nursing Process/Implementation
Content Area: Fundamental Skills
Reference: DeWit S: *Fundamental concepts and skills for nursing,* Philadelphia, 2001, WB Saunders, p. 559.

8. *Answer:* 4
Rationale: The catheter's balloon is behind the opening at the insertion tip. The catheter is inserted 2.5 to 5 cm after urine begins to flow to provide sufficient space to inflate the balloon. Inserting the catheter the extra distance will ensure that the balloon is inflated inside the bladder and not in the urethra. Inflating the balloon in the urethra could produce trauma.
Test-Taking Strategy: Visualize the proper procedure for inserting an indwelling urinary catheter to assist you in answering this question. Note the key words "urine begins to flow." Options 2 and 3 can easily be eliminated. Eliminate option 1 next because of the word "immediately." Review the procedure for bladder catheterization if you had difficulty with this question.
Level of Cognitive Ability: Application
Client Needs: Physiological Integrity
Integrated Concept/Process: Nursing Process/Implementation
Content Area: Fundamental Skills
Reference: DeWit S: *Fundamental concepts and skills for nursing,* Philadelphia, 2001, WB Saunders, p. 560.

9. *Answer:* 3
Rationale: The presence of fluctuation of the fluid level in the water seal chamber indicates a patent drainage system. With normal breathing, the water level rises with inspiration and falls with expiration. The apparatus and all connections must remain airtight at all times and the drainage is never emptied. Encouraging the client to deep breathe is unrelated to this observation. The client is not told to hold the breath.
Test-Taking Strategy: Focusing on the issue of the question, fluctuation of the fluid level in the water seal chamber, will assist in eliminating options 1, 2, and 4. Review expected and unexpected findings when caring for a client with a chest tube if you had difficulty with this question.
Level of Cognitive Ability: Application
Client Needs: Physiological Integrity
Integrated Concept/Process: Nursing Process/Implementation
Content Area: Fundamental Skills
Reference: DeWit S: *Fundamental concepts and skills for nursing,* Philadelphia, 2001, WB Saunders, p. 532.

10. *Answer:* 4
Rationale: When the chest tube is removed, the client is asked to perform the Valsalva maneuver (take a deep breath, exhale, and bear down), the tube is quickly withdrawn, and an airtight dressing is taped in place. An alternative instruction is to ask the client to take a deep breath and hold the breath while the tube is removed. Options 1, 2, and 3 are incorrect client instructions.
Test-Taking Strategy: Use the process of elimination. Visualize the procedure and the client instructions in each option as you answer the question. If you had difficulty with this question, review the procedure for removal of a chest tube.
Level of Cognitive Ability: Application
Client Needs: Physiological Integrity
Integrated Concept/Process: Nursing Process/Implementation
Content Area: Fundamental Skills
Reference: DeWit S: *Fundamental concepts and skills for nursing,* Philadelphia, 2001, WB Saunders, p. 536.

11. *Answer:* 2
Rationale: It is best to have two people help change the ties at the tracheostomy. The movement of the tube can easily cause the client to cough and expel the tube from the stoma. Removing the old ties, cleaning the site, then applying the new ties is not appropriate because if the client coughs, the tube could be expelled. This procedure is a nursing procedure; therefore it is not appropriate to call the physician. The respiratory therapist can assist in changing the ties, but it is not necessary to specifically call the therapist for the procedure.
Test-Taking Strategy: Visualize this procedure. Eliminate option 1 knowing that this action can create a risk of the tube being expelled if the client coughs. Eliminate option 3 next knowing that this is a nursing procedure. For the remaining options, select option 2 because it is the most global option. Review care to the client with a tracheostomy if you had difficulty with this question.
Level of Cognitive Ability: Application
Client Needs: Safe, Effective Care Environment
Integrated Concept/Process: Nursing Process/Planning
Content Area: Fundamental Skills
Reference: DeWit S: *Fundamental concepts and skills for nursing,* Philadelphia, 2001, WB Saunders, p. 537.

12. *Answer:* 4
Rationale: When a tube feeding is administered, the head of the bed is elevated 30 to 45 degrees to allow gravity to help the flow of formula, to prevent reflux, and to prevent aspiration. Options 1, 2, and 3 are inappropriate positions during a tube feeding.
Test-Taking Strategy: Use the process of elimination. Eliminate options 1 and 2 first because they are similar. Recalling the risks associated with administering a tube feeding will easily direct you to option 4. Review the procedure for administering tube feedings if you had difficulty with this question.
Level of Cognitive Ability: Application
Client Needs: Physiological Integrity
Integrated Concept/Process: Nursing Process/Implementation
Content Area: Fundamental Skills
Reference: DeWit S: *Fundamental concepts and skills for nursing,* Philadelphia, 2001, WB Saunders, p. 506.

13. *Answer:* 3
Rationale: When more than 150 mL of residual formula is obtained, the feeding is held and the physician is notified because it is an indication that the feeding is not being absorbed. Elevating the head of the bed to 90 degrees and flushing the tubing are not appropriate actions.
Test-Taking Strategy: Use the process of elimination. Eliminate options 1 and 4 first because they are similar. Recalling that the feeding is held when more that 150 mL of residual is obtained will easily direct you to option 3. Review this procedure if you had difficulty with this question.
Level of Cognitive Ability: Application
Client Needs: Physiological Integrity
Integrated Concept/Process: Nursing Process/Implementation
Content Area: Fundamental Skills
Reference: DeWit S: *Fundamental concepts and skills for nursing,* Philadelphia, 2001, WB Saunders, p. 501.

14. *Answer:* 1
Rationale: Feeding can be hung at room temperature for a period of 4 hours. If 100 mL per hour is prescribed, the nurse would fill the feeding bag with a maximum amount of 400 mL. Feeding hung longer than 4 hours at room temperature creates the risk of bacterial invasion in the formula.
Test-Taking Strategy: Use the process of elimination. Eliminate options 3 and 4 first because they are similar. From the remaining options, recalling that feeding can be hung at room temperature for 4 hours will easily direct you to option 1. Review the procedure for administering tube feedings if you had difficulty with this question.
Level of Cognitive Ability: Application
Client Needs: Safe, Effective Care Environment
Integrated Concept/Process: Nursing Process/Planning
Content Area: Fundamental Skills
Reference: DeWit S: *Fundamental concepts and skills for nursing,* Philadelphia, 2001, WB Saunders, p. 502.

15. *Answer:* 4
Rationale: Suction is not placed on the catheter when the catheter is introduced into the tracheostomy tube. Suction

draws out oxygen and placing suction on the catheter at this time could traumatize tracheal tissue. Options 1, 2, and 3 are appropriate components of the plan of care for suctioning.
Test-Taking Strategy: Use the process of elimination. Note the key word "avoids." Attempt to visualize the procedure recalling the risks associated with this procedure. Review the procedure for suctioning if you had difficulty with this question.
Level of Cognitive Ability: Application
Client Needs: Physiological Integrity
Integrated Concept/Process: Nursing Process/Implementation
Content Area: Fundamental Skills
Reference: DeWit S: *Fundamental concepts and skills for nursing,* Philadelphia, 2001, WB Saunders, p. 537.

16. *Answer:* 1
Rationale: During suctioning, the nurse would apply suction during the withdrawal of the catheter for a period of 5 to 10 seconds. Suction applied longer than this time can cause hypoxia in the client.
Test-Taking Strategy: Attempt to visualize this procedure and recall the complications associated with suctioning. Note the key words "no greater than." It is best to select the option that identifies the least amount of time. Review the procedure for suctioning if you had difficulty with this question.
Level of Cognitive Ability: Application
Client Needs: Physiological Integrity
Integrated Concept/Process: Nursing Process/Planning
Content Area: Adult Health/Respiratory
Reference: DeWit S: *Fundamental concepts and skills for nursing,* Philadelphia, 2001, WB Saunders, p. 537.

17. *Answer:* 2
Rationale: Fenestrated tubes have a small opening in the outer cannula that allows some air to escape through the larynx. This type of tube enables the client to speak.
Test-Taking Strategy: Knowledge regarding the design and purpose of a fenestrated tracheostomy tube will easily direct you to option 2. Review the purpose of a fenestrated tube if you had difficulty with this question.
Level of Cognitive Ability: Comprehension
Client Needs: Physiological Integrity
Integrated Concept/Process: Nursing Process/Planning
Content Area: Fundamental Skills
Reference: DeWit S: *Fundamental concepts and skills for nursing,* Philadelphia, 2001, WB Saunders, p. 536.

18. *Answer:* 4
Rationale: Removal of chest tubes can be uncomfortable for a client. The nurse should medicate the client 30 to 60 minutes before the chest tube is removed. Options 1, 2, and 3 are inappropriate actions and would not be performed by the nurse.
Test-Taking Strategy: Use the process of elimination and Maslow's Hierarchy of Needs theory to answer the question. Option 4 is the only client-centered nursing action and this option addresses physiological integrity. Review care to the client in preparation for chest tube removal if you had difficulty with this question.
Level of Cognitive Ability: Application
Client Needs: Physiological Integrity
Integrated Concept/Process: Nursing Process/Implementation
Content Area: Fundamental Skills
Reference: DeWit S: *Fundamental concepts and skills for nursing,* Philadelphia, 2001, WB Saunders, p. 542.

19. *Answer:* 3
Rationale: Chest tube tubing is never pinned to bed clothing because it presents the risk of accidental dislodgement of the tube when the client moves. Options 1, 2, and 4 are appropriate interventions in the plan of care for a client with a chest tube.
Test-Taking Strategy: Note the key word "inappropriate" in the stem of the question. Use the process of elimination recalling the complications associated with a chest tube. Review care to the client with a chest tube if you had difficulty with this question.
Level of Cognitive Ability: Application
Client Needs: Physiological Integrity
Integrated Concept/Process: Nursing Process/Implementation
Content Area: Fundamental Skills
Reference: DeWit S: *Fundamental concepts and skills for nursing,* Philadelphia, 2001, WB Saunders, p. 536.

20. *Answer:* 2
Rationale: Subcutaneous emphysema is also known as crepitus. It presents as a "puffed-up" appearance caused by leakage of air into the subcutaneous tissues. It is monitored by palpating and feels like bubble-wrap when palpated. Although options 1, 3, and 4 may be a component of the plan of care for a client with a chest tube, these actions will not identify subcutaneous emphysema.
Test-Taking Strategy: Use the process of elimination. Note the similarity between the words "subcutaneous emphysema" in the question and "subcutaneous tissues" in the correct option. Review this complication if you had difficulty with this question.
Level of Cognitive Ability: Application
Client Needs: Physiological Integrity
Integrated Concept/Process: Nursing Process/Data Collection
Content Area: Fundamental Skills
Reference: Black J, Hawks J, Keene A: *Medical-surgical nursing: clinical management for positive outcomes,* ed 6, Philadelphia, 2001, WB Saunders, p. 1655.

REFERENCES

Black J, Hawks J, Keene A: *Medical-surgical nursing: Clinical management for positive outcomes,* ed 6, Philadelphia, 2001, WB Saunders.

DeWit S: *Fundamental concepts and skills for nursing,* Philadelphia, 2001, WB Saunders.

National Council of State Boards of Nursing, editors: *Test plan for the National Council Licensure Examination for Practical/Vocational Nurses,* Chicago, 2001, Author.

Potter P, Perry A: *Fundamentals of nursing,* ed 5, St Louis, 2001, Mosby.

UNIT V

Growth and Development Across the Life Span

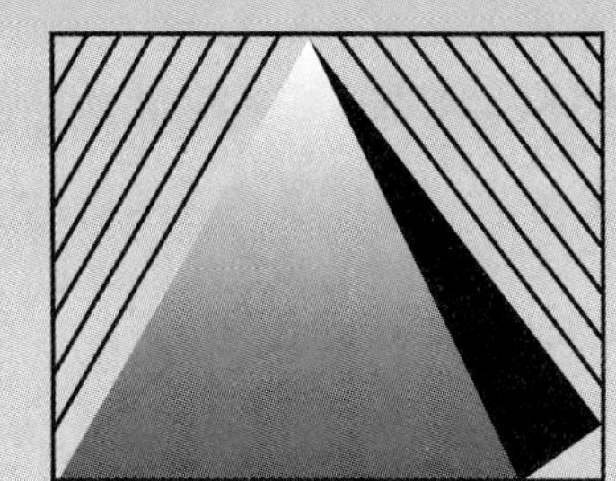

PYRAMID TERMS

Conscious Includes all experiences that are within an individual's awareness and that the individual is able to control.

Ego One's "sense of self"; provides such functions as problem solving, mobilization of defense mechanisms, reality testing, and the capability of functioning independently. The mediator between the id and the superego.

Id Source of all primitive drives and instincts and is thought of as a reservoir of all psychic energy.

Subconscious Often called the preconscious and includes experiences, thoughts, feelings, or desires that might not be in the immediate awareness but can be recalled to consciousness; helps repress unpleasant thoughts or feelings.

Superego Representative of the values, ideals, and moral standards of society.

Unconscious Memories, feelings, thoughts, or wishes are repressed and are not available to the conscious mind.

PYRAMID TO SUCCESS

Normal growth and development proceeds in an orderly, systematic, and predictable pattern. It provides a basis for identifying an individual's abilities. Understanding the path of growth and development across the life span assists the nurse in identifying appropriate expected human behavior. The Pyramid to Success focuses on the basic concepts of Sigmund Freud's theory of psychosexual development, Jean Piaget's theory of cognitive development, Erik Erikson's psychosocial theory, and Lawrence Kohlberg's theory of moral development. The Integrated Concepts and Processes addressed in this unit include Caring, Clinical Problem-Solving Process (Nursing Process), Communication and Documentation, Cultural Awareness, Self-Care, and Teaching/Learning.

CLIENT NEEDS

Safe, Effective Care Environment

Advocacy
Caring
Client rights
Confidentiality
Consultations and referrals
Establishing priorities
Ethical practice and legal responsibilities

Health Promotion and Maintenance

Aging process
Communication
Developmental stages and transitions
Family planning
Health care beliefs
Health promotion programs
Lifestyle choices

Psychosocial Integrity

Communication
Coping mechanisms
Cultural heritage
Mental health concepts
Religious and spiritual influences on health
Support systems

Physiological Integrity

Basic care and comfort
Health care preferences

Incorporating interventions compatible with client's cultural, religious, and health care beliefs, education level, and language

Practices or restrictions related to procedures and treatments

Providing care using a nonjudgmental approach

REFERENCES

DeWit S: *Fundamental concepts and skills for nursing,* Philadelphia, 2001, WB Saunders.

Hill S, Bauer B: *Mental health nursing,* Philadelphia, 2000, WB Saunders.

Hill S, Howlett H: *Success in practical/vocational nursing: from student to Leader,* ed 4, Philadelphia, 2001, WB Saunders.

Lewis S, Heitkemper M, Dirksen S: *Medical-surgical nursing: assessment and management of clinical problems,* ed 5, St Louis, 2000, Mosby.

Lowdermilk D, Perry S, Bobak I: *Maternity and women's health care,* ed 7, St Louis, 2000, Mosby.

McKinney E et al: *Maternal-child nursing,* Philadelphia, 2000, WB Saunders.

National Council of State Boards of Nursing, editors: *Test plan for the National Council Licensure Examination for Practical/Vocational Nurses,* Chicago, 2001, Author.

Potter P, Perry A: *Fundamentals of nursing,* ed 5, St Louis, 2001, Mosby.

Riley J: *Communication in nursing,* ed 4, St Louis, 2000, Mosby.

Schulte E, Price D, Gwin J: *Thompson's pediatric nursing,* ed 8, Philadelphia, 2001, WB Saunders.

Varcarolis E: *Foundations of psychiatric-mental health nursing,* ed 4, Philadelphia, 2002, WB Saunders.

Theories of Growth and Development

I. PSYCHOSOCIAL DEVELOPMENT AND ERIK ERIKSON

A. The theory
  1. Describes the human life cycle as a series of eight **ego** developmental stages spanning from birth to death
  2. Each stage presents a psychosocial crisis the goal of which is to integrate physical, maturation, and societal demands
  3. Focuses on psychosocial tasks that are accomplished throughout the life cycle
  4. **Ego** development is influenced by family, social, and developmental factors

B. Psychosocial development
  1. A lifelong series of conflicts affected by social and cultural factors
  2. Each conflict must be resolved for the child or adult to progress emotionally
  3. Unsuccessful resolution leaves the individual emotionally handicapped

C. Stages of psychosocial development (Table 19-1)

II. COGNITIVE DEVELOPMENT AND JEAN PIAGET

A. The theory: defines cognitive acts as ways in which the mind organizes and adapts to its environment

B. Stages of cognitive development
  1. Sensorimotor stage
    a. 0 to 2 years
    b. Development proceeds from reflex activity to imagining and solving problems through the senses and movement
  2. Preoperational stage
    a. 2 to 7 years
    b. Learning to think in terms of the past, present, and future
    c. The child moves from knowing the world through sensation and movement to prelogical thinking and finding solutions to problems
  3. Concrete operational
    a. 7 to 11 years
    b. Able to classify, order, and sort facts
    c. The child moves from prelogical thought to solving concrete problems through logic
  4. Formal operations
    a. 11 years to adulthood
    b. Able to think abstractly and logically
    c. Logical thinking is expanded to include solving abstract and concrete problems

III. MORAL DEVELOPMENT AND LAWRENCE KOHLBERG

A. Moral development
  1. A complicated process involving the acceptance of the values and rules of society in a way that shapes behavior
  2. Classified in a series of levels and behaviors

B. Levels of moral development (Box 19-1)

IV. PSYCHOSEXUAL DEVELOPMENT AND SIGMUND FREUD

A. Components of the theory
  1. Levels of awareness
  2. Agencies of the mind (**id**, **ego**, **superego**)
  3. Concept of anxiety and defense mechanisms
  4. Psychosexual stages of development

B. Levels of awareness
  1. **Conscious** level of awareness

TABLE 19-1

Erik Erikson's Stages of Psychosocial Development

Age	Psychosocial Crisis	Task
Infancy (0-18 months)	Trust vs. mistrust	Attachment to the mother
Resolution of Crisis: Trust in people; faith and hope about the environment and the future		
Unsuccessful Resolution of Crisis: General difficulties relating to people effectively; suspicion; trust-fear conflict, fear of the future		
Age	**Psychosocial Crisis**	**Task**
Early childhood (18 months to 3 years)	Autonomy vs. shame and doubt	Gaining some basic control over self and environment
Resolution of Crisis: Sense of self-control and adequacy; willpower		
Unsuccessful Resolution of Crisis: Independence-fear conflict; severe feelings of self-doubt		
Age	**Psychosocial Crisis**	**Task**
Late childhood (3-6 years)	Initiative vs. guilt	Becoming purposeful and directive
Resolution of Crisis: Ability to initiate one's own activities; sense of purpose		
Unsuccessful Resolution of Crisis: Aggression-fear conflict; sense of inadequacy or guilt		
Age	**Psychosocial Crisis**	**Task**
School Age (6-12 years)	Industry vs. inferiority	Developing social, physical and school skills
Resolution of Crisis: Competence; ability to learn and work		
Unsuccessful Resolution of Crisis: Sense of inferiority; difficulty learning and working		
Age	**Psychosocial Crisis**	**Task**
Adolescence (12-20 years)	Identity vs. role confusion	Developing sense of identity
Resolution of Crisis: Sense of personal identity		
Unsuccessful Resolution of Crisis: Confusion about who one is; identity submerged in relationships or group memberships		
Age	**Psychosocial Crisis**	**Task**
Early adulthood (20-35 years)	Intimacy vs. isolation	Establishing intimate bonds of love and friendship
Resolution of Crisis: Ability to love deeply and commit oneself		
Unsuccessful Resolution of Crisis: Emotional isolation, egocentricity		
Age	**Psychosocial Crisis**	**Task**
Middle adulthood (35-65 years)	Generativity vs. stagnation	Fulfilling life goals that involve family, career, and society
Resolution of Crisis: Ability to give and care for others		
Unsuccessful Resolution of Crisis: Self-absorption; inability to grow as a person		
Age	**Psychosocial Crisis**	**Task**
Later years (65 years to death)	Integrity vs. despair	Looking back over one's life and accepting its meaning
Resolution of Crisis: Sense of integrity and fulfillment		
Unsuccessful Resolution of Crisis: Dissatisfaction with life		

a. Includes all experiences that are within an individual's awareness and that the individual is able to control
b. Includes all information that is easily remembered and immediately available to an individual
2. Preconscious level of awareness
a. Called the **subconscious**
b. Includes experiences, thoughts, feelings, or desires that might not be in the immediate awareness but can be recalled to consciousness
c. The **subconscious** can help repress unpleasant thoughts or feelings and can examine and censor certain wishes and thinking
3. **Unconscious** level of awareness
a. Memories, feelings, thoughts, or wishes are repressed and are not available to the **conscious** mind
b. These repressed memories, thoughts, or feelings, if made prematurely **conscious**, can cause anxiety

C. Agencies of the mind
1. **Id**, **ego**, and **superego**
a. The three systems of personality
b. In a mature and well-adjusted personality, they work together as a team under the leadership of the **ego**
2. The **id**
a. Source of all drives

BOX 19-1

Moral Development and Lawrence Kohlberg's

LEVEL ONE: PRECONVENTIONAL

Stage 0 (0-2 years)

The infant has no awareness of right or wrong.

Stage 1 (2-3 years)

At this stage children cannot reason as mature members of society.

Children view the world in a selfish way, with no real understanding of right or wrong.

The child obeys rules and demonstrates acceptable behavior to avoid punishment, to avoid displeasing those who are in power, and because he or she fears punishment from a superior force such as a parent.

A toddler typically is at the first substage of the preconventional stage; the toddler makes judgments on the basis of avoiding punishment or obtaining a reward.

Physical punishment and withholding privileges tend to give the toddler a negative view of morals.

Withdrawing love and affection as punishment leads to feelings of guilt in the toddler.

Appropriate discipline includes providing simple explanations of why certain behaviors are unacceptable, praising appropriate behavior, and using distractions when the toddler is headed for danger.

Stage 2 (4-7 years)

The child conforms to rules to obtain rewards or have favors returned.

A preschooler is in the preconventional stage of moral development.

In this stage, conscience emerges and the emphasis is on external control.

LEVEL TWO: CONVENTIONAL

The child conforms to rules to please others.

The child has increased awareness of others' feelings.

A concern for social order begins to emerge.

A child views good behavior as that which those in authority will approve.

If the behavior is not acceptable, the child feels guilty.

Stage 3 (7-10 years)

Conformity occurs to avoid disapproval or dislike by others.

This stage involves living up to what is expected by individuals close to you or what individuals generally expect of others in their role as son, brother, friend, and so on.

Stage 4 (10-12 years)

Child has more concern with society as a whole.

Emphasis is on obeying laws to maintain social order.

The school-aged child is at the conventional level of the role conformity stage and has an increased desire to please others.

The child observes and to some extent internalizes the standards of others.

The child wants to be considered "good" by those individuals whose opinions matter to the child.

LEVEL THREE: POSTCONVENTIONAL

The individual focuses on individual rights and principles of conscience.

The focus is a concern regarding what is best for all.

Stage 5

Being aware that people hold a variety of values and opinions and that most values and rules are relative to the group.

The adolescent in this stage gives as well as takes, and does not expect to get something without paying for it.

Stage 6

This stage involves following self-chosen ethical principles.

The development of the postconventional level of morality occurs in the adolescent at about age 13, marked by the development of an individual conscience and a defined set of moral values.

The adolescent can now acknowledge a conflict between two socially accepted standards and try to decide between them.

b. Is present at birth
c. Includes genetic inheritance, reflexes, capacities to respond, instincts, basic drives, needs, and wishes that motivate an individual
d. The **id** does not tolerate uncomfortable states and seeks to discharge the tension and return to a more comfortable constant level of energy
e. The **id** acts immediately in an impulsive, irrational way and pays no attention to the consequences of its actions, and therefore often behaves in ways harmful to self and others
f. The "primary" process is a psychological activity in which the **id** attempts to reduce tension
g. The "primary" process can include hallucinating or forming an image of the object that will satisfy its needs and remove the tension
h. The "primary" process by itself is not capable of reducing tension; therefore a "secondary" psychological process must develop if the individual is to survive; when this occurs, the structure of the second system of the personality, the **ego**, begins to take form

3. The **ego**
   a. The functions of the **ego** include reality testing and problem solving
   b. Begins its development during the fourth or fifth month of life
   c. The **ego** merges out of the **id** and acts as an intermediary between the **id** and the external world
   d. Emerges because the needs, wishes, and demands of the **id** require appropriate exchanges with the outside world of reality
   e. Reality testing is a function of the **ego**, and the **ego** uses realistic thinking
4. The **superego**
   a. A necessary part of socialization that develops during the phallic stage during 3 to 5 years of age
   b. It develops from the interactions with one's parents during the extended period of childhood dependency
   c. It includes the internalization of the values, ideals, and moral standards of society
   d. The **superego** consists of the conscience and the **ego** ideal
   e. The conscience refers to the capacity for self-evaluation and criticism; when moral codes are violated, the conscience punishes the individual by instilling guilt
   f. The **superego** strives for perfection rather than pleasure and represents the ideal rather than the real

D. Anxiety and defense mechanisms
   1. The **ego** develops defenses or defense mechanisms to fight off anxiety
   2. Defense mechanisms operate on an **unconscious** level, except for suppression, so the individual is not aware of their operation
   3. Defense mechanisms deny, falsify, or distort reality to make it less threatening
   4. An individual cannot survive without defense mechanisms; however, if they become too extreme in distorting reality, then interference in healthy adjustment and personal growth may occur

E. Psychosexual stages of development (Box 19-2)
   1. Each stage is associated with a particular conflict that must be resolved before the child can move successfully to the next stage
   2. Experiences during the early stages determine an individual's adjustment patterns and the personality traits that an individual has as an adult

PRACTICE QUESTIONS

1. A nurse is reinforcing instructions to a new mother regarding the psychosocial development of the infant. Using Erikson's psychosocial development theory, the nurse would instruct the mother to:
   1. Allow the infant to signal a need
   2. Anticipate all of the needs of the infant
   3. Avoid the infant during the first 10 minutes of crying
   4. Attend to the infant immediately when crying
2. A mother of a 3-year-old tells the nurse that the child is constantly rebelling and having temper tantrums. The most appropriate instruction to the mother is to:
   1. Punish the child every time the child says "no," to change the behavior
   2. Allow the behavior, because this is normal at this age period
   3. Set limits on the child's behavior
   4. Ignore the child when this behavior occurs
3. A nurse employed in long-term care facility is caring for a 70-year-old woman. The client reminisces about past life experiences in a positive way. The nurse interprets this behavior as:
   1. A normal psychosocial response
   2. Requiring a psychiatric consultation
   3. A mental status alteration
   4. A sensory deficit requiring social activities
4. A mother of an 8-year-old child tells the nurse that she is concerned about the child because the child seems to be more attentive to friends than anything

BOX 19-2

Freud's Psychosexual Stages of Development

ORAL STAGE (0-1 YEARS)

During this stage the infant is concerned with his or her own gratification.

The infant is all id and striving for immediate gratification of needs.

When the infant experiences gratification of basic needs, a sense of trust and security begins.

The ego begins to emerge as the infant begins to see self as separate from the mother; this marks the beginning of the development of a sense of self.

ANAL STAGE (1-3 YEARS)

Toilet training occurs during this period, and the child gains pleasure both from the elimination of the feces and from their retention.

The conflict of this stage is between those demands from society and the parents and the sensations of pleasure associated with the anus.

The child begins to gain a sense of control over instinctive drives and learns to delay immediate gratification to gain a future goal.

PHALLIC STAGE (3-6 YEARS)

The child experiences both pleasurable and conflicting feelings associated with the genital organs.

The pleasures of masturbation and the fantasy life of children set the stage for the Oedipus Complex.

The child's unconscious sexual attraction to and wish to possess the parent of the opposite sex, the hostility and desire to remove the parent of the same sex, and the subsequent guilt for these wishes are the conflicts the child faces.

The conflicts are resolved when the child identifies with the parent of the same sex.

The emergence of the superego is both the solution to and the result of these intense impulses.

LATENCY STAGE (6-12 YEARS)

A tapering off of conscious biological and sexual urges.

The sexual impulses are channeled and elevated into a more culturally accepted level of activity.

Growth of ego functions and the ability to care about and relate to others outside the home are the tasks of this stage of development.

GENITAL STAGE (12 YEARS AND BEYOND)

Emerges at adolescence with the onset of puberty when the genital organs mature.

The individual gains gratification from his or her own body.

During this stage, the individual develops satisfying sexual and emotional relationships with members of the opposite sex.

The individual plans life goals and gains a strong sense of personal identity.

else. The most appropriate nursing response would be which of the following?

1. "You need to be concerned."
2. "You need to monitor the child's behavior closely."
3. "At this age, the child is developing his or her own personality."
4. "You need to provide more praise to the child to stop this behavior."

5. A mother of a 4-year-old child tells the nurse that she is concerned because the child has been masturbating. The most appropriate response by the nurse is which of the following?
   1. "The child is very young to begin this behavior and should be brought to the mental health clinic."
   2. "This is not normal behavior and the child should be brought to the mental health clinic."
   3. "This is a normal behavior at this age."
   4. "Children usually begin this behavior at age 8 years."
6. A nursing instructor asks a nursing student to present a clinical conference to peers regarding Freud's psychosexual stages of development, specifically the anal stage. The nursing student prepares for the conference knowing that which of the following most appropriately relates to this stage of development?
   1. This stage is associated with toilet training
   2. This stage is associated with pleasurable and conflicting feelings about the genital organs
   3. This stage is characterized by a tapering-off of conscious biological and sexual urges
   4. This stage is characterized by the gratification of self
7. A mother of a 5-year-old child tells the nurse that the child scolds the floor or a table if the child hurts herself on the object. According to Piaget's theory of cognitive development, this behavior is identified as:
   1. Object permanence
   2. Egocentric speech
   3. Animism
   4. Global organization
8. A nursing instructor asks a nursing student to describe the formal operations stage of Piaget's cognitive developmental theory. The most appropriate response by the nursing student is:
   1. "The child has the ability to think abstractly."

2. "The child develops logical thought patterns."
3. "The child has difficulty separating fantasy from reality."
4. "The child begins to understand the environment."

9. According to Kohlberg's theory of moral development, in the preconventional level, moral development is thought to be motivated by which of the following?
1. The parents' behavior
2. Peer pressure
3. Social pressures
4. Punishment and reward

10. A nursing instructor asks a nursing student about Kohlberg's theory of moral development. The instructor determines that the student needs to further research this theory if the student states that a component of the theory includes which of the following?
1. Moral development progresses in relationship to cognitive development
2. Individuals move through all six stages in a sequential fashion
3. It provides a framework for understanding how individuals determine a moral code to guide their behavior
4. A person's ability to make moral judgments develops over a period of time

ANSWERS

1. *Answer:* 1
Rationale: According to Erikson, the caregiver should not try to anticipate the infant's needs at all times but must allow the infant to signal needs. If an infant is not allowed to signal a need, he or she will not learn how to control the environment. Erikson believed that a delayed or prolonged response to an infant's signal would inhibit the development of trust and lead to mistrust of others.
Test-Taking Strategy: Use the process of elimination. Eliminate options 3 and 4 first because of the words "avoid" and "immediately." Additionally, option 2 can be eliminated because of the absolute word "all." Review Erikson's psychosocial development theory if you had difficulty with this question.
Level of Cognitive Ability: Application
Client Needs: Psychosocial Integrity
Integrated Concept/Process: Teaching/Learning
Content Area: Child Health
Reference: Schulte E, Price D, Gwin J: *Thompson's pediatric nursing*, ed 8, Philadelphia, 2001, WB Saunders, p. 204.

2. *Answer:* 3
Rationale: According to Erikson, the child focuses on independence between ages 1 and 3 years. Gaining independence often means that the child has to rebel against the parents' wishes. Saying things like "no" or "mine" and having temper tantrums are common during this period of development. Being consistent and setting limits on the child's behavior are necessary elements.
Test-Taking Strategy: Use the process of elimination. Options 2 and 4 can be eliminated first because they are similar. Eliminate option 1 next because this action is likely to produce a negative response during this normal developmental pattern. Review psychosocial development of the toddler according to Erikson if you had difficulty with this question.
Level of Cognitive Ability: Application
Client Needs: Psychosocial Integrity
Integrated Concept/Process: Nursing Process/Implementation
Content Area: Child Health
Reference: Schulte E, Price D, Gwin J: *Thompson's pediatric nursing*, ed 8, Philadelphia, 2001, WB Saunders, p. 162.

3. *Answer:* 1
Rationale: According to Erikson, the later years are 65 years to death. The adult reminisces about past life experiences, viewing them in a positive way. The adult needs to feel good about accomplishments, see successes in life, and feel that he or she has made a contribution to society.
Test-Taking Strategy: Use knowledge regarding Erikson's theory of psychosocial development of late adulthood to answer the question. Note the similarity in options 2, 3, and 4. This will direct you to option 1. Review psychosocial development if you had difficulty with this question.
Level of Cognitive Ability: Comprehension
Client Needs: Psychosocial Integrity
Integrated Concept/Process: Nursing Process/Data Collection
Content Area: Fundamental Skills
Reference: DeWit S: *Fundamental concepts and skills for nursing*, Philadelphia, 2001, WB Saunders, p. 133.

4. *Answer:* 3
Rationale: According to Erikson, during middle childhood (ages 7 to 12 years), the child begins to move for support toward peers and friends and away from the parents. The child also begins to develop special interests that reflect his or her own developing personality instead of the parents.
Test-Taking Strategy: Use Erikson's psychosocial development theory related to middle childhood to assist in eliminating options 1 and 2. Eliminate option 4 next because although praising the child for accomplishments is important at this age, the behavior that the child is exhibiting is normal. Review Erikson's psychosocial development theory if you had difficulty with this question.

Level of Cognitive Ability: Application
Client Needs: Psychosocial Integrity
Integrated Concept/Process: Caring
Content Area: Child Health
Reference: Schulte E, Price D, Gwin J: *Thompson's pediatric nursing*, ed 8, Philadelphia, 2001, WB Saunders, p. 214.

5. *Answer:* 3
Rationale: According to Freud's psychosexual stages of development, between the ages of 3 and 6 years the child is in the phallic stage. At this time, the child devotes much energy to examining their genitalia, masturbating, and expressing interest in sexual concerns.
Test-Taking Strategy: Use the process of elimination. Eliminate options 1 and 2 because they are similar. From the remaining options, use Freud's psychosexual stages of development to direct you to option 3. If you had difficulty with this question, review Freud's psychosocial stages of development.
Level of Cognitive Ability: Application
Client Needs: Psychosocial Integrity
Integrated Concept/Process: Nursing Process/Implementation
Content Area: Child Health
Reference: Schulte E, Price D, Gwin J: *Thompson's pediatric nursing*, ed 8, Philadelphia, 2001, WB Saunders, p. 214.

6. *Answer:* 1
Rationale: Generally, toilet training occurs during this period. According to Freud, the child gains pleasure both from the elimination of feces and from its retention. Option 2 relates to the phallic stage. Option 3 relates to the latency period. Option 4 relates to the oral stage.
Test-Taking Strategy: Use the process of elimination. Note the relationship between the words "anal" in the question and "toilet training" in the correct option. If you had difficulty with this question, review Freud's psychosocial stages of development.
Level of Cognitive Ability: Comprehension
Client Needs: Psychosocial Integrity
Integrated Concept/Process: Nursing Process/Planning
Content Area: Child Health
Reference: Schulte E, Price D, Gwin J: *Thompson's pediatric nursing*, ed 8, Philadelphia, 2001, WB Saunders, p.161.

7. *Answer:* 3
Rationale: Animism means that all inanimate objects are given living meaning. Object permanence, the realization that something out of sight still exists, occurs in the later stages of the sensorimotor stage of development. Egocentric speech occurs when the child talks just for fun and cannot see another's point of view. Global organization means that if any part of an object or situation changes, the whole thing has changed. Options 2 and 4 occur during the preoperational stage.
Test-Taking Strategy: Use the process of elimination. Attempt to make a relationship with the behavior identified in the question and the correct option. This will direct you to option 3. If you had difficulty with this question, review the concepts of Piaget's theory of cognitive development.
Level of Cognitive Ability: Comprehension
Client Needs: Psychosocial Integrity
Integrated Concept/Process: Nursing Process/Data Collection
Content Area: Child Health
Reference: Schulte E, Price D, Gwin J: *Thompson's pediatric nursing*, ed 8, Philadelphia, 2001, WB Saunders, p. 203.

8. *Answer:* 1
Rationale: In the formal operation stage, the child has the ability to think abstractly and solve hypotheses. Option 2 identifies the concrete operations stage. Option 3 identifies the preoperational stage. Option 4 identifies the sensorimotor stage.
Test-Taking Strategy: Knowledge regarding the characteristics of Piaget's cognitive developmental theory is required to answer this question. If you had difficulty with this question, review these concepts.
Level of Cognitive Ability: Comprehension
Client Needs: Psychosocial Integrity
Integrated Concept/Process: Teaching/Learning
Content Area: Child Health
Reference: Schulte E, Price D, Gwin J: *Thompson's pediatric nursing*, ed 8, Philadelphia, 2001, WB Saunders, p. 204.

9. *Answer:* 4
Rationale: In the preconventional stage, morals are thought to be motivated by punishment and reward. If the child is obedient and is not punished, then he or she is being moral. The child sees actions as either good or bad. If the child's actions are good, the child is praised. If the child's actions are bad, the child is punished.
Test-Taking Strategy: Use the process of elimination. Eliminate options 2 and 3 because they are similar. Knowledge that the preconventional stage occurs between the ages of 2 and 7 years will assist in directing you to option 4. If you had difficulty with this question, review Kohlberg's theory of moral development.
Level of Cognitive Ability: Comprehension
Client Needs: Psychosocial Integrity
Integrated Concept/Process: Nursing Process/Implementation
Content Area: Child Health
Reference: Schulte E, Price D, Gwin J: *Thompson's pediatric nursing*, ed 8, Philadelphia, 2001, WB Saunders, p. 161.

10. *Answer:* 2
Rationale: Kohlberg's theory states that individuals move through the six stages of development in a sequential fashion but that not everyone reaches stages 5 and 6 in their development of personal morality. Options 1, 3, and 4 are correct statements regarding Kohlberg's theory.
Test-Taking Strategy: Note the key words "needs to further research." Also, note the absolute word "all" in option 2. If you had difficulty with this question, review Kohlberg's theory.
Level of Cognitive Ability: Comprehension
Client Needs: Psychosocial Integrity
Integrated Concept/Process: Teaching/Learning
Content Area: Fundamental Skills
Reference: Schulte E, Price D, Gwin J: *Thompson's pediatric nursing*, ed 8, Philadelphia, 2001, WB Saunders, p. 204.

REFERENCES

DeWit, S: *Fundamental concepts and skills for nursing,* Philadelphia, 2001, WB Saunders.

Hill S, Bauer B: *Mental health nursing,* Philadelphia, 2000, WB Saunders.

Potter P, Perry A: *Fundamentals of nursing,* ed 5, St Louis, 2001, Mosby.

Schulte E, Price D, Gwin J: *Thompson's pediatric nursing,* ed 8, Philadelphia, 2001, WB Saunders.

Varcarolis E: *Foundations of psychiatric-mental health nursing,* ed 4, Philadelphia, 2002, WB Saunders.

UNIT VI

Maternity Nursing

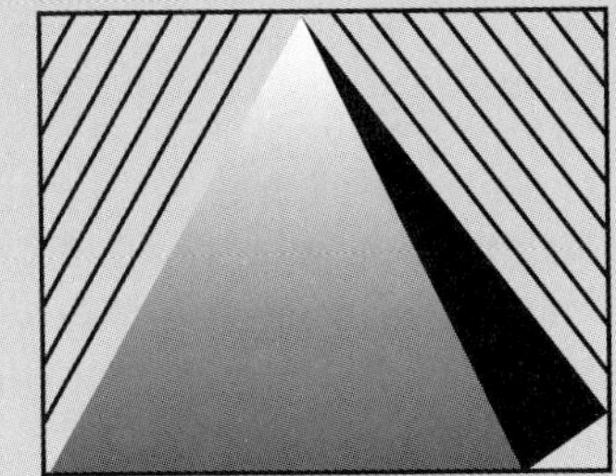

PYRAMID TERMS

Amniotic Fluid Fluid that surrounds and protects the fetus; consists of 500 to 1000 mL in amount by the end of pregnancy. The fetus floats in the amniotic fluid, which serves as a cushion against injury from sudden blows or movements and helps maintain a constant body temperature for the fetus.

Ballottement Rebounding of the fetus against the examiner's finger on palpation. When the cervix is tapped, the fetus floats upward in the amniotic fluid. A rebound is felt by the examiner when the fetus falls back.

Chadwick's Sign Bluish coloration of the mucous membranes of cervix, vagina, and vulva.

Delivery Actual event of birth; the expulsion or extraction of the neonate and fetal membranes at birth.

Fertilization Takes place when sperm and ovum unite. Occurs within 12 hours of ovulation and within 2 to 3 days of insemination, the average duration of viability for the ovum and sperm.

Goodell's Sign Softening of the cervix; occurs at the beginning of the second month of gestation and is a probable sign of pregnancy.

Gravida A pregnant woman; called gravida I (primigravida) during the first pregnancy, gravida II (secundigravida) during the second, and so on.

Hegar's Sign Compressibility and softening of the lower uterine segment; occurs at about week six of gestation; a probable sign of pregnancy.

Implantation Zygote propels toward the uterus and implants in the uterine wall 6 to 8 days after ovulation.

Infant A baby born alive; also from 28 days of age until the first birthday.

Labor Coordinated sequence of involuntary uterine contractions resulting in effacement and dilation of cervix, followed by expulsion of the products of conception.

Lochia Discharge from the uterus that consists of blood from the vessels of the placental site and debris from the decidua.

Nagele's Rule Determines the estimated date of confinement (EDC). Add 7 days to the first day of last menstrual period (LMP). Subtract 3 months and add 1 year.

Neonate A human offspring from the time of birth to the 28th day of life; also called a newborn.

Newborn A human offspring from the time of birth to the 28th day of life; also called a neonate.

Parity The number of pregnancies that have been carried to viability.

Placenta Provides for the exchange of nutrients and waste products between the fetus and mother. Develops by the third month of gestation; also called afterbirth.

Quickening First perception of fetal movement appearing usually in the 16th to 18th week of pregnancy.

PYRAMID TO SUCCESS

The Pyramid to Success focuses on the physiological and psychosocial aspects related to the experience of pregnancy. Pyramid points begin with instructing the pregnant client in measures that will promote a healthy environment for both the mother and fetus. Focus on the importance of antenatal follow-up care, nutrition, and the interventions for common discomforts that occur during pregnancy. Review the purpose of the commonly prescribed diagnostic tests and procedures in the antenatal period. Focus on disorders that can occur during pregnancy, particularly pregnancy-induced hypertension (PIH) and diabetes. Review the labor and delivery process and the immediate interventions when the mother or fetal status is compromised, such as prolapsed cord or altered fetal heart rate. Review fetal effects from the mother with acquired immunodeficiency syndrome or the substance abuse mother. Focus on the normal expectations of the postpartum period and the complications that can occur. Pyramid points also focus on the normal physical assessment findings in the newborn and the early identification of disorders in the newborn. The Integrated Concepts and Processes addressed in this unit include Caring, Clinical Problem-Solving Process (Nursing Process), Communication and Documentation, Cultural Awareness, Self-Care, and Teaching/Learning.

CLIENT NEEDS

Safe, Effective Care Environment

Asepsis
Confidentiality
Continuity of care
Establishing priorities
Handling infectious materials
Informed consent for procedures
Parent rights
Standard (Universal) precautions when delivering care

Health Promotion and Maintenance

Antenatal, intrapartum, and postpartum care
Expected body image changes
Family interaction patterns
Family planning
Growth and development and health care screening
Health and wellness
Lifestyle choices
Reproduction and human sexuality

Psychosocial Integrity

Communication
Coping mechanisms
Cultural and religious influences regarding birth and motherhood
Role changes
Support systems

Physiological Integrity

Alterations in body systems
Commonly prescribed diagnostic tests and procedures
Interventions for unexpected events during the pregnancy
Labor and delivery process
Normal expectations during pregnancy
Nutrition
Physiological changes that occur during pregnancy
Risk identification during pregnancy

REFERENCES

Burroughs A, Leifer G: *Maternity nursing,* ed 8, Philadelphia, 2002, WB Saunders.

Hill S, Bauer B: *Mental health nursing,* Philadelphia, 2000, WB Saunders.

Hill S, Howlett H: *Success in practical/vocational nursing: from student to leader,* ed 4, Philadelphia, 2001, WB Saunders.

Lowdermilk D, Perry S, Bobak I: *Maternity and women's health care,* ed 7, St Louis, 2000, Mosby.

McKinney E et al: *Maternal-child nursing,* Philadelphia, 2000, WB Saunders.

National Council of State Boards of Nursing, editors: *Test plan for the National Council Licensure Examination for Practical/Vocational Nurses,* Chicago, 2001, Author.

Riley J: *Communication in nursing,* ed 4, St Louis, 2000, Mosby.

Schulte E, Price D, Gwin J: *Thompson's pediatric nursing,* ed 8, Philadelphia, 2001, WB Saunders.

Varcarolis E: *Foundations of psychiatric-mental health nursing,* ed 4, Philadelphia, 2002, WB Saunders.

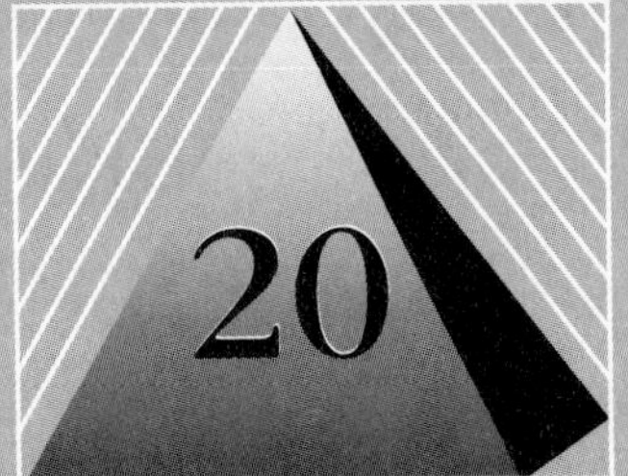

Female Reproductive System

I. ORGANS

A. Ovaries
  1. Formation and expulsion of ova
  2. Secretes estrogen and progesterone

B. Fallopian tubes
  1. Muscular tubes (oviducts) approximate to the ovaries and connect to the uterus
  2. Propels the ova from the ovaries to the uterus

C. Uterus
  1. Organ in which the fetus develops
  2. Organ from which menstruation occurs

D. Cervix
  1. Internal os opens into the body of the uterine cavity
  2. Cervical canal is located between the internal os and external os
  3. External os opens into the vagina

E. Vagina
  1. Passageway for menstrual blood
  2. Organ of copulation
  3. Passageway for fetus

II. MENSTRUAL CYCLE (Table 20-1)

A. Ovarian hormones
  1. Includes the follicle-stimulating hormone (FSH) and luteinizing hormone (LH)
  2. Released by the anterior pituitary gland
  3. Produce changes in the ovaries
  4. Secretion of ovarian hormones lead to changes in the endometrium
  5. Menstrual cycle: the regularly recurring physiological changes in the endometrium that culminate in its shedding; may vary in length, with the average length of approximately 28 days

B. Ovarian changes
  1. Preovulatory phase
  2. Luteal phase

C. Uterine changes
  1. Menstrual phase
  2. Proliferative phase
  3. Secretory phase

III. FEMALE PELVIS AND MEASUREMENTS

A. True pelvis
  1. Lies below pelvic brim
  2. Consists of the pelvic inlet, mid pelvis, and pelvic outlet

B. False pelvis
  1. Shallow portion above the pelvic brim
  2. Supports the abdominal viscera

C. Types of pelvis (Figure 20-1)
  1. Gynecoid
    a. Normal female pelvis
    b. Transversely rounded or blunt
    c. Most favorable for successful **labor** and birth
  2. Android
    a. Wedge-shaped or angulated
    b. Seen in males
    c. Not favorable for **labor**
    d. Narrow pelvic planes can cause slow descent and midpelvis arrest
  3. Anthropoid
    a. Oval-shaped
    b. The outlet is adequate, with a normal or moderately narrow pubic arch
  4. Platypelloid
    a. Flat shaped with an oval inlet

TABLE 20-1

Menstrual Cycle

OVARIAN CHANGES

Preovulatory Phase	Luteal Phase
The hypothalamus releases gonadotropin-releasing hormone (GnRH) through the portal system to the anterior pituitary system. Secretion of FSH by the anterior lobe of the pituitary gland stimulates growth of follicles. Most follicles die, leaving one to mature into a large graafian follicle. Estrogen produced by the follicle stimulates increased secretions of LH by the anterior lobe of the pituitary gland. The follicle ruptures and releases an ovum into the peritoneal cavity.	Begins with ovulation. Body temperature drops and then rises by 0.5° F to 1° F around the time of ovulation. Corpus luteum is formed from follicle cells that remain in the ovary after ovulation. Corpus luteum secretes estrogen and progesterone during remaining 14 days of cycle. Corpus luteum degenerates if the ovum is not fertilized, and secretion of estrogen and progesterone declines. Estrogen and progesterone inhibit secretions of FSH and LH. Once corpus luteum degenerates, pituitary secretion of estrogen and progesterone decreases and ovarian cycle begins again.

UTERINE CHANGES

Menstrual Phase	Proliferative Phase	Secretory Phase
Consists of 4 to 6 days of bleeding as endometrium breaks down owing to the decreased amount of estrogen and progesterone. FSH rises, enabling the beginning of a new cycle.	Estrogen stimulates proliferation and growth of endometrium. This phase lasts about 9 days. As estrogen increases, it suppresses secretion of FSH and increases secretion of LH. LH stimulates ovulation and the development of the corpus luteum. Ovulation occurs between day 12 and day 16. Estrogen is high and progesterone is low.	This phase lasts about 12 days. Follows ovulation. Initiated in response to the increase of LH. Graafian follicle replaced by corpus luteum. Corpus luteum secretes progesterone and estrogen. Progesterone prepares endometrium for pregnancy should a fertilized ovum be implanted.

b. Transverse diameter is wide but anteroposterior diameter is short, making the outlet inadequate

D. Pelvic inlet diameters
1. Anteroposterior diameters
   a. Diagonal conjugate: distance from the lower margin of the symphysis pubis to the sacral promontory; is at least 11.5 cm
   b. True conjugate or conjugate vera: distance from the upper margin of the symphysis pubis to the sacral promontory; is 1.5 cm less than diagonal conjugate
   c. Obstetric conjugate: the smallest front-to-back distance through which the fetal head must pass in moving through the pelvic inlet; is 1.5 to 2 cm less than diagonal conjugate
2. Transverse diameter: the largest of the pelvic inlet diameters; is located at right angles to the true conjugate and is about 13.5 cm
3. Oblique (diagonal) diameter: cannot be measured clinically

E. Pelvic cavity (midplane/midpelvis) diameters
   1. Anteroposterior diameter: 12 cm
   2. Transverse diameter: 10.5 cm

F. Pelvic outlet diameters
   1. Bi-ischial or intertuberous diameter: 11 cm
   2. Anteroposterior diameter: 11.5 cm
   3. Posterior sagittal diameter: 7.5 cm

IV. FERTILIZATION AND IMPLANTATION

A. **Fertilization**
   1. Occurs in the upper region of the fallopian tubes
   2. Occurs within 12 hours of ovulation and within 2 to 3 days of insemination, the average duration of viability for the ovum and sperm
   3. Takes place when sperm and ovum unite
   4. Once **fertilized**, the membrane of the ovum undergoes changes that prevent the entry of other sperm
   5. Each reproductive cell carries 23 chromosomes
   6. Sperm carry an X and Y chromosome; XY: male, XX: female

B. **Implantation**
   1. Zygote propelled toward uterus
   2. Implants 6 to 8 days after ovulation
   3. Blastocyst secretes chorionic gonadotropin to ensure that the corpus luteum remains viable and secretes estrogen and progesterone for the first 2 to 3 months of gestation

V. FETAL DEVELOPMENT (Table 20-2)

A. Embryonic stage: from conception to 12 weeks

B. Fetal period: from third month to gestation

VI. FETAL ENVIRONMENT

A. Amnion
   1. Encloses the amniotic cavity
   2. Inner membrane that forms about the second week of embryonic development
   3. Forms a fluid-filled sac that surrounds the embryo and later the fetus

B. Chorion
   1. Outer membrane
   2. Becomes vascularized and forms the fetal part of the **placenta**

C. **Amniotic fluid**
   1. Consists of 500 to 1000 mL by the end of pregnancy

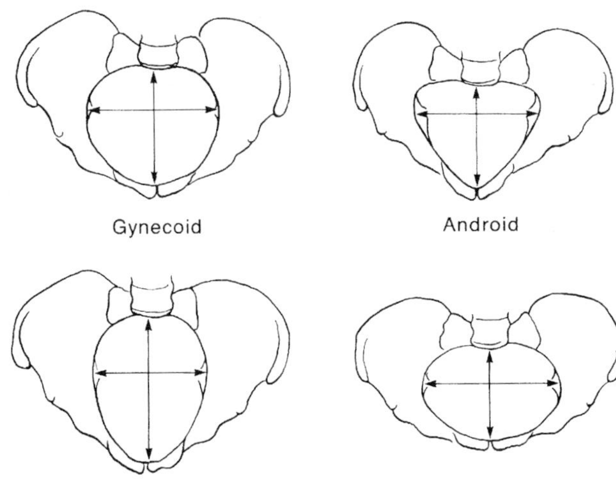

FIG. 20-1 Four basic types of pelves. (From Burroughs A, Leifer G: *Maternity nursing*, ed 8, Philadelphia, 2002, WB Saunders.)

   2. Surrounds, cushions, and protects the fetus and allows for fetal movement
   3. Maintains body temperature of the fetus
   4. Consists largely of fetal urine and is therefore a measure of fetal kidney function
   5. The fetus drinks, swallows, and urinates the **amniotic fluid** and breathes the **amniotic fluid** into its lungs

D. **Placenta**
   1. Provides for exchange of nutrients and waste products between fetus and mother
   2. Develops by the third month
   3. Dependent on maternal circulation
   4. Produces hormones to maintain pregnancy and assumes full responsibility for the production of these hormones by the 12th week of gestation
   5. Large particles such as bacteria cannot pass through the **placenta**
   6. In addition to nutrients, drugs, antibodies, and viruses can pass through the **placenta**
   7. In the third trimester, transfer of maternal immunoglobulin provides fetus passive immunity to certain diseases for the first few months after birth
   8. By week 8, genetic testing can be done

TABLE 20-2

Fetal Development

Embryonic Stage

WEEK 1
Free-floating blastocyst

WEEK 2 TO 3
2 mm long
Groove formed along middle of back
Beginning of blood circulation
Heart tubular in shape

WEEK 4
4 to 6 mm long
0.4 g in weight
Double heart chambers visible
Heart beginning to beat
Limb buds

WEEK 8
3 cm long
2 g in weight
Eyelids begin to fuse
Circulatory system through umbilical cord well established
Every organ system present

WEEK 12
8 cm long
45 g in weight
Face well formed
Limbs long and slender
Kidneys begin to form urine
Spontaneous movements occur
Heart tones detected by electronic devices between 8 and 12 weeks
Sex visually recognizable

Fetal Period

WEEK 16
Active movements are present
Fetal skin is transparent
Lanugo hair begins to develop
Skeletal ossification occurs
Sex of fetus can be determined

WEEK 20
19 cm long
465 g in weight
Lanugo covers the entire body
Fetus has nails
Muscles developed
Enamel and dentin depositing
Heart beat detected by fetoscope

WEEK 24
28 cm long
780 g in weight
Hair on head well formed
Skin reddish and wrinkled
Reflex hand grasp
Vernix caseosa covers entire body
Has ability to hear

WEEK 28
38 cm long
1200 g in weight
Limbs are well flexed
Brain develops rapidly
Eyelids open and close
Lungs sufficiently developed to provide gas exchange (lecithin forming)
If born, neonate can breathe at this time

WEEK 32
30 cm long
2000 g (5.5 lb) in weight
Bones are fully developed
Subcutaneous fat collected
L/S (lecithin/sphingomyelin) ratio switching to 1.2:1

WEEK 36
42 to 48 cm long
2500 g in weight
Skin pink, body rounded
Less wrinkled
Lanugo disappearing
L/S (lecithin/sphingomyelin) ratio $\geq$ 2:1

WEEK 40
48 to 52 cm long
3000 to 3600 g in weight
Skin pinkish and smooth
Lanugo present in upper arms and shoulders
Vernix caseosa decreases
Fingernails extend beyond fingertips
Sole (plantar) creases down to heel
Testes in scrotum
Labia major well developed

VII. FETAL CIRCULATION

A. Umbilical cord
   1. Contains two arteries and one vein
   2. Arteries carry deoxygenated blood and waste products from the fetus
   3. The vein carries oxygenated blood and provides oxygen and nutrients to the fetus

B. Fetal heart rate
   1. 120 to 160 beats per minute
   2. Approximately twice the maternal heart rate

C. Fetal circulation bypass
   1. Present because of nonfunctioning lungs
   2. Bypasses must close after birth to allow blood to flow through the lungs and the liver
   3. Ductus arteriosus connects the pulmonary artery to aorta, bypassing the lungs
   4. Ductus venosus connects the umbilical vein and inferior vena cava, bypassing the liver
   5. Foramen ovale is the opening between the right and left atria of heart, bypassing the lungs

PRACTICE QUESTIONS

1. A pregnant client asks the nurse about the hormone that causes milk production. The nurse tells the client that the primary hormone that stimulates the secretion of milk is:
   1. Testosterone
   2. Oxytocin
   3. Prolactin
   4. Progesterone
2. A licensed practical nurse (LPN) is assisting a high school nurse in conducting a session with female adolescents regarding the menstrual cycle. The LPN tells the adolescents that the normal duration of the menstrual cycle is about:
   1. 14 days
   2. 28 days
   3. 30 days
   4. 45 days
3. A maternity nursing instructor asks a nursing student to identify the hormones that are produced by the ovaries. Which of the following, if identified by the student, indicates an understanding of the hormones produced by this endocrine gland?
   1. Estrogen and progesterone
   2. Follicle stimulating hormone (FSH)
   3. Luteinizing hormone (LH)
   4. Oxytoxin
4. A nurse midwife is conducting a session on the process of fertilization with a group of nursing students. The nurse midwife asks a student to identify the structure where fertilization of an ovum takes place. Which of the following, if identified by the student, indicates an understanding of this process?
   1. Fallopian tube
   2. Fundus of the uterus
   3. In the ovary
   4. In the corpus of the uterus
5. A nursing student is conducting a clinical conference regarding the hormones that are related to pregnancy. The instructor asks the student about the function of progesterone. Which of the following responses, if made by the student, indicates an understanding of the function of this hormone?
   1. "It softens the muscles and joints of the pelvis."
   2. "It is the primary hormone of milk production."
   3. "It increases during pregnancy to stimulate the basal metabolic rate."
   4. "It maintains the uterine lining for implantation and relaxes all smooth muscle including the uterus."
6. A nurse is reinforcing teaching to a pregnant woman about the physiological effects and hormone changes that occur in pregnancy. The woman asks the nurse about the purpose of estrogen. The nurse bases the response on which of the following purposes of estrogen?
   1. It maintains the uterine lining for implantation
   2. It stimulates metabolism of glucose and converts the glucose to fat
   3. It prevents the involution of the corpus luteum and maintains the production of progesterone until the placenta is formed
   4. It stimulates uterine development to provide an environment for the fetus and stimulates the breasts to prepare for lactation
7. A maternity nurse is describing the ovarian cycle to a group of nursing students. The instructor asks a nursing student to identify the phases of the cycle. Which phase, if stated by the nursing student, indicates a need to further research this area?
   1. Follicular phase
   2. Ovulatory phase
   3. Luteal phase
   4. Proliferative phase
8. A nursing student is asked to describe the size of the uterus in a nonpregnant client. Which of the following responses, if made by the student, indicates an understanding of the anatomy of this structure?
   1. "The uterus weighs about 2 ounces."
   2. "The uterus weighs about 2.2 pounds."
   3. "The uterus has a capacity of about 50 mL."
   4. "The uterus is round in shape and weighs approximately 1000 grams."

9. A nurse is collecting data from a pregnant client. The client asks the nurse about the purpose of the fallopian tubes. The nurse responds to the client knowing that the fallopian tubes:
   1. Secrete estrogen and progesterone
   2. Are the organ of copulation
   3. Are where the fetus develops
   4. Are where fertilization occurs
10. A nursing student is assigned to care for an adolescent female client in the health care clinic. The instructor reviews the menstrual cycle with the student. The instructor determines that the student understands the process of secretion of the follicle-stimulating hormone (FSH) and the luteinizing hormone (LH) if the student states:
   1. "FSH and LH are released from the anterior pituitary gland."
   2. "FSH and LH are secreted by the corpus luteum of the ovary."
   3. "FSH and LH are secreted by the adrenal glands."
   4. "FSH and LH stimulate the formation of milk during pregnancy."
11. A nurse working in a prenatal clinic reviews a client's chart and notes that the physician documents that the client has a gynecoid pelvis. Based on this documentation, the nurse determines that this type of pelvis is:
   1. Not favorable for labor
   2. Seen in 25% of women
   3. A wide pelvis with a short diameter
   4. The most favorable for labor and birth
12. A client asks the nurse about the purpose of the placenta. The nurse plans to respond to the client knowing that the placenta:
   1. Prevents antibodies and viruses from passing to the fetus
   2. Cushions and protects the fetus
   3. Provides an exchange of nutrients and waste products between the mother and fetus
   4. Maintains the body temperature of the fetus
13. A nurse is describing the process of fetal circulation to a client during a prenatal visit. The nurse tells the client that fetal circulation consists of:
   1. Two umbilical veins and one umbilical artery
   2. Two umbilical arteries and one umbilical vein
   3. Arteries carrying oxygenated blood to the fetus
   4. Veins carrying deoxygenated blood to the fetus
14. A nursing student is assigned to a client in labor. The nursing instructor asks the student to describe fetal circulation, specifically the ductus venosus. The instructor determines that the student understands the structure of the ductus venosus if the student states that it:
   1. Connects the pulmonary artery to the aorta
   2. Is an opening between the right and left atria
   3. Connects the umbilical artery to the inferior vena cava
   4. Connects the umbilical vein to the inferior vena cava
15. During the prenatal visit, the nurse checks the fetal heart rate (FHR) using a fetoscope. The nurse determines that the FHR is normal if which of the following heart rates is noted?
   1. 80 beats per minute
   2. 100 beats per minute
   3. 150 beats per minute
   4. 180 beats per minute

ANSWERS

1. *Answer:* 3

Rationale: Prolactin stimulates the secretion of milk, called lactogenesis. Oxytocin stimulates contractions during birth and stimulates postpartum contractions to compress uterine vessels and control bleeding. Testosterone is produced by the adrenal glands in the female and induces the growth of pubic and axillary hair at puberty. Progesterone stimulates the secretions of the endometrial glands and causes the endometrial vessels to become dilated and tortuous in preparation for possible embryo implantation.

Test-Taking Strategy: Use the process of elimination. Knowledge regarding the functions of the various hormones in the female reproductive system is required to answer this question. Note the relationship between "secretion of milk" in the question and the hormone "prolactin" in the correct option. Review the functions of the various hormones of the reproductive system if you had difficulty with this question.

Level of Cognitive Ability: Application
Client Needs: Physiological Integrity
Integrated Concept/Process: Teaching/Learning
Content Area: Maternity
Reference: Murray S, McKinney E, Gorrie T: *Foundations of maternal-newborn nursing,* ed 3, Philadelphia, 2002, WB Saunders, p. 581.

2. *Answer:* 2

Rationale: The normal duration of the menstrual cycle is about 28 days, although it may range from 20 to 45 days. The first day of the menstrual period is counted as day 1 of the woman's cycle.

Test-Taking Strategy: Knowledge regarding the duration of the menstrual cycle is required to answer this question. Note the key words "normal duration" in the question. This will assist in eliminating options 1, 3, and 4. Review the physiology related to the menstrual cycle if you had difficulty with this question.

Level of Cognitive Ability: Application
Client Needs: Physiological Integrity
Integrated Concept/Process: Teaching/Learning
Content Area: Maternity
Reference: Murray S, McKinney E, Gorrie T: *Foundations of maternal-newborn nursing,* ed 3, Philadelphia, 2002, WB Saunders, p. 66.

3. *Answer:* 1
Rationale: The ovaries are the endocrine glands that produce estrogen and progesterone. The FSH and LH are produced by the anterior pituitary gland. Oxytoxin is produced by the posterior pituitary gland and stimulates the uterus to produce contractions during birth.
Test-Taking Strategy: Knowledge regarding the various hormones and the production and secretion of the hormones is required to answer this question. Review this information if you had difficulty with this question.
Level of Cognitive Ability: Comprehension
Client Needs: Physiological Integrity
Integrated Concept/Process: Teaching/Learning
Content Area: Maternity
Reference: Murray S, McKinney E, Gorrie T: *Foundations of maternal-newborn nursing,* ed 3, Philadelphia, 2002, WB Saunders, p. 61.

4. *Answer:* 1
Rationale: Fallopian tubes, also called oviducts, are 8 to 14 cm long and are quite narrow. The fallopian tubes are a pathway for the ovum between the ovary and the uterus. Fertilization occurs in the fallopian tube. Options 2, 3, and 4 are incorrect.
Test-Taking Strategy: Knowledge regarding the process of fertilization and the area in which fertilization occurs is required to answer this question. Review this information if you had difficulty with this question.
Level of Cognitive Ability: Comprehension
Client Needs: Physiological Integrity
Integrated Concept/Process: Teaching/Learning
Content Area: Maternity
Reference: Murray S, McKinney E, Gorrie T: *Foundations of maternal-newborn nursing,* ed 3, Philadelphia, 2002, WB Saunders, p. 62.

5. *Answer:* 4
Rationale: Progesterone maintains the uterine lining for implantation and relaxes all smooth muscle including the uterus. Relaxin is the hormone that softens the muscles and joints of the pelvis. Thyroxine increases during pregnancy to stimulate basal metabolic rates, and prolactin is the primary hormone of milk production.
Test-Taking Strategy: Knowledge regarding the function of the various hormones related to pregnancy is required to answer this question. Review the functions of these hormones if you had difficulty with this question.
Level of Cognitive Ability: Comprehension
Client Needs: Physiological integrity
Integrated Concept/Process: Teaching/Learning
Content Area: Maternity
Reference: Murray S, McKinney E, Gorrie T: *Foundations of maternal-newborn nursing,* ed 3, Philadelphia, 2002, WB Saunders, p. 122.

6. *Answer:* 4
Rationale: Estrogen stimulates uterine development to provide an environment for the fetus, and stimulates the breasts to prepare for lactation. Progesterone maintains the uterine lining for implantation and relaxes all smooth muscle. Human placental lactogen stimulates the metabolism of glucose and converts the glucose to fat. Human chorionic gonadotropin prevents involution of the corpus luteum and maintains the production of progesterone until the placenta is formed.
Test-Taking Strategy: Knowledge regarding the functions of various hormones related to pregnancy is required to answer this question. Review these various hormones if you had difficulty with this question.
Level of Cognitive Ability: Application
Client Needs: Physiological Integrity
Integrated Concept/Process: Teaching/Learning
Content Area: Maternity
Reference: Murray S, McKinney E, Gorrie T: *Foundations of maternal-newborn nursing,* ed 3, Philadelphia, 2002, WB Saunders, p. 130.

7. *Answer:* 4
Rationale: The ovarian cycle consists of three phases: the follicular, ovulatory, and luteal. The proliferative phase is a phase of the endometrial cycle.
Test-Taking Strategy: Note the key words "indicates a need to further research." Knowledge regarding the ovarian cycle and the phases included in the cycle will direct you to option 4. Review the ovarian cycle if you had difficulty with this question.
Level of Cognitive Ability: Comprehension
Client Needs: Physiological Integrity
Integrated Concept/Process: Teaching/Learning
Content Area: Maternity
Reference: Murray S, McKinney E, Gorrie T: *Foundations of maternal-newborn nursing,* ed 3, Philadelphia, 2002, WB Saunders, p. 68.

8. *Answer:* 1
Rationale: Before conception, the uterus is a small pear-shaped organ contained entirely in the pelvic cavity. Before pregnancy, the uterus weighs approximately 60 grams (2 oz) and has a capacity of about 10 mL (one third of an ounce). At the end of pregnancy, the uterus weighs approximately 1000 g (2.2 pounds) and has a sufficient capacity for the fetus, placenta, and amniotic fluid.
Test-Taking Strategy: Knowledge regarding the structure of the uterus is required to answer this question. Note the key word "nonpregnant" and visualize each of the items identified in the options to assist in directing you to the correct option. Review the anatomy of the uterus if you had difficulty with this question.
Level of Cognitive Ability: Comprehension
Client Needs: Physiological Integrity
Integrated Concept/Process: Teaching/Learning

Content Area: Maternity
Reference: Murray S, McKinney E, Gorrie T: *Foundations of maternal-newborn nursing,* ed 3, Philadelphia, 2002, WB Saunders, p. 64.

9. *Answer:* 4
Rationale: Each fallopian tube is a hollow muscular tube that transports a mature oocyte for final maturation and fertilization. Fertilization typically occurs near the boundary between the ampulla and isthmus of the tube. Estrogen is a hormone produced by the ovarian follicles, corpus luteum, adrenal cortex, and placenta during pregnancy. Progesterone is a hormone secreted by the corpus luteum of the ovary, adrenal glands, and placenta during pregnancy. The vagina is the organ of copulation, and the fetus develops in the uterus.
Test-Taking Strategy: Knowledge of the anatomy and physiology of the female reproductive system is required to answer this question. Review this information if you had difficulty with this question.
Level of Cognitive Ability: Comprehension
Client Needs: Physiological Integrity
Integrated Concept/Process: Nursing Process/Implementation
Content Area: Maternity
Reference: Burroughs A, Leifer G: *Maternity nursing,* ed 8, Philadelphia, 2002, WB Saunders, p. 15.

10. *Answer:* 1
Rationale: FSH and LH are released from the anterior pituitary gland to stimulate follicular growth and development, growth of the graafian follicle, and the production of progesterone. Options 2, 3, and 4 are incorrect.
Test-Taking Strategy: Use the process of elimination to answer the question. Option 4 can be eliminated because the case of the question does not address pregnancy. From this point, use your knowledge related to the menstrual cycle to select the correct option. Review the menstrual cycle if you had difficulty with this question.
Level of Cognitive Ability: Comprehension
Client Needs: Physiological Integrity
Integrated Concept/Process: Teaching/Learning
Content Area: Maternity
Reference: Burroughs A, Leifer G: *Maternity nursing,* ed 8, Philadelphia, 2002, WB Saunders, p. 43.

11. *Answer:* 4
Rationale: A gynecoid pelvis is a normal female pelvis and is the most favorable for successful labor and birth. An android pelvis, seen in 20% of women, would not be favorable for labor because of the narrow pelvic planes. An anthropoid pelvis has an outlet that is adequate, with a normal or moderately narrow pubic arch, and is seen in 25% of women. The platypelloid pelvis, seen in 5% of women, has a wide transverse diameter, but the anteroposterior diameter is short, making the outlet inadequate.
Test-Taking Strategy: Knowledge regarding pelvic types is required to answer this question. Remember that the gynecoid pelvis is the normal female pelvis. Review pelvic types if you had difficulty with this question.
Level of Cognitive Ability: Comprehension
Client Needs: Physiological Integrity
Integrated Concept/Process: Nursing Process/Data Collection
Content Area: Maternity
Reference: Burroughs A, Leifer G: *Maternity nursing,* ed 8, Philadelphia, 2002, WB Saunders, p. 17.

12. *Answer:* 3
Rationale: The placenta provides an exchange of nutrients and waste products between the mother and fetus. The amniotic fluid surrounds, cushions, and protects the fetus and maintains the body temperature of the fetus.
Test-Taking Strategy: Knowledge regarding the purpose of the placenta and amniotic fluid is required to answer this question. Remember that the placenta provides nutrients. Review the structure and function of the placenta and amniotic fluid if you had difficulty with this question.
Level of Cognitive Ability: Comprehension
Client Needs: Physiological Integrity
Integrated Concept/Process: Nursing Process/Planning
Content Area: Maternity
Reference: Burroughs A, Leifer G: *Maternity nursing,* ed 8, Philadelphia, 2002, WB Saunders, p. 30.

13. *Answer:* 2
Rationale: Blood pumped by the fetus' heart leaves the fetus through two umbilical arteries. Once oxygenated, the blood is then returned by one umbilical vein. Arteries carry deoxygenated blood and waste products from the fetus and veins carry oxygenated blood and provide oxygen and nutrients to the fetus.
Test-Taking Strategy: Knowledge regarding fetal circulation is required to answer this question. Remember that there are three umbilical vessels within an umbilical cord (two arteries and one vein). Review fetal circulation if you had difficulty with this question.
Level of Cognitive Ability: Application
Client Needs: Physiological Integrity
Integrated Concept/Process: Nursing Process/Implementation
Content Area: Maternity
Reference: Burroughs A, Leifer G: *Maternity nursing,* ed 8, Philadelphia, 2002, WB Saunders, p. 140.

14. *Answer:* 4
Rationale: The ductus venosus connects the umbilical vein to the inferior vena cava. The foramen ovale is a temporary opening between the right and left atria. The ductus arteriosus joins the aorta and the pulmonary artery.
Test-Taking Strategy: Knowledge regarding fetal circulation is required to answer this question. Review fetal circulation if you had difficulty with this question.
Level of Cognitive Ability: Comprehension
Client Needs: Physiological Integrity
Integrated Concept/Process: Teaching/Learning
Content Area: Maternity
Reference: Burroughs A, Leifer G: *Maternity nursing,* ed 8, Philadelphia, 2002, WB Saunders, p. 141.

15. *Answer:* 3
Rationale: The normal fetal heart rate is 120 to 160 beats per minute. If the fetal heart rate is less than 100 or more than 160 beats per minute with the uterus at rest, the fetus may be in distress.
Test-Taking Strategy: Knowledge regarding normal fetal heart rate is required to answer this question. Review fetal heart rate if you had difficulty with this question.
Level of Cognitive Ability: Comprehension
Client Needs: Physiological Integrity
Integrated Concept/Process: Nursing Process/Data Collection
Content Area: Maternity
Reference: Burroughs A, Leifer G: *Maternity nursing,* ed 8, Philadelphia, 2002, WB Saunders, p. 83.

REFERENCES

Burroughs A, Leifer G: *Maternity nursing,* ed 8, Philadelphia, 2002, WB Saunders.

Lowdermilk D, Perry S, Bobak I: *Maternity and women's health care,* ed 7, St Louis, 2000, Mosby.

McKinney E, Ashwill J, Murray S, James S, Gorrie T, Droske S: *Maternal-child nursing,* Philadelphia, 2000, WB Saunders.

Obstetrical Assessment

I. GESTATION

A. Estimated date of confinement (EDC)
B. Lasts approximately 280 days
C. **Nagele's rule** for estimating EDC (Box 21-1)
   1. For **Nagele's rule** to be accurate requires that the woman have a regular 28-day menstrual cycle
   2. Add 7 days to the first day of the last menstrual period (LMP), subtract 3 months, and then add 1 year to that date

II. GRAVIDITY AND PARITY

A. **Gravidity**
   1. **Gravida** refers to a pregnant woman
   2. **Gravidity** refers to the number of pregnancies
   3. **Nulligravida** is a woman who has never been pregnant
   4. **Primigravida** is a woman who is pregnant for the first time
   5. **Multigravida** is a woman in at least her second pregnancy
B. **Parity**
   1. **Parity** is the number of births (not the number of fetuses, e.g., twins) past 20 weeks' gestation, whether or not the fetus was born alive
   2. **Nullipara** is a woman who has not had a birth at more than 20 weeks of gestation
   3. **Primipara** is a woman who has had one birth that occurs after the 20th week of gestation
   4. **Multipara** is a woman who has had two or more pregnancies resulting in viable offspring

BOX 21-1

Nagele's Rule for Estimating EDC

First day of LMP: September 11, 2003
Add 7 days: September 18, 2003
Subtract 3 months: June 18, 2003
Add 1 year: June 18, 2004
EDC: June 18, 2004

III. PREGNANCY SIGNS

A. Presumptive signs
   1. Amenorrhea
   2. Nausea and vomiting
   3. Increased size and increased feeling of fullness in breasts
   4. Pronounced nipples
   5. Urinary frequency
   6. **Quickening**: First perception of fetal movement; may occur as early as the 14th to 16th week of gestation
   7. Fatigue
   8. Discoloration and thickening of vaginal mucosa
B. Probable signs
   1. Uterine enlargement
   2. **Hegar's sign**: Softening of the uterus that occurs about week 6
   3. **Goodell's sign**: Softening of the cervix that occurs at the beginning of the second month
   4. **Chadwick's sign**: Bluish coloration of the mucous membranes of cervix, vagina, and vulva
   5. **Ballottement**: Rebounding of the fetus against the examiner's fingers on palpation
   6. Braxton Hicks contractions
   7. Positive pregnancy test measuring for human chorionic gonadotropin (hCG)

C. Positive signs
   1. Fetal heart rate by Doppler ultrasound at 8 to 12 weeks and by fetoscope at 20 weeks
   2. Active fetal movements palpable
   3. Outline of fetus via ultrasound

IV. FUNDAL HEIGHT (Box 21-2)
   A. Performed to evaluate gestational age of fetus
   B. Between 18 and 32 weeks, fundal height in centimeters equals the fetus's age in weeks
   C. At 16 weeks, the fundus can be found halfway between the symphysis pubis and the umbilicus
   D. At 20 to 22 weeks, the fundus is at the umbilicus
   E. At 36 weeks, the fundus is at the xiphoid process

V. MATERNAL RISK FACTORS
   A. German measles (rubella)
      1. The risk of maternal and fetal or congenital infection is related to the trimester of placental infection
      2. Maternal infection during the first 8 weeks of gestation carries the highest rate of maternal and fetal infection
   B. Sexually transmitted diseases
      1. Syphilis
         a. May cross the **placenta**
         b. Usually leads to spontaneous abortions
         c. Increases the incidence of mental subnormality and physical deformities in the fetus
      2. Genital herpes
         a. May cross **placenta**
         b. Fetus contaminated after membranes rupture or with vaginal **delivery**
      3. Gonorrhea
         a. The fetus is contaminated at the time of **delivery**
         b. May result in postpartum infection
         c. Risks to the neonate include ophthalmia neonatorum, pneumonia, sepsis
   C. Human immunodeficiency virus (HIV)
      1. The virus is transmitted through blood, blood products, and other bodily fluids such as urine, semen, and vaginal fluid
      2. Repeated exposure to HIV during pregnancy through unsafe sex practices or intravenous drug use can increase the risk of transmission to the fetus
   D. Substance abuse
      1. Many substances cross the **placenta**; therefore no drugs, including over-the-counter medications, should be taken unless prescribed by physician
      2. Substances commonly abused include alcohol, cocaine, crack, marijuana, amphetamines, barbiturates, and heroin
      3. Substance abuse threatens normal fetal growth and successful term completion of the pregnancy
      4. Substance abuse places the pregnancy at risk for fetal growth retardation, **abruptio placentae**, and fetal bradycardia
      5. Physical signs of drug abuse may include dilated or contracted pupils, fatigue, track marks, skin abscesses, inflamed nasal mucosa, and inappropriate behavior by the mother
      6. Alcohol during pregnancy may lead to fetal alcohol syndrome and can cause jitteriness, physical abnormalities, congenital anomalies, and growth deficits
      7. Smoking leads to low birth weights, a higher incidence of birth defects, and stillbirths
   E. Adolescent pregnancy
      1. Factors that result in adolescent pregnancy include the early onset of menarche, changing sexual behaviors in this age group, faulty family development, poverty, and the lack of knowledge of reproduction and birth control
      2. The major concerns related to adolescent pregnancy include poor nutritional status, emotional and behavioral difficulties, lack of support systems, increased risk of stillbirth, low-birth-weight newborn infants, fetal mortality, cephalopelvic disproportion, and the increased risks of maternal complications such as hypertension, anemia, prolonged **labor**, and infections

BOX 21-2

Measuring Fundal Height

1. Place the client in a supine position.
2. Place the end of the tape measure at the level of the symphysis pubis.
3. Stretch the tape to the top of the uterine fundus.
4. Note and record measurement.

PRACTICE QUESTIONS

1. A client arrives at the prenatal clinic for the first prenatal assessment. The client tells the nurse that the first day of her last menstrual period was September 19, 2003. Using Nagele's rule, the nurse determines the estimated date of confinement as:
   1. July 26, 2004
   2. June 12, 2004
   3. June 26, 2004
   4. July 12, 2004

2. A client is in her second trimester of pregnancy. During her routine prenatal visit, she tells the primary health care provider that she frequently has calf pain when she walks. The nurse reviews the health record to note documentation of which of the following that will differentiate the origin of the discomfort?
   1. Chadwick's sign
   2. Leopold's sign
   3. Homan's sign
   4. Kernig's sign
3. A nurse is collecting data during an admission assessment on a client, pregnant with twins. The client also has a 5-year-old child. The nurse would document which gravida and para status on this client?
   1. Gravida III, Para II
   2. Gravida II, Para II
   3. Gravida I, Para I
   4. Gravida II, Para I
4. A primipara is being evaluated in the clinic during her second trimester of pregnancy. Which of the following would indicate an abnormal physical finding necessitating further testing?
   1. Consistent increase in fundal height
   2. Fetal heart rate of 180 beats per minute
   3. Braxton Hicks contractions
   4. Quickening
5. A nurse is providing instructions to a pregnant client with genital herpes about the measures that need to be implemented to protect the fetus. The nurse tells the client that:
   1. Daily administration of acyclovir (Zovirax) is necessary during the entire pregnancy
   2. Total abstinence from sexual intercourse is necessary during the entire pregnancy
   3. Sitz baths need to be taken every 4 hours while awake if vaginal lesions are present
   4. A Cesarean section will be necessary if vaginal lesions are present at the time of labor
6. A nurse is collecting data on a pregnant client who is at 28 weeks of gestation. The nurse measures the fundal height in centimeters and expects the findings to be which of the following?
   1. 22 cm
   2. 28 cm
   3. 36 cm
   4. 40 cm
7. A pregnant client is seen in the health care clinic for a regular prenatal visit. The client tells the nurse that she is experiencing irregular contractions. The nurse determines that the client is experiencing Braxton Hicks contractions. Based on this finding, which nursing action is most appropriate?
   1. Instruct the client to maintain bed rest for the remainder of the pregnancy
   2. Instruct the client that these are common and may occur throughout the pregnancy
   3. Contact the physician
   4. Call the maternity unit and inform them that the client will be admitted in a prelabor condition
8. A nurse is reviewing the record of a client who has just been told that a pregnancy test is positive. The physician has documented the presence of Goodell's sign. The nurse determines that this sign is indicative of:
   1. A softening of the cervix
   2. A soft blowing sound that corresponds to the maternal pulse while auscultating the uterus
   3. The presence of human chorionic gonadotropin (hCG) in the urine
   4. The presence of fetal movement
9. A nursing instructor asks a nursing student to describe the process of quickening. Which of the following statements, if made by the student, indicates an understanding of this term?
   1. "It is the irregular, painless contractions that occur throughout pregnancy."
   2. "It is the soft blowing sound that can be heard when the uterus is auscultated."
   3. "It is the fetal movement that is felt by the mother."
   4. "It is the thinning of the lower uterine segment."
10. A pregnant client asks the nurse in the clinic when she will be able to start feeling the fetus move. The nurse responds by telling the mother that fetal movements will be noted between:
    1. 6 to 8 weeks of gestation
    2. 8 to 10 weeks of gestation
    3. 10 to 12 weeks of gestation
    4. 14 to 16 weeks of gestation

ANSWERS

1. *Answer:* 3

Rationale: Accurate use of Nagele's rule requires that the woman have a regular 28-day menstrual cycle. Add 7 days to the first day of the last menstrual period (LMP), subtract 3 months, and then add 1 year to that date. First day of the LMP: September 19, 2003; add 7 days: September 26, 2003; subtract 3 months: June 26, 2003; add 1 year: June 26, 2004.

Test-Taking Strategy: Knowledge regarding the use of Nagele's rule is required to answer this question. Use caution when following steps to determine the estimated date of confinement. Avoid taking short cuts, particularly when math is involved. Review Nagele's rule if you had difficulty with this question.

Level of Cognitive Ability: Comprehension

Client Needs: Physiological Integrity

Integrated Concept/Process: Nursing Process/Data Collection

Content Area: Maternity

Reference: Burroughs A, Leifer G: *Maternity nursing*, ed 8, Philadelphia, 2002, WB Saunders, p. 40.

2. *Answer:* 3

Rationale: Chadwick's sign is a cervical change and is a presumptive sign of pregnancy. Leopold's sign is a fictitious term. Leopold's maneuvers are a series of abdominal palpation maneuvers that provide information regarding fetal presentation, position, presenting part, attitude, and descent. Kernig's sign tests for meningeal irritability. Homan's sign tests for venous thrombosis of the lower extremity. Pain in the calf during walking could indicate venous thrombosis.

Test-Taking Strategy: Use the process of elimination. Knowledge of the signs related to pregnancy and signs indicating a potential problem are required to answer this question. Review the signs identified in options 1, 3, and 4 if you had difficulty with this question.

Level of Cognitive Ability: Application

Client Needs: Physiological Integrity

Integrated Concept/Process: Nursing Process/Data Collection

Content Area: Maternity

Reference: Burroughs A, Leifer G: *Maternity nursing*, ed 8, Philadelphia, 2002, WB Saunders, p. 41.

3. *Answer:* 4

Rationale: Gravida is a term that refers to a woman who is or has been pregnant regardless of the duration of the pregnancy. Para is a term that means the number of pregnancies that have progressed past 20 weeks' gestation. Parity does not reflect the number of fetuses or infants. Option 1, 2, and 3 are incorrect based on the above definition.

Test-Taking Strategy: Knowledge of the terms *gravida* and *para* is necessary to answer this question correctly. Review the description of these terms if you had difficulty with this question.

Level of Cognitive Ability: Application

Client Needs: Physiological Integrity

Integrated Concept/Process: Communication and Documentation

Content Area: Maternity

Reference: Burroughs A, Leifer G: *Maternity nursing*, ed 8, Philadelphia, 2002, WB Saunders, p. 40.

4. *Answer:* 2

Rationale: The fetal heart rate should be 120 to 160 beats per minute throughout pregnancy. Options 1, 3, and 4 are normal expected findings.

Test-Taking Strategy: Use the process of elimination. Note the key words "indicates an abnormal physical finding." Recalling that the normal fetal heart rate is 120 to 160 beats per minute will easily direct you to option 2. Review normal assessment findings in pregnancy, if you had difficulty with this question.

Level of Cognitive Ability: Comprehension

Client Needs: Physiological Integrity

Integrated Concept/Process: Nursing Process/Data Collection

Content Area: Maternity

Reference: Burroughs A, Leifer G: *Maternity nursing*, ed 8, Philadelphia, 2002, WB Saunders, p. 83.

5. *Answer:* 4

Rationale: For women with active lesions, either recurrent or primary at the time of labor, delivery should be by Cesarean section to prevent the fetus from being in contact with the genital herpes. The safety of acyclovir has not been established during pregnancy and should be used only when a life-threatening infection is present. Clients should be advised to abstain from sexual contact while the lesions are present. If this is an initial infection, they should continue to abstain until they become culture-negative because prolonged viral shedding may occur in such cases. Keeping the genital area clean and dry will promote healing.

Test-Taking Strategy: Use the process of elimination. Eliminate options 1 and 2 first because of the absolute word "entire" in these options. From the remaining options, recalling that the lesions should be kept clean and dry to promote healing will assist in eliminating option 3. If you had difficulty with this question, review the content related to genital herpes as a maternal risk factor.

Level of Cognitive Ability: Application

Client Needs: Safe, Effective Care Environment

Integrated Concept/Process: Teaching/Learning

Content Area: Maternity

Reference: Burroughs A, Leifer G: *Maternity nursing*, ed 8, Philadelphia, 2002, WB Saunders, p. 242.

6. *Answer:* 2

Rationale: During the second and third trimesters (weeks 18 to 30), fundal height in centimeters approximately equals the fetus's age in weeks ± 2 cm. At 16 weeks, the fundus can be located halfway between the symphysis pubis and the umbilicus. At 20 to 22 weeks, the fundus is at the umbilicus and at 36 weeks, the fundus is at the xiphoid process.

Test-Taking Strategy: Use the process of elimination. Remember that during the second and third trimesters (weeks 18 to 30), fundal height in centimeters approximately equals the fetus's age in weeks ± 2 cm. If you are unfamiliar with this data collection technique, review this content area.

Level of Cognitive Ability: Comprehension

Client Needs: Health Promotion and Maintenance

Integrated Concept/Process: Nursing Process/Data Collection

Content Area: Maternity

Reference: Lowdermilk D, Perry S, Bobak I: *Maternity and women's health care*, ed 7, St Louis, 2000, Mosby, p. 401.

7. *Answer:* 2
Rationale: Braxton Hicks contractions are irregular, painless contractions that may occur intermittently throughout pregnancy. Since Braxton Hicks contractions may occur and are normal in some pregnant women during pregnancy, options 1, 3, and 4 are unnecessary and inappropriate actions.
Test-Taking Strategy: Use the process of elimination. Options 3 and 4 are similar and can be eliminated first. From the remaining options, knowing that Braxton Hicks contractions are common and can occur throughout pregnancy will assist in directing you to option 2. If you had difficulty with this question, review the physiology associated with Braxton Hicks contractions.
Level of Cognitive Ability: Application
Client Needs: Health Promotion and Maintenance
Integrated Concept/Process: Teaching/Learning
Content Area: Maternity
Reference: Lowdermilk D, Perry S, Bobak I: *Maternity and women's health care,* ed 7, St Louis, 2000, Mosby, p. 339.

8. *Answer:* 1
Rationale: In the early weeks of pregnancy, the cervix becomes softer as a result of pelvic vasoconstriction, which causes Goodell's sign. Cervical softening is noted by the examiner during pelvic examination. A soft blowing sound that corresponds to the maternal pulse may be auscultated over the uterus and is due to blood circulation through the placenta. hCG is noted in maternal urine in a positive urine pregnancy test. Goodell's sign does not indicate the presence of fetal movement.
Test-Taking Strategy: Use the process of elimination and knowledge regarding the physiological findings in Goodell's sign to answer this question. Remember that Goodell's sign refers to a softening of the cervix. If you had difficulty with this question, review the changes in the cervix that occurs during pregnancy.
Level of Cognitive Ability: Comprehension
Client Needs: Health Promotion and Maintenance
Integrated Concept/Process: Nursing Process/Data Collection
Content Area: Maternity
Reference: Lowdermilk D, Perry S, Bobak I: *Maternity and women's health care,* ed 7, St Louis, 2000, Mosby, p. 339.

9. *Answer:* 3
Rationale: Quickening is fetal movement and may occur as early as the 14th to 16th weeks of gestation, and the expectant mother first notices subtle fetal movements that gradually increase in intensity. A soft blowing sound that corresponds to the maternal pulse may be auscultated over the uterus and this is known as uterine souffle. This sound is due to the blood circulation to the placenta and corresponds to the maternal pulse. Braxton Hicks contractions are irregular, painless contractions that may occur throughout pregnancy. A thinning of the lower uterine segment occurs about the sixth week of pregnancy and is called Hegar's sign.
Test-Taking Strategy: Use the process of elimination and knowledge regarding the term *quickening* to answer this question. Remember that quickening is fetal movement. If you are unfamiliar with this sign associated with pregnancy, review this content area.
Level of Cognitive Ability: Comprehension
Client Needs: Health Promotion and Maintenance
Integrated Concept/Process: Teaching/Learning
Content Area: Maternity
Reference: Lowdermilk D, Perry S, Bobak I: *Maternity and women's health care,* ed 7, St Louis, 2000, Mosby, p. 340.

10. *Answer:* 4
Rationale: Quickening is fetal movement and may occur as early as the 14th to 16th weeks of gestation. The expectant mother first notices subtle fetal movements during this time that gradually increase in intensity. Options 1, 2, and 3 are incorrect.
Test-Taking Strategy: Use the process of elimination and knowledge regarding the occurrence of quickening. In this situation, it is best to select the option that indicates the greatest length of gestational time. Review the process of quickening if you had difficulty with this question.
Level of Cognitive Ability: Application
Client Needs: Health Promotion and Maintenance
Integrated Concept/Process: Teaching/Learning
Content Area: Maternity
Reference: Lowdermilk D, Perry S, Bobak I: *Maternity and women's health care,* ed 7, St Louis, 2000, Mosby, p. 340.

REFERENCES

Burroughs A, Leifer G: *Maternity nursing,* ed 8, Philadelphia, 2002, WB Saunders.

Lowdermilk D, Perry S, Bobak I: *Maternity and women's health care,* ed 7, St Louis, 2000, Mosby.

McKinney E et al: *Maternal-child nursing,* Philadelphia, 2000, WB Saunders.

Prenatal Period and Risk Conditions

I. PHYSIOLOGICAL MATERNAL CHANGES

A. Cardiovascular system
   1. Circulating blood volume increases
   2. Heart is elevated upward and to the left because of displacement of the diaphragm as the uterus enlarges
   3. Pulse may increase about 10 beats per minute; blood pressure may decline in the second trimester
   4. Iron requirements are increased

B. Respiratory system
   1. Oxygen consumption increases
   2. Diaphragm is elevated as a result of the enlarged uterus
   3. Respiratory rate remains unchanged
   4. Shortness of breath may be experienced

C. Gastrointestinal (GI) system
   1. Nausea and vomiting may occur as a result of the secretion of human chorionic gonadotropin (hCG), which subsides by the third month
   2. Constipation resulting from decreased GI motility or pressure of the uterus
   3. Flatulence and heartburn resulting from decreased GI motility and slow emptying of the stomach
   4. Hemorrhoids resulting from increased venous pressure

D. Renal system
   1. Decreased bladder tone is caused by hormonal changes
   2. Renal threshold for glucose may be reduced

E. Endocrine system: basal metabolic rate rises

F. Reproductive system
   1. Uterus
      a. Uterus enlarges from 60 to 1000 g
      b. Irregular contractions occur
   2. Cervix
      a. Becomes shorter, more elastic, and larger in diameter
      b. Endocervical glands secrete a thick mucus plug, which is expelled from the canal when dilation begins
      c. Increased vascularization causes a softening and blue-purple discoloration **(Chadwick's sign)**
   3. Ovaries: cease ovum production
   4. Vagina
      a. Hypertrophy and thickening of muscle
      b. Increase in vaginal secretions; secretions are usually thick, white, and acidic
   5. Breast
      a. Breast size increases
      b. Nipples become more pronounced and areola becomes darker
      c. Colostrum may appear from the breast

G. Skin
   1. A dark streak down the midline of the abdomen may appear (linea nigra)
   2. Chloasma (melasma), or mask of pregnancy, may occur over the forehead, cheeks, and nose
   3. Reddish purple stretch marks (striae) may occur on the abdomen, breasts, thighs, and upper arms

H. Skeletal system: postural changes occur as the increased weight of the uterus causes a forward pull of the bony pelvis

I. Metabolism
   1. The average expected weight gain during pregnancy is 2 to 4 pounds in the first trimester and approximately 1 pound per week in the second and third trimesters
   2. Water retention is increased, which can contribute to weight gain

II. PSYCHOLOGICAL MATERNAL CHANGES

A. Ambivalence
   1. Occurs early in pregnancy even when the pregnancy is planned
   2. Mother may experience dependency-independence conflict and ambivalence related to role changes
   3. Father may experience ambivalence related to the new role he is assuming, increased financial responsibilities, and sharing wife's attention with the child

B. Acceptance
   1. Factors that may be related to acceptance of the pregnancy are the woman's readiness for the experience and her identification with the motherhood role
   2. When the mother plans and expects the pregnancy, she tends to display pleasure and experience fewer physical discomforts

C. Emotional lability
   1. May be manifested by frequency in the change of emotional states or extremes in emotional states
   2. These emotional changes are common, but the mother may feel that these changes are abnormal

D. Body image changes: changes in a woman's perception of her image during pregnancy occur gradually and may be either positive or negative

III. DISCOMFORTS OF PREGNANCY

A. Nausea and vomiting
   1. Occurs in the first trimester
   2. Caused by elevated hCG levels and changes in carbohydrate metabolism
   3. Implementation
      a. Eating dry crackers before arising
      b. Eating small, frequent, low-fat meals during the day
      c. Drinking liquids between meals

B. Syncope
   1. Usually occurs in the first trimester
   2. May be hormonally triggered or caused by the increased blood volume, anemia, fatigue, or sudden position changes
   3. Implementation
      a. Sitting with the feet up
      b. Changing positions slowly
      c. Changing the position to the left side to relieve the pressure of the uterus on the inferior vena cava

C. Urinary urgency and frequency
   1. Usually occurs in first and third trimesters
   2. Caused by pressure of the uterus on the bladder
   3. Implementation
      a. Drinking 2 quarts of fluid per day, limiting fluid intake in the evening
      b. Voiding at regular intervals
      c. Wearing perineal pads if necessary

D. Breast tenderness
   1. Can occur from the first through the third trimester
   2. Caused by increased levels of estrogen and progesterone
   3. Implementation
      a. Encouraging the use of a supportive bra with nonelastic straps
      b. Avoiding the use of soap on the nipples and areola area to prevent drying

E. Increased vaginal discharge
   1. Can occur from the first through the third trimester
   2. Caused by hyperplasia of vaginal mucosa and increased mucus production
   3. Implementation
      a. Wearing cotton underwear
      b. Avoiding douching
      c. Using proper cleansing and hygiene techniques
      d. Advising the client to consult the physician or health care provider if infection is suspected

F. Nasal stuffiness
   1. Occurs during the first through the third trimester
   2. Occurs because of increased estrogen that causes swelling of the nasal tissues and dryness
   3. Implementation
      a. Encouraging the use of humidifier
      b. Avoiding the use of nasal sprays or antihistamines

G. Fatigue
   1. Occurs usually in the first and third trimester
   2. Is usually due to hormonal changes
   3. Implementation
      a. Arranging frequent rest periods throughout the day
      b. Obtaining regular exercise

H. Heartburn
   1. Occurs in the second and third trimester
   2. Results from increased progesterone levels, decreased GI motility and esophageal reflux, and displacement of the stomach by the enlarging uterus
   3. Implementation
      a. Eating small, frequent meals, and avoiding fatty and spicy food

b. Sitting upright for 30 minutes after a meal
c. Drinking milk between meals

I. Ankle edema
1. Usually occurs in the second and third trimester
2. Occurs because of vasodilation, venous stasis, and increased venous pressure below the uterus
3. Implementation
a. Elevating the legs during the day
b. Sleeping on the left side
c. Avoiding sitting or standing in one position for long periods

J. Varicose veins
1. Usually occurs in the second and third trimesters
2. Occurs because of weakening walls of the veins or valves and venous congestion
3. Implementation
a. Wearing support hose
b. Sitting or lying with the feet and hips elevated
c. Avoiding leg crossing
d. Avoiding long periods of standing or sitting
e. Avoiding constricting articles of clothing

K. Headaches
1. Usually occurs in the second and third trimesters
2. Occurs as a result of changes in blood volume and vascular tone
3. Implementation
a. Changing position slowly
b. Applying a cool cloth to the forehead
c. Using acetaminophen (Tylenol) sparingly only if prescribed by the physician

L. Hemorrhoids
1. Usually occurs in the second and third trimesters
2. Occurs because of increased venous pressure and/or constipation
3. Implementation
a. Soaking in a warm sitz bath
b. Eating a high-fiber diet, drinking sufficient fluids, and avoiding constipation
c. Increasing exercise such as walking
d. Applying ointments, suppositories, or compresses as prescribed

M. Constipation
1. Usually occurs in the second and third trimesters
2. Occurs because of decreased intestinal motility, displacement of the intestines, and from taking iron supplements
3. Implementation
a. Eating high-fiber foods such as fresh fruits, vegetables, and bran
b. Drinking plenty of fluids
c. Exercising regularly

N. Backache
1. Usually occurs in the second and third trimesters
2. Occurs from an exaggerated lumbosacral curve because of the enlarged uterus
3. Implementation
a. Encouraging rest and sleeping on a firm mattress
b. Using good body mechanics
c. Wearing low-heeled shoes
d. Performing pelvic tilt exercises and exercises such as squatting, sitting, and pelvic rocking

O. Leg cramps
1. Usually occur in the second and third trimesters
2. Occurs because of an altered calcium-phosphorus balance and pressure of the uterus on nerves, or from fatigue
3. Implementation
a. Getting regular exercise, especially walking
b. Elevating the feet and dorsiflexing the feet when resting
c. Increasing calcium intake

P. Shortness of breath
1. Can occur in the second and third trimesters
2. Occurs as a result of pressure on the diaphragm
3. Implementation
a. Allowing frequent rest periods and avoiding overexertion
b. Sleeping with the head elevated or on the side

IV. LABORATORY TESTS (Box 22-1)

A. Blood type and Rh factor
1. ABO typing is performed to determine the woman's blood type
2. Rh typing is done to determine the presence or absence of Rh antigen (Rh-positive or Rh-negative)
3. If the client is Rh negative and has a negative antibody screen, the client will need repeat antibody screens and should receive Rh immune globulin at 28 weeks' gestation

BOX 22-1

Prenatal Visits

Every 4 weeks from 28 to 32 weeks
Every 2 weeks from 32 to 36 weeks
Every week from 36 to 40 weeks

B. Rubella titer
   1. If the client has a negative titer, indicating susceptibility to the rubella virus, the client should receive the appropriate immunization postpartum
   2. The client must be using effective birth control at the time of the immunization and counseled not to become pregnant for 3 months after immunization
C. Hemoglobin and hematocrit levels
   1. Hemoglobin and hematocrit levels will drop during gestation as a result of increased plasma volume
   2. An increase in the hematocrit level may indicate the development of pregnancy-induced hypertension (PIH)
   3. A decrease in the hemoglobin level below 10 g/dL or in the hematocrit level below 30 g/dL indicates anemia
D. Papanicolaou smear: done during the initial prenatal examination to screen for cervical neoplasia
E. Gonorrhea culture: done during the initial prenatal examination to screen for gonorrhea; may be repeated during the third trimester in high-risk clients
F. Syphilis screening: done during the initial prenatal examination to screen for syphilis; may be repeated during the third trimester in high-risk clients
G. Herpes cultures
   1. Indicated for clients with a positive history or those with active lesions
   2. Performed to determine the route of **delivery**
   3. Weekly cultures may be done at the 35th or 36th week of pregnancy until delivery
H. Chlamydia culture
   1. Indicated if the client is in a high-risk group
   2. Indicated if **infants** from previous pregnancies have developed neonatal conjunctivitis or pneumonia
I. Sickle cell screening
   1. Indicated for clients at risk for sickle cell disease
   2. A positive test may indicate need for further screening
J. Tuberculin skin test
   1. The health care provider may prefer to perform this skin test after **delivery**
   2. A positive skin test indicates the need for chest radiograph (using an abdominal lead shield) to rule out active disease
   3. In a pregnant client, chest radiograph will not be performed until after 20 weeks of gestation (after fetal organs are formed)
   4. Converters to positive may be referred for treatment with medication after **delivery**
K. Hepatitis B surface antigens
   1. Recommended for all women because of the prevalence of the disease in the general population
   2. Vaccination for hepatitis B antigen may be specifically indicated for:
      a. Health care workers
      b. Clients born in Asia, Africa, Haiti, or the Pacific islands
      c. Clients with previously undiagnosed jaundice or chronic liver disease
      d. IV drug abusers
      e. Clients with tattoos
      f. Clients with histories of blood transfusions
      g. Clients with histories of multiple episodes of sexually transmitted diseases
      h. Clients who have been previously rejected as blood donors
      i. Clients with histories of dialysis or renal transplantation
      j. Clients from households having hepatitis B-infected members or clients undergoing hemodialysis
L. Urinalysis and urine culture
   1. A urine specimen for glucose and protein determinations should be obtained at every prenatal visit
   2. Glycosuria is a common result of decreased renal threshold that occurs during pregnancy
   3. If glycosuria persists, this may indicate diabetes
   4. White blood cells in the urine may indicate infection
   5. Ketonuria may result from insufficient food intake or vomiting
   6. Protein levels of 2+ to 4+ in the urine may indicate infection or PIH

V. DIAGNOSTIC TESTS

A. Ultrasound
   1. Outlines and identifies fetal and maternal structures
   2. Assists to confirm gestational age and estimated date of **delivery**
   3. May be done abdominally or transvaginally during pregnancy
   4. Implementation
      a. If the abdominal ultrasound is being performed, the woman usually needs to have a full bladder to obtain a better image of the fetus
      b. Inform the client that the test presents no known risks to the client or fetus

B. Alpha-fetoprotein screening (AFP)
   1. Assesses the quantity of fetal serum proteins; if elevated, is associated with open neural tube and abdominal wall defects
   2. Can detect spina bifida and Down syndrome
   3. Implementation
      a. Explain that the level is determined by a single maternal blood sample drawn at 15 to 18 weeks of gestation
      b. If the level is elevated and the gestation is less than 18 weeks, a second sample is drawn
      c. An ultrasound is performed for elevated levels to rule out fetal abnormalities or multiple gestation

C. Chorionic villus sampling (CVS)
   1. Aspiration of a small sample of chorionic villus tissue at 8 to 12 weeks' gestation
   2. Test is performed for the purpose of detecting genetic abnormalities; obtain informed consent
   3. Implementation
      a. Instruct the client to drink water to fill the bladder before the procedure, to aid in positioning the uterus for catheter insertion
      b. Instruct the client to report bleeding, infection, or leakage of fluid at the insertion site after the procedure
      c. Rh-negative women may be given RhoGAM for risks related to the procedure

D. Kick counts (fetal movement counting)
   1. Mother sits quietly or lies down on the left side for 1 hour after meals and counts fetal kicks for 30 minutes
   2. Instruct the client to notify the physician or health care provider if there are fewer than 3 kicks in 1 hour

E. Amniocentesis
   1. Aspiration of **amniotic fluid** done from 14 weeks of pregnancy or thereafter
   2. Performed to determine genetic disorders, sex of the fetus, and fetal lung maturity
   3. Risks
      a. Maternal hemorrhage
      b. Infection
      c. Rh isoimmunization
      d. Abruptio placentae
      e. **Amniotic fluid** emboli
   4. Implementation
      a. Obtain informed consent
      b. Instruct the client to empty the bladder before the procedure
      c. Prepare the client for ultrasound, which is performed to locate the **placenta**
      d. Obtain baseline vital signs and fetal heart rate (FHR), and monitor every 15 minutes
      e. Place the client in the supine position
      f. Instruct the client to notify the physician or health care provider if chills, fever, leakage of fluid at the needle insertion site, decreased fetal movement, or uterine contractions occur

F. Fern test
   1. A microscopic slide test to determine the presence of **amniotic fluid** leakage
   2. By use of sterile technique, a specimen is obtained from the external os of the cervix and vaginal pool
   3. Fluid is examined on a slide under a microscope
   4. A fernlike pattern occurring from the salts of **amniotic fluid** indicates the presence of **amniotic fluid**
   5. Implementation
      a. Place the client in the dorsal lithotomy position
      b. Instruct the client to cough to cause the fluid to leak from the uterus if the membranes are ruptured

G. Nitrazine test
   1. Use of a Nitrazine test strip to detect the presence of **amniotic fluid** in vaginal secretions
   2. Vaginal secretions have a pH of 4.5 to 5.5 and do not affect the yellow Nitrazine strip or swab
   3. **Amniotic fluid** has a pH of 7.0 to 7.5 and turns the yellow Nitrazine strip or swab blue

   4. Implementation
      a. Place the client in the dorsal lithotomy position
      b. Touch the test tape to the fluid
      c. Assess the test tape for a blue-green, blue-gray, or deep blue color, which indicates that the membranes are probably ruptured

H. Nonstress test (Box 22-2)

I. Contraction stress test (Box 22-3)

VI. NUTRITION (Box 22-4)

A. General guidelines
   1. The average expected weight gain during pregnancy is 2 to 4 pounds in the first trimester, and approximately 1 pound per week in the second and third trimesters
   2. Instruct the client to choose foods from the Food Guide Pyramid
   3. An increase of about 300 calories per day is needed during pregnancy

BOX 22-2
Nonstress Test (NST)

DESCRIPTION

Performed to assess placental function and oxygenation

Determines fetal well-being

Evaluates fetal heart rate (FHR) in response to fetal movement

IMPLEMENTATION

External ultrasound transducer and the tocodynamometer (toco) are applied to the mother, and a tracing of at least 20 minutes' duration is obtained so that the FHR and the uterine activity can be observed

Obtain baseline blood pressure (BP) and monitor BP frequently

Place mother in the left lateral position to avoid vena cava compression

The mother may be asked to press a button every time she feels fetal movement; the monitor records a mark at each point of fetal movement, which is used as a reference point to assess FHR response

RESULTS

Reactive Nonstress Test (Normal/Negative)

Indicates a healthy fetus

Two or more FHR accelerations of at least 15 beats per minute, lasting at least 15 seconds from the beginning of the acceleration to the end, in association with fetal movement, during a 20-minute period

Nonreactive Nonstress Test (Abnormal)

No accelerations or accelerations of less than 15 beats per minute or lasting less than 15 seconds in duration for a 40-minute observation

Unsatisfactory

Cannot be interpreted because of the poor quality of the FHR tracing

BOX 22-3
Contraction Stress Test

DESCRIPTION

Assesses placental oxygenation and function

Determines fetal ability to tolerate labor and determines fetal well-being

Fetus is exposed to the stressor of contractions to assess the adequacy of placental perfusion under simulated labor conditions

Performed if the nonstress test is abnormal

IMPLEMENTATION

The external fetal monitor is applied to the mother, and a 20- to 30-minute baseline strip is recorded

The uterus is stimulated to contract either by the administration of a dilute dose of oxytocin (Pitocin) or by having the mother use nipple stimulation until three palpable contractions with a duration of 40 seconds or more in a 10-minute period have been achieved

Frequent maternal BP readings are done, and the mother is monitored closely while increasing doses of oxytocin are given

RESULTS

Negative Contraction Stress Test

Represented by no late or variable decelerations of the FHR

Positive Contraction Stress Test (Abnormal)

Represented by late or variable decelerations of the FHR with 50% or more of the contractions in the absence of hyperstimulation of the uterus

Equivocal

Contains decelerations but with less than 50% of the contractions, or the uterine activity shows a hyperstimulated uterus

Unsatisfactory

Adequate uterine contractions cannot be achieved, or the FHR tracing is not of sufficient quality for adequate interpretation

4. A diet consisting of 2500 calories per day, depending on age, should meet the nutritional demands of pregnancy
5. Calorie needs are greater in the last two trimesters than in the first
6. An increase of about 500 calories per day is needed during lactation
7. Encourage a diet high in folic acid with folic acid supplements
8. A diet rich in folic acid is necessary for all women of child-bearing age to prevent neural tube defect in the fetus during the first trimester of pregnancy
9. Increase calories, proteins, vitamins, calcium, and other minerals as required
10. Drink at least 8 to 10 (8-oz) glasses of fluid each day, of which 4 to 6 glasses are water
11. Sodium is not restricted unless specifically prescribed by the physician or health care provider

BOX 22-4

Cultural Considerations in Nutrition

ASIAN, CHINESE, AND JAPANESE

Important foods in diet include seafood, rice, vegetables, and fresh fruits

Milk and cheese are used infrequently

ORTHODOX JEWISH

Poultry and some meat of cattle, sheep, goats, and deer are permissible; pork and pork products are not permissible

Milk and cheese may not be eaten with, or within 6 hours of, a meat meal

MEXICAN

Food products include corn, chili peppers, and beans

Milk is used infrequently

B. Vegetarianism
1. During pregnancy, it is necessary to obtain ample and complete proteins from dairy products and eggs
2. An adequate pure vegetarian diet contains protein from unrefined grains such as brown rice and whole wheat; legumes such as beans, split peas, and lentils; nuts in large quantities; and a variety of cooked and fresh vegetables and fruits
3. Seeds may provide protein if consumed in large enough quantities
4. Vegetarians do not eat any animal products; therefore a daily supplement of 4 μg of vitamin B_{12} is necessary
5. Complete protein may be obtained by eating any of the following food combinations at the same time:
a. Legumes and whole grain cereals
b. Nuts and whole grain cereals
c. Nuts and legumes

C. Lactose intolerance
1. Lactose consumed by an individual with an intolerance can cause abdominal distention, discomfort, nausea, vomiting, cramps, and loose stools
2. Milk may be tolerated in cooked form, such as in custards, or fermented dairy products
3. Cheese and yogurt are sometimes tolerated
4. Lactase, an enzyme, may be prescribed and is available as a tablet to be chewed before ingesting milk or milk products or as a liquid to add to milk
5. Lactase-treated milk or lactose-free products are also available commercially

D. Pica
1. Defined as eating substances that are not ordinarily considered edible or to have nutritive value
2. Practiced in poverty-stricken areas where diets tend to be inadequate, but pica may also be found at other socioeconomic levels
3. Substances most commonly ingested are dirt, clay, starch, and freezer frost
4. Iron deficiency anemia occurs as a result of pica

VII. ABORTION

A. Description: termination of pregnancy before the fetus is viable (20 weeks or a weight of 500 g)

B. Data collection
1. Spontaneous vaginal bleeding
2. Passage of clots and tissue through vagina
3. Low uterine cramping and contractions

C. Implementation
1. Maintain bed rest and vital signs
2. Count perineal pads to evaluate blood loss
3. Save expelled tissues and clots
4. Monitor IV fluids as prescribed to prevent shock
5. Prepare the client for dilation and curretage as prescribed for incomplete abortion

VIII. ACQUIRED IMMUNODEFICIENCY SYNDROME (AIDS)

A. Description
1. The human immunodeficiency virus (HIV) is a causative factor in the development of AIDS
2. HIV infection is a progressive, severe weakening of the immune system that makes an individual highly susceptible to other infections and certain types of cancer
3. The virus attacks the lymphocytes and produces immune deficiency by destroying the T-helper lymphocytes; this interferes with cell-mediated immunity
4. Develops slowly over years
5. Women infected with HIV virus may first demonstrate symptoms at the time of pregnancy or possibly develop life-threatening infections because normal pregnancy involves some suppression of the maternal immune system
6. Zidovudine (AZT) is recommended for the prevention of maternal-fetal HIV transmission and reduces the transmission risk if given late in pregnancy, during **labor**, and to the **newborn infant** for the first 6 weeks of life; zidovudine is administered orally at 14 to 34 weeks' gestation, intravenously during **labor**, and in the form of syrup to the **neonate** after birth

B. Transmission
   1. All body fluids from an infected host, except perspiration, have been shown to contain the virus
   2. Blood, semen, and breast milk have higher concentrations of the virus than urine, saliva, vomitus, and stool
   3. HIV can cross some membranes such as the **placental** barrier, the blood-brain barrier, vaginal mucosa, and (in the **neonate**) the walls of the GI tract
   4. Sexual contact
   5. Transfusion with blood or blood products
   6. Occupational exposure, such as in health care workers
   7. Shared needles during drug use and use of dirty needles
   8. Perinatal transmission from infected mother to fetus or **newborn** via transplacental transmission, via contamination with maternal blood during birth, or through breast milk

C. Risks to the mother
   1. The mother with HIV is managed as high-risk
   2. Frequent complaints of fatigue, shortness of breath, nausea, back pain, urinary frequency, and headaches
   3. More vulnerable to postpartum infections
   4. May need longer courses of antibiotics for infection

D. Diagnosis
   1. Client may be infected with the virus but has not yet produced antibodies, thereby testing negative, but being capable of infecting others
   2. Clients who by history may be at risk for possible HIV but test negative for the HIV antibody should be retested; it usually takes 6 to 12 weeks for a host to manufacture detectable HIV antibodies
   3. Enzyme-linked immunosorbent assay (ELISA) screening test for AIDS antibody is a very sensitive test but not highly specific; a positive ELISA test indicates the need for further testing using the Western blot

E. Data collection (Table 22-1)

F. Implementation
   1. Prenatal period
      a. Prevention of opportunistic infections
      b. Instruct the client on good handwashing procedure
      c. Avoid persons who are ill
      d. Avoid exposure to cat feces, cat or dog litter, or fish tanks
      e. Avoid undercooked meats, raw eggs, and unpasteurized milk
      f. Prevent further exposure to HIV through sexual contact or the use of needles
      g. Initiate recovery from substance abuse
      h. Avoid procedures that increase the risk of perinatal transmission, such as amniocentesis and fetal scalp sampling
   2. Intrapartal period
      a. Note that if the fetus has not been exposed to HIV in utero, the highest risk exists during **delivery** through the birth canal
      b. Never use scalp electrodes
      c. Avoid episiotomy to decrease the amount of maternal blood in and around the birth canal
      d. Avoid the administration of oxytocin (Pitocin) since oxytocin contractions can be strong, inducing vaginal tears or necessitating the need for episiotomy
      e. Minimize the **neonate's** exposure to maternal blood and body fluids
      f. Place heavy absorbent pads under the mother's hips to absorb **amniotic fluid** and maternal blood
      g. Promptly remove the **neonate** from the mother's blood after delivery
      h. Suction the **infant** promptly
      i. Prepare to administer AZT intravenously as prescribed during **labor** and **delivery**

TABLE 22-1

Stages of AIDS

Stage 1	Stage 2	Stage 3	Stage 4
Fever Myalgia Lymphadenopathy Headache	Active but asymptomatic and may remain so for years. May experience an outbreak of herpes zoster (shingles). May experience a transient thrombocytopenia.	Symptomatic; evidence of immune dysfunction. All body systems can present with signs of immune dysfunction. Integumentary and gynecological problems are common.	Advanced HIV infection. Vulnerable to common bacterial infections. Development of opportunistic infections. Serious immune compromise.

3. Postpartum period
   a. Monitor for signs of infection such as an increased temperature and white blood cell (WBC) count
   b. Place the mother in protective isolation to prevent infection if the mother is experiencing a suppressed immune response
   c. Restrict breastfeeding
   d. Instruct the mother how to take the temperature and to identify symptoms necessitating immediate follow-up care
   e. Urge the mother to refrain from donating blood or body organs
   f. Advise the mother to avoid sharing toothbrushes, razors, or other materials potentially contaminated with blood

G. The **neonate** and HIV
1. Description
   a. The fetus of an HIV antibody-positive woman should be monitored closely throughout the pregnancy
   b. Serial ultrasound screenings should be done to identify intrauterine growth restriction
   c. Weekly nonstress testing after 32 weeks of gestation and biophysical profiles may be necessary
   d. **Neonates** born to HIV-positive clients may test positive because the mother's positive antibodies may persist for as long as 18 months after birth
   e. The use of antiviral medication, reduction of **neonate** exposure to maternal blood and body fluids, and early identification of HIV in pregnancy reduce the risk of transmission to the **neonate**
   f. All **neonates** acquire maternal antibody to HIV infection, but not all acquire infection
2. Transmission
   a. Across the **placental** barrier
   b. During the process of **labor** and **delivery**
   c. Via breast milk
3. Implementation
   a. Bathe **neonate** carefully before any invasive procedure, such as the administration of vitamin K, heel sticks, or venipunctures
   b. **Neonate** can room with mother
   c. Prepare to administer AZT to the **newborn infant** as prescribed for the first 6 weeks of life
   d. All HIV-exposed **newborn infants** should be treated with medication to prevent infection by *Pneumocystis carinii*
   e. Note that an HIV culture is recommended at age 1 month and after 4 months; **infants** at risk for HIV infection should be seen by the physician at birth, 1 week, 2 weeks, 1 month, and 2 months of life
   f. **Infants** at risk for HIV infection need to receive all recommended immunizations at the regular schedule; no live immunizations should be administered
   g. Note that the **neonate** may be asymptomatic for the first several years of life; monitor for early signs of immune deficiency, such as an enlarged spleen or liver, lymphadenopathy, and impairment in growth and development

IX. ANEMIA

A. Description
1. Condition that can develop as a result of iron deficiency, with a hemoglobin below 10 g/dL or a hematocrit level below 30%
2. Anemia predisposes the client to postpartum infection and hemorrhage

B. Data collection
1. Fatigue
2. Headache
3. Pallor
4. Tachycardia
5. Hemoglobin below 10 g/dL and hematocrit below 30%

C. Implementation
1. Hemoglobin and hematocrit levels may be monitored every 2 weeks
2. Instruct client about iron and folic acid supplements
3. Instruct client to take iron with a source of vitamin C and to avoid taking iron with tea
4. Instruct client to eat foods high in iron, folic acid, and protein

X. CARDIAC DISEASE

A. Description: Inability to cope with the added plasma volume and the increased cardiac output

B. Data collection
1. Dyspnea and fatigue
2. Cough
3. Peripheral edema
4. Anginal-type pain
5. Palpitations and tachycardia

C. Implementation
1. Monitor vital signs, fetal heart rate, and condition of fetus
2. Plan activity level and emphasize the need for sufficient rest
3. Encourage adequate nutrition to prevent anemia

4. Maintain bed rest for client as prescribed during the last weeks of pregnancy
5. During **labor**
   a. Monitor vital signs frequently
   b. Place client on a cardiac monitor and on external fetal monitor
   c. Maintain bed rest with the mother lying on her side or in semirecumbent position
   d. Administer oxygen as prescribed
   e. Monitor for signs of pulmonary edema and heart failure
   f. Provide emotional support

XI. CHRONIC HYPERTENSION

A. Description
1. Hypertension that occurs before pregnancy, is diagnosed before the 20th week of gestation, or is diagnosed for the first time during pregnancy and persists beyond the 42nd day postpartum
2. The condition predisposes the client to PIH
3. Can cause **abruptio placentae** and intrauterine growth retardation

B. Data collection
1. Headaches
2. Visual changes
3. BP of 140/90 mm Hg or greater

C. Implementation
1. Monitor blood pressure
2. Monitor fetal activity and fetal growth
3. Encourage frequent rest periods, instructing the client to lie in the left lateral position
4. Administer antihypertensive medications as prescribed for diastolic pressures greater than 100 mm Hg
5. Monitor intake and output (I&O)

XII. DIABETES MELLITUS

A. Description
1. Chronic metabolic disease caused by a disturbance in normal production of insulin
2. Pregnancy places demands on carbohydrate metabolism and causes insulin requirements to increase

B. Insulin-dependent diabetes mellitus
1. Maternal glucose crosses the **placenta** but insulin does not
2. During the first trimester, maternal insulin needs decrease
3. Fetus produces its own insulin and pulls glucose from the mother, which predisposes the mother to hypoglycemic reactions
4. During the second and third trimesters, increases in **placental** hormones cause an insulin-resistant state, requiring an increase in the client's insulin dose
5. After **placental delivery**, **placental** hormone levels drop abruptly and insulin requirements decrease

C. Diabetes mellitus in pregnancy
1. Diabetes mellitus is more difficult to control during pregnancy
2. Premature **delivery** is more frequent
3. The **newborn infant** of a diabetic mother may be large in size but will have functions related to gestational age rather than size
4. The **newborn infant** of a diabetic mother is subject to hypoglycemia, hyperbilirubinemia, respiratory distress syndrome, and congenital anomalies
5. Stillborn and neonatal mortality rates are higher in pregnancies of a diabetic woman
6. Conditions that can occur as a result of diabetes mellitus include:
   a. Acidosis
   b. Infection
   c. PIH
   d. Hemorrhage
   e. Polyhydramnios
   f. Fetal death

D. Gestational diabetes mellitus
1. Occurs during the second or third trimester
2. Occurs in pregnancy in clients not previously diagnosed as diabetic and occurs when the pancreas cannot respond to the demand for more insulin
3. Pregnant women should be screened for glucose levels at the 26th week of gestation
4. A 3-hour glucose tolerance test will be performed to confirm diabetes mellitus
5. Oral hypoglycemic agents are never used during pregnancy
6. Frequently can be treated by diet alone; however, insulin may be needed for some clients
7. Most clients with gestational diabetes convert to normal after **delivery**; however, these individuals have an increased risk of developing diabetes mellitus in their lifetime

E. Predisposing conditions to gestational diabetes
1. Over age 35
2. Obesity
3. Multiple gestation
4. Family history of diabetes mellitus

F. Data collection
1. Excessive thirst
2. Hunger
3. Weight loss
4. Blurred vision
5. Frequent urination

6. Recurrent urinary tract infections and vaginal yeast infections
7. Glycosuria and ketonuria
8. Signs of pregnancy-induced hypertension
9. Polyhydramnios
10. Fetus large for gestational age

G. Implementation
1. Screen clients between the 24th and 28th weeks of pregnancy
2. Prenatal visits bimonthly for 6 months and weekly thereafter
3. The goal of therapy is to maintain the blood glucose in a narrow, low range of 65 to 130 mg/dL
4. Monitor for signs of hypoglycemia; episodes of mild or moderate hypoglycemia can be treated with oral intake of 10 to 15 g of simple carbohydrate
5. Observe for signs of hyperglycemia
6. Assess insulin needs
7. Monitor and maintain blood glucose levels according to gestational week
8. Monitor for glycosuria and ketonuria
9. Monitor weight
10. Insulin administration if blood glucose levels cannot be controlled by diet
11. Monitor for signs of preeclampsia, which include hypertension, proteinuria, and edema
12. Check for increased temperature and signs of infection
13. Instruct the client to report burning and pain on urination or vaginal discharge or itching
14. Monitor fetal status and for signs of premature **labor**
15. Monitor for signs of polyhydramnios
16. Increase calorie intake to 2200 to 2500 daily as prescribed, with adequate insulin therapy so that glucose will move into the cells
17. Calories in diet should consist of 50% to 60% carbohydrates, 12% to 20% protein, and 20% to 30% fat

H. Implementation during **labor**
1. Monitor fetal status continuously for signs of distress and, if noted, prepare the client for immediate cesarean section
2. Insulin is carefully regulated and IV glucose is administered as prescribed, as **labor** depletes glycogen

I. Implementation during the postpartum period
1. Observe the client closely for an insulin reaction; a precipitous drop in insulin requirements is usual
2. The client may not require insulin for the first 24 hours
3. Reregulate insulin needs as prescribed after the first day, according to blood glucose testing
4. Monitor dietary needs based on blood glucose and insulin requirements
5. Monitor for signs of infection or postpartum hemorrhage

XIII. DISSEMINATED INTRAVASCULAR COAGULATION (DIC)

A. Description
1. Condition in the mother's body that results in an exaggerated clotting process that increases the formation of clots in microcirculation
2. The rapid and extensive formation of clots results in bleeding and the potential vascular occlusion of organs from thromboembolus formation

B. Predisposing conditions
1. Abruptio placentae
2. Intrauterine fetal death
3. **Amniotic fluid** embolism
4. Pregnancy-induced hypertension
5. Liver disease
6. Sepsis

C. Data collection
1. Uncontrolled bleeding
2. Bruising, purpura, petechiae, and ecchymosis
3. Hematuria, hematemesis, or vaginal bleeding

D. Implementation
1. Monitor vital signs
2. Administer oxygen as prescribed
3. Monitor for bleeding and for signs of shock
4. Heparin may be prescribed to prevent clot formation

XIV. ECTOPIC PREGNANCY

A. Description: pregnancy that occurs in an other than uterine site, with **implantation** usually occurring in the fallopian tubes

B. Data collection
1. Pain unilaterally, with cramping and tenderness
2. Mass in the adnexa or cul-de-sac
3. Slight, dark vaginal bleeding
4. Fever
5. Low hemoglobin and hematocrit, elevated erythrocyte sedimentation rate
6. Profound shock if rupture occurs

C. Implementation
1. Obtain vital signs
2. Monitor for bleeding and signs of rupture
3. Obtain a blood specimen for type and crossmatch
4. Prepare the client for administration of methotrexate if prescribed, for masses smaller than 4 cm, to induce abortion and preserve the fallopian tube

5. Prepare the client for laparotomy and removal of pregnancy and tube, if necessary, or repair of tube

XV. ENDOMETRITIS

A. Description
1. Infection of the lining of the uterus after **delivery;** caused by bacteria that invade the uterus at the **placental** site
2. The infection may spread and involve the entire endometrium and cause peritonitis, pelvic thrombophlebitis, or cellulitis

B. Data collection
1. Chills and fever
2. Increased pulse
3. Decreased appetite
4. Headache
5. Backache
6. Prolonged, severe afterpains
7. Tender, large uterus
8. Foul odor to **lochia** or reddish-brown **lochia**
9. Ileus
10. Elevated WBC

C. Implementation
1. Monitor vital signs
2. Place the mother in Fowler's position to facilitate drainage of **lochia**
3. Provide a private room for the mother
4. Inform the mother that it is not necessary to isolate the **newborn infant** from the mother
5. Instruct the mother in proper handwashing techniques
6. Initiate wound and skin precautions as necessary
7. Monitor I&O and encourage fluids
8. IV antibiotics may be prescribed
9. Administer comfort measures such as back rubs and positioning changes, and pain medications as prescribed
10. Oxytoxic medications may be prescribed to improve uterine tone

XVI. FETAL DEATH IN UTERO (FDIU)

A. Description
1. Death of a fetus after the 20th week of gestation and before birth
2. DIC can develop if the dead fetus is retained in uterus for 3 to 4 weeks or more

B. Data collection
1. Absence of fetal movement
2. Absence of fetal heart tones
3. Maternal weight loss
4. Lack of fetal growth or decrease in fundal height
5. Lack of cardiac activity and other characteristics suggestive of fetal death noted on the ultrasound

C. Implementation
1. Prepare for **delivery** of the fetus
2. Support the client's decision about **labor**, birth, and the postpartum period
3. Facilitate the grieving process
4. Allow parents to hold **infant** after birth
5. Allow parents to name the **infant**
6. Accept such behaviors as anger and hostility from parents
7. Refer parents to an appropriate support group

XVII. HEPATITIS B

A. Description
1. An inflammation of the liver caused by the hepatitis B virus
2. Maternal fetal risk in uncomplicated hepatitis B is not generally increased unless infection occurs in the third trimester or in the immediate postpartum period
3. Intrapartum risks include increased risk for prematurity, premature **delivery,** and vertical fetal transmission

B. Transmission to fetus and **neonate**
1. Transplacental
2. Intrapartum exposure to infected blood, **amniotic fluid**, or vaginal secretions
3. Through postpartum exposure
4. Through breastfeeding

C. Risk to fetus and **neonate**
1. Infections in early life are usually asymptomatic
2. The **neonate** is identified as an HBsAg carrier
3. Chronic hepatitis
4. Associated with glomerulonephritis and nephritis

D. Implementation
1. Minimize the number of vaginal examinations
2. Minimize the risk for intrapartum ascending infections
3. Double-glove for extended periods of blood contact
4. Antibiotics may be prescribed during **labor** to decrease risk of transmission to the **neonate**, especially if the membranes are ruptured
5. Remove maternal blood from the **neonate** immediately after birth
6. Protect **neonate's** scalp integrity
7. Suction **neonate** immediately after birth
8. Bathe **neonate** before invasive procedures
9. Clean and dry the face and eyes before instilling eye prophylaxis

10. Discourage kissing until the mother and **neonate** have been treated
11. Support breastfeeding after maternal and neonatal treatment; breastfeeding is not contraindicated if an infected mother and **newborn infant** are treated
12. Immune globulin and vaccine are given to all HbsAg-positive **neonates** within 2 to 12 hours of **delivery**, at least before 24 hours, and not more than 7 days after birth
13. Inform the mother that HBV vaccine will be administered to the **neonate**, with the first dose given before the **newborn infant** leaves the hospital, the second dose at 1 month, and the third dose at 6 months
14. If the mother is identified positive more than 1 month after **delivery**, her HbsAg-negative **infant** should be treated

XVIII. HYDATIDIFORM MOLE

A. Description
   1. Developmental anomaly of the **placenta** that changes chorionic villi into a mass of clear vesicles
   2. Presents as an edematous grapelike cluster that may be nonmalignant or may develop into choriocarcinoma

B. Data collection
   1. Fetal heart rate not detectable
   2. Vaginal bleeding, which usually occurs by week 12, of bright red or dark brown color; may be slight, profuse, or intermittent
   3. Symptoms of PIH, such as an elevated blood pressure, edema, and proteinuria, which may be present before week 20
   4. Fundal height is greater than expected for date
   5. Elevated human chorionic gonadotropin (hCG) levels
   6. Ultrasound shows a characteristic snowstorm pattern

C. Implementation
   1. Monitor vital signs
   2. Prepare the mother for uterine evacuation or induced abortion
   3. Prepare for hysterectomy if necessary
   4. Monitor for postprocedure hemorrhage and infection
   5. Instruct the parents regarding birth control measures so that pregnancy can be prevented during the 1-year follow-up examination

XIX. HYPEREMESIS GRAVIDARUM

A. Description: intractable nausea and vomiting that persists beyond the first trimester and causes disturbances in nutrition, electrolytes, and fluid balance

B. Data collection
   1. Nausea most pronounced on arising; however, can occur at other times during the day
   2. Persistent vomiting
   3. Signs of dehydration and electrolyte imbalances

C. Implementation
   1. Monitor vital signs
   2. Monitor fetal heart rate and fetal activity
   3. Monitor for signs of dehydration and electrolyte imbalances
   4. Monitor daily weight
   5. Monitor I&O and calorie count
   6. Restrict PO intake until vomiting subsides; begin on a dry diet, alternating liquids and solids in small quantities, and advance the diet slowly
   7. IV fluids, electrolytes, and antiemetics may be prescribed

XX. INCOMPETENT CERVIX

A. Description
   1. Premature dilation of cervix, which occurs in the 4th or 5th month of pregnancy
   2. Is associated with cervical trauma as a result of a previous surgery or birth
   3. Treatment is surgical

B. Data collection
   1. Vaginal bleeding at 18 to 28 weeks of gestation
   2. Fetal membranes visible through the cervix

C. Implementation
   1. Monitor vital signs
   2. Monitor fetal heart rate
   3. Provide bed rest
   4. Prepare the client for surgery as prescribed

XXI. INFECTIONS

A. Toxoplasmosis (protozoa)
   1. Produces symptoms of acute, flulike infection in the mother
   2. Transmitted through raw meat or handling cat litter of infected cats
   3. Organism is transmitted across the **placenta**
   4. Spontaneous abortion likely to occur early in pregnancy

B. Rubella
   1. Organism is transmitted across **placenta**
   2. Extremely teratogenic in first trimester
   3. Causes congenital defects of eyes, heart, ears, and brain

4. Women with low titers should be vaccinated at least 3 months before becoming pregnant or after a **delivery**

C. Cytomegalovirus (CMV)
1. Produces flulike or mononucleosis-like symptoms in the mother
2. Transmitted through the respiratory or sexual route
3. Organism is transmitted across the **placenta,** or the fetus may be infected through birth canal
4. May cause fetal death, retardation, heart defects, deafness
5. No effective treatment available

D. Genital herpes
1. Affects the external genitalia, vagina, and cervix
2. Causes draining, painful vesicles
3. Viral is lethal to the fetus if it is inoculated during vaginal **delivery**
4. **Delivery** of the fetus is usually by cesarean section if active lesions are present in the vagina; **delivery** may be performed vaginally if the lesions are in the anal, perineal, or inner thigh area (strict precautions are necessary to protect the fetus during delivery)
5. No vaginal examinations are done in the presence of active vaginal herpetic lesions
6. Maintain isolation procedures during hospitalization if the disease is active
7. **Neonate** and mother may be separated during the active period or other special precautionary measures may be used to avoid transmission to neonate

XXII. MULTIPLE GESTATION

A. Description: results from double ovulation (fraternal or dizygotic) or a splitting of the fertilized egg (identical or monozygotic)

B. Data collection
1. Excessive fetal activity
2. Uterus large for gestational age
3. Palpation of three or four large parts in the uterus
4. Auscultation of more than one fetal heart rate
5. Excessive weight gain

C. Implementation
1. Monitor vital signs
2. Monitor fetal heart rate and fetal activity
3. Monitor for cervical changes
4. Assess fetal growth
5. Administer supplemental iron and vitamins as prescribed for anemia
6. Monitor for preterm **labor**
7. Prepare the client for ultrasound as prescribed
8. Prepare the client for cesarean section for abnormal presentation as prescribed
9. Oxytoxic medications may be prescribed after **delivery** to prevent postpartum hemorrhage from uterine overdistention

XXIII. PREGNANCY-INDUCED HYPERTENSION (PIH) 

A. Description
1. Acute hypertensive state that develops after the 20th week of gestation
2. The condition can be mild or severe and can progress to seizures (eclampsia) (Box 22-5)

B. Predisposing conditions
1. Primigravida
2. Teenagers and women over 35 years old
3. Poor nutrition
4. Low socioeconomic status
5. Chronic hypertension
6. Diabetes mellitus
7. Chronic renal disease
8. History of PIH

C. Complications of PIH
1. Abruptio placentae
2. DIC
3. Thrombocytopenia
4. **Placental** insufficiency
5. Intrauterine fetal death

D. Mild preeclampsia
1. Data collection
   a. Hypertension of 15 to 30 mm Hg above baseline
   b. Weight gain of 1 lb or more per week in the last trimester
   c. Mild, generalized edema
   d. Proteinuria of 1+
2. Implementation
   a. Provide bed rest and place the client in left lateral position
   b. Monitor blood pressure and weight
   c. Monitor neurological status, as changes can indicate cerebral hypoxia or impending seizure

BOX 22-5

Signs of Worsening PIH or Impending Seizures

BP 160/110 mm Hg or above
Epigastric pain
Decreased urinary output
Visual changes
Headache
Excessive proteinuria

d. Deep tendon reflexes are monitored for presence of clonus, as hyperreflexia indicates increased central nervous system irritability (Box 22-6)
e. Provide adequate fluids
f. Monitor I&O; a urinary output of 30 mL per hour indicates adequate renal perfusion
g. Increase dietary protein and carbohydrates with no added salt as prescribed
h. Administer medications as prescribed to lower the blood pressure to prevent a cerebrovascular accident; however, blood pressure should not be lowered drastically because **placental** perfusion can be compromised

E. Severe preeclampsia
1. Data collection
a. Severe hypertension, 30 to 40 mm Hg above baseline while on bed rest
b. Massive, generalized edema and weight gain
c. Proteinuria 4+
d. Less than 400 mL urine output in 24 hours
e. Severe headache
f. Dizziness
g. Blurred vision and spots before eyes
h. Nausea and vomiting
i. Epigastric pain
j. Central nervous system irritability
2. Implementation
a. Magnesium sulfate may be prescribed
b. Antihypertensive medications may be prescribed to prevent cerebrovascular accident
c. Prepare the client for induction of **labor**
d. Plan for administration of magnesium sulfate for 24 to 48 hours postpartum as prescribed

F. Eclampsia
1. Data collection
a. Severe edema
b. Proteinuria 4+
c. Sudden large increase in weight
d. Blood pressure greater than 160/110 mm Hg
e. Cyanosis
f. Fetal distress
g. Convulsions
h. Coma
2. Implementation
a. Protect the client from injury
b. Administer oxygen as prescribed
c. Monitor fetal heart rate and contractions
d. Initiate seizure precautions
e. Anticonvulsants may be prescribed
f. Prepare for **delivery** after stabilization of client

XXIV. SEXUALLY TRANSMITTED DISEASES (STD)

A. Chlamydia
1. Description
a. Common, sexually transmitted pathogen associated with an increased risk for premature births, stillborns, neonatal conjunctivitis, and **newborn** chlamydial pneumonia
b. In the nonpregnant state, it can cause salpingitis, pelvic abscesses, chronic pelvic pain, and infertility

BOX 22-6

Checking the Reflexes

PATELLAR

Client is positioned with legs dangling over the edge of the examining table or lying on the back with legs slightly flexed.
Strike patellar tendon just below the kneecap with the percussion hammer.
Normal Response: Extension or kicking out of leg.

BICEPS

The thumb is positioned over the client's biceps tendon supporting the client's elbow with the palm of the hand.
Strike a downward blow over the examiner's thumb with the percussion hammer.
Normal Response: Flexion of the arm at the elbow.

CLONUS

Position the client with the legs dangling over the edge of the examining table.
The leg is supported with one hand; sharply dorsiflex the client's foot with the other hand.
A dorsiflexed position is maintained for a few seconds; then the foot is released.
Normal Response: Negative clonus response.
Foot will remain steady in the dorsiflexed position.
No rhythmic oscillations or jerking of the foot will be felt.
When released, the foot will drop to a plantar flexed position with no oscillations.
Abnormal Response: Positive clonus response.
Rhythmic oscillations when the foot is dorsiflexed.
Similar oscillations will be noted when the foot drops to the plantar flexed position.

c. Incubation period is 5 to 10 days or longer, up to 28 days
d. Diagnostic test is culture for *Chlamydia trachomatis*

2. Data collection
a. Increased vaginal discharge and itching
b. Low-grade temperature
c. Right upper quadrant abdominal pain
d. Bleeding between periods
e. Pain with coitus
f. Dysuria
g. Rectal pain or discharge
h. Mucopurulent cervicitis
i. Cervix that bleeds easily
j. In the **newborn**, conjunctivitis and pneumonia

3. Implementation
a. Screen client to determine whether high risk; instruct client in the importance of rescreening, because reinfection can occur as the client nears term
b. Instruct client about the prescribed medication for treatment of the STD
c. Instruct mother about medication for the **neonate** if prescribed
d. Administer appropriate eye prophylaxis to the **neonate** as prescribed
e. Monitor **neonate** for signs and symptoms of pneumonia if at risk
f. Ensure that the sexual partner is treated

B. Syphilis
1. Description
a. A chronic infectious disease caused by the organism *Treponema pallidum*
b. Transmission is by intimate physical contact with syphilitic lesions, which are usually found on the skin or mucous membranes of the mouth and genitals
c. The incubation period is 2 to 6 weeks after exposure
d. Infection may cause abortion or premature **labor** and is passed to the fetus after the 4th month of pregnancy as congenital syphilis

2. Data collection (Table 22-2)
3. Implementation
a. Obtain serum test for syphilis on first prenatal visit; prepare to repeat the test just before the fourth month, as the disease may be acquired after the initial visit
b. Instruct client that treatment of her partner is necessary if infection occurs
c. Prepare to administer procaine penicillin G to the mother as prescribed

C. Gonorrhea
1. Description
a. Infection caused by *Neisseria gonorrhoeae*, that causes inflammation of the mucous membranes of the genital and urinary tract
b. Transmission of organism is by sexual intercourse
c. Infection may be transmitted to the baby's eyes during **delivery** causing blindness (ophthalmia neonatorum)

2. Data collection
a. Female: usually asymptomatic; vaginal discharge, urinary frequency, and pain possible
b. Male: fever, painful urination, pelvic pain, epididymitis with pain, tenderness, and swelling

3. Implementation
a. Obtain culture for gonorrhea on the first prenatal visit; prepare to repeat culture, as infection may occur during pregnancy
b. Administer prophylactic antibiotics: erythromycin or 1% silver nitrate to the **newborn infant** as prescribed
c. Instruct client that treatment of her partner is necessary if infection occurs

TABLE 22-2

Stages of Syphilis

Primary Stage	Secondary Stage	Tertiary Stage
Most infectious stage Appearance of ulcerative, painless lesions produced by spirochetes at point of entry into the body.	Highly infectious stage Lesions appear about 3 weeks after primary may occur anywhere on skin and mucous membranes. Generalized lymphadenopathy occurs.	Spirochetes enter the internal organs and causes permanent damage; symptoms may occur 10 to 30 years after occurrence of an untreated primary lesion. Invades the central nervous system, causing meningitis, ataxia, general paresis, and progressive mental deterioration. Affects the aortic valve and aorta.

D. Genital warts
   1. Description
      a. Caused by human papillomavirus (HPV) and affects the cervix, urethra, penis, scrotum, and anus
      b. Appears 1 to 2 months after exposure
      c. Transmitted through sexual contact
      d. There is no cure for HPV
   2. Data collection
      a. Small to large wartlike growths on genitals
      b. Cervical cell changes noted because HPV is associated with cervical malignancies
   3. Implementation
      a. Encourage yearly Papanicolaou smear
      b. Limit sexual contacts and use condoms
      c. Instruct client regarding potential treatment, including cytotoxic, cryotherapy, electrocautery, and surgical excision to remove the lesions

XXV. TUBERCULOSIS (TB)

A. Description
   1. Highly communicable disease caused by *Mycobacterium tuberculosis*
   2. Transmitted by the airborne route
   3. Tuberculosis has an insidious onset, and many clients are not aware of symptoms until the disease is well advanced
   4. A multidrug-resistant strain (MDR-TB) of TB can exist as a result of improper compliance or noncompliance with treatment programs and the development of mutations in the tubercle bacilli
B. Transmission
   1. Transplacental transmission is rare
   2. Can occur during birth through aspiration of infected **amniotic fluid**
   3. **Neonate** can become infected from contact with infected individuals
C. Risk to mother: active disease during pregnancy has been associated with an increase in hypertensive disorders of pregnancy
D. Diagnosis
   1. If a chest radiograph is required for the mother, it is done only after 20 weeks' gestation, and a lead shield to the abdomen is required
   2. TB skin testing is safe during pregnancy
   3. Many immigrants have false-positive PPDs as a result of the immunizations received in their home countries; therefore immigrants are more likely to require a chest radiograph after 20 weeks' gestation to assist in confirming the diagnosis
E. Data collection
   1. Maternal
      a. May be asymptomatic
      b. Fever and chills
      c. Night sweats
      d. Weight loss
      e. Fatigue
      f. Cough, hemoptysis, or green or yellow sputum
      g. Dyspnea
      h. Pleural pain
   2. **Neonate**
      a. Fever
      b. Lethargy
      c. Poor feeding
      d. Failure to thrive
      e. Respiratory distress
      f. Hepatosplenomegaly
      g. Meningitis
      h. Disease may spread to all major organs
F. Implementation
   1. Mother
      a. Administration of isoniazid (INH), ethambutol (Myambutol), and rifampin (Rifadin) for 6 to 12 months during and after pregnancy
      b. Pyridoxine should be administered with INH to pregnant women to prevent development of peripheral neuropathy caused by the INH
      c. Note that teratogenicity is unknown with rifampin
      d. Promote breastfeeding only if the mother is noninfectious
      e. Breastfeeding is not contraindicated with INH, ethambutol, or rifampin
      f. Note that pregnancy and immunosuppression are contraindications to bacille Calmette-Guérin (BCG) administration
   2. **Neonate**
      a. If born to a mother with active TB, should be treated with INH for 3 months
      b. **Neonates** born to infected mothers with active disease can be vaccinated with BCG; note that Mantoux test results will be positive after BCG is given
      c. Isolate and separate the **neonate** from the mother during active disease until the mother is known to be noninfectious, after a minimum of 3 weeks of medication therapy

PRACTICE QUESTIONS

1. A client is in her second trimester of pregnancy. She complains of frequent low back pain and ankle edema at the end of the day. The nurse recommends which measure to help relieve both discomforts?
   1. Lie on the floor with the legs elevated onto a couch or padded chair, with the hips and knees at a right angle
   2. Lie on the left side with the feet dorsiflexed
   3. Soak the feet in hot water after performing 10 pelvic tilt exercises
   4. Lie on the right side with the feet elevated on pillow and a heating pad to back
2. A client beginning week 30 of gestation comes to the clinic for a routine visit. Which of the following observations by the nurse indicates a need for teaching?
   1. The client is wearing panty hose
   2. The client is wearing shoes with arch supports
   3. The client is wearing nonslip shoes
   4. The client is wearing knee-high hose
3. The plan of care for a pregnant teen should include teaching regarding which of the following concerning dental care?
   1. Use toothpaste with baking soda to decrease plaque build-up
   2. Avoid the use of local anesthetics during dental work
   3. Expect to lose at least one tooth because of calcium and phosphorus leaving the teeth to nourish the fetus
   4. Tell the dentist office staff that she is pregnant
4. A pregnant woman complains of being awakened frequently by leg cramps. The nurse reinforces instructions to the client's partner and tells the partner to:
   1. Dorsiflex the client's foot while flexing the knee
   2. Dorsiflex the client's foot while extending the knee
   3. Plantarflex the client's foot while flexing the knee
   4. Plantarflex the client's foot while extending the knee
5. A nurse is providing instructions to a pregnant client with heartburn regarding measures that will alleviate the discomfort. The nurse instructs the client to:
   1. Lie down for 30 minutes after eating
   2. Drink decaffeinated coffee and tea
   3. Substitute salt in cooking for other spices
   4. Eliminate between-meal snacks
6. A nurse is reinforcing instructions to a pregnant woman who is complaining of low back pain. The nurse instructs the woman:
   1. To wear an abdominal support
   2. In the technique of pelvic tilt
   3. To relax abdominal muscles when standing
   4. To wear at least a 2-inch heel on her shoes
7. A client of 28 weeks' gestation is Rh negative and Coombs' antibody negative. The nurse determines that the client understands what the nurse has taught her about Rh sensitization when the client states:
   1. "I know I can never have another child."
   2. "I will have to have an injection once a month until the baby is born."
   3. "I will tell the nurse at the hospital that I had RhoGAM during pregnancy."
   4. "I am glad I won't have to have these shots if I have another child."
8. While assisting with the measurement of fundal height, the client (36 weeks' gestation) states she is feeling light-headed. Based on the nurse's knowledge of pregnancy, the nurse determines that this is most likely due to:
   1. Emotional instability
   2. Compression of the vena cava
   3. A full bladder
   4. Insufficient iron intake
9. A nurse is providing information to a pregnant woman about food items high in folic acid. Which of the following mid-afternoon snacks would be recommended to supply folic acid?
   1. 1 medium banana
   2. Nuts and green leafy vegetables
   3. 1 cup milk with 2 graham crackers
   4. 1 cup yogurt
10. A contraction stress test is scheduled for a client. The woman asks the nurse about the test. The most accurate description of the test includes which of the following?
    1. "Small amounts of oxytocin (Pitocin) are administered during internal fetal monitoring to stimulate uterine contractions."
    2. "An internal fetal monitor is attached and you will ambulate on a treadmill until contractions begin."
    3. "The uterus is stimulated to contract by either small amounts of oxytocin (Pitocin) or by nipple stimulation."
    4. "Uterine contractions are stimulated by Leopold's maneuvers."
11. A client at 38 weeks of pregnancy is admitted to the birthing center in early labor. The client is carrying twins and one of the fetuses is a breech presentation. The nurse assists in planning care for the client and identifies which of the following as the lowest priority in the care of this client?
    1. Attach electronic fetal monitoring
    2. Prepare the client for a possible cesarean section
    3. Measure fundal height
    4. Gather equipment for starting an IV

12. A stillborn was delivered in the birthing suite a few hours ago. After the birth, the family has remained together, holding and touching the baby. Which statement by the nurse would further assist the family in their initial period of grief?
    1. "Don't worry, there is nothing you could do to prevent this from happening."
    2. "We need to take the baby from you now so that you can get some sleep."
    3. "What have you named your lovely baby?"
    4. "We will see to it that you have an early discharge so that you don't have to be reminded of this experience."
13. A nurse is collecting data from a prenatal client. The nurse determines that which of the following places the client into the high-risk category for contracting human immunodeficiency virus (HIV)?
    1. Living in an area where HIV infections are minimal
    2. A history of IV drug use in the past year
    3. A history of one sexual partner within the past 10 years
    4. A spouse who is heterosexual and had only 1 sexual partner in the past 10 years
14. A perinatal client is admitted to the obstetric unit during an exacerbation of a heart condition. When planning for the nutritional requirements of the client, the nurse would consult with the dietitian to ensure which of the following?
    1. A low-calorie diet to ensure absence of weight gain
    2. A diet low in fluids and fiber to decrease blood volume
    3. A diet high in fluids and fiber to decrease constipation
    4. Unlimited sodium intake to increase circulating blood volume
15. A perinatal client is at risk for toxoplasmosis. The nurse would teach the client which of the following to prevent exposure to this disease?
    1. Wash hands only before meals
    2. Eat raw meats
    3. Avoid exposure to litter boxes used by cats
    4. Use topical corticosteroid treatments prophylactically
16. A nurse caring for a client with abruptio placentae is monitoring the client for signs of disseminated intravascular coagulopathy (DIC). The nurse would suspect DIC if the nurse observes:
    1. Pain and swelling of the calf of one leg
    2. Rapid clotting times
    3. Laboratory values indicating increased platelets
    4. Petechiae, oozing from injection sites, and hematuria
17. A nurse has a teaching session with a malnourished client regarding iron supplementation to prevent anemia during pregnancy. Which of the following statements, if made by the client, would indicate successful learning?
    1. "The iron is needed for the red blood cells."
    2. "Meat does not provide iron and should be avoided."
    3. "Iron supplements will give me diarrhea."
    4. "My body has all the iron it needs and I don't need to take supplements."
18. During a prenatal visit, a nurse is explaining dietary management to a client with diabetes mellitus. The nurse determines that the teaching has been effective when the client states:
    1. "I can eat more sweets now because I need more calories."
    2. "I need more fat in my diet so the baby can gain enough weight."
    3. "I need to eat a high-protein, low-carbohydrate diet now to control my blood glucose."
    4. "I need to increase the fiber in my diet to control my blood glucose and prevent constipation."
19. A nurse is assigned to assist in caring for a client at risk for eclampsia. When a client progresses from preeclampsia to eclampsia, the nurse's first action should be to:
    1. Prepare for the administration of IV magnesium sulfate
    2. Check the blood pressure and fetal heart tones
    3. Clear and maintain an open airway
    4. Administer oxygen by facemask
20. A nurse is doing a 48-hour postpartum check on a client with mild pregnancy-induced hypertension (PIH). Which of the following data indicate that the PIH is not resolving?
    1. Blood pressure reading has returned to the prenatal baseline
    2. Urinary output has increased
    3. The client complains of a headache and blurred vision
    4. There is no evidence of dependent edema

ANSWERS

1. *Answer:* 1

Rationale: The position described in option 1 will produce the posture of the pelvic tilt while countering gravity as the force that leads to edema of the lower extremities. Although the other options might seem useful, options 3 and 4 identify heat, which should be prescribed by the physician. Option 2 will not relieve back pain and ankle edema.

Test-Taking Strategy: Use the process of elimination. Focus on the issue of the question, back pain and ankle edema. Eliminate options 3 and 4 because the application of heat needs to be prescribed by the physician. From the remaining options, focus on the issue to direct you to option 1. Review measures that will reduce these discomforts if you had difficulty with this question.

Level of Cognitive Ability: Application

Client Needs: Physiological Integrity

Integrated Concept/Process: Nursing Process/Implementation

Content Area: Maternity

Reference: Burroughs A, Leifer G: *Maternity nursing,* ed 8, Philadelphia, 2002, WB Saunders, p. 69.

2. *Answer:* 4

Rationale: Varicose veins often develop in the lower extremities during pregnancy. Any constricting clothing such as knee-high hose impedes venous return from the lower legs and thus places the client at higher risk for developing varicosities. Clients should be encouraged to wear support (panty) hose. Flat, nonslip shoes with proper support are important to assist the pregnant woman to maintain proper posture, balance, and minimize fall risks.

Test-Taking Strategy: Note the key words "need for teaching." Use the process of elimination, seeking the option that will cause complications. Recalling that knee-high hose impedes venous return from the lower legs will direct you to option 4. Review these measures if you had difficulty with this question.

Level of Cognitive Ability: Comprehension

Client Needs: Health Promotion and Maintenance

Integrated Concept/Process: Nursing Process/Data Collection

Content Area: Maternity

Reference: Burroughs A, Leifer G: *Maternity nursing,* ed 8, Philadelphia, 2002, WB Saunders, p. 56.

3. *Answer:* 4

Rationale: Baking soda may irritate gums, which are more likely to bleed because of hormonal changes of pregnancy. Local anesthetics for minor dental work should not have adverse effects on the fetus. Option 3 is inaccurate information. The dental staff needs to know about the pregnancy so that care is taken during examinations and x-ray studies are avoided.

Test-Taking Strategy: Use the process of elimination. Focus on the safety of the unseen client (fetus). Option 4 is the most global option. Review client teaching points related to pregnancy if you had difficulty with this question.

Level of Cognitive Ability: Application

Client Needs: Safe, Effective Care Environment

Integrated Concept/Process: Nursing Process/Planning

Content Area: Maternity

Reference: Burroughs A, Leifer G: *Maternity nursing,* ed 8, Philadelphia, 2002, WB Saunders, p.58.

4. *Answer:* 2

Rationale: Leg cramps often occur when the pregnant woman stretches the leg and plantarflexes the foot. Dorsiflexion of the foot while extending the knee stretches the gastrocnemius muscle, prevents the muscle from contracting, and halts the cramping.

Test-Taking Strategy: Use the process of elimination. Knowledge regarding the actions that will alleviate muscle cramps will assist you in answering the question. Attempt to visualize each of the descriptions in the options to assist in directing you to the correct option. Review these measures if you had difficulty with this question.

Level of Cognitive Ability: Application

Client Needs: Health Promotion and Maintenance

Integrated Concept/Process: Teaching/Learning

Content Area: Maternity

Reference: Burroughs A, Leifer G: *Maternity nursing,* ed 8, Philadelphia, 2002, WB Saunders, p. 57.

5. *Answer:* 2

Rationale: Lying down after meals is likely to lead to reflux of stomach contents. Spices tend to trigger heartburn. Salt leads to the retention of fluid. Eating smaller, more frequent portions is preferable to eating three large meals to control heartburn. Caffeine, like spices, may cause heartburn.

Test-Taking Strategy: Use the process of elimination recalling those items that will cause heartburn. This will direct you to option 2. Review measures to alleviate heartburn if you had difficulty with this question.

Level of Cognitive Ability: Application

Client Needs: Health Promotion and Maintenance

Integrated Concept/Process: Self-Care

Content Area: Maternity

Reference: Burroughs A, Leifer G: *Maternity nursing,* ed 8, Philadelphia, 2002, WB Saunders, p. 56.

6. *Answer:* 2

Rationale: Pelvic tilt exercises decrease strain to the muscles of the abdomen and lower back caused by the added weight of the abdomen and the shift in the center of gravity. An abdominal support should be worn only if recommended by the physician. Relaxing abdominal muscles will add to the problem. Wearing 2-inch heels on shoes will add to the strain on the muscles and will exaggerate the shift in the center of gravity.

Test-Taking Strategy: Focus on the issue and use the process of elimination. Visualize each of the instructions in the options and think about its effect on relieving low back pain. Review the measures to relieve low back pain in the pregnant client if you had difficulty with this question.

Level of Cognitive Ability: Application

Client Needs: Physiological Integrity

Integrated Concept/Process: Teaching/Learning

Content Area: Maternity

Reference: Burroughs A, Leifer G: *Maternity nursing,* ed 8, Philadelphia, 2002, WB Saunders, p. 57.

7. *Answer:* 3

Rationale: It is accepted practice to administer RhoGam at 28 weeks of gestation to a woman as described in the question,

with a second injection within 72 hours of delivery. This prevents sensitization, which could jeopardize a future pregnancy. For subsequent pregnancies or abortions, the injections must be repeated because immunity is passive. Options 1, 2, and 4 are inaccurate information.
Test-Taking Strategy: Note the key words "that the client understands." Recalling the guidelines regarding the administration of RhoGam will direct you to option 3. Review Rh sensitization if you had difficulty with this question.
Level of Cognitive Ability: Comprehension
Client Needs: Physiological Integrity
Integrated Concept/Process: Nursing Process/Evaluation
Content Area: Maternity
References: Burroughs A, Leifer G: *Maternity nursing,* ed 8, Philadelphia, 2002, WB Saunders, p. 229.

8. *Answer:* 2
Rationale: Compression of the inferior vena cava and aorta by the uterus may cause supine hypotension syndrome in pregnancy. Having the woman turn onto her left side or elevating the left buttock during fundal height measurement will prevent or correct the problem. Options 1, 3, and 4 are not the cause of the client's problem described in the question.
Test-Taking Strategy: Focus on the data in the question and recall the complications associated with pregnancy. Use the ABCs—airway, breathing, and circulation—to direct you to option 2. Review vena cava syndrome if you had difficulty with this question.
Level of Cognitive Ability: Comprehension
Client Needs: Physiological Integrity
Integrated Concept/Process: Nursing Process/Data Collection
Content Area: Maternity
Reference: Burroughs A, Leifer G: *Maternity nursing,* ed 8, Philadelphia, 2002, WB Saunders, p. 57.

9. *Answer:* 2
Rationale: Folic acid is needed during pregnancy for healthy cell growth and repair. A pregnant woman should have at least four daily servings of foods rich in folic acid. The food items in option 2 contain folic acid. Bananas provide potassium. Milk and yogurt supply calcium.
Test-Taking Strategy: Knowledge regarding food sources high in folic acid is required to answer the question. Remembering that green leafy vegetable are high in folic acid will direct you to option 2. Review the foods high in folic acid if you had difficulty with this question.
Level of Cognitive Ability: Application
Client Needs: Physiological Integrity
Integrated Concept/Process: Nursing Process/Implementation
Content Area: Maternity
Reference: Burroughs A, Leifer G: *Maternity nursing,* ed 8, Philadelphia, 2002, WB Saunders, p. 65.

10. *Answer:* 3
Rationale: A contraction stress test assesses placental oxygenation and function, determines fetal ability to tolerate labor, determines fetal well-being, and is performed if the nonstress test is abnormal. The fetus is exposed to the stressor of contractions to assess the adequacy of placental perfusion under simulated labor conditions. An external fetal monitor is applied to the mother and a 20- to 30-minute baseline strip is recorded. The uterus is stimulated to contract either by the administration of a dilute dose of oxytocin (Pitocin) or by having the mother use nipple stimulation until three palpable contractions with a duration of 40 seconds or more in a 10-minute period have occurred. Frequent maternal blood pressure readings are done and the client is monitored closely while increasing doses of oxytocin are given.
Test-Taking Strategy: Knowledge regarding the contraction stress test is required to answer the question. Remember that in both the nonstress test and the contraction stress test, external monitoring is performed. Review this test if you had difficulty with this question.
Level of Cognitive Ability: Application
Client Needs: Physiological Integrity
Integrated Concept/Process: Nursing Process/Implementation
Content Area: Maternity
Reference: Burroughs A, Leifer G: *Maternity nursing,* ed 8, Philadelphia, 2002, WB Saunders, p. 75.

11. *Answer:* 3
Rationale: Option 3 is a low priority because fundal height should be measured at each antepartal clinic visit and not as a priority of care in the intrapartum period. Options 1, 2, and 4 are all high priorities. The twins should be monitored by dual electronic fetal monitoring and in so doing, any signs of distress need to be reported. Many physicians choose to perform a cesarean birth if either of the twins is breech. The mother should have an IV in place in case fluid or blood replacement is required.
Test-Taking Strategy: Note the key words "lowest priority." Use Maslow's Hierarchy of Needs theory and the ABCs—airway, breathing, and circulation—to prioritize and direct you to option 3. Review care to the pregnant client with a breech presentation if you had difficulty with this question.
Level of Cognitive Ability: Application
Client Needs: Physiological Integrity
Integrated Concept/Process: Nursing Process/Planning
Content Area: Maternity
Reference: Burroughs A, Leifer G: *Maternity nursing,* ed 8, Philadelphia, 2002, WB Saunders, p. 260.

12. *Answer:* 3
Rationale: Nurses should explore measures that assist the family to create memories of an infant so that the existence of the child is confirmed and so that parents can complete the grieving process. Option 3 meets this goal and also demonstrates a caring and empathetic response. Options 1, 2, and 4 are blocks to communication and devalue parents' feelings.
Test-Taking Strategy: Use therapeutic communication techniques and always focus on the client's feelings first. Option 3 demonstrates a caring and empathetic response by the nurse and addresses the grieving process. Review the grief process if you had difficulty with this question.
Level of Cognitive Ability: Application
Client Needs: Psychosocial Integrity
Integrated Concept/Process: Caring
Content Area: Maternity
Reference: Burroughs A, Leifer G: *Maternity nursing,* ed 8, Philadelphia, 2002, WB Saunders, p. 6.

13. *Answer:* **2**
Rationale: HIV is transmitted by intimate sexual contact and the exchange of body fluids, exposure to infected blood, and the transmission from an infected woman to her fetus. Women who fall into the high-risk category for HIV infection include those with persistent and recurrent sexually transmitted diseases or a history of multiple sexual partners, and those who use or have used IV drugs. Options 1, 3, and 4 are not situations that contribute to the incidence of contracting HIV.
Test-Taking Strategy: Knowledge regarding risk factors for HIV is necessary to answer the question. Use the process of elimination recalling that IV drug use places the client at high risk for contracting the disease. Review these risk factors if you had difficulty with this question.
Level of Cognitive Ability: Comprehension
Client Needs: Health Promotion and Maintenance
Integrated Concept/Process: Nursing Process/Data Collection
Content Area: Maternity
Reference: Burroughs A, Leifer G: *Maternity nursing,* ed 8, Philadelphia, 2002, WB Saunders, p. 363.

14. *Answer:* **3**
Rationale: Constipation causes the client to use the Valsalva maneuver. This causes blood to rush to the heart and overload the cardiac system. Absence of weight gain is not recommended during pregnancy. Diets low in fluid and fiber would cause a decrease in blood volume, which in turn deprives the fetus of nutrients. Too much sodium could cause an overload to the circulating blood volume and contribute to the cardiac condition.
Test-Taking Strategy: Use the process of elimination and try to relate the situation to something you are familiar with. Look for options that would apply to any heart condition and think about the needs of a pregnant client. Then, use the process of elimination. Review dietary measures for the client with cardiac disease if you had difficulty with question.
Level of Cognitive Ability: Application
Client Needs: Physiological Integrity
Integrated Concept/Process: Nursing Process/Planning
Content Area: Maternity
Reference: Burroughs A, Leifer G: *Maternity nursing,* ed 8, Philadelphia, 2002, WB Saunders, p. 56.

15. *Answer:* **3**
Rationale: Infected house cats transmit toxoplasmosis through feces. Handling litter boxes can transmit the disease to the maternity client. Meats that are undercooked can harbor microorganisms that can cause infection. Hands should be washed throughout the day when items that could be contaminated are handled. Topical corticosteroid treatment is not the pharmacological treatment of choice for toxoplasmosis.
Test-Taking Strategy: Use the process of elimination. Eliminate option 1 because of the absolute word "only." Option 2 also represents an extreme statement and should be eliminated. From the remaining options, recalling the causes and treatment for toxoplasmosis will direct you to option 3. Review the causes of toxoplasmosis if you had difficulty with this question.
Level of Cognitive Ability: Application
Client Needs: Health Promotion and Maintenance
Integrated Concept/Process: Teaching/Learning
Content Area: Maternity
Reference: Burroughs A, Leifer G: *Maternity nursing,* ed 8, Philadelphia, 2002, WB Saunders, p. 242.

16. *Answer:* **4**
Rationale: DIC is a state of diffuse clotting in which clotting factors are consumed. This leads to widespread bleeding. Platelets are decreased because they are consumed by the process; coagulation studies show no clot formation (and are thus prolonged); and fibrin plugs may clog the microvasculature diffusely, rather than in an isolated area.
Test-Taking Strategy: Use the process of elimination. Eliminate option 1 based on the knowledge that DIC is a widespread problem, not a localized one. Eliminate options 2 and 3 next because they are similar. Review the signs related to DIC if you had difficulty with this question.
Level of Cognitive Ability: Comprehension
Client Needs: Physiological Integrity
Integrated Concept/Process: Nursing Process/Data Collection
Content Area: Maternity
Reference: Burroughs A, Leifer G: *Maternity nursing,* ed 8, Philadelphia, 2002, WB Saunders, p. 229.

17. *Answer:* **1**
Rationale: A nutritional supplement commonly needed during pregnancy is iron. Anemia of pregnancy is primarily caused by iron deficiency. Iron supplements usually cause constipation. Meats are an excellent source of iron. Iron for the fetus comes from the maternal serum.
Test-Taking Strategy: Use the process of elimination. Note the key word "malnourished." Eliminate options 2 and 4 because of the absolute terminology "not" and "all." Knowledge regarding the effects of iron supplements would assist in eliminating option 3. Review the relationship of nutrition to anemia if you had difficulty with this question.
Level of Cognitive Ability: Comprehension
Client Needs: Physiological Integrity
Integrated Concept/Process: Teaching/Learning
Content Area: Maternity
Reference: Burroughs A, Leifer G: *Maternity nursing,* ed 8, Philadelphia, 2002, WB Saunders, p. 63.

18. *Answer:* **4**
Rationale: An increase in calories is needed with pregnancy, but concentrated sugars should be avoided because they may cause hyperglycemia. The fat intake should be at 20% to 30% of the total calories. The client with diabetes needs about 50% to 60% of the diet from carbohydrates and about 12% to 20% from protein. High-fiber foods will control blood glucose levels and prevent constipation.
Test-Taking Strategy: Note the key words "teaching has been effective." Use the process of elimination and knowledge regarding diabetes mellitus and diet therapy to direct you to the correct option. Review these components of the diabetic diet if you had difficulty with this question.
Level of Cognitive Ability: Comprehension
Client Needs: Health Promotion and Maintenance
Integrated Concept/Process: Nursing Process/Evaluation
Content Area: Maternity

Reference: Burroughs A, Leifer G: *Maternity nursing,* ed 8, Philadelphia, 2002, WB Saunders, p. 61.

19. *Answer:* 3
Rationale: The first action is to maintain an open airway and prevent injuries to the client. Options 1, 2, and 4 may be components of care but are not the first action.
Test-Taking Strategy: Note the key word "first." Use the ABCs—airway, breathing, and circulation—to answer the question. Airway is the first priority. Review care to the client with eclampsia if you had difficulty with this question.
Level of Cognitive Ability: Application
Client Needs: Physiological Integrity
Integrated Concept/Process: Nursing Process/Implementation
Content Area: Maternity
Reference: Burroughs A, Leifer G: *Maternity nursing,* ed 8, Philadelphia, 2002, WB Saunders, p. 230.

20. *Answer:* 3
Rationale: Options 1, 2, and 4 are all signs that the PIH is being resolved. Option 3 is a symptom of worsening of the PIH.
Test-Taking Strategy: Note the key word "not resolving." Recalling the signs of worsening PIH will direct you to the correct option. Review these signs if you had difficulty with this question.
Level of Cognitive Ability: Analysis
Client Needs: Physiological Integrity
Integrated Concept/Process: Nursing Process/Evaluation
Content Area: Maternity
Reference: Burroughs A, Leifer G: *Maternity nursing,* ed 8, Philadelphia, 2002, WB Saunders, p. 231.

REFERENCES

Burroughs A, Leifer G: *Maternity nursing,* ed 8, Philadelphia, 2002, WB Saunders.

Lowdermilk D, Perry S, Bobak I: *Maternity and women's health care,* ed 7, St Louis, 2000, Mosby.

McKinney E et al: *Maternal-child nursing,* Philadelphia, 2000, WB Saunders.

Murray S, McKinney E, Gorrie T: *Foundations of maternal-newborn nursing,* ed 3, Philadelphia, 2002, WB Saunders.

Labor and Delivery and Associated Complications

I. THE PROCESS OF LABOR

A. Labor
  1. Coordinated sequence of involuntary uterine contractions
  2. Results in effacement and dilation of cervix, followed by expulsion of products of conception
B. Delivery: actual event of birth
C. Passenger: the fetus
D. Attitude
  1. The relationship of the fetal body parts to one another
  2. Normal intrauterine attitude is flexion, in which the fetal back is rounded, the head is forward on the chest, and the arms and legs are folded in against the body
E. Lie
  1. Relationship of the spine of the fetus to the spine of the mother
  2. Longitudinal or vertical: Fetal spine is parallel with the mother's spine; fetus is either cephalic or breech presentation
  3. Transverse or horizontal:
    a. Fetal spine is at a right angle or perpendicular to the mother's spine
    b. Presenting part is the shoulder
    c. **Delivery** by cesarean section
  4. Oblique
    a. Fetal spine is at a slight angle from a true horizontal lie
    b. **Delivery** is by cesarean section if uncorrectable
F. Presentation
  1. Presenting part: portion of the fetus that enters the pelvis first
  2. Cephalic
    a. The most common presentation
    b. Fetal head presents first
  3. Breech
    a. Buttocks present first
    b. **Delivery** by cesarean section may be required, although it is often possible to deliver vaginally
  4. Shoulder
    a. Fetus is in a transverse lie, or the arm, back, abdomen, or side could present
    b. If the fetus does not spontaneously rotate or if it is not possible to manually turn the fetus, a cesarean section may be performed
G. Position: relationship of the assigned area of the presenting part or landmark to the maternal pelvis (Box 23-1)
H. Station
  1. The measurement of the progress of descent in centimeters above or below the midplane from the presenting part to the ischial spines
  2. Station o: at ischial spine
  3. Minus station: above ischial spine
  4. Plus station: below ischial spine

BOX 23-1

Fetal Positions

ROA—Right occiput anterior
LOA—Left occiput anterior
ROP—Right occiput posterior
LOP—Left occiput posterior
ROT—Right occiput transverse
LOT—Left occiput transverse
RMA—Right mentum anterior
LMA—Left mentum anterior
RMP—Right mentum posterior
LSA—Left sacrum anterior
LSP—Left sacrum posterior

I. Powers
  1. The forces acting to expel the fetus
  2. Effacement: shortening and thinning of the cervix during the first stage of **labor**
  3. Dilation: enlargement of cervical os and cervical canal during first stage

II. MECHANISMS OF LABOR (Box 23-2)

A. Data collection
  1. Lightening or dropping: fetus descends into the pelvis about 2 weeks before **delivery**
  2. Braxton Hicks contractions increase
  3. Show
  4. Vaginal mucosa congested and vaginal mucus increases
  5. Brownish or blood-tinged cervical mucus passed
  6. Cervix ripens, becomes soft and partly effaced, and may begin to dilate
  7. Sudden burst of energy
  8. Loss of 1 to 3 lb from water loss resulting from fluid shifts produced by changes in progesterone and estrogen levels
  9. Spontaneous rupture of membranes

B. False **labor**
  1. Exaggeration of normal contractions
  2. Does not produce dilation, effacement, or descent
  3. Contractions are irregular without progression
  4. Walking has no effect on contractions and often relieves false **labor**

C. True **labor**
  1. Contractions increase in duration and intensity
  2. Cervical dilation and effacement are progressive

III. LEOPOLD'S MANEUVERS

A. Description: to determine position, presentation, and engagement

B. Preparation
  1. Ask the mother to empty her bladder
  2. Hands are warmed and applied to the abdomen with firm and gentle pressure

C. First maneuver
  1. Determines which part of the fetus is in the fundus
  2. The palms are placed on each side of the upper abdomen and palpation around the fundus is done
  3. If the head is in fundus, the examiner feels a hard, round, movable object
  4. The buttocks will feel soft and have an irregular shape and are more difficult to move

D. Second maneuver
  1. The hands are moved downward over each side of the abdomen, applying firm, even pressure

BOX 23-2

Mechanisms of Labor

ENGAGEMENT
Mechanism by which the fetus nestles into the pelvis
Also termed as lightening or dropping

DESCENT
The process that the fetal head undergoes as it begins its journey through the pelvis
A continuous process from the time of engagement until birth and is assessed by the measurement called station

FLEXION
Process of the fetal head nodding forward toward the fetal chest

INTERNAL ROTATION
Internal rotation of the fetus; most commonly from the occiput transverse position assumed at engagement into the pelvis, to the occiput anterior position while continuously descending

EXTENSION
Enables the head to be born when the fetus is in a cephalic position
Begins after the head is crowned
Is complete when the head passes under the symphysis pubis and the occiput, and the anterior fontanel, brow, face, and chin pass over the sacrum and coccyx and are over the perineum

RESTITUTION
Realignment of the fetal head with the body after the head emerges

EXTERNAL ROTATION
The shoulders externally rotate after the head is born and restitution occurs, so that the shoulders are in the anteroposterior diameter of the pelvis

EXPULSION
The birth of the entire body

2. The fetus's back, which is a smooth, hard surface, should be felt on one side of the abdomen
3. Irregular knobs and lumps (the hands, feet, elbows, and knees) will be felt on the opposite side of the abdomen

E. Third maneuver
1. To confirm fetal position
2. A hand is placed above the symphysis pubis
3. The thumb and fingers are brought together to grasp the part of fetus between them, either the head or buttocks

F. Fourth maneuver
1. Used in the late stage to determine how far the fetus has descended into the pelvic inlet
2. Hands are placed on the sides of the lower abdomen, close to the midline
3. Hands are slid downward and pressed inward
4. If it has been determined that the buttocks are in the fundus, then the examiner feels for the head
5. If the head cannot be felt, it has probably descended

IV. BREATHING TECHNIQUES

A. Abdominal breathing
1. Used until **labor** is more advanced
2. The abdomen moves outward during inhalation and downward during exhalation
3. The rate remains slow, with approximately 6 to 9 breaths per minute

B. Pant-pant-blow
1. Used in advanced **labor**
2. A more rapid pattern, consisting of two short blows from the mouth followed by a longer blow
3. All exhalations are a blowing motion

V. FETAL MONITORING

A. Description
1. Displays the fetal heart rate (FHR)
2. Monitors uterine activity, frequency, duration, and intensity of contractions
3. Monitors the FHR in relation to maternal contractions
4. Baseline FHR is measured between contractions; the normal FHR is 120 to 160 beats per minute

B. External fetal monitoring
1. Noninvasive and performed by the use of a tocotransducer or Doppler ultrasonic transducer
2. Leopold's maneuvers are performed to determine on which side the fetal back is located; the ultrasonic transducer is placed over this area (fasten with a belt)
3. The tocotransducer is placed over the fundus of the uterus where contractions feel the strongest (fasten with a belt)
4. Allow the client to assume a comfortable position, avoiding vena cava compression

C. Internal fetal monitoring
1. Invasive and requires rupturing of the membranes and attaching an electrode to presenting part of the fetus
2. Mother must be dilated 2 to 3 cm to perform internal monitoring

D. Patterns
1. Fetal bradycardia
   a. Less than 120 beats per minute
   b. Change position of the mother and administer oxygen as prescribed
   c. The physician is notified
2. Fetal tachycardia
   a. Greater than 160 beats per minute
   b. Change position of the mother and administer oxygen as prescribed
   c. The physician is notified
3. Variability
   a. A change in the baseline FHR in response to fetal sleep, wake states, medications, and hypoxia
   b. A FHR that fluctuates 6 to 25 beats per minute at the baseline indicates a well-oxygenated functioning central nervous system (CNS)
4. Acceleration
   a. A transient rise in FHR of more than 15 beats per minute for more than 15 seconds
   b. May or may not be related to uterine contractions
   c. Marked acceleration (more than 180 beats per minute) may be related to prematurity, maternal fever, hypoxia, fetal infection, or medications
5. Decelerations: A transient decrease in the FHR
6. Early deceleration
   a. Decrease in the FHR below baseline
   b. Can be due to head compression
7. Variable deceleration
   a. An abrupt decrease in FHR that is variable in duration, intensity, and timing
   b. Can be due to cord compression
8. Late deceleration
   a. Decrease in the FHR below baseline
   b. Due to uteroplacental insufficiency
9. Hyperstimulation: increasing resting tone or peak contraction pressures
10. Implementation for altered patterns
    a. The physician is notified

b. Check for cord prolapse
c. Maintain the client in left lateral position
d. Administer oxygen as prescribed
e. Oxytocin infusion is discontinued as prescribed
f. Fetal scalp pH is done to determine a blood pH value
g. Intravenous (IV) fluids are increased as prescribed
h. Monitor and maintain blood pressure if hypotension occurs
i. Prepare the client for cesarean **delivery as prescribed**

VI. STAGES OF LABOR

A. Stage I latent phase
1. Data collection
a. Cervical dilation of 1 to 4 cm
b. Uterine contractions every 15 to 30 minutes; 15 to 30 seconds' duration of mild intensity
c. The mother talkative and eager to be in **labor**
2. Implementation
a. Encourage the mother and partner to participate in care
b. Assist with comfort measures, changes of position, and ambulation
c. Keep the mother and partner informed of progress
d. Offer fluids and ice chips
e. Encourage voiding every 1 to 2 hours

B. Stage I active phase
1. Data collection
a. Cervical dilation of 4 to 7 cm
b. Uterine contractions every 3 to 5 minutes, 30 to 60 seconds' duration of moderate intensity
c. The mother may experience feelings of helplessness
d. The mother becomes restless and anxious as contractions become stronger
2. Implementation
a. Encourage maintenance of effective breathing patterns
b. Provide a quiet environment
c. Keep the mother and partner informed of progress
d. Promote comfort with backrubs, sacral pressure, pillow support, and position changes
e. Instruct the partner in effleurage
f. Offer ointment for dry lips
g. Offer fluids and ice chips
h. Encourage voiding every 1 to 2 hours

C. Stage I transition phase
1. Data collection
a. Cervical dilation of 8 to 10 cm
b. Uterine contractions every 2 to 3 minutes, 45 to 90 seconds' duration of strong intensity
c. The mother becomes tired, is restless and irritable, and feels out of control
2. Implementation
a. Encourage rest between contractions
b. Wake the mother at beginning of contraction so she can begin breathing pattern
c. Keep the mother and partner informed of progress
d. Provide privacy
e. Offer ointment for dry lips
f. Offer fluids and ice chips
g. Encourage voiding every 1 to 2 hours

D. Implementation throughout stage I
1. Monitor maternal vital signs
2. Monitor FHR before, during, and after a contraction, noting that the normal FHR is 120 to 160 beats per minute
3. Monitor uterine contractions by palpation or monitor, determining frequency, duration, and intensity
4. Assist with monitoring the status of cervical dilation and effacement
5. Assist with monitoring the fetal station presentation and position by Leopold's maneuvers
6. Assist with the pelvic examination and prepare for a Nitrazine test and a fern test
7. Monitor the color of the **amniotic fluid** if the membranes have ruptured, because meconium stained fluid can indicate fetal distress

E. Stage 2
1. Data collection
a. Cervical dilation is complete
b. Progressive **labor** continues, with cervical dilation of 1 cm per hour for primigravidas and 1.5 cm per hour for multigravidas
c. Fetal descent occurring and demonstrated by change in fetal station
d. Uterine contractions occur every 2 to 3 minutes lasting 60 to 75 seconds, and the intensity is strong
e. Increase in bloody show occurs
f. The mother may feel out of control, helpless, and panicky
g. The mother feels urge to bear down; assist her in pushing efforts
2. Implementation
a. Monitor maternal vital signs
b. Monitor the FHR before, during, and after a contraction

c. Monitor uterine contractions by palpation or monitor, determining frequency, duration and intensity
d. Provide the mother with encouragement and praise
e. Keep the mother and partner informed of progress
f. Maintain privacy
g. Provide ice chips
h. Assist the mother into position that promotes comfort and assists pushing efforts as lithotomy, semisitting, kneeling, side lying, or squatting
i. Monitor for signs of approaching birth, such as perineal bulging or visualization of the fetal head
j. Prepare for birth

F. Stage 3
1. Data collection
a. Contractions occur until the **placenta** is born
b. **Placental** separation and expulsion occurs
c. Birth of **placenta** occurs 5 to 30 minutes after birth of baby
d. Schultze's mechanism: center portion of the **placenta** separates first and its shiny fetal surface emerges from the vagina
e. Duncan's mechanism: margin of the **placenta** separates, and a dull, red, rough maternal surface emerges from the vagina first
2. Implementation
a. Monitor maternal vital signs and uterine status
b. After birth of the **placenta**, the uterine fundus remains firm and is located 2 fingerbreadths below the umbilicus
c. Examine the **placenta** for cotyledons and membranes
d. Monitor the mother for shivering and provide warmth
e. Promote parental-**newborn** attachment
f. Assist with **newborn** assessment and Apgar Score

G. Stage 4
1. Description: The period from 1 to 4 hours after **delivery**
2. Data collection
a. Blood pressure returns to prelabor level
b. Pulse is slightly lower than during **labor**
c. Fundus remains contracted, in midline, 1 to 2 fingerbreadths below the umbilicus
d. **Lochia** is moderate or scant and is red
3. Implementation
a. Monitor maternal vital signs frequently
b. Provide warm blankets
c. Provide icepacks to the perineum
d. Massage the uterus if needed as prescribed

VII. ANESTHESIA

A. Local anesthesia
1. Used for blocking pain during episiotomy
2. Administered just before birth of the baby
3. No effect on the fetus

B. Paracervical block
1. Used in the first stage of **labor**
2. Provides a rapid block of uterine pain
3. No effect on the perineal area
4. No effect on the ability to bear down
5. May cause fetal bradycardia

C. Pudendal block
1. Administered just before the birth of the baby
2. Injection site is at pudendal nerve through a transvaginal route
3. Blocks perineal area for episiotomy
4. Effects last about 30 minutes
5. No effects on contractions or fetus

D. Epidural block
1. Injection site in epidural space at L3-L4
2. Administered after **labor** is established or just before a scheduled cesarean birth
3. Relieves pain from contractions and numbs vagina and perineum
4. May cause hypotension
5. Does not cause headache because the dura mater is not penetrated
6. Monitor maternal blood pressure
7. Maintain the mother in the side-lying position or place a rolled blanket beneath the right hip to displace the uterus from the vena cava
8. IV fluids are administered and increased as prescribed if hypotension occurs

E. Spinal block
1. Injection site in spinal subarachnoid space at L3-L5
2. Administered just before birth
3. Relieves uterine and perineal pain and numbs vagina, perineum, and lower extremities
4. May cause maternal hypotension
5. May cause postpartum headache
6. The mother must lie flat 8 to 12 hours after spinal injection
7. Place a rolled blanket under the right hip to displace the uterus from vena cava
8. IV fluids are administered as prescribed

F. General anesthesia
1. May be used for some surgical interventions
2. The mother is not awake
3. Presents a danger of respiratory depression and vomiting

VIII. OBSTETRICAL PROCEDURES

A. Bishop score (Box 23-3)
   1. Used to determine maternal readiness for **labor**
   2. Evaluates cervical status and fetal position
   3. Indicated before the induction of **labor**
   4. The five factors are assigned a score of 0 to 3, and the total score is calculated
   5. A score of 6 or more indicates a readiness for **labor** induction

B. Induction
   1. A deliberate initiation of uterine contractions that stimulates **labor**
   2. Elective induction may be accomplished by oxytocin (Pitocin) infusion
   3. IV dosage of oxytocin is increased as prescribed only after assessing contractions, FHR, and maternal blood pressure and pulse
   4. The rate of oxytocin is not increased once the desired contraction pattern is obtained (contraction frequency of 2 to 3 minutes lasting 60 seconds)
   5. Oxytocin infusion is discontinued as prescribed if contraction frequency is less than 2 minutes or duration is more than 90 seconds, or if fetal distress is noted

C. Amniotomy
   1. Artificial rupture of membranes (AROM); performed by the physician to stimulate **labor**
   2. Increases the risk of prolapsed cord and infection
   3. Monitor FHR before and after AROM
   4. Record time of AROM, FHR, and characteristics of fluid
   5. Meconium stained **amniotic fluid** may be associated with fetal distress
   6. Bloody **amniotic fluid** may indicate abruptio placentae or fetal trauma
   7. An unpleasant odor to **amniotic fluid** is associated with infection
   8. Limit maternal activity after AROM if prescribed

D. External version
   1. External manipulation of the fetus from an abnormal position into a normal presentation
   2. Indicated for an abnormal presentation that exists after the 34th week
   3. If mother is Rh-negative, ensure that RH immune globulin was given at 28 weeks' gestation
   4. A nonstress test may be performed to evaluate fetal well-being
   5. IV fluids and tocolytic therapy may be administered to relax the uterus and permit easier manipulation of fetus
   6. Ultrasound is used during the procedure to evaluate fetal position and **placental** placement and guide direction to the fetus
   7. Abdominal wall is manipulated to direct the fetus into a cephalic presentation if possible
   8. Monitor blood pressure to identify vena cava compression
   9. Monitor for unusual pain
   10. After the procedure
       a. A nonstress test is performed to evaluate fetal well-being
       b. Monitor for uterine activity, bleeding, ruptured membranes, and decreased fetal activity
       c. With Rh-negative clients, a Kleihauer-Betke test is performed as prescribed to detect the presence and amount of fetal blood in the maternal circulation and to identify clients who need additional Rh immune globulin

E. Episiotomy
   1. Incision made into perineum to enlarge the vaginal outlet and facilitate **delivery**
   2. Check episiotomy site
   3. Institute measures to relieve pain
   4. Provide ice pack during the first 24 hours
   5. Instruct the mother in the use of sitz baths
   6. Apply analgesic spray or ointment as prescribed
   7. Provide perineal care, using clean technique
   8. Instruct the mother in the proper care of the incision
   9. Instruct the mother to dry the perineal area from front to back and to blot the area rather than wipe it
   10. Instruct the mother to shower rather than bathe in a tub
   11. Apply a peripad without touching the inside surface of the pad
   12. Report any bleeding or discharge

F. Forceps **delivery**
   1. Two double-crossed, spoonlike articulated blades that are used to assist in the **delivery** of the fetal head
   2. Reassure the mother and explain the need for forceps

BOX 23-3

Factors of the Bishop Score

Dilation of cervix
Effacement of cervix
Consistency of cervix
Position of cervix
Station of presenting part

3. Check **neonate** and mother after **delivery** for any possible injury
4. Assist with repair of any lacerations

G. Vacuum extraction
1. A caplike suction device is applied to the fetal head to facilitate extraction
2. Suction is used to assist in **delivery** of the fetal head
3. Traction is applied during uterine contraction until descent of the fetal head is achieved
4. The suction device should not be kept in place longer than 25 minutes
5. Monitor FHR every 5 minutes if external fetal monitoring is not used
6. Monitor **newborn** at birth and throughout the postpartum period for signs of cerebral trauma
7. Monitor for developing cephalohematoma
8. Caput succedaneum is normal and will resolve in 24 hours

H. Cesarean **delivery**
1. **Delivery** of the fetus through a transabdominal, low segment incision of the uterus
2. Preoperative
   a. If planned, prepare the mother and partner
   b. If an emergency, quickly explain the need and procedure to the mother and partner
   c. Obtain informed consent
   d. Make sure that the preoperative diagnostic tests are done, including the Rh factor
   e. Prepare the mother for insertion of an IV line and a Foley catheter
   f. Prepare the abdomen as prescribed
   g. Monitor the mother and fetus continuously for signs of **labor**
   h. Provide emotional support
   i. Administer preoperative medications as prescribed
3. Postoperative
   a. Monitor vital signs
   b. Provide pain relief
   c. Encourage turning, coughing, and deep breathing
   d. Encourage ambulation
   e. Monitor for signs of infection and bleeding
   f. Burning and pain on urination may indicate a bladder infection
   g. A tender uterus and foul-smelling **lochia** may indicate endometritis
   h. A productive cough or chills may indicate pneumonia
   i. A positive Homans' sign, pain, or edema of an extremity may indicate thrombophlebitis

IX. DYSTOCIA

A. Description
1. Difficult **labor** that is prolonged or more painful
2. Occurs because of problems caused by uterine contractions, the fetus, or the bones and tissues of the maternal pelvis
3. Contractions may be hypotonic or hypertonic
4. Fetus may be excessively large, malpositioned, or in an abnormal presentation

B. Data collection
1. Excessive abdominal pain
2. Abnormal contraction pattern
3. Fetal distress
4. Elevated maternal temperature
5. Maternal or fetal tachycardia
6. Lack of progress in **labor**
7. Ketonuria
8. Decreased urine output

C. Implementation
1. Monitor FHR and for fetal distress
2. Monitor uterine contractions, maternal temperature, and heart rate
3. Assist with pelvic examination, measurements, ultrasounds, and other procedures
4. Oxytocin infusion may be prescribed; prophylactic antibiotics may be prescribed to prevent infection
5. Monitor IV fluids, I&O, and for signs of dehydration
6. Instruct the mother in breathing techniques and relaxation exercises
7. Monitor color of **amniotic fluid**
8. Provide comfort as with a normal **delivery** such as backrubs and position changes
9. Monitor the mother's fatigue and pain and administer sedatives and pain medications as prescribed
10. Monitor for prolapse of the cord after rupture of the membranes
11. If prolapse occurs
    a. Place the mother in Trendelenburg or knee-chest position to minimize pressure on the cord
    b. Administer oxygen as prescribed
    c. The physician is notified
    d. Prepare the mother for emergency cesarean section

X. PRECIPITOUS LABOR AND DELIVERY

A. Description: **labor** lasts less than 3 hours

B. Implementation
1. Stay with the mother at all times

2. Provide emotional support and keep the mother calm
3. Encourage the mother to pant between contractions
4. Prepare the mother for rupturing membranes when the head crowns, if not already ruptured
5. Do not try to keep the fetus from being delivered
6. Gentle pressure is applied to the fetal head upward toward the vagina to prevent damage to the head and vaginal lacerations
7. Fetus is delivered between contractions, checking for the cord around the neck
8. If outside of the hospital, the cord is clamped in two places and cut between with a clean knife or scissors after the cord stops pulsating, the **placenta** is allowed to separate naturally, and the **newborn** is placed on the mother's abdomen or breast to induce uterine contractions

XI. PRETERM LABOR

A. Description
1. **Labor** occurring after the 20th week but before the 37th week
2. Contractions occurring at least once every 10 minutes and lasting 30 seconds or longer
3. Documented cervical change or cervical effacement of 80% or dilation of 2 cm

B. Data collection
1. Increased or bloody discharge
2. Backache, pressure, and cramping
3. Palpable uterine contractions
4. Diarrhea

C. Implementation
1. Maintain bed rest, a quiet environment, and a lateral recumbent position
2. Tocolytic medications may be prescribed to suppress **labor**
3. Betamethasone (Celestone) may be administered to stimulate fetal lung maturity when preterm **delivery** appears inevitable
4. When magnesium sulfate is administered
   a. Monitor effects of medications on **labor** and fetus; monitor FHR
   b. Reflexes are monitored
   c. Have antidote (calcium gluconate) available at the bedside
   d. Monitor vital signs and for signs of maternal hypotension
   e. Monitor for increased respiratory rate, which may indicate pulmonary edema
   f. Monitor for signs of fluid overload

XII. RUPTURE OF THE UTERUS

A. Description: complete or incomplete separation of the uterine tissue due to rupture of the uterus from the stress of **labor**

B. Complete rupture of the uterus
1. Pain, which is shearing, excruciating, diffuse, or localized
2. Contractions may stop or fail to progress
3. Relaxation between contractions is incomplete
4. Rigid abdomen
5. Signs of maternal shock
6. Absent FHR
7. Fetus palpated outside the uterus

C. Incomplete rupture of the uterus
1. Abdominal pain that occurs during contractions
2. Cervix fails to dilate
3. Slight vaginal bleeding
4. Absent FHR

D. Implementation
1. Monitor maternal and fetal vital signs
2. Prepare the client for cesarean section or hysterotomy with hysterectomy
3. Provide emotional support for the client and partner
4. Monitor for and treat signs of shock as prescribed

XIII. PLACENTA PREVIA

A. Description
1. Improperly implanted **placenta** in the lower uterine segment near or over the internal os of the cervix
2. Complete, total, or central: internal os covered by **placenta** when cervix is fully dilated
3. Partial: incomplete coverage of os, marginal or low-lying with only the edge of the **placenta** approaching the internal os

B. Data collection
1. Painless bleeding as early as 7 months
2. Bleeding may range from mild to hemorrhage
3. Soft uterus
4. Abnormal fetal position of breech or transverse lie
5. High presenting part
6. Uterine contractions

C. Implementation
1. Monitor maternal vital signs, FHR, and fetal activity
2. Monitor bleeding, including amount and quality
3. Maintain bed rest and position the mother in left lateral position

4. Monitor IV fluids as prescribed and for signs of shock
5. Avoid a vaginal examination if bleeding is occurring
6. Prepare for ultrasound for **placenta**l localization
7. Prepare to administer Rh immune globulin if the mother is Rh negative and has not been given the injection at 28 weeks' gestation
8. Prepare for premature birth or cesarean section

XIV. ABRUPTIO PLACENTAE

A. Description: premature separation of the **placenta** from the uterine wall after 20th week of gestation and before the fetus is delivered

B. Data collection
1. Painful vaginal bleeding
2. Hypertonic to tetanic, enlarged uterus
3. Boardlike rigidity of abdomen
4. Abnormal or absent fetal heart tones
5. Bloody **amniotic fluid**
6. Rising fundal height from blood trapped behind the **placenta**
7. Signs of shock

C. Implementation
1. Monitor maternal vital signs and FHR
2. Monitor for vaginal bleeding, abdominal pain, and increase in fundal height
3. Maintain bed rest
4. Administer oxygen as prescribed
5. Monitor and report any uterine activity
6. Monitor IV fluids as prescribed
7. Monitor I&O, because a urine output of less than 30 mL per hour indicates decreased renal perfusion
8. Prepare for the **delivery** of the fetus as quickly as possible with vaginal **delivery** preferable if the fetus is healthy and stable, and the presenting part is in the pelvis
9. Prepare for emergency cesarean section if the fetus is alive but shows signs of distress
10. Monitor for signs of disseminated intravascular coagulation (DIC), particularly in the postpartum period

XV. PROLAPSED CORD

A. Description: umbilical cord is displaced, either between the presenting part and the amnion or else protruding through the cervix, and causes compression of the cord, compromising fetal circulation

B. Data collection
1. A feeling that something is coming through the vagina
2. Umbilical cord is seen or palpated
3. FHR is irregular and slow
4. If fetal hypoxia is severe, violent fetal activity may occur and then cease

C. Implementation
1. Relieve cord pressure immediately
2. Place the mother in knee-chest or Trendelenburg position
3. Elevate the fetal presenting part that is lying on the cord by applying finger pressure with a sterile gloved hand
4. Do not attempt to push the cord into the uterus
5. Monitor FHR and for signs of fetal hypoxia
6. Administer oxygen by face mask to the mother as prescribed
7. Prepare for cesarean birth

XVI. INVERTED UTERUS

A. Description: uterus turns inside out usually during **delivery** of the **placenta**

B. Data collection
1. Hemorrhage
2. Severe pain
3. Signs of shock

C. Implementation
1. Monitor vital signs
2. Monitor for signs of shock
3. Prepare the client for a return of the uterus to the correct position via the vagina

XVII. AMNIOTIC FLUID EMBOLISM

A. Description
1. The escape of **amniotic fluid** into the maternal circulation
2. The debris containing **amniotic fluid** deposits in the pulmonary arterioles and is usually fatal to the mother

B. Data collection
1. Dyspnea
2. Sudden chest pain
3. Cyanosis
4. Pulmonary edema

C. Implementation
1. Institute emergency measures to maintain life
2. Monitor vital signs
3. Administer oxygen as prescribed
4. Monitor for uncontrolled hemorrhage
5. Assist with the administration of medications as prescribed
6. Prepare for forceps **delivery** if the cervix is dilated

XVIII. VENA CAVA SYNDROME (SUPINE HYPOTENSIVE SYNDROME) (Figure 23-1)

A. Description
   1. Occurs when the venous return to the heart is impaired by the weight of uterus
   2. Results in partial occlusion of the vena cava

B. Data collection
   1. Signs of shock
   2. Hypotension
   3. Tachycardia
   4. Sweating
   5. Nausea and vomiting
   6. Fetal distress

C. Implementation
   1. Monitor vital signs
   2. Monitor FHR
   3. Administer oxygen as prescribed
   4. Position the mother by turning her to a lateral recumbent position to shift the weight of the fetus off the inferior vena cava
   5. Monitor for signs of shock caused by reduced cardiac output

XIX. HEMATOMA

A. Description
   1. The formation of a hematoma after the escape of blood into the tissues of the reproductive sac after the **delivery**
   2. Predisposing conditions include operative **delivery** with forceps or injury to a blood vessel
   3. A life-threatening condition

B. Data collection
   1. Abnormal severe pain and pressure in the perineal area
   2. Sensitive, palpable tumor in perineal area with discolored skin
   3. Inability to void
   4. Decreased hemoglobin and hematocrit
   5. Signs of shock such as pallor, tachycardia, and hypotension if significant blood loss has occurred

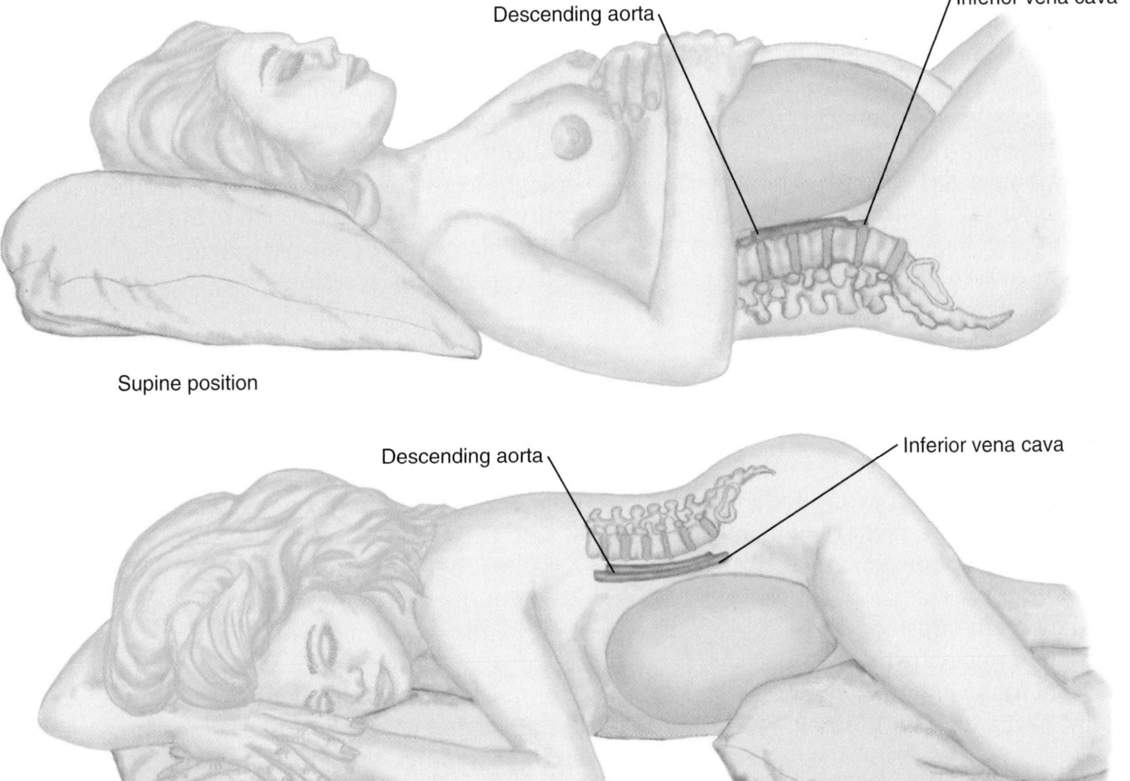

FIG. 23-1 Supine hypotensive syndrome. When the woman is in the supine position, the weight of the gravid uterus partially occludes the vena cava and the descending aorta. A lateral recumbent position corrects supine hypotension. (From Murray S, McKinney E, Gorrie T: *Foundations of maternal-newborn nursing*, ed 3, Philadelphia, 2002, WB Saunders.)

C. Implementation
1. Monitor vital signs
2. Monitor the mother for abnormal pain, especially when forceps **delivery** has occurred
3. Place ice to the hematoma site
4. Administer analgesics as prescribed
5. Monitor I&O
6. Encourage fluids
7. Encourage voiding
8. Prepare for urinary catheterization if the mother is unable to void
9. Monitor for signs of infection such as increased temperature, pulse rate, and white blood cell count
10. Prepare for incision and evacuation of hematoma if necessary

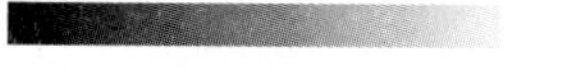

XX. FETAL DISTRESS

A. Data collection
1. FHR is above 160 or below 120 beats per minute
2. Meconium-stained fluid
3. Fetal hyperactivity
4. Fetal pH below 7.2

B. Implementation
1. Position the mother by turning her to her left side; elevate legs
2. Administer oxygen via face mask as prescribed
3. Oxytocin infusion is discontinued as prescribed
4. IV may be increased to treat hypotension
5. Monitor vital signs
6. Prepare for emergency cesarean section

PRACTICE QUESTIONS

1. The nurse is assigned to assist in caring for a client admitted to the labor unit. The client is dilated 9 cm and is experiencing precipitous labor. A priority nursing action is to:
   1. Prepare for an oxytocin infusion
   2. Keep the client in a side-lying position
   3. Prepare the client for an epidural anesthesia
   4. Encourage the client to start pushing with the contractions
2. A client is admitted to the labor suite complaining of painless vaginal bleeding. The nurse assists with the examination of the client knowing that a routine labor procedure that is contraindicated with this client's situation is:
   1. Leopold maneuvers
   2. External electronic fetal heart rate monitoring
   3. A manual pelvic examination
   4. Hemoglobin and hematocrit evaluation
3. A nurse is assigned to assist in caring for a client with abruptio placentae who is experiencing vaginal bleeding. The nurse collects data from the client knowing that abruptio placentae is accompanied by which additional finding?
   1. Abdomen soft upon palpation
   2. No complaints of abdominal pain
   3. Lack of uterine irritability or tetanic contractions
   4. Uterine tenderness upon palpation
4. A nurse is assigned to work in the delivery room and is assisting in caring for a client who has just delivered a newborn infant. The nurse is monitoring for signs of placental separation knowing that which of the following indicates that the placenta has separated?
   1. Shortening of the umbilical cord
   2. Decrease in blood loss from the introitus
   3. Change in the uterine contour
   4. Sudden sharp abdominal pain
5. A nurse is assisting in caring for a client with abruptio placentae. While caring for the client, the nurse notes that the client begins to develop signs of shock. A first priority nursing action would be to:
   1. Turn the client onto her side
   2. Monitor the maternal pulse
   3. Monitor urinary output
   4. Monitor the maternal blood pressure
6. A client being prepared for a cesarean delivery is brought to the delivery room. To maintain optimal perfusion of oxygenated blood to the fetus, the nurse would plan to place the client in a:
   1. Trendelenburg position
   2. Semi-Fowler's position
   3. Supine position with a wedge under the right hip
   4. Prone position
7. A nurse is asked to assist the primary health care provider in performing Leopold maneuvers on a client. Which priority nursing intervention should be implemented before this procedure is performed?
   1. Locate fetal heart tones
   2. Have the client drink 8 ounces of water
   3. Warm the sonogram gel
   4. Have the client empty her bladder
8. A woman in active labor has contractions every 2 to 3 minutes lasting 45 seconds. The fetal heart rate between contraction is 100 beats per minute. Based on these findings, the priority nursing intervention is to:
   1. Notify the registered nurse (RN) immediately
   2. Encourage relaxation and breathing techniques between contractions
   3. Continue monitoring labor and fetal heart rate
   4. Monitor maternal vital signs
9. A nurse is assigned to assist in caring for a client being admitted to the birthing center in early labor. On admission, the nurse would initially:

1. Check pelvic adequacy
2. Administer an analgesic
3. Estimate fetal size
4. Determine maternal and fetal vital signs

10. Leopold's maneuvers will be performed on a pregnant client. The client asks the nurse about this procedure. The nurse responds knowing that this procedure:
    1. Determines the "lie" and "attitude" of the fetus
    2. Is a systemic method for palpating the fetus through the maternal back
    3. Is a systemic method for palpating the fetus through the maternal abdominal wall
    4. Measures the height of the maternal fundus
11. A nurse is assigned to care for a client who is in early labor. When collecting data from the client, it is most important for the nurse to first determine which of the following?
    1. Intensity of contractions
    2. Frequency of contractions
    3. Baseline fetal heart rate
    4. Maternal blood pressure
12. A nurse is caring for a client in labor. The nurse rechecks the client's blood pressure and notes that it has dropped. To decrease the incidence of supine hypotension, the nurse should encourage the client to remain in which position?
    1. Left lateral
    2. Semi-Fowler's
    3. Squatting
    4. Tailor sitting
13. A nurse instructs a client in active relaxation techniques to help her cope with the discomfort of contractions. The nurse determines teaching has been effective when the client tells the nurse that active relaxation includes:
    1. Assuming a state of mind that is open to suggestions from a coach
    2. Believing that a supreme power can help relieve the discomfort of contractions
    3. Relaxing uninvolved muscles while the uterus contracts
    4. Understanding that the origin of contraction discomfort is more psychological than physical
14. A primigravida's membranes rupture spontaneously. The nurse's first action is to:
    1. Monitor contraction pattern
    2. Determine the fetal heart rate
    3. Note the amount, color, and odor of the amniotic fluid
    4. Prepare for immediate delivery
15. After a client vaginally delivers a viable newborn, the nurse observes the umbilical cord lengthen and a spurt of blood from the vagina. The nurse recognizes these findings as signs of:
    1. Abruptio placentae
    2. Placenta previa
    3. Placental separation
    4. Uterine atony

ANSWERS

1. *Answer:* 2

Rationale: Priority care of this client includes promotion of fetal oxygenation. Precipitous labor progresses quickly with frequent contractions and short periods of relaxation between contractions. This does not allow for maximal reperfusion of the placenta with oxygenated blood. A side-lying position can assist in blood flow to the uterus by preventing vena cava and abdominal aorta compression. Further stimulation with oxytocin is contraindicated. There may not be enough time to administer an epidural anesthesia before delivery with such quick progression. Pushing with contractions is not indicated, especially with this type of labor. Controlled delivery of the fetus is essential to prevent maternal and fetal injury.
Test-Taking Strategy: Note the key words "precipitous" and "priority." Use the ABCs—airway, breathing, and circulation—when prioritizing and include the baby's needs as well as the mother's. Option 2 will promote fetal oxygenation. Review care to the client with precipitous labor if you had difficulty with this question.
Level of Cognitive Ability: Application
Client Needs: Physiological Integrity
Integrated Concept/Process: Nursing Process/Implementation
Content Area: Maternity
Reference: Burroughs A, Leifer G: *Maternity nursing,* ed 8, Philadelphia, 2002, WB Saunders, p. 258.

2. *Answer:* 3

Rationale: Painless vaginal bleeding is a sign of a possible placenta previa. Digital examination of the cervix can lead to maternal and fetal hemorrhage. Leopold maneuver's can reveal a nonengaged presenting part or malpresentation, both of which often accompany placenta previa as a result of the placenta filling the lower uterine segment. Hemoglobin and hematocrit values help to estimate the amount of blood loss. Electronic fetal monitoring (external) is crucial in evaluating the status of the fetus, who is at risk for severe hypoxia. Options 1, 2, and 4 are procedures that would not place the client at further risk.
Test-Taking Strategy: Use the process of elimination and note the key word "contraindicated." Option 3 is the only procedure that is invasive to the pregnancy and endangers the physiological safety of the client and fetus. Review care to the client with placenta previa if you had difficulty with this question.

Level of Cognitive Ability: Comprehension
Client Needs: Physiological Integrity
Integrated Concept/Process: Nursing Process/Data Collection
Content Area: Maternity
Reference: Burroughs A, Leifer G: *Maternity nursing,* ed 8, Philadelphia, 2002, WB Saunders, p. 226.

3. *Answer:* 4
Rationale: Vaginal bleeding in a pregnant client most often is caused by placenta previa or a placental abruption. Uterine tenderness accompanies abruptio placentae, especially with a central abruption and trapped blood behind the placenta. The abdomen will feel hard and boardlike on palpation as the blood penetrates the myometrium and causes uterine irritability. A sustained tetanic contraction can occur if the client is in labor and the uterine muscle cannot relax.
Test-Taking Strategy: Note the issue of the question, abruptio placentae. It can be easy to confuse a placenta previa and abruption. Remember, the difference involves the presence of uterine pain and tenderness with an abruptio placentae as opposed to painless bleeding with a placenta previa. Options 1, 2, and 3 describe the absence of a sign or symptom of abruptio placentae, whereas option 4 is the only one that describes the presence of one. Review the signs of abruptio placentae if you had difficulty with this question.
Level of Cognitive Ability: Comprehension
Client Needs: Physiological Integrity
Integrated Concept/Process: Nursing Process/Data Collection
Content Area: Maternity
Reference: Burroughs A, Leifer G: *Maternity nursing,* ed 8, Philadelphia, 2002, WB Saunders, p. 228.

4. *Answer:* 3
Rationale: Signs of placental separation include lengthening of the umbilical cord, a sudden gush of dark blood from the introitus, a firmly contracted uterus, and the uterus changing from a discoid to globular shape. The client may experience vaginal fullness, but not sudden and sharp abdominal pain.
Test-Taking Strategy: Use the process of elimination. Thinking about what one would expect to occur when the placenta separates will assist in eliminating options 1 and 2. Option 4 is eliminated because of the words "sudden, sharp." Review the signs of placental separation if you had difficulty with this question.
Level of Cognitive Ability: Comprehension
Client Needs: Physiological Integrity
Integrated Concept/Process: Nursing Process/Data Collection
Content Area: Maternity
Reference: Burroughs A, Leifer G: *Maternity nursing,* ed 8, Philadelphia, 2002, WB Saunders, p. 123.

5. *Answer:* 1
Rationale: With a client in shock, the nurse would want to increase perfusion to the placenta. A simple way to achieve this that requires no equipment is to turn the mother on her side. This would increase blood flow to the placenta by relieving pressure from the gravid uterus on the great vessels. The nurse would immediately contact the registered nurse who would then contact the physician. The other options would follow quickly.
Test-Taking Strategy: Note the key word "first." Eliminate options 2 and 4 because they are similar. Recalling that positioning will affect the status of blood flow will assist in directing you to option 1 from the remaining options. Review care to the client in shock if you had difficulty with this question.
Level of Cognitive Ability: Application
Client Needs: Physiological Integrity
Integrated Concept/Process: Nursing Process/Implementation
Content Area: Maternity
Reference: McKinney E et al: Maternal-child nursing, Philadelphia, 2000, WB Saunders, p. 644.

6. *Answer:* 3
Rationale: Vena cava and descending aorta compression by the pregnant uterus impedes blood return from the lower trunk and extremities, thereby decreasing cardiac return, cardiac output, and blood flow to the uterus and subsequently the fetus. The best position to prevent this would be side lying with the uterus displaced off the abdominal vessels. Positioning for abdominal surgery necessitates a supine position; however, a wedge placed under the right hip provides displacement of the uterus. Trendelenburg positioning places pressure from the pregnant uterus on the diaphragm and lungs, decreasing respiratory capacity and oxygenation. A semi-Fowler's or prone position is not practical for this type of abdominal surgery.
Test-Taking Strategy: Note the key words "maintain optimal perfusion." Use the process of elimination and visualize each of the positions and their effect on the fetus. Review client positioning if you had difficulty with this question.
Level of Cognitive Ability: Application
Client Needs: Physiological Integrity
Integrated Concept/Process: Nursing Process/Planning
Content Area: Maternity
Reference: Burroughs A, Leifer G: *Maternity nursing,* ed 8, Philadelphia, 2002, WB Saunders, p. 96.

7. *Answer:* 4
Rationale: An empty bladder contributes to a woman's comfort during the examination. Drinking water to fill the bladder and warming sonogram gel may be done before a sonogram (ultrasound). Often the Leopold maneuvers are performed to aid the examiner in locating the fetal heart tones.
Test-Taking Strategy: Use the process of elimination. Eliminate option 1 because Leopold maneuvers are often used to help locate fetal heart tones. Eliminate options 2 and 3 because sonogram gel is used for an ultrasound and not during Leopold maneuvers. Also, a client is requested to have a full bladder before ultrasonography. Review the preparation of a client for this procedure if you had difficulty with this question.
Level of Cognitive Ability: Application
Client Needs: Physiological Integrity
Integrated Concept/Process: Nursing Process/Implementation
Content Area: Maternity
Reference: Burroughs A, Leifer G: *Maternity nursing,* ed 8, Philadelphia, 2002, WB Saunders, p. 109.

8. *Answer:* 1
Rationale: Fetal bradycardia between contractions may indicate the need for immediate medical management. The nurse would immediately contact the registered nurse who in turn would contact the physician. Options 2, 3, and 4 will delay necessary and immediate interventions.
Test-Taking Strategy: Use the ABCs—airway, breathing, and circulation. Note that the woman is in active labor and that the fetal heart rate is below normal. It is imperative that the circulation in the fetus be restored to normal limits. Review care to the client in active labor if you had difficulty with this question.
Level of Cognitive Ability: Application
Client Needs: Physiological Integrity
Integrated Concept/Process: Nursing Process/Implementation
Content Area: Maternity
Reference: Burroughs A, Leifer G: *Maternity nursing,* ed 8, Philadelphia, 2002, WB Saunders, p. 148.

9. *Answer:* 4
Rationale: To evaluate a woman's physical well-being, the temperature, pulse, respirations, and blood pressure, as well as the fetal heart beat, are checked. Option 2 is incorrect because it would be too premature for an analgesic. Medication given too early tends to slow or stop labor contractions. Options 1 and 3 are incorrect. These assessments should be done by the physician or a nurse midwife during prenatal visits.
Test-Taking Strategy: Use the ABCs—airway, breathing, and circulation. This will easily direct you to option 4. Remember, measuring vital signs is the priority. Review care to the client in labor if you had difficulty with this question.
Level of Cognitive Ability: Application
Client Needs: Physiological Integrity
Integrated Concept/Process: Nursing Process/Implementation
Content Area: Maternity
Reference: Burroughs A, Leifer G: *Maternity nursing,* ed 8, Philadelphia, 2002, WB Saunders, p. 113.

10. *Answer:* 3
Rationale: Leopold's maneuvers is a systemic method for palpating the fetus through the maternal abdominal wall. Options 1, 2, and 4 are incorrect.
Test-Taking Strategy: Knowledge of the purpose and procedure for Leopard's maneuvers is required to answer this question. Visualizing this procedure will assist in directing you to option 3. Review Leopold's maneuvers if you had difficulty with this question.
Level of Cognitive Ability: Comprehension
Client Needs: Physiological Integrity
Integrated Concept/Process: Nursing Process/Implementation
Content Area: Maternity
Reference: Burroughs A, Leifer G: *Maternity nursing,* ed 8, Philadelphia, 2002, WB Saunders, p. 109.

11. *Answer:* 3
Rationale: The nurse should first determine the baseline fetal heart rate. Although options 1, 2, and 4 will be a component of the data collection process, the fetal heart rate is the priority.
Test-Taking Strategy: Note the key word "first." Use the ABCs when selecting an answer. Remember the order of priority of airway, breathing, and circulation. Fetal heart rate reflects the ABCs. Review care to the client in labor if you had difficulty with this question.
Level of Cognitive Ability: Application
Client Needs: Physiological Integrity
Integrated Concept/Process: Nursing Process/Implementation
Content Area: Maternity
Reference: Burroughs A, Leifer G: *Maternity nursing,* ed 8, Philadelphia, 2002, WB Saunders, p. 83.

12. *Answer:* 1
Rationale: Pressure from the enlarged uterus and the aorta and vena cava when the woman is supine can result in hypotension. This can be relieved by having the woman lie on her left side. Options 2, 3, and 4 are incorrect.
Test-Taking Strategy: Use the process of elimination and knowledge of the anatomy of the pregnant uterus and the physiological response caused by pressure on the large abdominal vessels. Note that options 2, 3, and 4 are all similar in that the client is upright. Review nursing measures when the pregnant client becomes hypotensive if you had difficulty with this question.
Level of Cognitive Ability: Application
Client Needs: Physiological Integrity
Integrated Concept/Process: Nursing Process/Implementation
Content Area: Maternity
Reference: Burroughs A, Leifer G: *Maternity nursing,* ed 8, Philadelphia, 2002, WB Saunders, p. 42.

13. *Answer:* 3
Rationale: Active relaxation techniques include specific relaxation exercises and conditioned responses such as distraction from the discomfort of labor. The woman is an active participant in the use of the technique, which focuses on relaxing uninvolved muscles while the uterus contracts. Options 1, 2, and 4 are incorrect.
Test-Taking Strategy: Note the key words "active relaxation techniques." Use the process of elimination noting that option 3 contains an active verb and is different from other options. Review the purpose of active relaxation techniques if you had difficulty with this question.
Level of Cognitive Ability: Comprehension
Client Needs: Physiological Integrity
Integrated Concept/Process: Teaching/Learning
Content Area: Maternity
Reference: Burroughs A, Leifer G: *Maternity nursing,* ed 8, Philadelphia, 2002, WB Saunders, p. 68.

14. *Answer:* 2
Rationale: When the membranes rupture, the nurse immediately assesses the fetal heart rate to detect changes associated with prolapse or compression of the umbilical cord. Monitoring the contraction pattern and noting the amount, color, and odor of the amniotic fluid may be done but would not be the first action. There is no information in the question that indicates the necessity to prepare the client for immediate delivery.
Test-Taking Strategy: Note the key word "first." Use the ABCs—airway, breathing, and circulation. Fetal heart rate is associated with fetal breathing and circulation. Review the

initial nursing interventions when the membranes rupture if you had difficulty with this question.
Level of Cognitive Ability: Application
Client Needs: Physiological Integrity
Integrated Concept/Process: Nursing Process/Implementation
Content Area: Maternity
Reference: Burroughs A, Leifer G: *Maternity nursing,* ed 8, Philadelphia, 2002, WB Saunders, p. 91.

15. *Answer:* 3
Rationale: As the placenta separates, it settles downward into the lower uterine segment, the umbilical cord lengthens, and a sudden trickle or spurt of blood appears. The clinical manifestations identified in the question are not related to options 1, 2, and 4.
Test-Taking Strategy: Use the process of elimination. Note the similarity between options 1, 2, and 4 in that they represent complications associated with pregnancy. Option 3 indicates a normal finding after vaginal delivery of the newborn. Review this stage of labor if you had difficulty with this question.
Level of Cognitive Ability: Comprehension
Client Needs: Physiological Integrity
Integrated Concept/Process: Nursing Process/Data Collection
Content Area: Maternity
Reference: Burroughs A, Leifer G: *Maternity nursing,* ed 8, Philadelphia, 2002, WB Saunders, pp. 90, 123.

REFERENCES

Burroughs A, Leifer G: *Maternity nursing,* ed 8, Philadelphia, 2002, WB Saunders.

Lowdermilk D, Perry S, Bobak I: *Maternity and women's health care,* ed 7, St Louis, 2000, Mosby.

McKinney E et al: *Maternal-child nursing,* Philadelphia, 2000, WB Saunders.

Murray S, McKinney E, Gorrie T: *Foundations of maternal-newborn nursing,* ed 3, Philadelphia, 2002, WB Saunders.

24 The Postpartum Period and Associated Complications

I. POSTPARTUM

A. Description: period when the reproductive tract returns to the normal, nonpregnant state

B. Postpartum period: starts immediately after **delivery** and is completed usually by week 6 after **delivery**

II. PHYSIOLOGICAL MATERNAL CHANGES

A. Involution (Figure 24-1)

1. Description

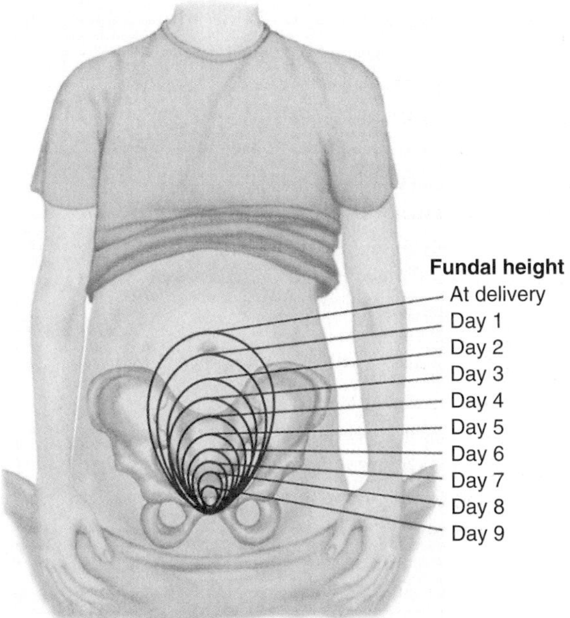

FIG. 24-1 Involution of the uterus. Height of the uterine fundus decreases by approximately 1 cm per day. (From Murray S, McKinney E, Gorrie T: *Foundations of maternal-newborn nursing*, ed 3, Philadelphia, 2002, WB Saunders.)

a. The rapid decrease in the size of the uterus as it returns to the nonpregnant state

b. Clients who breastfeed may experience a more rapid involution

2. Data collection

a. Weight of the uterus decreases from 2 lb to 2 oz in 6 weeks

b. Fundus steadily descends into pelvis; the fundal height decreases about one fingerbreadth (1 cm) per day

c. By 10 days' postpartum, the uterus cannot be palpated abdominally

d. A flaccid fundus indicates uterine atony

e. A tender fundus indicates an infection

B. **Lochia** (Figure 24-2)

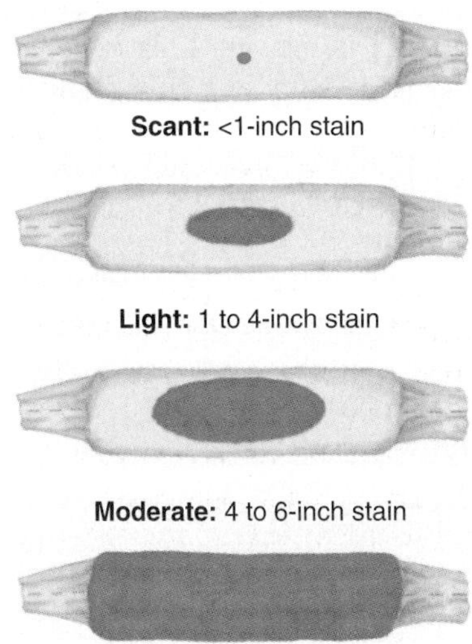

FIG. 24-2 Guidelines for assessing the amount of lochia on the perianal pad. (From Murray S, McKinney E, Gorrie T: *Foundations of maternal-newborn nursing*, ed 3, Philadelphia, 2002, WB Saunders.)

1. Description: discharge from the uterus that consists of blood from the vessels of the **placental** site and debris from the decidua
2. Data collection
   a. Rubra: bright red discharge that occurs from **delivery** day to day 3 postpartum
   b. Serosa: brownish-pink discharge that occurs from days 4 to 10 postpartum
   c. Alba: white discharge that occurs from days 10 to 14 postpartum
   d. Normally, the discharge has a fleshy odor
   e. Discharge decreases daily in amount
   f. Discharge increases with ambulation

C. Cervix: cervical involution; after 1 week the muscle begins to regenerate

D. Vagina: vaginal distention decreases, although muscle tone is never restored completely to the pregravid state

E. Ovarian function and menstruation
1. Menstrual flow resumes within 8 weeks in nonbreastfeeding mothers
2. Menstrual flow usually resumes within 3 to 4 months in breastfeeding mothers
3. Breastfeeding mothers may experience amenorrhea during the entire period of lactation
4. A woman may ovulate without menstruating, so breastfeeding should not be considered a form of birth control

F. Breasts
1. A decrease of estrogen and progesterone levels after **delivery** stimulates increased prolactin levels, which promotes breast milk production
2. Breasts become distended with milk on the third day
3. Engorgement occurs in 48 to 72 hours in nonbreastfeeding mothers; breastfeeding will relieve engorgement

G. Urinary tract
1. May have urinary retention because of loss of elasticity and tone and loss of sensation in the bladder from trauma, medications, anesthesia, and lack of privacy
2. Diuresis usually begins within the first 12 hours after **delivery**

H. Gastrointestinal tract
1. Women are usually very hungry after **delivery**
2. Constipation can occur
3. Hemorrhoids are common

I. Vital signs
1. Temperature may be elevated during the first 24 hours because of dehydration
2. Bradycardia is common during the first week, with a range of 50 to 70 beats per minute
3. Blood pressure remains unchanged

III. POSTPARTUM IMPLEMENTATION

A. Data collection
1. Monitor vital signs
2. Monitor height, consistency, and location of the fundus
3. Monitor color, amount, and odor of **lochia**
4. Check breasts for engorgement
5. Monitor perineum for swelling or discoloration; episiotomy for healing
6. Check incisions or dressings of cesarean birth client
7. Monitor input and output (I&O)
8. Monitor bowel status
9. Encourage frequent voiding
10. Encourage ambulation
11. RhoGam is prescribed to be administered within 72 hours postpartum to the Rh-negative client who has given birth to an Rh-positive **neonate**
12. Monitor parent-**newborn** bonding
13. Monitor emotional status

B. Client teaching
1. Demonstrate **newborn** care skills as necessary
2. Provide the opportunity for the mother to bathe the **newborn**
3. Instruct on feeding technique
4. Instruct the mother to avoid heavy lifting for at least 3 weeks
5. Instruct the mother to plan at least one rest period per day
6. Instruct the mother that contraception should begin after **delivery** or with the initiation of intercourse
7. Instruct the mother on the importance of follow-up care, which should be scheduled at 4 to 6 weeks postpartum
8. Instruct the mother to report immediately any signs of chills, fever, increased **lochia**, or depressed feelings to the physician

IV. POSTPARTUM DISCOMFORTS

A. Afterbirth pains
1. Occur because of contractions of the uterus
2. Are more common in multiparas, breastfeeding mothers, clients treated with oxytocin (Pitocin), and clients who had an overdistended uterus during pregnancy

B. Perineal discomfort
1. Apply ice packs to the perineum as prescribed during the first 24 hours to reduce swelling
2. After the first 24 hours, apply warmth by sitz baths as prescribed

C. Episiotomy

1. Instruct the client to administer perineal care after each voiding
2. Encourage the use of analgesic spray as prescribed
3. Administer analgesics as prescribed if comfort measures are unsuccessful

D. Breast discomfort from engorgement
1. Encourage wearing a support bra at all times, even while sleeping
2. Encourage the use of ice packs if not breastfeeding
3. Encourage the use of warm soaks before feeding for a breastfeeding mother
4. Administer analgesics as prescribed if comfort measures are unsuccessful

E. Postpartum blues
1. The condition may be caused by physiological or emotional stress
2. Weepiness, mood changes, anxiety, and irritability in the first few days after childbirth
3. Verbalization should be encouraged
4. If unresolved, postpartum blues may progress to postpartum depression

V. NUTRITION

A. Nutritional needs depend on prepregnancy weight, ideal weight for height, and whether the mother is breastfeeding

B. If the mother is breastfeeding, calorie needs increase by approximately 500 calories per day, and the mother may require increased fluids and the continuance of prenatal vitamins and minerals

VI. BREASTFEEDING

A. General principles/considerations
1. Put the baby to breast as soon as the mother and baby's condition are stable (on **delivery** table if possible)
2. Stay with the mother each time she nurses until she feels secure and confident with the baby and her feelings
3. Uterine cramping may occur the first day after **delivery** while nursing, when oxytocin simulation causes the uterus to contract
4. Use general hygiene and wash the breasts once daily
5. Do not use soap on the breasts because it tends to remove natural oils and increases the chances of cracking
6. Bra should be well fitted and supporting
7. Breasts may leak between feedings or during coitus; place a breast pad in bra
8. Calories should be increased by 500 per day, and the diet should include additional fluids; prenatal vitamins should be taken as prescribed
9. Baby's stools will be light yellow, watery, and frequent
10. Medications should be avoided unless prescribed
11. Gas-producing foods and caffeine should be avoided
12. Hormonal contraceptives may cause a decrease in the milk supply and are best avoided during the first 6 weeks after birth
13. Oral contraceptives containing estrogen are not recommended for breastfeeding mothers; progestin-only birth control pills are less likely to interfere with the milk supply
14. Baby will develop his or her own feeding schedule

B. Breastfeeding procedure for mother
1. Wash hands and assume a comfortable position
2. Start with the breast that the last feeding ended with (baby sucks more vigorously at the beginning of a feeding)
3. Brush the **newborn** infant's lower lip with nipple
4. Tickle the lips to have the baby open the mouth wide
5. Guide the nipple and surrounding areola into the baby's mouth
6. After the baby has nursed, release suction by depressing the **newborn's** chin or inserting a clean finger into the baby's mouth
7. Burp the baby after the first breast
8. Repeat the procedure on the second breast until the baby stops nursing
9. Burp the baby again
10. Instruct the mother to listen for audible sucking and swallowing during feeding

C. Engorgement
1. Breastfeed frequently
2. Apply warm packs before feeding
3. Apply ice packs between feedings

D. Cracked nipples
1. Expose nipples to air for 10 to 20 minutes after feeding
2. Rotate the position of the baby for each feeding
3. Be sure that the baby is latched on to the areola, not just the nipple

VII. CYSTITIS

A. Description: an infection of the bladder

B. Data collection

1. Burning and pain on urination
2. Lower abdominal pain
3. Increased frequency of urination
4. Fever
5. Proteinuria, hematuria, bacteriuria, white blood cells (WBCs) in the urine

C. Implementation
1. Palpate the bladder for distention
2. Palpate the fundus for position
3. Obtain a urine specimen for culture and sensitivity if prescribed
4. Institute measures to assist the client to void
5. Encourage frequent and complete emptying of the bladder
6. Force fluids to 3000 mL per day
7. Administer antibiotics as prescribed after the urine culture is obtained

VIII. HEMATOMA

A. Description
1. Occurs after the escape of blood into the tissues of the reproductive sac after the **delivery**
2. Predisposing conditions include operative **delivery** with forceps or injury to a blood vessel
3. Can be a life-threatening condition

B. Data collection
1. Abnormal, severe pain and pressure in perineal area
2. Inability to void
3. Palpable tumor
4. Decreased hemoglobin and hematocrit (H&H)
5. Signs of shock such as pallor, tachycardia, and hypotension if significant blood loss has occurred

C. Implementation
1. Monitor vital signs
2. Monitor the client for abnormal pain, especially when forceps **delivery** has occurred
3. Place ice to the hematoma site
4. Administer analgesics as prescribed
5. Monitor I&O; encourage fluids
6. Monitor for signs of infection such as increased temperature, pulse rate, and WBC count
7. Prepare the client for incision and evacuation of hematoma if necessary

IX. HEMORRHAGE

A. Description: bleeding of 500 mL or more after **delivery**

B. Data collection
1. Early
   a. Hemorrhage occurs during the first 24 hours after **delivery**
   b. Caused by uterine atony, lacerations, or inversion of uterus
2. Late
   a. Hemorrhage occurs later than the first 24 hours after **delivery**
   b. Caused by retained **placental** fragments

C. Implementation
1. Massage fundus, with care not to overmassage
2. Physician or health care provider is notified if hemorrhage occurs; monitor vital signs and fundus every 5 to 15 minutes
3. Monitor and estimate blood loss by pad count
4. Maintain asepsis because hemorrhage predisposes to infection
5. Monitor level of consciousness
6. Oxytocin (Pitocin) may be administered
7. H&H is monitored; blood transfusions may be administered

X. INFECTION

A. Description: any infection of the reproductive organs that occurs within 28 days of **delivery** or abortion

B. Data collection
1. Fever and chills
2. Pelvic discomfort or pain
3. Vaginal discharge
4. Elevated WBC count

C. Implementation
1. Monitor vital signs and temperature every 2 to 4 hours
2. Make the mother as comfortable as possible; position for comfort and to promote drainage
3. Keep the mother warmed if chilled
4. Isolate the baby from the mother only if the mother is infected
5. Provide a nutritious high-caloric, protein diet
6. Force fluids to 3000 to 4000 mL per day, if not contraindicated
7. Encourage frequent voiding; monitor I&O
8. Monitor culture results if cultures were prescribed
9. Administer antibiotics as prescribed

XI. MASTITIS

A. Description
1. Inflammation of the breast as a result of infection
2. Primarily seen in breastfeeding mothers 2 to 3 weeks after **delivery** but may occur at any time during lactation

B. Data collection

1. Localized heat and swelling
2. Pain
3. Elevated temperature
4. Complaints of flulike symptoms

C. Implementation
1. Instruct the mother in good handwashing and breast hygiene techniques
2. Apply heat or cold to site as prescribed
3. Maintain lactation in breastfeeding mothers
4. Encourage manual expression of breast milk or use of breast pump every 4 hours
5. Encourage the mother to support the breasts with a supportive bra
6. Administer analgesics or antibiotics as prescribed

XII. PULMONARY EMBOLISM

A. Description: the passage of thrombus, often originating in one of the uterine or other pelvic veins, into the lungs, where it disrupts the circulation of blood

B. Data collection
1. Dyspnea, tachypnea, and tachycardia
2. Cough and rales
3. Hemoptysis
4. Pleuritic chest pain
5. Feeling of impending doom

C. Implementation
1. Administer oxygen as prescribed
2. Position the client with the head of the bed elevated to promote comfort
3. Monitor vital signs frequently
4. Frequently monitor respiratory rate
5. Monitor for signs of respiratory distress and for signs of hypoxemia, such as tachypnea, tachycardia, restlessness, cool and clammy skin, cyanosis, and the use of accessory muscles
6. Increased IV fluids may be prescribed
7. Anticoagulants may be prescribed

XIII. SUBINVOLUTION

A. Description: incomplete involution or failure of the uterus to return to its normal size and condition

B. Data collection
1. Uterine pain on palpation
2. Uterus is larger than expected
3. Greater than normal vaginal bleeding

C. Implementation
1. Monitor vital signs
2. Monitor uterus and fundus and for vaginal bleeding
3. Elevate the legs to promote venous return
4. Encourage frequent voiding
5. H&H is monitored
6. Methylergonovine maleate (Methergine) may be prescribed

XIV. THROMBOPHLEBITIS

A. Description
1. A condition in which a clot forms in a vessel wall as a result of inflammation of the vessel wall
2. A partial obstruction of the vessel can occur
3. Increased blood-clotting factors in the postpartum period place the client at risk

B. Data collection (Table 24-1)
1. Superficial thrombophlebitis
2. Femoral thrombophlebitis
3. Pelvic thrombophlebitis

C. Implementation
1. Assess lower extremities for edema, tenderness, varices, and increased skin temperature
2. Evaluate legs for Homans' sign by extending the legs with the knees slightly flexed and dorsiflexing the foot
3. Maintain bed rest
4. Elevate the affected leg

TABLE 24-1

Data Collection: Types of Thrombophlebitis

Superficial	Femoral	Pelvic
Tenderness and pain in the affected lower extremity Warm and pinkish-red color over thrombus area Palpable thrombus that feels bumpy and hard	Chills and fever Malaise Pain, stiffness, and swelling of the affected leg Shiny, white skin over the affected area Positive Homans' sign Diminished peripheral pulses	Severe chills Dramatic body temperature changes Occurrence of pulmonary embolism may be the first sign

5. Apply a bed cradle and keep bedclothes off the affected leg
6. Never massage the leg
7. Monitor for manifestations of pulmonary embolism
8. Superficial thrombophlebitis
    a. Provide rest
    b. Apply hot packs to the affected site as prescribed
    c. Apply elastic stockings
    d. Administer analgesics as prescribed
9. Femoral thrombophlebitis
    a. Provide bed rest
    b. Elevate the affected leg
    c. Apply moist heat continuously to affected area if prescribed to alleviate discomfort
    d. Administer analgesics as prescribed
    e. Administer antibiotics if prescribed
    f. Intravenous heparin sodium may be prescribed to prevent further thrombus formation
10. Pelvic thrombophlebitis
    a. Provide bed rest
    b. Administer analgesics as prescribed
    c. Administer antibiotics if prescribed
    d. Intravenous heparin sodium may be prescribed to prevent further thrombus formation

D. Client teaching (Box 24-1)

PRACTICE QUESTIONS

1. A nurse palpates the fundus and checks the character of the lochia of a postpartum client in the fourth stage of labor. The nurse expects the lochia to be:
    1. White
    2. Pink
    3. Serosanguinous
    4. Red
2. After episiotomy and delivery of a newborn, the nurse performs a perineal check on the mother. The nurse notes a trickle of bright red blood coming from the perineum. The nurse checks the fundus and notes that it is firm. The nurse determines that:
    1. This is a normal expectation after episiotomy
    2. The perineal assessment should be performed more frequently
    3. The bright red bleeding is abnormal and should be reported
    4. The mother should be allowed bathroom privileges only
3. A nurse is assigned to care for a client in the postpartum period. The client asks the nurse what the term involution means. The nurse responds to the client knowing that involution is:
    1. A progressive descent of the uterus into the pelvic cavity occurring approximately 1 cm per day
    2. The gradual reversal of the uterine muscle into the abdominal cavity
    3. The descent of the uterus into the pelvic cavity occurring at a rate of 2 cm a day
    4. The inverted uterus returning to normal
4. A mother is breastfeeding her newborn baby and experiences breast engorgement. The nurse encourages the mother to do which of the following measures to provide comfort for the engorgement?
    1. Breastfeed only during the daytime hours
    2. Apply cold compresses to the breast
    3. Massage the breasts before feeding to stimulate let-down
    4. Avoid the use of a bra while the breasts are engorged
5. A nurse is assisting in developing a plan of care for a client in the fourth stage of labor. Which of the following problems is most likely to occur during this stage?
    1. Pain because of the process of labor or birth
    2. Anxiety related to childbirth
    3. Fatigue resulting from physical exertion during labor
    4. Urinary retention caused by the loss of sensation to void and rapid bladder filling
6. After delivery, a nurse checks the height of the uterine fundus. The nurse expects that the position of the fundus would most likely be noted:
    1. At the level of the umbilicus
    2. Above the level of the umbilicus
    3. One fingerbreadth above the symphysis pubis
    4. To the right of the abdomen
7. A nurse is caring for a postpartum client. Four hours postpartum, the client's temperature is 102° F. The most appropriate nursing action would be to:
    1. Continue to monitor the temperature
    2. Notify the registered nurse who will then contact the physician
    3. Apply cool packs to the abdomen
    4. Remove the blanket from the client's bed

BOX 24-1

Client Education for Thrombophlebitis

Avoid pressure behind the knees
Avoid prolonged sitting
Avoid constrictive clothing
Avoid crossing the legs
Avoid massaging the leg
Know how to apply support hose if prescribed
Understand the importance of anticoagulant therapy as prescribed
Understand the importance of follow-up monitoring with the health care provider

8. A nurse is assigned to care for a client in the immediate postpartum period who received epidural anesthesia for delivery. The nurse monitors the client for complications. Which of the following would best identify an indicator of a hematoma?
   1. Complaints of a tearing sensation
   2. Complaints of lower abdominal discomfort
   3. Changes in vital signs
   4. Signs of heavy bruising
9. A nurse is assisting in planning care for the postpartum woman who has small vulvar hematomas. To assist in reducing the swelling, the nurse suggests to:
   1. Check the vital signs every 4 hours
   2. Prepare a heat pack for application to the area
   3. Measure the fundal height every 4 hours
   4. Prepare an ice pack for application to the area
10. A client received epidural anesthesia during labor and had a forceps delivery after pushing for 2 hours. At 6 hours postpartum, the client's systolic blood pressure (BP) drops 20 points, the diastolic BP drops 10 points, and the pulse is 120 beats per minute. The client is very anxious and restless. The nurse is told that the client has a vulvar hematoma. Based on this diagnosis, the nurse would most appropriately plan to:
    1. Monitor fundal height
    2. Apply perineal pressure
    3. Prepare the client for surgery
    4. Reassure the client
11. A nurse is assigned to care for a client after cesarean section. To prevent thrombophlebitis, the nurse encourages the woman to:
    1. Ambulate frequently
    2. Apply warm moist packs to the legs
    3. Remain on bed rest with the legs elevated
    4. Wear support stockings
12. A postpartum client has developed thrombophlebitis. The nurse knows that the affected extremity should be elevated by:
    1. Elevating it on a pillow
    2. Elevating the foot of the bed
    3. Placing the bed in reverse Trendelenburg position
    4. Placing the bed in Trendelenburg position
13. A nurse is caring for a postpartum client with a diagnosis of thrombophlebitis. The client suddenly complains of chest pain and dyspnea. The nurse would initially check:
    1. Level of consciousness (LOC)
    2. Fundal height
    3. Presence of Homans' sign
    4. Vital signs
14. A nurse suspects that a client has a pulmonary embolism. The most important nursing action is to:
    1. Administer oxygen by facemask as prescribed
    2. Elevate the head of the bed
    3. Increase the IV rate
    4. Monitor vital signs
15. A nurse notes that the 4-hour postpartum client has cool, clammy skin, and is restless and excessively thirsty. The nurse immediately notifies the registered nurse and then:
    1. Encourages ambulation
    2. Checks vital signs
    3. Begins fundal massage
    4. Encourages the client to drink fluids
16. A new mother attempting breastfeeding for the first time has developed mastitis. She states, "My breasts look terrible and I think that I will stop breastfeeding." The nurse plans care knowing that the client's statement relates to:
    1. Body image
    2. Newborn nutrition
    3. Feelings of inadequacy
    4. Infection
17. Breastfeeding instructions for the postpartum mother should include avoidance of soaps on the nipples, frequent changing of breast pads, intermittent exposure of nipples to air, and handwashing before handling the breast and before breastfeeding. The nurse understands that these measures are specific to the prevention of:
    1. Engorgement
    2. Newborn colic
    3. "Let-down" reflex
    4. Mastitis
18. The new breastfeeding mother is being discharged from the hospital after being treated for mastitis. The nurse knows that the mother needs further teaching when the mother states:
    1. "I need to change my breast pads when they are wet."
    2. "I will wash my breasts gently with plain water."
    3. "My left breast is sore, so I will offer the right breast frequently for breastfeeding."
    4. "When my breasts feel engorged, I will use an ice pack for the pain."
19. A postpartum client with a pulmonary embolism has been separated from her newborn infant for 2 days. Which observation by the nurse indicates a potential client need?
    1. The client nurses her newborn infant in the side-lying position
    2. The client needs the head of the bed elevated for comfort
    3. The newborn infant prefers the bottle over breast milk
    4. The client turns herself from side to side

20. A nurse is assisting in caring for a postpartum client experiencing uterine hemorrhage. In planning to meet the psychosocial needs of the client, the nurse would:
   1. Keep the client and her family members informed of progress
   2. Monitor vital signs every 2 hours
   3. Maintain strict bed rest
   4. Perform firm fundal massage every 2 hours

ANSWERS

1. *Answer:* 4
Rationale: The color of the lochia during the fourth stage of labor is bright red. This may last from 1 to 3 days. The color of the lochia then changes to a pinkish brown that lasts 4 to 10 days. Finally, the lochia changes to a creamy white color that lasts approximately 10 to 14 days.
Test-Taking Strategy: Knowledge regarding the color, amount, and consistency of lochia after delivery is required to answer the question. Focus on the key words "fourth stage of labor." Review postpartum expected findings if you had difficulty with this question.
Level of Cognitive Ability: Comprehension
Client Needs: Physiological Integrity
Integrated Concept/Process: Nursing Process/Data Collection
Content Area: Maternity
Reference: Burroughs A, Leifer G: *Maternity nursing,* ed 8, Philadelphia, 2002, WB Saunders, p. 203.

2. *Answer:* 3
Rationale: Lochial flow should be distinguished from bleeding originating from a laceration or episiotomy, which is usually brighter red than lochia and presents as a continuous trickle of bleeding even though the fundus of the uterus is firm. This bright red bleeding is abnormal and needs to be reported.
Test-Taking Strategy: Use the process of elimination. Note the key words "bright red." This should be an indication that the flow is not normal. Review lochial flow and complications associated with episiotomy if you had difficulty with this question.
Level of Cognitive Ability: Analysis
Client Needs: Physiological Integrity
Integrated Concept/Process: Nursing Process/Data Collection
Content Area: Maternity
Reference: Burroughs A, Leifer G: *Maternity nursing,* ed 8, Philadelphia, 2002, WB Saunders, p. 203.

3. *Answer:* 1
Rationale: Involution is a progressive descent of the uterus into the pelvic cavity. After birth, descent occurs approximately 1 fingerbreadth, or approximately 1 cm per day.
Test-Taking Strategy: Knowledge regarding the definition and process of involution is required to answer this question. Use medical terminology to assist you in defining the word "involution." This will assist in directing you to the correct option. Review the process of involution if you had difficulty with this question.
Level of Cognitive Ability: Comprehension
Client Needs: Physiological Integrity
Integrated Concept/Process: Nursing Process/Implementation
Content Area: Maternity
Reference: Burroughs A, Leifer G: *Maternity nursing,* ed 8, Philadelphia, 2002, WB Saunders, p. 425.

4. *Answer:* 3
Rationale: Comfort measures for breast engorgement include massaging the breasts before feeding to stimulate let-down, wearing a supportive well-fitting bra at all times, taking a warm shower or applying warm compresses just before feeding, and alternating breasts during feeding.
Test-Taking Strategy: Use the process of elimination to answer the question. Eliminate option 1 because of the absolute word "only." From the remaining options, recalling the self-care measures to promote comfort to the mother with breast engorgement will assist in directing you to option 3. Review these measures if you had difficulty with this question.
Level of Cognitive Ability: Application
Client Needs: Health Promotion and Maintenance
Integrated Concept/Process: Self-Care
Content Area: Maternity
Reference: Murray S, McKinney E, Gorrie T: *Foundations of maternal-newborn nursing,* ed 3, Philadelphia, 2002, WB Saunders, p. 593.

5. *Answer:* 4
Rationale: The fourth stage of labor is composed of the first hour postpartum when the woman's body begins to readjust and relax. Options 1 and 2 relate to the first stage of labor. Option 3 relates to the second stage of labor. Option 4 is related to the third and fourth stages of labor.
Test-Taking Strategy: Use the process of elimination. Focus on the key words "fourth stage of labor." Remembering that the fourth stage of labor is the last stage will direct you toward the correct option. Review the stages of labor if you had difficulty with this question.
Level of Cognitive Ability: Comprehension
Client Needs: Physiological Integrity
Integrated Concept/Process: Nursing Process/Planning
Content Area: Maternity
Reference: Murray S, McKinney E, Gorrie T: *Foundations of maternal-newborn nursing,* ed 3, Philadelphia, 2002, WB Saunders, p. 280.

6. *Answer:* 1
Rationale: Immediately after delivery, the uterine fundus should be at the level of the umbilicus or 1 to 3 fingerbreadths below it and in the midline of the abdomen. If the fundus is above the umbilicus, this may indicate that there are blood clots in the uterus that need to be expelled by fundal

massage. If the fundus is noted to the right of the abdomen, it may indicate a full bladder.
Test-Taking Strategy: Knowledge regarding normal postdelivery findings in the mother and normal anatomy is required to answer this question. Review expected postdelivery findings if you had difficulty with this question.
Level of Cognitive Ability: Comprehension
Client Needs: Physiological Integrity
Integrated Concept/Process: Nursing Process/Data Collection
Content Area: Maternity
Reference: Murray S, McKinney E, Gorrie T: *Foundations of maternal-newborn nursing,* ed 3, Philadelphia, 2002, WB Saunders, p. 325.

7. *Answer:* 2
Rationale: In the postpartum period, the mother's temperature may be elevated during the first 24 hours as a result of dehydration. However, if the temperature is greater than 2° F above normal, this may indicate infection and the physician will need to be notified.
Test-Taking Strategy: Use the process of elimination. Focus on the key words "4 hours" and "102° F." Noting that the temperature is extreme compared with the normal temperature will direct you to option 2. Review the expected findings in the postpartum period if you had difficulty with this question.
Level of Cognitive Ability: Application
Client Needs: Physiological Integrity
Integrated Concept/Process: Nursing Process/Implementation
Content Area: Maternity
Reference: Burroughs A, Leifer G: *Maternity nursing,* ed 8, Philadelphia, 2002, WB Saunders, p. 210.

8. *Answer:* 3
Rationale: Changes in vital signs indicate hypovolemia in the anesthetized postpartum woman with vulvar hematoma. Options 1 and 2 are inaccurate for a client who is anesthetized. Heavy bruising may be noted, but vital sign changes are most likely to indicate the presence of a hematoma.
Test-Taking Strategy: Use the process of elimination. Eliminate options 1 and 2 first. Because the woman is anesthetized, she cannot feel pain or lower abdominal discomfort. Option 4 (heavy bruising) may be visualized, but vital sign changes indicate hematoma caused by blood collection in the perineal tissues. Review the signs of a hematoma if you had difficulty with this question.
Level of Cognitive Ability: Analysis
Client Needs: Physiological Integrity
Integrated Concept/Process: Nursing Process/Data Collection
Content Area: Maternity
Reference: Burroughs A, Leifer G: *Maternity nursing,* ed 8, Philadelphia, 2002, WB Saunders, p. 301.

9. *Answer:* 4
Rationale: Application of ice will reduce swelling caused by hematoma formation in the vulvar area. Options 1, 2, and 3 will not reduce the swelling.
Test-Taking Strategy: Use the process of elimination. Focus on the issue of the question "reducing the swelling." This will assist in eliminating options 1 and 3. Recalling the principles related to heat and cold will direct you to option 4 from the remaining options. Review nursing care to the client with a hematoma if you had difficulty with this question.
Level of Cognitive Ability: Application
Client Needs: Physiological Integrity
Integrated Concept/Process: Nursing Process/Implementation
Content Area: Maternity
Reference: Burroughs A, Leifer G: *Maternity nursing,* ed 8, Philadelphia, 2002, WB Saunders, p. 301.

10. *Answer:* 3
Rationale: The information provided in the question indicates that the client is experiencing blood loss. Surgery would be indicated for this complication to stop the bleeding. Options 1, 2, and 4 would not assist in controlling the bleeding in this emergency situation.
Test-Taking Strategy: Use the process of elimination. Focus on the information provided in the question. Noting the signs and symptoms in the question will indicate the presence of bleeding. This should direct you to option 3. Review nursing interventions related to vulvar hematomas if you had difficulty with this question.
Level of Cognitive Ability: Analysis
Client Needs: Physiological Integrity
Integrated Concept/Process: Nursing Process/Planning
Content Area: Maternity
Reference: Burroughs A, Leifer G: *Maternity nursing,* ed 8, Philadelphia, 2002, WB Saunders, p. 302.

11. *Answer:* 1
Rationale: Stasis is believed to be a major predisposing factor in the development of thrombophlebitis. Because cesarean delivery poses a risk factor, the client should ambulate early and frequently to promote circulation and prevent stasis. Options 2, 3, and 4 are implemented if thrombophlebitis occurs.
Test-Taking Strategy: Focus on the issue of the question, prevention of thrombophlebitis. Use the process of elimination. Options 2, 3, and 4 are implemented if thrombophlebitis occurs. Ambulating frequently (option 1) is a preventive measure. Review content related to the prevention of thrombophlebitis in the postoperative period if you had difficulty with this question
Level of Cognitive Ability: Application
Client Needs: Physiological Integrity
Integrated Concept/Process: Nursing Process/Implementation
Content Area: Maternity
Reference: Burroughs A, Leifer G: *Maternity nursing,* ed 8, Philadelphia, 2002, WB Saunders, p. 236.

12. *Answer:* 4
Rationale: Placing the bed in Trendelenburg position rather than flexing the leg at the hip promotes venous drainage. The reverse Trendelenburg position will not aid in promoting venous return. Elevating the extremity by using a pillow, or elevating the foot of the bed will cause flexion at the hip, thus impeding venous drainage.
Test-Taking Strategy: Focus on the issue of the question and use the process of elimination. Recalling that flexion at the hip area restricts venous flow will direct you to option 4. Review these concepts if you had difficulty answering this question.

Level of Cognitive Ability: Comprehension
Client Needs: Physiological Integrity
Integrated Concept/Process:Nursing Process/Implementation
Content Area: Maternity
Reference: Burroughs A, Leifer G: *Maternity nursing*, ed 8, Philadelphia, 2002, WB Saunders, p. 305.

13. ***Answer:*** 4
Rationale: Pulmonary embolism is a complication of thrombophlebitis. Vital signs will be one of the first changes to occur with pulmonary embolism as pulmonary blood flow is compromised. LOC may change as the condition worsens and would indicate hypoxia. Homans' sign is an indicator of thrombophlebitis. Fundal height is unrelated to the issue of the question.
Test-Taking Strategy: Note the key word "initially." Use the ABCs—airway, breathing, and circulation—to assist in directing you to option 4. Review the complications of thrombophlebitis if you had difficulty with this question.
Level of Cognitive Ability: Application
Client Needs: Physiological Integrity
Integrated Concept/Process: Nursing Process/Data Collection
Content Area: Maternity
Reference: Burroughs A, Leifer G: *Maternity nursing*, ed 8, Philadelphia, 2002, WB Saunders, p. 305.

14. ***Answer:*** 1
Rationale: Because pulmonary circulation is compromised in the presence of an embolus, cardiorespiratory support is initiated by oxygen administration. Options 2 and 4 may be a component of the plan of care but are not the most important action. The nurse would not increase the IV rate without a physician's order to do so.
Test-Taking Strategy: Note the key words "most important" and use the ABCs—airway, breathing, and circulation. This will direct you to option 1. Review care to the client in the event of a pulmonary embolism if you had difficulty with this question.
Level of Cognitive Ability: Application
Client Needs: Physiological Integrity
Integrated Concept/Process: Nursing Process/Implementation
Content Area: Maternity
Reference: Burroughs A, Leifer G: *Maternity nursing*, ed 8, Philadelphia, 2002, WB Saunders, p. 305.

15. ***Answer:*** 2
Rationale: Symptoms of hypovolemia include cool, clammy, pale skin; sensations of anxiety; restlessness; and thirst. The nurse would check the vital signs. The nurse would not ambulate the client or encourage fluids until specific orders are given to do so. There is no information in the question to indicate the need for fundal massage.
Test-Taking Strategy: Focus on the symptoms in the question. Use the ABCs—airway, breathing, and circulation—to assist in directing you to option 2. Review nursing care for the client with hypovolemia if you had difficulty with this question.
Level of Cognitive Ability: Application
Client Needs: Physiological Integrity
Integrated Concept/Process: Nursing Process/Implementation
Content Area: Maternity
Reference: Murray S, McKinney E, Gorrie T: *Foundations of maternal-newborn nursing*, ed 3, Philadelphia, 2002, WB Saunders, p. 439.

16. ***Answer:*** 1
Rationale: Inflammation and engorgement are symptoms of mastitis that may alter the new breastfeeding mother's body image. The client's statement does not relate to a problem with newborn nutrition, inadequacy, or infection.
Test-Taking Strategy: Focus on the information in the question and use the process of elimination. Noting the key words, "My breasts look terrible" will direct you to option 1. Review the psychosocial issues related to mastitis if you had difficulty with this question.
Level of Cognitive Ability: Comprehension
Client Needs: Psychosocial Integrity
Integrated Concept/Process: Nursing Process/Planning
Content Area: Maternity
Reference: Burroughs A, Leifer G: *Maternity nursing*, ed 8, Philadelphia, 2002, WB Saunders, p. 298.

17. ***Answer:*** 4
Rationale: Mastitis is an infection frequently associated with a break in the skin surface of the nipple. The measures described in the question are personal hygiene measures to help prevent mastitis.
Test-Taking Strategy: Use the process of elimination and knowledge of the cause and prevention of mastitis to answer this question. Focusing on the data in the question will assist in directing you to option 4. Review the preventive measures for mastitis if you had difficulty with this question.
Level of Cognitive Ability: Comprehension
Client Needs: Health Promotion and Maintenance
Integrated Concept/Process: Teaching/Learning
Content Area: Maternity
Reference: Burroughs A, Leifer G: *Maternity nursing*, ed 8, Philadelphia, 2002, WB Saunders, p. 308.

18. ***Answer:*** 3
Rationale: Failure to nurse equally on both sides will decrease the flow of milk through the breast, causing engorgement of the breast offered less frequently. Options 1, 2, and 4 are appropriate measures.
Test-Taking Strategy: Note the key words "needs further teaching." Use knowledge regarding the treatment for mastitis and the process of elimination to select the correct option. Review the concepts related to breastfeeding and mastitis if you had difficulty with this question.
Level of Cognitive Ability: Comprehension
Client Needs: Health Promotion and Maintenance
Integrated Concept/Process: Nursing Process/Evaluation
Content Area: Maternity
Reference: Burroughs A, Leifer G: *Maternity nursing*, ed 8, Philadelphia, 2002, WB Saunders, p. 307.

19. ***Answer:*** 3
Rationale: Breastfeeding will be compromised and the newborn infant may begin to prefer the bottle over the breast if the mother and newborn are separated for an extended period. When the mother's condition is stable after being separated,

reestablishing breastfeeding should be a nursing priority. Options 1, 2, and 4 do not indicate the need for intervention.
Test-Taking Strategy: Use the process of elimination focusing on the key words "separated from her newborn infant for 2 days." This should easily direct you to option 3. Review the concepts related to maternal-infant bonding if you had difficulty with this question.
Level of Cognitive Ability: Comprehension
Client Needs: Psychosocial Integrity
Integrated Concept/Process: Nursing Process/Evaluation
Content Area: Maternity
Reference: Murray S, McKinney E, Gorrie T: *Foundations of maternal-newborn nursing,* ed 3, Philadelphia, 2002, WB Saunders, p. 476.

20. ***Answer:*** 1
Rationale: Keeping the client and her family informed of her condition will help minimize fear and apprehension. Options 2, 3, and 4 identify physiological interventions.
Test-Taking Strategy: Use the process of elimination. Focus on the key words "meet the psychosocial needs." Option 1 is the only option that addresses psychosocial needs. Review the interventions that will meet the psychosocial needs of a client if you had difficulty with this question.
Level of Cognitive Ability: Application
Client Needs: Psychosocial Integrity
Integrated Concept/Process: Nursing Process/Implementation
Content Area: Maternity
Reference: Burroughs A, Leifer G: *Maternity nursing,* ed 8, Philadelphia, 2002, WB Saunders, p. 5.

REFERENCES

Burroughs A, Leifer G: *Maternity nursing,* ed 8, Philadelphia, 2002, WB Saunders.
Lowdermilk D, Perry S, Bobak I: *Maternity and women's health care,* ed 7, St Louis, 2000, Mosby.
McKinney E et al: *Maternal-child nursing,* Philadelphia, 2000, WB Saunders.
Murray S, McKinney E, Gorrie T: *Foundations of maternal-newborn nursing,* ed 3, Philadelphia, 2002, WB Saunders.

Care of the Newborn

I. INITIAL CARE OF THE NEWBORN

A. Data collection
   1. Observe or assist with initiation of respirations
   2. Assess Apgar score
   3. Note characteristics of cry
   4. Obtain vital signs
   5. Monitor for nasal flaring, grunting, retractions, and abnormal respirations
   6. Observe **newborn** for signs of hypothermia or hyperthermia
   7. Monitor for gross anomalies

B. Implementation
   1. Suction the mouth then nares with bulb syringe
   2. Dry the **newborn** and stimulate crying by rubbing
   3. Maintain temperature stability
   4. Wrap the **newborn** in warm blankets
   5. Place a stockinette cap on the **newborn's** head
   6. Keep the **newborn** with the mother to facilitate bonding
   7. Place the **newborn** at the mother's breast if breastfeeding is planned or place on the mother's abdomen
   8. Place the **newborn** in warmer
   9. Position the **newborn** on the side or abdomen or modified Trendelenburg position to facilitate drainage of mucus
   10. Ensure the **newborn's** proper identification
   11. Footprint the **newborn** and fingerprint the mother on identification sheet
   12. Place matching identification bracelets on the mother and **newborn**

C. Apgar scoring system
   1. Perform and record Apgar score at 1 minute and 5 minutes
   2. If the score is less than 7 at 5 minutes, the Apgar score should be performed at 10 minutes
   3. Assess each of the five items to be scored and assign a value of 0 (very poor) to 2 (excellent) for each item
   4. Add the points to determine the **newborn's** total score
      a. A score of 7 to 10 indicates a healthy **newborn**
      b. A score of 3 to 6 is considered moderately depressed
      c. A score of 0 to 2 is severely depressed
   5. Five vital indicators (Table 25-1)
      a. Heart rate

TABLE 25-1

Apgar Scoring

Indicator	0 Points	1 Point	2 Points
Heart rate	Absent	Less than 100	More than 100
Respiratory rate	Absent	Slow, irregular weak cry	Good vigorous cry
Muscle tone	Flaccid, limp	Some flexion of extremities	Good flexion, active motion
Reflex irritability	No response	Weak cry and grimace	Vigorous cry, cough, sneeze
Skin color	Blue	Body skin normal, extremities blue	Body and extremity skin color normal

b. Respiratory rate
c. Muscle tone
d. Reflex irritability
e. Skin color
6. Implementation (Table 25-2)

II. INITIAL PHYSICAL EXAMINATION

A. General guidelines
1. Keep the **newborn** warm during the examination
2. Begin with general observations and proceed to detailed findings
3. Perform assessments that are least disturbing to the **newborn** first
4. Initiate nursing interventions for abnormal findings
5. Document all abnormal findings

B. Vital signs
1. Heart rate: 120 to 160 beats per minute (apical); assess for a full minute because of irregularities after birth
2. Respirations: 30 to 60 breaths per minute; assess for a full minute
3. Axillary temperature: 36.4° C to 37° C (97.6° F to 98.6° F)
4. Blood pressure: 60/40 to 80/50 mm Hg

C. Body measurements
1. Length: 45 to 55 cm (18 to 22 inches)
2. Weight: 2500 to 4300 g (5.5 to 9.5 lb)
3. Head circumference: 33 to 35.5 cm (13 to 14 inches)
4. Chest circumference: 30 to 33 cm (12 to 13 inches) and should be equal to or 2 to 3 cm less than the head circumference

D. Head
1. 25% of the body length (cephalocaudal development)
2. Bones of the skull are not fused
3. Palpable sutures (connective tissue between the skull bones)
4. Fontanelles: unossified membranous tissue at the junction of the sutures (Table 25-3)
5. Molding
   a. Asymmetry of head resulting from pressure in the birth canal
   b. Disappears in about 72 hours
6. Masses from birth trauma
   a. Caput succedaneum: edema of the soft tissue over bone (crosses over suture line); subsides within a few days
   b. Cephalhematoma: swelling caused by bleeding into an area between the bone and its periosteum (does not cross over suture line); usually absorbed within 6 weeks with no treatment
7. Head lag
   a. Common when pulling the **newborn** to a sitting position
   b. When prone, the **newborn** should be able to lift the head slightly and turn from side to side

E. Eyes
1. Slate gray (light skin) or brown-gray (dark skin) in color
2. Symmetrical and clear
3. Pupils equal, round, react to light by accommodation
4. Blink reflex present
5. Eyes cross because of weak extraocular muscles

TABLE 25-2

Apgar Score Implementation

Score	Implementation
7 to 10	Rarely need resuscitation
3 to 6	Require resuscitation Suction Dry quickly Maintain warmth Ventilate 30 to 50 times a minute until heart rate is above 100, color is pink, and spontaneous respirations begin Provide oxygen Careful observation during the first few days of life
0 to 2	Requires intensive resuscitation Clear airway Insert endotracheal tube Use Ambu bag if necessary Ventilate with 100% oxygen at 40 to 60 breaths per minute Initiate full CPR as needed Maintain body temperature Support parents

TABLE 25-3

Fontanelles

Fontanelle	Characteristics	Closure
Anterior	Soft, flat diamond-shaped 3 to 4 cm wide x 2 to 3 cm long	Closes between 12 and 18 months
Posterior	Triangular 0.5 to 1 cm wide Located between occipital and parietal bones	Closes between birth and 2 to 3 months of age

6. Able to track and fixate momentarily
7. Red reflex present
8. Eyelids often edematous because of pressure during the birth process and the effects of eye medication

F. Ears
1. Symmetrical
2. Firm cartilage with recoil
3. Pinna should be on or above line drawn from the canthus of the eye
4. Low-set ears are associated with Down syndrome

G. Nose
1. Flat, broad, and in the center of face
2. Obligatory nose breathing
3. Occasional sneezing to remove obstructions

H. Mouth
1. Pink moist gums
2. Soft and hard palates intact
3. Epstein's pearls (small, white cysts) may be present on hard palate
4. Uvula in midline
5. Tongue moves freely, is symmetrical, and has a short frenulum
6. Sucking and crying movements are symmetrical
7. Able to swallow
8. Gag reflex is present

I. Neck
1. Short and thick
2. Head held in midline
3. Trachea on midline
4. Raises head momentarily when prone
5. Good range of motion and is able to flex and extend

J. Chest
1. Appears circular because anteroposterior and lateral diameters are about equal
2. Respirations appear diaphragmatic
3. Bronchial sounds heard on auscultation
4. Nipples prominent and often edematous
5. Milky secretion (witch's milk) common
6. Breast tissue present
7. Clavicles need to be palpated to assess for fractures

K. Skin
1. Pinkish-red (light-skinned **newborn**) to pinkish-brown or pinkish-yellow (dark-skinned **newborn**
2. Vernix caseosa
3. Lanugo
4. Milia
5. Dry, peeling skin
6. Dark red color common in premature **newborns**
7. Cyanosis common with hypothermia, infection, hypoglycemia, and with cardiac, respiratory, or neurological abnormalities
8. Acrocyanosis is not uncommon and may be due to immature peripheral circulation
9. Assess for ecchymosis and petechiae resulting from trauma of birth
10. Assess skin turgor over the abdomen to determine hydration status
11. Observe for forceps marks
12. Harlequin sign
   a. Deep red color develops over one side of the **newborn's** body, whereas the other side remains pale as a result of vasomotor disturbance
   b. Skin resembles a clown's suit
13. Birthmarks (Table 25-4)

L. Abdomen
1. Umbilical cord
   a. Three vessels, two arteries, and one vein in cord; if less than three vessels are noted, the physician is notified
   b. Small, thin cord may be associated with poor fetal growth
   c. Assess for intact cord and ensure that the clamp is secured

TABLE 25-4

Birthmarks

Birthmark	Characteristics
Telangiectatic nevi (stork bites)	Pale pink or red, flat, dilated capillaries On eyelids, nose, lower occipital bone, and nape of neck Blanch easily More noticeable during crying periods Disappear by age 2 years
Nevus flammeus (port-wine stain)	Capillary angioma directly below epidermis Nonelevated, sharply demarcated, red to purple, dense areas of capillaries Commonly appears on face Does not fade with time May require surgery in the future
Nevus vasculosus (strawberry mark)	Capillary hemangioma Raised, clearly delineated, dark red, with a rough surface Common in head region Disappear by age 7 to 9 years
Mongolian spots	Bluish black pigmentation On lumbar dorsal area and buttocks Gradually fade during first and second years of life Common in Asian and dark-skinned races

d. Cord should be clamped for at least the first 24 hours after birth; clamp can be removed when the cord is dried and occluded
e. Note any bleeding or drainage from the cord
f. Triple dye may be applied for initial cord care because it minimizes microorganisms and promotes drying; use a cotton-tipped applicator to paint the dye, one time, on the cord and on 1 inch of surrounding skin
g. Application of 70% isopropyl alcohol to the cord minimizes microorganisms and promotes drying
h. If symptoms of infection such as moistness, oozing, discharge, and a reddened base occur, antibiotic treatment is prescribed

2. Gastrointestinal
a. Monitor the cord for meconium staining
b. Assess for umbilical hernia
c. Note abdominal depression associated with a diaphragmatic hernia
d. Monitor for abdominal distention associated with obstruction, mass, or sepsis
e. Monitor bowel sounds, which should occur within 1 to 2 hours after birth

3. Anus
a. Anal opening patent
b. First stool meconium should pass within first 24 hours

M. Genitals
1. Female
a. Labia edematous, clitoris enlarged
b. Smegma present (thick white mucus discharge)
c. Pseudomenstruation possible (blood-tinged mucus)
d. Hymen tag may be visible
e. First voiding should occur within 24 hours

2. Male
a. Prepuce (foreskin) covers glans penis
b. Scrotum edematous
c. Meatus at tip of penis
d. Testes descended but may retract on cold
e. Assess for hernia or hydrocele
f. First voiding should occur within 24 hours

N. Spine
1. Straight
2. Posture flexed
3. Supports head momentarily when prone
4. Arms and legs flexed
5. Chin flexed on upper chest
6. Sporadic movements that are well coordinated
7. Degree of hypotonicity or hypertonicity is indicative of central nervous system (CNS) damage

O. Extremities
1. Flexed
2. Full range of motion (ROM)
3. Movements symmetrical
4. Fists clenched
5. Fingers and toes should be 10 each in number and separate
6. Legs bowed
7. Major gluteal folds even
8. Creases on soles of feet
9. Assess for hip dysplasia
10. When thighs are rotated outward, no clicks should be heard
11. Pulses (radial, brachial, femoral) palpable
12. Assess for fractures (especially clavicle) or dislocations (hip)
13. Slight tremors are common but may be a sign of hypoglycemia or drug withdrawal

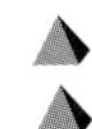

III. BODY SYSTEMS

A. Cardiovascular
1. Keep the **newborn** warm
2. Take the apical heart rate for 1 full minute
3. Listen for murmurs
4. Palpate pulses
5. Assess for cyanosis
6. Blanch skin on the trunk and extremities to assess circulation
7. Observe cord stump for bleeding
8. Document inability to feed without cardiac distress

B. Respiratory
1. Position **newborn** on the side
2. Suction as necessary
a. Use a bulb syringe for upper airway suctioning (compress bulb before insertion)
b. Use a French catheter for deeper suctioning
3. Observe for respiratory distress and hypoxemia
a. Nasal flaring
b. Increasingly severe retractions
c. Grunting
d. Cyanosis
e. Bradycardia
f. Low body temperature
g. Periods of apnea lasting longer than 15 seconds
4. Administer oxygen per hood if necessary as prescribed

C. Hepatic
1. Normal or physiological jaundice appears after the first 24 hours in full-term **neonates** and after the first 48 hours in premature **neonates**; jaundice occurring before this

time (pathological jaundice) may indicate early hemolysis of red blood cells (RBCs) and must be reported to the physician
2. Physiological jaundice peaks about the fifth day of life (indirect bilirubin levels: 6 to 7 mg/dL)
3. Monitor serum bilirubin levels
4. Feed early to stimulate intestinal activity and to keep the bilirubin level low
5. If the **neonate** is being breastfed, temporarily discontinue breastfeeding for 48 hours if bilirubin levels exceed 15 to 20 mg/dL, and if prescribed by the physician
6. Prevent chilling, as hypothermia can cause acidosis that interferes with bilirubin conjugation and excretion
7. Liver stores iron passed from the mother for 5 to 6 months
8. Glycogen storage occurs in the liver
9. **Newborn** is at risk for hemorrhagic disorders; coagulation factors synthesized in the liver are dependent on vitamin K, which is not synthesized until intestinal bacteria is present
10. Handle **newborn** carefully and monitor for any bruising or bleeding episodes
11. Watch for meconium stool and subsequent stools
12. Administer one dose of vitamin K (AquaMEPHYTON) 0.5 to 1.0 mg IM to the **neonate** in the vastus lateralis muscle as prescribed, to aid in blood coagulation
13. Assess the **newborn's** hemoglobin and blood glucose level

D. Renal
1. The immature kidneys are unable to concentrate urine
2. A weight loss of 5% to 15% during the first week of life occurs as a result of voiding and limited intake
3. Weigh the **newborn** daily
4. Monitor intake and output (I&O)
5. Weigh the diapers if necessary
6. Measure specific gravity if necessary
7. Monitor for signs of dehydration
   a. Dry mucous membranes
   b. Sunken eyeballs
   c. Poor skin turgor
   d. Sunken fontanelles

E. Immune
1. Passive immunity via the **placenta** (immunoglobulin G, IgG)
2. Passive immunity from colostrum (IgA)
3. Elevations in IgM indicate infection in utero
4. Use aseptic technique when caring for the **newborn**
5. Observe universal (standard) precautions when handling the **newborn**
6. Ensure meticulous hand washing
7. Wear gowns when caring for the **newborn**
8. Ensure that an infection-free staff cares for the **newborn**
9. Monitor the **newborn's** temperature
10. Observe for any cracks or openings in the skin
11. Administer eye medication within 1 hour after birth to prevent ophthalmia neonatorum
   a. Eye prophylaxis may be delayed until an hour or so after birth so that eye contact and parent-**infant** attachment and bonding are facilitated
   b. Erythromycin (0.5%) and tetracycline (1%) ophthalmic ointment or drops are both bacteriostatic and bactericidal and provide prophylaxis against *Neisseria gonorrhoeae* and *Chlamydia trachomatis*
   c. Silver nitrate (1%) solution may be prescribed, but its use is minimal because it does not protect against chlamydial infection and can cause chemical conjunctivitis
12. Provide cord care
   a. Umbilical clamp can be removed after 24 hours
   b. Teach mother how to perform cord care
   c. Keep the cord clean and dry by wiping with alcohol after each diaper change and at least two to three times a day
   d. Keep diaper from covering cord; fold diaper below cord
   e. Assess cord for odor, swelling, or discharge
   f. Sponge bathe the **newborn** until the cord falls off (within 2 weeks)
13. Provide circumcision care
   a. Apply petroleum jelly gauze to the penis except when a Plastibell is used
   b. Remove petroleum jelly gauze, if applied, after first voiding following circumcision
   c. Observe for swelling, infection, or bleeding from the circumcision site
   d. Teach mother care of circumcision site
   e. Cleanse the penis after each voiding by squeezing warm water over the penis
   f. A milky covering over the glans penis is normal and should not be disrupted
   g. Monitor for urinary retention

F. Metabolic and gastrointestinal
1. **Newborns** are able to digest simple carbohydrates but unable to digest fats because of the lack of lipase
2. Proteins may be only partially broken down and thus may serve as antigens and provoke an allergic reaction

3. The **newborn** has a small stomach capacity (about 90 mL) with rapid intestinal peristalsis (bowel emptying time is 2.5 to 3 hours)
4. Breastfeeding can usually begin immediately after birth; bottle-fed **newborns** may be offered a few milliliters of sterile water or 5% dextrose 1 to 4 hours after birth before a feeding with formula
5. Observe feeding reflexes, such as rooting, sucking, and swallowing
6. Assist the mother with breastfeeding or formula-feeding
7. Burp **newborn** during and after feeding
8. Assess for regurgitations or vomiting
9. Position **newborn** on right side after feeding
10. Observe for normal stool and the passage of meconium
    a. Meconium stool, which is greenish-black with a thick, sticky, tarlike consistency, is usually passed within the first 24 hours of life
    b. Transitional stool, the second type of stool excreted by the **newborn**, is greenish-brown and of looser consistency than meconium
    c. Soft, yellow stools are noted in breast-fed **newborns**; seedy, yellow stools in formula-fed **newborns**
11. Phenylketonuria (PKU) screening test is done before discharge and as an outpatient after sufficient protein intake occurs; the **newborn** should be on formula or breast milk for 24 hours before screening, and screening must be repeated in 7 to 14 days

G. Neurological
1. **Newborn** head size is proportionally larger than that of adults because of cephalocaudal development
2. Myelinization of nerve fibers is incomplete, so primitive reflexes are present
3. Fontanelles open to allow for brain growth
4. Assess for an abnormal size and bulging or depressed anterior fontanelle
5. Measure and graph head circumference in relation to chest circumference and length
6. Assess the **newborn's** movements, noting symmetry, posture, and abnormal movements
7. Observe for jitteriness, marked tremors, and seizures
8. Test the **newborn's** reflexes
9. Assess for lethargy
10. Assess pitch of cry

H. Thermoregulatory
1. **Newborns** do not shiver to produce heat
2. **Newborns** have brown fat deposits that produce heat
3. Heat is dissipated through vasodilation
4. Prevent heat loss resulting from evaporation by keeping the **newborn** dry and well wrapped with a blanket
5. Prevent heat loss resulting from radiation by keeping the **newborn** away from cold objects and outside walls
6. Prevent heat loss resulting from convection by shielding the **newborn** from drafts
7. Prevent heat loss resulting from conduction by performing all treatments on a warm, padded surface
8. Keep the room temperature warm
9. Take the **newborn's** axillary temperature every hour for the first 4 hours of life, every 4 hours for the remainder of the first 24 hours, and then every shift

I. Reflexes
1. Sucking and rooting
    a. Touch the **newborn's** lip, cheek, or corner of the mouth with a nipple
    b. **Newborn** turns head toward the nipple, opens the mouth, takes hold of the nipple, and sucks
    c. Usually disappears after 3 to 4 months but may persist for up to 1 year
2. Swallowing reflex
    a. Occurs spontaneously after sucking and obtaining fluids
    b. **Newborn** swallows in coordination with sucking without gagging, coughing, or vomiting
3. Tonic neck or fencing
    a. While the **newborn** is falling asleep or sleeping, gently and quickly turn the head to one side
    b. As the **newborn** faces the left side, the left arm and leg extend outward while the right arm and leg flex
    c. When turned to the right side, the right arm and leg extend outward while the left arm and leg flex
    d. Usually disappears within 3 to 4 months
4. Palmar-plantar grasp
    a. Place a finger in the palm of the **newborn's** hand; then place a finger at the base of the toes
    b. The **newborn's** fingers curl around the examiner's fingers, and the **newborn's** toes curl downward
    c. Palmar response lessens within 3 to 4 months
    d. Plantar response lessens within 8 months
5. Moro reflex
    a. Hold the newborn in a semisitting position; then allow the head and trunk to fall backward to at least a 30-degree angle

b. The **newborn** symmetrically abducts and extends the arms
c. The **newborn** fans the fingers out and forms a C with the thumb and the forefinger
d. The **newborn** adducts the arms to an embracing position and returns to a relaxed flexion state
e. Present at birth; a complete response may occur up to 8 weeks
f. A body jerk motion occurs from 8 to 18 weeks
g. No response may be noted by 6 months as long as neurological maturation has not been delayed
h. A persistent response lasting more than 6 months may indicate the occurrence of brain damage during pregnancy

6. Startle reflex
   a. The response is best elicited if the **newborn** is a least 24 hours old
   b. The examiner makes a loud noise or claps hands to elicit the response
   c. The **newborn's** arms adduct while the elbows flex
   d. The hands stay clenched
   e. The reflex should disappear within 4 months
7. Pull-to-sit
   a. Pull the **newborn** up from the wrist while the **newborn** is in the prone position
   b. The head will lag until the **newborn** is in an upright position; then the head will be level with the chest and shoulders momentarily before falling forward
   c. The head will then lift for a few minutes
   d. The response depends on the **newborn's** general muscle tone and condition as well as maturity levels
8. Babinski sign-plantar
   a. Beginning at the heel of the foot, gently stroke upward along the lateral aspect of the sole; then the examiner moves the finger along the ball of the foot
   b. The **newborn's** toes hyperextend while the big toe dorsiflexes
   c. Reflex disappears after the **newborn** is 1 year old
   d. Absence of this reflex indicates the need for a neurological examination
9. Stepping or walking
   a. Hold the **newborn** in a vertical position, allowing one foot to touch a table surface
   b. The **newborn** simulates walking, alternately flexing and extending the feet
   c. The reflex is usually present for 3 to 4 months
10. Crawling
    a. Place the **newborn** on the abdomen
    b. The **newborn** begins making crawling movements with the arms and legs
    c. The reflex usually disappears after about 6 weeks

IV. PARENT TEACHING

A. Formula feeding
   1. Teach sterilization techniques if the water supply is located in areas where the purification process of the water is questionable
   2. Remind the mother not to heat the bottle of formula in the microwave oven
   3. Inform the mother that formula is a sufficient diet for the first 4 to 6 months
   4. Assess the mother's ability to burp the **newborn**

B. Breastfeeding
   1. Assess the **newborn's** ability to attach to the mother's breast and suck
   2. Teach the mother about engorgement
   3. Teach the mother how to pump her breasts and how to store breast milk properly
   4. Inform the mother that breast milk is a sufficient and superior diet for the first 4 to 6 months
   5. Give the mother the phone number of the local organizations that offer support to breastfeeding mothers

C. Bathing
   1. Bathe the **newborn** in a warm room before feeding
   2. Have all equipment for bathing available
   3. Use a mild soap (not on the face)
   4. Proceed from the cleanest area to the dirtiest
   5. Clean eyes from the inner canthus outward
   6. Special care should be taken to clean under the folds of the neck, underarms, groin, and genitals
   7. Make bath time enjoyable for both the **newborn** and mother

D. Clothing
   1. Assess diaper and clothing needs for the **newborn** with the mother
   2. Instruct the mother that the **newborn's** head should be covered in cold weather to prevent heat loss
   3. Instruct the mother to layer the **newborn's** clothing in cooler weather

E. Cord care: refer to cord care under body systems

F. Circumcision: refer to circumcision care under body systems

G. Uncircumcised **newborn**

1. Inform the mother that the foreskin and glans are two similar layers of cells that separate from each other and that the separation process is normally complete between 3 and 5 years of age
2. Instruct the mother not to pull back the foreskin but to allow for the natural separation to occur
3. Inform the mother that as the process of separation occurs, sterile sloughed cells build up between the layers of the foreskin and the glans, and when retraction occurs, daily gentle washing of the glans with soap and water is sufficient to maintain adequate cleanliness

V. PRETERM NEWBORN

A. Description
1. A **neonate** born before 37 weeks' gestation
2. The primary concern relates to immaturity of all body systems

B. Data collection
1. Respirations irregular with periods of apnea
2. Body temperature is below normal
3. The **newborn** has poor suck and swallow reflexes
4. Bowel sounds are diminished
5. Increased or decreased urinary output
6. Extremities are thin with minimal creasing on soles and palms
7. The **newborn** extends extremities and does not maintain flexion
8. Lanugo, on skin and on the **newborn's** head, is present in woolly patches
9. Skin is thin with visible blood vessels and minimal subcutaneous fat pads
10. Skin may appear jaundiced
11. Testes are undescended in male
12. Labia is narrow in female

C. Implementation
1. Monitor vital signs every 2 to 4 hours
2. Maintain cardiopulmonary functions
3. Administer oxygen and humidification as prescribed
4. Monitor I&O and electrolyte balance
5. Monitor daily weight
6. Maintain **newborn** in warming device
7. Position every 1 to 2 hours and handle **newborn** carefully
8. Avoid exposure to infections
9. Provide **newborn** with appropriate stimulation as touch

VI. POSTTERM NEWBORN

A. Description: a **neonate** born after 42 weeks of gestation

B. Data collection
1. Hypoglycemia
2. Parchmentlike skin (dry and cracked) without lanugo
3. Fingernails long and extended over ends of fingers
4. Profuse scalp hair
5. Body is long and thin
6. Extremities show wasting of fat and muscle
7. Meconium staining may be present on nails and umbilical cord

C. Implementation
1. Provide normal **newborn** care
2. Monitor for hypoglycemia
3. Maintain **newborn's** temperature
4. Monitor for meconium aspiration

VII. SMALL FOR GESTATIONAL AGE

A. Description: a **neonate** who is plotted at or below the 10th percentile on the intrauterine growth curve

B. Data collection
1. Fetal distress
2. Gestational age and physical maturity
3. Lowered or elevated body temperature
4. Physical abnormalities
5. Hypoglycemia
6. Signs of polycythemia
   a. Ruddy appearance
   b. Cyanosis
   c. Jaundice
7. Signs of infection
8. Signs of aspiration of meconium

C. Implementation
1. Maintain airway
2. Maintain body temperature
3. Observe for signs of respiratory distress
4. Monitor for signs of infection
5. Monitor glucose levels and for signs of hypoglycemia
6. Initiate early feedings and monitor for signs of aspiration
7. Provide stimulation, such as touch and cuddling

VIII. LARGE FOR GESTATIONAL AGE

A. Description: a **neonate** who is plotted at or above the 90th percentile on the intrauterine growth curve

B. Data collection
1. Gestational age
2. Birth trauma or injury
3. Respiratory distress
4. Hypoglycemia

C. Implementation
1. Monitor vital signs
2. Monitor glucose levels and for signs of hypoglycemia
3. Initiate early feedings
4. Monitor for infection
5. Provide stimulation, such as touch and cuddling

IX. RESPIRATORY DISTRESS SYNDROME (RDS)

A. Description: a serious lung disorder caused by immaturity and inability to produce surfactant, resulting in hypoxia and acidosis

B. Data collection
1. Tachypnea
2. Flaring nares
3. Expiratory grunting
4. Retractions
5. Decreased breath sounds
6. Apnea
7. Pallor and cyanosis
8. Hypothermia
9. Poor muscle tone

C. Implementation
1. Monitor color, respiratory rate, and degree of effort in breathing
2. Support respirations as prescribed
3. Monitor arterial blood gases (ABGs) and oxygen saturation levels (ABGs from umbilical artery)
4. Monitor ABGs so that oxygen administered to the **newborn** is at the lowest possible concentration necessary to maintain adequate arterial oxygenation
5. Schedule any premature **newborn** who required oxygen support for an eye examination before discharge to assess for retinal damage
6. Suction every 2 hours or more often as necessary
7. Position **newborn** on side or back, with neck slightly extended
8. Anticipate that the newborn will receive surfactant replacement therapy (instilled into the endotracheal tube)
9. Administer respiratory therapy (percussion and vibration) as prescribed; use padded small plastic cup or small oxygen mask for percussion; use padded electric toothbrush for vibration
10. Provide nutrition
11. Support bonding
12. Prepare parents for short- to long-term period of oxygen dependency if necessary
13. Encourage mother to pump breasts for future breastfeeding if she so desires
14. Encourage as much participation in **newborn's** care as condition allows

X. HYPERBILIRUBINEMIA

A. Description
1. At any serum bilirubin level, the appearance of jaundice during the first day of life indicates a pathological process
2. Evaluation is indicated when serum levels are more than 12 mg/dL in the term **newborn**
3. Therapy is aimed at preventing kernicterus, which results in permanent neurological damage resulting from the deposition of bilirubin in the brain cells

B. Data collection
1. Jaundice
2. Elevated serum bilirubin levels
3. Enlarged liver
4. Poor muscle tone
5. Lethargy
6. Poor sucking reflex

C. Implementation
1. Monitor for presence of jaundice
   a. Examine the **newborn's** skin color in natural light
   b. Press finger over a bony prominence or tip of the **newborn's** nose to press out capillary blood from the tissues
   c. Note that jaundice starts at the head first, spreads to the chest, then the abdomen, then the arms and legs, followed by the hands and feet, which are the last to be jaundiced
2. Keep the **newborn** well hydrated to maintain blood volume
3. Facilitate early, frequent feeding to hasten passage of meconium and encourage excretion of bilirubin
4. Report any signs of jaundice in the first 24 hours and any abnormal signs and symptoms
5. Prepare for phototherapy, and monitor the **newborn** closely during the treatment

D. Phototherapy
1. Description
   a. Use of intense florescent lights to reduce serum bilirubin levels in the **newborn**
   b. Injury from treatment, such as eye damage, dehydration, or sensory deprivation, can occur
2. Implementation
   a. Expose as much of the **newborn's** skin as possible

b. Cover the genital area, and monitor genital area for skin irritation or breakdown
c. Cover the **newborn's** eyes with eye shields or patches; make sure eyelids are closed when shields or patches are applied
d. Remove the shields or patches at least once per shift to inspect the eyes for infection or irritation and to allow eye contact
e. Measure the quantity of light every 8 hours
f. Monitor skin temperature closely
g. Increase fluids to compensate for water loss
h. Expect loose green stools and green urine
i. Monitor the **newborn's** skin color with the florescent light turned off, every 4 to 8 hours
j. Monitor the skin for bronze baby syndrome, a grayish-brown discoloration of the skin
k. Reposition **newborn** every 2 hours
l. Provide stimulation
m. After treatment, continue monitoring for signs of hyperbilirubinemia, as rebound elevations are normal after therapy is discontinued

XI. ERYTHROBLASTOSIS FETALIS

A. Description
1. Destruction of RBCs that results from an antigen-antibody reaction
2. Characterized by hemolytic anemia or hyperbilirubinemia
3. Exchange of fetal and maternal blood takes place primarily when the **placenta** separates at birth
4. Rh antigens from the baby's blood enters the maternal bloodstream
5. The mother's produces anti-Rh antibodies against the fetal blood cells
6. Antibodies are harmless to the mother but attach to the erythrocytes in the fetus and cause hemolysis
7. Sensitization is rare with the first pregnancy
8. ABO incompatibility is usually less severe

B. Data collection
1. Anemia
2. Jaundice that develops rapidly after birth and before 24 hours
3. Edema

C. Implementation
1. Administer Rho(D) immune globulin to the mother during the first 72 hours after **delivery** if the Rh-negative mother delivers an Rh-positive fetus but remains unsensitized
2. Assist with exchange transfusion after birth or intrauterine transfusion as prescribed
3. The baby's blood is replaced with Rh-negative blood to stop the destruction of the baby's RBCs; the Rh-negative blood is replaced gradually with the baby's own blood
4. Reassure the mother that the **newborn** will not experience any untoward effects from the condition

XII. SEPSIS

A. Description: generalized infection resulting from the presence of bacteria in the blood

B. Data collection
1. Pallor
2. Tachypnea, tachycardia
3. Poor feeding
4. Abdominal distention
5. Temperature instability

C. Implementation
1. Monitor for periods of apnea or irregular respirations
2. If apnea is present, stimulate by gently rubbing chest or foot
3. Administer oxygen as prescribed
4. Monitor vital signs
5. Maintain warmth in an Isolette
6. Provide isolation as necessary
7. Monitor for a fever
8. Monitor I&O and obtain daily weight
9. Monitor for diarrhea
10. Monitor feeding and sucking reflex, which may be poor
11. Monitor for jaundice
12. Monitor for irritability and lethargy
13. Administer antibiotics as prescribed and observe carefully for toxicity, because a **newborn's** liver and kidney are immature

XIII. TORCH SYNDROME

A. Description
1. Refers to infections of the fetus or **newborn**
2. Caused by one of the following
   a. **T**oxoplasmosis
   b. **O**ther viruses
   c. **R**ubella
   d. **C**ytomegalovirus
   e. **H**erpes

B. Infections (Table 25-5)

XIV. SYPHILIS

A. Description
1. Sexually transmitted disease

TABLE 25-5

Infections Included in TORCH Syndrome

Infection	Characteristics
Toxoplasmosis	Protozoan infection Produces no serious effects in the mother Can be transmitted to the fetus Can result in severe physical and developmental abnormalities Common carriers include cat feces and raw beef
Other Infections	Such as syphilis
Rubella	Systemic viral infection Causes congenital rubella syndrome, which includes congenital heart disease, cataracts, growth retardation, and pneumonia if the mother becomes infected within the first trimester Deafness and some learning disabilities can occur if the mother becomes infected during the first trimester
Cytomegalovirus	A viral infection that persists in the body indefinitely, with periods of reactivation without symptoms Can infect the fetus or infant during delivery or after birth through breast milk, blood transfusions, or contact with infected secretions May cause microcephaly, blindness, deafness, and mental and motor retardation
Herpes simplex	Sexually transmitted disease caused by a virus Periods of reactivation Neonate is commonly infected during delivery by direct contact with lesions in the genital tract Can cause neurological impairment or death

2. Congenital syphilis can result in premature **delivery**, skin lesions, abnormal skeletal development
3. The organism *Treponema pallidum*, a spirochete, is able to cross the **placenta** throughout pregnancy and infect the fetus, usually after 18 weeks' gestation
4. Risks include preterm birth, still birth, and low birth weight
5. Congenital effects are irreversible and may include CNS damage and hearing loss

B. Data collection
1. Hepatosplenomegaly
2. Joint swelling
3. Rash
4. Anemia
5. Jaundice
6. Snuffles
7. Ascites
8. Pneumonitis
9. Cerebrospinal fluid changes

C. Implementation
1. Monitor **newborn** for signs of syphilis
2. Monitor for palmar rash and snuffles
3. Prepare **newborn** for serological testing if prescribed
4. Administer antibiotic therapy as prescribed
5. Use universal (standard) precautions and drainage/secretion precautions with suspected congenital syphilis
6. Wear gloves when handling **neonate** until 24 hours of antibiotic therapy has been administered
7. Provide psychological support to the mother and provide instructions regarding follow-up care to the **newborn**

XV. THE ADDICTED NEWBORN

A. Description: **newborn** who has become passively addicted to drugs that have passed through the **placenta**

B. Common addicting drugs
1. Heroin
   a. **Newborn** may appear normal at birth with a low birth weight
   b. Withdrawal occurs within 12 to 24 hours and may last 5 to 7 days
2. Methadone
   a. Withdrawal occurs within 1 to 2 days to 1 week or more, is most evident 48 to 72 hours, and may last 6 days to 8 weeks
   b. **Newborn** appears very ill
   c. May develop jaundice as a result of prematurity
3. Cocaine
   a. Causes decreased interactive behavior
   b. Feeding problems are present
   c. Irregular sleep patterns and diarrhea occur

C. Data collection
1. Irritability
2. Tremors
3. Hyperactivity and hypertonicity
4. Respiratory distress
5. Vomiting
6. High-pitched cry
7. Sneezing
8. Fever
9. Diarrhea
10. Excessive sweating
11. Poor feeding
12. Extreme sucking of fists
13. Convulsions

D. Implementation
1. Monitor respiratory and cardiac status frequently
2. Monitor temperature and vital signs
3. Hold **newborn** firm and close to the body during feeding and when giving care
4. Initiate seizure precautions
5. Pad sides of crib
6. Provide small, frequent feedings and allow a longer period for feeding
7. Monitor I&O
8. Administer IV hydration if prescribed
9. Protect **neonate's** skin from injury that can be caused by the constant rubbing from hyperactive jitters
10. Swaddle **newborn**
11. Place **newborn** in a quiet room and reduce stimulation
12. Allow mother to ventilate feelings of anxiety and guilt
13. Refer mother for treatment of substance abuse problem

XVI. FETAL ALCOHOL SYNDROME

A. Description
1. Caused by maternal alcohol use during pregnancy
2. Most serious cause of teratogenesis
3. Causes mental and physical retardation

B. Data collection
1. Facial changes
   a. Short palpebral fissures
   b. Hypoplastic philtrum
   c. Short, upturned nose
   d. Flat midface
   e. Thin upper lip
   f. Low nasal bridge
2. Abnormal palmar creases
3. Respiratory distress (apnea, cyanosis)
4. Congenital heart disorders
5. Irritability, hypersensitivity to stimuli
6. Tremors
7. Poor feeding
8. Seizures

C. Implementation
1. Monitor for respiratory distress
2. Position **newborn** on side to facilitate drainage of secretions
3. Keep resuscitation equipment at the bedside
4. Monitor for hypoglycemia
5. Monitor suck and swallow reflex
6. Administer small feedings and burp well
7. Suction as necessary
8. Monitor I&O
9. Monitor weight and head circumference
10. Decrease environmental stimuli

XVII. HUMAN IMMUNODEFICIENCY VIRUS (HIV)

A. Description
1. The fetus of an HIV antibody-positive woman should be monitored closely throughout the pregnancy
2. Serial ultrasound screenings should be done to identify intrauterine growth restriction
3. Weekly nonstress testing after 32 weeks of gestation and biophysical profiles may be necessary during pregnancy
4. **Neonates** born to HIV-positive clients may test positive because the mother's positive antibodies may persist for as long as 18 months after birth
5. The use of antiviral medication, the reduction of **neonate** exposure to maternal blood and body fluids, and the early identification of HIV in pregnancy reduces the risk of transmission to the **newborn**
6. All **neonates** born to HIV-positive mothers acquire maternal antibody to HIV infection, but not all acquire the infection
7. The **neonate** may be asymptomatic for the first several years of life

B. Transmission
1. Across **placental** barrier
2. During **labor** and **delivery**
3. Breast milk

C. Data collection
1. May have no outward signs for the first several months of life
2. Signs of immune deficiency
3. Hepatomegaly
4. Splenomegaly
5. Lymphadenopathy
6. Impairment in growth and development

D. Implementation
1. Cleanse **newborn's** skin carefully before any invasive procedure such as the administration of vitamin K, heel sticks, or venipunctures
2. Circumcisions are not done on **newborns** with HIV-positive mothers until the **newborn's** status is determined
3. **Newborn** can room with mother
4. All HIV-exposed **newborns** should be treated with medication to prevent infection by *Pneumocystis carinii*
5. Zidovudine (AZT) may be prescribed for the first 6 weeks of life
6. Monitor for early signs of immune deficiency, such as enlarged spleen or liver, lymphadenopathy, and impairment in growth and development
7. **Newborns** at risk for HIV infection should be seen by the physician at birth, 1 week, 2 weeks, 1 month, and 2 months of life

8. Inform the mother that an HIV culture is recommended at age 1 month and after 4 months of age

E. Immunizations
1. **Newborns** at risk for HIV infection need to receive all recommended immunizations at the regular schedule
2. Immunizations with live vaccines, such as oral polio and measles-mumps-rubella (MMR), should not be done until the **newborn's, infant's,** or child's status is confirmed
3. If a child is infected, live vaccine is not given

XVIII. NEWBORN OF DIABETIC MOTHER

A. Description
1. **Neonate** born to an insulin-dependent mother or gestational diabetic mother
2. High incidence of congenital anomalies
3. High incidence of hypoglycemia, respiratory distress, hypocalcemia, and hyperbilirubinemia

B. Data collection
1. Excessive size and weight resulting from excess fat and glycogen in tissues
2. Edema or puffiness in the face and cheeks
3. Signs of hypoglycemia, such as twitching, difficulty in feeding, lethargy, apnea, seizures, and cyanosis
4. Hyperbilirubinemia
5. Signs of respiratory distress, such as tachypnea, cyanosis, retractions, grunting, nasal flaring

C. Implementation
1. Monitor for signs of respiratory distress
2. Monitor bilirubin and blood glucose levels
3. Monitor weight
4. Feed early, with 10% glucose in water, breast milk, or formula
5. IV glucose may be prescribed if necessary
6. Monitor for edema
7. Monitor for tremors, seizures, apnea, and acidosis

XIX. HYPOGLYCEMIA

A. Description
1. Abnormally low level of glucose in the blood (less than 30 mg/dL in the first 72 hours or below 45 mg/dL after the first 3 days of life)
2. Normal blood glucose level is 40 to 60 mg/dL in a 1-day-old **neonate** and 50 to 90 mg/dL in a **neonate** older than 1 day

B. Data collection
1. Increased respiratory rate
2. Twitching, nervousness, or tremors
3. Unstable temperature
4. Cyanosis

C. Implementation
1. Prevent low blood glucose through early feedings
2. Administer glucose orally or IV as prescribed
3. Monitor blood glucose values as prescribed
4. Monitor for feeding problems
5. Evaluate apneic periods
6. Monitor for shrills or intermittent cries
7. Evaluate lethargy and poor muscle tone

PRACTICE QUESTIONS

1. A nurse is reinforcing measures regarding the care of the newborn. To bathe a newborn, a mother should be taught to:
   1. Start with the dirtiest area first
   2. Begin with the eyes and face
   3. Begin with the feet and work upward
   4. Only wash the diaper area, as this is the only part of the baby that gets soiled
2. After birth, the nurse prevents hypothermia due to evaporation in the newborn by:
   1. Warming the crib pad
   2. Turning on the overhead radiant warmer
   3. Closing the doors to the room
   4. Drying the baby with a warm blanket
3. A nurse is planning to teach cord care to a new mother. The nurse understands that which of the following principles is of greatest importance?
   1. Cord care is done only at birth to control bleeding
   2. Alcohol is the best agent used to clean the cord
   3. The process of keeping the cord clean and dry will decrease bacterial growth
   4. It takes 21 days for the cord to dry up and fall off
4. A male neonate has just been circumcised. The nurse would expect the surgical site to appear:
   1. Pink, without drainage
   2. Reddened, with a small amount of bloody drainage
   3. Reddened with a large amount of bloody drainage that requires a dressing change every 30 minutes
   4. Reddened with a small amount of yellow exudate on the glans
5. The parents of a male neonate that is not circumcised request information on how to clean the newborn's penis. The best response to the parents would be:
   1. "Retract the foreskin and cleanse the glans when bathing the neonate."
   2. "Do not retract the foreskin to cleanse because this may cause adhesions."
   3. "Retract the foreskin no farther than it will easily go and replace it over the glans after cleaning."
   4. "Retract the foreskin and cleanse with every diaper change."

6. Preterm newborns are at risk for developing respiratory distress syndrome (RDS). The nurse monitors for the clinical signs associated with RDS knowing that these signs include:
   1. Cyanosis, tachypnea, retractions, and expiratory grunt
   2. Acrocyanosis, apnea, pnuemothorax, and grunting
   3. Barrel-shaped chest, hypotension, bradycardia
   4. Acrocyanosis, emphysema, and interstitial edema
7. A 4-day-old newborn will be receiving phototherapy at home for a bilirubin level of 14 mg/dL. The nurse plans to include which of the following in the instructions to the parents regarding the newborn?
   1. Have minimal contact with the newborn to prevent stimulation
   2. Limit newborn oral intake during phototherapy
   3. Apply lotions to the exposed newborn skin
   4. Assess skin integrity and fluid and electrolyte status of the newborn
8. A pregnant HIV-positive woman delivers a baby. The nurse provides guidance to help the client in decision making regarding newborn care. The nurse avoids telling the mother to:
   1. Be sure to wash hands before and after bathroom use
   2. Be sure to wash hands before feeding the newborn
   3. Breastfeed, especially for the first 6 weeks postpartum
   4. Administer the prescribed antiviral medication to the newborn for the first 6 weeks after delivery
9. A pregnant woman has a positive history of genital herpes, but has not had lesions during this pregnancy. The nurse plans to provide which of the following information to the client?
   1. "You will be isolated from your newborn after delivery."
   2. "You will be evaluated at the time of delivery for herpetic genital tract lesions; if present, a cesarean delivery will be needed."
   3. "There is little risk to your neonate during this pregnancy, birth, and after delivery."
   4. "Vaginal deliveries can reduce neonatal infection risks even if you have an active lesion at birth."
10. A nurse administers erythromycin ointment (0.5%) to the eyes of the newborn. The mother asks the nurse why this is performed. The nurse tells the client that this is routinely done to:
    1. Minimize spread of microorganisms to the neonate from invasive procedures during labor
    2. Protect the neonate's eyes from possible infections acquired while hospitalized
    3. Prevent ophthalmia neonatorum from occurring postdelivery to a neonate born to a woman with an untreated gonococcal infection
    4. Prevent cataracts in the neonate born to a woman who is rubella susceptible
11. A client asks the nurse why her newborn baby needs an injection of vitamin K. The best response by the nurse would be:
    1. "Your newborn needs vitamin K to develop immunity."
    2. "The vitamin K will protect your newborn from becoming jaundiced."
    3. "Newborns are deficient in vitamin K. This injection prevents your baby from abnormal bleeding."
    4. "Newborns have sterile bowels and the vitamin K will colonize the bowel with the necessary bacteria."
12. A nurse is assigned to assist in caring for a neonate born to a mother with acquired immunodeficiency syndrome (AIDS). The nurse understands that which of the following should be included in the plan of care?
    1. Instruct breastfeeding mothers regarding treatment of their nipples with an antifungal cream
    2. Monitor the neonate's vital signs routinely
    3. Maintain universal (standard) precautions at all times while caring for the neonate
    4. Initiate referral to evaluate for blindness, deafness, learning, or behavioral problems in the neonate
13. A nurse in the newborn nursery receives a telephone call to prepare for the admission of a 43-week-gestation newborn infant with Apgar scores of 1 and 4. In planning for admission of this infant, the nurse's highest priority should be to:
    1. Connect the resuscitation bag to the oxygen outlet
    2. Turn on the apnea and cardiorespiratory monitor
    3. Set up the intravenous line with 5% dextrose in water
    4. Set up the radiant warmer control temperature at 36.5° C (97.6° F)
14. A nurse is caring for a postterm neonate immediately after admission to the nursery. The priority nursing action would be to monitor:
    1. Urinary output
    2. Total bilirubin levels
    3. Blood glucose levels
    4. Hemoglobin and hematocrit
15. A nurse is reinforcing instructions to a new mother about cord care and how to monitor for infection. The nurse tells the mother that which of the following are signs of infection?
    1. A darkened, drying stump
    2. A moist cord with discharge
    3. A purple stump that shows pinkness around the base
    4. A purple stump that shows some moistness at the base

ANSWERS

1. *Answer:* 2
Rationale: Bathing should start at the eyes and face, usually the cleanest area. Next, the external ear and behind the ears are cleansed. The newborn's neck should be washed because formula, lint, or breast milk will often accumulate in the folds of the neck. Hands and arms are then washed. The baby's legs are washed, and the diaper area is washed last.
Test-Taking Strategy: Use the basic techniques of bathing a client to answer the question. Remember when bathing an adult or baby, start with the cleanest part of the body and proceed to the dirtiest part. Options 1, 3, and 4 are incorrect. Review the techniques for bathing a newborn if you had difficulty with this question.
Level of Cognitive Ability: Application
Client Needs: Health Promotion and Maintenance
Integrated Concept/Process: Nursing Process/Implementation
Content Area: Maternity
Reference: Burroughs A, Leifer G: *Maternity nursing*, ed 8, Philadelphia, 2002, WB Saunders, p. 172.

2. *Answer:* 4
Rationale: Evaporation occurs when moisture from the newborn's wet body surface dissipates heat along with moisture. By keeping the newborn dry (by drying the wet newborn at birth), evaporation is prevented. Conduction occurs when the newborn is on a cold surface, such as a pad. Convection occurs as air moves across the newborn's skin from an open door and heat is transferred to the air. Radiation occurs when heat from the newborn radiates to a colder surface.
Test-Taking Strategy: Recalling the methods of preventing heat loss in a newborn and focusing on the issue, evaporation, will direct you to option 4. Review these methods if you had difficulty with this question.
Level of Cognitive Ability: Application
Client Needs: Physiological Integrity
Integrated Concept/Process: Nursing Process/Implementation
Content Area: Maternity
Reference: Burroughs A, Leifer G: *Maternity nursing*, ed 8, Philadelphia, 2002, WB Saunders, p. 142.

3. *Answer:* 3
Rationale: The cord should be kept clean and dry to decrease bacterial growth. This includes keeping the diaper folded below the cord to keep urine away from the cord. The cord should be cleansed two to three times a day. It usually falls off within 7 to 14 days.
Test-Taking Strategy: Use the process of elimination. Eliminate option 1 noting the absolute word "only" and because cord care is required until the cord dries up and falls off. Option 2 is eliminated next because agents other than alcohol may be used on the cord. Option 4 is incorrect because the cord should fall off between 7 and 14 days. Option 3 is the most global option. Review the concepts of cord care if you had difficulty answering the question.
Level of Cognitive Ability: Comprehension
Client Needs: Physiological Integrity
Integrated Concept/Process: Teaching/Learning
Content Area: Maternity
Reference: Burroughs A, Leifer G: *Maternity nursing*, ed 8, Philadelphia, 2002, WB Saunders, p. 174.

4. *Answer:* 2
Rationale: The glans penis is normally dark red. After circumcision, a small amount of bloody drainage is expected. During the normal healing process, the glans become covered with a yellow exudate. If excessive bleeding is noted from the circumcision, the nurse applies gentle pressure to the site of bleeding with a sterile gauze pad. If bleeding is not controlled, the physician is notified because a blood vessel may need to be ligated.
Test-Taking Strategy: Use the process of elimination and focus on the issue, an expected appearance. Remember, a small amount of bloody drainage is expected. Review the expected findings after circumcision if you had difficulty with this question.
Level of Cognitive Ability: Comprehension
Client Needs: Physiological Integrity
Integrated Concept/Process: Nursing Process/Data Collection
Content Area: Maternity
Reference: Burroughs A, Leifer G: *Maternity nursing*, ed 8, Philadelphia, 2002, WB Saunders, p. 178.

5. *Answer:* 2
Rationale: In newborn males, prepuce is continuous with the epidermis of the glans and is nonretractable. Forced retraction may cause adhesions to develop. Separation should be allowed to occur naturally, which will take place between 3 and 5 years of age. Most foreskins are retractable by 3 years of age and should be pushed back gently for cleaning once a week.
Test-Taking Strategy: Use the process of elimination and note the similarities between options 1, 3, and 4. Options 1, 3, and 4 are incorrect because retracting the foreskin is not recommended in an uncircumcised male. Option 2 is the only different option stating that the foreskin should not be retracted. Review care to the neonate who is uncircumcised if you had difficulty with this question.
Level of Cognitive Ability: Application
Client Needs: Physiological Integrity
Integrated Concept/Process: Teaching/Learning
Content Area: Maternity
Reference: Burroughs A, Leifer G: *Maternity nursing*, ed 8, Philadelphia, 2002, WB Saunders, p. 178.

6. *Answer:* 1
Rationale: The neonate with RDS may present with clinical signs of cyanosis, tachypnea or apnea, nasal flaring, chest wall retractions, or an audible expiratory grunt. Acrocyanosis, the bluish discoloration of the hands or feet, can be a normal finding in a newborn.
Test-Taking Strategy: Use the process of elimination. Recalling that acrocyanosis can be a normal sign in a newborn will assist in eliminating options 2 and 4. From the remaining options, select option 1 because all of the signs present in this option are related to the respiratory system. Review the signs of RSD if you had difficulty with this question.
Level of Cognitive Ability: Application
Client Needs: Physiological Integrity

Integrated Concept/Process: Nursing Process/Data Collection
Content Area: Maternity
Reference: Burroughs A, Leifer G: *Maternity nursing*, ed 8, Philadelphia, 2002, WB Saunders, p. 274.

7. *Answer:* 4
Rationale: Safe care for the newborn during phototherapy requires shielding the eyes using a soft eye shield to prevent retinal damage, keeping the newborn's skin exposed except for a diaper, and changing the newborn's position frequently. No lotions are used on the skin. Adequate oral fluids are essential to prevent dehydration, as diarrhea is a common side effect of therapy. Contact with the newborn is important.
Test-Taking Strategy: Recall the principles related to phototherapy. Remember that these include maintaining adequate skin integrity, fluid and electrolyte balance, and parental bonding. Recalling these principles allows you to eliminate each of the incorrect options. Review these principles if you had difficulty with this question.
Level of Cognitive Ability: Application
Clients Needs: Safe, Effective Care Environment
Integrated Concept/Process: Nursing Process/Planning
Content Area: Maternity
Reference: Burroughs A, Leifer G: *Maternity nursing*, ed 8, Philadelphia, 2002, WB Saunders, p. 291.

8. *Answer:* 3
Rationale: The mode of perinatal transmission of HIV to the fetus or neonate of an HIV-positive woman can occur during the antenatal, intrapartal, or postpartum periods. HIV transmission can occur during breastfeeding; thus HIV-positive clients are encouraged to bottle feed their neonates. Antiviral medications will be prescribed for the neonate for the first 6 weeks of life. The principles related to handwashing need to be taught to the mother.
Test-Taking Strategy: Use the process of elimination and note the key word "avoids." Options 1 and 2 can be eliminated first because they are similar. From the remaining options, recalling the modes of transmission of HIV from the mother to the newborn will direct you to option 3. Review these modes of transmission if you had difficulty with this question.
Level of Cognitive Ability: Application
Clients Needs: Safe, Effective Care Environment
Integrated Concept/Process: Teaching/Learning
Content Area: Maternity
Reference: Burroughs A, Leifer G: *Maternity nursing*, ed 8, Philadelphia, 2002, WB Saunders, p. 363.

9. *Answer:* 2
Rationale: If herpetic genital lesions are present at the time of delivery, a cesarean delivery will be necessary to reduce the risk of infecting the neonate. In the absence of herpetic genital lesions, a vaginal delivery may be indicated unless there are other reasons for performing a cesarean delivery. Maternal isolation is not necessary, but potentially exposed neonates should be cultured on the day of delivery.
Test-Taking Strategy: Use the process of elimination. Focusing on the issue of the question, a positive history of genital herpes, and recalling the risks to the neonate will direct you to option 2. Review the methods of transmission of genital herpes to the neonate if you had difficulty with this question.
Level of Cognitive Ability: Application
Clients Needs: Safe, Effective Care Environment
Integrated Concept/Process: Nursing Process/Implementation
Content Area: Maternity
Reference: Burroughs A, Leifer G: *Maternity nursing*, ed 8, Philadelphia, 2002, WB Saunders, p. 242.

10. *Answer:* 3
Rationale: Erythromycin ophthalmic ointment (Ilotycin ophthalmic) 0.5% is used as a prophylactic treatment of ophthalmia neonatorum, which is caused by the bacteria *Neisseria gonorrhoeae.* Preventive treatment of gonorrhea is required by law. Options 1, 2, and 4 are not the purposes of administering this medication to the newborn infant.
Test-Taking Strategy: Use the process of elimination and knowledge of the purpose of administering erythromycin ophthalmic ointment to the newborn infant. If you had difficulty with this question, review initial care to the newborn infant.
Level of Cognitive Ability: Application
Clients Needs: Safe, Effective Care Environment
Integrated Concept/Process: Nursing Process/Implementation
Content Area: Maternity
Reference: Burroughs A, Leifer G: *Maternity nursing*, ed 8, Philadelphia, 2002, WB Saunders, p. 361.

11. *Answer:* 3
Rationale: Vitamin K is necessary for the body to synthesize coagulation factors. Vitamin K is administered to the newborn infant to prevent abnormal bleeding. It promotes liver formation of the clotting factors II, VII, IX, and X. Newborn infants are vitamin K deficient because the bowel does not have the bacteria necessary for synthesizing fat-soluble vitamin K. The normal flora in the intestinal tract produces vitamin K. The newborn infant's bowel does not support the normal production of vitamin K until bacteria adequately colonize it. The bowel becomes colonized by bacteria as food is ingested. Vitamin K does not promote the development of immunity or prevent the infant from becoming jaundiced.
Test-Taking Strategy: Use the process of elimination. Note the key word "best." Because jaundice and immunity are not related to the action of vitamin K, eliminate options 1 and 2. From the remaining options, recall the action of vitamin K to direct you to option 3. If you had difficulty with this question, review the purpose of vitamin K injection.
Level of Cognitive Ability: Application
Client's Needs: Psysiological Integrity
Integrated Concept/Process: Nursing Process/Implementation
Content Area: Maternity
Reference: Burroughs A, Leifer G: *Maternity nursing*, ed 8, Philadelphia, 2002, WB Saunders, p. 169.

12. *Answer:* 3
Rationale: The neonate born to a mother with AIDS must be cared for with strict attention to standard (universal) precautions. This prevents the transmission of the infection from the neonate, if infected, to others, and prevents the transmission of other infectious agents to the possibly immunocompromised

neonate. A mother with AIDS should not breastfeed. Options 2 and 4 are not specifically associated with the care of a potentially AIDS-infected neonate.
Test-Taking Strategy: Use the process of elimination and knowledge regarding care to a neonate born to a woman with AIDS. Eliminate options 2 and 4 first because they are not specifically associated with the care of a potentially infected neonate. Recalling that AIDS-infected mothers should not breastfeed will easily direct you to option 3. Review care to a neonate born to a woman with AIDS if you had difficulty with this question.
Level of Cognitive Ability: Application
Client Needs: Safe, Effective Care Environment
Integrated Concept/Process: Nursing Process/Planning
Content Area: Maternity
Reference: Burroughs A, Leifer G: *Maternity nursing,* ed 8, Philadelphia, 2002, WB Saunders, p. 363.

13. *Answer:* 1
Rationale: The highest priority on admission to the nursery for a newborn with low Apgar scores is airway, which would involve preparing respiratory resuscitation equipment. The remaining options are also important, although they are of somewhat lower priority. The newborn infant will be placed on a cardiorespiratory monitor. Setting up an IV with 5% dextrose in water would provide circulatory support. The radiant warmer will provide an external heat source, which is necessary to prevent further respiratory distress.
Test-Taking Strategy: Use the process of elimination and note the key words "highest priority." This question asks you to prioritize care based on information about a newborn infant's condition. Use the ABCs—airway, breathing, and circulation. A method of planning for airway support is to have the resuscitation bag connected to an oxygen source. Review care to the newborn infant with low Apgar scores if you had difficulty with this question.
Level of Cognitive Ability: Application
Client Needs: Physiological Integrity
Integrated Concept/Process: Nursing Process/Planning
Content Area: Maternity
Reference: Burroughs A, Leifer G: *Maternity nursing,* ed 8, Philadelphia, 2002, WB Saunders, p. 123.

14. *Answer:* 3
Rationale: The most common metabolic complication in the postterm newborn is hypoglycemia, which can produce CNS abnormalities and mental retardation if not corrected immediately. Urinary output, although important, is not the highest priority action. Hemoglobin and hematocrit levels are monitored because the postterm neonate exhibits polycythemia, although this also does not require immediate attention. The polycythemia contributes to increased bilirubin levels, usually beginning on the second day after delivery.
Test-Taking Strategy: Use the process of elimination and note the key word "priority." Recalling that hypoglycemia is a primary concern in the postterm newborn will direct you to option 3. Review the postterm newborn content if you had difficulty with this question.
Level of Cognitive Ability: Application
Client Needs: Physiological Integrity
Integrated Concept/Process: Nursing Process/Data Collection
Content Area: Maternity
Reference: Burroughs A, Leifer G: *Maternity nursing,* ed 8, Philadelphia, 2002, WB Saunders, p. 273.

15. *Answer:* 2
Rationale: Signs of infection at the umbilical cord are moistness, oozing, discharge, and a reddened base. If signs of infection occur, the health care provider is notified. Antibiotic treatment may be necessary.
Test-Taking Strategy: Use the process of elimination. Options 1 and 3 identify normal signs and are eliminated first. From the remaining options, noting the word "discharge" in option 2 will direct you to this option. Review the signs and symptoms of infection if you had difficulty with this question.
Level of Cognitive Ability: Application
Client Needs: Health Promotion and Maintenance
Integrated Concept/Process: Teaching/Learning
Content Area: Maternity
Reference: Burroughs A, Leifer G: *Maternity nursing,* ed 8, Philadelphia, 2002, WB Saunders, p. 174.

REFERENCES

Burroughs A, Leifer G: *Maternity nursing,* ed 8, Philadelphia, 2002, WB Saunders.
Lowdermilk D, Perry S, Bobak I: *Maternity and women's health care,* ed 7, St Louis, 2000, Mosby.
McKinney E et al: *Maternal-child nursing.* Philadelphia, 2000, WB Saunders.
Murray S, McKinney E, Gorrie T: *Foundations of maternal-newborn nursing,* ed 3, Philadelphia, 2002, WB Saunders.

26 Maternity and Newborn Medications

I. OXYTOCIC MEDICATION: OXYTOCIN (PITOCIN)

A. Description
1. Stimulates the smooth muscle of the uterus and induces contraction of the myocardium
2. Promotes milk let-down
3. Routes of administration include intranasal, intramuscular (IM), or intravenous (IV)
4. Minimal cervical change is usually noted until the active phase of labor is achieved

B. Uses
1. Induce or augment **labor**
2. Control postpartum bleeding
3. Promote milk let-down and facilitate breastfeeding (intranasal route)
4. Induce or complete an abortion

C. Adverse reactions and contraindications
1. Rare, but may include allergies, dysrhythmias, changes in blood pressure (BP), uterine rupture, and water intoxication; intranasal administration may cause nasal vasoconstriction
2. May produce uterine hypertonicity resulting in fetal or maternal injury
3. High doses may cause hypotension with rebound hypertension
4. Postpartum hemorrhage can occur because the uterus may become atonic when the medication wears off
5. Should not be used in a client who cannot deliver vaginally or in a client with hypertonic uterine contractions

D. Implementation
1. Monitor maternal vital signs (every 15 minutes) especially the BP and heart rate, weight, intake and output (I&O), level of consciousness (LOC), and lung sounds
2. Monitor frequency, duration, force of contractions, and resting uterine tone every 15 minutes
3. Monitor fetal heart rate (FHR) every 15 minutes and notify the registered nurse if significant changes occur
4. Administered by IV infusion via an infusion monitoring device; dose administered is monitored carefully
5. Do not leave the client unattended while the oxytocin is infusing
6. Administer oxygen if prescribed
7. Monitor for hypertonic contractions
8. The medication is stopped if uterine hyperstimulation or a nonreassuring FHR occurs; if these occur, notify the registered nurse, turn the client on her side, and administer oxygen via facemask
9. Notify the registered nurse if contractions last less than 1 minute, occur more frequently than every 2 minutes, or stop
10. Monitor for signs of water intoxication
11. Have emergency equipment available
12. Keep the family informed of the client's progress

II. ERGOT ALKALOIDS (Box 26-1)

A. Description
1. Directly stimulate uterine muscle and increase the force and frequency of contractions

BOX 26-1

Ergot Alkaloids

Ergonovine (Ergotrate)
Methylergonovine (Methergine)

2. Produce a firm tetanic contraction of the uterus
3. Produce arterial vasoconstriction and can cause vasospasm of the coronary arteries
4. Not administered before the **delivery** of the **placenta**

B. Uses
1. Postpartum hemorrhage
2. Postabortal hemorrhage resulting from atony or involution

C. Adverse reactions and contraindications
1. Nausea
2. Uterine cramping
3. Can cause bradycardia, dysrhythmias, myocardial infarction, and severe hypertension
4. High doses are associated with peripheral vasospasm or vasoconstriction, angina, miosis, confusion, respiratory depression, seizures, or unconsciousness; uterine tetany can occur
5. Contraindicated during pregnancy
6. Contraindicated in clients with significant cardiovascular disease, peripheral vascular disease, hypertension, eclampsia, or preeclampsia

D. Implementation
1. Monitor maternal vital signs, weight, I&O, LOC, and lung sounds
2. Monitor the BP closely; the medication produces vasoconstriction, and if a rise in BP is noted, withhold the medication and notify the registered nurse
3. Monitor uterine contractions (frequency, strength, and duration)
4. Assess for chest pain, headache, shortness of breath, itching, pale or cold hands or feet, nausea, diarrhea, or dizziness
5. Notify the registered nurse if chest pain occurs
6. Assess the extremities for color, warmth, movement, and pain
7. Assess vaginal bleeding
8. Administer analgesics as prescribed; may be required because the medication produces painful uterine contractions

III. UTERINE RELAXANTS (Box 26-2)

A. Description
1. Produce uterine relaxation
2. Ritodrine is the preferred medication of choice to control premature **labor**
3. Ritodrine may be used orally or IV
4. Ritodrine is usually administered IV when premature **labor** begins; when contractions have been controlled for 12 to 24 hours, the client may be started on oral ritodrine, and the IV infusion may be discontinued
5. Contractions may resume when client is on oral therapy

B. Uses
1. Ritrodrine is used to halt spontaneous **labor** when it appears after the 20th week of pregnancy and before the 36th week
2. Terbutaline, primarily used to control bronchospasm, is an alternate medication for the control of premature **labor**

C. Adverse reactions and contraindications
1. Ritodrine
   a. Heart palpitations, tachycardia, nausea and vomiting, trembling, flushing, and headache
   b. Fetal heart stimulation
   c. High doses can cause cardiovascular symptoms and pulmonary edema
   d. Contraindicated in clients with preexisting cardiac disease
2. Terbutaline
   a. Hypokalemia, pulmonary edema, and hypoglycemia may occur if given during **labor**
   b. Hypoglycemia may be found in **neonate**

D. Implementation
1. Monitor vital signs, uterine contractions, and FHR every 5 minutes when initiating therapy, every 15 to 30 minutes when the client is stable, and every 4 hours when the client is taking oral maintenance doses
2. An infusion monitoring device is used when administered by IV
3. Monitor for pulmonary edema; check lung sounds for rales
4. Potassium and glucose levels are monitored
5. Instruct the client to contact the health care provider if 4 to 6 contractions per hour occur

IV. PROSTAGLANDINS (Box 26-3)

A. Description
1. Potent stimulators of the myometrium

BOX 26-2

Uterine Relaxants

Ritodrine (Yutopar)
Terbutaline (Bricanyl)

BOX 26-3

Prostaglandins

Carboprost (Hemabate)
Dinoprostone (Cervidil)

2. Dinoprostone is administered as a gel or suppository directly into the vagina
3. Carboprost can be administered by deep intramuscular (IM) injection

B. Uses
1. Abortifacient
2. Induce abortion during the second trimester, when the uterus is resistant to oxytocin
3. Dinoprostone is also used to soften and promote dilation of the cervix to facilitate vaginal **delivery**

C. Adverse reactions and contraindications
1. Significant gastrointestinal side effects, including diarrhea, nausea, vomiting, and stomach cramps
2. Fever, chills, and flushing
3. Anaphylaxis, dysrhythmias, bronchoconstriction, chest pain, hypertension, and peripheral vasoconstriction
4. Contraindicated in clients with significant cardiovascular disease or those with a history of asthma or pulmonary disease
5. High doses can cause uterine cramping and tetany

D. Implementation
1. Monitor maternal vital signs, especially the BP and heart rate, weight, I&O, LOC, and lung sounds
2. Monitor frequency, duration, force of uterine contractions, and resting uterine tone frequently; palpate the fundus
3. Monitor vaginal bleeding
4. Remain with the client for 30 minutes after administration to monitor for anaphylaxis; signs include shortness of breath or difficulty breathing, tachycardia, hives, tightness in the chest, or swelling of the face
5. Maintain the client in a supine position for 30 minutes after administration of the medication
6. Keep side rails up; have a suction machine at the bedside
7. Administer antidiarrheal and antiemetic medications as prescribed

V. MAGNESIUM SULFATE

A. Description
1. A central nervous system (CNS) depressant and anticonvulsant
2. Causes smooth muscle relaxation
3. Antidote: calcium gluconate

B. Uses
1. Prevent and control seizures in preeclamptic and eclamptic client
2. Treat preterm **labor**

C. Adverse reactions and contraindications
1. Can cause reduced respiratory rate, decreased reflexes, flushing, hypotension, and decreased heart rate
2. A continuous IV infusion increases the risk of magnesium toxicity in the **neonate;** an IV infusion should not be used 2 hours preceding **delivery**
3. Magnesium sulfate is continued for the first 12 to 24 hours postpartum if it is used for preeclampsia
4. High doses can cause loss of deep tendon reflexes, heart block, respiratory paralysis, and cardiac arrest
5. Contraindicated in the client with heart block, myocardial damage, or renal failure
6. Used with caution in the client with severe renal impairment

D. Implementation
1. Monitor maternal vital signs, especially respirations, every 30 to 60 minutes
2. Notify the registered nurse if respirations are fewer than 12, indicating respiratory depression
3. Renal and cardiac function is monitored closely
4. Magnesium levels are monitored closely and the target range is 4 to 7 mEq/L; if a rise in the magnesium level occurs, the health care provider is notified immediately
5. Administered by IV infusion via an infusion monitoring device
6. Keep calcium gluconate on hand in case of a magnesium sulfate overdose, because calcium gluconate antagonizes the effect of magnesium sulfate
7. Deep tendon reflexes are monitored hourly for signs of developing toxicity
8. Monitor I&O hourly; output should be maintained at 30 mL per hour because the medication is eliminated through the kidneys

VI. MEPERIDINE HYDROCHLORIDE (DEMEROL)

A. Description
1. Narcotic analgesic
2. Administered by IM or IV route
3. Antidote: naloxone (Narcan)

B. Use: Relieve moderate to severe pain associated with **labor**

C. Adverse reactions and contraindications
1. Dizziness, nausea, vomiting, sedation, decreased BP, decreased respirations, diaphoresis, flushed face, decreased urination
2. May be administered with promethazine (Phenergan) to prevent nausea

3. High dosages may result in respiratory depression, skeletal muscle flaccidity, cold, clammy skin, cyanosis, extreme somnolence progressing to convulsions, stupor, and coma
4. Used cautiously in clients delivering preterm **infants**
5. Not administered in early **labor** because it may slow the **labor** process
6. Not administered in advanced **labor** (within 1 hour of **delivery**) if the **neonate** is to be delivered before the medication is adequately removed from the fetal circulation (may cause respiratory depression)
7. Regular use of opiates during pregnancy may produce withdrawal symptoms in the **neonate** (irritability, excessive crying, tremors, hyperactive reflexes, fever, vomiting, diarrhea, yawning, sneezing, and seizures)

D. Implementation
1. Monitor vital signs, particularly respiratory status; if respirations are 12 per minute or lower, withhold medication and notify the registered nurse
2. Monitor for BP changes (hypotension); maintain in a recumbent position
3. Maintain in a recumbent position
4. Have antidote available

VII. Rho(D) IMMUNE GLOBULIN (RDIG)

A. Description
1. Prevention of anti-Rh (D) antibody formation is most successful if the medication is administered twice: at 28 weeks of gestation and again within 72 hours after **delivery**
2. Should be administered within 72 hours after potential or actual exposure to Rh-positive blood; must be given with each subsequent exposure or potential exposure to Rh-positive blood
3. Of no benefit once the client has developed a positive antibody titer to the Rh antigen

B. Use: prevent isoimmunization in Rh-negative clients who are exposed or potentially exposed to Rh-positive red blood cells by transfusion, termination of pregnancy, amniocentesis, chorionic villus sampling (CVS), abdominal trauma, or bleeding during pregnancy or the birth process

C. Adverse reactions and contraindications
1. Slight rise in temperature
2. Tenderness at the injection site
3. Contraindicated for Rh-positive women
4. Contraindicated in clients with a history of systemic allergic reactions to preparations containing human immunoglobulins
5. Not administered to a **newborn infant**

D. Implementation
1. Administer to mother by IM injection within 72 hours after **delivery**
2. Monitor for temperature elevation
3. Monitor injection site for tenderness

VIII. BETAMETHASONE (CELESTONE)

A. Description
1. Corticosteroid
2. Increases production of surfactant

B. Use: for client in preterm **labor** between 28 and 32 weeks whose **labor** can be inhibited for 48 hours without jeopardizing mother or fetus

C. Adverse reactions and contraindications
1. Decreases mother's resistance to infection
2. Breastfeeding is contraindicated during medication administration

D. Implementation
1. Monitor maternal vital signs
2. Monitor mother for signs of infection
3. White blood cell count is monitored

IX. LUNG SURFACTANTS (Box 26-4)

A. Description
1. Replenish surfactant and restore surface activity to the lungs
2. Administered by the intratracheal route

B. Use: prevent or treat respiratory distress syndrome (hyaline membrane disease) in premature **infants**

C. Adverse reactions and contraindications
1. Side effects include transient bradycardia and oxygen desaturation
2. Administered with caution in those at risk for circulatory overload

D. Nursing implementation
1. The medication is instilled through a catheter inserted into **infant's** endotracheal tube; avoid suctioning for at least 2 hours after administration
2. Monitor for bradycardia and decreased oxygen saturation during administration
3. Check the lung sounds for rales and moist breath sounds

BOX 26-4

Lung Surfactants

Beractant (Survanta)
Colfosceril palmitate (Exosurf)

X. EYE PROPHYLAXIS FOR THE NEONATE

A. Description
1. Erythromycin (0.5% Ilotycin) and tetracycline (1%) ophthalmic ointment or drops are both bacteriostatic and bactericidal and provide prophylaxis against *Neisseria gonorrhoeae* and *Chlamydia trachomatis*
2. Silver nitrate (1%) solution may be prescribed, but its use is minimal because it does not protect against chlamydial infection and can cause chemical conjunctivitis
3. Preventive treatment of gonorrhea is required by law

B. Use: as a prophylactic measure to protect against *N. gonorrhoeae* and *C. trachomatis*

C. Adverse reaction: silver nitrate (1%) solution can cause chemical conjunctivitis

D. Implementation
1. Cleanse the **neonate's** eyes before instilling drops or ointment
2. Instill into each of the **neonate's** conjunctival sacs within 1 hour after **delivery;** eye prophylaxis may be delayed until an hour or so after birth so that eye contact and parent-**infant** attachment and bonding are facilitated
3. Do not flush the eyes after instillation

XI. VITAMIN K (AquaMEPHYTON)

A. Description
1. Necessary for aiding in the production of active prothrombin
2. **Newborns** are deficient in vitamin K for the first 5 to 8 days of life because of the lack of intestinal flora that is necessary to absorb vitamin K

B. Use: for prophylaxis and to treat hemorrhagic disease of the **newborn**

C. Adverse reaction: can cause hyperbilirubinemia in the **newborn**

D. Implementation
1. Protect the medication from light
2. Administer during the early neonatal period
3. Administer in the vastus lateralis muscle of the thigh
4. Monitor for bruising at the injection site and for bleeding from the cord
5. Monitor for jaundice; the bilirubin level is monitored because the medication can cause hyperbilirubinemia in the **newborn**

PRACTICE QUESTIONS

1. Epidural analgesia is administered to a woman for pain relief after a cesarean birth. The nurse assisting in caring for the woman ensures that which medication is readily available if respiratory depression occurs?
   1. Betamethasone (Celestone)
   2. Morphine sulfate
   3. Merperidine hydrochloride (Demerol)
   4. Naloxone (Narcan)
2. Rho(D) immune globulin (RDIG) is prescribed for a woman after delivery of a newborn infant and the nurse provides information to the woman about the purpose of the medication. The nurse determines that the woman understands the purpose of the medication if the woman states that it will protect her next baby from which of the following?
   1. Being affected by Rh incompatibility
   2. Having Rh-positive blood
   3. Developing a rubella infection
   4. Developing physiological jaundice
3. Methylergonovine (Methergine) is prescribed for a postpartum woman to treat postpartum hemorrhage. The nurse assisting in caring for the woman collects data regarding which priority item before the administration of the medication?
   1. Amount of lochia
   2. Blood pressure
   3. Deep tendon reflexes
   4. Uterine tone
4. A nurse is assisting with the administration of beractant (Survanta) to a premature infant who has respiratory distress syndrome (hyaline membrane disease). The nurse understands that the medication will be administered by which of the following routes?
   1. Subcutaneous
   2. Intratracheal
   3. Intramuscular
   4. Intradermal
5. A nurse is assisting in caring for a client who is receiving pitocin (Oxytocin) for the induction of labor. The nurse notifies the registered nurse if which of the following is noted in the client?
   1. Drowsiness
   2. Fatigue
   3. Fetal heart rate of 140 beats per minute
   4. Uterine hyperstimulation
6. A pregnant client is receiving magnesium sulfate for the management of preeclampsia. The nurse assisting in caring for the client identifies that the client has developed an unwanted outcome if which of the following is noted?
   1. Presence of deep tendon reflexes
   2. Serum magnesium level of 6 mEq/L
   3. Proteinuria of +3
   4. Respirations of 10 breaths per minute
7. A woman with preeclampsia is receiving magnesium sulfate. The nurse assisting in caring for the client

determines that the magnesium sulfate therapy is effective if:
1. Ankle clonus is noted
2. The blood pressure decreases
3. Seizures do not occur
4. Scotomas are present

8. Methylergonovine (Methergine) is prescribed for a client with postpartum hemorrhage. The nurse assisting in caring for the client notifies the registered nurse if which of the following conditions were documented in the client's medical history?
   1. Peripheral vascular disease
   2. Hypothyroidism
   3. Hypotension
   4. Diabetes mellitus

9. Vitamin K (AquaMEPHYTON) is prescribed for the neonate. The nurse prepares the medication and selects which muscle site to administer the medication?
   1. Deltoid
   2. Tricep
   3. Vastus lateralis
   4. Bicep

10. A nursing instructor asks a nursing student to describe the procedure for administering erythromycin (0.5% Ilotycin) ointment to the eyes of the neonate. The instructor determines that the student needs to further research this procedure if the student states:
    1. "I will cleanse the neonate's eyes before instilling ointment."
    2. "I will flush the eyes after instilling the ointment."
    3. "I will instill the eye ointment into each of the neonate's conjunctival sacs within 1 hour after birth."
    4. "Administration of the eye ointment may be delayed until an hour or so after birth so that eye contact and parent-infant attachment and bonding can occur."

ANSWERS

1. *Answer:* 4

Rationale: Narcotics are used for epidural analgesia. An adverse reaction of epidural analgesia is a delayed respiratory depression. Naloxone (Narcan) is a narcotic antagonist that reverses the effects of narcotics and is given for respiratory depression. Morphine sulfate and meperidine hydrochloride are narcotics. Celestone is a corticosteroid administered to enhance fetal lung maturity.

Test-Taking Strategy: Use the process of elimination focusing on the issue of the question, the antidote for respiratory depression. Eliminate options 2 and 3 first knowing that these medications are narcotics. Next eliminate option 1 knowing that this medication is a corticosteroid. Review the purpose and actions of these medications if you had difficulty with this question.

Level of Cognitive Ability: Application
Client's Needs: Physiological Integrity
Integrated Concept/Process: Nursing Process/Implementation
Content Area: Maternity
Reference: Hodgson B, Kizior R: *Saunders nursing drug handbook 2002*, Philadelphia, 2002, WB Saunders, p. 771.

2. *Answer:* 1

Rationale: Rh incompatibility can occur when an Rh-negative mother becomes sensitized to the Rh antigen. Sensitization may develop when an Rh-negative woman becomes pregnant with a fetus who is Rh positive. During pregnancy and at delivery, some of the baby's Rh-positive blood can enter the maternal circulation, causing the woman's immune system to form antibodies against Rh-positive blood. Administration of RDIG prevents the woman from developing antibodies against Rh-positive blood by providing passive antibody protection against the Rh antigen.

Test-Taking Strategy: Use the process of elimination. Options 3 and 4 can be easily eliminated first because they are unrelated to the medication. From the remaining options, note the relationship between the name of the medication, Rho (D) immune globulin, and the word "incompatibility" in the correct option. Review the purpose of this medication if you had difficulty with this question.

Level of Cognitive Ability: Comprehension
Client's Needs: Health Promotion and Maintenance
Integrated Concept/Process: Teaching/Learning
Content Area: Maternity
Reference: Hodgson B, Kizior R: *Saunders nursing drug handbook 2002*, Philadelphia, 2002, WB Saunders, p. 614.

3. *Answer:* 2

Rationale: Methylergonovine, an ergot alkaloid, is an agent that is used to prevent or control postpartum hemorrhage by contracting the uterus. It causes continuous uterine contractions and may elevate the blood pressure. A priority assessment before the administration of the medication is to check the blood pressure. The physician should be notified if hypertension is present. Although options 1, 3, and 4 may be a component of the postpartum data collection, option 2, blood pressure, is specifically related to the administration of this medication.

Test-Taking Strategy: Use the process of elimination. Eliminate options 1 and 4 first because they are similar and relate to one another. From the remaining options, use the

ABCs—airway, breathing, and circulation. Blood pressure is a method of checking circulation. Review the adverse effects of this medication if you had difficulty with this question.
Level of Cognitive Ability: Application
Client's Needs: Physiological Integrity
Integrated Concept/Process: Nursing Process/Data Collection
Content Area: Maternity
Reference: Hodgson B, Kizior R: *Saunders nursing drug handbook 2002*, Philadelphia, 2002, WB Saunders, p. 713.

4. *Answer:* 2
Rationale: Respiratory distress is common in premature neonates and may be due to lung immaturity as a result of surfactant deficiency. The mainstay of treatment is the administration of exogenous surfactant. It is administered by the intratracheal route. Options 1, 3, and 4 are not routes of administration for this medication.
Test-Taking Strategy: Use the process of elimination. Note the relationship between the diagnosis "respiratory distress syndrome" and the correct option "intratracheal." Review this medication if you had difficulty with this question.
Level of Cognitive Ability: Comprehension
Client's Needs: Physiological Integrity
Integrated Concept/Process: Nursing Process/Planning
Content Area: Maternity
Reference: Burroughs A, Leifer G: *Maternity nursing*, ed 8, Philadelphia, 2002, WB Saunders, p. 338.

5. *Answer:* 4
Rationale: Pitocin stimulates uterine contractions and is one of the most common pharmacological methods to induce labor. An adverse reaction associated with administration of the medication is hyperstimulation of uterine contractions. Therefore pitocin infusion must be stopped when there are any signs of uterine hyperstimulation. Drowsiness and fatigue may be due to the labor experience. The normal fetal heart rate is 120 to 160 beats per minute.
Test-Taking Strategy: Use the process of elimination focusing on the issue, an adverse reaction to pitocin. Options 1 and 2 can be easily eliminated first because they are similar. From the remaining options, recalling the normal fetal heart rate will direct you to option 4. Review the nursing responsibilities associated with this medication if you had difficulty with this question.
Level of Cognitive Ability: Application
Client Need: Physiological Integrity
Integrated Concept/Process: Nursing Process/Implementation
Content Area: Maternity
Reference: Hodgson B, Kizior R: *Saunders nursing drug handbook 2002*, Philadelphia, 2002, WB Saunders, p. 838.

6. *Answer:* 4
Rationale: Magnesium toxicity can occur from magnesium sulfate therapy. Signs of magnesium sulfate toxicity relate to central nervous system (CNS) depressant effects of the medication and include respiratory depression, loss of deep tendon reflexes, sudden drop in fetal heart rate, and/or maternal heart rate and blood pressure. Therapeutic serum levels of magnesium are 4 to 7 mEq/L. Proteinuria of 3+ is likely to be noted in a client with preeclampsia.
Test-Taking Strategy: Use the process of elimination and eliminate option 1 first because it is a normal finding. Next eliminate option 2 knowing that the therapeutic serum level of magnesium is between 4 and 7 mEq/L. From the remaining options, recalling that proteinuria of 3+ would be noted in a client with preeclampsia will direct you to the correct option. Review the adverse effects of magnesium sulfate if you had difficulty with this question.
Level of Cognitive Ability: Analysis
Client Needs: Physiological Integrity
Integrated Concept/Process: Nursing Process/Data Collection
Content Area: Maternity
Reference: Hodgson B, Kizior R: *Saunders nursing drug handbook 2002*, Philadelphia, 2002, WB Saunders, p. 674.

7. *Answer:* 3
Rationale: For a client with preeclampsia, the goal of care is directed at preventing eclampsia (seizures). Magnesium sulfate is an anticonvulsant; it is not an antihypertensive agent. Although a decrease in blood pressure may be noted initially, this effect is usually transient. Ankle clonus indicates hyperreflexia and may precede the onset of eclampsia. Scotomas are areas of complete or partial blindness. Visual disturbances, such as scotomas, often precede an eclamptic seizure.
Test-Taking Strategy: Use the process of elimination. Knowing that magnesium sulfate is an anticonvulsant will easily direct you to option 3. Review this medication if you had difficulty with this question.
Level of Cognitive Ability: Analysis
Client's Needs: Physiological Integrity
Integrated Concept/Process: Nursing Process/Evaluation
Content Area: Maternity
Reference: Hodgson B, Kizior R: *Saunders nursing drug handbook 2002*, Philadelphia, 2002, WB Saunders, p. 674.

8. *Answer:* 1
Rationale: Methylergonovine is an ergot alkaloid used for postpartum hemorrhage. Ergot alkaloids are avoided in clients with significant cardiovascular disease, peripheral disease, hypertension, eclampsia, or preeclampsia. These conditions are worsened by the vasoconstrictive effects of the ergot alkaloids. Options 2, 3, and 4 are not contraindications related to the use of ergot alkaloids.
Test-Taking Strategy: Use the process of elimination. Recalling that ergot alkaloids produce vasoconstriction will direct you to option 1. Review the effects of this medication and the associated contraindications if you had difficulty with this question.
Level of Cognitive Ability: Application
Client's Needs: Safe, Effective Care Environment
Integrated Concept/Process: Nursing Process/Implementation
Content Area: Maternity
Reference: Hodgson B, Kizior R: *Saunders nursing drug handbook 2002*, Philadelphia, 2002, WB Saunders, p. 713.

9. *Answer:* 3
Rationale: Newborns are deficient in vitamin K for the first 5 to 8 days of life because of the lack of intestinal flora that is necessary to absorb vitamin K. Vitamin K is administered to the neonate to aid in the production of active prothrombin

and to prevent hemorrhagic disease. It is administered in the vastus lateralis muscle. Options 1, 2, and 4 are incorrect administration sites.
Test-Taking Strategy: Use the process of elimination. Visualize the procedure for administering an injection to a neonate to assist in directing you to option 3. Review this procedure if you had difficulty with this question.
Level of Cognitive Ability: Application
Client's Needs: Physiological Integrity
Integrated Concept/Process: Nursing Process/Implementation
Content Area: Maternity
Reference: Hodgson B, Kizior R: *Saunders nursing drug handbook 2002*, Philadelphia, 2002, WB Saunders, p. 1158.

10. *Answer:* 2
Rationale: Eye prophylaxis protects the neonate against *N. gonorrhoeae* and *C. trachomatis.* The eyes are not flushed after instilling the medication because the flush will wash away the administered medication. Options 1, 3, and 4 are correct statements regarding the procedure for administering eye medication to the neonate.
Test-Taking Strategy: Use the process of elimination noting the key words "needs to further research." Eliminate options 3 and 4 first because they are similar. From the remaining options, visualize the effect of each. This will direct you to option 2. Review the procedure for administering eye medication to the neonate if you had difficulty with this question.
Level of Cognitive Ability: Analysis
Client's Needs: Safe, Effective Care Environment
Integrated Concept/Process: Teaching/Learning
Content Area: Maternity
Reference: Burroughs A, Leifer G: *Maternity nursing*, ed 8, Philadelphia, 2002, WB Saunders, p. 171.

REFERENCES

Burroughs A, Leifer G: *Maternity nursing*, ed 8, Philadelphia, 2002, WB Saunders.

Clark J, Queener S, Karb V: *Pharmacologic basis of nursing practice*, ed 6, St Louis, 2000, Mosby.

Hodgson B, Kizior R: *Saunders nursing drug handbook 2002*, Philadelphia, 2002, WB Saunders.

Lowdermilk D, Perry S, Bobak I: *Maternity and women's health care*, ed 7, St Louis, 2000, Mosby.

McKinney E et al: *Maternal-child nursing*, Philadelphia, 2000, WB Saunders.

Murray S, Mckinney E, Gorrie T: *Foundations of maternal-newborn nursing*, ed 3, Philadelphia, 2002, WB Saunders.

Schulte E, Price D, Gwin J: *Thompson's pediatric nursing*, ed 8, Philadelphia, 2001, WB Saunders.

Wong D: *Whaley and Wong's nursing care of infants and children*, ed 6, St Louis, 1999, Mosby.

UNIT VII

Pediatric Nursing

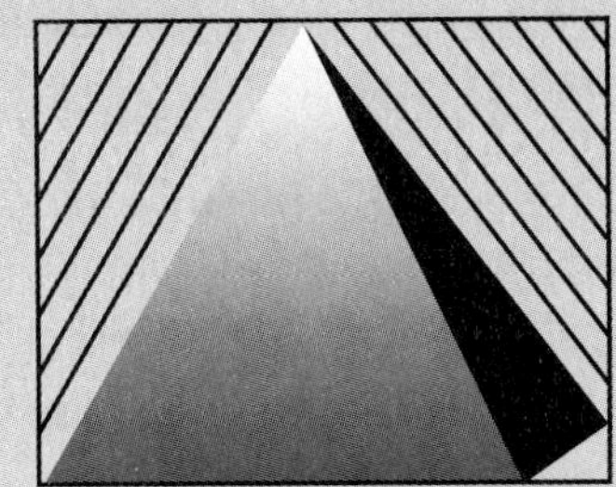

PYRAMID TERMS

Abuse Includes nonaccidental physical injury or the nonaccidental act of omission by a parent or person responsible for the care of the child.

Active Immunity The protection that can last months, years, or even a lifetime that forms in response to exposure to antigens in nature or vaccines.

Atresia Congenital absence or closure of a body orifice.

Attenuated Vaccines Vaccines derived from microorganisms or viruses whose virulence has been weakened due to passage through another host.

Cephalocaudal Growth and development that proceeds from head to toe.

Chronological Age Age in years.

Developmental Age Age based on functional behavior and ability to adapt to the environment. It does not necessarily correspond to chronological age.

Functional Age The age equivalent at which the child is actually able to perform specific self-care or related tasks.

Growth Measurable physical and physiological changes that occur over time.

Growth Spurts Brief periods of rapid increase in growth rate.

Hereditary The transmission of genetic characteristics from parent to offspring.

Inactivated Vaccines Vaccines that contain killed microorganisms.

Intelligence What an individual can do relative to learning, thinking, and problem solving.

Learning Behavior changes that occur as a result of both maturation and experience with the environment.

Nasal Flaring A serious sign of air hunger. A widening of the nares to enable the child to take in more oxygen.

Passive Immunity Antibody transfer from a person with active immunity to a person who does not have that antibody.

Puberty The period of time during which the adolescent experiences a growth spurt, develops secondary sex characteristics, and achieves reproductive maturity.

Regression Behavior that is more appropriate to an earlier stage of development and is often used to cope with stress or anxiety.

Regurgitation An abnormal backward flow of body fluid.

Retractions An abnormal movement of the chest wall during inspiration.

Separation Anxiety Distress and apprehension caused by being removed from parents, home, or familiar surroundings.

Shunt Abnormal blood flow from one side of the heart to the other.

Stenosis The narrowing or constriction of an opening.

Stridor A shrill harsh sound heard during inspiration or expiration, or both, that is produced by the flow of air through a narrowed segment of the respiratory tract.

Wheezing High-pitched musical whistles heard with or without a stethoscope.

PYRAMID TO SUCCESS

Pyramid points focus on the stages of growth and development. Growth and development includes physical characteristics, nutritional behaviors, skills, play, and specific safety measures relevant to a particular age group. Pyramid points focus on safety and the age-appropriate measures to ensure a safe and hazard free environment for the child. Additional pyramid points focus on acute disorders that can occur in children. Focus on specific feeding techniques, positioning techniques, and interventions that will provide and maintain adequate airway, breathing, and circulation patterns in the child. On NCLEX-PN, be alert to the age of the client, if the age is presented in a question. The Integrated Concepts and Processes addressed in this unit include Caring, Clinical Problem-Solving Process (Nursing Process), Communication and Documentation, Cultural Awareness, Self-Care, and Teaching/Learning.

CLIENT NEEDS

Safe, Effective Care Environment

Accident prevention
Confidentiality

Continuity of care
Environmental and personal safety related to the developmental age of the child
Informed consent in regard to minors
Parent and child rights
Priorities of care
Protective measures
Spread and control of infectious agents, particularly with regard to communicable diseases

Health Promotion and Maintenance

Communicable diseases
Developmental stages
Disease prevention
Family interaction patterns
Health promotion programs
Immunizations
Instructions to the child and parents regarding care at home
Protection of the child and other contacts to prevent illness

Psychosocial Integrity

Child abuse and neglect
Communication
Cultural, religious, and spiritual differences
Family and support systems
Play

Physiological Integrity

Age-appropriate normal body structure and function
Comfort measures
Elimination
Intrusive procedures
Medication administration
Nutrition
Responses to therapies
Rest and sleep

REFERENCES

Burroughs A, Leifer G: *Maternity nursing*, ed 8, Philadelphia, 2002, WB Saunders.

Hill S, Bauer B: *Mental health nursing*, Philadelphia, 2000, WB Saunders.

Hill S, Howlett H: *Success in practical/vocational nursing: from student to leader*, ed 4, Philadelphia, 2001, WB Saunders.

Lowdermilk D, Perry S, Bobak I: *Maternity and women's health care*, ed 7, St Louis, 2000, Mosby.

McKinney E et al: *Maternal-child nursing*, Philadelphia, 2000, WB Saunders.

Murray S, McKinney E, Gorrie T: *Foundations of maternal-newborn nursing*, ed 3, Philadelphia, 2002, WB Saunders.

National Council of State Boards of Nursing, editors: *Test plan for the National Council Licensure Examination for Practical/Vocational Nurses*, Chicago, 2001, Author.

Riley J: *Communication in nursing*, ed 4, St Louis, 2000, Mosby.

Schulte E, Price D, Gwin J: *Thompson's pediatric nursing*, ed 8, Philadelphia, 2001, WB Saunders.

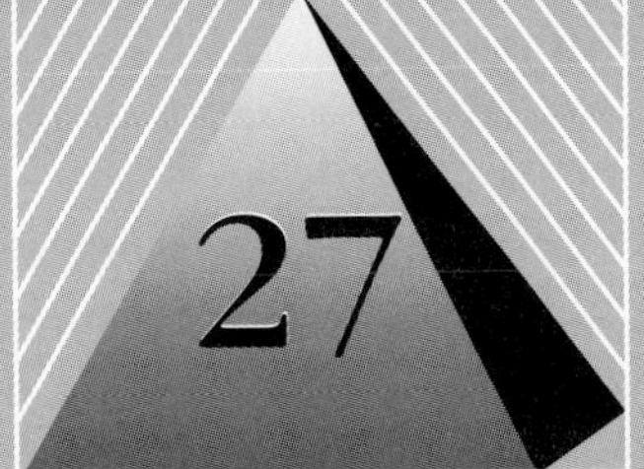

Growth and Development

I. THE HOSPITALIZED INFANT AND TODDLER

A. Separation anxiety
  1. Protest
    a. Cries, screams, searches for a parent; avoids and rejects contact with strangers
    b. Verbal attack on others
    c. Physical fighting; kicks, fights, hits, pinches
  2. Despair
    a. Withdrawn, depressed, disinterested in the environment
    b. Loss of newly learned skills
  3. Detachment
    a. Is uncommon and is sometimes called denial
    b. Superficially, the toddler appears to have adjusted to the loss
    c. During this phase, the toddler again becomes more interested in the environment, plays with others, and seems to form new relationships; this behavior is a form of resignation and is not a sign of contentment
    d. The toddler may detach from the parents in an effort to escape the emotional pain of desiring the parents' presence
    e. The toddler copes by forming shallow relationships with others, becoming increasingly self-centered, and attaching primary importance to material objects
    f. This is the most serious phase because reversal of the potential adverse effects is less likely to occur once detachment is established; in most situations, the temporary separation imposed by hospitalization does not cause such prolonged parental absence that the toddler enters into detachment

B. Fear of injury and pain: Affected by previous experiences, separation from parents, and preparation for the experience

C. Loss of control
  1. Hospitalization with its own set of rituals and routines can severely disrupt the life of a toddler
  2. Lack of control is often exhibited in behaviors related to feeding, toileting, playing, and bedtime
  3. The toddler may demonstrate **regression**

D. Implementation
  1. Provide swaddling and soft talking to the infant
  2. Provide opportunities for sucking and oral stimulation for the infant using a pacifier if the infant is NPO
  3. Provide stimulation if appropriate for the infant, using objects of contrasting colors and textures
  4. Provide routines and rituals as close as possible to what the toddler is used to at home
  5. Provide choices as much as possible to the toddler, to provide some control
  6. Approach the toddler with a positive attitude
  7. Allow the toddler to express feelings of protest
  8. Encourage the toddler to talk about parents or others in their lives
  9. Accept regressive behavior without ridiculing the toddler
  10. Provide the toddler with favorite and comforting objects
  11. Allow the toddler as much mobility as possible
  12. Anticipate temper tantrums from the toddler, and maintain a safe environment for physical acting out

13. Use pain-reduction techniques as appropriate

II. THE HOSPITALIZED PRESCHOOLER

A. Separation anxiety
   1. Generally less obvious and less serious than in the toddler
   2. As stress increases, the preschooler's ability to separate from the parents decreases
   3. Protest
      a. Less direct and aggressive than the toddler
      b. May displace feelings onto others
   4. Despair
      a. Similar to the toddler
      b. Quietly withdrawn, depressed, disinterested in the environment
      c. Loss of newly learned skills
      d. The preschooler becomes generally uncooperative, refusing to eat or take medication
      e. The preschooler repeatedly asks when the parents will be visiting
   5. Detachment: similar to the toddler

B. Fear of injury and pain
   1. The preschooler has a general lack of understanding of body integrity
   2. Fears invasive procedures and mutilation
   3. Imagines things to be much worse than they are
   4. Preschoolers believe that they are ill because of something they did or thought

C. Loss of control
   1. Likes familiar routines and rituals and may show **regression** if not allowed to maintain some control
   2. Has attained a good deal of independence and self-care at home and may expect that to continue in the hospital

D. Implementation
   1. Provide a safe and secure environment
   2. Take time for communication
   3. Allow the preschooler to express anger
   4. Acknowledge fears and anxieties
   5. Accept regressive behavior; assist the preschooler in moving from regressive to appropriate behaviors according to age
   6. Encourage rooming-in or leave favorite toy
   7. Allow mobility and provide play and diversional activities
   8. Place the preschooler with other children of the same age if possible
   9. Encourage the preschooler to be independent
   10. Explain procedures simply, on the preschooler's level
   11. Avoid intrusive procedures when possible
   12. Allow wearing underpants

III. THE HOSPITALIZED SCHOOL-AGED CHILD

A. Separation anxiety
   1. Accustomed to periods of separation from the parents, but as stressors are added the separation becomes more difficult
   2. More concerned with missing school and the fear that their friends will forget them
   3. Usually do not see the stage of behavior of protest, despair, and detachment with school-aged children

B. Fear of injury and pain
   1. Fear bodily injury and pain
   2. Fear of illness itself, disability, death, and intrusive procedures in genital areas
   3. Uncomfortable with any type of sexual examination
   4. Groans or whines, holds rigidly still, communicates about pain

C. Loss of control
   1. Are usually highly social, independent, and involved with activities
   2. Seeks information and asks relevant questions about tests and procedures and their illness
   3. Associates his or her actions with the cause of the illness
   4. May feel helpless and dependent if physical limitations occur

D. Implementation
   1. Encourage rooming-in
   2. Focus on the school-aged child's abilities and needs
   3. Encourage the school-aged child to become involved with his or her own care
   4. Accept **regression** but encourage independence
   5. Provide choices to the school-aged child
   6. Allow expression of feelings both verbally and nonverbally
   7. Acknowledge fears and concerns and allow for discussion
   8. Explain all procedures, using body diagrams or outlines
   9. Provide privacy
   10. Avoid intrusive procedures if possible 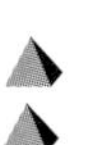
   11. Allow the school-aged child to wear underpants
   12. Involve the school-aged child in activities appropriate to developmental level and conditions
   13. Provide individualized recreation
   14. Encourage the school-aged child to contact friends
   15. Provide for educational needs
   16. Use appropriate interventions to relieve pain

IV. THE HOSPITALIZED ADOLESCENT

A. Separation anxiety
  1. Not sure whether they want their parents with them when they are hospitalized
  2. Separation from friends is a source of anxiety
  3. Become upset if friends go on with their lives, excluding them

B. Fear of injury and pain
  1. Fear of being different from others and their peers
  2. May give the impression that they are not afraid even though they are terrified
  3. Become guarded when any areas related to sexual development are examined

C. Loss of control
  1. Behaviors exhibited include anger, withdrawal, and uncooperativeness
  2. Seek help and then reject it

D. Implementation
  1. Encourage questions about appearance and effects of the illness on the future
  2. Explore feelings about the hospital and significance the illness might have for relationships
  3. Encourage to wear own clothes and perform normal grooming
  4. Allow favorite foods to be brought in to the hospital if possible
  5. Provide privacy
  6. Use medical terminology and body diagrams to prepare for procedures
  7. Introduce to other adolescents in the nursing unit
  8. Encourage maintaining contact with peer groups
  9. Provide for educational needs
  10. Identify formation of future plans
  11. Help develop positive coping mechanisms

V. COMMUNICATION APPROACHES

A. General guidelines
  1. Allow the child to feel comfortable with the nurse
  2. Communicate through the use of objects
  3. Allow the child to express fears and concerns
  4. Speak clearly in a quiet, unhurried voice
  5. Offer choices when possible
  6. Be honest with the child
  7. Set limits with the child as appropriate

B. Infant
  1. Infants respond to nonverbal communication behaviors of adults, such as holding, rocking, patting, and touching
  2. Use a slow approach and allow the infant to get to know the nurse
  3. Use a calm, soft, soothing voice
  4. Be responsive to cries
  5. Talk and read to infants
  6. Allow security objects such as blankets and pacifiers if the infant has them

C. Toddler
  1. Approach toddler cautiously
  2. Remember that toddlers accept verbal communications of others literally
  3. Learn the toddler's words for common items and use them in conversations
  4. Use short, concrete terms
  5. Prepare the toddler for procedures immediately before the event
  6. Repeat explanations and descriptions
  7. Use play for demonstrations
  8. Use visual aids such as picture books, puppets, and dolls
  9. Allow the toddler to handle the equipment or instruments; explain what the equipment or instrument does and how it feels
  10. Encourage the use of comfort objects

D. Preschooler
  1. Seek opportunities to offer choices
  2. Speak in simple sentences
  3. Be concise and limit the length of explanations
  4. Allow asking questions
  5. Describe procedures as they are about to be performed
  6. Use play to explain procedures and activities
  7. Allow handling the equipment or instruments, which will ease fear and help to answer questions

E. School-aged child
  1. Establish limits
  2. Provide reassurance to help in alleviating fears and anxieties
  3. Engage in conversations that encourage thinking
  4. Use medical play techniques
  5. Use photographs, books, dolls, and videos to explain procedures
  6. Explain in clear terms
  7. Allow time for composure and privacy

F. Adolescent
  1. Remember that the adolescent may be preoccupied with body image
  2. Encourage and support independence
  3. Provide privacy
  4. Use photographs, books, and videos to explain procedures
  5. Engage in conversations about adolescents' interests

6. Avoid becoming too abstract, too detailed, and too technical
7. Avoid responding to less than desirable social behaviors by prying, confrontation, or judgmental attitudes

VI. DEVELOPMENTAL CHARACTERISTICS

A. Infant
   1. Physical
      a. Height increases by ¾ inch per month
      b. Weight is doubled at 5 to 6 months and tripled at 12 months
      c. At birth, head circumference is 2 cm greater than chest circumference
      d. By 1 to 2 years of age, head circumference and chest circumference are equal
      e. Anterior fontanelle (soft and flat in a normal infant) closes at 12 to 18 months
      f. Posterior fontanelle (soft and flat in a normal infant) closes by 2 to 3 months
      g. 10 upper and 10 lower deciduous teeth by 1 to 2 years of age
      h. Lower central incisors present by 6 to 8 months
      i. Reflexes such as rooting, tonic neck, palmar grasp, Moro, and stepping disappear by 4 months of age, with sucking lasting through infancy
      j. Sleeps most of the time
   2. Vital signs (Table 27-1)
   3. Nutrition
      a. The infant may breastfeed or bottle-feed depending on the mother's choice
      b. Calorie requirements are 110 to 120 kcal/kg/day
      c. Give no more than 30 oz of formula per day
      d. Iron stores from birth are depleted by 4 months
      e. Do not give skim milk, because fatty acids are required

TABLE 27-1

Vital Signs

Newborn Infant	1-Year-Old
Temperature: axillary, 96.8°F to 99° F	Temperature: axillary 96.8° F to 99° F
Apical rate: 100 to 170 beats per minute	Apical rate: 90 to 130 beats per minute
Respirations: 30 to 80 breaths per minute	Respirations: 20 to 40 breaths per minute
Blood pressure: average, 73/55 mm Hg	Blood pressure: average, 90/56 mm Hg

      f. Introduce solid foods at 4 to 6 months
      g. Introduce solid foods one at a time, with sequence as follows: rice cereal; fruits and vegetables, starting with yellow and then green; meats; and then egg yolks, avoiding egg whites
      h. Avoid nuts, foods with seeds, raisins, and popcorn
      i. Never mix food and/or medications with formula
      j. Avoid adding honey to milk or water to prevent botulism
      k. By 12 to 14 months the child should drink from a cup
   4. Skills (Table 27-2)
   5. Play
      a. Solitary
      b. Birth to 3 months: verbal, visual, and tactile stimuli
      c. 4 to 6 months: initiates actions and recognizes new experiences
      d. 6 to 12 months: aware of self, imitates, repeats pleasurable actions
      e. Enjoys soft stuffed animals, crib mobiles with contrasting colors, squeeze toys, rattles, musical toys, water toys during the bath, large picture books, and push toys after he or she begins to walk
   6. Safety
      a. Baby-proof home
      b. Infants who weigh up to 20 pounds should be restrained in a car seat in a semireclined, rear-facing position
      c. Use safety straps for infant seats
      d. Guard infant when on bed or changing table
      e. Use gates to protect infant from stairs
      f. Never shake or vigorously jiggle a baby's head
      g. Be sure that bath water is not hot; do not leave unattended in bath
      h. Do not hold infant while drinking or working near hot liquids
      i. Cool vaporizers should be used instead of steam, to prevent burn injuries
      j. Avoid food that is round in shape and similar to the size of the airway, to prevent choking
      k. Be sure toys have no small pieces
      l. Hanging toys or mobiles over the crib should be well out of reach, to prevent strangulation
      m. Avoid placing large toys in the crib because an older infant may use them as steps to climb

TABLE 27-2

Infant Skills

2-3 Months	4-5 Months	6-7 Months
Smiles Turns head side to side Cries Follows objects Holds head in midline	Grasps objects Switches objects from hands Rolls over for the first time Enjoys social interaction Begins to show memory Aware of unfamiliar surroundings	Creeps Sits with support Imitates Exhibits fear of strangers Holds arms out Frequent mood swings Waves bye-bye
8-9 Months	**10-11 Months**	
Sits steadily unsupported Crawls May stand while holding on Begins to stand without help	Can change from prone to sitting position Walks holding onto furniture Stands securely Entertains self for periods of time	
12-13 Months	**14-15 Months**	
Walks with one hand held Can take a few steps without falling	Walks alone Can crawl upstairs Shows emotions such as anger and affection Will explore away from mother in familiar surroundings	

n. Cribs should be positioned away from curtains and blind cords
o. Cover electrical outlets
p. Remove hazardous objects from low, reachable places
q. Remove chemicals, poisons, and plants from infant's reach
r. Keep syrup of Ipecac and the poison control number available

B. Toddler
1. Physical
a. Height and weight increase in a steplike fashion, reflecting **growth spurts** and lags
b. Head circumference increases about 1 inch between ages 1 and 2 years; thereafter, head circumference increases about ½ inch per year until age 5 years
c. Anterior fontanelle closes between ages 12 and 18 months
d. Weight gain is slower than in infancy; by age 2 years, the average weight is 27 pounds
e. Normal height changes include a **growth** of about 3 inches per year; average height of the toddler is 34 inches at age 2 years
f. Lordosis is evident, with a "pot belly"
g. The toddler should see a dentist soon after the first teeth erupt, usually around 1 year of age; flouride supplements may be necessary if the water is not fluoridated
h. A toddler should never be allowed to fall asleep with a bottle containing milk, juice, soda pop, or sweetened water because of the risk of bottle-mouth caries; if a bottle is allowed at nap time or bedtime, it should contain only water
i. Typically sleeps through the night and has one daytime nap; discontinues the daytime nap at about age 3
j. A consistent bedtime ritual helps prepare the toddler for sleep
k. Security objects at bedtime may assist in sleep

2. Vital signs (Box 27-1)
3. Nutrition
a. Calorie requirements are 100 kcal/kg/day
b. Most toddlers prefer to feed themselves
c. The toddler generally does best by eating several small nutritious meals each day rather than three large meals

BOX 27-1

The Toddler's Vital Signs

Temperature: axillary, 97.5° F to 98.6° F
Apical rate: 80 to 120 beats per minute
Respirations: 20 to 30 breaths per minute
Blood pressure: average, 92/55 mm Hg

d. Offer a limited number of foods at any one time
e. Limit concentrated sweets and empty calories
f. At risk for aspiration of small foods that are not easily chewed, such as peanuts and popcorn
g. Physiological anorexia is normal, owing to the alternating periods of fast and slow **growth**
h. Sit the toddler in a high chair at the family table
i. Allow sufficient time to eat, but remove food when the toddler begins playing with it
j. The toddler drinks well from a cup held with both hands
k. The toddler is skillful at handling finger foods
l. Avoid using food as a reward or punishment

4. Skills
   a. The toddler begins to walk with one hand held by age 12 to 13 months
   b. Runs by age 2 years and walks backward and hops on one foot by age 3 years
   c. The toddler usually cannot alternate feet when climbing stairs
   d. The toddler begins to master fine-motor skills for building, undressing, and drawing lines
   e. Often uses "no" even when the toddler means "yes," to assert independence
   f. Begins to use short sentences and has a vocabulary of about 300 words by age 2
   g. Tends to ask many "why" questions
5. Bowel and bladder control
   a. Signs that a toddler is ready for toilet training include muscle coordination with walking, communicating with parents, awareness of a wet or soiled diaper, holding urine for 2 hours, and interest in pleasing parents
   b. Bowel control develops before bladder control
   c. By age 3, the toddler achieves fairly good bowel and bladder control
   d. The toddler may stay dry during the day but may need a diaper at night until about age 4
6. Play
   a. The major socializing mechanism is parallel play, and therapeutic play can begin at this age
   b. Has a short attention span causing the toddler to change toys often
   c. Explores body parts of self and others
   d. Typical toys include push/pull toys, blocks, sand, finger paints and bubbles, large balls, crayons, trucks and dolls, containers, Play-Doh, toy telephones, cloth books, wooden puzzles
7. Safety
   a. Toddlers are eager to explore the world around them
   b. The toddler should be supervised at play
   c. Once toddlers are able to sit up alone, they should be restrained in an upright, forward-facing position in a car seat when they reach a body weight of 9 kg (20 pounds), and a car seat should be used until they weigh at least 40 pounds, regardless of age
   d. Lock car doors
   e. Use back burners on the stove to prepare a meal, and turn pot handles inward and toward the middle of the stove
   f. Keep dangling cords from small appliances away from toddlers
   g. Place inaccessible locks on windows and doors, and keep furniture away from windows
   h. Secure screens on all windows
   i. Place gates at stairways
   j. Do not permit to sleep or play in an upper bunk bed
   k. Never leave the toddler alone near a bathtub, pail of water, swimming pool, or any other body of water
   l. Keep toilet lids closed
   m. Keep all medicines, poisons, household plants, and toxic products high and locked out of reach
   n. Keep syrup of Ipecac and the poison control number available

C. Preschooler
1. Physical
   a. Grows 2 ½ to 3 inches per year
   b. Average height is 37 inches at age 3, 40 ½ inches at age 4, and 43 inches at age 5
   c. Gains 5 pounds per year; average weight of 42 pounds at age 5
   d. Requires about 12 hours of sleep each day
   e. A security object and night light assist with sleeping
   f. At the beginning of the preschool period, the eruption of the deciduous (primary) teeth is complete
   g. Dental care is essential, and the preschooler requires assistance with brushing and flossing of teeth; fluoride supplements may be necessary if the water is not fluoridated

2. Vital signs (Box 27-2)
3. Nutrition
   a. Daily calorie requirement is about 1700 kcal/per day
   b. Exhibits food fads and strong taste preferences
   c. By 5 years old, tends to focus on social aspects of eating, table conversations, manners, and willingness to try new foods
4. Skills
   a. Has good posture
   b. Develops fine motor coordination
   c. Can hop, skip, and run more smoothly
   d. Athletic abilities begin to develop
   e. Demonstrates increased skills in balancing
   f. Alternates feet when climbing stairs
   g. Can tie shoelaces
   h. May talk continuously and ask many "why" questions
   i. Vocabulary increases to about 900 words by age 3 and 2100 words by age 5
   j. By age 3 usually talks in three- or four-word sentences and speaks in short phrases
   k. By age 4 speaks five- or six-word sentences and by age 5 speaks in longer sentences that contain all parts of speech
   l. Can be readily understood by others and can clearly understand what others are saying
5. Bowel and bladder control
   a. By age 4, the preschooler has daytime control of bowel and bladder but may experience bed-wetting accidents at night
   b. By age 5, the preschooler achieves both bowel and bladder control, although accidents may occur in stressful situations
6. Play
   a. Cooperative
   b. Imaginary playmates
   c. Likes to build and create things, and play is simple and imaginative
   d. Understands sharing and is able to interact with peers
   e. Requires regular socialization with age mates
   f. Play activities include a large space for running and jumping
   g. Likes dress-up clothes, paints, paper, and crayons for creative expressions
   h. Swimming and sports aid with **growth** development
   i. Puzzles and toys aid with fine motor development
7. Safety
   a. Preschoolers are active and inquisitive
   b. Because of their magical thinking, they may believe that daring feats seen in cartoons are possible and they may attempt them
   c. Can learn simple safety practices because they can follow simple and verbal directions and their attention span is lengthened
   d. Once the child has outgrown the car safety seat (weight more than 40 pounds), the preschooler should be placed and restrained in a booster seat (until the preschooler weighs 60 pounds or his or her head is higher than the back of the seat), which raises the child high enough to allow the car seat belt to be correctly positioned over the child's chest and pelvis
   e. Teach the preschooler basic safety rules to ensure safety when playing in a playground near swings and ladders
   f. Never allow the preschooler to play with matches or lighters
   g. The preschooler should be taught what to do in the event of a fire or if clothes catch fire; fire drills should be practiced with preschooler
   h. Guns should be stored unloaded and secured under lock and key; the preschooler should be taught to leave an area immediately if a gun is seen, and to tell an adult
   i. The preschooler should be taught never to point a toy gun at another person
   j. Teach the preschooler that if another person touches his or her body in an inappropriate way to tell an adult
   k. Teach the preschooler to avoid speaking to strangers and never to accept a ride, toys, or gifts from a stranger
   l. Teach the preschooler his or her full name, address, parents' name, and telephone number
   m. Keep syrup of Ipecac and the poison control number available
   n. Teach the preschooler how to dial 911 in an emergency situation

D. School-aged child
   1. Physical

BOX 27-2

The Preschooler's Vital Signs

Temperature: axillary, 97.5° F to 98.6° F
Apical rate: 70 to 110 beats per minute
Respirations: 16 to 22 breaths per minute
Blood pressure: average, 95/57 mm Hg

a. Girls usually grow faster than boys
b. **Growth** of about 2 inches per year between ages 6 and 12
c. Height ranges from 45 inches at age 6 to 59 inches at age 12
d. Weight gain of 4 ½ to 6 ½ pounds per year
e. Average weight of 46 pounds at age 6 and 88 pounds at age 12
f. The first permanent (secondary) teeth erupt around age 6, and deciduous teeth are gradually lost
g. Regular dentist visits are necessary, and the school-aged child needs to be supervised with brushing and flossing teeth; fluoride supplements may be necessary if the water is not fluoridated
h. For school-aged children with mixed and permanent dentition, the best toothbrush is one with soft nylon bristles and an overall length of about 6 inches
i. Sleep requirements range from 10 to 12 hours a night

2. Vital signs (Box 27-3)
3. Nutrition
   a. Increased **growth** needs
   b. Balanced diet from foods in the Food Group Pyramid
   c. May still be a picky eater but willing to try new foods
4. Skills
   a. Refinement of fine motor skills
   b. Continued development of gross motor skills
   c. Increase in strength and endurance
5. Play
   a. Play is more competitive
   b. Rules and rituals are important aspects of play and games
   c. Enjoys drawing, collecting items, dolls, pets, guessing games, board games, listening to the radio, TV, reading, and videos and computer games
   d. Participation in team sports
   e. Participates in secret clubs, gang activities, scout organizations

BOX 27-3

The School-Aged Child's Vital Signs

Temperature: oral, 97.5° F to 98.6° F
Apical rate: 60 to 100 beats per minute
Respirations: 16 to 20 breaths per minute
Blood pressure: average, 107/64 mm Hg

6. Safety
   a. Experiences less fear in play activities and frequently imitates real life by using tools and household items
   b. Adjust car seat belts so that the lap belt fits snugly over the bony pelvis and the shoulder harness is positioned across the chest
   c. Place the shoulder harness of the seat belt behind the shoulder if it crosses the face or soft tissue of the neck
   d. Major causes of injuries include bicycles, skateboards, and team sports as the child is increasing motor abilities and independence
   e. Children should always wear a helmet when riding a bike or using inline skates or skateboards
   f. Teach the school-aged child water safety rules
   g. Instruct the school-aged child to avoid teasing or playing rough with animals
   h. Never allow the school-aged child to play with matches or lighters
   i. The school-aged child should be taught what to do in the event of a fire or if clothes catch fire; fire drills should be practiced with the school-aged child
   j. Guns should be stored unloaded and secured under lock and key; the school-aged child should be taught to leave an area immediately if a gun is seen, and to tell an adult
   k. Teach the school-aged child that if another person touches his or her body in an inappropriate way to tell an adult
   l. Teach the school-aged child to avoid speaking to strangers and never to accept a ride, toys, or gifts from a stranger
   m. Teach the school-aged child traffic safety rules
   n. Teach the school-aged child how to dial 911 in an emergency situation
   o. Keep syrup of Ipecac and the poison control number available

E. Adolescent
1. Physical
   a. In girls, **puberty** begins between ages 8 and 14 years
   b. In boys, **puberty** begins between the ages of 9 and 16 years
   c. Body mass increases to adult size
   d. Sebaceous and sweat glands become active and fully functional
   e. Body hair distribution occurs
   f. Increase in height, weight, breast development, and pelvic girth in girls

g. Menstrual periods occur about 2 ½ years after the onset of **puberty**
h. In boys, increase in height, weight, muscle mass, and penis and testicle size
i. Voice deepens in boys
j. Normal weight gain during **puberty**: girls gain 15 to 55 pounds; boys gain 15 to 65 pounds
k. Careful brushing and care of the teeth are important, and many adolescents must wear braces
l. Sleep patterns include a tendency to stay up late; therefore, in an attempt to catch up on missed sleep, adolescents sleep late at every opportunity

2. Vital signs (Box 27-4)
3. Nutrition
   a. Average daily requirements in girls: 38 to 48 kcal/kg/day
   b. Average daily requirements in boys: 42 to 60 kcal/kg/day
   c. Teaching about the Food Guide Pyramid is important
   d. Typically eat whenever they have a break in activities
   e. Calcium and protein needed to aid in bone and muscle **growth**
4. Skills
   a. Gross and fine motor skills are well developed
   b. Strength and endurance increase
5. Play
   a. Games and athletics are the most common forms of play
   b. Competition and strict rules are important
   c. Enjoy activities such as sports, videos, movies, reading, parties, hobbies, computer games, music, and experimenting as with makeup and hairstyles
6. Safety
   a. Risk takers
   b. Have a natural urge to experiment and be independent
   c. Instruct in the dangers related to drugs and alcohol
   d. Help to recognize that there are choices when difficult or potentially dangerous situations arise
   e. Advocate the use of seat belts
   f. Instruct in the consequences of injuries that motor vehicle accidents can cause
   g. Instruct in water safety and emphasize that they should enter the water feet first as opposed to diving, especially when the depth of the water is unknown
   h. Instruct about the dangers associated with violence and gangs

BOX 27-4

The Adolescent's Vital Signs

Temperature: oral, 97.5° F to 98.6° F
Apical rate: 55 to 90 beats per minute
Respirations: 12 to 20 breaths per minute
Blood pressure: average, 121/70 mm Hg

PRACTICE QUESTIONS

1. The parents of a 2-year-old arrive at the hospital to visit the child. The child is in the play room and ignores the parents during the visit. This 2-year-old behavior indicates:
   1. The child is withdrawn
   2. The child is more interested in playing with other children
   3. The child has adjusted to the hospitalized setting
   4. A normal pattern
2. The most appropriate toy to provide to a 3-year-old is which of the following?
   1. A farm set
   2. A golf set
   3. A puzzle
   4. A wagon
3. A nurse reinforces instructions to the parents of a newborn regarding car travel and safety seats. Which of the following is the most appropriate information related to the safety of the infant?
   1. Restrain in a car seat in the front seat in a semireclined, rear-facing position
   2. Restrain in a car seat in the front seat in a semireclined, face-forward position
   3. Restrain in a car seat in the back seat in a semireclined, rear-facing position
   4. Restrain in a car seat in the back seat in a semireclined, face-forward position
4. A nurse is assigned to monitor a 3-month-old infant for increased intracranial pressure. On palpation of the fontanelles, the nurse notes that the anterior fontanelle has not closed and is soft and flat. Which of the following actions should the nurse take?
   1. Elevate the head of the bed to 90 degrees
   2. Notify the registered nurse (RN)
   3. Increase oral fluids
   4. Document the findings
5. A nurse is caring for a 5-year-old who has been placed in traction after experiencing a fracture to the femur. Which of the following is the most appropriate activity for this child?
   1. Large picture books
   2. A radio
   3. A sports video
   4. Finger paints

6. The mother of a 16-year-old tells the nurse that she is concerned because the child sleeps until noon every weekend, and whenever the child has a day off from school. The most appropriate nursing response is which of the following?
   1. "The child should have a blood test to check for anemia."
   2. "Adolescents love to sleep late in the morning."
   3. "The child shouldn't be staying up so late at night."
   4. "If the child eats properly, that shouldn't be happening."
7. A 16-year-old is admitted to the hospital for acute appendicitis and an appendectomy is performed. Which of the following interventions is most appropriate to facilitate normal growth and development?
   1. Allow the family to bring in favorite computer games
   2. Encourage the parents to room-in with the child
   3. Encourage the child to rest and read
   4. Allow the child to participate in activities with other individuals in the same age group when the condition permits
8. A 2-year-old is treated in the emergency room for a burn to the chest and abdomen. The child sustained the burn from grabbing a cup of hot coffee that was left on the kitchen counter. The nurse reinforces safety principles with the parents before discharge. Which of the following statements, if made by the parents, indicates an understanding of the measures to provide safety in the home?
   1. "I guess my children need to understand what the word 'hot' means."
   2. "We will install a safety gate as soon as we get home so the children can't get into the kitchen."
   3. "We will be sure that the children stay in their rooms when we work in the kitchen."
   4. "We will be sure not to leave hot liquids unattended."
9. A mother of a 4-year-old expresses concern because her hospitalized child began sucking his or her thumb. The mother states that this behavior began 2 days after hospital admission. The most appropriate nursing response is which of the following?
   1. "A 4-year-old is too old for this type of behavior."
   2. "Your child is acting like a baby."
   3. "The doctor will need to notified."
   4. "It is best to ignore the behavior."
10. The mother of a toddler asks the nurse when it is safe to place the car safety seat in a face-forward position. The best nursing response is which of the following?
   1. Once the toddler is able to sit up alone and weighs 20 pounds
   2. The seat should not be placed forward unless there are safety locks in the car
   3. The seat should never be placed in a face-forward position because of the risk of the child unbuckling the harness
   4. When the height of the toddler is 27 inches

ANSWERS

1. *Answer:* 4
Rationale: The toddler is particularly vulnerable to separation. A toddler often shows anger at being left by ignoring the parent or by pretending to be more interested in play than in going home. Parents of hospitalized toddlers are frequently distressed by such behavior. The toddler engages in parallel play and plays along side, but not with other children. Options 1, 2, and 3 are incorrect.
Test-Taking Strategy: Use concepts of growth and development. Option 3 can be easily eliminated first. There are no data in the question to support option 1. From the remaining options, knowledge regarding separation anxiety in the toddler will direct you to option 4. Review these concepts if you had difficulty with this question.
Level of Cognitive Ability: Comprehension
Client Needs: Psychosocial Integrity
Integrated Concept/Process: Nursing Process/Data Collection
Content Area: Child Health
Reference: McKinney E et al: *Maternal-child nursing,* Philadelphia, 2000, WB Saunders, p. 905.

2. *Answer:* 4
Rationale: Toys for the toddler must be strong, safe, and too large to swallow or place in the ear or nose. Toddlers need supervision at all times. Push/pull toys, large balls, coloring with large crayons, trucks, and dolls are some of the appropriate toys. A farm set and a golf set may contain items that the child could swallow. A large puzzle only is appropriate.
Test-Taking Strategy: Use the process of elimination. Options 1 and 2 can be easily eliminated because they contain items that the child could swallow. From the remaining options, the most appropriate toy is a wagon. Remember that large and strong toys are safest for the toddler. Review the safety measures for the toddler if you had difficulty with this question.
Level of Cognitive Ability: Comprehension
Client Needs: Safe, Effective Care Environment
Integrated Concept/Process: Nursing Process/Implementation
Content Area: Child Health
Reference: McKinney E et al: *Maternal-child nursing,* Philadelphia, 2000, WB Saunders, p. 116.

3. *Answer:* 3
Rationale: Infants should be placed in a car seat in a semireclined rear facing position in the back seat until they weigh 20 pounds. Infants should never face forward or ride in the front seat.
Test-Taking Strategy: Visualize each of the descriptions in the options with a focus of safety in mind. This should easily direct you to option 3. Review safety measures for the infant if you had difficulty with this question.
Level of Cognitive Ability: Application
Client Needs: Safe, Effective Care Environment
Integrated Concept/Process: Teaching/Learning
Content Area: Child Health
Reference: McKinney E et al: *Maternal-child nursing*, Philadelphia, 2000, WB Saunders, p. 96.

4. *Answer:* 4
Rationale: The anterior fontanelle is diamond-shaped and located on the top of the head. It should be soft and flat in a normal infant, and it normally closes by 12 to 18 months of age. The posterior fontanelle closes by 2 to 3 months of age.
Test-Taking Strategy: Use the process of elimination. Note the key words "soft and flat." This should provide you with the clue that this is a normal finding. A bulging or tense fontanelle may result from crying or increased intracranial pressure. Review normal findings in the infant if you had difficulty with this question.
Level of Cognitive Ability: Application
Client Needs: Physiological Integrity
Integrated Concept/Process: Nursing Process/Implementation
Content Area: Child Health
Reference: McKinney E et al: *Maternal-child nursing*, Philadelphia, 2000, WB Saunders, p. 533.

5. *Answer:* 4
Rationale: In the preschooler, play is simple and imaginative, and includes activities such as dressing up, finger paints, clay, pasting, and simple board and card games. Large picture books are most appropriate for the infant. A radio and sports video are most appropriate for the adolescent.
Test-Taking Strategy: Note the age of the child and think about the age-related activity that would be most appropriate. Eliminate options 2 and 3 knowing that they are most appropriate for the adolescent. From the remaining options, the word "large" in option 1 should provide you with the clue that this activity would be more appropriate for a child younger than age 5. Review the appropriate activities for a preschooler if you had difficulty with this question.
Level of Cognitive Ability: Application
Client Needs: Psychosocial Integrity
Integrated Concept/Process: Nursing Process/Implementation
Content Area: Child Health
Reference: McKinney E et al: *Maternal-child nursing*, Philadelphia, 2000, WB Saunders, p. 107.

6. *Answer:* 2
Rationale: Sleep patterns in the adolescent vary according to individual need. Adolescents love to sleep late in the morning, but they should be encouraged to be responsible for waking themselves, particularly in time to get ready for school. Options 1, 3, and 4 are incorrect.
Test-Taking Strategy: Use the process of elimination. The question asks for the most appropriate nursing response. Options 3 and 4 can be eliminated first because they are inappropriate responses. From the remaining options, there is no indication that a physiological alteration is present; therefore option 2 is most appropriate. Review adolescent sleep patterns if you had difficulty with this question.
Level of Cognitive Ability: Application
Client Needs: Physiological Integrity
Integrated Concept/Process: Nursing Process/Implementation
Content Area: Child Health
Reference: Schulte E, Price D, Gwin J: *Thompson's pediatric nursing*, ed 8, Philadelphia, 2001, WB Saunders, p. 302.

7. *Answer:* 4
Rationale: Adolescents often are not sure whether they want their parents with them when they are hospitalized. Because of the importance of the peer group, separation from friends is a source of anxiety. Ideally, the peer group will support their ill friend. Options 1, 2, and 3 isolate the child from the peer group.
Test-Taking Strategy: Consider the psychosocial needs of the adolescent when answering the question. Options 1, 2, and 3 are similar in that they isolate the child from their own peer group. Review the psychosocial needs of the adolescent if you had difficulty with this question.
Level of Cognitive Ability: Application
Client Needs: Psychosocial Integrity
Integrated Concept/Process: Nursing Process/Implementation
Content Area: Child Health
Reference: Schulte E, Price D, Gwin J: *Thompson's pediatric nursing*, ed 8, Philadelphia, 2001, WB Saunders, p. 305.

8. *Answer:* 4
Rationale: Toddlers, with their increased mobility and developing of motor skills, can reach hot water, open fires, or hot objects placed on counters and stoves above their eye level. Parents should be encouraged to remain in the kitchen when preparing a meal and reminded to use the back burners on the stove, and to turn pot handles inward and toward the middle of the stove. Hot liquids should never be left unattended and the toddler should always be supervised. Options 1, 2, and 3 do not reflect an adequate understanding of the principles of safety.
Test-Taking Strategy: Use the process of elimination. Option 1 can be easily eliminated. Options 2 and 3 are similar in that they isolate the child from the environment. Review safety principles for the toddler if you had difficulty with this question.
Level of Cognitive Ability: Comprehension
Client Needs: Safe, Effective Care Environment
Integrated Concept/Process: Nursing Process/Evaluation
Content Area: Child Health
Reference: Schulte E, Price D, Gwin J: *Thompson's pediatric nursing*, ed 8, Philadelphia, 2001, WB Saunders, p. 164.

9. *Answer:* 4
Rationale: In the hospitalized preschooler, it is best to accept regression if it occurs. Regression is most often due to the

stress of the hospitalization. Parents may be overly concerned about regression and should be told that their child may continue the behavior at home. There is no need to call the physician. Options 1 and 2 are inappropriate.
Test-Taking Strategy: Use the process of elimination. Note the key words "most appropriate." Options 1, 2, and 3 will cause additional stress and concern in the parent. Review the psychosocial issues related to the hospitalized preschooler if you had difficulty with this question.
Level of Cognitive Ability: Application
Client Needs: Psychosocial Integrity
Integrated Concept/Process: Nursing Process/Implementation
Content Area: Child Health
Reference: Schulte E, Price D, Gwin J: *Thompson's pediatric nursing*, ed 8, Philadelphia, 2001, WB Saunders, p. 351.

10. ***Answer:*** **1**
Rationale: Once a toddler is able to sit up alone and weighs 20 pounds, car safety seats can be adjusted to face forward in an upright position. The car safety seat is suitable for the growing toddler until the toddler reaches the weight of 40 pounds. Options 2, 3, and 4 are incorrect.
Test-Taking Strategy: Knowledge regarding car safety and the toddler is required to answer this question. Review these safety principles if you had difficulty with this question.
Level of Cognitive Ability: Application
Client Needs: Safe, Effective Care Environment
Integrated Concept/Process: Nursing Process/Implementation
Content Area: Child Health
Reference: Schulte E, Price D, Gwin J: *Thompson's pediatric nursing*, ed 8, Philadelphia, 2001, WB Saunders, p. 171.

REFERENCES

Burroughs A, Leifer G:. *Maternity nursing*, ed 8, Philadelphia, 2002, WB Saunders.

McKinney E et al: *Maternal-child nursing*, Philadelphia, 2000, WB Saunders.

Murray S, McKinney E, Gorrie T: *Foundations of maternal-newborn nursing*, ed 3, Philadelphia, 2002, WB Saunders.

Riley J: *Communication in nursing*, ed 4, St Louis, 2000, Mosby.

Schulte E, Price D, Gwin J: *Thompson's pediatric nursing*, ed 8, Philadelphia, 2001, WB Saunders.

Neurological, Cognitive, and Psychosocial Disorders

I. HEAD INJURY

A. Description
1. The pathological result of any mechanical force to the skull, scalp, meninges, or brain
2. Manifestations depend on the type of injury and the subsequent amount of increased intracranial pressure (ICP)

B. Data collection (ICP)
1. Early signs
    a. Headache
    b. Visual disturbances, diplopia
    c. Nausea and vomiting
    d. Dizziness or vertigo
    e. Slight change in vital signs
    f. Change in pupillary response or quality
    g. Sunsetting eyes
    h. Slight change in level of consciousness (LOC)
    i. Infant: bulging fontanelle; wide sutures, increased head circumference; dilated scalp veins; high-pitched cry
2. Late signs
    a. Significant decrease in LOC
    b. Cushing's triad: increased systolic blood pressure and widened pulse pressure; bradycardia; and irregular respirations
    c. Decorticate posturing: Adduction of the arms at the shoulders, the arms being flexed on the chest with the wrists flexed and the hands fisted, and the lower extremities being extended and adducted; seen with severe dysfunction of the cerebral cortex (Figure 28-1)
    d. Decerebrate posturing: Rigid extension and pronation of the arms and legs; a sign of dysfunction at the level of the midbrain (Figure 28-1)
    e. Fixed and dilated pupils

C. Implementation
1. Monitor the airway
2. Check for injuries; immobilize the neck if a cervical injury is suspected
3. Monitor vital signs and neurological function
4. Monitor for decreased responsiveness to pain (a significant sign of altered LOC)
5. Initiate seizure precautions
6. Maintain an NPO status or provide clear liquids if prescribed, until it is determined that vomiting will not occur

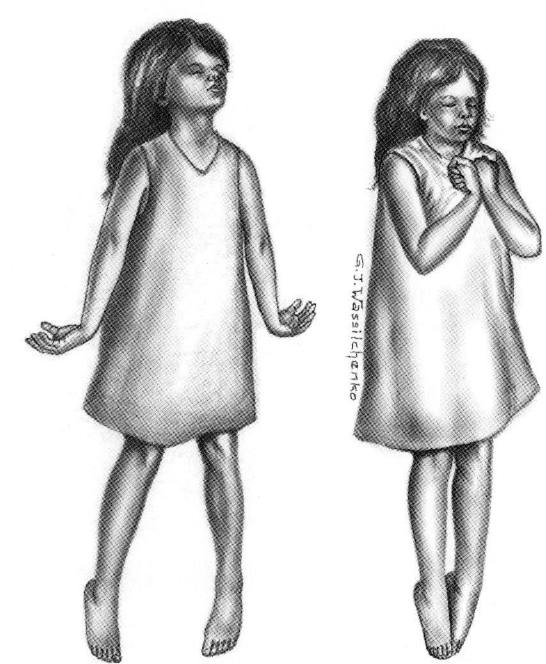

FIG. 28-1 Decerebrate posturing and decorticate posturing. (From Wong D: *Whaley and Wong's nursing care of infants and children*, ed 6, St Louis, 1999, Mosby. p. 1773.)

7. Administer oxygen and intravenous (IV) fluids as prescribed
8. Monitor IV fluids carefully to avoid aggravating any cerebral edema and to minimize the possibility of overhydration
9. Elevate the head of the bed 15 to 30 degrees if not contraindicated
10. Position so that the head is maintained midline to facilitate venous drainage and avoid jugular vein compression; turning the head side to side is contraindicated because of the risk of jugular vein compression
11. Check wound dressings for the presence of drainage and monitor for nose or ear drainage, which could indicate leakage of cerebrospinal fluid (CSF); drainage that is positive for glucose indicates leakage of CSF from a skull fracture
12. Administer tepid sponge baths or place on a hypothermia blanket if hyperthermia occurs
13. Suctioning through the nares is contraindicated because of the high risk of a secondary infection and the probability of the catheter entering the brain through a fracture
14. As prescribed, administer acetaminophen (Tylenol) for headache; antiepileptics for seizures; antibiotics if a laceration is present; and tetanus toxoid as appropriate
15. Sedating medications are withheld during the acute phase of the injury
16. Monitor for signs of brainstem involvement (Box 28-1)
17. Epidural hematoma: monitor for asymmetric pupils (one dilated, unreactive pupil in a comatose child is a neurosurgical emergency that may require evacuation of the hematoma)

II. HYDROCEPHALUS

A. Description
1. An imbalance of CSF absorption or production, caused by malformations, tumors, hemorrhage, infections, or trauma
2. Results in head enlargement and increased ICP

B. Types
1. Communicating
   a. Occurs as a result of impaired absorption within the subarachnoid space
   b. No interference of CSF within the ventricular system occurs
2. Noncommunicating: obstruction of CSF flow within the ventricular system occurs

C. Data collection
1. Infant
   a. Increased head circumference; bones of head are thin and widely separated and scalp veins are dilated
   b. Anterior fontanelle tense, bulging, and nonpulsating
   c. Frontal bossing and sunsetting eyes
2. Child
   a. Behavior changes such as irritability and lethargy
   b. Headache on awakening
   c. Nausea and vomiting
   d. Ataxia and nystagmus
   e. High shrill cry and seizure activity are late signs

D. Surgical implementation
1. The goal of surgical treatment is to prevent further CSF accumulation by bypassing the blockage and draining the fluid from the ventricles, where it may be reabsorbed
2. Ventriculoperitoneal **shunt** (VP **shunt**): CSF drains into the peritoneal cavity from the lateral ventricle (Figure 28-2)
3. Atrioventricular **shunt** (AV **shunt**): CSF drains into right atrium of the heart from the lateral ventricle bypassing the obstruction

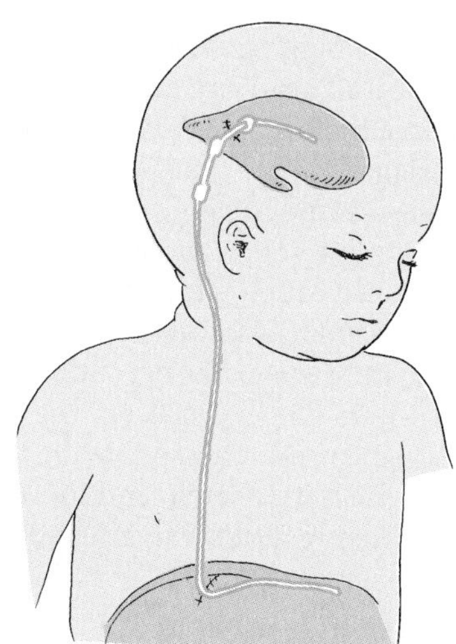

FIG. 28-2 Ventriculoperitoneal shunt (From Wong D: *Whaley and Wong's nursing care of infants and children*, ed 6, St Louis, 1999, Mosby. p. 500.)

BOX 28-1

Signs of Brainstem Involvement

Deep, rapid, or intermittent and gasping respirations
Wide fluctuations or noticeable slowing of the pulse
Widening pulse pressure or extreme fluctuations in blood pressure

E. Postoperative implementation
   1. Monitor vital signs
   2. Monitor for signs of infection and check dressings for drainage
   3. For the first 2 days, position on the nonoperated side as prescribed so that no weight is placed on the valve
   4. The child is kept flat as prescribed to avoid rapid reduction of intracranial fluid
   5. Observe for increased ICP; if increased ICP occurs, elevate the head of the bed 15 to 30 degrees to enhance gravity flow through the **shunt**
   6. Measure head circumference
   7. Monitor input and output (I&O)
   8. Provide comfort measures
   9. Administer medications as prescribed, which may include diuretics, antibiotics, or anticonvulsants
   10. Reinforce instructions to parents regarding how to recognize **shunt** infection or malfunction

III. SPINA BIFIDA

A. Description
   1. Central nervous system (CNS) defect that occurs as a result of neural tube failure to close during embryonic development
   2. Associated deficits include sensory or motor disturbance, dislocated hips, club feet, and hydrocephalus
   3. Defect closure usually done during infancy

B. Types
   1. Spina bifida occulta
      a. Spinal cord remains intact and usually is not visible
      b. Meninges are not exposed on skin surface
      c. Neurological deficits are not usually present
   2. Spina bifida cystica
      a. Protrusion of the spinal cord and/or its meninges
      b. Results in incomplete closure of the vertebral and neural tubes, causing saclike protrusion in the lumbar or sacral area with varying degrees of nervous tissue involvement
      c. Can include meningocele, myelomeningocele, lipomeningocele, and lipomeningomyelocele
   3. Meningocele
      a. Protrusion involves meninges and a saclike cyst that contains CSF in the midline of the back, usually in the lumbosacral area
      b. No involvement of spinal cord and neurological deficits are usually not present
   4. Myelomeningocele
      a. Protrusion of meninges, CSF, nerve roots, and a portion of the spinal cord
      b. The sac is covered by a thin membrane that is prone to leakage or rupture
      c. Neurological deficits evident

C. Data collection
   1. Depends on spinal cord involvement
   2. Visible spinal defect
   3. Flaccid paralysis of legs and hip and joint deformities
   4. Altered bladder and bowel function

D. Implementation
   1. Evaluate sac and measure the lesion
   2. Monitor the neurological status and for signs of increased ICP
   3. Measure the head circumference and check the anterior fontanelle for fullness
   4. Protect the sac and cover with a sterile saline dressing to maintain the moisture of the sac and contents as prescribed
   5. Place the child in a prone position to avoid stress or pressure on the sac
   6. Monitor the sac for redness or clear or purulent drainage; change the dressing whenever soiled using aseptic technique to prevent infection
   7. Assess for physical impairments
   8. Prepare the child and family for surgery
   9. Antibiotics may be prescribed to prevent infection, anticholinergics to improve urinary continence, antispasmodics to control bladder spasms, and laxatives to achieve bowel continence as prescribed

IV. REYE'S SYNDROME

A. Description
   1. Acute encephalopathy characterized by a viral infection leading to hepatic, metabolic, and neurological failure
   2. The exact cause in not clear
   3. It is recommended that aspirin not be administered to children with varicella or influenza because of its association with Reye's syndrome; acetaminophen (Tylenol) is considered the medication of choice for pediatric clients
   4. The goal of treatment is to maintain effective cerebral perfusion and control increasing ICP

B. Data collection
   1. History of systemic viral illness 4 to 7 days before the onset of symptoms

2. Malaise, nausea, and vomiting
3. Progressive neurological deterioration

C. Implementation
1. Monitor neurological status and for signs of ICP
2. Monitor cardiac and respiratory status
3. Monitor hydration status and maintain fluid and electrolyte balance
4. Monitor for signs of bleeding, which can occur with hepatic involvement

V. MENINGITIS

A. Description
1. An infectious process of the CNS caused by bacteria and viruses that may be acquired as a primary disease or as a result of complications of neurosurgery, trauma, infection of the sinus or ears, or systemic infections
2. Diagnosis is made by testing CSF obtained by lumbar puncture, which shows increased pressure, cloudy CSF, high protein, and low glucose
3. Meningococcal meningitis is transmitted primarily by droplet infection
4. Viral meningitis is associated with viruses such as mumps, paramyxovirus, herpes virus, and enterovirus

B. Data collection
1. Signs and symptoms vary depending on the age of the child and the duration of the preceding illness, and there is no one classic sign or symptom
2. Fever
3. Poor feeding, anorexia, and vomiting,
4. Diarrhea
5. Headache
6. Poor or high-pitched cry
7. Altered level of consciousness such as lethargy or irritability
8. Nuchal rigidity
9. Bulging anterior fontanelle in the infant
10. Kernig's sign and Brudzinski's sign in children and adolescents
11. Muscle or joint pain

C. Implementation
1. Provide isolation and maintain for at least 24 hours after antibiotics are initiated
2. Antibiotics are prescribed as necessary
3. Monitor neurological status and for personality changes and irritability
4. Monitor I&O and nutritional status
5. Close contacts of the child are determined because they will need prophylactic treatment

VI. SEIZURES

A. Description
1. Sudden, transient alterations in brain function resulting from excessive levels of electrical activity in the brain
2. Classified as either partial or generalized, depending on the area of the brain involved

B. Data collection
1. Obtain information from the parents about the time of onset, precipitating events, and behavior before and after the seizure
2. Determine child's history related to seizures

C. Seizure precautions (Box 28-2)

D. Implementation (Box 28-3)

BOX 28-2

Seizure Precautions

Raise the side rails when the child is sleeping or resting
Pad the side rails and other hard objects
Place a waterproof mattress or pad on the bed or crib
Instruct the child to wear or carry medical identification
Instruct the child in precautions to take during potentially hazardous activities
Instruct the child to swim with a companion
Instruct the child to use a protective helmet and padding during bicycle riding, skateboarding, in-line skating
Alert caregivers to the need for any special precautions

BOX 28-3

Emergency Treatment for Seizures

Ensure airway patency
Time the seizure episode
If the child is standing or sitting, ease the child down to the floor
Place a pillow or folded blanket under the child's head; if no bedding is available, place own hands under the child's head or place the child's head in own lap
Loosen restrictive clothing
Remove eyeglasses from the child if present
Clear area of any hazards or hard objects
Allow seizure to proceed and end without interference
If vomiting occurs, turn child to one side as a unit
Do not restrain the child, place anything in the child's mouth, or give any food or liquids to the child
Prepare to administer medications as prescribed
Remain with the child until the child fully recovers
Observe for incontinence, which may have occurred during the seizure
Document the occurrence

VII. CEREBRAL PALSY (CP)

A. Description
1. Disorder characterized by impaired movement and posture resulting from an abnormality in the extrapyramidal or pyramidal motor system
2. The most common clinical type is spastic CP, which represents an upper motor neuron type of muscle weakness

B. Data collection
1. Extreme irritability and crying
2. Feeding difficulties
3. Stiff and rigid arms or legs
4. Delayed gross development
5. Abnormal motor performance
6. Alterations of muscle tone
7. Abnormal posturing, such as opisthotonic (exaggerated arching of the back)
8. Persistence of primitive infantile reflexes

C. Implementation
1. The goal of management is early recognition and intervention to maximize the child's abilities
2. A multidisciplinary team approach is implemented to meet the many needs of the child
3. Therapeutic management includes physical therapy, occupational therapy, speech therapy, education, and recreation
4. Assess the child's developmental level and **intelligence**
5. Encourage early intervention and participation in school programs
6. Prepare for using mobilizing devices to help prevent or reduce deformities
7. Encourage communication and interaction with the child on a functional level, not **chronological age** level
8. Provide a safe environment such as removing sharp objects, using a protective helmet if the child falls frequently, and implementing seizure precautions if necessary
9. Provide safe, appropriate toys for age and developmental level
10. Position upright after meals
11. Administer medications as prescribed to decrease spasticity
12. Surgical interventions are reserved for the child who does not respond to more conservative measures or for the child whose spasticity causes progressive deformity

VIII. MENTAL RETARDATION

A. Description
1. Subaverage general intellectual functioning along with a deficit in adaptation in behavior
2. Down syndrome is a congenital condition that results in moderate to severe retardation and has been linked to an extra group G chromosome, chromosome 21 (trisomy 21)

B. Data collection
1. Deficits in cognitive skills and level of adaptive functioning
2. Delays in fine- and gross-motor skills
3. Speech delays
4. Decreased spontaneous activity
5. Nonresponsiveness
6. Irritability
7. Poor eye contact during feeding

C. Implementation
1. Medical strategies are focused at correcting structural deformities and treating associated behaviors
2. Implement community and educational services using a multidisciplinary approach
3. Promote care skills as much as possible
4. Assist with communication and socialization skills
5. Facilitate appropriate playtime
6. Initiate safety precautions as necessary
7. Assist the family with decisions regarding care
8. Provide information regarding support services and community agencies

IX. AUTISM

A. Description
1. A severe mental disorder beginning in infancy or during the toddler stage
2. Apparent to the parents before the age of 3 years
3. Characterized by impairment in reciprocal social interaction and in verbal and nonverbal communication
4. The cause is unknown and the prognosis may be poor
5. Diagnosis is established on the basis of symptoms and through the use of specialized autism assessment tools
6. Also called infantile autism

B. Data collection
1. Disturbance in the rate and appearance of physical, social, and language skills
2. Abnormal responses of body sensations
3. Abnormal ways of relating to people, objects, and events; the child is self-absorbed and unable to relate to others
4. There are no delusions, hallucinations, or incoherence, and the facies is intelligent and responsive

5. The child may play happily alone for hours, but have temper tantrums if interrupted
6. Language disturbance often includes repetition of previously heard speech and reversal of the pronouns "I" and "you"
7. If the child can talk, he or she uses speech not for communication but to repeat words or phrases meaninglessly
8. The child may develop an unusual attachment to a significant object and display frequent rocking, spinning, twirling, or other bizarre behaviors

C. Implementation
1. Determine the child's routines, habits, and preferences, and maintain consistency as much as possible
2. Determine the specific ways in which the child communicates
3. Facilitate communication through the use of picture boards
4. Evaluate the child for safety
5. Implement safety precautions as necessary for self-injurious behaviors such as head banging
6. Monitor for stress and anxiety
7. Avoid placing demands on the child
8. Initiate referrals to special programs as required
9. Provide support to parents

X. ATTENTION-DEFICIT HYPERACTIVITY DISORDER (ADHD)

A. Description
1. A developmental disorder characterized by developmentally inappropriate degrees of inattention, overactivity, and impulsivity
2. One of the most common reasons for referral of children to mental health services
3. Childhood problems include lowered intellectual development, some minor physical abnormalities, sleeping disturbances, behavioral or emotional disorders, and difficulty in social relationships
4. Diagnosis is established on the basis of self-reports, parent and teacher reports, and psychological assessments

B. Data collection
1. Fidgets with hands or feet or squirms in the seat
2. Easily distracted with external or internal stimuli
3. Difficulty with following through on instructions
4. Poor attention span
5. Shifts from one uncompleted activity to another
6. Talks excessively
7. Interrupts or intrudes upon others
8. Engages in physically dangerous activities without considering the possible consequences

C. Implementation
1. Provide environmental and physical safety measures
2. Enhance capabilities and self-esteem
3. Encourage support groups for parents
4. Administer prescribed medication; the most commonly prescribed medications include methylphenidate hydrochloride (Ritalin), pemoline (Cylert), and dextroamphetamine sulfate (Dexadrine)
5. Instruct the child and parents regarding medication administration
6. Inform the child and parents that positive effects of the medication may be seen within 1 to 2 weeks if taken as prescribed

XI. TOURETTE'S DISORDER

A. Description: Appears between ages 2 and 15 and is characterized by recurrent involuntary and rapid movements affecting various parts of the body accompanied by vocal noises such as barks, grunts, or profanities

B. Implementation
1. Establish a trusting one-to-one relationship
2. Protect the child from harm by providing a helmet or protective padding
3. Allow the child to have a favorite toy or other object
4. Provide positive reinforcement for appropriate behaviors
5. Maintain eye contact
6. Assess suicide potential
7. Remove dangerous objects from the environment
8. Set limits on socially inappropriate or manipulative behaviors
9. Encourage the child to confront tension and frustration before they emerge as inappropriate behaviors
10. Provide noncompetitive group situations

XII. CHILD ABUSE

A. Description: Involves emotional or physical **abuse** or neglect, as well as sexual exploitation or molestation by caretakers or other individuals

B. Data collection
1. Physical **abuse**
   a. Unexplained bruises, burns, or fractures
   b. Bald spots on the scalp

c. Apprehensive child
d. Extreme aggressiveness or withdrawal
e. Fear of parents
f. Lack of crying when approached by a stranger

2. Physical neglect
a. Inadequate weight gain
b. Poor hygiene
c. Consistent hunger
d. Inconsistent school attendance
e. Constant fatigue
f. Reports of lack of child supervision
g. Delinquency

3. Emotional **abuse**
a. Speech disorders
b. Habit disorders such as sucking, biting, and rocking
c. Psychoneurotic reactions
d. **Learning** disorders
e. Suicide attempts

4. Sexual **abuse**
a. Difficulty walking or sitting
b. Torn, stained, or bloody underclothing
c. Pain, swelling, or itching of the genitals
d. Bruises, bleeding, or lacerations in the genital or anal area
e. Unwillingness to change clothes or unwillingness to participate in gym activities
f. Poor peer relations
g. Delinquency
h. Changes in sleep performance
i. Self-disruptive behavior

C. Implementation
1. Support the child during a thorough physical assessment
2. Check the child for injuries
3. Report case of suspected **abuse**
4. Place the child in an environment that is safe, thereby preventing further injury
5. Document in an objective manner information related to the suspected **abuse**
6. Assess parents' strengths and weaknesses, normal coping mechanisms, and presence or absence of support systems
7. Assist the family in identifying stressors, support systems, and resources
8. Refer the family to appropriate support groups

PRACTICE QUESTIONS

1. A nurse is assisting in collecting data on a 6-month-old infant with a diagnosis of hydrocephalus. The nurse checks for the major symptom associated with hydrocephalus when the nurse:
   1. Tests the urine for protein
   2. Takes the apical pulse
   3. Palpates the anterior fontanelle
   4. Takes the blood pressure

2. A mother arrives at the emergency room with her 5-year-old child. The mother states that the child fell off a bunk bed. A head injury is suspected. The nurse checks the child for signs of increased intracranial pressure (ICP). Which of the following is a late sign of increased ICP?
   1. Bulging fontanelle
   2. Altered level of consciousness
   3. Nausea
   4. Widening pulse pressure

3. A nurse is caring for a child with Reye's syndrome. The nurse checks for the major symptom associated with Reye's syndrome when the nurse notes:
   1. Persistent vomiting
   2. Protein in the urine
   3. A history of a staphylococcus infection
   4. Symptoms of hyperglycemia

4. A child is diagnosed with Reye's syndrome. The nurse assists in preparing a nursing care plan for this child and suggests to include:
   1. Providing a quiet atmosphere with dimmed lights
   2. Checking for hearing loss
   3. Monitoring output
   4. Changing body position every 2 hours

5. Which of the following data if noted by the nurse would indicate a potential complication associated with a tonic-clonic seizure?
   1. Blood on the pillow
   2. Blanched toenails
   3. Migraine headaches
   4. High-pitched cry

6. A nurse plans for a safe environment when caring for an infant at risk for a seizure. In the plan of care, the seizure precautions would most appropriately include placing which of the following items at the bedside?
   1. A suction apparatus and an airway
   2. Oxygen with a tracheotomy set
   3. Emergency cart
   4. Airway and a tracheotomy set

7. A nurse is reinforcing instructions with an adolescent with a history of seizures, who is on an anticonvulsant medication. Which of the following statements, if made by the adolescent, indicates an understanding of the instructions?
   1. "I will never be able to drive a car."
   2. "My anticonvulsant medication will clear up my skin."
   3. "I can't drink alcohol while I am taking my medication."
   4. "If I forget my morning medication, I can take just 2 pills at bedtime."

8. A nurse is collecting data on a child admitted to the hospital with a diagnosis of seizures. The nurse checks for causes of the seizure activity when the nurse:
   1. Tests the child's urine for specific gravity
   2. Obtains a family history of psychiatric illness
   3. Obtains a history of any factors that might precipitate seizure activity
   4. Asks the child what happens during a seizure
9. A nurse is caring for a child recently diagnosed with cerebral palsy. The parents of the child ask the nurse about the disorder. The nurse bases the response to the parents on the understanding that cerebral palsy is:
   1. A chronic disability characterized by a difficulty in controlling the muscles
   2. An infectious disease of the central nervous system
   3. An inflammation of the brain as a result of a viral illness
   4. A congenital condition that results in moderate to severe retardation
10. A nurse is caring for a child with cerebral palsy. The primary goal to be included in the plan of care is to:
   1. Eliminate the cause of the disease
   2. Prevent the occurrence of emotional disturbances
   3. Maximize the child's assets and minimize the limitations caused by the disease
   4. Improve muscle control and coordination
11. A nurse is assigned to care for an 8-year-old child with a basilar skull fracture. Which of the following physician orders would the nurse question?
   1. Restrict fluid intake
   2. Keep an IV line patent
   3. Insert an indwelling urinary catheter
   4. Suction as needed
12. A lumbar puncture is performed on a child suspected of having bacterial meningitis. Cerebrospinal fluid (CSF) is obtained for analysis. The nurse understands that which of the following results would verify the diagnosis?
   1. Cloudy CSF with low protein and low glucose
   2. Cloudy CSF with high protein and low glucose
   3. Clear CSF with high protein and low glucose
   4. Decreased pressure and cloudy CSF with high protein
13. A nurse is caring for a child with meningococcal meningitis. Based on the mode of transmission of this infection, which of the following would be included in the plan of care?
   1. No precautions are required as long as antibiotics have been started
   2. Maintain enteric precautions
   3. Maintain isolation precautions for at least 24 hours after the initiation of antibiotics
   4. Maintain neutropenic precautions
14. A nurse is observing a child diagnosed with autism. The nurse knows that the primary characteristic(s) of autism include which of the following?
   1. Consistent imitation of others actions
   2. Normal social play
   3. Lack of social interaction and awareness
   4. Normal verbal but abnormal nonverbal communication
15. An emergency room nurse is collecting data on a child suspected of being sexually abused. Which of the following data would most likely indicate this suspicion?
   1. Poor hygiene
   2. Bald spots on the scalp
   3. Fear of the parents
   4. Swelling of the genitals

ANSWERS

1. *Answer:* 3

Rationale: An elevated or bulging anterior fontanelle indicates an increase in CSF collection in the cerebral ventricle. Proteinuria, apical pulse, and blood pressure changes are not specifically associated with increasing CSF in the brain tissue.

Test-Taking Strategy: Use the principles associated with excessive fluid buildup in the cranial cavity and note the age of the infant. Additionally, correlate "hydrocephalus" in the question, with "anterior fontanelle" in option 3. Review the symptoms associated with hydrocephalus if you had difficulty with this question.

Level of Cognitive Ability: Application

Client Needs: Physiological Integrity

Integrated Concept/Process: Nursing Process/Data Collection

Content Area: Child Health

Reference: Schulte E, Price D, Gwin J: *Thompson's pediatric nursing*, ed 8, Philadelphia, 2001, WB Saunders, p. 48.

2. *Answer:* 4

Rationale: Late signs of increased ICP include tachycardia leading to bradycardia, apnea, systolic hypertension, widening pulse pressure, and posturing. A bulging fontanelle is a sign of increased ICP in an infant. Nausea and altered level of consciousness are signs of increased ICP in a child. Options 1, 2, and 3 are not late signs.

Test-Taking Strategy: Note the age of the child and that the question asks for the "late" sign. Option 1 can be eliminated because the fontanelles are closed in a child. Knowledge of the early and late signs will direct you to the correct option from those remaining. Review these signs if you had difficulty with this question.

Level of Cognitive Ability: Comprehension

Client Needs: Physiological Integrity

Integrated Concept/Process: Nursing Process/Data Collection

Content Area: Child Health

Reference: Schulte E, Price D, Gwin J: *Thompson's pediatric nursing,* ed 8, Philadelphia, 2001, WB Saunders, p. 222.

3. ***Answer:*** 1
Rationale: Persistent vomiting is a major symptom associated with intracranial pressure. ICP and encephalopathy are major symptoms of Reye's syndrome. Options 2, 3, and 4 are incorrect. Protein is not present in the urine. Reye's syndrome is related to a history of viral infections, and hypoglycemia is a symptom of this disease.
Test-Taking Strategy: Use the process of elimination and knowledge related to the symptoms associated with Reye's syndrome to answer this question. Recalling that increased ICP is an associated characteristic will direct you to option 1. Review the symptoms of Reye's syndrome and the signs of increased ICP if you had difficulty with this question.
Level of Cognitive Ability: Application
Client Needs: Physiological Integrity
Integrated Concept/Process: Nursing Process/Data Collection
Content Area: Child Health
Reference: Schulte E, Price D, Gwin J: *Thompson's pediatric nursing,* ed 8, Philadelphia, 2001, WB Saunders, p. 81.

4. ***Answer:*** 1
Rationale: The major elements of care are to maintain effective cerebral perfusion and control ICP. Decreasing stimuli in the environment would decrease the stress on the cerebral tissue and neuron responses. Cerebral edema is a progressive part of this disease process. Hearing loss and output are not affected. Changing the body position every 2 hours would not affect the cerebral edema and ICP directly. The child should be in a head-elevated position to decrease the progression of the cerebral edema and promote drainage of CSF.
Test-Taking Strategy: Use the process of elimination and knowledge regarding the pathophysiology associated with Reye's syndrome to answer the question. Recalling the effects of environmental stimuli, the responses of the brain cells to stimuli, and how cerebral edema can result will direct you to option 1. Review the symptoms of Reye's syndrome and the signs of increased ICP if you had difficulty with this question.
Level of Cognitive Ability: Application
Client Needs: Physiological Integrity
Integrated Concept/Process: Nursing Process/Planning
Content Area: Child Health
Reference: Schulte E, Price D, Gwin J: *Thompson's pediatric nursing,* ed 8, Philadelphia, 2001, WB Saunders, p. 222.

5. ***Answer:*** 1
Rationale: The complications associated with seizures include airway compromise, extremity and teeth injuries, and tongue lacerations. Night seizures can cause the child to bite down on the tongue. Cyanosis can occur during the tonic-clonic part of the seizure activity, but blanching does not occur. Migraine headaches are not common in children with seizures. Seizures do not cause a high-pitched cry, unless a tumor or intracranial pressure is the cause of the seizure diagnosis.
Test-Taking Strategy: Use knowledge of tonic-clonic activity and the involuntary tightening of all the body muscles that occurs during seizure activity when answering this question. Recall that the tongue can get easily caught by the child's teeth when the seizure activity occurs. This causes injury, swelling, and bleeding of the tongue tissue. Review the complications associated with seizures if you had difficulty with this question.
Level of Cognitive Ability: Comprehension
Client Needs: Physiological Integrity
Integrated Concept/Process: Nursing Process/Data Collection
Content Area: Child Health
Reference: Schulte E, Price D, Gwin J: *Thompson's pediatric nursing,* ed 8, Philadelphia, 2001, WB Saunders, p. 223.

6. ***Answer:*** 1
Rationale: Seizures cause tightening of all body muscles followed by tremors. Obstructive airway and increased oral secretions are the major complications during and after the seizure. Option 2 and 4 are incorrect because inserting a tracheostomy is not done. Suctioning is helpful to prevent choking and cyanosis. Option 3 is incorrect because this cart would not be left at the bedside, but would be available in the treatment room or on the nursing unit.
Test-Taking Strategy: Use the process of elimination. Recalling that seizures produce excessive oral secretions and airway obstruction will direct you to option 1. Review the plan of care associated with seizure precautions if you had difficulty with this question.
Level of Cognitive Ability: Application
Client Needs: Safe, Effective Care Environment
Integrated Concept/Process: Nursing Process/Planning
Content Area: Child Health
Reference: Schulte E, Price D, Gwin J: *Thompson's pediatric nursing,* ed 8, Philadelphia, 2001, WB Saunders, p. 223.

7. ***Answer:*** 3
Rationale: Alcohol will lower the seizure threshold and should be avoided. The adolescent can attain a driver's license, in most states, when they are seizure-free for 1 year. Anticonvulsants cause acne and oily skin; therefore a dermatologist may need to be consulted. If an anticonvulsant medication is missed, the physician should be notified.
Test-Taking Strategy: Use the process of elimination and note the key words "indicates an understanding." Using general principles related to medication instructions will direct you to option 3. Review teaching points related to anticonvulsants if you had difficulty with this question.
Level of Cognitive Ability: Comprehension
Client Needs: Health Promotion and Maintenance
Integrated Concept/Process: Nursing Process/Evaluation
Content Area: Child Health
Reference: Schulte E, Price D, Gwin J: *Thompson's pediatric nursing,* ed 8, Philadelphia, 2001, WB Saunders, p. 223.

8. ***Answer:*** 3
Rationale: Fever and infections raise the body metabolism. This can cause seizure activity in children less than 5 years old. Dehydration and electrolyte imbalance can also contribute to the occurrence of a seizure. Falls can cause head injury, which would increase intracranial pressure or cerebral edema. Some medications could cause seizures. Specific gravity would not be a reliable test because it varies depending on the existing

condition. Psychiatric illness has no impact on seizure occurrence or cause. Children do not remember what happened during the seizure itself.
Test-Taking Strategy: Use the process of elimination and focus on the issue, the cause of the seizure activity. Recalling the causes and precipitating factors associated with seizures will direct you to option 3. Review the precipitating factors associated with seizures if you had difficulty with this question.
Level of Cognitive Ability: Application
Client Needs: Physiological Integrity
Integrated Concept/Process: Nursing Process/Data Collection
Content Area: Child Health
Reference: Schulte E, Price D, Gwin J: *Thompson's pediatric nursing*, ed 8, Philadelphia, 2001, WB Saunders, p. 223.

9. ***Answer:*** **1**
Rationale: Cerebral palsy is a chronic disability characterized by difficulty in controlling the muscles because of an abnormality in the extrapyramidal or pyramidal motor system. Meningitis is an infectious process of the central nervous system. Encephalitis is an inflammation of the brain that occurs as a result of viral illness or central nervous system infection. Down syndrome is an example of a congenital condition that results in moderate to severe retardation.
Test-Taking Strategy: Use the process of elimination. Eliminate options 2 and 3 first noting that they are similar. From the remaining options, noting the relationship between "palsy" in the question and "muscles" in option 1 will direct you to this option. Review the characteristics associated with cerebral palsy if you had difficulty with this question.
Level of Cognitive Ability: Comprehension
Client Needs: Physiological Integrity
Integrated Concept/Process: Nursing Process/Implementation
Content Area: Child Health
Reference: Schulte E, Price D, Gwin J: *Thompson's pediatric nursing*, ed 8, Philadelphia, 2001, WB Saunders, p. 186.

10. ***Answer:*** **3**
Rationale: The goal of managing the child with cerebral palsy is early recognition and intervention to maximize the child's abilities. The cause of the disease cannot be eliminated. It is best to minimize emotional disturbances if possible, but not to prevent them because it is healthy for the child to express emotions. Improvement of muscle control and coordination is a component of the plan, but the primary goal is to maximize the child's assets and minimize the limitations caused by the disease.
Test-Taking Strategy: Use the process of elimination. Eliminate options 1 and 2 first because the cause of the disease cannot be eliminated and emotional disturbances cannot be prevented. From the remaining options, identify the option that is the most global, option 3. Review the goals of care for the child with cerebral palsy if you had difficulty with this question.
Level of Cognitive Ability: Application
Client Needs: Psychosocial Integrity
Integrated Concept/Process: Nursing Process/Planning
Content Area: Child Health
Reference: Schulte E, Price D, Gwin J: *Thompson's pediatric nursing*, ed 8, Philadelphia, 2001, WB Saunders, p. 187.

11. ***Answer:*** **4**
Rationale: Nasotracheal suctioning is contraindicated in a child with a basilar skull fracture. Because of the nature of the injury, the suction catheter may be introduced into the brain. The child may need a urinary catheter for accurate monitoring of I&O. Fluids are restricted to prevent fluid overload. An IV line is maintained to administer fluids or medications if necessary.
Test-Taking Strategy: Use the process of elimination and note the key words "does the nurse question." Note that options 1, 2, and 3 are similar in that they all address the issue of fluid intake or output. Review care to the child with this type of skull fracture if you had difficulty with this question.
Level of Cognitive Ability: Comprehension
Client Needs: Safe, Effective Care Environment
Integrated Concept/Process: Nursing Process/Implementation
Content Area: Child Health
Reference: Schulte E, Price D, Gwin J: *Thompson's pediatric nursing*, ed 8, Philadelphia, 2001, WB Saunders, p. 188.

12. ***Answer:*** **2**
Rationale: A diagnosis of meningitis is made by testing CSF obtained by lumbar puncture. In the case of bacterial meningitis, findings usually include increased pressure, cloudy CSF, high protein, and low glucose.
Test-Taking Strategy: Use the process of elimination and knowledge regarding the diagnostic findings in meningitis. Eliminate options 3 and 4 first because clear CSF and decreased pressure are not likely to be found if an infectious process such as meningitis is suspected. From this point, knowledge that a high protein level indicates a possible diagnosis of meningitis will direct you to option 2. Review the findings in meningitis if you had difficulty with this question.
Level of Cognitive Ability: Comprehension
Client Needs: Physiological Integrity
Integrated Concept/Process: Nursing Process/Data Collection
Content Area: Child Health
Reference: Schulte E, Price D, Gwin J: *Thompson's pediatric nursing*, ed 8, Philadelphia, 2001, WB Saunders, p. 148.

13. ***Answer:*** **3**
Rationale: Meningococcal meningitis is transmitted primarily by droplet infection. Isolation is begun and maintained for at least 24 hours after antibiotics are given. Options 1, 2, and 4 are incorrect.
Test-Taking Strategy: Use the process of elimination to rule out options 2 and 4 first. Both enteric and neutropenic precautions are unrelated to the mode of transmission of meningococcal meningitis. Knowledge that it takes approximately 24 hours for antibiotics to reach a therapeutic blood level will assist in directing you to option 3 from the remaining options. Review the mode of transmission of meningococcal meningitis if you had difficulty with this question.
Level of Cognitive Ability: Application
Client Needs: Safe, Effective Care Environment
Integrated Concept/Process: Nursing Process/Planning
Content Area: Child Health
Reference: Schulte E, Price D, Gwin J: *Thompson's pediatric nursing*, ed 8, Philadelphia, 2001, WB Saunders, p. 148.

14. ***Answer:*** 3
Rationale: Autism is a severe developmental disorder that begins in infancy or during the toddler stage. The primary characteristic is lack of social interaction and awareness. Social behaviors in autism include lack of or abnormal imitation of others' actions and the lack of or abnormal social play. Additional characteristics include lack of or impaired verbal communication and markedly abnormal nonverbal communication.
Test-Taking Strategy: Use the process of elimination. Eliminate options 2 and 4 first because they address normal behaviors. From the remaining options, recalling that the autistic child lacks social interaction and awareness will direct you to option 3. Review the characteristics associated with autism if you had difficulty with this question.
Level of Cognitive Ability: Comprehension
Client Needs: Psychosocial Integrity
Integrated Concept/Process: Nursing Process/Data Collection
Content Area: Child Health
Reference: McKinney E et al: *Maternal-child nursing,* Philadelphia, 2000, WB Saunders, p. 1552.

15. ***Answer:*** 4
Rationale: The most likely findings in sexual abuse include difficulty walking or sitting; torn, stained, or bloody underclothing; pain, swelling, or itching of the genitals; and bruises, bleeding, or lacerations in the genital or anal area. Poor hygiene may be indicative of physical neglect. Bald spots on the scalp and fear of the parents are most likely associated with physical abuse.
Test-Taking Strategy: Use the process of elimination. Note the key words "sexually abused." The only option that specifically addresses a finding related to sexual abuse is option 4. Review the findings in a child suspected of abuse if you had difficulty with this question.
Level of Cognitive Ability: Comprehension
Client Needs: Physiological Integrity
Integrated Concept/Process: Nursing Process/Data Collection
Content Area: Child Health
Reference: McKinney E et al: *Maternal-child nursing,* Philadelphia, 2000, WB Saunders, p. 1054.

REFERENCES

Burroughs A, Leifer G: *Maternity nursing,* ed 8, Philadelphia, 2002, WB Saunders.

McKinney E et al: *Maternal-child nursing,* Philadelphia, 2000, WB Saunders.

Murray S, McKinney E, Gorrie T: *Foundations of maternal-newborn nursing,* ed 3, Philadelphia, 2002, WB Saunders.

Schulte E, Price D, Gwin J: *Thompson's pediatric nursing,* ed 8, Philadelphia, 2001, WB Saunders.

Wong D: *Whaley and Wong's nursing care of infants and children,* ed 6, St. Louis, 1999, Mosby.

Eye, Ear, Throat, and Respiratory Disorders

I. STRABISMUS

A. Description
1. Called "squint" or "lazy eye"
2. A condition in which the eyes are not aligned because of lack of coordination of the extraocular muscles
3. Most often due to muscle imbalance or paralysis of extraocular muscles, but may also result from conditions such as a brain tumor, myasthenia gravis, or infection
4. Normal in the young infant but should not be present after about age 4 months

B. Data collection
1. Amblyopia or permanent loss of vision if not treated early
2. Loss of binocular vision
3. Impairment of depth perception
4. Frequent headaches
5. Squints or tilts head to see

C. Implementation
1. Corrective lenses as indicated
2. Instruct the parents regarding eye patching (occlusion therapy) of the "good" eye to strengthen the weak eye
3. Prepare for botulinum toxin (Botox) injection into the eye muscle, which produces temporary paralysis and allows muscles opposite the paralyzed muscle to straighten the eye
4. Inform the parents the injection of botulinum toxin wears off in about 2 months, and if successful, correction will occur
5. Prepare for surgery to realign the weak muscles as prescribed if nonsurgical interventions are unsuccessful
6. Instruct the parents in the need for follow-up visits

II. CONJUNCTIVITIS

A. Description
1. Also known as "pink eye"
2. Inflammation of the conjunctiva
3. Usually caused by either allergy, infection, or trauma
4. Bacterial and viral conjunctivitis is extremely contagious
5. Chlamydial conjunctivitis is rare in older children and if diagnosed in a nonsexually active child, the child should be assessed for possible sexual **abuse**

B. Data collection
1. Itching, burning, or scratchy eyelids
2. Redness, edema, discharge

C. Implementation
1. Instruct in infection control measures such as good handwashing and not sharing towels and washcloths
2. Administer antibiotic or antiviral eye drops or ointment as prescribed if infection is present
3. Administer antihistamines as prescribed if an allergy is present
4. Instruct the child and parents in the administration of the prescribed medications
5. Instruct the parents that the child should be kept home from school or day care until antibiotic eye drops have been administered for 24 hours
6. Instruct the child to avoid rubbing the eye to prevent injury
7. Instruct the child wearing contact lenses to discontinue wearing them and to obtain new lenses to eliminate the chance of reinfection
8. Instruct the adolescent that eye makeup should be discarded and replaced

9. Instruct in the use of cool compresses to lessen irritation, and in wearing dark glasses for photophobia

III. OTITIS MEDIA

A. Description
  1. Infection of the middle ear occurring from a blocked eustachian tube, which prevents normal drainage
  2. Otitis media is a common complication of an acute respiratory infection
  3. Infants and children are more prone to otitis media because their eustachian tubes are shorter, wider, and straighter

B. Data collection
  1. Fever, irritability, restlessness
  2. Earache or pain
  3. Rolling of the head from side to side
  4. Pulling or rubbing the ear
  5. Loss of appetite
  6. Hearing loss
  7. Purulent drainage
  8. Red, opaque, bulging, or retracting tympanic membrane

C. Implementation
  1. Encourage fluids
  2. Teach the parents to feed infants in an upright position
  3. Instruct the child to avoid chewing during the acute period because chewing increases pain
  4. Provide local heat and have the child lie with the affected ear down
  5. Instruct the parents in the appropriate procedure to clean drainage from the ear with sterile cotton swabs
  6. Instruct the parents in the administration of analgesics or antipyretics such as acetaminophen (Tylenol) to decrease fever and pain
  7. Instruct the parents in the administration of the prescribed antibiotics, emphasizing that the 10- to 14-day period is necessary to eradicate positive organisms
  8. Instruct the parents that screening for hearing loss may be necessary
  9. If ear drops are prescribed, instruct the parents that the auditory canal is straightened by pulling the pinna down and back in children younger than 3 years old, and by pulling the pinna up and back for a child older than 3 years

D. Myringotomy
  1. Description: insertion of tympanoplasty tubes into the middle ear to equalize pressure and keep the ear aerated
  2. Implementation postoperatively
    a. Instruct the parents and child to keep the ears dry
    b. Earplugs should be worn during bathing, shampooing, and swimming
    c. Diving and submerging under water is not allowed

IV. TONSILLECTOMY AND ADENOIDECTOMY

A. Description
  1. Tonsillitis is a term commonly used to describe an inflammation and infection of the tonsils
  2. Adenoiditis refers to infection and inflammation of the adenoids

B. Data collection
  1. Persistent or recurrent sore throat
  2. Enlarged bright red tonsils, which may be covered with white exudate
  3. Difficulty swallowing
  4. Mouth breathing and an unpleasant mouth odor
  5. Fever
  6. Cough
  7. Enlarged adenoids may cause nasal quality of speech, mouth breathing, hearing difficulty, snoring, or obstructive sleep apnea

C. Preoperative implementation
  1. Monitor for signs of active infection
  2. Monitor bleeding and clotting studies because the throat is very vascular
  3. Prepare the child for postoperative sore throat and inform child of the need to drink liquids
  4. Check for any loose teeth to decrease the risk of aspiration during surgery

D. Postoperative implementation
  1. Position prone or side-lying to facilitate drainage
  2. Have suction equipment available, but do not suction unless there is an airway obstruction
  3. Monitor for signs of hemorrhage; if hemorrhage occurs, turn the child to the side and notify the registered nurse who will contact the physician
  4. Discourage coughing or clearing the throat
  5. Provide clear, cool, noncitrus, and noncarbonated fluids
  6. Avoid milk products initially because they will coat the throat
  7. Avoid red liquids, which will indicate the appearance of blood if the child vomits
  8. Do not give the child any straws, forks, or sharp objects that can be put in the mouth
  9. Administer acetaminophen (Tylenol) for sore throat as prescribed

10. Instruct the parents to notify the physician if bleeding, persistent earache, or fever occurs
11. Instruct the parents to keep child away from crowds until healing has occurred

V. EPIGLOTTITIS

A. Description
   1. A bacterial form of croup
   2. An inflammation of the epiglottis, which may be caused by *Haemophilus influenzae* type B or *Streptococcus pneumoniae*
   3. Occurs most frequently in age group 2 to 5 years
   4. The onset is abrupt and the condition occurs most often in the winter
   5. Considered an emergency situation

B. Data collection
   1. High fever
   2. Sore, red, and inflamed throat
   3. Absence of spontaneous cough
   4. Drooling
   5. Difficulty swallowing
   6. Muffled voice
   7. Inspiratory **stridor**
   8. Agitation
   9. Tripod positioning; while supporting the body with the hands, the child thrusts the chin forward and opens the mouth in an attempt to widen the airway

C. Implementation
   1. Maintain a patent airway
   2. Assess respiratory status and breath sounds, noting **nasal flaring**, the use of accessory muscles, and the presence of **stridor**
   3. Assess temperature by the axillary route, not the oral route
   4. To prevent spasm of the epiglottis and airway occlusion, NO attempts should be made to visualize the posterior pharynx or to obtain a throat culture
   5. Prepare the child for lateral neck films to confirm the diagnosis
   6. Maintain NPO status
   7. Do not leave the child unattended
   8. Do not force the child to lie down
   9. Do not restrain the child
   10. Administer intravenous (IV) fluids and antibiotics as prescribed
   11. Administer analgesics and antipyretics (acetaminophen [Tylenol]) to reduce fever and throat pain as prescribed
   12. Provide cool-mist oxygen therapy as prescribed
   13. Provide high humidification to cool the airway and decrease swelling
   14. Have resuscitation equipment available and prepare for endotracheal intubation or tracheotomy for severe respiratory distress
   15. Question the physician regarding the need for immunization (*Haemophilus* type B)

VI. LARYNGOTRACHEOBRONCHITIS (LTB)

A. Description
   1. Inflammation of larynx, trachea, and bronchi
   2. Most common type of croup and may be viral or bacterial
   3. Has a gradual onset and may be preceded by an upper respiratory infection

B. Data collection
   1. Fever
   2. Irritability, restlessness
   3. Hoarse voice, seal bark, and brassy cough
   4. Inspiratory **stridor** and labored respirations
   5. Use of accessory muscles for breathing
   6. Anorexia, nausea, and vomiting
   7. Cyanosis

C. Implementation
   1. Maintain a patent airway
   2. Assess respiratory status, monitoring for **nasal flaring**, sternal retraction, and inspiratory **stridor**
   3. Monitor for pallor or cyanosis
   4. Elevate head of the bed and provide bed rest
   5. Provide humidified oxygen via cool-mist tent for the hospitalized child
   6. Instruct the parents to use a cool-air vaporizer or humidifier at home; other measures include having the child breathe in the cool night air or the air from an open freezer, or taking the child to a cool basement or garage
   7. Provide and encourage fluid intake; IVs may be prescribed to maintain hydration status if the child is unable to take oral fluids
   8. Administer acetaminophen (Tylenol) as prescribed to reduce fever
   9. Avoid cough syrups and cold medicines, which may dry and thicken secretions
   10. Administer bronchodilators if prescribed to relax smooth muscle and relieve **stridor**
   11. Administer corticosteroids if prescribed for the antiinflammatory effect
   12. Administer nebulized epinephrine (racemic epinephrine) as prescribed for children with severe disease, **stridor** at rest, **retractions**, or difficulty breathing
   13. Administer antibiotics as prescribed, noting that they are not indicated unless a bacterial infection is present
   14. Have resuscitation equipment available

VII. BRONCHITIS

A. Description: Infection of the major bronchi that may be referred to as tracheobronchitis

B. Data collection
1. Fever
2. Dry, hacking, and nonproductive cough that is worse at night and becomes productive in 2 to 3 days

C. Implementation
1. Monitor for respiratory distress
2. Provide cool, humidified air
3. Monitor for signs of dehydration, such as a sunken fontanelle, poor skin turgor, and decreased and concentrated urinary output
4. Increased fluid intake
5. Administer acetaminophen (Tylenol) for fever as prescribed

VIII. BRONCHIOLITIS/RESPIRATORY SYNCYTIAL VIRUS (RSV)

A. Description
1. An inflammation of the bronchioles that causes a thick production of mucus that occludes bronchiole tubes and small bronchi
2. RSV is a common cause of bronchiolitis
3. RSV, although not airborne, is highly communicable and is usually transferred by the hands

B. Data collection
1. Upper respiratory infection (URI) symptoms such as rhinorrhea and low-grade fever
2. Lethargy, poor feeding, and irritability in infants
3. Tachypnea
4. Increased difficulty in breathing
5. **Nasal flaring** and **retractions**
6. Expiratory wheeze and grunt
7. Diminished breath sounds

C. Implementation
1. Maintain a patent airway
2. Position the child at a 30- to 40-degree angle with the neck slightly extended to maintain an open airway and decrease pressure on the diaphragm
3. Provide cool, humidified oxygen
4. Encourage fluids; IV fluid may be necessary until the acute stage has passed
5. Assess for signs of dehydration

D. The child with RSV
1. Isolate in a single room or place in a room with another RSV child
2. Maintain good handwashing procedures
3. Ensure that nurses caring for these children do not care for other high-risk children
4. Wear gowns when soiling of clothing may occur during care
5. Administer ribavirin (Virazole), an antiviral respiratory medication, if prescribed
6. Ribavirin is administered via aerosol by hood, tent, mask, or through ventilator tubing; pregnant health care providers should not care for a child receiving ribavirin
7. The nurse wearing contact lenses should wear goggles when coming in contact with ribavirin because the mist may dissolve soft lenses
8. Prepare for the administration of respiratory syncytial virus immune globulin (RSV-IGIV or RespiGam)
   a. Used prophylactically to prevent RSV in high-risk infants
   b. RespiGam is an IV preparation of immunoglobulin G and is administered before the RSV epidemic season (November through April); subsequent doses are given every month to maintain protection
   c. Not administered to infants or children with congenital heart disease (CHD) or with cyanotic CHD

IX. ASTHMA

A. Description
1. Chronic inflammatory disease of the airways
2. Is commonly caused by physical and chemical irritants as foods, pollens, dust mites, cockroaches, smoke, animal dander, temperature changes, respiratory infection, activity, and stress
3. The allergic reaction in the airways can cause an immediate reaction, with obstruction occurring, and it can precipitate a late bronchial obstructive reaction several hours after the initial exposure
4. A common symptom is coughing in the absence of respiratory infection, especially at night
5. Status asthmaticus
   a. Child displays respiratory distress despite vigorous treatment measures
   b. A medical emergency that can result in respiratory failure and death if left untreated

B. Data collection
1. Episodes of **wheezing**, breathlessness, dyspnea, chest tightness, and cough, particularly at night and/or in the early morning
2. Itching localized at the front of the neck or over the upper part of the back
3. Exacerbations are episodes of progressively worsening shortness of breath, cough,

wheezing, chest tightness, decreases in expiratory airflow because of bronchospasm, mucosal edema, and mucus plugging; air is trapped behind occluded or narrow airways, and hypoxemia can occur

4. Asthmatic episode
    a. Begins with irritability, restlessness, headache, feeling tired, or chest tightness
    b. Respiratory symptoms include a hacking, irritable, nonproductive cough, caused by bronchial edema
    c. Accumulated secretions stimulate the cough, and the cough becomes rattling and productive of frothy, clear, gelatinous sputum
    d. Child may be pale or flushed and the lips may have a deep, dark red color that may progress to cyanosis observed in the nail beds and skin, especially around the mouth
    e. Restlessness, apprehension, and diaphoresis occurs
    f. Younger children assume the tripod sitting position; older children sit upright with the shoulders in a hunched-over position, with the hands on the bed or a chair, and arms braced to facilitate the use of accessory muscles of breathing (child refuses to lie down)
    g. Child speaks in short, broken phrases
    h. **Retractions**
    i. Breath sounds are coarse and loud, with crackles and coarse rhonchi and inspiratory and expiratory **wheezing**; expiration is prolonged
5. Exercise-induced bronchospasm (EIB): cough, shortness of breath, chest pain or tightness, **wheezing**, and endurance problems during exercise
6. Severe spasm or obstruction: breath sounds and crackles may become inaudible, and the cough is ineffective (represents a lack of air movement)
7. Ventilatory failure and asphyxia: shortness of breath, with air movement in the chest restricted to the point of absent breath sounds accompanied by a sudden rise in the respiratory rate

C. Implementation: acute episode
1. Assess airway patency
2. Administer humidified oxygen by nasal prongs or facemask as prescribed
3. Administer quick-relief (rescue) medications as prescribed
4. Continuously monitor respiratory status, pulse oximetry, and color; be alert to decreased **wheezing** or a silent chest, which may signal the inability to move air
5. An IV line is initiated; prepare to correct dehydration, acidosis, or electrolyte imbalances
6. Prepare the child for a chest x-ray study
7. Arterial blood gases and serum electrolytes will be obtained

D. Medications
1. Quick-relief (rescue medications)
    a. To treat symptoms and exacerbations
    b. Short-acting B_2-agonists: for acute exacerbations (albuterol [Proventil HFA, Ventolin], metaproterenol sulfate [Alupent], and terbutaline sulfate [Brethaire, Brethine, Bricanyl])
    c. Anticholinergics: for relief of acute bronchospasm (atropine sulfate, ipratropium bromide [Atrovent])
    d. Systemic corticosteroids: antiinflammatory action to treat reversible airflow obstruction
2. Long-term control (preventer medications)
    a. Achieve and maintain control of inflammation
    b. Corticosteroids: antiinflammatory action to reduce bronchial hyperactivity
    c. Cromolyn sodium (Intal): a nonsteroidal antiinflammatory (NSAID) that inhibits acute airway narrowing
    d. Nedocromil sodium (Tilade): An antiallergic and antiinflammatory used for maintenance therapy
    e. Long-acting B_2-agonists: for the prevention of EIB (albuterol [Proventil HFA, Ventolin], metaproterenol sulfate [Alupent], and terbutaline sulfate [Brethaire, Brethine, Bricanyl])
    f. Methylxanthines: for bronchodilation
    g. Leukotriene modifiers: to prevent bronchospasm and inflammatory cell infiltration (zafirlukast [Accolate] and zileuton [Zyflo]); used in children older than 12 years
    h. Long-acting bronchodilator: used for long-term prevention of symptoms, especially nocturnal symptoms (salmeterol [Serevent])
3. Nebulizer, metered-dose inhaler (MDI), or peak flow expiratory meters (PEFMs)
    a. Used to deliver many of the medications to treat asthma
    b. A nonchlorofluorocarbon (CFC) is available for albuterol (Proventil Hydrofluoroalkane [HFA])
    c. Turbuhaler (CFC-free MDI) delivers inhaled powder and eliminates the need

for coordination of the device with inhalation and holding the breath
   d. If the child has difficulty using the MDI, medication can be administered by nebulization (medication is mixed with saline and then nebulized with compressed air by a machine)

E. Chest physiotherapy (CPT)
   1. Includes breathing exercises and physical training
   2. Not recommended during an acute exacerbation

F. Allergen control
   1. Prevents and reduces exposure to airborne allergens
   2. Skin testing to identify allergens; immunotherapy is not recommended for allergens that can be eliminated effectively
   3. Dust mites: maintain the humidity in the house under 50%
   4. Cockroaches: exterminating, cleaning kitchen floors and cabinets, putting food away quickly after eating, taking the trash out in the evening

G. Home care measures
   1. Instruct in measures to eliminate allergens
   2. Avoid extremes of environmental temperature; in cold temperatures, instruct the child to breathe through the nose, not the mouth, and to cover the nose and mouth with a scarf
   3. Avoid exposure to individuals with a viral respiratory infection
   4. Instruct the child how to recognize early symptoms of an asthma attack
   5. Instruct the child in the administration of medications as prescribed
   6. Instruct the child in the use of a nebulizer, MDI, or PEFM
   7. Instruct the child in the cleaning of devices used for inhaled medications (oral candidiasis can occur with the use of aerosolized steroids)
   8. Encourage adequate rest, sleep, and a well-balanced diet
   9. Instruct the child in the importance of adequate fluid intake to liquefy secretions
   10. Assist in developing an exercise program
   11. Instruct the child in the procedure for respiratory treatments and exercises as prescribed
   12. Encourage the child to cough effectively
   13. Encourage the parents to keep immunizations up to date; annual influenza vaccinations are recommended
   14. Inform other health care providers and school personnel of the asthma condition
   15. Allow the child to take control of self-care measures based on age appropriateness

X. PNEUMONIA

A. Description
   1. Inflammation of the alveoli caused by a virus, mycoplasmal agents, bacteria, or the aspiration of foreign substances
   2. The causative agent is usually introduced into the lungs through inhalation or from the bloodstream
   3. Viral pneumonia occurs more frequently than bacterial and is often associated with a viral URI
   4. Primary atypical pneumonia (*M. pneumoniae*) is the most common cause of pneumonia in children between 5 and 12 years; occurs primarily in the fall and winter months and is more prevalent in crowded living conditions
   5. Bacterial pneumonia is often a serious infection; hospitalization is indicated when pleural effusion or empyema accompanies the disease, and is mandatory for children with staphylococcal pneumonia
   6. Aspiration pneumonia occurs when food, secretions, liquids, or other materials enter the lung and cause inflammation and a chemical pneumonitis; classic symptoms include an increasing cough or fever with foul-smelling sputum, deteriorating results on chest x-ray films, and other signs of airway involvement

B. Viral pneumonia
   1. Data collection
      a. Mild fever, slight cough, and malaise, to high fever, severe cough, and prostration
      b. Nonproductive or productive cough of small amounts of whitish sputum
      c. Wheezes or fine crackles
   2. Implementation
      a. Administer oxygen with cool mist as prescribed
      b. Increase fluid intake
      c. Administer antipyretics for fever as prescribed
      d. Administer chest physiotherapy and postural drainage as prescribed
      e. Antimicrobial therapy is reserved for children in whom the presence of infection is demonstrated by cultures

C. Primary atypical pneumonia
   1. Data collection
      a. Fever, chills, anorexia, headache, malaise, and muscle pain
      b. Rhinitis, sore throat, and dry, hacking cough
      c. Cough is nonproductive initially; then produces seromucoid sputum that becomes mucopurulent or blood-streaked

2. Implementation: symptomatic

D. Bacterial pneumonia
1. Data collection
a. Acute onset, fever, toxic appearance
b. Infant: irritability, lethargy, poor feeding; abrupt fever (may be accompanied by seizures); respiratory distress (air hunger, tachypnea, and circumoral cyanosis)
c. Older child: headache, chills, abdominal pain, chest pain, meningeal symptoms (meningism)
d. Hacking, nonproductive cough
e. Diminished breath sounds or scattered crackles
f. As the infection resolves, coarse crackles and **wheezing** are heard and the cough becomes productive with purulent sputum
2. Implementation
a. Antimicrobial therapy is initiated as soon as the diagnosis is suspected
b. Administer oxygen (via hood, mist tent, or nasal cannula) for respiratory distress as prescribed
c. Place the child in a mist tent as prescribed; cool humidification moistens the airways and assists in temperature reduction
d. Suction the infant to maintain a patent airway if the infant is unable to handle secretions
e. Administer chest physiotherapy and postural drainage every 4 hours as prescribed
f. Promote bed rest to conserve energy
g. Encourage the child to lie on the affected side (if pneumonia is unilateral) to splint the chest and reduce the discomfort caused by pleural rubbing
h. Provide liberal fluid intake (administer cautiously to prevent aspiration); IV fluids may be necessary
i. Administer antipyretics for fever as prescribed; monitor temperature frequently because of the risk for febrile seizures
j. Institute isolation precautions with pneumococcal and staphylococcal pneumonia (according to agency policy)
k. Administer antitussives as prescribed before rest times and meals if the cough is disturbing
l. Continuous closed chest drainage may be instituted if purulent fluid is present (usually noted in staphylococcus infections)
m. Fluid accumulation in the pleural cavity may be removed by thoracentesis; thoracentesis also provides a means for obtaining fluid for culture and for instilling antibiotics directly into the pleural cavity

XI. CYSTIC FIBROSIS (CF) (Figure 29-1)

A. Description
1. A chronic multisystem disorder (autosomal recessive trait disorder) characterized by exocrine gland dysfunction
2. The mucus produced by the exocrine glands is abnormally thick, causing obstruction of the small passageways of the affected organs
3. The most common symptoms are pancreatic enzyme deficiency resulting from duct blockage, progressive chronic lung disease associated with infection, and sweat gland dysfunction resulting in increased sodium and chloride sweat concentrations
4. An increase in sodium and chloride in both sweat and saliva forms the basis for the most reliable diagnostic test, the sweat chloride test

B. Respiratory system
1. Symptoms are produced by the stagnation of mucus in the airway, leading to bacterial colonization and destruction of lung tissue
2. Emphysema and atelectasis occur as the airways become increasingly obstructed
3. Chronic hypoxemia causes contraction and hypertrophy of the muscle fibers in pulmonary arteries and arterioles, leading to pulmonary hypertension and eventual cor pulmonale
4. Pneumothorax from ruptured bullae and hemoptysis from erosion of the bronchial wall through an artery occur as the disease progresses
5. **Wheezing** and dry nonproductive cough
6. Dyspnea
7. Cyanosis
8. Clubbing of the fingers and toes (Figure 29-2)
9. Repeated episodes of bronchitis and pneumonia

C. Gastrointestinal system
1. Meconium ileus in the neonate
2. Intestinal obstruction (distal intestinal obstructive syndrome) caused by thick intestinal secretions; signs include pain, abdominal distention, nausea, and vomiting
3. Steatorrhea (frothy, foul-smelling stools)
4. Deficiency of the fat-soluble vitamins A, D, E, and K, which causes easy bruising and anemia
5. Malnutrition and failure to thrive; demonstrate hypoalbuminemia from diminished absorption of protein resulting in generalized edema
6. Rectal prolapse can occur as a result of the large, bulky stools, and lack of the supportive fat pads around the rectum

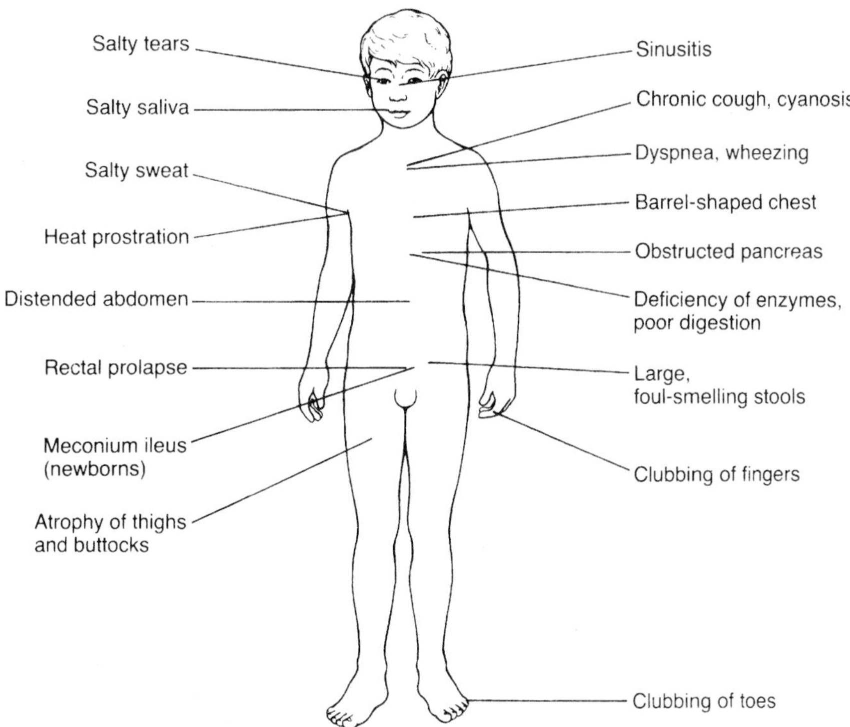

FIG. 29-1 Manifestations of cystic fibrosis. (From Thompson ED: *Introduction to maternity and pediatric nursing*, ed 2 Philadelphia, 1995, WB Saunders.)

D. Integumentary system
   1. Abnormally high concentrations of sodium and chloride in sweat
   2. Parents report that the infant tastes "salty" when kissed
   3. Dehydration and electrolyte imbalances especially during hyperthermic conditions

E. Reproductive system
   1. Delayed **puberty** in females
   2. Fertility can be inhibited by highly viscous cervical secretions, which act as a plug and block sperm entry
   3. Males are usually sterile, caused by the blockage of the vas deferens by abnormal secretions or by failure of normal development of duct structures

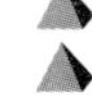

F. Diagnostic tests
   1. Quantitative sweat chloride test
      a. The production of sweat is stimulated (pilocarpine iontophoresis), the sweat is collected, and the sweat electrolytes are measured (a minimum of 50 mg of sweat is needed)
      b. Normally, sweat chloride concentration is less than 40 mEq/L
      c. A chloride concentration greater than 60 mEq/L is a positive test result
      d. Chloride concentrations of 40 to 60 mEq/L is highly suggestive of CF and requires a repeat test
   2. Chest x-ray study: reveals atelectasis and obstructive emphysema
   3. Pulmonary function tests: provide evidence of abnormal small airway function
   4. Stool/fat and/or enzyme analysis: a 72-hour stool sample is collected to check the fat and/or enzyme (trypsin) content (food intake is recorded during the collection)

G. Implementation
   1. Respiratory system
      a. Goals of treatment include preventing and treating pulmonary infection by improving aeration, removing secretions, and administering antimicrobial medications
      b. Chest physiotherapy (percussion and postural drainage) on awakening and in the evening (more frequently during pulmonary infection)
      c. Chest physiotherapy should not be performed before or immediately after a meal
      d. Bronchodilator medication by aerosol to open the bronchi for easier expectoration (administered before the CPT when the child has reactive airway disease or is **wheezing**)

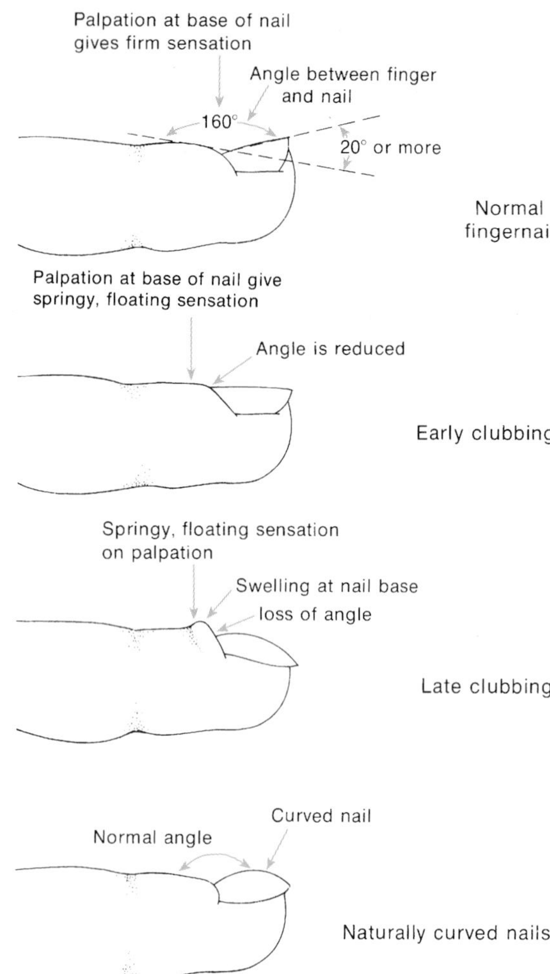

FIG. 29-2 Clubbing of fingers. (From Schulte E, Price D, Gwin J: *Thompson's pediatric nursing*, ed 8, Philadelphia, 2001, WB Saunders.)

e. Use of a flutter mucus clearance device (a small, hand-held plastic pipe with a stainless-steel ball on the inside that facilitates removal of mucus); store away from small children because if the device separates, the steel ball poses a choking hazard
f. Use of a ThAIRapy vest device that provides high-frequency chest wall oscillation to help loosen secretions
g. Administration of recombinant human deoxyribonuclease (DNase), known generically as dornase alfa (Pulmozyme), which decreases the viscosity of mucus
h. Instruct the parents not to give cough suppressants, as they will inhibit expectoration of secretions and promote infection
i. Teach the child forced expiratory technique (huffing) to mobilize secretions
j. Develop a physical exercise program with the aim of establishing a good habitual breathing pattern
k. Administer antibiotics as prescribed, which may be prescribed prophylactically or when pulmonary symptoms develop
l. Aerosolized antibiotics may be prescribed and are administered after CPT is performed, or IV antibiotics may be prescribed and administered at home through a central venous access device
m. Administer oxygen as prescribed during acute episodes; monitor closely for oxygen narcosis
n. Monitor for hemoptysis; greater than 300 mL in 24 hours for the older child (less for a younger child) needs to be treated immediately
o. Hemoptysis may be controlled by bed rest, cough suppressants, antibiotics, and vitamin K; if hemoptysis persists, the site of bleeding may be cauterized or embolized
p. Lung transplantation is a final therapeutic option for the end-stage child

2. Gastrointestinal system
   a. The goal of treatment for pancreatic insufficiency is to replace pancreatic enzymes; administered with meals and snacks (or within 30 minutes of eating meals and snacks) to ensure that digestive enzymes are mixed with food in the duodenum
   b. The amount of pancreatic enzymes administered is adjusted to achieve normal **growth** and a decrease in the number of stools to two to three per day
   c. Pancreatic enzymes should not be given if the child is NPO
   d. Enteric-coated pancreatic enzymes should not be crushed or chewed
   e. Enzyme powder should be mixed with nonfat, nonprotein foods such as applesauce
   f. Enzyme powder is not to be mixed with hot foods or foods containing tapioca or other starches; the enzymes are inactivated by heat and are partially degraded by gastric acids
   g. Encourage a well-balanced, high-protein, high-calorie diet; multivitamins and vitamins A, D, E, and K are also administered
   h. Assess weight and monitor for failure to thrive
   i. Monitor for constipation and intestinal obstruction
   j. Supplement the child's diet with salt during extremely hot weather or if the child

has a fever; include fluids such as Gatorade or Exceed, which provide an adequate supply of electrolytes

H. Home care
1. Instruct the parents about the prescribed treatment measures and their importance
2. Instruct the parents to be sure immunizations are up to date
3. Inform the parents that the child should be vaccinated yearly for pneumococcus and influenza
4. Inform the parents about the Cystic Fibrosis Foundation

XII. SUDDEN INFANT DEATH SYNDROME (SIDS)

A. Description
1. Unexpected death of an apparently healthy infant under age 1 year for which a thorough autopsy fails to demonstrate an adequate cause of death
2. The cause is not known

B. Characteristics
1. Maternal risk factors
   a. Maternal smoking
   b. Substance **abuse**
   c. Younger mothers
2. Birth risk factors
   a. Prematurity
   b. Low-birth-weight infants
   c. Multiple births
   d. Infants with central nervous system problems
3. Time of year: most frequently during winter months
4. Time of death: usually occurs during sleep
5. Age: most frequently occurs from 2 months to 4 months of life
6. Sex and race
   a. Higher in males
   b. Higher in Native Americans and Blacks
7. Sleep risk habits
   a. Prone position
   b. Use of soft bedding
   c. Overheating (thermal stress)
   d. Possibly: sleeping with an adult

C. Appearance when found
1. Apneic, blue, lifeless
2. Frothy blood-tinged fluid in the nose and mouth
3. May be found in any position but is typically found in a disheveled bed, with blankets over the head, and huddled in a corner
4. May be clutching bedding
5. Diaper is wet and full of stool

D. Prevention
1. Healthy infants should be placed in the supine position for sleep
2. Infants with gastroesophageal reflux and other airway anomalies that predispose to airway obstruction may be placed in a prone sleeping position
3. Soft moldable mattresses and bedding, such as pillows or quilts, should not be used under the infant for bedding
4. Stuffed animals should be removed from the crib while the infant is sleeping

XIII. TUBERCULOSIS (TB) IN CHILDREN

A. Description
1. A contagious disease caused by *Mycobacterium tuberculosis*, an acid-fast bacillus
2. Children are susceptible to the human *M. tuberculosis* and the *Mycobacterium bovis*
3. *M. bovis* is common in parts of the world where TB is not controlled or pasteurization of milk is not practiced; the organism can be ingested via infected milk
4. Multidrug-resistant strains of *M. tuberculosis* occurs because of client or family noncompliance with therapeutic regimens
5. The route of transmission of *M. tuberculosis* is through inhalation of droplets from an individual with active TB
6. Most children are infected by a family member or by another individual with whom they have frequent contact, such as a baby sitter

B. Data collection
1. May be asymptomatic or develop symptoms such as malaise, fever, cough, weight loss, anorexia, and lymphadenopathy
2. Specific symptoms related to the site of infection, such as the lungs, brain, or bone may be present

C. Mantoux test
1. Will produce a positive reaction 2 to 10 weeks after the initial infection
2. Determines whether the child has been infected and has developed a sensitivity to the protein of the tubercle bacillus; a positive reaction does not confirm the presence of active disease
3. Once the child reacts positively, the child will always react positively; a positive reaction in a previously negative test indicates that the child has been infected since the last test
4. TB testing should not be done at the same time as measles immunization; viral interference from the measles vaccine may cause a false-negative reaction

5. Induration measuring 15 mm or greater is considered to be a positive reaction in children 4 years of age or older who do not have any risk factors
6. Induration measuring 10 mm or greater is considered to be a positive reaction in children younger than 4 years old and in those with chronic illness or at high risk for exposure to TB
7. Induration measuring 5 mm or greater is considered to be positive for the highest risk groups, such as children with immunosuppressive conditions or human immunodeficiency syndrome (HIV)

D. Sputum culture
1. A definitive diagnosis is made by demonstrating the presence of mycobacteria in a culture
2. Because an infant or young child often swallows sputum rather than expectorates, gastric washings (aspiration of lavaged contents from the fasting stomach) may be done to obtain a specimen; specimen is obtained in the early morning before breakfast

E. Implementation
1. Medications
   a. Include isoniazid (INH), rifampin (Rifadin), and pyrazinamide
   b. A 9-month course of INH is prescribed to prevent a latent infection from progressing to clinically active TB and to prevent initial infection in children in high-risk situations; a 12-month course is prescribed for the HIV-infected child
   c. Recommendation for the child with clinically active TB: INH, rifampin, and pyrazinamide daily for 2 months; then, INH and rifampin twice weekly
2. Place children with infectious disease on isolation precautions until medications have been initiated, sputum cultures demonstrate a diminished number of organisms, and cough is improving
3. Wear a mask if the child is coughing and does not reliably cover his or her mouth
4. Maintain airborne precautions with family members until they are demonstrated not to have infectious TB
5. Bacillus Calmette-Guérin (BCG) vaccine
   a. Produces limited immunity (definite although incomplete protection against TB)
   b. Positive tuberculin reactions develop after inoculation
   c. Not generally recommended; however, may be used for long-term protection of infants and children who are at high risk for continuing exposure to persons with infectious TB
6. Stress the importance of adequate rest and adequate diet
7. Instruct the child and family in measures to prevent transmission of TB

PRACTICE QUESTIONS

1. A day care nurse is observing a 2-year-old child. The nurse suspects that the child may have strabismus. Which of the following observations may be indicative of this condition?
   1. The child consistently tilts the head to see
   2. The child consistently turns the head to see
   3. The child does not respond when spoken to
   4. The child has difficulty hearing
2. A nurse has provided instructions to a mother of a child diagnosed with bacterial conjunctivitis. Which of the following, if stated by the mother, would indicate a need for further instructions?
   1. "I need to wash my hands frequently."
   2. "I need to clean the eye as prescribed."
   3. "I need to give the eye drops as prescribed."
   4. "It is OK to share towels and washcloths."
3. A nurse provides instructions to parents regarding the methods that will decrease the risk of recurrent otitis media in infants. Which of the following would be included in the instructions?
   1. Feed the infant in an upright position
   2. Allow the infant to have a bottle during nap time
   3. Maintain bottle-feeding as long as possible
   4. Discontinue breastfeeding as soon as possible
4. A nurse is assigned to care for a child after myringotomy with insertion of tympanostomy tubes. The nurse notes a small amount of reddish drainage from the child's ear after the surgery. Which of the following is the most appropriate nursing action?
   1. Notify the registered nurse (RN)
   2. Change the ear tubes so that they do not become blocked
   3. Document the findings
   4. Check the ear drainage for the presence of cerebrospinal fluid (CSF)
5. A nurse prepares a teaching plan regarding administration of eardrops for the parents of a 2-year-old child. Which of the following would be included in the plan?
   1. Pull the ear up and back before instilling the eardrops
   2. Wear gloves when administering the eardrops
   3. Hold the child in a sitting position when administering the eardrops
   4. Pull the ear down and back before instilling the eardrops

6. A child is scheduled for a tonsillectomy. Which of the following would present the highest risk of aspiration during surgery?
   1. Difficulty swallowing
   2. The presence of loose teeth
   3. Bleeding during surgery
   4. Exudate in the throat area
7. The most appropriate child position after a tonsillectomy is which of the following?
   1. Supine
   2. Trendelenburg
   3. Side-lying
   4. High-Fowler's
8. After tonsillectomy, the child begins to vomit bright red blood. The initial nursing action would be to:
   1. Administer the prescribed antiemetic
   2. Turn the child to the side
   3. Notify the registered nurse (RN)
   4. Maintain an NPO status
9. After tonsillectomy, which of the following fluid or food items would be appropriate to offer to the child?
   1. Cool cherry Kool-Aid
   2. Vanilla pudding
   3. Cold ginger ale
   4. Jell-O
10. A nurse is reinforcing instructions to the mother of an 8-year-old child who had a tonsillectomy. The mother tells the nurse that the child loves tacos and asks when the child can safely eat one. The most appropriate response would be:
    1. "In 1 week."
    2. "In 3 weeks."
    3. "Two days after surgery."
    4. "When the physician says it's OK."
11. A nurse reinforces instructions to the mother of a child with croup about the measures to take if an acute spasmodic episode occurs. Which statement by the mother indicates a need for further instructions?
    1. "I will place a steam vaporizer in my child's room."
    2. "I will place my child in a closed bathroom and allow my child to inhale mist from the warm running water."
    3. "I will place a cool-mist humidifier in my child's room."
    4. "I will take my child out into the cool humid night air."
12. A nurse reinforces instructions to the mother of a child hospitalized with croup. Which of the following statements, if made by the mother, would indicate a need for further instruction?
    1. "I will give my child cough syrup if a cough develops."
    2. "I will be sure that my child drinks at least 3 to 4 glasses of fluids every day."
    3. "I will give acetaminophen (Tylenol) if my child develops a fever."
    4. "Sips of warm fluid will help if my child develops a croup attack."
13. A nurse working in the emergency room is caring for a child diagnosed with epiglottitis. Indications that the child may be experiencing airway obstruction include which of the following?
    1. The child is leaning backward supporting self with the hands and arms
    2. A low-grade fever and complaints of a sore throat
    3. The child is leaning forward with the chin thrust out
    4. Nasal flaring and bradycardia
14. A nurse is caring for a hospitalized infant with bronchiolitis. Diagnostic tests have confirmed respiratory syncytial virus (RSV). Based on this finding, which of the following would be the most appropriate nursing action?
    1. Plan to move the infant to another room with another RSV child
    2. Leave the infant in the present room because RSV is not contagious
    3. Wear a mask when caring for the child
    4. Initiate strict enteric precautions
15. A child is brought to the emergency room for treatment of an acute asthma attack. The nurse prepares to administer which of the following medications first?
    1. A leukotriene modifier
    2. A nonsteroidal antiinflammatory
    3. Oral corticosteroids
    4. Albuterol (Proventil HFA, Ventolin)
16. A nursing student is asked to discuss sudden infant death syndrome (SIDS) at the clinical conference being held at the end of the clinical day. The student plans to include which of the following in the discussion during the conference?
    1. SIDS usually occurs during sleep and is more common in premature infants
    2. SIDS usually occurs during sleep and is more common in girls
    3. SIDS usually occurs during sleep and most frequently occurs between 8 and 10 months of age
    4. SIDS usually occurs during sleep and is more common in high-birth weight infants
17. A nurse is instructing a mother of a child with cystic fibrosis (CF) about the appropriate dietary measures. Which of the following diets will be included in the instructions?
    1. Low-calorie, low-fat diet
    2. High-calorie, high-protein diet
    3. High-calorie, low-protein diet
    4. Low-calorie, restricted fat

18. A nurse prepares to administer a pancreatic enzyme powder to the child with cystic fibrosis (CF). Which of the following food items will the nurse mix with the medication?
   1. Applesauce
   2. Tapioca
   3. Mashed potatoes
   4. Hot oatmeal
19. A nurse reviews the results of a Mantoux test performed on a 3-year-old child. The results indicate an area of induration measuring 10 mm. The nurse would interpret these results as:
   1. Negative
   2. Positive
   3. Inconclusive
   4. Definitive requiring a repeat test
20. Isoniazid (INH) is prescribed for a 2-year-old child with a positive Mantoux test. The mother of the child asks the nurse how long the child will need to take the medication. The most appropriate response is:
   1. 6 months
   2. 9 months
   3. 15 months
   4. 18 months

ANSWERS

1. *Answer:* 1
Rationale: The nurse may suspect strabismus in a child when the child complains of frequent headaches, squints, or tilts the head to see. Options 2, 3, and 4 are not indicative of this condition.
Test-Taking Strategy: Use the process of elimination. Begin by eliminating options 3 and 4 because they are similar and refer to hearing. From the remaining options, recalling the signs of this condition will assist in directing you to option 1. Review these signs if you had difficulty with this question.
Level of Cognitive Ability: Comprehension
Client Needs: Physiological Integrity
Integrated Concept/Process: Nursing Process/Data Collection
Content Area: Child Health
Reference: Schulte E, Price D, Gwin J: *Thompson's pediatric nursing*, ed 8, Philadelphia, 2001, WB Saunders, p. 219.

2. *Answer:* 4
Rationale: Bacterial conjunctivitis is highly contagious and infection control measures should be taught. These include frequent hand washing and not sharing towels and washcloths. Options 1, 2, and 3 are correct treatment measures.
Test-Taking Strategy: Note the key words "indicates a need for further instructions." Recalling that bacterial conjunctivitis is highly contagious will easily direct you to option 4. Review infection control measures for bacterial conjunctivitis if you had difficulty with this question.
Level of Cognitive Ability: Comprehension
Client Needs: Health Promotion and Maintenance
Integrated Concept/Process: Teaching/Learning
Content Area: Child Health
Reference: Schulte E, Price D, Gwin J: *Thompson's pediatric nursing*, ed 8, Philadelphia, 2001, WB Saunders, p.37.

3. *Answer:* 1
Rationale: To decrease the risk of recurrent otitis media, parents should be encouraged to breastfeed during infancy, discontinue bottle-feeding as soon as possible, feed the infant in an upright position, and instructed not to give the infant a bottle in bed. Parents should be told not to smoke in the child's presence because passive smoking increases the incidence of otitis media.
Test-Taking Strategy: Use the process of elimination. Option 2 can be eliminated first recalling the principles related to bottle-feeding. Recalling that breastfeeding offers some protection by providing maternal antibodies will assist in eliminating options 3 and 4. Review measures that will assist in preventing otitis media if you had difficulty with this question.
Level of Cognitive Ability: Application
Client Needs: Health Promotion and Maintenance
Integrated Concept/Process: Nursing Process/Implementation
Content Area: Child Health
Reference: Schulte E, Price D, Gwin J: *Thompson's pediatric nursing*, ed 8, Philadelphia, 2001, WB Saunders, p. 127.

4. *Answer:* 3
Rationale: After myringotomy with insertion of tympanostomy tubes, the child is monitored for ear drainage. A small amount of reddish drainage is normal for the first few days after surgery. Any heavy bleeding or bleeding that occurs after 3 days should be reported. The nurse would document the findings. Options 1, 2, and 4 are not necessary.
Test-Taking Strategy: Use the process of elimination. Note the key words "small amount." Considering both the anatomical location of the surgery and these key words will direct you to the correct option. Review postoperative findings after this type of surgery if you had difficulty with this question.
Level of Cognitive Ability: Application
Client Needs: Physiological Integrity
Integrated Concept/Process: Nursing Process/Implementation
Content Area: Child Health
Reference: Schulte E, Price D, Gwin J: *Thompson's pediatric nursing*, ed 8, Philadelphia, 2001, WB Saunders, p. 127.

5. *Answer:* 4
Rationale: To administer eardrops in a child younger than age 3 years, the ear should be pulled down and back. In children older than 3 years, the ear is pulled up and back. Parents do not need to wear gloves, but they do need to wash their hands before and after the procedure. The child needs to be in a side-

lying position with the affected ear facing upward to facilitate the flow of medication down the ear canal by gravity.
Test-Taking Strategy: Use the process of elimination. Visualizing this procedure will assist in eliminating options 2 and 3 first. From the remaining options, recalling the anatomy of the child's ear canal will direct you to option 4. Review this procedure if you had difficulty with this question.
Level of Cognitive Ability: Application
Client Needs: Health Promotion and Maintenance
Integrated Concept/Process: Nursing Process/Planning
Content Area: Child Health
Reference: Schulte E, Price D, Gwin J: *Thompson's pediatric nursing*, ed 8, Philadelphia, 2001, WB Saunders, p. 362.

6. *Answer:* 2
Rationale: In the preoperative period, the child should be observed for the presence of loose teeth to decrease the risk of aspiration during surgery. Options 1 and 4 are incorrect. Bleeding during surgery will be controlled via packing and suction as needed.
Test-Taking Strategy: The issue of the question relates to aspiration. Note the key word "highest." Options 1 and 4 can be easily eliminated because they are similar. Recalling that the tonsillar area is vascular, anticipation of bleeding during surgery is expected and would be controlled. Review preoperative assessment procedures related to tonsillectomy if you had difficulty with this question.
Level of Cognitive Ability: Comprehension
Client Needs: Physiological Integrity
Integrated Concept/Process: Nursing Process/Data Collection
Content Area: Child Health
Reference: Schulte E, Price D, Gwin J: *Thompson's pediatric nursing*, ed 8, Philadelphia, 2001, WB Saunders, p. 220.

7. *Answer:* 3
Rationale: The child should be placed in a prone or side-lying position after tonsillectomy to facilitate drainage. Options 1, 2, and 4 will not achieve this goal.
Test-Taking Strategy: Use the process of elimination. Visualize each of the positions described in the options. Keeping in mind that the goal is to facilitate drainage will direct you to option 3. Review positioning procedures after tonsillectomy if you had difficulty with this question.
Level of Cognitive Ability: Application
Client Needs: Physiological Integrity
Integrated Concept/Process: Nursing Process/Implementation
Content Area: Child Health
Reference: Schulte E, Price D, Gwin J: *Thompson's pediatric nursing*, ed 8, Philadelphia, 2001, WB Saunders, p. 220.

8. *Answer:* 2
Rationale: After tonsillectomy, if bleeding occurs, the child is turned to the side and the RN is notified; the RN then contacts the physician. An NPO status would be maintained and an antiemetic may be prescribed; however, the initial nursing action would be to turn the child to the side.
Test-Taking Strategy: Note the key word "initial." Although all of the options may be appropriate, to maintain physiological integrity, the initial action is to turn the child to the side. Review care to the child after tonsillectomy if you had difficulty with this question.
Level of Cognitive Ability: Application
Client Needs: Physiological Integrity
Integrated Concept/Process: Nursing Process/Implementation
Content Area: Child Health
Reference: Schulte E, Price D, Gwin J: *Thompson's pediatric nursing*, ed 8, Philadelphia, 2001, WB Saunders, p. 220.

9. *Answer:* 4
Rationale: After tonsillectomy, clear, cool liquids should be administered. Citrus, carbonated, and extremely hot or cold liquids need to be avoided because they may irritate the throat. Red liquids need to be avoided because they give the appearance of blood if the child vomits. Milk and milk products (pudding) are avoided because they coat the throat and cause the child to clear the throat, thus increasing the risk of bleeding.
Test-Taking Strategy: Use the process of elimination. Remember, avoiding foods and fluids that may irritate or cause bleeding is the concern. This will assist in eliminating options 2 and 3. The word "cherry" in option 1 should be the clue that this is not an appropriate food item. Review dietary measures after tonsillectomy if you had difficulty with this question.
Level of Cognitive Ability: Application
Client Needs: Physiological Integrity
Integrated Concept/Process: Nursing Process/Implementation
Content Area: Child Health
Reference: Schulte E, Price D, Gwin J: *Thompson's pediatric nursing*, ed 8, Philadelphia, 2001, WB Saunders, p. 220.

10. *Answer:* 2
Rationale: Rough, scratchy foods or spicy foods are to be avoided for 3 weeks. Citrus juices, which irritate the throat, need to be avoided for 10 days. Red liquids are avoided because they will give the appearance of blood if the child vomits. The mother is instructed to add full liquids on the second day and soft foods as the child tolerates them.
Test-Taking Strategy: Use the process of elimination and knowledge regarding the specific instructions related to food and fluids after tonsillectomy to answer this question. Eliminate option 4 because it places the mother's question on hold and is not a therapeutic response. From the remaining options, focus on the issue, when the child can safely eat a taco, and select option 2 because it is the most lengthy time period after surgery. Review these dietary instructions if you had difficulty with this question.
Level of Cognitive Ability: Application
Client Needs: Health Promotion and Maintenance
Integrated Concept/Process: Nursing Process/Implementation
Content Area: Child Health
Reference: Schulte E, Price D, Gwin J: *Thompson's pediatric nursing*, ed 8, Philadelphia, 2001, WB Saunders, p. 220.

11. *Answer:* 1
Rationale: Mist from warm running water in a closed bathroom and cool mist from a bedside humidifier are effective in reducing mucosal edema. Cool-mist humidifiers are recommended over steam vaporizers, which present a danger of

scald burns. Taking the child out into the cool humid night air may also relieve mucosal swelling. Remember, however, that a cold mist may precipitate bronchospasm.
Test-Taking Strategy: Note the key words "need for further instructions" and focus on the issue, to reduce mucosal edema and to provide a safe environment. Option 1 is the option that would provide an unsafe environment for the child. Review management of acute spasmodic croup if you had difficulty with this question.
Level of Cognitive Ability: Comprehension
Client Needs: Safe, Effective Care Environment
Integrated Concept/Process: Teaching/Learning
Content Area: Child Health
Reference: Schulte E, Price D, Gwin J: *Thompson's pediatric nursing*, ed 8, Philadelphia, 2001, WB Saunders, p. 183.

12. *Answer:* 1
Rationale: Cough syrups and cold medicines are not to be given because they may dry and thicken secretions. Adequate hydration of 500 to 1000 mL of fluids daily is important in thinning secretions. Acetaminophen is used if a fever develops. Sips of warm fluids during a croup attack help relax the vocal cords and thin mucus.
Test-Taking Strategy: Use the process of elimination. Note the key words "a need for further instruction." Knowledge of the pathophysiology related to croup will assist in eliminating options 2 and 3 first. Recalling that warm fluids can relax membranes and thin secretions will assist in directing you to option 1 from the remaining options. Review the effects of cough medicines if you had difficulty with this question.
Level of Cognitive Ability: Comprehension
Client Needs: Physiological Integrity
Integrated Concept/Process: Teaching/Learning
Content Area: Child Health
Reference: Schulte E, Price D, Gwin J: *Thompson's pediatric nursing*, ed 8, Philadelphia, 2001, WB Saunders, p. 184.

13. *Answer:* 3
Rationale: Clinical manifestations suggestive of airway obstruction include tripod positioning (leaning forward supported by arms, chin thrust out, mouth open), nasal flaring, tachycardia, a high fever, and sore throat.
Test-Taking Strategy: Use the process of elimination. Eliminate option 4 first because tachycardia rather than bradycardia will occur in a child experiencing respiratory distress. Eliminate option 2 next knowing that a high fever occurs with epiglottitis. From the remaining options, visualize the descriptions in each, and determine which position would best assist a child experiencing respiratory distress. Review tripod position if you had difficulty with this question.
Level of Cognitive Ability: Comprehension
Client Needs: Physiological Integrity
Integrated Concept/Process: Nursing Process/Data Collection
Content Area: Child Health
Reference: Schulte E, Price D, Gwin J: *Thompson's pediatric nursing*, ed 8, Philadelphia, 2001, WB Saunders, p. 357.

14. *Answer:* 1
Rationale: RSV is a highly communicable disorder. It is not transmitted via the airborne route. It is usually transferred by the hands and meticulous handwashing is necessary to decrease the spread of organisms. The infant with RSV is isolated in a single room or placed in a room with another RSV child. Enteric precautions are not necessary; however, the nurse should wear a gown when soiling of clothing may occur.
Test-Taking Strategy: Knowledge regarding the transmission of RSV will easily direct you to option 1. Review care of the child with RSV if you had difficulty with this question.
Level of Cognitive Ability: Application
Client Needs: Safe, Effective Care Environment
Integrated Concept/Process: Nursing Process/Implementation
Content Area: Child Health
Reference: Schulte E, Price D, Gwin J: *Thompson's pediatric nursing*, ed 8, Philadelphia, 2001, WB Saunders, p. 129.

15. *Answer:* 4
Rationale: In treating an acute asthma attack, a short-acting B_2-agonist such as albuterol will be given to produce bronchodilation. Options 1, 2, and 3 are long-term control (preventer) medications.
Test-Taking Strategy: Use the process of elimination and note the key words "acute asthma attack." Recalling that asthma is a reversible obstructive airway disease should assist in directing you to option 4. It would seem logical that the first action would be to dilate the bronchi. Review the treatment for an acute asthma attack if you had difficulty with this question.
Level of Cognitive Ability: Application
Client Needs: Physiological Integrity
Integrated Concept/Process: Nursing Process/Planning
Content Area: Child Health
Reference: Schulte E, Price D, Gwin J: *Thompson's pediatric nursing*, ed 8, Philadelphia, 2001, WB Saunders, p. 271.

16. *Answer:* 1
Rationale: SIDS usually occurs during sleep. It most frequently occurs between the second and fourth months of life. It is more common in boys, low-birth weight infants, and in the premature infant.
Test-Taking Strategy: Use the process of elimination and knowledge regarding the characteristics related to the etiology and the incidence of SIDS. Review this information if you are unfamiliar with it.
Level of Cognitive Ability: Application
Client Needs: Health Promotion and Maintenance
Integrated Concept/Process: Teaching/Learning
Content Area: Child Health
Reference: Schulte E, Price D, Gwin J: *Thompson's pediatric nursing*, ed 8, Philadelphia, 2001, WB Saunders, p. 52.

17. *Answer:* 2
Rationale: Children with CF are managed with a high-calorie, high-protein diet. Pancreatic enzyme replacement therapy and fat-soluble vitamin supplements are administered. Fats are not restricted unless steatorrhea cannot be controlled by increased pancreatic enzymes.
Test-Taking Strategy: Use the process of elimination. Eliminate options 1 and 4 first because of the words "low-calorie." From the remaining options, recalling the appropriate diet in the child with CF will direct you to option 2. Review the treatment measures in CF if you had difficulty with this question.

Level of Cognitive Ability: Application
Client Needs: Physiological Integrity
Integrated Concept/Process: Nursing Process/Implementation
Content Area: Child Health
Reference: Schulte E, Price D, Gwin J: *Thompson's pediatric nursing,* ed 8, Philadelphia, 2001, WB Saunders, p. 142.

18. *Answer:* 1
Rationale: Pancreatic enzyme powders are not to be mixed with hot foods or foods containing tapioca or other starches. Enzyme powder should be mixed with nonfat, nonprotein foods such as applesauce. Pancreatic enzymes are inactivated by heat and are partially degraded by gastric acids.
Test-Taking Strategy: Use the process of elimination. Eliminate option 4 first because of the word "hot" and option 2 because of the probable temperature of mashed potatoes. From the remaining options, recalling that enzyme powder should be mixed with nonfat, nonprotein foods will direct you to option 1. Review the procedure for administering pancreatic enzyme powder if you had difficulty with this question.
Level of Cognitive Ability: Application
Client Needs: Physiological Integrity
Integrated Concept/Process: Nursing Process/Implementation
Content Area: Child Health
Reference: Schulte E, Price D, Gwin J: *Thompson's pediatric nursing,* ed 8, Philadelphia, 2001, WB Saunders, p. 143.

19. *Answer:* 2
Rationale: Induration measuring 10 mm or greater is considered to be a positive result in children younger that 4 years old and in those with chronic illness or high-risk for environmental exposure to tuberculosis. A reaction of 5 mm or greater is considered to be a positive result for the highest risk groups.
Test-Taking Strategy: Use the process of elimination and knowledge regarding a positive Mantoux test in children to answer this question. Option 4 can be easily eliminated first. Note the child's age in the question to determine the correct option from the remaining three. Review analysis of a Mantoux test in children if you had difficulty with this question.
Level of Cognitive Ability: Comprehension
Client Needs: Physiological Integrity
Integrated Concept/Process: Nursing Process/Data Collection
Content Area: Child Health
Reference: Schulte E, Price D, Gwin J: *Thompson's pediatric nursing,* ed 8, Philadelphia, 2001, WB Saunders, p. 102.

20. *Answer:* 2
Rationale: INH is given to prevent TB infection from progressing to active disease. A chest x-ray film is obtained before initiation of preventive therapy. In infants and children, the recommended duration of INH therapy is 9 months. For children with human immunodeficiency virus infection, a minimum of 12 months is recommended.
Test-Taking Strategy: Knowledge regarding treatment with INH in a 2-year-old child is required to answer this question. Review the recommended treatment plans for a child with TB if you had difficulty with this question.
Level of Cognitive Ability: Application
Client Needs: Health Promotion and Maintenance
Integrated Concept/Process: Nursing Process/Implementation
Content Area: Child Health
Reference: Schulte E, Price D, Gwin J: *Thompson's pediatric nursing,* ed 8, Philadelphia, 2001, WB Saunders, p. 103.

REFERENCES

Burroughs A, Leifer G: *Maternity nursing,* ed 8, Philadelphia, 2002, WB Saunders.
McKinney E et al: *Maternal-child nursing,* Philadelphia, 2000, WB Saunders.
Murray S, McKinney E, Gorrie T: *Foundations of maternal-newborn nursing,* ed 3, Philadelphia, 2002, WB Saunders.
Schulte E, Price D, Gwin J: *Thompson's pediatric nursing,* ed 8, Philadelphia, 2001, WB Saunders.
Wong D: *Whaley and Wong's nursing care of infants and children,* ed 6, St Louis, 1999, Mosby.

Cardiovascular Disorders

I. CONGESTIVE HEART FAILURE (CHF)

A. Description
   1. Inability of the heart to pump sufficiently to meet the metabolic needs of the body
   2. In infants and children, inadequate cardiac output is most commonly caused by congenital heart defects that produce an excessive volume or pressure load on the myocardium
   3. In infants and children, a combination of both left-sided and right-sided heart failure is usually present
   4. The goals of treatment are to improve cardiac function, remove accumulated fluid and sodium, decrease cardiac demands, improve tissue oxygenation, and decrease oxygen consumption

B. Data collection of early signs
   1. Tachycardia, especially during rest and slight exertion
   2. Tachypnea
   3. Profuse scalp sweating, especially in infants
   4. Fatigue and irritability
   5. Sudden weight gain
   6. Respiratory distress

C. Implementation
   1. Monitor vital signs closely and for the early signs of CHF
   2. Monitor for respiratory distress (count respirations for 1 full minute)
   3. Monitor apical pulse (count pulse for 1 full minute) and monitor for dysrhythmias
   4. Monitor temperature for hyperthermia and for other signs of infection, particularly respiratory infection
   5. Monitor I&O; weigh diapers
   6. Monitor daily weight to assess for fluid retention; a weight gain of 0.5 kg (1 pound) in 1 day is due to the accumulation of fluid
   7. Monitor for facial or peripheral edema and report abnormal findings
   8. Elevate the head of the bed (semi-Fowler's position)
   9. Maintain a neutral thermal environment to prevent cold stress in infants
   10. Provide rest; decrease environmental stimuli
   11. Administer cool, humidified oxygen as prescribed; use an oxygen hood for young infants and a nasal cannula or face tent for older infants and children
   12. Organize nursing activities to allow for uninterrupted sleep
   13. Maintain adequate nutritional status
   14. Feed when hungry and soon after awakening (crying exhausts the limited energy supply) accommodating the infant's sleep and wake patterns; the infant should be well rested before feeding
   15. Provide small, frequent feedings, which will be less tiring
   16. Administer sedation as prescribed during the acute stage to promote rest
   17. Administer digoxin (Lanoxin) as prescribed; digoxin levels are monitored for signs of digoxin toxicity, especially bradycardia and vomiting
   18. Monitor apical heart rate for 1 minute before administering digoxin
   19. Check regarding parameters for withholding digoxin; generally, digoxin is withheld if the pulse is below 90 to 110 beats per minute in infants and young children or below 70 beats per minute in older children

20. Note that infants rarely receive more than 1mL (50 μg, or 0.05 mg) of digoxin in one dose
21. Angiotensin-converting enzyme (ACE) inhibitors such as captopril (Capoten) or enalapril (Vasotec) may be prescribed
22. Monitor for hypotension, renal dysfunction, and cough when angiotensin-converting enzyme (ACE) inhibitors are administered
23. Administer diuretics as prescribed; monitor for hypokalemia with furosemide (Lasix) and with the thiazide diuretics
24. Administer potassium supplements and provide dietary sources of potassium as prescribed
25. Monitor serum electrolytes, particularly the potassium level
26. Restrict fluids as prescribed in the acute stage; monitor for dehydration
27. Check the physician's orders regarding sodium restriction; note that most infant formulas have slightly more sodium than does breast milk
28. Instruct the parents regarding the description of the diagnosis and administration of medications (Box 30-1)
29. Instruct the parents in cardiopulmonary resuscitation (CPR)

II. DEFECTS WITH INCREASED PULMONARY BLOOD FLOW (Box 30-2)

A. Description

BOX 30-1

Home Care Instructions for Administering Digoxin

Administer as prescribed
Administer 1 hour before or 2 hours after feedings
Use a calendar to mark off the dose administered
Do not mix the medication with foods or fluid
If a dose is missed and more than 4 hours have elapsed, withhold the dose and give the next dose at the scheduled time; if less than 4 hours have elapsed, administer the missed dose
If the child vomits, do not administer a second dose
If more than two consecutive doses have been missed, notify the physician; do not increase or double the dose for missed doses
If the child has teeth, give water after the medication; if possible, brush the teeth to prevent tooth decay from the sweetened liquid
If the child becomes ill, notify the physician
Keep the medication in a locked cabinet
Call the poison control center immediately if accidental overdose occurs

BOX 30-2

Defects with Increased Pulmonary Blood Flow

Atrial septal defect (ASD)
Ventricular septal defect (VSD)
Atrioventricular canal (AVC) defect
Patent ductus arteriosus (PDA)

1. Intracardiac communications along the septum or an abnormal connection between the great arteries allows blood to flow from the high-pressure left side of the heart to the low-pressure right side of the heart
2. The infant typically demonstrates signs and symptoms of CHF

B. Atrial septal defect (ASD)
1. Abnormal opening between the atria that causes an increased flow of oxygenated blood into the right side of the heart
2. Right atrial and ventricular enlargement occurs
3. Infant may be asymptomatic or may develop CHF
4. Nonsurgical treatment: ASD may be closed using devices during a cardiac catheterization
5. Surgical treatment: open repair with cardiopulmonary bypass is usually performed before school age

C. Ventricular septal defect (VSD)
1. Abnormal opening between the right and left ventricles
2. Many VSDs close spontaneously during the first year of life in children having small or moderate defects
3. A characteristic murmur is present; CHF is common
4. Nonsurgical treatment: device closure during cardiac catheterization may be possible
5. Surgical treatment: open repair with cardiopulmonary bypass

D. Atrioventricular canal (AVC) defect
1. Incomplete fusion of the endocardial cushions
2. Most common cardiac defect in Down syndrome
3. A characteristic murmur is present
4. The infant usually has mild to moderate CHF; mild cyanosis increases with crying
5. Surgical treatment is usually necessary

E. Patent ductus arteriosus (PDA)
1. Failure of the fetal ductus arteriosus (artery connecting the aorta and pulmonary artery) to close within the first weeks of life
2. A characteristic machinery-like murmur is present; asymptomatic or may show signs of CHF

3. A widened pulse pressure and bounding pulses are present
4. Medical management: indomethacin (prostaglandin inhibitor) may be administered to close patent ductus in premature infants and some newborns
5. Nonsurgical management may include occluding the PDA during cardiac catheterization or surgical treatment may be necessary

III. OBSTRUCTIVE DEFECTS (Box 30-3)

A. Description
   1. Blood exiting the heart meets an area of anatomic narrowing (**stenosis**) causing obstruction to blood flow
   2. The location of narrowing is usually near the valve of the obstructive defect
   3. Infants and children exhibit signs of CHF
   4. Children with mild obstruction may be asymptomatic

B. Coarctation of the aorta (COA)
   1. Localized narrowing near the insertion of the ductus arteriosus
   2. Collateral circulation develops during fetal life to maintain flow from the ascending to the descending aorta
   3. Signs of CHF in infants
   4. High blood pressure and bounding pulses in the arms, weak or absent femoral pulses, and cool lower extremities may be present
   5. Children may experience headaches, dizziness, fainting, and epistaxis resulting from hypertension
   6. Nonsurgical management may include balloon angioplasty during cardiac catheterization, or surgical treatment may be necessary

C. Aortic **stenosis** (AS)
   1. Narrowing or stricture of the aortic valve, causing resistance to blood flow in the left ventricle, decreased cardiac output, left ventricular hypertrophy, and pulmonary vascular congestion
   2. A characteristic murmur is present
   3. Infants with severe defects demonstrate signs of decreased cardiac output with faint pulses, hypotension, tachycardia, and poor feeding
   4. Children show signs of exercise intolerance, chest pain, and dizziness when standing for long periods
   5. Nonsurgical management may include balloon angioplasty during cardiac catheterization to dilate the narrowed valve, or surgical treatment may be necessary

D. Pulmonic **stenosis** (PS)
   1. Narrowing at the entrance to the pulmonary artery
   2. Resistance to blood flow causes right ventricular hypertrophy and decreased pulmonary blood flow; the right ventricle may be hypoplastic
   3. Pulmonary **atresia** is the extreme form of PS in that there is total fusion of the commissures and no blood flows to the lungs
   4. A characteristic murmur is present
   5. May be asymptomatic; mild cyanosis or CHF occurs
   6. Newborns with severe narrowing will be cyanotic
   7. If PS is severe, CHF occurs
   8. Nonsurgical management may include balloon angioplasty during cardiac catheterization to dilate the narrowed valve, or surgical treatment may be necessary

IV. DEFECTS WITH DECREASED PULMONARY BLOOD FLOW (Box 30-4)

A. Description
   1. Obstructed pulmonary blood flow and an anatomic defect (ASD or VSD) between the right and left sides of the heart
   2. Pressure on the right side of the heart increases, exceeding left-sided pressure, which allows desaturated blood to **shunt** right to left, causing desaturation in the left side of the heart and in the systemic circulation
   3. Typically hypoxemia and cyanosis appear

B. Tetralogy of Fallot (TOF)
   1. Includes four defects: VSD, PS, overriding aorta, and right ventricular hypertrophy
   2. If pulmonary vascular resistance is higher than systemic resistance, the **shunt** is from right to left; if systemic resistance is higher than pulmonary resistance, the **shunt** is left to right

BOX 30-3

Obstructive Defects

Coarctation of the aorta (COA)
Aortic stenosis (AS)
Pulmonary stenosis (PS)

BOX 30-4

Defects with Decreased Pulmonary Blood Flow

Tetralogy of Fallot (TOF)
Tricuspid atresia

3. Infants
   a. May be acutely cyanotic at birth or may have mild cyanosis that progresses over the first year of life as the pulmonic **stenosis** worsens
   b. A characteristic murmur is present
   c. Acute episodes of cyanosis and hypoxia (hypercyanotic spells), called blue spells or tet spells, occur when the infant's oxygen requirements exceed the blood supply (usually during crying or after feeding)
4. Children: with increasing cyanosis, there may be clubbing of the fingers, squatting, and poor **growth**
5. Surgical treatment may include a palliative **shunt** or complete repair

C. Tricuspid **atresia**
1. Failure of the tricuspid valve to develop
2. There is no communication from the right atrium to the right ventricle
3. Blood flows through an ASD or a patent foramen ovale to the left side of the heart and through a VSD to the right ventricle and out to the lungs
4. Often associated with pulmonic **stenosis** and transposition of the great arteries
5. Complete mixing of unoxygenated and oxygenated blood in the left side of the heart, resulting in systemic desaturation, pulmonary obstruction, and decreased pulmonary blood flow
6. Cyanosis, tachycardia, and dyspnea are seen in the newborn
7. Older children exhibit signs of chronic hypoxemia and clubbing
8. Surgical treatment is necessary; for the neonate whose pulmonary blood flow depends on the patency of the ductus arteriosus, a continuous infusion of prostaglandin E_1 is initiated until surgery

V. MIXED DEFECTS (Box 30-5)

A. Description
1. Fully saturated systemic blood flow mixes with the desaturated blood flow, causing a desaturation of the systemic blood flow

BOX 30-5

Mixed Defects

Transposition of the great arteries (TGA) or transposition of the great vessels (TGV)
Total anomalous pulmonary venous connection (TAPVC)
Truncus arteriosus (TA)
Hypoplastic left heart syndrome (HLHS)

2. Pulmonary congestion occurs and cardiac output decreases
3. Signs of CHF; symptoms depend on the degree of desaturation

B. Transposition of the great arteries (TGA) or transposition of the great vessels (TGV)
1. The pulmonary artery leaves the left ventricle, and the aorta exits from the right ventricle
2. No communication between the systemic and pulmonary circulation
3. Infants with minimal communication are severely cyanotic and depressed at birth
4. Infants with large septal defects or a patent ductus arteriosus may be less severely cyanotic but may have symptoms of CHF
5. Cardiomegaly is evident a few weeks after birth
6. Nonsurgical management includes balloon atrial septostomy during cardiac catheterization, or surgical treatment may be required

C. Total anomalous pulmonary venous connection (TAPVC)
1. Failure of the pulmonary veins to join the left atrium
2. Results in mixed blood being returned to the right atrium and shunted from the right to the left through an ASD
3. The right side of the heart hypertrophies, whereas the left side of the heart may remain small
4. CHF develops
5. Cyanosis worsens with pulmonary vein obstruction; once obstruction occurs, the infant's condition deteriorates rapidly
6. Surgical treatment is necessary

D. Truncus arteriosus (TA)
1. Failure of normal septation and division of the embryonic bulbar trunk into the pulmonary artery and the aorta, resulting in a single vessel that overrides both ventricles
2. Blood from both ventricles mixes in the common great artery, causing desaturation and hypoxemia
3. A characteristic murmur is present
4. The infant exhibits moderate to severe CHF and variable cyanosis, poor **growth**, and activity intolerance
5. Surgical treatment is necessary

E. Hypoplastic left heart syndrome (HLHS)
1. Underdevelopment of the left side of the heart, resulting in a hypoplastic left ventricle and aortic **atresia**
2. Mild cyanosis and signs of CHF occur until the ductus arteriosus closes; then, progressive deterioration with cyanosis and decreased cardiac output occurs, leading to cardiovascular collapse

3. Fatal in the first few months of life without intervention
4. Surgical treatment is necessary

VI. IMPLEMENTATION: CARDIOVASCULAR DEFECTS

A. Monitor for signs of a defect in the infant and child
B. Monitor vital signs closely
C. Monitor respiratory status for the presence of **nasal flaring** and use of accessory muscles; the physician is notified if any changes occur
D. Breath sounds are monitored for crackles, rhonchi, or rales
E. If respiratory effort is increased, place the child in reverse Trendelenburg (elevate head and upper body) to decrease the work of breathing
F. Administer humidified oxygen as prescribed
G. Endotracheal tube and ventilator care may be necessary; restrain the hands of an intubated child
H. Monitor for hypercyanotic spells (Box 30-6)
I. Monitor for signs of CHF such as fluid retention in the eyes, hands, feet, and chest
J. Monitor peripheral pulses
K. Monitor I&O and weigh diapers; the physician is notified if a decrease in urine output occurs
L. Obtain daily weight
M. Maintain fluid restriction if prescribed
N. Provide adequate nutrition (high calorie requirements) as prescribed
O. Administer medications as prescribed
P. Keep the child as stress free as possible; plan interventions to allow maximal rest for the child
Q. Prepare parents and child, if appropriate, for surgery
R. Allow parents and child to verbalize feelings and concerns regarding the disorder
S. Familiarize parents and child with hospital procedures and equipment

VII. CARDIAC SURGERY

A. Postoperative implementation
1. Monitor vital signs frequently
2. Monitor temperature; the physician is notified if a fever occurs
3. Monitor for signs of sepsis, such as fever, chills, diaphoresis, lethargy, and altered levels of consciousness
4. Maintain aseptic technique
5. Assist with monitoring lines, tubes, or catheters that are in place and prepare to remove promptly as prescribed when no longer needed to prevent infection
6. Monitor for signs of discomfort such as irritability, changes in heart rate, respiratory rate, and blood pressure, and the inability to sleep
7. Administer pain medications as prescribed noting effectiveness
8. Administer antibiotics and antipyretics as prescribed
9. Encourage rest periods
10. Facilitate parent-child contact as soon as possible

B. Postoperative home care (Box 30-7)

VIII. RHEUMATIC FEVER (Figure 30-1)

A. Description
1. An inflammatory autoimmune disease that affects the connective tissues of the heart, joints, subcutaneous tissues and/or blood vessels of the central nervous system (CNS)
2. The most serious complication is rheumatic heart disease, which affects the cardiac valves

BOX 30-6

Treatment for Hypercyanotic Spells

Place the infant in a knee-chest position
Administer 100% oxygen by facemask
Morphine sulfate may be prescribed
IV fluids may be prescribed

BOX 30-7

Home Care After Cardiac Surgery

Omit play outside for several weeks
Avoid activities in which the child could fall, such as bike riding, for 2 to 4 weeks
Avoid crowds for 2 weeks after discharge
Follow a no-added-salt diet if prescribed
Do not add any new foods to the infant's eating schedule
Do not place creams, lotions, or powders on the incision until completely healed
The child may return to school the third week after discharge, starting with half days
No physical education for 2 months
Instruct the parents to discipline the child normally
Instruct the parents about the importance of the 2-week follow-up appointment
Avoid immunizations, invasive procedure, and dental visits for 2 months
Advise the parents regarding the importance of a dental visit every 6 months after age 3 years and to inform the dentist of the cardiac problem so that antibiotics can be prescribed if necessary
Inform the parents to call the physician when coughing, tachypnea, cyanosis, vomiting, diarrhea, anorexia, pain, fever, or any swelling, redness, or drainage occurs at the site of the incision

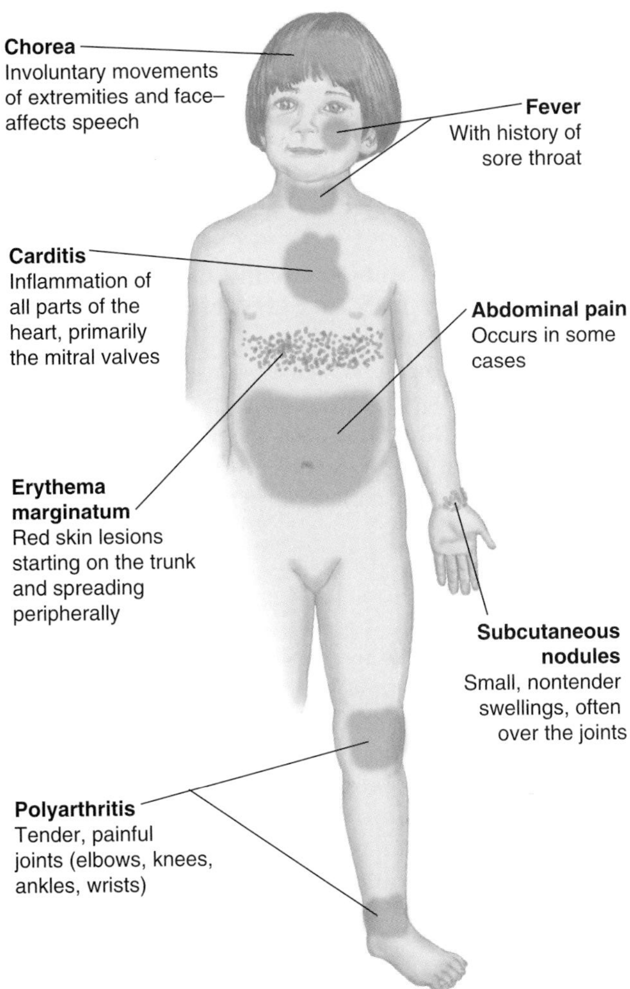

FIG. 30-1 Clinical manifestations of rheumatic fever. (From McKinney E et al: *Maternal-child nursing*, Philadelphia, 2000, WB Saunders.)

3. Presents 2 to 6 weeks after an untreated or partially treated group A beta hemolytic streptococcal infection of the upper respiratory tract
4. Jones criteria are used in determining the diagnosis

B. Data collection
1. Aschoff bodies (lesions): found in the heart, blood vessels, brain, and serous surfaces of the joints and pleura
2. Signs of carditis: shortness of breath, edema of the face, abdomen or ankles, and precordial pain
3. Signs of polyarthritis: edema, inflammation of large joints, and joint pain
4. Erythema marginatum: erythematous macular rash on the trunk and extremities
5. Subcutaneous nodules found in crops over the bony prominences
6. Chorea: sudden, aimless, irregular movements of the extremities, involuntary facial grimaces, speech disturbances, emotional lability, and muscle weakness
7. Fever: low-grade that spikes in the late afternoon
8. Elevated antistreptolysin-O titer
9. Elevated sedimentation rate
10. Elevated C-reactive protein

C. Implementation
1. Monitor vital signs
2. Control joint pain and inflammation with massage and alternating hot and cold applications as prescribed
3. Provide bed rest during acute febrile phase
4. Limit physical exercise in the child with carditis
5. Administer antibiotics (penicillin) as prescribed
6. Administer salicylates and antiinflammatory agents as prescribed (should not be instituted before the diagnosis is confirmed because these medications mask the polyarthritis)
7. Initiate seizure precautions if the child is experiencing chorea
8. Instruct the parents about the importance of follow-up care, and the need for antibiotic prophylaxis for dental work, infection, and invasive procedures
9. Advise the child to inform the parents if anyone in school develops a streptococcal throat infection

IX. KAWASAKI DISEASE

A. Description
1. Known as mucocutaneous lymph node syndrome and is an acute systemic inflammatory illness
2. The cause is unknown but may be associated with an infection from an organism or toxin
3. Cardiac involvement is the most serious complication; aneurysms can develop

B. Data collection
1. Acute stage
   a. Fever
   b. Conjunctival hyperemia
   c. Red throat
   d. Swollen hands, rash, and enlargement of the cervical lymph nodes
2. Subacute stage
   a. Cracking lips and fissures
   b. Desquamation of the skin on the tips of the fingers and toes
   c. Joint pain
   d. Cardiac manifestations

e. Thrombocytosis
3. Convalescent stage: child appears normal but signs of inflammation may be present

C. Implementation
1. Monitor temperature frequently
2. Monitor heart sounds and rhythm
3. Monitor extremities for edema, redness, and desquamation
4. Examine eyes for conjunctivitis
5. Monitor mucous membranes for inflammation
6. Monitor dietary and fluid intake (I&O)
7. Administer soft foods and liquids that are neither too hot nor too cold
8. Weigh daily
9. Provide passive range-of-motion exercises to facilitate joint movement
10. Administer acetylsalicylic acid (aspirin) as prescribed for its antipyretic and antiplatelet effect
11. IV immune globulin (IVIG) may be prescribed to reduce the duration of the fever and the incidence of coronary artery lesions and aneurysms
12. Instruct the parents in the administration of prescribed medications, the need to monitor for bleeding, and the need for follow-up care to monitor for cardiac complications

PRACTICE QUESTIONS

1. A nurse caring for an infant with congenital heart disease is monitoring the infant closely for signs of congestive heart failure (CHF). The nurse monitors the infant closely for which early sign of CHF?
   1. Cough
   2. Tachycardia
   3. Slow and shallow breathing
   4. Pallor
2. A physician has prescribed oxygen PRN for the child with congestive heart failure (CHF). In which of the following situations does the nurse administer oxygen to the child?
   1. During feeding
   2. When the mother is holding the child
   3. When changing the child's diapers
   4. When drawing blood for electrolyte values
3. An infant with congestive heart failure (CHF) is receiving diuretic therapy and the nurse is closely monitoring the intake and output (I&O). The nurse uses which most appropriate method to monitor the urine output?
   1. Inserting a Foley catheter
   2. Weighing the diapers
   3. Comparing intake with output
   4. Measuring the amount of water added to formula
4. A nurse is monitoring the daily weight of an infant with congestive heart failure (CHF). Which of the following alerts the nurse to suspect fluid accumulation and the need to notify the registered nurse?
   1. Bradypnea
   2. Diaphoresis
   3. Decreased blood pressure (BP)
   4. A weight gain of 1 pound in 1 day
5. A nurse provides home care instructions to the parents of a child with congestive heart failure (CHF) regarding the procedure for the administration of digoxin (Lanoxin). Which statement, if made by a parent, indicates the need for further instruction?
   1. "If my child vomits after medication administration, I will repeat the dose."
   2. "I will take my child's pulse before administering the medication."
   3. "I will not mix the medication with food."
   4. "If more than one dose is missed, I will call the physician."
6. A nurse is assigned to care for an infant with a diagnosis of tricuspid atresia. The nurse plans care knowing that in this disorder:
   1. There is no communication from the systemic and pulmonary circulation
   2. Frequent episodes of hypercyanotic spells occur
   3. There is no communication from the right atrium to the right ventricle
   4. A single vessel overrides both ventricles
7. Prostaglandin E_1 is prescribed for a child with transposition of the great arteries. The mother of the child asks the nurse why the child needs the medication. The most appropriate response would be to tell the mother that the medication:
   1. Maintains an adequate hormonal level
   2. Maintains the position of the great arteries
   3. Provides adequate oxygen saturation and maintains cardiac output
   4. Prevents hypercyanotic spells
8. A nurse reviews the record of a child just seen by the physician. The physician has documented a diagnosis of suspected aortic stenosis. The nurse expects to note documentation of which of the following clinical manifestations specifically found in this disorder?
   1. Hyperactivity
   2. Exercise intolerance
   3. Pallor
   4. Gastrointestinal disturbances
9. A nurse has reinforced home care instructions to the mother of a child who is being discharged after cardiac surgery. Which statement made by the mother indicates a need for further instructions?
   1. "Large crowds of people need to be avoided for at least 2 weeks after surgery."
   2. "I can apply lotion or powder to the incision if it is itchy."

3. "A balance of rest and exercise is important."
4. "Activities where the child could fall need to be avoided for 2 to 4 weeks."

10. A nurse is caring for an infant with tetralogy of Fallot. The nurse recognizes that the infant is experiencing a hypercyanotic episode. The initial nursing action is to:
    1. Ask the unit secretary to call the physician
    2. Place the infant in a knee-chest position
    3. Elevate the head of the bed
    4. Monitor the infant

11. A nurse is told that a child with rheumatic fever (RF) will be arriving to the nursing unit for admission. On admission, the nurse prepares to ask the mother which question to elicit information specific to the development of RF?
    1. "Did the child have a sore throat or an unexplained fever within the last 2 months?"
    2. "Has the child had any nausea or vomiting?"
    3. "Has the child complained of headaches?"
    4. "Has the child complained of back pain?"

12. Acetylsalicylic acid (aspirin) is prescribed for the child with rheumatic fever. The nurse would question this order if the child had documented evidence of which of the following?
    1. A viral infection
    2. Joint pain
    3. Facial edema
    4. Arthralgia

13. A nurse is caring for a child with a suspected diagnosis of rheumatic fever (RF). The nurse reviews the laboratory results knowing that which laboratory study would assist in confirming the diagnosis of RF?
    1. White blood cell count
    2. Red blood cell count
    3. Immunoglobulin
    4. Anti-streptolysin O titer

14. A nurse is caring for a child with a diagnosis of Kawasaki disease. The mother of the child asks the nurse about the disorder. The nurse tells the mother that:
    1. It is an acquired cell-mediated immunodeficiency disorder
    2. It is an inflammatory autoimmune disease that affects the connective tissue of the heart, joints, and subcutaneous tissues
    3. It is a chronic multisystem autoimmune disease characterized by the inflammation of connective tissue
    4. Is also called mucocutaneous lymph node syndrome and is a febrile generalized vasculitis of unknown etiology

15. A nurse assists in admitting a child with a diagnosis of acute stage Kawasaki disease. On data collection, the nurse expects to note which clinical manifestation of the acute stage of the disease?
    1. Conjunctival hyperemia
    2. Cracked lips
    3. Desquamation of the skin
    4. A normal appearance

ANSWERS

1. *Answer:* 2

Rationale: The early signs of CHF include tachycardia, tachypnea, profuse scalp sweating, fatigue and irritability, sudden weight gain, and respiratory distress. A cough may occur in CHF as a result of mucosal swelling and irritation, but it is not an early sign. Pallor may be noted in the infant with CHF, but is also not an early sign.

Test-Taking Strategy: Use the process of elimination and note the key word "early." Think about the physiology and the effects on the heart when fluid overload occurs. These concepts will assist in directing you to option 2. If you had difficulty with this question, review the early signs of CHF in an infant.

Level of Cognitive Ability: Application

Client Needs: Physiological Integrity

Integrated Concept/Process: Nursing Process/Data Collection

Content Area: Child Health

Reference: Schulte E, Price D, Gwin J: *Thompson's pediatric nursing,* ed 8, Philadelphia, 2001, WB Saunders, p. 89.

2. *Answer:* 4

Rationale: Oxygen administration may be ordered for stressful periods, especially during bouts of crying or invasive procedures. Drawing blood is an invasive procedure that would likely cause the child to cry.

Test-Taking Strategy: Use the process of elimination. Read the option and recall the situations that would place stress and an increased workload on the heart. This concept should easily direct you to option 4. Review care to the child with CHF if you had difficulty with this question.

Level of Cognitive Ability: Application

Client Needs: Physiological Integrity

Integrated Concept/Process: Nursing Process/Implementation

Content Area: Child Health

Reference: Schulte E, Price D, Gwin J: *Thompson's pediatric nursing,* ed 8, Philadelphia, 2001, WB Saunders, p. 89.

3. *Answer:* 2

Rationale: The most appropriate method to monitor urine output in an infant on diuretic therapy is to weigh the diapers. Comparing intake with output would not provide an accurate measure of urine output. Measuring the amount of water added to formula is unrelated to the amount of output. Although Foley catheter drainage is most accurate in determining output, it is not the most appropriate method in an infant, and it places the infant at risk for infection.

Test-Taking Strategy: Use the process of elimination. Eliminate options 3 and 4 first because they will not provide an indication of urine output. From the remaining options, note the words "most appropriate" in the stem of the question. These words will direct you to option 2. Review care to the infant receiving diuretic therapy if you had difficulty with this question.
Level of Cognitive Ability: Application
Client Needs: Physiological Integrity
Integrated Concept/Process: Nursing Process/Data Collection
Content Area: Child Health
Reference: Schulte E, Price D, Gwin J: *Thompson's pediatric nursing*, ed 8, Philadelphia, 2001, WB Saunders, p. 353.

4. *Answer:* 4
Rationale: A weight gain of 0.5 kg (1 pound) in 1 day is due to the accumulation of fluid. The nurse should monitor urine output, monitor for evidence of facial or peripheral edema, check the lung sounds, and report the weight gain. Tachypnea and an increased BP would occur with fluid accumulation. Diaphoresis is a sign of CHF but is not specific to fluid accumulation, and usually occurs with exertional activities.
Test-Taking Strategy: Use the process of elimination and focus on the issue, fluid accumulation. Note the relationship between "fluid accumulation" in the question and "weight gain" in the correct option. Review the indications of fluid accumulation in an infant with CHF if you had difficulty with this question.
Level of Cognitive Ability: Comprehension
Client Needs: Physiological Integrity
Integrated Concept/Process: Nursing Process/Data Collection
Content Area: Child Health
Reference: Schulte E, Price D, Gwin J: *Thompson's pediatric nursing*, ed 8, Philadelphia, 2001, WB Saunders, p. 89.

5. *Answer:* 1
Rationale: The parents need to be instructed that if the child vomits after the digoxin is administered, they are not to repeat the dose. Options 2, 3, and 4 are accurate instructions regarding the administration of this medication. Additionally, the parents should be instructed that if a dose is missed and it is not identified until 4 hours later, the dose should not be administered.
Test-Taking Strategy: Use the process of elimination. Note the key words "need for further instruction." General knowledge regarding digoxin administration will assist in eliminating option 2. Principles related to administering medications to children will assist in eliminating option 3. From the remaining options, select option 1 over option 4 because if the child vomits it would be difficult to determine if the medication was also vomited or absorbed by the body. Review home care instructions regarding the administration of digoxin if you had difficulty with this question.
Level of Cognitive Ability: Comprehension
Client Needs: Health Promotion and Maintenance
Integrated Concept/Process: Teaching/Learning
Content Area: Child Health
Reference: Schulte E, Price D, Gwin J: *Thompson's pediatric nursing*, ed 8, Philadelphia, 2001, WB Saunders, p. 397.

6. *Answer:* 3
Rationale: In tricuspid atresia, there is no communication from the right atrium to the right ventricle. Option 1 describes transposition of the great arteries. Frequent episodes of hypercyanotic spells occur in tetralogy of Fallot. Option 4 describes truncus arteriosus.
Test-Taking Strategy: Use the process of elimination. Note the relationship between "tricuspid atresia" and the description in option 3. Recalling that the tricuspid valve is located between the right atrium and the right ventricle will direct you to this option. Review the characteristics of tricuspid atresia if you had difficulty with this question.
Level of Cognitive Ability: Comprehension
Client Needs: Physiological Integrity
Integrated Concept/Process: Nursing Process/Planning
Content Area: Child Health
Reference: Wong D: *Whaley and Wong's nursing care of infants and children*, ed 6, St Louis, 1999, Mosby, p. 1615.

7. *Answer:* 3
Rationale: A child with transposition of the great arteries may receive prostaglandin E_1 temporarily to increase blood mixing if systemic and pulmonary mixing is inadequate to provide an oxygen saturation of 75% or to maintain cardiac output. Options 1, 2, and 4 are incorrect. Additionally, hypercyanotic spells occur in tetralogy of Fallot.
Test-Taking Strategy: Use the ABCs—airway, breathing, and circulation—to answer the question. Option 3 addresses circulation. Review the purpose of this medication in this condition if you had difficulty with this question.
Level of Cognitive Ability: Application
Client Needs: Physiological Integrity
Integrated Concept/Process: Nursing Process/Implementation
Content Area: Child Health
Reference: Wong D: *Whaley and Wong's nursing care of infants and children*, ed 6, St Louis, 1999, Mosby, p. 1617.

8. *Answer:* 2
Rationale: The child with aortic stenosis shows signs of exercise intolerance, chest pain, and dizziness when standing for long periods. Pallor may be noted, but is not specific to this type of disorder alone. Options 1 and 4 are not related to this disorder.
Test-Taking Strategy: Use the process of elimination focusing on the disorder. Options 1 and 4 can be eliminated first because they are not associated with a cardiac disorder. From the remaining options, noting the word "specifically" in the stem of the question will direct you to option 2. Review the manifestations associated with aortic stenosis if you had difficulty with this question.
Level of Cognitive Ability: Comprehension
Client Needs: Physiological Integrity
Integrated Concept/Process: Communication and Documentation
Content Area: Child Health
Reference: Wong D: *Whaley and Wong's nursing care of infants and children*, ed 6, St Louis, 1999, Mosby, p. 1613.

9. *Answer:* 2
Rationale: The mother should be instructed that lotions and powders should not be applied to the incision site. Options 1,

3, and 4 are accurate instructions regarding home care after cardiac surgery.
Test-Taking Strategy: Use the process of elimination. Note the key words "indicates a need for further instructions" in the stem of the question. Using general principles related to post-operative incisional site care will direct you to option 2. Review home care instructions after cardiac surgery if you had difficulty with this question.
Level of Cognitive Ability: Comprehension
Client Needs: Health Promotion and Maintenance
Integrated Concept/Process: Teaching/Learning
Content Area: Child Health
Reference: Wong D, Hockenberry-Eaton M: *Wong's essentials of pediatric nursing,* ed 6, St Louis, 2001, Mosby, p. 963.

10. *Answer:* 2
Rationale: If a hypercyanotic episode occurs, the infant is placed in a knee-chest position and then the physician is notified. This position is thought to increase pulmonary blood flow by increasing systemic vascular resistance. This position also improves systemic arterial oxygen saturation by decreasing venous return, so that smaller amounts of highly saturated blood reach the heart. Toddlers and children squat to obtain this position and relieve chronic hypoxia.
Test-Taking Strategy: Use the process of elimination. Note the key word "initial." Eliminate option 4 first. Next, eliminate option 1 because a nursing intervention is required before notifying the physician. Remembering that a toddler or a child squats to achieve this position will assist in directing you to option 2. Review the initial nursing interventions when a hypercyanotic episode occurs in an infant if you had difficulty with this question.
Level of Cognitive Ability: Application
Client Needs: Physiological Integrity
Integrated Concept/Process: Nursing Process/Implementation
Content Area: Child Health
Reference: Schulte E, Price D, Gwin J: *Thompson's pediatric nursing,* ed 8, Philadelphia, 2001, WB Saunders, p. 85.

11. *Answer:* 1
Rationale: RF characteristically presents 2 to 6 weeks after an untreated or partially treated group A beta-hemolytic streptococcal infection of the upper respiratory tract. Initially, the nurse determines if the child had a sore throat or an unexplained fever within the past 2 months. Options 2, 3, and 4 are unrelated to RF.
Test-Taking Strategy: Use the process of elimination. Note the similarity between rheumatic "fever" in the question and the word "fever" in the correct option. If you had difficulty with this question, review the etiology related to RF.
Level of Cognitive Ability: Application
Client Needs: Physiological Integrity
Integrated Concept/Process: Nursing Process/Data Collection
Content Area: Child Health
Reference: Schulte E, Price D, Gwin J: *Thompson's pediatric nursing,* ed 8, Philadelphia, 2001, WB Saunders, p. 276.

12. *Answer:* 1
Rationale: Antiinflammatory agents including aspirin may be prescribed for the child with RF. Aspirin should not be given to a child who has chickenpox or other viral infections such as the flu. Options 2 and 4 are clinical manifestations of RF. Facial edema may be associated with the development of a cardiac complication.
Test-Taking Strategy: Use the process of elimination. Options 2 and 4 can be eliminated because they are similar. Recalling that facial edema may indicate a cardiac complication will assist in eliminating this option. Review the contraindications related to the use of aspirin if you had difficulty with this question.
Level of Cognitive Ability: Application
Client Needs: Safe, Effective Care Environment
Integrated Concept/Process: Nursing Process/Implementation
Content Area: Child Health
Reference: Hodgson B, Kizior R: *Saunders nursing drug handbook 2002,* Philadelphia, 2002, WB Saunders, p. 82.

13. *Answer:* 4
Rationale: A diagnosis of RF is confirmed by the presence of two major manifestations or one major and two minor manifestations from the Jones criteria. Additionally, evidence of a recent streptococcal infection is confirmed by a positive anti-streptolysin-O titer, streptozyme, or an anti-DNAase B assay. Options 1, 2, and 3 will not assist in confirming the diagnosis of RF.
Test-Taking Strategy: Use the process of elimination. Recalling that RF is characteristically associated with streptococcal infection will easily direct you to option 4. If you had difficulty with this question, review RF.
Level of Cognitive Ability: Comprehension
Client Needs: Physiological Integrity
Integrated Concept/Process: Nursing Process/Data Collection
Content Area: Child Health
Reference: Schulte E, Price D, Gwin J: *Thompson's pediatric nursing,* ed 8, Philadelphia, 2001, WB Saunders, p. 276.

14. *Answer:* 4
Rationale: Kawasaki disease, also called mucocutaneous lymph node syndrome, is a febrile generalized vasculitis of unknown etiology. Option 1 describes human immunodeficiency virus (HIV) infection. Option 2 describes rheumatic fever. Option 3 describes systemic lupus erythematosus.
Test-Taking Strategy: Knowledge regarding the description of Kawasaki disease is required to answer this question. Review the characteristics of this disorder if you are unfamiliar with it.
Level of Cognitive Ability: Application
Client Needs: Physiological Integrity
Integrated Concept/Process: Nursing Process/Implementation
Content Area: Child Health
Reference: Wong D: *Whaley and Wong's nursing care of infants and children,* ed 6, St Louis, 1999, Mosby, p. 1631.

15. *Answer:* 1
Rationale: In the acute stage, the child presents with fever, conjunctival hyperemia, a red throat, swollen hands, a rash, and enlargement of the cervical lymph nodes. In the subacute stage, cracking lips and fissures, desquamation of the skin on the tips of the fingers and toes, joint pain, cardiac manifestations, and thrombocytosis occurs. In the convalescent stage, the child appears normal but signs of inflammation may be present.

Test-Taking Strategy: Use the process of elimination. Noting the key words "acute stage" in the question will assist in directing you to option 1. Review the clinical manifestations associated with each stage of Kawasaki disease if you had difficulty with this question.
Level of Cognitive Ability: Comprehension
Client Needs: Physiological Integrity
Integrated Concept/Process: Nursing Process/Data Collection
Content Area: Child Health
Reference: Wong D: *Whaley and Wong's nursing care of infants and children*, ed 6, St Louis, 1999, Mosby, p. 1631.

REFERENCES

Burroughs A, Leifer G: *Maternity nursing*, ed 8, Philadelphia, 2002, WB Saunders.

Hodgson B, Kizior R: *Saunders nursing drug handbook 2002*, Philadelphia, 2002, WB Saunders.

McKinney E et al: *Maternal-child nursing*, Philadelphia, 2000, WB Saunders.

Murray S, McKinney E, Gorrie T: *Foundations of maternal-newborn nursing*, ed 3, Philadelphia, 2002, WB Saunders.

Schulte E, Price D, Gwin J: *Thompson's pediatric nursing*, ed 8, Philadelphia, 2001, WB Saunders.

Wong D: *Whaley and Wong's nursing care of infants and children*, ed 6, St Louis, 1999, Mosby.

Metabolic, Endocrine, and Gastrointestinal Disorders

I. FEVER

A. Description

1. An abnormal body temperature elevation
2. A child's temperature can vary depending on activity, emotional stress, the type of clothing the child is wearing, and the temperature of the environment
3. Findings associated with the fever provide important indications of the seriousness of the fever

B. Data collection

1. Temperature elevation, increased heart rate
2. Flushed skin
3. Diaphoresis
4. Chills
5. Restlessness or lethargy

C. Implementation

1. Monitor vital signs
2. Administer a sponge bath with lukewarm water for 20 to 30 minutes
3. Administer antipyretics such as acetaminophen (Tylenol) as prescribed
4. Do not administer aspirin (acetylsalicylic acid, ASA) because of the risk of Reye's syndrome
5. Retake temperature 30 to 60 minutes after the antipyretic is administered
6. Provide adequate fluid intake as tolerated and as prescribed
7. Monitor for dehydration and fluid and electrolyte imbalance
8. Instruct the parents how to take the temperature, how to safely medicate their child, and when it is necessary to call the physician

II. DEHYDRATION

A. Description

1. Dehydration is the most common fluid and electrolyte imbalance in children
2. Infants and children are more vulnerable to fluid-volume deficit because a greater amount of their body water is in the extracellular fluid compartment
3. In infants and children, the organs that conserve water are immature, placing them at risk for fluid-volume deficit
4. The causes can include decreased fluid intake, diaphoresis, vomiting, diarrhea, diabetic ketoacidosis, burns, or other serious injuries

B. Data collection

1. Tachycardia
2. Dry skin and mucous membranes
3. Sunken eyeballs and fontanelles
4. Decreased urine output and increased urine specific gravity
5. Changes in level of consciousness and responses to stimuli
6. Signs of circulatory failure, such as coolness and mottling of the extremities
7. Loss of skin elasticity and turgor
8. Delayed capillary filling time
9. Weight loss
10. Decreased blood pressure
11. Thirst
12. Absence of tears

C. Implementation

1. Monitor vital signs
2. Monitor for signs of dehydration

3. Monitor weight and monitor for changes including fluid gains and losses
4. Monitor input and output (I&O) and urine for specific gravity
5. Monitor level of consciousness
6. Monitor skin turgor and mucous membranes for dryness
7. Provide oral rehydration therapy with solutions as prescribed if the child is able to take fluids orally
8. Intravenous (IV) fluids and electrolyte replacements may be prescribed if the child is unable to take sufficient fluids orally
9. Introduce a regular diet as prescribed when rehydrated
10. Provide instructions to the parents about the types and amounts of fluid to encourage, the signs of dehydration, and the indications of the need to notify the physician

III. VOMITING

A. Description
   1. The major concerns when a child is vomiting are the risk of dehydration, the loss of fluid and electrolytes, and the development of metabolic alkalosis
   2. Additional concerns include aspiration, atelectasis, and the development of pneumonia

B. Data collection
   1. Signs of aspiration
   2. Character of vomitus
   3. Pain and abdominal cramping
   4. Dehydration and fluid and electrolyte imbalances
   5. Metabolic alkalosis

C. Implementation
   1. Maintain a patent airway
   2. Position the child on side to prevent aspiration
   3. Monitor vital signs
   4. Monitor the character, amount, and frequency of vomiting
   5. Monitor the force of the vomiting, as projectile vomiting is indicative of pyloric **stenosis** or increased intracranial pressure
   6. Monitor intake and output (I&O) and for signs of dehydration
   7. Monitor electrolyte levels
   8. Provide oral rehydration therapy as tolerated and as prescribed; start feeding slowly with small amounts of fluid at frequent intervals
   9. Monitor for diarrhea or abdominal pain
   10. Advise the parents to inform the physician when signs of dehydration, blood in vomitus, forceful vomiting, or abdominal pain are present

IV. DIARRHEA

A. Description: The major concerns when a child is having diarrhea are the risk of dehydration, the loss of fluid and electrolytes, and the development of metabolic acidosis

B. Data collection
   1. Character of stools
   2. Pain and abdominal cramping
   3. Dehydration
   4. Fluid and electrolyte imbalances
   5. Metabolic acidosis

C. Implementation
   1. Monitor vital signs (avoid rectal temperatures)
   2. Monitor the character, amount, and frequency of diarrhea
   3. Monitor skin integrity
   4. Monitor I&O and for signs of dehydration
   5. Monitor electrolyte levels
   6. For mild to moderate dehydration, provide oral rehydration therapy; avoid carbonated beverages and those containing high amounts of sugar
   7. For severe dehydration, maintain NPO status to place the bowel at rest and provide fluid and electrolyte replacement by IV as prescribed; if potassium is prescribed by IV, monitor urine output
   8. Reintroduce a normal diet once rehydration is achieved
   9. Provide enteric isolation as required
   10. Instruct the parents in good handwashing technique

V. PHENYLKETONURIA (PKU)

A. Description
   1. Genetic disorder that results in central nervous system (CNS) damage from toxic levels of phenylalanine in the blood
   2. An autosomal recessive disorder
   3. PKU is characterized by blood phenylalanine levels greater than 8 mg/dL (normal level is less than 2 mg/dL 2 to 5 days after birth)
   4. All 50 states require routine screening of all newborn infants for PKU

B. Data collection
   1. In all children
      a. Digestive problems and vomiting
      b. Seizures
      c. Musty or mousy odor of the urine
      d. Mental retardation

2. In older children
   a. Eczema
   b. Hypertonia
   c. Hypopigmentation of the hair, skin, and irises
   d. Hyperactive behavior

C. Implementation
1. Screening of newborn infants for PKU; the infant should have begun formula or breast milk feeding before specimen collection
2. If initial screening is positive, a repeat test is performed and further diagnostic evaluation is required to verify the diagnosis
3. Rescreen infants by 14 days of age if the initial screening was done before 48 hours of age
4. If PKU is diagnosed:
   a. Restrict phenylalanine intake; high-protein foods (meats and dairy products) and aspartame are avoided because they contain large amounts of phenylalanine
   b. Monitor physical, neurological, and intellectual development
   c. Stress the importance of follow-up treatment
   d. Encourage the parents to express feelings about the diagnosis and the risk of PKU in future children

VI. TYPE 1 DIABETES MELLITUS (TYPE 1 DM)

A. Description
1. Type 1 DM is also known as insulin-dependent diabetes mellitus (IDDM); the majority of children with diabetes mellitus have type 1
2. Type 1 DM is caused by the partial or complete lack of secretory capacity of the beta cells of the pancreas, resulting in insulin deficiency
3. Complete insulin deficiency requires the use of exogenous insulin to promote appropriate glucose use and to prevent complications related to elevated blood glucose levels, such as hyperglycemia, diabetic ketoacidosis, and death
4. Diagnosis is based on the presence of classic symptoms and an elevated blood glucose level (normal blood glucose level is 80 to 120 mg/dL)

B. Data collection
1. Polyuria, polydipsia, polyphagia
2. Hyperglycemia
3. Weight loss
4. Unexplained fatigue or lethargy
5. Headaches
6. Stomach aches
7. Occasional enuresis in a previously toilet-trained child
8. Vaginitis in adolescent girls (caused by *Candida*, which thrives in hyperglycemic tissues)
9. Fruity odor to breath
10. Dehydration
11. Blurred vision
12. Slow wound healing
13. Changes in level of consciousness (LOC)

C. Long-term effects
1. Failure to grow at a normal rate
2. Delayed maturation
3. Recurrent infections
4. Neuropathy
5. Cardiovascular disease
6. Retinal microvascular disease
7. Renal microvascular disease

D. Complications
1. Hypoglycemia
2. Hyperglycemia
3. Diabetic ketoacidosis
4. Coma
5. Hypokalemia
6. Hyperkalemia
7. Microvascular changes
8. Cardiovascular changes

E. Diet
1. Total amount of calories are individualized on the basis of the child's age and **growth** expectations
2. As prescribed by the physician, the child may be instructed to follow the food exchange from the American Diabetic Association diet or the dietary guidelines for Americans (Food Guide Pyramid) issued by the U.S. Departments of Agriculture and Health and Human Services
3. Dietary intake should include three meals per day, eaten at consistent intervals, plus a mid-afternoon carbohydrate snack and a bedtime snack high in protein; a consistent intake of carbohydrates at each meal and snack is needed
4. Instruct the child and the parents that the child should carry candy with him or her at all times
5. Incorporate the diet into individual child's needs, likes and dislikes, lifestyle, cultural, and socioeconomic patterns
6. Allow the child to participate in making food choices, to provide a sense of control

F. Exercise
1. Instruct the child in dietary adjustments when exercising
2. Extra food needs to be consumed for increased activity, usually 10 to15 g of carbohydrate for every 30 to 45 minutes of activity

3. Instruct the child to monitor blood glucose before exercising
4. Plan with the child an appropriate exercise regimen, incorporating the developmental stage

G. Insulin
1. Diluted insulin may be required for some infants to provide small enough dosages to avoid hypoglycemia
2. Diluted insulin should be clearly labeled to avoid dosage errors
3. To prevent dosage errors, be certain that there is a match of the insulin concentration with the calibration of units on the insulin syringe
4. A pen-shaped device that contains an insulin- filled cartridge may be prescribed for the adolescent
5. Laboratory evaluation of glycosylated hemoglobin should be performed every 3 months
6. Illness, infection, and stress increase the need for insulin, and insulin should not be withheld during illness, infection, or stress because hyperglycemia and ketoacidosis can result
7. When the child is NPO for a special procedure, verify with the physician about the need to withhold the morning insulin, and when food, fluids, and insulin are to be given
8. Instruct the child and parents in the administration of the insulin
9. Instruct the child and parents to recognize symptoms of hypoglycemia and hyperglycemia
10. Instruct the parents on the administration of intramuscular (IM) or subcutaneous (SC) glucagon if the child has a hypoglycemic reaction and is unable to consume sugar-containing items orally
11. Instruct the child and parents to always have a spare bottle of insulin available
12. Advise the parents to obtain a Medic-Alert bracelet indicating the type and daily insulin dosage prescribed for the child

H. Blood glucose monitoring
1. Results provide information needed to maintain good glycemic control
2. More accurate than urine testing
3. Requires that the child pricks himself or herself several times a day as prescribed
4. Instruct the child and parents in the proper procedure for obtaining the blood glucose level
5. Inform the child and parents that the procedure must be done precisely to obtain accurate results
6. Stress the importance of handwashing before and after performing the procedure, to prevent infection
7. Stress the importance of following the manufacturer's instructions for the blood glucose monitoring device
8. Instruct the child and parents to calibrate the monitor as instructed by the manufacturer
9. Instruct the child and parents to check the expiration date on the test strips used for the blood glucose monitoring
10. Instruct the child and parents that if the blood glucose results do not seem reasonable, reread the instructions, reassess technique, check the expiration date of the test strips, and perform the procedure again to verify results

I. Urine testing
1. Instruct the parents and child in the procedure for testing urine for ketones and glucose
2. Teach the child that the second voided urine specimen is most accurate
3. The presence of ketones may indicate impending ketoacidosis
4. Urine glucose testing is not recommended as the only means of monitoring control in the child taking insulin, because it is a less reliable indicator as compared with blood glucose monitoring

J. Hypoglycemia
1. Description
   a. A blood glucose level below 60 mg/dL
   b. Occurs as a result of too much insulin, not enough food, or excessive activity
2. Implementation (Box 31-1)
   a. If able to, confirm with a blood glucose reading
   b. Administer glucose immediately in the form of a carbohydrate-containing snack or drink, cake frosting, glucose tablets, or glucose paste
   c. Give an extra snack if the next meal is not planned for more than 30 minutes or if activity is planned

BOX 31-1

Carbohydrates to Treat Hypoglycemia

1/2 cup (120 mL) of orange juice or a sugar-sweetened carbonated beverage
1 small box of raisins
3 to 4 hard candies
1 candy bar
2 or 3 glucose tablets

d. If the child becomes unconscious, squeeze cake frosting or glucose paste onto the gums and retest the blood glucose level if the child does not improve within 15 to 20 minutes; if the reading remains low, administer additional sugar
e. If the child remains unconscious, it may be necessary to administer glucagon
f. In the hospital setting, prepare to administer IV dextrose

K. Hyperglycemia
1. Description: elevated blood glucose level over 200 mg/dL
2. Implementation: Instruct the parents to notify the physician when blood glucose results are greater than 200 mg/dL, when moderate or high ketonuria is present, when the child is unable to take food or fluids, and when illness persists (Box 31-2)

L. Diabetic ketoacidosis (DKA)
1. Description
a. A complication of diabetes mellitus that develops when a severe insulin deficiency occurs
b. DKA is a life-threatening condition
c. Hyperglycemia that progresses to metabolic acidosis occurs
d. It develops over a period of several hours to days
e. The blood glucose level is greater than 300 mg/dL and urine and serum ketones are positive
2. Implementation
a. Restore circulating volume and protect against cerebral, coronary, or renal hypoperfusion
b. Dehydration is corrected with IV infusions of 0.9%, or 0.45% normal saline as prescribed
c. Hyperglycemia is corrected with IV Regular insulin administration as prescribed
d. Monitor vital signs, urine output, and mental status closely
e. Correct acidosis and electrolyte imbalances
f. Administer oxygen as prescribed
g. Monitor blood glucose level frequently
h. The potassium level is monitored closely because when the child receives insulin to lower the blood glucose level, the serum potassium will decrease as the acidosis improves, and potassium replacement may be required
i. Monitor the child closely for signs of fluid overload
j. IV dextrose is added as prescribed when the blood glucose reaches an appropriate level
k. Treat the cause of hyperglycemia

BOX 31-2

Sick Day Rules for the Diabetic Child

Always give insulin even if the child does not have an appetite, or contact the physician for specific instructions
Test blood glucose levels at least every 4 hours
Test for urinary ketones with each voiding
Notify the physician if moderate or large amounts of urinary ketones are present
Follow the child's usual meal plan
Encourage calorie-free liquids to aid in clearing ketones
Encourage rest, especially if urinary ketones are present
Notify the physician if vomiting, fruity odor to the breath, deep rapid respirations, decreasing level of consciousness, or persistent hyperglycemia occurs

VII. CLEFT LIP AND CLEFT PALATE (Figure 31-1)

A. Description
1. A congenital anomaly that occurs due to failure of soft tissue or bony structure to fuse during embryonic development
2. Involves abnormal openings in the lip or palate that may occur unilaterally or bilaterally and are readily apparent at birth
3. Causes include genetic, **hereditary,** and environmental factors; exposure to radiation or rubella virus; chromosome abnormalities; and teratogenic factors
4. Closure of cleft lip defect precedes that of the palate and is performed usually during the first weeks of life
5. Cleft palate repair is performed sometime between 12 and 18 months of age to allow for the palatal changes that take place with normal **growth**; a cleft palate is closed before the child develops faulty speech habits

B. Data collection
1. Cleft lip can range from a slight notch to a complete separation from the floor of the nose
2. Cleft palate can include nasal distortion, midline or bilateral cleft, with various extension from the uvula and soft and hard palate

C. Implementation
1. Monitor the ability to suck, swallow, handle normal secretions, and breathe without distress
2. Monitor fluid and calorie intake daily and monitor weight
3. Modify feeding techniques; plan to use specialized feeding techniques, obturators, and special nipples and feeders

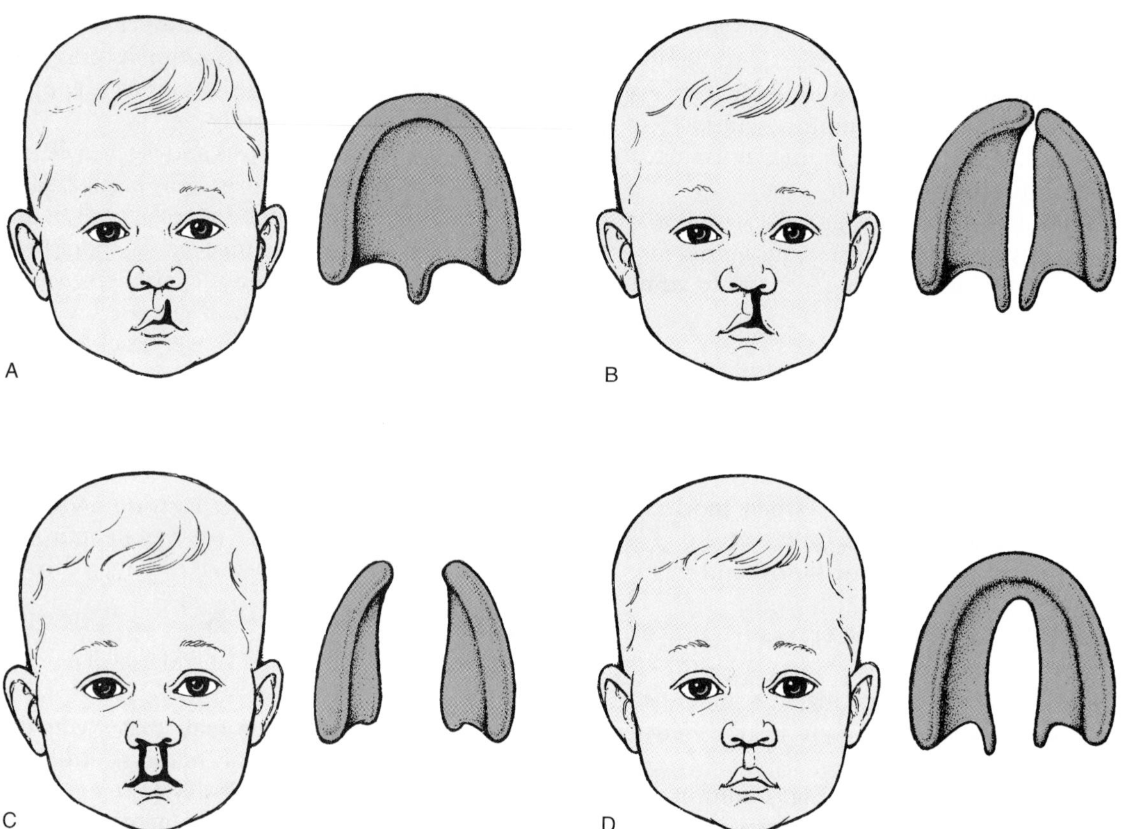

FIG. 31-1 Variations in cleft lip and palate at birth. (From Wong D, Hockenberry-Eaton M: *Wong's essentials of pediatric nursing*, ed 6, St Louis, 2001, Mosby.)

4. Hold the child in an upright position and direct the formula to the side and back of the mouth to prevent aspiration; feed small amounts gradually and burp frequently
5. Position on side after feeding
6. Keep suction equipment and bulb syringe at bedside
7. Encourage breastfeeding if appropriate
8. Teach the parents special feeding or suctioning techniques
9. Teach the parents the ESSR (enlarge, stimulate sucking, swallow, rest) method of feeding (Box 31-3)
10. Encourage the parents to describe their feelings related to deformity

BOX 31-3

ESSR Method of Feeding

ENLARGE the nipple
STIMULATE the suck reflex
SWALLOW
REST to allow the child to finish swallowing what has been placed in the mouth

D. Postoperative implementation
   1. Cleft lip repair
      a. A lip protector device may be taped securely to the cheeks to prevent trauma to the suture line
      b. Position the child on the side lateral to the repair; avoid the prone position to prevent rubbing of the surgical site on the mattress
      c. After feeding cleanse the suture line of formula or serosanguineous drainage with a cotton-tipped swab dipped in saline; apply antibiotic ointment if prescribed
   2. Cleft palate repair
      a. Child is allowed to lie on the abdomen
      b. Feedings are resumed by bottle, breast, or cup
      c. Oral packing may be secured to the palate (removed in 2 to 3 days)
      d. Do not allow the child to brush his or her teeth
      e. Instruct the parents to avoid offering hard food items to the child, such as toast or cookies

3. Soft elbow or jacket restraints may be used (check agency policies and procedures) to keep the child from touching the repair site; remove restraints at least every 2 hours to check skin integrity and allow for exercising the arms
4. Avoid contact with sharp objects near the surgical site
5. Avoid the use of oral suction or placing objects in the mouth such as a tongue depressor, thermometer, straws, spoons, forks, or pacifiers
6. Provide analgesics for pain
7. Instruct the parents in feeding techniques and in the care of the surgical site
8. Instruct the parents to monitor for signs of infection at the surgical site, such as redness, swelling, or drainage
9. Encourage the parents to hold the child
10. Initiate appropriate referrals for speech impairment or language-based **learning** difficulties

VIII. ESOPHAGEAL ATRESIA AND TRACHEOESOPHAGEAL FISTULA

A. Description
1. The esophagus terminates before it reaches the stomach and/or a fistula is present that forms an unnatural connection with the trachea
2. The condition causes oral intake to enter the lungs or a large amount of air to enter the stomach; and choking, coughing, and severe abdominal distention can occur
3. Aspiration pneumonia and severe respiratory distress will develop, and death will occur without surgical intervention
4. Treatment includes maintenance of a patent airway, prevention of pneumonia, gastric or blind pouch decompression, supportive therapy, and surgical repair

B. Data collection
1. Frothy saliva in the mouth and nose, and drooling
2. Coughing and choking during feedings
3. Unexplained cyanosis
4. **Regurgitation** and vomiting
5. Abdominal distention
6. Inability to pass an orogastric feeding tube via the mouth into the stomach

C. Preoperative implementation
1. Infant may be placed in an incubator or radiant warmer and humidified oxygen is administered (intubation and mechanical ventilation may be necessary if respiratory distress occurs)
2. Maintain an NPO status
3. Maintain IV fluids as prescribed
4. Suction accumulated secretions from the mouth and pharynx
5. A double-lumen catheter is placed into the upper esophageal pouch and attached to intermittent or continuous low suction to keep the pouch empty of secretions; it is irrigated with normal saline as prescribed to prevent clogging
6. Maintain in an upright position to facilitate drainage and to prevent aspiration of gastric secretions
7. A gastrostomy tube may be placed and is left open so that air entering the stomach through the fistula can escape, minimizing the danger of **regurgitation**
8. Broad-spectrum antibiotics may be prescribed because of the high risk for aspiration pneumonia

D. Postoperative implementation
1. Monitor respiratory status
2. Maintain IV fluids, antibiotics, and parenteral nutrition as prescribed
3. Monitor I&O and weight daily
4. Inspect surgical site
5. Provide care to the chest tube if in place
6. Monitor for signs of pain
7. Monitor for dehydration and possible fluid overload
8. Monitor for anastomotic leaks as evidenced by purulent chest drainage, increased temperature, and an increased white blood cell count
9. The double-lumen catheter placed preoperatively is attached to low-suction
10. If a gastrostomy tube is present, it is attached to gravity drainage until the infant can tolerate feedings (usually the 5th to 7th postoperative day)
11. Before oral feedings and removal of the chest tube, a barium swallow is performed to verify the integrity of the esophageal anastomosis
12. Before feeding, the gastrostomy tube is elevated and secured above the level of the stomach to allow gastric secretions to pass to the duodenum and swallowed air to escape through the open gastrostomy tube
13. Feedings through the gastrostomy tube may be prescribed until the anastomosis is healed
14. Oral feedings are begun with sterile water followed by frequent small feedings of formula
15. The gastrostomy tube may be removed before discharge or may be maintained for supplemental feedings at home

16. If the infant is awaiting esophageal replacement, a cervical esophagostomy may be performed
17. Check the cervical esophagostomy site for redness, breakdown, or exudate (continued discharge or saliva can cause skin breakdown); remove drainage frequently and apply a protective ointment, a barrier dressing, and/or a collection device
18. If the infant is awaiting esophageal replacement, nonnutritive sucking is provided by a pacifier; infants who remain NPO for extended periods and have not received oral stimulation frequently may have difficulty eating by mouth after surgery and develop oral hypersensitivity and food aversion
19. Reinforce instructions to the parents in the techniques of suctioning, gastrostomy tube care and feedings, and skin site care as appropriate
20. Instruct the parents to identify behaviors that indicate the need for suctioning, signs of respiratory distress, and signs of a constricted esophagus (poor feeding, dysphagia, drooling, or regurgitated undigested food)

IX. GASTROESOPHAGEAL REFLUX (GER)

A. Description
1. Backflow of gastric contents into the esophagus, as a result of relaxation or incompetence of the lower esophageal or cardiac sphincter
2. Complications include esophagitis, esophageal strictures, aspiration of gastric contents, and aspiration pneumonia
3. Most infants with GER have a mild problem that improves in about 1 year and requires only medical therapy
4. Treatment includes diet, positioning, medications, and surgery; however, surgery is performed only in children with severe complications from the GER

B. Data collection
1. Passive **regurgitation** or emesis
2. Poor weight gain
3. Hematemesis and melena
4. Irritability
5. Heartburn (in older children)
6. Anemia from blood loss

C. Implementation
1. Monitor amount and characteristics of emesis
2. Monitor the relation of vomiting to the time of feedings and infant activity
3. Monitor respiratory status before and after feedings
4. Place suction equipment at the bedside
5. Monitor I&O and for signs and symptoms of dehydration
6. Maintain IV fluids as prescribed

D. Positioning: place in either the flat prone position or the head-elevated prone position after feedings and at night

E. Diet
1. Provide small, frequent feedings to decrease the amount of **regurgitation**; nasogastric (NG) tube feedings are indicated if severe **regurgitation** and poor **growth** are present
2. For infants, thicken formula by adding 1 tablespoon of rice cereal per 6 ounces of formula and crosscut the nipple; monitor for coughing during feeding
3. Breastfeeding may continue and the mother may provide more frequent feeding times or express milk for thickening with rice cereal
4. Burp the infant frequently when feeding and handle the infant minimally after feedings
5. For toddlers, feed solids first, followed by liquids
6. The parents are instructed to avoid feeding the child fatty foods, chocolate, tomato products, carbonated liquids, fruit juices, citrus products, and spicy foods
7. Avoid vigorous play after feeding and avoid feeding just before bedtime

F. Medications
1. Administer antacids and histamine-receptor antagonists as prescribed to reduce the amount of acid present in gastric secretions and to prevent esophagitis
2. Administer prokinetic agents to accelerate gastric emptying and decrease reflux
3. Administer acetaminophen (Tylenol) as prescribed to relieve reflux pain

G. Surgery
1. If surgery is prescribed, it will require a procedure known as fundoplication, in which a wrap to the stomach fundus is made around the distal esophagus (restores the competence of the lower esophageal sphincter)
2. A gastrostomy may be performed at the same time as the fundoplication for postoperative decompression of the stomach
3. Fundoplication may be combined with pyloroplasty in children with GER who also have delayed gastric emptying
4. Postoperative care is similar to that for other types of abdominal surgery
5. Instruct the parents in the potential postoperative problems, such as bloating symptoms or discomfort after consuming large, solid meals

X. HYPERTROPHIC PYLORIC STENOSIS (Figure 31-2)

A. DESCRIPTION
1. Hypertrophy of the circular muscles of the pylorus causes narrowing of the pyloric canal between the stomach and duodenum
2. Usually develops in the first few weeks of life, causing projectile vomiting, dehydration, metabolic alkalosis, and failure to thrive

B. Data collection
1. Vomiting that progresses from mild **regurgitation** to forceful and projectile and usually occurs after a feeding
2. Vomitus contains gastric contents such as milk or formula; may contain mucus, may be blood-tinged, and does not usually contain bile
3. Hunger and irritability
4. Peristaltic waves visible from left to right across the epigastrium during or immediately after a feeding
5. Olive-shaped mass in the epigastrium just right of the umbilicus
6. Dehydration and malnutrition
7. Electrolyte imbalances
8. Metabolic alkalosis

C. Implementation
1. Monitor vital signs
2. Monitor I&O and weight
3. Monitor for signs of dehydration and electrolyte imbalances
4. Prepare the child and parents for pyloromyotomy if prescribed

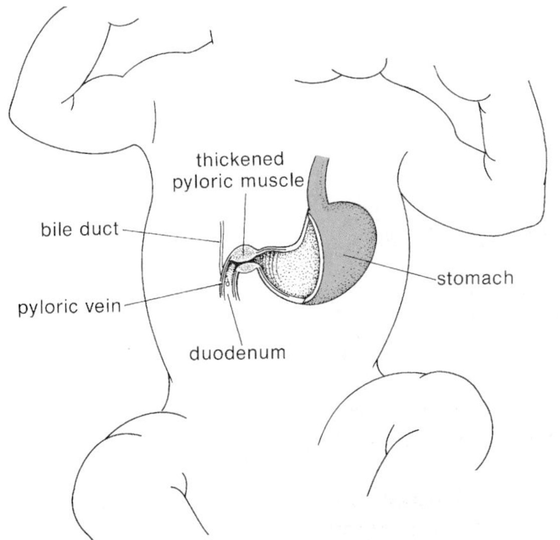

FIG. 31-2 Pyloric stenosis. (From Schulte E et al: *Thompson's pediatric nursing: an introductory text*, ed 7, Philadelphia, 1997, WB Saunders.)

D. Pyloromyotomy
1. Description: an incision through the muscle fibers of the pylorus; may be performed by laparoscopy
2. Preoperative implementation
   a. Monitor hydration status by daily weights, I&O, and urine for specific gravity
   b. Correct fluid and electrolyte imbalances; IV fluids will be administered as prescribed for rehydration
   c. Maintain NPO status
   d. Monitor the number and character of stools
   e. Maintain patency of the NG tube placed for stomach decompression
3. Postoperative implementation
   a. Monitor I&O
   b. Maintain IV fluids until the infant is taking and retaining adequate amounts by mouth
   c. Begin small, frequent feedings of glucose, water, or electrolyte solution after 4 to 6 postoperative hours as prescribed; advance the diet to formula after 24 hours as prescribed
   d. Gradually increase amount and interval between feedings until a full feeding schedule is reinstated, usually by 48 postoperative hours
   e. Feed infant slowly, burping frequently; handle the infant minimally after feedings
   f. Monitor for abdominal distention
   g. Monitor the surgical wound and for signs of infection
   h. Instruct the parents about wound care and feeding

XI. LACTOSE INTOLERANCE

A. Description: inability to tolerate lactose as a result of an absence or deficiency of lactase, an enzyme found in the secretions of the small intestine that is required for the digestion of lactose

B. Data collection
1. Symptoms occur after the ingestion of milk products
2. Diarrhea
3. Abdominal distention
4. Crampy, abdominal pain
5. Excessive flatus

C. Implementation
1. Eliminate the offending dairy product or administer an enzyme replacement
2. Provide information to parents about enzyme tablets (Lactaid, Lactrase, Dairy Ease) that predigest the lactose in milk or supplement the body's own lactase

3. Provide calcium and vitamin D supplements to prevent deficiency
4. Limit milk consumption to one glass at a time
5. If milk is consumed, drink with other foods rather than alone
6. Encourage consumption of hard cheese, cottage cheese, or yogurt (contains inactive lactase enzyme) instead of drinking milk
7. Encourage consumption of small amounts of dairy foods daily to help colonic bacteria adapt to ingested lactose
8. Instruct the parents about the importance of calcium and vitamin D supplements
9. Instruct the parents about the foods that contain lactose, including hidden sources

XII. CELIAC DISEASE (GLUTEN-SENSITIVITY ENTEROPATHY)

A. Description
1. Intolerance to gluten, the protein component of wheat, barley, rye, and oats
2. It results in the accumulation of the amino acid glutamine, which is toxic to intestinal mucosal cells
3. Intestinal villi atrophy, which affects absorption of ingested nutrients
4. Symptoms of the disorder occur most often between the ages of 1 and 5 years; there is usually an interval of several months between the introduction of gluten in the diet and the onset of symptoms
5. Strict dietary avoidance of gluten minimizes the risk of developing malignant lymphoma of the small intestine and other GI malignancies

B. Data collection
1. Acute or insidious diarrhea; stools are watery and pale with an offensive odor
2. Anorexia
3. Abdominal pain and distention
4. Muscle wasting, particularly in the buttocks and extremities
5. Vomiting
6. Anemia
7. Irritability

C. Celiac crisis
1. Precipitated by infection, fasting, and ingestion of gluten
2. Can lead to electrolyte imbalance, rapid dehydration, and severe acidosis
3. Causes profuse watery diarrhea and vomiting

D. Implementation
1. Gluten-free diet and substituting corn, rice, and millet as a grain source
2. Lifelong elimination of gluten sources such as wheat, rye, oats, and barley
3. Mineral and vitamin supplements, including iron, folic acid, and fat-soluble supplements A, D, E, and K
4. Teach the parents about a gluten-free diet and to read food labels carefully for hidden sources of gluten (Box 31-4)
5. Instruct the parents in the measures to prevent celiac crisis
6. Inform the parents about the Celiac Sprue Association/United States of America

XIII. APPENDICITIS

A. Description
1. Inflammation of the appendix
2. When the appendix becomes inflamed or infected, perforation may occur within a matter of hours, leading to peritonitis and sepsis
3. Treatment is surgical removal of the appendix before perforation occurs

B. Data collection
1. Pain in periumbilical area that descends to the right lower quadrant
2. Abdominal pain that is most intense at McBurney's point
3. Referred pain indicating the presence of peritoneal irritation
4. Rebound tenderness and abdominal rigidity
5. Elevated white blood cell (WBC) count
6. Side-lying position with abdominal guarding (legs flexed)
7. Difficulty walking and pain in the right hip
8. Low-grade fever
9. Anorexia, nausea, and vomiting after the pain develops
10. Diarrhea

BOX 31-4

Basics of a Gluten-Free Diet

FOODS ALLOWED

Meat such as beef, pork, and poultry, fish, eggs, milk and dairy products, vegetables, fruits, grains, rice, corn, gluten-free wheat flour, puffed rice, cornflakes, cornmeal, precooked gluten-free cereals

FOODS PROHIBITED

Commercially prepared ice cream; malted milk; prepared puddings; grains, including anything made from wheat, rye, oats, or barley such as breads, rolls, cookies, cakes, crackers, cereal, spaghetti, macaroni noodles, beer, and ale

C. Peritonitis (perforated appendix)
1. Data collection
a. Increased fever
b. Sudden relief of pain after the perforation; then, a subsequent increase in pain accompanied by right guarding of the abdomen occurs
c. Progressive abdominal distention
d. Tachycardia and tachypnea
e. Pallor
f. Chills
g. Restlessness and irritability

D. Appendectomy
1. Description: surgical removal of the appendix
2. Preoperative implementation
a. Maintain NPO status
b. IV fluids and electrolytes may be prescribed to prevent dehydration and correct electrolyte imbalances
c. Monitor for signs of ruptured appendix and peritonitis
d. Antibiotics may be prescribed
e. Monitor for changes in the level of pain
f. Monitor bowel sounds
g. Position in right side-lying or low to semi-Fowler's position to promote comfort
h. Apply ice packs to the abdomen for 20 to 30 minutes every hour if prescribed
i. Avoid the application of heat to abdomen
j. Avoid laxatives or enemas
3. Postoperative implementation
a. Monitor temperature for signs of infection
b. Maintain NPO status until bowel function has returned; advance diet gradually as tolerated and as prescribed when bowel sounds return
c. Check incision for signs of infection, such as redness, swelling, drainage, and pain
d. If perforation of the appendix had occurred, expect a drain (Penrose drain) to be inserted or the incision may be left open to heal from the inside out
e. Expect that drainage from the drain may be profuse for the first 12 hours
f. Position the client in right side-lying or low to semi-Fowler's position with legs flexed to facilitate drainage
g. Change the dressing as prescribed, and record type and amount of drainage
h. Perform wound irrigations if prescribed
i. Maintain NG tube suction and patency of tube if present
j. Administer antibiotics and analgesics as prescribed

XIV. HIRSCHSPRUNG'S DISEASE (Figure 31-3)

A. Description
1. A congenital anomaly also known as congenital aganglionosis or megacolon
2. Occurs as the result of an absence of ganglion cells in the rectum and upward in the colon
3. Results in mechanical obstruction from inadequate motility in an intestinal segment
4. May be a familial congenital defect or may be associated with other anomalies, such as Down syndrome and genital urinary abnormalities
5. A rectal biopsy demonstrates histologic evidence of the absence of ganglionic cells
6. The most serious complication is enterocolitis; signs include fever, severe prostration, GI bleeding, or explosive watery diarrhea
7. Treatment for mild or moderate disease is based on relieving the chronic constipation with stool softeners and rectal irrigations; however, most children require surgery
8. Treatment for moderate to severe disease involves a two-step surgical procedure
9. Initially, in the neonatal period, the obstruction is relieved by a temporary colostomy to relieve obstruction and allow the normally innervated, dilated bowel to return to its normal size
10. A complete surgical repair is performed, when the child weighs approximately 9 kg (20 pounds), via a pull-through procedure to excise portions of the bowel; at this time, the colostomy is closed

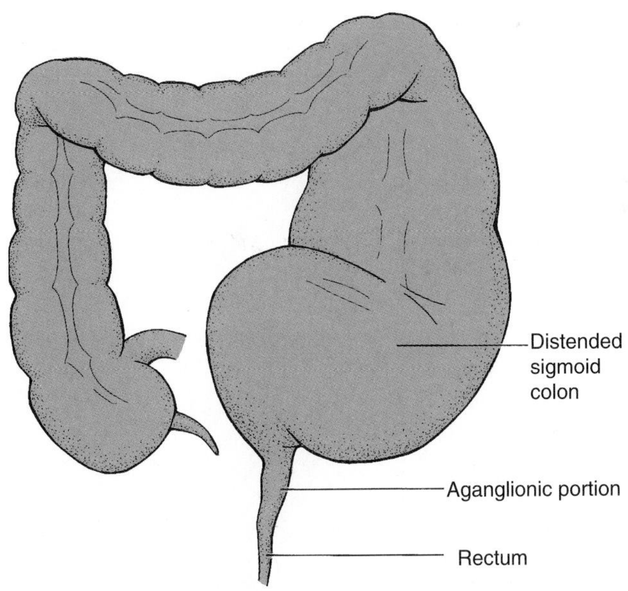

FIG. 31-3 Hirschsprung's disease. (From Wong D: *Whaley & Wong's nursing care of infants and children*, ed 6, St Louis, 1999, Mosby.)

B. Data collection
   1. Newborn infants
      a. Failure to pass meconium stool
      b. Refusal to suck
      c. Abdominal distention
      d. Bile-stained vomitus
   2. Children
      a. Failure to gain weight and delayed **growth**
      b. Abdominal distention
      c. Vomiting
      d. Constipation alternating with diarrhea
      e. Ribbon-like and foul-smelling stools

C. Implementation: medical management
   1. Dietary management
   2. Stool softeners
   3. Daily rectal irrigations with normal saline to promote adequate elimination and prevent obstruction

D. Surgical management: preoperative implementation
   1. Monitor bowel function and administer bowel preparation as prescribed
   2. Maintain NPO status
   3. Monitor hydration and fluid and electrolyte status; IV fluids may be prescribed for hydration
   4. Antibiotics may be prescribed to clear the bowel of bacteria
   5. Monitor I&O and weight
   6. Measure abdominal girth
   7. Avoid rectal temperatures
   8. Monitor for respiratory distress associated with abdominal distention

E. Postoperative implementation
   1. Monitor vital signs, avoiding rectal temperatures
   2. Measure abdominal girth
   3. Check the surgical site for redness, swelling, and drainage
   4. Monitor the stoma for bleeding or skin breakdown
   5. Check the anal area for the presence of stool, redness, or discharge
   6. Maintain NPO status until bowel sounds return or flatus is passed; bowel sounds usually return within 48 to 72 hours
   7. Maintain the NG tube to intermittent suction until peristalsis returns
   8. Maintain the IV until the child tolerates appropriate oral intake; begin the diet with clear liquids, advancing to regular as tolerated and as prescribed
   9. Monitor for dehydration and fluid overload
   10. Monitor I&O and weight
   11. Monitor pain level and provide comfort measures as required
   12. Reinforce instructions with the parents regarding colostomy care and skin care
   13. Teach the parents about the appropriate diet and the need for adequate fluid intake

XV. INTUSSUSCEPTION (Figure 31-4)

A. Description
   1. Telescoping of one portion of the bowel into another portion

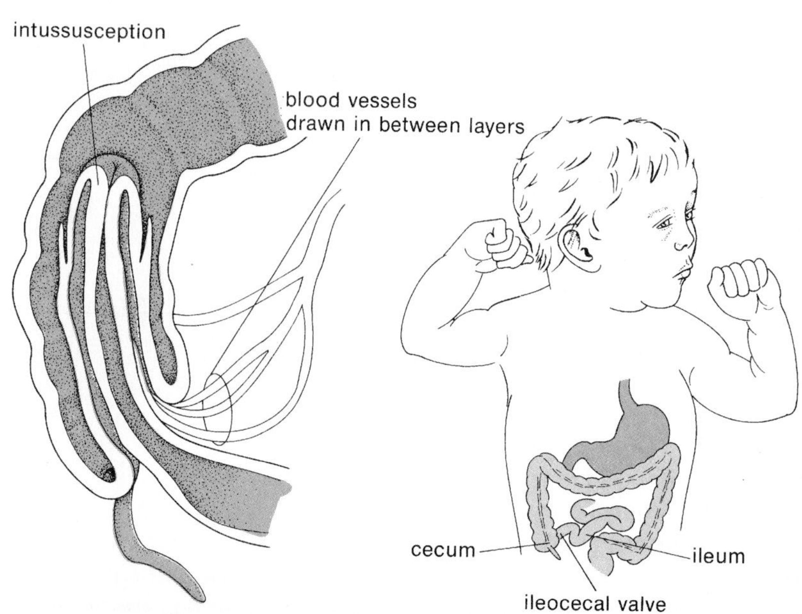

FIG. 31-4 Intussusception. (From Schulte E et al: *Thompson's pediatric nursing: an introductory text*, ed 7, Philadelphia, 1997, WB Saunders.)

2. Results in an obstruction to the passage of intestinal contents

B. Data collection
1. Colicky abdominal pain that causes the child to scream and draw the knees to the abdomen
2. Vomiting of gastric contents
3. Bile-stained fecal emesis
4. Currant jellylike stools containing blood and mucus
5. Hypoactive or hyperactive bowel sounds
6. Tender distended abdomen, possibly with a palpable sausage-shaped mass in the upper right quadrant

C. Implementation
1. Monitor for signs of perforation and shock as evidenced by fever, increased heart rate, changes in level of consciousness (LOC) or blood pressure, and respiratory distress, and report immediately
2. Prepare for hydrostatic reduction if prescribed (not performed if signs of perforation or shock occur)
   a. Antibiotics, IV fluids, and NG decompression may be prescribed
   b. Monitor for the passage of normal, brown stool, which indicates that the intussusception has reduced itself
3. After hydrostatic reduction:
   a. Monitor for the return of normal bowel sounds, for the passage of barium, and the characteristics of stool
   b. Administer clear fluids and advance the diet gradually as prescribed
4. If surgery is required, postoperative care is similar to that after any abdominal surgery

XVI. ABDOMINAL WALL DEFECTS

A. Omphalocele
1. Occurs when there is a herniation of the abdominal contents through the umbilical ring (hernia of the umbilical cord), usually with an intact peritoneal sac
2. The protrusion is covered by a translucent sac that may contain bowel or other abdominal organs
3. Rupture of the sac results in evisceration of the abdominal contents
4. Immediately after birth, the sac is covered with sterile gauze soaked in normal saline to prevent drying of abdominal contents; a layer of plastic wrap is placed over the gauze to provide additional protection against heat and moisture loss
5. Monitor vital signs every 2 to 4 hours, particularly temperature, because the infant can lose heat through the sac
6. Preoperative implementation: maintain NPO status, administer IVs as prescribed to maintain hydration and electrolyte balance, monitor for signs of infection, and handle the infant carefully to prevent rupture of the sac
7. Postoperative implementation: control pain, prevent infection, maintain fluid and electrolyte balance, and ensure adequate nutrition

B. Gastroschisis
1. Occurs when the herniation of the intestine is lateral to the umbilical ring
2. There is no membrane covering the exposed bowel
3. The exposed bowel is loosely covered in saline-soaked pads, and the abdomen is wrapped in a plastic drape; wrapping around the exposed bowel is contraindicated because if the exposed bowel expands, wrapping could cause pressure and necrosis
4. Preoperative implementation: care is similar to that for omphalocele; surgery is performed within several hours after birth because there is no membrane covering the sac
5. Postoperative implementation: most infants have a prolonged ileus and require mechanical ventilation and parenteral nutrition; otherwise, care is similar to that for omphalocele

XVII. UMBILICAL HERNIA, INGUINAL HERNIA, OR HYDROCELE (Figure 31-5)

A. Description
1. A hernia is a protrusion of the bowel through an abnormal opening in the abdominal wall
2. In children, a hernia most commonly occurs at the umbilicus and through the inguinal canal

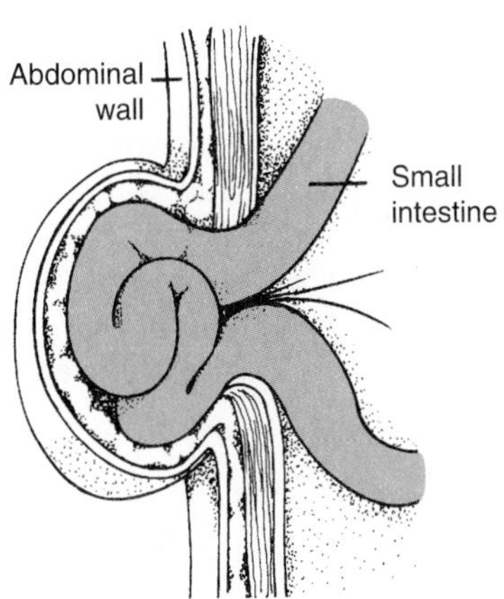

FIG. 31-5 Umbilical hernia. (From Schulte E et al: *Thompson's pediatric nursing: An introductory text*, ed 7, Philadelphia, 1997, WB Saunders.)

3. A hydrocele is the presence of abdominal fluid in the scrotal sac

B. Data collection
1. Umbilical hernia: soft swelling or protrusion around the umbilicus that is usually reducible with the finger
2. Inguinal hernia
   a. Painless inguinal swelling that is reducible
   b. Swelling may disappear during periods of rest and is most noticeable when the infant cries or coughs
3. Incarcerated hernia
   a. When the descended portion becomes tightly caught in the hernial sac, compromising blood supply
   b. A medical emergency requiring surgical repair
   c. Irritability
   d. Tenderness at site
   e. Anorexia
   f. Abdominal distention
   g. Difficulty defecating
   h. May lead to complete intestinal obstruction and gangrene
4. Noncommunicating hydrocele
   a. Occurs when residual peritoneal fluid is trapped with no communication to the peritoneal cavity
   b. Usually disappears by age 1 year
5. Communicating hydrocele
   a. Associated with a hernia that remains open from the scrotum to the abdominal cavity
   b. A bulge in the inguinal area or the scrotum that increases with crying or straining and decreases when the child is at rest

C. Postoperative implementation (hernia)
1. Monitor vital signs
2. Check for wound infection
3. Monitor for redness or drainage
4. Monitor I&O and hydration status
5. Advance the diet as tolerated
6. Administer analgesics as prescribed

D. Postoperative implementation (hydrocele)
1. Provide ice bags and a scrotal support to relieve pain and swelling
2. Instruct the child to avoid tub bathing until the incision heals
3. Instruct the child to avoid strenuous physical activities

XVIII. CONSTIPATION/ENCOPRESIS

A. Description
1. Constipation is the infrequent and difficult passage of dry, hard stools
2. Encopresis is fecal incontinence and children often complain that soiling is involuntary and occurs without warning
3. If the child does not have a neurological or anatomical disorder, encopresis is usually the result of fecal impaction and an enlarged rectum caused by chronic constipation

B. Data collection
1. Constipation
   a. Abdominal pain and cramping without distention
   b. Palpable, movable fecal masses
   c. Normal or decreased bowel sounds
   d. Malaise and headache
   e. Anorexia, nausea, and vomiting
2. Encopresis
   a. Evidence of soiling clothing
   b. Scratching or rubbing of the anal area
   c. Fecal odor
   d. Social withdrawal

C. Implementation
1. Simple constipation may resolve using only dietary changes or methods to change the habit of retention
2. Severe encopresis may require intervention to be continued over 3 to 6 months
3. Overcoming withholding
   a. Administer enemas as prescribed until the impaction is cleared
   b. Monitor for hypernatremia or hyperphosphatemia when administering repeated enemas
   c. Administer stool softener or laxative as prescribed
   d. Administer mineral oil, 30 to 75 mL twice a day as prescribed; administer chilled or mixed with cold drinks to disguise the taste
4. Dietary changes
   a. Increase water and fiber intake
   b. Decrease sugar and milk intake
   c. Administer fat-soluble vitamins during the use of mineral oil because the oil can interfere with vitamin absorption in the small intestine
5. Changing the retention habit: have the child sit on the toilet for 5 to 10 minutes approximately 20 to 30 minutes after breakfast and dinner to assist with defecation

XIX. IRRITABLE BOWEL SYNDROME

A. Description
1. Occurs as a result of increased motility that can lead to spasm and pain
2. The diagnosis is based on the elimination of pathology

3. It is a self-limiting, intermittent problem with no definitive treatment
4. Stress and emotional factors may contribute to its occurrence

B. Data collection
1. Diffuse abdominal pain unrelated to meals or activity
2. Alternating constipation and diarrhea with the presence of undigested food and mucus in the stool

C. Implementation
1. Reassure that the problem is self-limiting and intermittent and will resolve
2. Encourage the maintenance of a healthy, well-balanced, moderate-fiber diet
3. Encourage health promotion activities such as exercise and school activities
4. Inform the parents of psychosocial resources if required

XX. IMPERFORATE ANUS

A. Description: incomplete development or absence of the anus in its normal position in the perineum

B. Data collection
1. Failure to pass meconium stool
2. Absence or **stenosis** of the anorectal canal
3. Anal membrane
4. External fistula to the peritoneum

C. Implementation
1. Determine patency of the anus
2. Monitor for the presence of stool in the urine and vagina and report immediately

D. Postoperative implementation
1. Monitor the skin for signs of infection
2. Position side-lying with the legs flexed or in a prone position to keep the hips elevated to reduce edema and pressure on the surgical site
3. Keep the anal surgical incision clean and dry, and monitor for redness, swelling, or drainage
4. Maintain NPO status and NG tube if in place
5. Maintain IV fluids as prescribed until GI motility returns
6. Assist with providing colostomy care if prescribed
7. A fresh colostomy stoma will be red and edematous, but this should decrease with time
8. Reinforce instructions to the parents to perform anal dilation if prescribed to achieve and maintain bowel patency
9. Instruct parents to use only dilators supplied by the physician and a water-soluble lubricant, and to insert the dilator no more than 1 to 2 cm into the anus to prevent damage to the mucosa

XXI. HEPATITIS

A. This section contains specific information regarding hepatitis as it relates to infants and children; refer to Chapters 22 and 44 for additional information on hepatitis

B. Description: an acute or chronic inflammation of the liver that may be caused by a virus, medication reaction, or other disease process

C. Hepatitis A (HAV)
1. Highest incidence occurs among preschool or school-aged children under 15 years old
2. Many affected children are asymptomatic, but mild nausea, vomiting, and diarrhea may occur
3. Infected children who are asymptomatic can still spread HAV to others

D. Hepatitis B (HBV)
1. Most HBV in children is acquired perinatally
2. Newborn infants are at risk if the mother is infected with HBV or was a carrier of HBV during pregnancy
3. Possible routes of maternal-fetal (infant) transmission include leakage of the virus across the placenta late in pregnancy or during labor; ingestion of amniotic fluid or maternal blood; and breastfeeding, especially if the mother has cracked nipples
4. The severity in the infant varies from no liver disease to fulminant (severe, acute course) or chronic, active disease
5. In children and adolescents, HBV occurs in specific high-risk groups including children with hemophilia or other disorders who have received multiple blood transfusions, children or adolescents involved in drug abuse, institutionalized children, and preschool-aged children in endemic areas, and if involvement with heterosexual activity or sexual activity with homosexual males occurs
6. HBV infection can cause a carrier state and lead to eventual cirrhosis or hepatocellular carcinoma in adulthood

E. Hepatitis C (HCV)
1. Transmission is primarily by the parenteral route
2. Some children may be asymptomatic, but HCV often becomes a chronic condition and can cause cirrhosis and hepatocellular carcinoma

F. Hepatitis D (HDV)
1. Occurs in children already infected with HBV
2. Both acute and chronic forms tend to be more severe than HBV and can lead to cirrhosis

G. Hepatitis E (HEV)
1. Uncommon in children

2. Is not a chronic condition, does not cause chronic liver disease, and has no carrier state

H. Hepatitis G
1. Blood-borne and is similar to HCV
2. High-risk groups include transfusion recipients, IV drug users, and individuals infected with HCV
3. Individuals are often asymptomatic, and most infections are chronic

I. Data collection
1. Prodromal or anicteric phase
   a. Lasts 5 to 7 days
   b. Absence of jaundice
   c. Anorexia, malaise, lethargy, easy fatigability
   d. Fever (especially in adolescents)
   e. Nausea and vomiting
   f. Epigastric or right upper quadrant abdominal pain
   g. Arthralgia and skin rashes (more likely with HBV)
   h. Hepatomegaly
2. Icteric phase
   a. Jaundice, which is best assessed in the sclera, nail beds, and mucous membranes
   b. Dark urine and pale stools
   c. Pruritus

J. Diagnostic evaluation: refer to Chapter 10 for laboratory studies used to diagnose hepatitis

K. Prevention
1. Proper handwashing and standard precautions can prevent the spread of viral hepatitis
2. Prophylactic use of standard immune globulin (IG) to prevent HAV in situations of preexposure (such as anticipated travel to areas where HAV is prevalent) or within 2 weeks of exposure
3. Hepatitis B immune globulin (HBIG) is effective in preventing infection after one-time exposures, such as accidental needle punctures or other contact of contaminated material with mucous membranes, and should be given to newborns whose mothers are HbsAg positive; should be given within 72 hours of exposure
4. Hepatitis A vaccine is recommended for children 2 years and older who reside in communities with high endemic rates and for preexposure prophylaxis
5. Hepatitis B vaccine: refer to Chapter 36 for immunization schedule

L. Implementation
1. Strict handwashing
2. Hospitalization is required in the event of coagulopathy or fulminant hepatitis
3. Standard precautions are followed during hospitalization
4. Hospitalized child is not usually isolated in a separate room unless he or she is fecally incontinent and items are likely to become contaminated with feces
5. Children are discouraged from sharing toys
6. Instruct the child and parents on good handwashing techniques
7. Instruct the parents to thoroughly disinfect diaper-changing surfaces with 1/4 cup bleach to a gallon of water
8. Maintain comfort and provide adequate rest and sleep
9. Provide a low-fat balanced diet
10. Provide enteric precautions for at least 1 week after the onset of jaundice with HAV
11. Inform the parents that because hepatitis A is not infectious within 1 week after the onset of jaundice, the child may return to school at that time if he or she feels well enough
12. Inform the parents that jaundice may get worse before it resolves
13. Caution the parents about administering any medications to the child (liver is unable to detoxify and excrete medications)
14. Instruct the parents in the signs indicating a worsening of the child's condition, such as changes in the neurological status, bleeding, and fluid retention

XXII. INGESTION OF POISONS

A. Lead poisoning
1. Description: Excessive accumulation of lead in the blood
2. Causes
   a. The pathway for exposure may be in food, air, or water
   b. Dust and soil contaminated with lead may be a source of exposure
   c. Lead enters the child's body through ingestion or inhalation, or through placental transmission to an unborn child when the mother is exposed; the most common route is ingestion either from hand-to-mouth behavior from contaminated objects or from eating loose paint chips
   d. When lead enters the body, it affects the erythrocytes, bones and teeth, and organs and tissues, including the brain and nervous system; the most serious consequences are the effects on the CNS

3. Universal screening
   a. Recommended in high-risk areas at the ages of 1 to 2 years; children at high risk should be screened earlier
   b. Any child between the ages of 3 and 6 years who has not been screened should be tested
4. Targeted screening
   a. Acceptable in low-risk areas
   b. At the ages of 1 to 2 years (or a child between the ages of 3 and 6 years who has not been screened) may be targeted for screening if determined to be at risk
5. Blood lead level (BLL) test
   a. Used for screening and diagnosis
   b. BLL less than 10 μg/dL: reassess or rescreen in 1 year; sooner if exposure status changes
   c. BLL 10 to 14 μg/dL: Provide family lead education, follow-up testing, and social service referral if necessary
   d. BLL 15 to 19 μg/dL: Provide family lead education, follow-up testing, and social service referral if necessary
   e. BLL 20 to 44 μg/dL: A BLL greater than 20 μg/dL is considered acute; provide coordination of care, clinical management, including treatment, environmental investigation, and lead-hazard control (the child must not remain in a lead-hazardous environment if resolution is necessary)
   f. BLL 70 μg/dL or greater: Medical treatment is immediately provided, including coordination of care, clinical management, environmental investigation, and lead-hazard control
6. Erythrocyte protoporphyrin (EP) test
   a. An indicator of anemia
   b. Normal value for a child is 35 μg/100 mL of whole blood or less
7. Chelation therapy
   a. Removing lead from the circulating blood and from some organs and tissues
   b. Does not counteract any effects of the lead
   c. Medications: dimercaprol (BAL in oil); calcium disodium edetate (CaNa2EDTA); succimer (Chemet)
   d. Dimercaprol (BAL in oil) is contraindicated in children with an allergy to peanuts because the medication is prepared in a peanut oil solution
   e. Ensure adequate urinary output before administering medications
   f. Provide adequate hydration and monitor kidney function for nephrotoxicity when medication is given, because the medication is excreted via the kidneys
   g. Follow-up lead levels to monitor progress are essential
   h. Provide instructions to parents about safety from lead hazards, medication administration, and the need for follow-up care
   i. Confirm that the child will be discharged to home without lead hazards

B. Acetaminophen (Tylenol)
1. Description
   a. Seriousness of ingestion is determined by the amount ingested and the length of time before intervention
   b. Toxic dose is 150 mg/kg or greater in children
2. Data collection
   a. First 2 to 4 hours: malaise, nausea, vomiting, sweating, pallor, weakness
   b. Latent period: 24 to 36 hours; child improves
   c. Hepatic involvement: May last up to 7 days and be permanent; right upper quadrant pain, jaundice, confusion, stupor, elevated liver enzymes and bilirubin, prolonged prothrombin time
3. Implementation
   a. Administer antidote N-acetylcysteine (NAC)
   b. Dilute antidote in juice or soda because of its offensive odor
   c. Loading dose is followed by maintenance doses

C. Acetylsalicylic acid (Aspirin, ASA)
1. Description
   a. May be caused by acute ingestion or chronic ingestion
   b. Acute: Severe toxicity occurs with 300 to 500 mg/kg
   c. Chronic: More than 100 mg/kg/day for 2 days or more; can be more serious than acute ingestion
2. Data collection
   a. GI effects: nausea, vomiting, and thirst from dehydration
   b. CNS effects: hyperpnea, confusion, tinnitus, convulsions, coma, respiratory failure, circulatory collapse
   c. Renal effects: oliguria
   d. Hematopoietic effects: bleeding tendencies
   e. Metabolic effects: diaphoresis, dehydration, fever, hyponatremia, hypokalemia, dehydration, hypoglycemia
3. Implementation
   a. Induce vomiting with syrup of ipecac or perform gastric lavage
   b. Administer activated charcoal to decrease absorption of salicylate (important in early ASA toxicity)

c. IVs, sodium bicarbonate, electrolytes, or volume expanders may be prescribed
d. Vitamin K may be prescribed for bleeding tendencies
e. Administer glucose for hypoglycemia as prescribed
f. Prepare the child for dialysis as prescribed if the child is unresponsive to the therapy

PRACTICE QUESTIONS

1. A nurse is caring for an 18-month-old child who has been vomiting. The most appropriate position for the child during naps and sleep time is:
   1. Side-lying position
   2. Prone with the face turned to the side
   3. Supine
   4. Prone with the head elevated
2. A nurse is monitoring for signs of dehydration in a 1-year-old child who has been hospitalized for diarrhea. The nurse prepares to take the child's temperature. Which of the following methods of measurement would be avoided?
   1. Tympanic
   2. Axillary
   3. Rectal
   4. Electronic
3. An infant returns to the nursing unit after a surgical repair of a cleft lip located on the right side of the lip. The best position to place this infant at this time is:
   1. On the right side
   2. On the left side
   3. Prone
   4. Supine
4. A nurse reviews the record of an infant seen in the clinic. The nurse notes that a diagnosis of esophageal atresia with tracheoesophageal fistula (TEF) is suspected. The nurse expects to note which most likely sign of this condition documented in the record?
   1. Severe projectile vomiting
   2. Coughing at nighttime
   3. Choking with feedings
   4. Incessant crying
5. A nurse is reviewing the record of a child with a diagnosis of pyloric stenosis. Which of the following data would the nurse expect to note documented in the child's record?
   1. Vomiting large amounts of bile
   2. Watery diarrhea
   3. Increased urine output
   4. Projectile vomiting
6. A nurse reinforces instructions to the mother about dietary measures for a 5-year-old child with lactose intolerance. The nurse tells the mother that which of the following supplements will be required because of the necessity of lactose avoidance in the diet?
   1. Zinc
   2. Protein
   3. Calcium
   4. Fats
7. A nurse reinforces home care instructions to the parents of a child with celiac disease. Which of the following food items would the nurse advise the parents to include in the child's diet?
   1. Rice
   2. Rye toast
   3. Oatmeal
   4. Wheat bread
8. A nurse is caring for a child who is scheduled for an appendectomy. When the nurse reviews the physician's preoperative orders, which of the following would be questioned?
   1. Maintain IV fluids as prescribed
   2. Maintain NPO status
   3. Administer a Fleet enema
   4. Administer preoperative medication on call to the operating room
9. A nurse reviews the record of a 3-week-old infant and notes that the physician has documented a diagnosis of suspected Hirschsprung's disease. The nurse understands that which of the following symptoms most likely led the mother to seek health care for the infant?
   1. Diarrhea
   2. Projectile vomiting
   3. Regurgitation of feedings
   4. Foul-smelling ribbon-like stools
10. A nurse is caring for a child with a diagnosis of intussusception. Which of the following symptoms would the nurse expect to note in this child?
    1. Blood and mucus in the stools
    2. Profuse projectile vomiting
    3. Watery diarrhea
    4. Ribbon-like stools
11. A child with a diagnosis of umbilical hernia has been scheduled for surgical repair in 2 weeks. The nurse reinforces instructions to the parents about the signs of possible hernial strangulation. The nurse tells the parents that which of the following signs would require physician notification by the parents?
    1. Fever
    2. Diarrhea
    3. Constipation
    4. Vomiting
12. A nurse reinforces home care instructions to the parents of a child with hepatitis regarding care of the child and the prevention of transmission of the virus. Which statement by a parent indicates a need for further instruction?
    1. "Frequent handwashing is important."
    2. "I need to clean contaminated household surfaces with bleach."

3. "I need to provide a well-balanced, high-fat diet to my child."
4. "Diapers should not be changed near any surfaces used to prepare food."

13. A child is hospitalized with a diagnosis of lead poisoning. The nurse assisting in caring for the child would prepare to assist in administering which of the following medications?
1. Activated charcoal
2. Sodium bicarbonate
3. Ipecac syrup
4. Dimercaprol (BAL in oil)

14. An emergency nurse is caring for a child brought to the emergency room after the ingestion of approximately one-half bottle of acetylsalicylic acid (aspirin). The nurse anticipates that the most likely initial treatment will be:
1. The administration of syrup of ipecac
2. The administration of sodium bicarbonate
3. The administration of vitamin K
4. Dialysis

15. A nurse is gathering supplies in preparation to administer a tepid bath to a child with a fever. Which of the following items would not be needed for the bath?
1. Washcloths and towels
2. A bottle of alcohol
3. Toys
4. Lightweight pajamas

16. A cooling blanket is prescribed for a child with a fever. The nurse prepares to use the cooling blanket and avoids which of the following?
1. Placing the cooling blanket on the bed and covering it with a sheet
2. Checking the skin condition of the child before, during, and after the use of the cooling blanket
3. Keeping the child uncovered to assist in reducing the fever
4. Keeping the child dry while on the cooling blanket to prevent the risk of frostbite

17. A nursing instructor asks a nursing student about phenylketonuria (PKU). Which of the following statements, if made by the student, indicates an understanding of this disorder?
1. "PKU is an autosomal dominant disorder."
2. "Treatment includes dietary restriction of tyramine."
3. "All 50 states require routine screening of all newborns for PKU."
4. "PKU primarily affects the gastrointestinal system."

18. A school-aged child with type 1 diabetes mellitus has soccer practice three afternoons a week. The nurse reinforces instructions regarding how to prevent hypoglycemia during practice. The nurse most appropriately tells the child to:
1. Take half of the amount of prescribed insulin on practice days
2. Eat twice the amount normally eaten at lunchtime
3. Take the prescribed insulin at noontime rather than in the morning
4. Drink one-half cup of orange juice before soccer practice

19. The nurse is reinforcing instructions to an adolescent with type 1 diabetes mellitus regarding insulin administration and rotation sites. Which of the following statements, if made by the adolescent, would indicate effective teaching?
1. "I need to use one major site for the morning injection and another site for the evening injection for 2 to 3 weeks before changing major sites."
2. "I need to use a different site for each insulin injection."
3. "I need to use the same site for 1 month before rotating to another site."
4. "I should use only my stomach and my thighs for injections."

20. A mother of a 6-year-old with type 1 diabetes mellitus calls the clinic nurse and tells the nurse that the child has been sick. The mother reports that she checked the child's urine and it showed positive ketones. Which of the following would the nurse instruct the mother to do?
1. Come to the clinic immediately
2. Hold the next dose of insulin
3. Administer an additional dose of Regular insulin
4. Encourage the child to drink calorie-free liquids

ANSWERS

1. *Answer:* 1
Rationale: The vomiting child should be placed in an upright or side-lying position to prevent aspiration. Options 2, 3, and 4 will place the child at risk for aspiration if vomiting occurs.
Test-Taking Strategy: Use the process of elimination. Eliminate options 2 and 4 first because they are similar. Additionally, these positions would place the child at risk for aspiration if vomiting occurred. Visualize the remaining two positions. Option 3 is also inappropriate and would cause aspiration. Review appropriate positioning for the child who has been vomiting if you had difficulty with this question.
Level of Cognitive Ability: Application
Client Needs: Physiological Integrity
Integrated Concept/Process: Nursing Process/Implementation
Content Area: Child Health
Reference: Schulte E, Price D, Gwin J: *Thompson's pediatric nursing*, ed 8, Philadelphia, 2001, WB Saunders, p. 138.

2. *Answer:* 3
Rationale: Rectal temperature measurements should be avoided if diarrhea is present. Use of a rectal thermometer can stimulate peristalsis and cause more diarrhea. Axillary and tympanic measurements of temperature would be acceptable. Most measurements are done via electronic devices.
Test-Taking Strategy: Use the process of elimination and note the key word "avoided." Eliminate option 4 first because most methods of temperature measurement are done through an electronic device. Note the diagnosis stated in the question. This should easily direct you to option 3. Review interventions for the child with diarrhea if you had difficulty with this question.
Level of Cognitive Ability: Application
Client Needs: Physiological Integrity
Integrated Concept/Process: Nursing Process/Implementation
Content Area: Child Health
Reference: Schulte E, Price D, Gwin J: *Thompson's pediatric nursing*, ed 8, Philadelphia, 2001, WB Saunders, p. 101.

3. *Answer:* 2
Rationale: After cleft lip repair, the infant should be positioned on the side lateral to the repair to prevent the contact of the suture lines with the bed linens. It is best to place the infant on the left side rather than supine immediately after surgery to prevent the risk of aspiration if the infant vomits.
Test-Taking Strategy: Use the process of elimination. Consider the anatomical location of the surgical site and the key words "right side." You should be easily directed to the correct option using these concepts. Review postoperative positioning techniques if you had difficulty with this question.
Level of Cognitive Ability: Application
Client Needs: Physiological Integrity
Integrated Concept/Process: Nursing Process/Implementation
Content Area: Child Health
Reference: Schulte E, Price D, Gwin J: *Thompson's pediatric nursing*, ed 8, Philadelphia, 2001, WB Saunders, p. 90.

4. *Answer:* 3
Rationale: Any child who exhibits the "3 Cs," coughing and choking during feedings, and unexplained cyanosis should be suspected of having TEF. Options 1, 2, and 4 are not specifically associated with TEF.
Test-Taking Strategy: Use the process of elimination focusing on the diagnosis. Recalling the "3 Cs" associated with this disorder will assist in directing you to the correct option. Review the clinical manifestations associated with this disorder if you had difficulty with this question.
Level of Cognitive Ability: Comprehension
Client Needs: Physiological Integrity
Integrated Concept/Process: Communication and Documentation
Content Area: Child Health
Reference: Wong D, Hockenberry-Eaton M: *Wong's essentials of pediatric nursing*, ed 6, St Louis, 2001, Mosby, p. 918.

5. *Answer:* 4
Rationale: Clinical manifestations of pyloric stenosis include projectile, nonbilious vomiting, irritability, hunger and crying, constipation, and signs of dehydration including a decrease in urine output.
Test-Taking Strategy: Use the process of elimination. Considering the anatomical location of this disorder and its potential effects will assist in eliminating options 2 and 3. Recalling that a major clinical manifestation is projectile, nonbilious vomiting will assist in directing you to option 4. Review these clinical manifestations if you had difficulty with this question.
Level of Cognitive Ability: Comprehension
Client Needs: Physiological Integrity
Integrated Concept/Process: Nursing Process/Data Collection
Content Area: Child Health
Reference: Schulte E, Price D, Gwin J: *Thompson's pediatric nursing*, ed 8, Philadelphia, 2001, WB Saunders, p. 136.

6. *Answer:* 3
Rationale: Lactose intolerance is the inability to tolerate lactose, the sugar found in dairy products. Removing milk from the diet can provide relief from symptoms. Additional dietary changes may be required to provide adequate sources of calcium and, if the child is an infant, protein and calories.
Test-Taking Strategy: Knowledge that lactose is the sugar found in dairy products will easily direct you to option 3 because dairy products contain high sources of calcium. Review the dietary management for lactose intolerance if you had difficulty with this question.
Level of Cognitive Ability: Application
Client Needs: Health Promotion and Maintenance
Integrated Concept/Process: Nursing Process/Implementation
Content Area: Child Health
Reference: Wong D, Hockenberry-Eaton M: *Wong's essentials of pediatric nursing*, ed 6, St Louis, 2001, Mosby, p. 399.

7. *Answer:* 1
Rationale: Dietary management is the mainstay of treatment in celiac disease. All wheat, rye, barley, and oats should be eliminated from the diet and replaced with corn and rice. Vitamin supplements, especially fat-soluble vitamins and folate, may be needed in the early period of treatment to correct deficiencies. These restrictions are likely to be lifelong, although small amounts of grains may be tolerated after the ulcerations have healed.
Test-Taking Strategy: Use the process of elimination and knowledge regarding the dietary management in celiac disease to answer this question. Recalling that corn and rice are substitute food replacements in this disease will direct you to option 1. Review the dietary management in this disorder if you had difficulty with this question.
Level of Cognitive Ability: Application
Client Needs: Health Promotion and Maintenance
Integrated Concept/Process: Teaching/Learning
Content Area: Child Health
Reference: Wong D, Hockenberry-Eaton M: *Wong's essentials of pediatric nursing*, ed 6, St Louis, 2001, Mosby, p. 927.

8. *Answer:* 3
Rationale: In the preoperative period, enemas or laxatives should not be administered. No heat should be applied to the abdomen because this may increase the chance of perforation secondary to vasodilation. IV fluids would be started and the child would be NPO. Prescribed preoperative medications

most likely would be administered on call to the operating room.
Test-Taking Strategy: Use the process of elimination. Consider the anatomical location and the concern of rupture in this disorder. Options 1, 2, and 4 are standard preoperative measures. Option 3 would place the child at risk for a perforated appendix. Review preoperative care in the child with appendicitis if you had difficulty with this question.
Level of Cognitive Ability: Comprehension
Client Needs: Physiological Integrity
Integrated Concept/Process: Nursing Process/Implementation
Content Area: Child Health
Reference: Schulte E, Price D, Gwin J: *Thompson's pediatric nursing*, ed 8, Philadelphia, 2001, WB Saunders, p. 284.

9. *Answer:* 4
Rationale: Chronic constipation beginning in the first month of life resulting in ribbon-like or pelletlike stools that are foul-smelling is a clinical manifestation of this disorder. Delayed passage or absence of meconium stool in the neonatal period is the cardinal sign. Bowel obstruction, especially in the neonatal period, abdominal pain and distention, and failure to thrive are also clinical manifestations. Options 1, 2, and 3 are incorrect.
Test-Taking Strategy: Knowledge regarding the clinical manifestations associated with Hirschsprung's disease is required to answer this question. Review these manifestations if you had difficulty with this question.
Level of Cognitive Ability: Comprehension
Client Needs: Physiological Integrity
Integrated Concept/Process: Nursing Process/Data Collection
Content Area: Child Health
Reference: Schulte E, Price D, Gwin J: *Thompson's pediatric nursing*, ed 8, Philadelphia, 2001, WB Saunders, p. 57.

10. *Answer:* 1
Rationale: The child with intussusception classically presents with severe abdominal pain that is crampy and intermittent causing the child to draw in the knees to the chest. Vomiting may be present but it is not projectile. Bright red blood and mucus are passed through the rectum and are commonly described as currant jellylike stools. Ribbon-like stools are not a manifestation of this disorder.
Test-Taking Strategy: Knowledge related to the clinical manifestations associated with intussusception is required to answer this question. Recalling that a classic manifestation is current jelly stools will assist in directing you to option 1. Review this disorder if you had difficulty with this question.
Level of Cognitive Ability: Comprehension
Client Needs: Physiological Integrity
Integrated Concept/Process: Nursing Process/Data Collection
Content Area: Child Health
Reference: Schulte E, Price D, Gwin J: *Thompson's pediatric nursing*, ed 8, Philadelphia, 2001, WB Saunders, p. 137.

11. *Answer:* 4
Rationale: The parents of a child with an umbilical hernia need to be instructed in the signs of strangulation. These signs include vomiting, pain, and irreducible mass at the umbilicus. The parents should be instructed to contact the physician immediately if strangulation is suspected.
Test-Taking Strategy: Use the definition of the word "strangulation" to assist in answering this question. This will assist in eliminating options 1 and 2. From the remaining options, knowledge regarding the signs of strangulation will assist in answering the question. Review the signs of strangulation if you had difficulty with this question.
Level of Cognitive Ability: Application
Client Needs: Health Promotion and Maintenance
Integrated Concept/Process: Teaching/Learning
Content Area: Child Health
Reference: Schulte E, Price D, Gwin J: *Thompson's pediatric nursing*, ed 8, Philadelphia, 2001, WB Saunders, p. 135.

12. *Answer:* 3
Rationale: The child with hepatitis should consume a well-balanced, low-fat diet to provide rest to the liver. Options 1, 2, and 4 are components of the home care instructions to the family of a child with hepatitis.
Test-Taking Strategy: Use the process of elimination. Note the key words "need for further instruction." Options 1, 2, and 4 can be easily eliminated by using the basic principles related to standard precautions. Review home care instructions to the parents of a child with hepatitis if you had difficulty with this question.
Level of Cognitive Ability: Comprehension
Client Needs: Safe, Effective Care Environment
Integrated Concept/Process: Teaching/Learning
Content Area: Child Health
Reference: Schulte E, Price D, Gwin J: *Thompson's pediatric nursing*, ed 8, Philadelphia, 2001, WB Saunders, p. 243.

13. *Answer:* 4
Rationale: Dimercaprol (BAL in oil) is a chelating agent that is administered to remove lead from the circulating blood and from some tissues and organs for excretion in the urine. Sodium bicarbonate may be used in salicylate poisoning. Ipecac syrup is used in poisonings to induce vomiting. Activated charcoal is used to decrease absorption in certain poisoning situations.
Test-Taking Strategy: Knowledge regarding the treatment related to lead poisoning is required to answer this question. Review this treatment if you are unfamiliar with it.
Level of Cognitive Ability: Application
Client Needs: Physiological Integrity
Integrated Concept/Process: Nursing Process/Planning
Content Area: Child Health
Reference: Schulte E, Price D, Gwin J: *Thompson's pediatric nursing*, ed 8, Philadelphia, 2001, WB Saunders, p. 198.

14. *Answer:* 1
Rationale: Initial treatment of salicylate overdose includes inducing vomiting with syrup of ipecac, or gastric lavage. Activated charcoal may be administered to decrease absorption. IV fluids and sodium bicarbonate may be administered to enhance excretion but would not be the initial treatment. Dialysis is used in extreme cases if the child is unresponsive to therapy. Vitamin K is the antidote for warfarin (Coumadin) overdose.
Test-Taking Strategy: Note the key word "initial" in the stem of the question. This key word and knowledge regarding the

treatment for aspirin overdose will assist in directing you to option 1. Review the treatment for this overdose if you had difficulty with this question.
Level of Cognitive Ability: Comprehension
Client Needs: Physiological Integrity
Integrated Concept/Process: Nursing Process/Planning
Content Area: Child Health
Reference: Schulte E, Price D, Gwin J: *Thompson's pediatric nursing*, ed 8, Philadelphia, 2001, WB Saunders, p. 197.

15. *Answer:* 2
Rationale: Alcohol should never be used for bathing the child with a fever because it can cause rapid cooling, peripheral vasoconstriction, and chilling, thus elevating the temperature further. Washcloths can be used to squeeze water over the child's body. Towels are used to dry the child. Toys, especially water toys, can be used to provide distraction during the bath. Light-weight clothing should be placed on the child after the child is dried.
Test-Taking Strategy: Use the process of elimination. Note the key word "not." Options 1 and 4 can be easily eliminated first. From the remaining options, select option 2 because of the harmful effects of alcohol and the effect of potentially elevating the temperature. Review the procedure for administering a tepid bath if you had difficulty with this question.
Level of Cognitive Ability: Application
Client Needs: Physiological Integrity
Integrated Concept/Process: Nursing Process/Planning
Content Area: Child Health
Reference: Schulte E, Price D, Gwin J: *Thompson's pediatric nursing*, ed 8, Philadelphia, 2001, WB Saunders, p. 352.

16. *Answer:* 3
Rationale: While on a cooling blanket, the child should be covered lightly to maintain privacy and reduce shivering. Options 1, 2, and 4 are important interventions to prevent shivering, frostbite, and skin breakdown.
Test-Taking Strategy: Note the key word "avoids." Knowledge regarding the physiological response associated with fever will direct you to option 3. Review the procedure associated with the use of a cooling blanket if you had difficulty with this question.
Level of Cognitive Ability: Application
Client Needs: Physiological Integrity
Integrated Concept/Process: Nursing Process/Implementation
Content Area: Child Health
Reference: Wong D, Hockenberry-Eaton M: *Wong's essentials of pediatric nursing*, ed 6, St Louis, 2001, Mosby, p. 763.

17. *Answer:* 3
Rationale: PKU is an autosomal recessive disorder. Treatment includes dietary restriction of phenylalanine intake. PKU is a genetic disorder that results in CNS damage from toxic levels of phenylalanine in the blood. Option 3 is accurate.
Test-Taking Strategy: Use the process of elimination. Recalling that PKU is a recessive disorder will assist in eliminating option 1. Reading option 2 carefully will direct you to eliminate this option because tyramine is restricted in clients on monoamine oxidase inhibitors, not in PKU. Recalling that PKU affects the CNS will assist in directing you to option 3 from the remaining options. Review the characteristics associated with this disorder if you had difficulty with this question.
Level of Cognitive Ability: Comprehension
Client Needs: Physiological Integrity
Integrated Concept/Process: Teaching/Learning
Content Area: Child Health
Reference: Schulte E, Price D, Gwin J: *Thompson's pediatric nursing*, ed 8, Philadelphia, 2001, WB Saunders, p. 111.

18. *Answer:* 4
Rationale: An extra snack of 10 to 15 grams of carbohydrate eaten before activities and for every 30 to 45 minutes of activity will prevent hypoglycemia. One-half cup of orange juice will provide the needed carbohydrate. The child or parents should not be instructed to adjust the amount or time of insulin administration. Meal amounts should not be doubled.
Test-Taking Strategy: Use the process of elimination. Options 1 and 3 can be eliminated first because insulin dosages and times should not be adjusted. From the remaining options, recalling the manifestations and treatment associated with hypoglycemia will direct you to option 4. Review the treatment to prevent hypoglycemia if you had difficulty with this question.
Level of Cognitive Ability: Application
Client Needs: Health Promotion and Maintenance
Integrated Concept/Process: Self-Care
Content Area: Child Health
Reference: Schulte E, Price D, Gwin J: *Thompson's pediatric nursing*, ed 8, Philadelphia, 2001, WB Saunders, p. 292.

19. *Answer:* 1
Rationale: To help decrease variations in absorption from day to day, the child should use one location within a major site for the morning injection. The child should then rotate to another site for the evening injection, and a third site for the bedtime injection. The child should follow this pattern for 2 to 3 weeks before changing major sites.
Test-Taking Strategy: Use the process of elimination. Eliminate option 4 first because of the word "only." From the remaining options, it is necessary to know the physiology associated with absorption of insulin. Review insulin administration if you had difficulty with this question.
Level of Cognitive Ability: Comprehension
Client Needs: Physiological Integrity
Integrated Concept/Process: Self-Care
Content Area: Child Health
Reference: Schulte E, Price D, Gwin J: *Thompson's pediatric nursing*, ed 8, Philadelphia, 2001, WB Saunders, p. 289.

20. *Answer:* 4
Rationale: When the child is sick, the mother should test for urinary ketones with each voiding. If ketones are present, liquids are essential to aid in clearing. The child should be encouraged to drink calorie-free liquids. It is not necessary to bring the child to the clinic immediately. Insulin doses should not be adjusted or changed.
Test-Taking Strategy: Use the process of elimination. Eliminate options 2 and 3 first because insulin doses should not be adjusted or changed. From the remaining options, note the words "positive ketones." This finding does not require imme-

diate physician referral. Review home care instructions for the sick diabetic child if you had difficulty with this question.
Level of Cognitive Ability: Application
Client Needs: Health Promotion and Maintenance
Integrated Concept/Process: Nursing Process/Implementation
Content Area: Child Health
Reference: Schulte E, Price D, Gwin J: *Thompson's pediatric nursing,* ed 8, Philadelphia, 2001, WB Saunders, p. 295.

REFERENCES

Burroughs A, Leifer G: *Maternity nursing,* ed 8, Philadelphia, 2002, WB Saunders.

Hodgson B, Kizior R: *Saunders nursing drug handbook 2002,* Philadelphia, 2002, WB Saunders.

McKinney E et al: *Maternal-child nursing,* Philadelphia, 2002, WB Saunders.

Murray S, McKinney E, Gorrie T: *Foundations of maternal-newborn nursing,* ed 3, Philadelphia, 2002, WB Saunders.

Schulte E, Price D, Gwin J: *Thompson's pediatric nursing,* ed 8, Philadelphia, 2001, WB Saunders.

Wong D: *Whaley & Wong's Nursing care of infants and children,* ed 6, St. Louis, 1999, Mosby.

Wong D, Hockenberry-Eaton M: *Wong's essentials of pediatric nursing,* ed 6, St Louis, 2001, Mosby.

32 Renal and Urinary Disorders

I. GLOMERULONEPHRITIS

A. Description
1. A term that includes a variety of disorders, most of which are caused by an immunological reaction
2. Destruction, inflammation, and sclerosis of the glomeruli of both kidneys occurs, and loss of kidney function develops

B. Causes
1. Immunological or autoimmune diseases
2. Streptococcal infection, group A beta hemolytic
3. History of pharyngitis or tonsillitis 2 to 3 weeks before symptoms

C. Types
1. Acute: occurs 2 to 3 weeks after a streptococcal infection
2. Chronic: can occur after the acute phase or slowly over time

D. Data collection
1. Child is pale, irritable, and weak
2. Gross hematuria or dark, smoky, cola-colored or red-brown urine
3. Proteinuria that produces a persistent and excessive foam in the urine
4. Oliguria or anuria
5. Urinary debris, mid to high specific gravity, low urinary pH
6. Increased blood urea nitrogen (BUN) and creatinine
7. Azotemia
8. Abdominal or flank pain
9. Edema in the face and periorbital area, feet, or generalized
10. Hypertension
11. Increased antistreptolysin O titer (used to diagnose disorders caused by streptococcal infections)
12. Headache
13. Chills and fever
14. Anorexia, nausea, and vomiting

E. Implementation
1. Monitor vital signs, weight, intake and output (I&O), and the characteristics of urine
2. Limit activity; provide safety measures
3. Nutrition
   a. Restrictions depend on the stage and severity of the disease, especially the extent of the edema
   b. In uncomplicated cases, a regular diet is permitted but sodium is restricted to no added salt to foods
   c. Moderate sodium restriction is prescribed for the child with hypertension or edema
   d. Fluid and sodium intake is restricted as prescribed if edema is present and if urine output is significantly reduced
   e. Foods high in potassium are restricted during periods of oliguria
   f. Protein is restricted if the child has severe azotemia resulting from prolonged oliguria
4. Diuretics are prescribed if significant edema and fluid overload are present
5. Antihypertensives are prescribed for hypertension
6. Anticonvulsants are prescribed for seizures associated with hypertensive encephalopathy; initiate seizure precautions as indicated
7. Antibiotics are prescribed for the child with evidence of persistent streptococcal infections
8. Monitor for edema and signs of fluid overload
9. Monitor for signs of renal failure, cardiac failure, and hypertensive encephalopathy
10. Instruct the parents to report signs of bloody urine, headache, or edema

11. Instruct the parents that the child needs to obtain treatment for infections, specifically sore throats and upper respiratory infections

II. NEPHROTIC SYNDROME

A. Description: degenerative and noninflammatory disease of the kidneys, resulting in edema and large amounts of protein in the urine

B. Data collection
1. Pale, irritable, and fatigued child
2. Child gains weight (edema)
3. Decreased urine output
4. Dark, frothy urine; proteinuria
5. Abdominal ascites
6. Waxy pallor of the skin
7. BP normal or slightly decreased
8. Anorexia
9. Hypoalbuminemia
10. Hypercholesterolemia

C. Implementation
1. Monitor vital signs, I&O and daily weight
2. Monitor for edema
3. Monitor for signs of infection, particularly in the edematous child and in the child receiving corticosteroid therapy
4. Maintain bed rest if severe edema is present; activity is not restricted during remission
5. Nutrition
   a. A regular diet is prescribed if the child is in remission
   b. Sodium restriction is prescribed during periods of massive edema
   c. Normal protein intake is usually prescribed
6. Corticosteroid therapy is usually prescribed as soon as the diagnosis has been determined
7. Immunosuppressant therapy may be prescribed to reduce the relapse rate and induce long-term remission; may be administered in conjunction with the corticosteroid
8. A diuretic may be prescribed if edema interferes with breathing
9. Antibiotics may be prescribed for infection
10. Instruct the parents about testing the urine for protein, medication administration, and general care to the child
11. Instruct the parents regarding the signs of infection and the need to avoid contact with other children who may be infectious
12. Instruct the parents about the side effects of corticosteroid therapy

III. CRYPTORCHIDISM

A. Description: occurs when one or both testes fail to descend through the inguinal canal into the scrotal sac

B. Data collection: testes not palpable or easily guided into the scrotum

C. Implementation
1. Monitored during the first 12 months of life to determine if spontaneous descent occurs
2. After age 1, medical or surgical treatment may be instituted
3. Human chorionic gonadotropin (HCG), a pituitary hormone administered by injection that stimulates the production of testosterone, and hormone therapy with luteinizing hormone-releasing hormone (nasal spray) may be prescribed
4. Surgical correction, if needed, is done by orchiopexy before the child's second birthday (preferably between 1 and 2 years of age) if the testes do not descend spontaneously
5. Monitor for bleeding and infection postoperatively
6. Instruct the parents in postoperative home care measures, including preventing infection, pain control, and activity restrictions
7. Provide an opportunity for parental counseling if the parents are concerned about the future fertility of the child

IV. HYPOSPADIAS AND EPISPADIAS (Figure 32-1)

A. Description: congenital defects involving abnormal placement of the urethral orifice of the penis

B. Data collection
1. Hypospadias: urethral orifice located below the glans penis along the ventral surface
2. Epispadias: urethral orifice located on the dorsal surface of the penis; often occurs with exstrophy of the bladder

C. Surgical implementation
1. Done before the age of toilet training, preferably between 16 and 18 months of age
2. The child should not be circumcised because the foreskin may be used in surgical reconstruction

D. Postoperative implementation
1. The child will have a pressure dressing and may have some type of urinary diversion or a urinary stent (used to maintain patency of the urethral opening) while healing of the meatus occurs
2. Monitor vital signs
3. Encourage fluid intake to maintain adequate urine output and to maintain patency of the stent

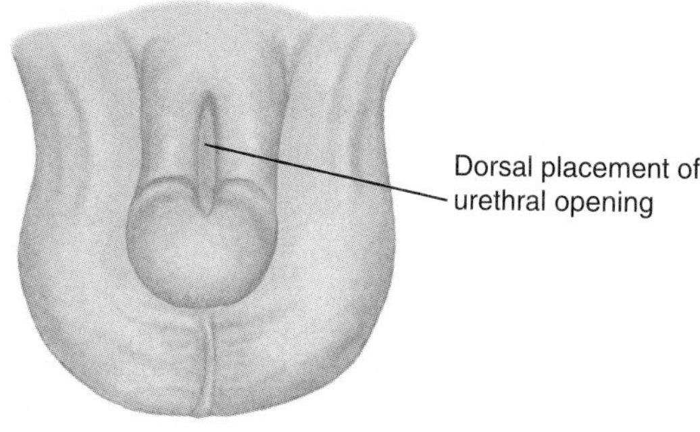

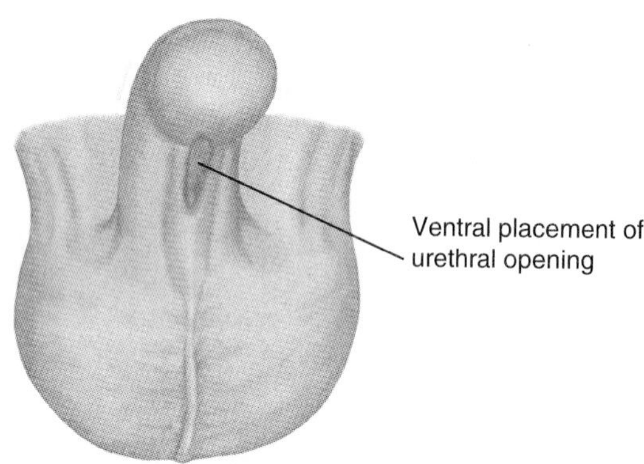

FIG. 32-1 Epispadias and hypospadias. (From McKinney E et al: *Maternal-child nursing*, Philadelphia, 2000, WB Saunders.)

4. Monitor I&O and the urine for cloudiness or a foul odor
5. The physician is notified if there is no urinary drainage for 1 hour, because this may indicate kinks in the system or obstruction by sediment
6. Provide pain medication (acetaminophen [Tylenol]) or medication to relieve bladder spasms (anticholinergic) as prescribed
7. Antibiotics may be prescribed
8. Reinforce instructions to the parents in the care of the urinary diversion or stent if present
9. Instruct the parents to avoid giving the child a tub bath until the stent, if present, is removed
10. Instruct the parents about fluid intake, medication administration, signs and symptoms of infection, and the need for physician follow-up visit for dressing removal approximately 4 days after surgery

V. BLADDER EXSTROPHY

A. Description
   1. A congenital anomaly characterized by the extrusion of the urinary bladder to the outside of the body through a defect in the lower abdominal wall
   2. The cause is not known
   3. Treatment requires surgical management and occurs in a series of staged reconstructions
   4. The initial surgery for closure of the abdominal defect should occur within the first few days of life
   5. The goal of subsequent surgeries is to reconstruct the bladder and genitalia and enable the child to achieve urinary continence

B. Data collection
   1. Exposed bladder mucosa
   2. Widened symphysis pubis
   3. Defects of the external genitalia

C. Implementation
   1. Monitor urinary output
   2. Monitor for signs of urinary tract or wound infection
   3. Maintain the integrity of the exposed bladder mucosa
   4. Prevent the bladder tissue from drying, while allowing the drainage of urine, until surgical closure is performed
      a. The bladder is covered with sterile nonadherent clear plastic wrap or a sterile thin film dressing without adhesive
      b. Petroleum jelly is avoided because it tends to dry out, adhere to the bladder mucosa, and damage the delicate tissues when the dressing is removed
   5. Monitor laboratory values and urinalysis to check renal function
   6. Antibiotics may be prescribed
   7. Provide emotional support to the parents and encourage verbalization of their fears and concerns

VI. ENURESIS

A. Description
   1. Refers to a condition in which the child is unable to control bladder function although the child has reached an age at which control of voiding is expected
   2. By age 5 years, most children are aware of bladder fullness and are able to control voiding

B. Primary nocturnal enuresis
   1. Bed-wetting in a child who has never been dry for extended periods
   2. Common in children, and most children will eventually outgrow bed-wetting without therapeutic intervention
   3. The child is not able to sense a full bladder and does not awaken to void

4. The child may have delayed maturation of the central nervous system (CNS)

C. Secondary or acquired enuresis
1. The onset of wetting after a period of established urinary continence
2. May occur during nighttime sleep (nocturnal), only during the waking hours (diurnal), or during both times of the day
3. The child may complain of dysuria, urgency, or frequency
4. The child should be assessed for urinary tract infections

D. Data collection
1. Normal voiding pattern
2. History of bed-wetting with no extended period of dryness in a child older than age 5 years

E. Implementation
1. Obtain urinalysis and urine culture as prescribed to rule out infection or existing disorder
2. Assist the family with identifying a treatment plan that will best fit their needs
3. Limit fluid intake at night, and encourage the child to void just before going to bed
4. Involve the child in caring for the wet sheets and changing the bed, to assist the child to take ownership of the problem
5. Provide reward systems as appropriate for the child
6. Incorporate behavioral conditioning techniques
7. Encourage follow-up visits to determine the effectiveness of the treatment

PRACTICE QUESTIONS

1. A nurse is reviewing the health record of a child recently diagnosed with glomerulonephritis. Which finding noted in the child's record is most often associated with the diagnosis of glomerulonephritis?
   1. Streptococcal throat infection 2 weeks before diagnosis
   2. Child fell off a bike onto the handlebars
   3. Nausea and vomiting for the last 24 hours
   4. Urticaria and itching for 1 week before diagnosis
2. A nurse is assigned to care for a child suspected of having glomerulonephritis. The nurse reviews the child's record and notes that which finding is associated with the diagnosis of glomerulonephritis?
   1. Low blood urea nitrogen (BUN)
   2. Hypotension
   3. Low urinary specific gravity
   4. Red-brown urine
3. A nurse is assisting in developing a plan of care for a 7-year-old child diagnosed with acute glomerulonephritis. The nurse includes which priority intervention in the plan of care?
   1. Encourage limited activity and provide safety measures
   2. Catheterize the child to strictly monitor intake and output
   3. Force oral fluids to prevent hypovolemic shock
   4. Encourage classmates to visit and to keep the child informed of school events
4. A nurse is assisting in performing an admission assessment on a 2-year-old child who has been diagnosed with nephrotic syndrome. The nurse collects data knowing that the most common characteristic associated with nephrotic syndrome is:
   1. Generalized edema
   2. Frank bright red blood in the urine
   3. Increased urinary output
   4. Hypertension
5. A 7-year-old child is seen in the clinic and the primary health care provider documents a diagnosis of primary nocturnal enuresis. The mother asks the nurse about the diagnosis. The nurse bases the response on the fact that primary nocturnal enuresis:
   1. Requires surgical intervention to improve the problem
   2. Is caused by a psychiatric problem
   3. Is common and most children will outgrow bed-wetting without therapeutic intervention
   4. Does not respond to treatment
6. A nurse is caring for an 8-month-old infant. A urinalysis has been ordered and the nurse plans to collect the specimen. The nurse performs which of the following most appropriate methods to collect the specimen?
   1. Catheterize the infant, using a No. 5 French Foley
   2. Obtain the specimen from the diaper, using a syringe, after the infant voids
   3. Attach a urinary collection device to the infant's perineum
   4. Monitor the urinary patterns and prepare to collect the specimen into a cup when the infant voids
7. The child with cryptorchidism is being discharged after orchiopexy, which was performed on an outpatient basis. The nurse informs the parents that which care measure should take priority in the plan of care at home?
   1. Administering anticholinergics
   2. Measuring intake and output
   3. Applying cold, wet compresses to the surgical site
   4. Preventing infection at the surgical site
8. A nurse is reinforcing discharge instructions to the mother of a 2-year-old child who has had an orchiopexy to correct cyptorchidism. Which of the following statements, if made by the mother of the child, indicates that further teaching is necessary?

1. "I'll check his temperature."
2. "I'll let him decide when to return to his play activities."
3. "I'll give him medication so he'll be comfortable."
4. "I'll check his voiding to be sure there are no problems."

9. A nurse collects a urine specimen from a child with epispadias who is scheduled for surgical repair. The nurse reviews the child's record for the laboratory results of the urine and would most likely expect to note which of the following?
   1. Hematuria
   2. Proteinuria
   3. Bacteriuria
   4. Glucosuria
10. A 1-year-old child with hypospadias is scheduled for surgery to correct this condition. A nurse is asked to assist in preparing a plan of care for this child and makes suggestions knowing that this surgery is taking place at a time when:
    1. Fears of separation and mutilation are great
    2. Sibling rivalry will cause regression to occur
    3. Embarrassment of voiding irregularities is common
    4. Concern over size and function of the penis is present
11. An 18-month-old child is being discharged after surgical repair of hypospadias. Which postoperative nursing care measure should the nurse stress to the parents as they prepare to take this child home?
    1. Encourage toilet training to ensure that flow of urine is normal
    2. Restrict fluid intake to reduce urinary output for the first few days
    3. Avoid tub baths until the stent has been removed
    4. Leave the diapers off to allow the site to heal
12. A nurse is reviewing the treatment plan with the parents of a newborn infant with hypospadias. Which statement by the parents indicates their understanding of the plan?
    1. "Circumcision has been delayed to save tissue for surgical repair."
    2. "Catheterization will be necessary if my infant does not void."
    3. "Caution should be used when straddling my infant on a hip."
    4. "Vital signs should be taken daily to check for bladder infection."
13. The parents of a newborn have been told that their child was born with bladder exstrophy. The parents ask the nurse about this condition. The nurse bases the response on knowledge that this condition is:
    1. Caused by the use of medications taken by the mother during pregnancy
    2. A hereditary disorder that occurs in every other generation
    3. A condition in which the urinary bladder is abnormally located in the pelvic cavity
    4. An extrusion of the urinary bladder to the outside of the body through a defect in the lower abdominal wall
14. The nurse assists in preparing a plan of care for the infant with bladder exstrophy. The nurse identifies which of the following nursing diagnoses as the priority for the infant?
    1. Alteration in elimination
    2. Impaired tissue integrity
    3. Parental knowledge deficit
    4. Potential for infection
15. A nurse is caring for an infant with a diagnosis of bladder exstrophy. To protect the exposed bladder tissue, the nurse plans to:
    1. Cover the bladder with petroleum jelly gauze
    2. Keep the bladder tissue dry by covering it with dry sterile gauze
    3. Cover the bladder with a nonadhering plastic wrap
    4. Apply sterile distilled water dressings over the bladder mucosa

ANSWERS

1. *Answer:* 1

Rationale: Group A beta-hemolytic streptococcal infection is a cause of glomerulonephritis. Often the child becomes ill with streptococcal infection of the upper respiratory tract and then develops symptoms of acute poststreptococcal glomerulonephritis after an interval of 1 to 2 weeks. The data in options 2, 3, and 4 are unrelated to a diagnosis of glomerulonephritis.

Test-Taking Strategy: Use knowledge regarding the causes of glomerulonephritis and the process of elimination to answer the question. Option 2 relates to a kidney injury. Options 3 and 4 are not related to the diagnosis of glomerulonephritis. Review the causes of glomerulonephritis if you had difficulty with this question.

Level of Cognitive Ability: Comprehension
Client Needs: Physiological Integrity
Integrated Concept/Process: Nursing Process/Data Collection
Content Area: Child Health
Reference: Schulte E, Price D, Gwin J: *Thompson's pediatric nursing,* ed 8, Philadelphia, 2001, WB Saunders, p. 236.

2. *Answer:* 4

Rationale: Gross hematuria resulting in dark, smoky, cola-colored or red-brown urine is a classic symptom of glomerulonephritis. Hypertension is also common. BUN levels may be elevated. A mid to high urinary specific gravity is associated with glomerulonephritis.

Test-Taking Strategy: Use the process of elimination. Eliminate options 2 and 3 first because hypertension and a high specific

gravity are most likely to occur in this kidney disorder. Knowledge that BUN levels elevate will assist in directing you to option 4 from the remaining options. If you had difficulty with this question, review the clinical manifestations associated with glomerulonephritis.
Level of Cognitive Ability: Comprehension
Client Needs: Physiological Integrity
Integrated Concept/Process: Nursing Process/Data Collection
Content Area: Child Health
Reference: Schulte E, Price D, Gwin J: *Thompson's pediatric nursing*, ed 8, Philadelphia, 2001, WB Saunders, p. 237.

3. *Answer:* 1
Rationale: Activity is limited and most children, because of fatigue, voluntarily restrict their activities during the active phase of the disease. Catheterization may cause a risk of infection. Fluids should not be forced. Visitors should be limited to allow for adequate rest.
Test-Taking Strategy: Use the process of elimination. Eliminate option 4 because rest is the priority over socialization. Eliminate option 2 next. Although monitoring I&O is essential, the risk of infection could occur with catheterization. From the remaining options, eliminate option 3 because of the words "force oral fluids." Review the appropriate nursing interventions for the child with glomerulonephritis if you had difficulty with this question.
Level of Cognitive Ability: Application
Client Needs: Physiological Integrity
Integrated Concept/Process: Nursing Process/Planning
Content Area: Child Health
Reference: Schulte E, Price D, Gwin J: *Thompson's pediatric nursing*, ed 8, Philadelphia, 2001, WB Saunders, p. 237.

4. *Answer:* 1
Rationale: Nephrotic syndrome is defined as massive proteinuria, hypoalbuminemia, hyperlipemia, and edema. Urine is dark, foamy, and frothy, and proteinuria may be present. Frank bright red blood in the urine does not occur. Urine output is decreased and hypertension does not occur.
Test-Taking Strategy: Use the process of elimination. Eliminate options 3 first because urine output is most likely to be decreased in a renal disorder. Eliminate option 4 because hypertension is not likely to occur in this disorder. Associate edema with nephrotic syndrome because this will be helpful to you if you encounter a similar question. If you had difficulty with this question, review the characteristics of nephrotic syndrome.
Level of Cognitive Ability: Application
Client Needs: Physiological Integrity
Integrated Concept/Process: Nursing Process/Data Collection
Content Area: Child Health
Reference: Schulte E, Price D, Gwin J: *Thompson's pediatric nursing*, ed 8, Philadelphia, 2001, WB Saunders, p. 192.

5. *Answer:* 3
Rationale: Primary nocturnal enuresis occurs in a child who has never been dry at night for extended periods. It is common in children and most children will eventually outgrow bed-wetting without therapeutic intervention. The child is not able to sense a full bladder and does not awaken to void. The child may have delayed maturation of the CNS. It is not caused by a psychiatric problem.
Test-Taking Strategy: Use the process of elimination. Note the relationship between the words "enuresis" in the question and "bed-wetting" in the correct option. If you had difficulty with this question, review the characteristics associated with enuresis.
Level of Cognitive Ability: Application
Client Needs: Physiological Integrity
Integrated Concept/Process: Nursing Process/Planning
Content Area: Child Health
Reference: Schulte E, Price D, Gwin J: *Thompson's pediatric nursing*, ed 8, Philadelphia, 2001, WB Saunders, p. 210.

6. *Answer:* 3
Rationale: Although many methods have been used to collect urine from an infant, the most reliable method is the urine collection device. This device is a plastic bag that has an opening that is lined with adhesive so that it may be attached to the perineum. Urine for certain tests, such as specific gravity, may be obtained from a diaper. Urinary catheterization is not to be done unless specifically prescribed, because of the risk of infection. It is not reasonable to monitor urinary patterns and attempt to collect the specimen in a cup when the infant voids.
Test-Taking Strategy: Use the process of elimination and note the key words "most appropriate." Eliminate option 4; this is unrealistic. Eliminate option 1 because catheterization is not prescribed and the risk of infection exists with this procedure. Eliminate option 2 because only certain tests can be obtained from the urine in a diaper. Review the procedure for collecting urine specimens from an infant if you had difficulty with this question.
Level of Cognitive Ability: Application
Client Needs: Physiological Integrity
Integrated Concept/Process: Nursing Process/Implementation
Content Area: Child Health
Reference: Schulte E, Price D, Gwin J: *Thompson's pediatric nursing*, ed 8, Philadelphia, 2001, WB Saunders, p. 353.

7. *Answer:* 4
Rationale: The most common complications associated with orchiopexy are bleeding and infection. The parents are instructed in postoperative home care measures including preventing infection, pain control, and activity restrictions. Anticholinergics are prescribed for the relief of bladder spasms and are not necessary after orchiopexy. Measurement of intake and output is not required. Cold wet compresses are not prescribed. Additionally, the moisture from a wet compress presents a potential for infection.
Test-Taking Strategy: Note the key word "priority" in the stem of the question. Use Maslow's Hierarchy of Needs theory to answer the question. Of the options presented, the potential for infection is the physiological priority. Review home care instructions after orchiopexy if you had difficulty with this question.
Level of Cognitive Ability: Application
Client Needs: Health Promotion and Maintenance
Integrated Concept/Process: Teaching/Learning
Content Area: Child Health
Reference: Schulte E, Price D, Gwin J: *Thompson's pediatric nursing*, ed 8, Philadelphia, 2001, WB Saunders, p. 149.

8. *Answer:* 2
Rationale: All vigorous activities should be restricted for 2 weeks after surgery to promote healing and prevent injury. This will prevent dislodging of the suture, which is internal. Normally, 2-year-olds will want to be very active; therefore, allowing the child to decide when to return to his play activities may prevent healing and cause injury. The parent should be taught to monitor the temperature, provide analgesics as needed, and monitor the urine output.
Test-Taking Strategy: Use the process of elimination. Note the key words "further teaching is necessary." Option 1 is an important action in order to recognize signs of infection. Option 3 is appropriate to keep pain to a minimum. Option 4 monitors voiding pattern, which is also important after this type of surgery. If you had difficulty with this question, review the discharge instructions after surgical correction of cryptorchidism.
Level of Cognitive Ability: Comprehension
Client Needs: Health Promotion and Maintenance
Integrated Concept/Process: Teaching/Learning
Content Area: Child Health
Reference: Schulte E, Price D, Gwin J: *Thompson's pediatric nursing,* ed 8, Philadelphia, 2001, WB Saunders, p. 150.

9. *Answer:* 3
Rationale: Epispadias is a congenital defect involving abnormal placement of the urethral orifice of the penis. The urethral opening is located anywhere on the dorsum of the penis. This anatomical characteristic leads to the easy access of bacterial entry into the urine. Options 1, 2, and 4 are not characteristically noted in this condition.
Test-Taking Strategy: Use knowledge regarding the anatomical characteristic of epispadias and the process of elimination to answer the question. Options 1, 2, and 4 do not relate to the potential for infection, which can be present in the condition of epispadias. If you had difficulty with this question, review the diagnostic findings associated with epispadias.
Level of Cognitive Ability: Comprehension
Client Needs: Physiological Integrity
Integrated Concept/Process: Nursing Process/Data Collection
Content Area: Child Health
Reference: Wong D, Hockenberry-Eaton M: *Wong's essentials of pediatric nursing,* ed 6, St Louis, 2001, Mosby, p. 220.

10. *Answer:* 1
Rationale: At the age of 1 year, a child's fears of separation and mutilation are great, because the child is facing the developmental task of trusting others. As the child gets older, fears about virility and reproductive ability may surface. The question does not provide enough data to determine that siblings exist. Options 3 and 4 may be issues if the child were older.
Test-Taking Strategy: Focus on the age of the child and use knowledge regarding the stages of growth and development to answer the question. Review the stages of growth and development if you had difficulty with this question.
Level of Cognitive Ability: Application
Client Needs: Psychosocial Integrity
Integrated Concept/Process: Nursing Process/Planning
Content Area: Child Health
Reference: Schulte E, Price D, Gwin J: *Thompson's pediatric nursing,* ed 8, Philadelphia, 2001, WB Saunders, p. 25.

11. *Answer:* 3
Rationale: After hypospadias repair, the parents are instructed to avoid giving the child a tub bath until the stent has been removed to prevent infection. Diapers are placed on the child to prevent contamination of the surgical site. Fluids should be encouraged to maintain hydration. Toilet training should not be an issue during this stressful period.
Test-Taking Strategy: Use the process of elimination. Option 1 is eliminated first since toilet training should not be initiated during times of stress, such as after surgery. Option 2 is inappropriate because fluids should be encouraged rather than restricted. Eliminate option 4 because this action can cause contamination of the surgical site. If you had difficulty with this question, review the postoperative care after surgical repair of hypospadias.
Level of Cognitive Ability: Application
Client Needs: Health Promotion and Maintenance
Integrated Concept/Process: Teaching/Learning
Content Area: Child Health
Reference: Wong D, Hockenberry-Eaton M: *Wong's essentials of pediatric nursing,* ed 6, St Louis, 2001, Mosby, p. 1042.

12. *Answer:* 1
Rationale: Hypospadias is a congenital defect involving abnormal placement of the urethral orifice of the penis. In hypospadias, the urethral orifice is located below the glans penis along the ventral surface. The infant should not be circumcised because the dorsal foreskin tissue will be used for surgical repair of the hypospadias. Options 2, 3, and 4 are unrelated to this disorder.
Test-Taking Strategy: Use the process of elimination. Note the key words "indicates their understanding." Recalling that hypospadias is a congenital defect involving abnormal placement of the urethral orifice of the penis will direct you to option 1. Review the treatment plan related to the repair of the hypospadias if you had difficulty with this question.
Level of Cognitive Ability: Comprehension
Client Needs: Health Promotion and Maintenance
Integrated Concept/Process: Teaching/Learning
Content Area: Child Health
Reference: Wong D, Hockenberry-Eaton M: *Wong's essentials of pediatric nursing,* ed 6, St Louis, 2001, Mosby, p. 1042.

13. *Answer:* 4
Rationale: Bladder exstrophy is a congenital anomaly characterized by the extrusion of the urinary bladder to the outside of the body through a defect in the lower abdominal wall. The cause in not known and a higher incidence occurs in males. Options 1, 2, and 3 are not characteristics of this disorder.
Test Taking Strategy: Use the process of elimination. If you are unfamiliar with this condition, note the relationship of "ex"strophy in the name of the disorder to the word "ex"trusion in the correct option. This should remind you that this condition is located external to the body. If you had difficulty with this question, review the characteristics of bladder exstrophy.
Level of Cognitive Ability: Comprehension
Client Needs: Physiological Integrity
Integrated Concept/Process: Nursing Process/Planning
Content Area: Child Health

Reference: McKinney E et al: *Maternal-child nursing,* Philadelphia, 2000, WB Saunders, p. 1175.

14. ***Answer:*** 2

Rationale: In bladder exstrophy, the bladder is exposed and external to the body. The highest priority is impaired tissue integrity related to the exposed bladder mucosa. Although the infant needs to be monitored for elimination patterns and kidney function, this is not the priority concern for this condition. Parental knowledge deficit related to the diagnosis and treatment of the condition will need to be addressed, but again is not the priority. Although infection related to the anatomically located defect is an appropriate nursing diagnosis, it is a potential problem and not an actual one.

Test-Taking Strategy: Use the process of elimination. Eliminate option 4 first because this addresses a potential problem rather than an actual one. Eliminate option 3 next because physiological needs take precedence over psychosocial needs. From the remaining options, knowledge that the bladder mucosa is exposed in this condition should direct you to the correct option. Review this disorder if you had difficulty with this question.

Level of Cognitive Ability: Analysis

Client Needs: Physiological Integrity

Integrated Concept/Process: Nursing Process/Planning

Content Area: Child Health

Reference: McKinney E et al: *Maternal-child nursing.* Philadelphia, 2000, WB Saunders, p. 1175.

15. ***Answer:*** 3

Rationale: In this disorder, care must be taken to protect the exposed bladder tissue from drying while allowing the drainage of urine. This is best accomplished by covering the bladder with a nonadhering plastic wrap. The use of petroleum jelly gauze should be avoided because this type of dressing can dry out, adhere to the mucosa, and damage the delicate tissue when removed. Dry sterile dressings and dressings soaked in solutions (that can dry out) also damage the mucosa when removed.

Test-Taking Strategy: Use the process of elimination. Also, note the key word "nonadherent" in the correct option. If you had difficulty with this question, review care to the infant with bladder exstrophy.

Level of Cognitive Ability: Application

Client Needs: Physiological Integrity

Integrated Concept/Process: Nursing Process/Planning

Content Area: Child Health

Reference: McKinney E et al: *Maternal-child nursing,* Philadelphia, 2000, WB Saunders, p. 1175.

REFERENCES

Burroughs A, Leifer G: *Maternity nursing,* ed 8, Philadelphia, 2002, WB Saunders.

Hodgson B, Kizior R: *Saunders nursing drug handbook 2002,* Philadelphia, 2002, WB Saunders.

McKinney E et al: *Maternal-child nursing,* Philadelphia, 2000, WB Saunders.

Murray S, McKinney E, Gorrie T: *Foundations of maternal-newborn nursing,* ed 3, Philadelphia, 2002, WB Saunders.

Schulte E, Price D, Gwin J: *Thompson's pediatric nursing,* ed 8, Philadelphia, 2001, WB Saunders.

Wong D: *Whaley & Wong's nursing care of infants and children,* ed 6, St Louis, 1999, Mosby.

Wong D, Hockenberry-Eaton M: *Wong's essentials of pediatric nursing,* ed 6, St Louis, 2001, Mosby.

33 Integumentary Disorders

I. ECZEMA (ATOPIC DERMATITIS)

A. Description
1. A superficial inflammatory process involving primarily the epidermis
2. A common allergic reaction in children; sometimes caused by an allergic sensitivity to foods such as milk, fish, or eggs
3. Childhood eczema often begins in infancy, and the rash appears on the face, neck, and folds of elbows and knees; may persist for several years or return after the child is older

B. Data collection
1. Redness and itching
2. Minute papules and vesicles
3. Weeping, oozing, and crusting of lesions

C. Implementation
1. Avoid exposure to skin irritants such as soaps, detergents, fabric softeners, diaper wipes, and powder
2. Improve skin hydration
3. Apply cool, wet compresses to soothe the skin
4. Administer antihistamines and topical corticosteroids as prescribed; corticosteroids are applied in a thin layer and are rubbed into the area thoroughly
5. Prevent or minimize scratching; keep the nails short and clean and place gloves or cotton socks over the hands
6. Eliminate conditions that increase itching such as heat, woolen clothes or blankets, rough fabrics, or furry stuffed animals
7. Instruct the mother to wash clothing in a mild detergent and rinse thoroughly; putting the clothes through a second complete wash cycle without detergent will minimize the amount of residue remaining on the fabric
8. Instruct the mother in the measures to prevent skin infections
9. Instruct the mother to monitor the lesions for signs of infection (honey-colored crusts with surrounding erythema)

II. IMPETIGO

A. Description
1. Incubation period: 7 to 10 days
2. Infectious period: during the course of the infection
3. Transmission: contact
4. Season: summer

B. Data collection
1. Small, red macules that progress to vesicles and rupture and release serous fluid
2. Located around the mouth and nose and may be present on the extremities

C. Implementation
1. Contact isolation; use standard (universal) precautions and implement agency-specific isolation procedures for the hospitalized child
2. Allow lesions to dry by air exposure
3. Assist the child with daily bathing with antibacterial soap, such as pHisoHex, as prescribed
4. Apply warm compresses to lesions two to three times per day as prescribed to remove crusts and to allow for healing
5. Apply and instruct the parents in the use of antibiotic ointments; the infection is communicable for 48 hours after antibiotic ointment treatment is begun
6. Administer oral antibiotics, which may be prescribed if there is no response to topical antibiotic treatment

7. Apply and instruct the parents in the use of emollients as prescribed to prevent skin cracking
8. Instruct the parents in the methods to prevent the spread of the infection, especially careful handwashing
9. Inform the parents that the child needs to use separate towels, linens, and dishes
10. Inform the parents that all linens and clothing should be washed separately with detergent in hot water

III. PEDICULOSIS CAPITIS (LICE)

A. Description
   1. Incubation period: eggs incubate for about 1 week and lice reach sexual maturity in about 2 weeks
   2. Infectious period: during infestation before treatment
   3. Transmission: direct contact with infected person and indirect contact with infected person's belongings
   4. Season: nonspecific, a common problem in schools

B. Data collection
   1. Adult lice are difficult to see and appear as small gray specks that may crawl very fast
   2. Nits are visible and firmly attached to the hair shaft near the scalp; they are tiny silver or gray specks resembling dandruff

C. Implementation
   1. Use of a pediculicide shampoo; the hair is towel dried, the nits are removed with a fine-toothed comb, and the treatment is repeated in 7 days
   2. Use of permethrin (Nix) rinse
      a. Apply to washed and towel-dried hair, leave in place for 10 minutes, then rinse
      b. After rinsing, towel dry the hair, and remove the nits with a fine-toothed comb
   3. Instruct the parents in the use of shampoo and rinse as prescribed
   4. Instruct the parents that bedding and clothing used by the child should be changed daily, laundered in hot water with detergent, and dried in a hot dryer for 20 minutes
   5. Instruct the parents that nonessential bedding and clothing can be stored in a tightly sealed bag for 10 days to 2 weeks and then washed
   6. Instruct the parents to seal toys that cannot be washed or dry cleaned in a plastic bag for 2 weeks
   7. Instruct the parents that hairbrushes or combs should be discarded or soaked in hot water 54.4° C [130° F] for 15 minutes
   8. Instruct the parents that furniture and carpets need to be vacuumed frequently
   9. Teach the child not to share clothing, headwear, or brushes and combs

IV. SCABIES

A. Description
   1. Incubation period
      a. Female mite burrows into epidermis, lays eggs, and dies in the burrow after 4 to 5 weeks
      b. The eggs hatch in 3 to 5 days and larvae migrate to the skin to mature and complete their life cycle
   2. Infectious period: during the course of the infestation
   3. Transmission: by close personal contact with infected person
   4. Season: any time of the year

B. Data collection
   1. Intense pruritis, especially at night
   2. Burrows (fine grayish thread-like red lines that may be difficult to see) on the skin

C. Implementation
   1. Topical application of a scabicide such as lindane cream (Kwell, Scabene), crotamiton (Eurax), or permethrin 5% (Elimite)
   2. Lindane cream (Kwell, Scabene) should not be used in children younger than age 2 years because of the risk of neurotoxicity and seizures
   3. Instruct the parents in the application of the scabicide
      a. Application should be preceded by a warm soap and water bath
      b. Skin must be cool and dry before the application of the lotion
      c. Lotion is left in place for 8 to 14 hours before it is washed off
   4. When permethrin 5% (Elimite) is used, the cream is thoroughly and gently massaged into all skin surfaces (not just the areas that have the rash); care should be taken to avoid contact with the eyes
   5. Household members and contacts of the infected child need to be treated at the same time
   6. Instruct the parents about the importance of frequent handwashing
   7. Instruct the parents that all clothing, bedding, and pillowcases used by the child need to be changed daily, washed in hot water with detergent, dried in a hot dryer, and ironed before reuse

8. Instruct the parents that nonwashable toys and other items should be sealed in plastic bags for 4 days

V. TINEA (RINGWORM)

A. Description
   1. Known as tinea capitis (scalp); tinea corporis (body); tinea pedis (feet)
   2. A fungal infection spread by direct contact

B. Data collection
   1. Papules and dry scales
   2. Itching

C. Implementation
   1. Provide meticulous skin care
   2. Apply antifungal ointments as prescribed
   3. Administer oral antifungal medications as prescribed

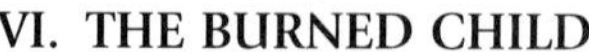

VI. THE BURNED CHILD

(Refer to Chapter 38 for additional information related to burns.)

A. Pediatric differences
   1. Very young children who have been severely burned have a higher mortality rate than older children and adults with comparable burns
   2. Lower burn temperatures and shorter exposure to heat can cause a more severe burn in a child than in an adult because a child's skin is thinner
   3. Severely burned children are at increased risk for fluid and heat loss, dehydration, and metabolic acidosis than an adult
   4. The higher proportion of body fluid to mass in children increases the risk of cardiovascular problems
   5. Burns involving more than 10% total body surface area (TBSA) require some form of fluid resuscitation
   6. Infants and children are at increased risk for protein and calorie deficiency because they have smaller muscle mass and lower body fat than adults
   7. Scarring is more severe in a child
   8. An immature immune system presents an increased risk of infection for infants and young children
   9. A delay in **growth** may occur after a burn

B. Extent of burn injury (Figure 33-1)
   1. The Rule of Nines gives an inaccurate estimate because of the differences in body proportion between children and adults

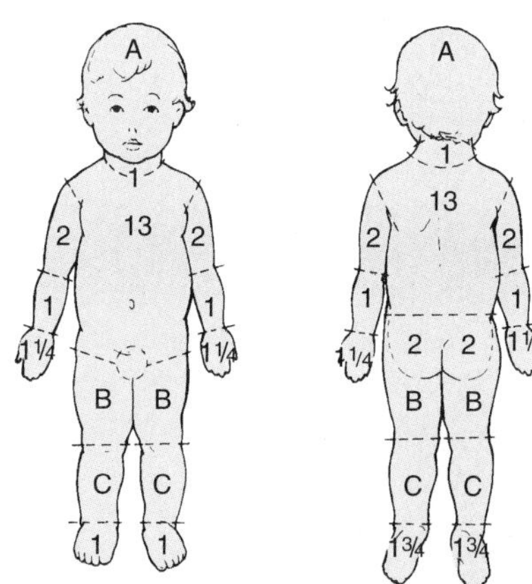

RELATIVE PERCENTAGES OF AREAS AFFECTED BY GROWTH

AREA	BIRTH	AGE 1 YR	AGE 5 YR
A = 1/2 of head	9 1/2	8 1/2	6 1/2
B = 1/2 of one thigh	2 3/4	3 1/4	4
C = 1/2 of one leg	2 1/2	2 1/2	2 3/4

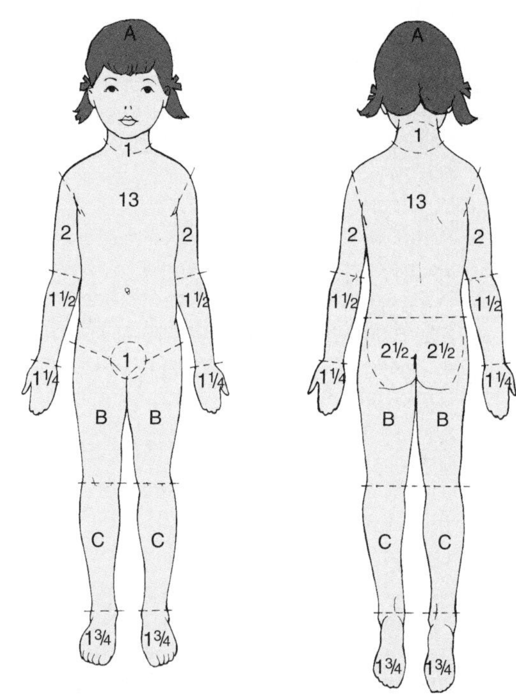

RELATIVE PERCENTAGES OF AREAS AFFECTED BY GROWTH

AREA	AGE 10 YR	AGE 15 YR	ADULT
A = 1/2 of head	5 1/2	4 1/2	3 1/2
B = 1/2 of one thigh	4 1/2	4 1/2	4 3/4
C = 1/2 of one leg	3	3 1/4	3 1/2

FIG. 33-1 Estimation of distribution of burns in children. (From Wong D, Hockenberry-Eaton M: *Wong's essentials of pediatric nursing*, ed 6, St Louis, 2001, Mosby.)

   2. A modified Rule of Nines may be used for the pediatric population

PRACTICE QUESTIONS

1. Corticream is prescribed by the physician for a child with atopic dermatitis (eczema) and the nurse instructs the mother how to appropriately apply the cream. The nurse tells the mother to:
   1. Avoid cleansing the area before applying the cream
   2. Apply the cream over the entire body
   3. Apply a thin layer of cream and rub into the area thoroughly
   4. Apply a thick layer of cream in affected areas only
2. A nurse assists in providing an instructional session to parents regarding impetigo. Which statement by a parent indicates a need for further instruction?
   1. "It is most common in humid weather."
   2. "It begins in an area of broken skin, such as an insect bite."
   3. "It is extremely contagious."
   4. "Lesions are most often located on the arms and chest."
3. A nurse provides instructions to the mother of a child with impetigo regarding the application of antibiotic ointment. The mother asks the nurse when the child can return to school. The most appropriate response is:
   1. 24 hours after using antibiotic ointment
   2. 48 hours after using antibiotic ointment
   3. 1 week after using antibiotic ointment
   4. 10 days after using antibiotic ointment
4. A nurse provides instructions regarding the use of permethrin 1% (Nix) to the parents of a child diagnosed with pediculosis (head lice). Which statement by a parent indicates a need for further instruction?
   1. "The medication can be obtained over-the-counter in a local pharmacy."
   2. "The medication is applied to the hair after shampooing and left on for 24 hours."
   3. "The medication is applied to the hair after shampooing, left on for 10 minutes, and then rinsed out."
   4. "The hair should not be shampooed for 24 hours after treatment."
5. A nurse prepares a list of home care instructions for the parents of schoolchildren diagnosed with pediculosis (head lice). Which of the following is included in this list?
   1. Use antilice sprays on all bedding and furniture
   2. Take all bedding and linens to the cleaners to be dry cleaned
   3. Boil combs and brushes in hot water for 2 hours
   4. Vacuum floors, play areas, and furniture to remove any hairs that might carry live nits
6. A mother of a 3-year-old child tells the nurse that the child has been continuously scratching the skin and has developed a rash. The nurse inspects the child and suspects the presence of scabies if which of the following is observed?
   1. Clusters of fluid-filled vesicles
   2. Fine thread-like lines
   3. Purple-colored lesions
   4. Thick, honey-colored crusts
7. Permethrin 5% (Elimite) is prescribed for a 4-year-old child with a diagnosis of scabies. The nurse instructs the mother regarding the use of this treatment and tells the mother to:
   1. Apply the lotion from head to toe
   2. Apply the lotion and leave it on for 4 hours
   3. Apply the lotion to cool, dry skin at least 1/2 hour after bathing
   4. Avoid clothing the child while the lotion is in place
8. A 2-year-old child is admitted to the burn unit with partial and full-thickness burns over 35% of the body. The nurse assisting in caring for the child plans care understanding that the priority nursing intervention is:
   1. Sedating the child with morphine sulfate
   2. Restricting IV fluids
   3. Inserting a nasogastric tube
   4. Inserting a Foley catheter
9. Griseofulvin (Fulvicin, Grisactin) is prescribed for a child with tinea capitis and the nurse provides instructions to the mother regarding administration of the medication. Which statement by the mother indicates a need for further instructions?
   1. "I need to administer the medication 2 hours before meals."
   2. "I need to shake the oral suspension before preparing the dose."
   3. "I need to continue the therapy as long as it is prescribed."
   4. "I need to keep my child out of the sun."
10. A nurse is providing home care instructions to an adolescent who has been diagnosed with tinea pedis. Which statement by the adolescent indicates a need for further instruction?
    1. "I need to dry my feet carefully especially between the toes."
    2. "I need to wear clean socks."
    3. "I need to wear shoes that are well ventilated."
    4. "I should wear plastic shoes as much as possible."

ANSWERS

1. *Answer:* 3
Rationale: Corticream is a topical corticosteroid. It should be applied sparingly and rubbed into the area thoroughly. The affected area should be cleansed gently before application. It should not be applied over extensive areas. Systemic absorption is more likely to occur with extensive application.
Test-Taking Strategy: Use the process of elimination. Eliminate option 1 because it does not make sense to avoid cleansing an affected area. Eliminate option 2 because cream should be applied only to the area that is affected. Eliminate option 4 because of the words "thick" and "only." Review the procedure for application of this cream if you had difficulty with this question.
Level of Cognitive Ability: Application
Client Needs: Health Promotion and Maintenance
Integrated Concept/Process: Teaching/Learning
Content Area: Child Health
Reference: Hodgson B, Kizior R: *Saunders nursing drug handbook 2002*, Philadelphia, 2002, WB Saunders, p. 68.

2. *Answer:* 4
Rationale: Impetigo is most common during hot, humid summer months. It begins in an area of broken skin, such as an insect bite. It may be caused by ***Staphylococcus aureus***, group A beta-hemolytic streptococci, or a combination of these bacteria. It is extremely contagious. Lesions are usually located around the mouth and nose, but may be present on the extremities.
Test-Taking Strategy: Use the process of elimination and note the key words "indicates a need for further instruction." Recalling that the lesions are most commonly located around the mouth and nose will direct you to option 4. Review this disorder if you had difficulty with this question.
Level of Cognitive Ability: Comprehension
Client Needs: Health Promotion and Maintenance
Integrated Concept/Process: Teaching/Learning
Content Area: Child Health
Reference: Schulte E, Price D, Gwin J: *Thompson's pediatric nursing*, ed 8, Philadelphia, 2001, WB Saunders, p. 153.

3. *Answer:* 2
Rationale: The child should not attend school for 24 to 48 hours after the initiation of systemic antibiotics or 48 hours after using antibiotic ointment. The school should be notified of the diagnosis.
Test-Taking Strategy: Use knowledge related to the administration of antibiotics to answer the question. Eliminate options 3 and 4 first because the time frames are closely related and rather lengthy. Note the key word "ointment" in the question; this should assist in directing you to option 2. Review the treatment measures for impetigo if you had difficulty with this question.
Level of Cognitive Ability: Application
Client Needs: Safe, Effective Care Environment
Integrated Concept/Process: Nursing Process/Implementation
Content Area: Child Health
Reference: Schulte E, Price D, Gwin J: *Thompson's pediatric nursing*, ed 8, Philadelphia, 2001, WB Saunders, p. 153.

4. *Answer:* 2
Rationale: Permethrin 1% is an over-the-counter antilice product that kills both lice and eggs with one application and has residual activity for 10 days. It is applied to the hair after shampooing and left for 10 minutes before rinsing out. The hair should not be shampooed for 24 hours after the treatment.
Test-Taking Strategy: Use the process of elimination and note the key words "need for further instruction" in the stem of the question. Recalling the treatment for the use of this medication will direct you to option 2. Review this treatment if you had difficulty with this question.
Level of Cognitive Ability: Comprehension
Client Needs: Health Promotion and Maintenance
Integrated Concept/Process: Teaching/Learning
Content Area: Child Health
Reference: Schulte E, Price D, Gwin J: *Thompson's pediatric nursing*, ed 8, Philadelphia, 2001, WB Saunders, p. 297.

5. *Answer:* 4
Rationale: Antilice sprays are unnecessary. Additionally, they should never be used on a child. Bedding and linens should be washed with hot water and dried on a hot setting. Items that cannot be washed should be dry cleaned or sealed in plastic bags in a warm place for 3 weeks. Combs and brushes should be boiled or soaked in antilice shampoo or hot water for 15 minutes. Thorough home cleaning is necessary to remove any remaining lice or nits.
Test-Taking Strategy: Use the process of elimination. Eliminate option 1 knowing that antilice sprays should not be used. Knowing that bedding and linens can be washed will eliminate option 2. The time for boiling in option 3 is rather lengthy; therefore, eliminate this option. Review home care instructions regarding pediculosis if you had difficulty with this question.
Level of Cognitive Ability: Application
Client Needs: Safe, Effective Care Environment
Integrated Concept/Process: Nursing Process/Implementation
Content Area: Child Health
Reference: Schulte E, Price D, Gwin J: *Thompson's pediatric nursing*, ed 8, Philadelphia, 2001, WB Saunders, p. 297.

6. *Answer:* 2
Rationale: Scabies appears as burrows or fine, grayish thread-like lines. They may be difficult to see if they are obscured by excoriation and inflammation. Clusters of fluid-filled vesicles are seen in herpes virus. Thick, honey-colored crusts are characteristic of impetigo. Purple-colored lesions may be indicative of various disorders, including systemic conditions.
Test-Taking Strategy: Use the process of elimination. Recalling that scabies infestation produces burrows will assist in directing you to option 2. Review the characteristics of scabies if you had difficulty with this question.
Level of Cognitive Ability: Comprehension
Client Needs: Physiological Integrity
Integrated Concept/Process: Nursing Process/Data Collection
Content Area: Child Health
Reference: Wong D, Hockenberry-Eaton M: *Wong's essentials of pediatric nursing*, ed 6, St Louis, 2001, Mosby, p. 1169.

7. *Answer:* 3
Rationale: Permethrin is applied from the neck downward, making sure that the soles of the feet, behind the ears, and under the toenails and fingernails are covered. The lotion should be kept on for 8 to 14 hours, and then the child should be given a bath. The lotion should not be applied for at least one-half hour after bathing and should be applied only to cool, dry skin. The child should be clothed during treatment.
Test-Taking Strategy: Use the process of elimination. Reading options 1 and 4 carefully will assist in eliminating these options. From the remaining options, recalling the treatment time for this medication will assist in directing you to option 3. Review this treatment if you had difficulty with this question.
Level of Cognitive Ability: Application
Client Needs: Safe, Effective Care Environment
Integrated Concept/Process: Teaching/Learning
Content Area: Child Health
Reference: Wong D, Hockenberry-Eaton M: *Wong's essentials of pediatric nursing,* ed 6, St Louis, 2001, Mosby, p. 1169.

8. *Answer:* 4
Rationale: A Foley catheter is inserted into the child's bladder so that urine output can be accurately measured on an hourly basis. Although pain medication may be required, the child should not be sedated. Intravenous fluids are not restricted and are administered at a rate sufficient to maintain adequate tissue perfusion. A nasogastric tube may or may not be required but would not be the priority intervention.
Test-Taking Strategy: Use the process of elimination and note the key word "priority." Option 1 can be eliminated first because the child should not be sedated. Eliminate option 2 next, knowing that fluid resuscitation is an important component of therapy to prevent burn shock. From the remaining options, recalling that urine output reflects adequate tissue perfusion will direct you to option 4. Review the treatment of burns if you had difficulty with this question.
Level of Cognitive Ability: Application
Client Needs: Physiological Integrity
Integrated Concept/Process: Nursing Process/Planning
Content Area: Child Health
Reference: Schulte E, Price D, Gwin J: *Thompson's pediatric nursing,* ed 8, Philadelphia, 2001, WB Saunders, p. 322.

9. *Answer:* 1
Rationale: Griseofulvin is given with or after meals to avoid gastrointestinal (GI) irritation and increase absorption. Oral suspensions should be shaken well. Parents are instructed to continue therapy as prescribed and not to miss a dose. Exposure to the sun is avoided during treatment.
Test-Taking Strategy: Use the process of elimination and note the key words "need for further instructions" in the stem of the question. Recalling that this medication causes GI irritation will direct you to option 1. Review this medication if you had difficulty with this question.
Level of Cognitive Ability: Comprehension
Client Needs: Physiological Integrity
Integrated Concept/Process: Teaching/Learning
Content Area: Child Health
Reference: Hodgson B, Kizior R: *Saunders nursing drug handbook 2002,* Philadelphia, 2002, WB Saunders, p. 520.

10. *Answer:* 4
Rationale: Plastic shoes retain heat and should be avoided because this condition is aggravated by heat and moisture. Options 1, 2, and 3 are appropriate measures to treat this condition.
Test-Taking Strategy: Use the process of elimination. Note the key words "a need for further instruction." Recalling that heat and moisture aggravate the condition will direct you to option 4. Review the measures to treat tinea pedis if you had difficulty with this question.
Level of Cognitive Ability: Comprehension
Client Needs: Health Promotion and Maintenance
Integrated Concept/Process: Teaching/Learning
Content Area: Child Health
Reference: Schulte E, Price D, Gwin J: *Thompson's pediatric nursing,* ed 8, Philadelphia, 2001, WB Saunders, p. 297.

REFERENCES

Burroughs A, Leifer G: *Maternity nursing,* ed 8, Philadelphia, 2002, WB Saunders.
Hodgson B, Kizior R: *Saunders nursing drug handbook* ***2002***, Philadelphia, 2002, WB Saunders.
McKinney E et al: *Maternal-child nursing,* Philadelphia, 2000, WB Saunders.
Murray S, McKinney E, Gorrie T: *Foundations of maternal-newborn nursing,* ed 3, Philadelphia, 2002, WB Saunders.
Schulte E, Price D, Gwin J: *Thompson's pediatric nursing,* ed 8, Philadelphia, 2001, WB Saunders.
Wong D: *Whaley & Wong's nursing care of infants and children,* ed 6, St Louis, 1999, Mosby.
Wong D, Hockenberry-Eaton M: *Wong's essentials of pediatric nursing,* ed 6, St Louis, 2001, Mosby.

Dysplasia of the Hip

I. DYSPLASIA OF THE HIP

A. Description
   1. A condition in which the head of the femur is improperly seated in the acetabulum or hip socket of the pelvis
   2. Can range from very mild to severely dislocated
   3. Can be congenital or develop after birth

B. Data collection (Figure 34-1)
   1. Neonates: laxity of the ligaments around the hip, which allows the femoral head to be displaced from the acetabulum upon manipulation
   2. Infants beyond the newborn period
      a. Asymmetry of the gluteal skinfolds when placed prone and the legs are extended against the examining table
      b. Limited range of motion (ROM) in the affected hip
      c. Asymmetrical abduction of the affected hip when placed supine with the knees and hips flexed
      d. Apparent short femur on the affected side (Galeazzi sign)
   3. The walking child: minimal to pronounced variations in gait with lurching toward the affected side
   4. Positive Barlow or Ortolani maneuver

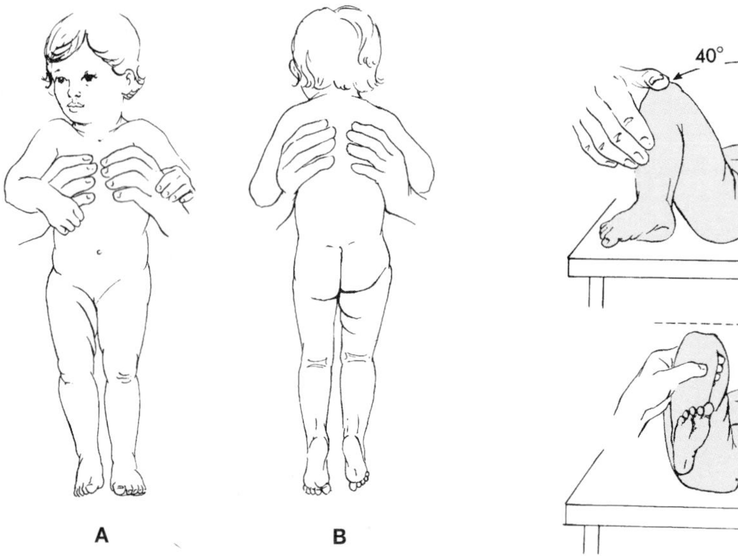

FIG. 34-1 The three classic signs of congenital hip dysplasia. (From Tachdjean M: *Pediatric Orthopedics*, Philadelphia, 1990, W.B. Saunders.)

C. Implementation
1. In the neonatal period, splinting of the hips with Pavlik harness to maintain flexion and abduction and external rotation
2. After the neonatal period, traction, and/or surgery to release muscles and tendons
3. Positioning and immobilization in a spica cast after surgery until healing is achieved
4. Osteotomy after traction in profoundly affected children
5. Instruct parents regarding proper care of a Pavlik harness or spica cast (Figures 34-2 and 34-3)

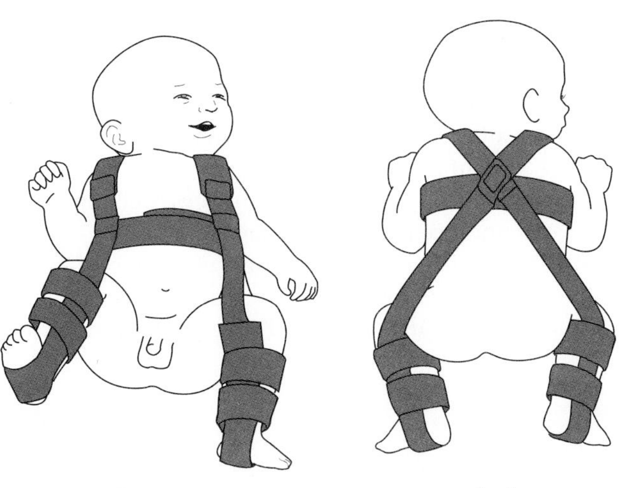

FIG. 34-2 Pavlik harness. (From Ball JW: *Mosby's pediatric patient teachings*, St Louis, 2001, Mosby.)

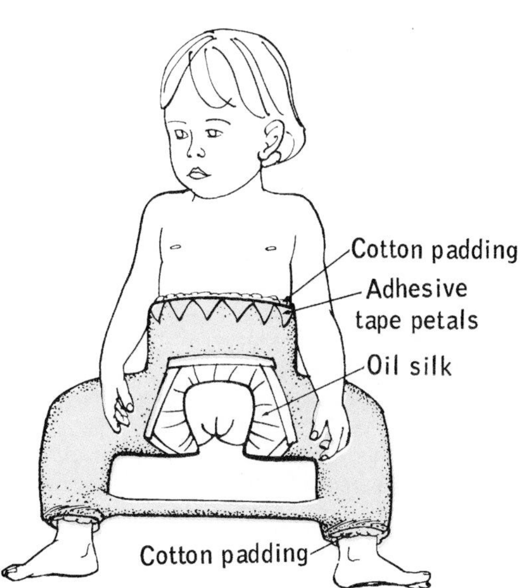

FIG. 34-3 Body (spica) cast. (From Leifer G: Principles and teachings in pediatric nursing, ed 4 Philadelphia, 1982, WB Saunders.)

II. CONGENITAL CLUBFOOT (Figure 34-4)

A. Description
1. A congenital malformation of the lower extremities
2. The defect may be unilateral or bilateral
3. Defects are rigid and cannot be manipulated into a neutral position
4. Long-term interval follow-up care is required until the child reaches skeletal maturity

B. Data collection: the foot is plantar flexed with an inverted heel and adducted forefoot

C. Implementation
1. Treatment begins as soon as possible after birth
2. Serial manipulation and casting are performed weekly, and if correction is not achieved in 3 to 6 months, surgery is indicated
3. Monitor for pain
4. Monitor neurovascular status of the toes
5. Instruct parents in cast care and signs of neurovascular impairment requiring physician notification

III. SCOLIOSIS

A. Description
1. A lateral curvature of the spine
2. Surgical and nonsurgical interventions are used and the type of treatment depends on the degree of curvature, the age of the child, and the amount of **growth** that is anticipated

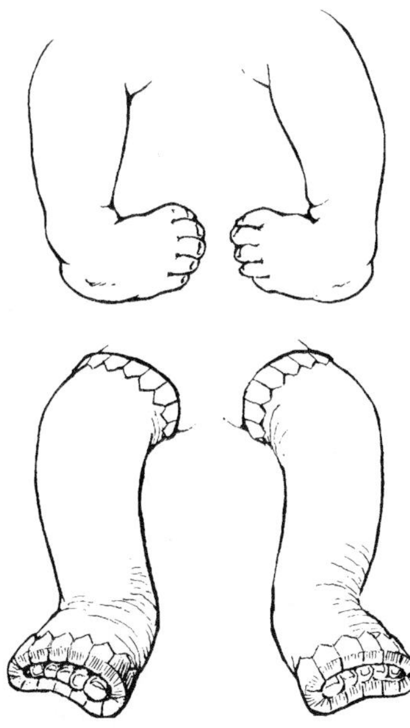

FIG. 34-4 Clubfoot. (From Leifer G: Principles and teachings in pediatric nursing, ed 4 Philadelphia, 1982, WB Saunders.)

3. Long-term monitoring is essential to detect any progression of the curve

B. Data collection
1. Visible curve fails to straighten when the child bends forward and hangs the arms down toward the feet
2. Hips, ribs, and shoulders are asymmetrical
3. Apparent leg length discrepancy

C. Implementation
1. Monitor progression of the curvature
2. Prepare the child for the use of a brace if prescribed
3. Prepare the child and parents for surgery (spinal fusion or internal instrumentation rods) if prescribed

D. Postoperative implementation
1. Maintain flat position
2. Logroll the child when turning to maintain alignment
3. Monitor extremities for neurovascular status
4. Encourage coughing and deep breathing and use of incentive spirometry
5. Monitor for pain and administer prescribed analgesics
6. Monitor for incontinence
7. Instruct the child in activity restrictions
8. Instruct the child to roll from a side-lying position to a sitting position and assist with ambulation

E. Braces
1. Instruct the child to wear the brace as prescribed
2. Inspect the skin for signs of redness or breakdown
3. Keep the skin clean and dry, avoiding lotions and powders
4. Advise the child to wear soft nonirritating clothing under the brace
5. Instruct in prescribed exercises
6. Encourage verbalization about body image

IV. JUVENILE RHEUMATOID ARTHRITIS (JRA)

A. Description
1. An autoimmune inflammatory disease affecting the joints; occurs most often in girls
2. The cause is unknown
3. Juvenile onset is diagnosed before age 16 years
4. Iridocyclitis is a unique complication of JRA
5. Treatment is supportive and directed toward preserving joint function, controlling inflammation, minimizing deformity, and reducing the impact that the disease may have on the development of the child
6. Therapy includes medications, physical and occupational therapies, and family education
7. Surgical intervention may be implemented when the child has problems with joint contractures and unequal growth of extremities

B. Data collection (Table 34-1)

C. Implementation
1. Facilitate social and emotional development
2. Instruct the parents and child in the administration of medications as prescribed, such as nonsteroidal antiinflammatory drugs (NSAIDs) and antirheumatic medications
3. Encourage normal performance of activities of daily living (ADL)
4. Assist the child with ROM and prescribed exercises
5. Instruct the parents and child in the use of hot or cold packs, splinting, and positioning the affected joint in a neutral position during painful episodes
6. Encourage and support prescribed physical and occupational therapy
7. Instruct in the importance of preventive eye care and reporting visual disturbances
8. Determine the child's perception regarding the chronic illness

V. FRACTURES

A. Description
1. A break in the continuity of the bone as a result of trauma, twisting, or bone decalcification
2. Fractures in children usually result from increased mobility and inadequate or immature motor and cognitive skills
3. Fractures in infancy are generally rare and warrant further investigation to rule out the possibility of child **abuse**
4. The most frequently seen fracture in children is in the forearm

TABLE 34-1

Characteristics of JRA

Systemic JRA	Pauciarticular JRA	Polyarticular JRA
Fever	Mild joint pain and swelling	Morning joint stiffness
Salmon-pink rash	Affects large joints	Low-grade fever
Affects five or more joints	Affects no more than 4 joints	Affects weight-bearing joints
May also have anorexia, anemia, fatigue	Iridocyclitis and visual disturbances	Affects five or more joints

B. Data collection
   1. Pain or tenderness over the involved area
   2. Loss of function
   3. Obvious deformity
   4. Crepitation
   5. Erythema, ecchymosis, and edema
   6. Muscle spasm
C. Initial care of a fracture
   1. Immobilize affected extremity
   2. If a compound fracture exists, splint the extremity and cover the wound with a sterile dressing
D. Implementation
   1. Reduction
      a. Restoring the bone to proper alignment
      b. Closed reduction: may require general anesthesia and is accomplished by manual alignment of the fragments followed by immobilization
      c. Open reduction: requires the surgical insertion of internal fixation devices such as rods, wires, or pins that help maintain alignment while healing occurs
   2. Retention: the application of traction or a cast to maintain alignment until healing occurs
E. Traction
   1. Russell skin traction
      a. Used to stabilize a fractured femur before surgery
      b. Similar to Buck's traction but provides a double pull with the use of a knee sling
      c. Traction pulls at the knee and foot
      d. Position the child with the foot of the bed slightly elevated
   2. Balanced suspension
      a. Used with skin or skeletal traction
      b. Used to approximate fractures of the femur, tibia, or fibula
      c. Produced by a counterforce other than the child
      d. Position the child in low-Fowler's position, either on the side or back
      e. Maintain a 20-degree angle from the thigh to the bed
      f. Protect the skin from breakdown
      g. Provide pin care if pins are used with the skeletal traction
      h. Clean pin site with normal saline and hydrogen peroxide or Betadine as prescribed
F. Casts
   1. Description
      a. Made of plaster or fiberglass to provide immobilization of bone and joints after a fracture or injury
      b. Fractures of the hip and knee may require a spica cast
   2. Implementation
      a. Examine the cast for pressure areas
      b. Monitor the extremity for circulatory impairment, such as pain, swelling, discoloration, tingling, numbness, or coolness or diminished pulse
      c. Notify the physician if circulatory impairment occurs
      d. Prepare for bivalving or cutting the cast if circulatory impairment occurs
      e. Instruct the child not to stick objects down the cast
      f. Teach the child to keep the cast clean and dry
      g. Instruct the child in isometric exercises to prevent muscle atrophy

PRACTICE QUESTIONS

1. A nurse is assisting a physician during the examination of an infant with hip dysplasia and the physician performs the Ortolani maneuver. The nurse understands that this maneuver is performed to:
   1. Push the unstable femoral head out of the acetabulum
   2. Reduce the dislocated femoral head back into the acetabulum
   3. Determine the extent of range of motion
   4. Check for asymmetry on the affected side
2. A 6-month-old infant is seen in the clinic and is diagnosed with unilateral hip dysplasia. The nurse reviews the health care record and understands that which of the following findings would not be noted in this condition?
   1. An apparent short femur on the affected side
   2. Limited range of motion in the affected hip
   3. Adduction of the affected hip when placed supine with the knees and hips flexed
   4. Asymmetry of the gluteal skin folds when the infant is placed prone and the legs are extended against the examining table
3. A nurse reinforces instructions to the parents of an infant with hip dysplasia regarding care of the Pavlik harness. The nurse tells the parents that the:
   1. Harness should be worn 12 hours a day
   2. Harness needs be removed for diaper changes and for feeding
   3. Harness should be removed to check the skin, and for bathing
   4. Infant should never be moved when out of the harness
4. A nurse provides information to the mother of a 2-week-old infant diagnosed at birth with clubfoot.

Which statement by the mother indicates a need for further instruction regarding this disorder?
  1. "I need to bring my child back to the clinic in 1 month for a new cast."
  2. "Treatment needs to be started as soon as possible."
  3. "I need to come to the clinic every week with my child for the casting."
  4. "I realize my child will require follow-up care until full grown."

5. A nurse is assigned to care for a child after spinal fusion for the treatment of scoliosis. The child complains of abdominal discomfort and begins to have episodes of vomiting. On further data collection, the nurse notes abdominal distention. Which of the following nursing actions would be most appropriate?
   1. Administer an antiemetic
   2. Place the child in a side-lying Sims' position
   3. Notify the registered nurse (RN)
   4. Increase the IV fluids
6. A nurse is providing instructions to the parents of a child with scoliosis regarding the use of a brace. Which statement by a parent indicates a need for further instruction?
   1. "I will apply lotion under the brace to prevent skin breakdown."
   2. "I need to avoid applying powder under the brace because it will cake."
   3. "I need to have my child wear a soft fabric under the brace."
   4. "I need to encourage my child to perform prescribed exercises."
7. The mother of a child with juvenile rheumatoid arthritis (JRA) calls the nurse because the child is experiencing a painful exacerbation of the disease. The mother asks the nurse if the child should perform the range of motion (ROM) exercises at this time. The most appropriate nursing response is:
   1. "The ROM exercises must be performed every day."
   2. "Avoid all exercise during painful periods."
   3. "Administer additional pain medication before performing ROM exercises."
   4. "Have the child perform simple isometric exercises during this time."
8. A 4-year-old child sustains a fall at home and is brought to the emergency room by the mother. After x-ray studies, it was determined that the child has a fractured arm and a plaster cast is applied. The nurse provides instructions to the mother regarding cast care for the child. Which statement by the mother indicates a need for further instruction?
   1. "The cast may feel warm as the cast dries."
   2. "If the cast becomes wet, a blow drier set on the cool setting may be used to dry the cast."
   3. "A small amount of white shoe polish can touch up a soiled white cast."
   4. "I can use lotion or powder around the cast edges to relieve itching."
9. A nurse is assigned to care for a child with a spica cast. The nurse avoids which of the following when caring for the child?
   1. Checks neurovascular status of the extremities
   2. Observes for nonverbal signs of pain
   3. Places the child on a stretcher and brings the child to the playroom
   4. Uses pillows to elevate the head and the shoulders
10. A child with a fractured femur is placed in Buck's skin traction. The nurse plans care knowing that this type of traction:
    1. Requires frequent pin care
    2. Places the child at risk for infection
    3. Is a type of skin traction that pulls the hip and leg into extension
    4. Uses skeletal traction and weights to provide a counterforce
11. A nurse is preparing to perform a neurovascular check for tissue perfusion in the child with an arm cast. Which of the following is the priority in performing this procedure?
    1. Taking the blood pressure
    2. Taking the temperature
    3. Checking the apical heart rate
    4. Checking the peripheral pulse in the affected arm
12. A nurse is checking the capillary refill in a child with a cast applied to the left arm. The nurse compresses the nail bed of a finger, and it returns to its original color in 2 seconds. Based on this finding, the most appropriate action is to:
    1. Notify the registered nurse (RN)
    2. Document the findings
    3. Prepare the child for bivalving the cast
    4. Elevate the extremity and recheck the capillary refill immediately
13. A nurse is performing a neurovascular check on a child with a cast applied to the lower leg. The child complains of tingling in the toes distal to the fracture site. The most appropriate nursing action is to:
    1. Ambulate the child with crutches
    2. Elevate the extremity
    3. Document the findings
    4. Notify the registered nurse (RN)
14. A nurse is assigned to care for a child in skeletal traction. The nurse avoids which of the following when caring for the child?
    1. Keeping the weights hanging freely
    2. Placing the bed linen on the traction ropes
    3. Ensuring that the ropes are in the pulleys
    4. Ensuring that the weights are out of the child's reach

15. The nurse is reinforcing information to the mother of a child about a synthetic cast that has been applied to the child for the treatment of a clubfoot. Which of the following information will the nurse provide to the mother?

1. The cast takes 24 hours to dry
2. The cast is heavier than a plaster cast
3. The cast is stronger than a plaster cast
4. The cast allows for greater mobility than a plaster cast

ANSWERS

1. *Answer:* 2
Rationale: In the Barlow maneuver, the examiner pushes the unstable femoral head out of the acetabulum. In the Ortolani maneuver the examiner reduces the dislocated femoral head back into the acetabulum. A positive effect of the Ortolani maneuver is a palpable clink on entry or exit of the femoral head over the acetabular ring. Options 3 and 4 are data collection techniques for identification of the clinical manifestations of hip dysplasia but do not describe the Ortolani maneuver.
Test-Taking Strategy: Use the process of elimination. Eliminate option 3 and 4 first because they are data collection techniques. From the remaining options, it is necessary to know the purpose of Ortolani maneuver. Review the purpose of this maneuver if you had difficulty with this question.
Level of Cognitive Ability: Comprehension
Client Needs: Physiological Integrity
Integrated Concept/Process: Nursing Process/Data Collection
Content Area: Child Health
Reference: Schulte E, Price D, Gwin J: *Thompson's pediatric nursing,* ed 8, Philadelphia, 2001, WB Saunders, p. 93.

2. *Answer:* 3
Rationale: Asymmetrical abduction of the affected hip, when placed supine with the knees and hips flexed, would be a finding in hip dysplasia in infants beyond the newborn period. Options 1, 2, and 4 are accurate assessment findings in this disorder.
Test-Taking Strategy: Use the process of elimination and note the key word "not." Attempt to visualize each of the findings described in the options. This will assist in directing you to option 3. Review the findings in hip dysplasia if you had difficulty with this question.
Level of Cognitive Ability: Comprehension
Client Needs: Physiological Integrity
Integrated Concept/Process: Nursing Process/Data Collection
Content Area: Child Health
Reference: Schulte E, Price D, Gwin J: *Thompson's pediatric nursing,* ed 8, Philadelphia, 2001, WB Saunders, p. 93.

3. *Answer:* 3
Rationale: The harness should be worn 23 hours a day and should be removed only to check the skin, and for bathing. The hips and buttocks should be supported carefully when the infant is out of the harness. The harness does not need to be removed for diaper changes or feedings.
Test-Taking Strategy: Attempt to visualize this harness to answer the question. This will assist in eliminating options 2 and 4. Select option 3 over option 1 because the timeframe in option 1 is rather low. Review home care instruction regarding this harness if you had difficulty with this question.
Level of Cognitive Ability: Application
Client Needs: Health Promotion and Maintenance
Integrated Concept/Process: Teaching/Learning
Content Area: Child Health
Reference: Schulte E, Price D, Gwin J: *Thompson's pediatric nursing,* ed 8, Philadelphia, 2001, WB Saunders, p. 93.

4. *Answer:* 1
Rationale: Treatment for clubfoot is started as soon as possible after birth. Serial manipulation and casting are performed at least weekly. If sufficient correction is not achieved in 3 to 6 months, surgery is usually indicated. Because clubfoot can recur, all children with clubfoot require long-term follow-up care until they reach skeletal maturity to ensure an optimal outcome.
Test-Taking Strategy: Use the process of elimination and focus on the issue, the treatment plan for clubfoot. Note the key words "indicates a need for further instruction" to assist in eliminating options 2 and 4. Recalling that serial manipulations and casting are required weekly will assist in directing you to option 1. Review these treatment procedures if you had difficulty with this question.
Level of Cognitive Ability: Comprehension
Client Needs: Physiological Integrity
Integrated Concept/Process: Teaching/Learning
Content Area: Child Health
Reference: Schulte E, Price D, Gwin J: *Thompson's pediatric nursing,* ed 8, Philadelphia, 2001, WB Saunders, p. 92.

5. *Answer:* 3
Rationale: A complication after surgical treatment of scoliosis is superior mesenteric artery syndrome. This disorder is caused by mechanical changes in the position of the child's abdominal contents, resulting from lengthening of the child's body. It results in a syndrome of emesis and abdominal distention similar to that which occurs with intestinal obstruction or paralytic ileus. Postoperative vomiting in children with body casts or those who have undergone spinal fusion warrants attention because of the possibility of superior mesenteric artery syndrome.
Test-Taking Strategy: Use the process of elimination. Eliminate option 4 first because it should not be implemented without a prescribed order. Eliminate option 2 next because this child requires logrolling and the Sims' position may cause injury after surgery. From the remaining options, note the signs and symptoms in the question. These should alert you that the RN needs to be notified. Review superior mesenteric artery syndrome if you had difficulty with this question.

Level of Cognitive Ability: Application
Client Needs: Physiological Integrity
Integrated Concept/Process: Nursing Process/Implementation
Content Area: Child Health
Reference: Schulte E, Price D, Gwin J: *Thompson's pediatric nursing,* ed 8, Philadelphia, 2001, WB Saunders, p. 319.

6. *Answer:* 1
Rationale: Both the use of lotions or powders should be avoided because they can become sticky or cake under the brace causing irritation. Options 2, 3, and 4 are appropriate statements regarding care to a child with a brace.
Test-Taking Strategy: Use the process of elimination and note the key words "need for further instruction." Recalling that lotions and powders need to be avoided will assist in directing you to option 1. Review home care instructions regarding the care of a child in a brace if you had difficulty with this question.
Level of Cognitive Ability: Comprehension
Client Needs: Health Promotion and Maintenance
Integrated Concept/Process: Teaching/Learning
Content Area: Child Health
Reference: Schulte E, Price D, Gwin J: *Thompson's pediatric nursing,* ed 8, Philadelphia, 2001, WB Saunders, p. 321.

7. *Answer:* 4
Rationale: During painful episodes, hot or cold packs, and splinting and positioning the affected joint in a neutral position help reduce the pain. Although resting the extremity is appropriate, it is important to begin simple isometric or tensing exercises as soon as the child is able. These exercises do not involve joint movement.
Test-Taking Strategy: Use the process of elimination. Eliminate options 1, 2, and 3 because of the words "must," "all," and "additional" in each of these options. Review pain management and care during exacerbations if you had difficulty with this question.
Level of Cognitive Ability: Application
Client Needs: Physiological Integrity
Integrated Concept/Process: Nursing Process/Implementation
Content Area: Child Health
Reference: Schulte E, Price D, Gwin J: *Thompson's pediatric nursing,* ed 8, Philadelphia, 2001, WB Saunders, p. 282.

8. *Answer:* 4
Rationale: The mother needs to be instructed not to use lotion or powders on the skin around the cast edges or inside the cast. Lotions or powders can become sticky or caked and cause skin irritation. Options 1, 2, and 3 are appropriate instructions.
Test-Taking Strategy: Use the process of elimination and note the key words "indicates a need for further instruction." Recalling the principles related to routine cast care should direct you to option 4. Review home care instructions regarding cast care if you had difficulty with this question.
Level of Cognitive Ability: Comprehension
Client Needs: Health Promotion and Maintenance
Integrated Concept/Process: Teaching/Learning
Content Area: Child Health
Reference: Wong D, Hockenberry-Eaton M: *Wong's essentials of pediatric nursing,* ed 6, St Louis, 2001, Mosby, p. 1214.

9. *Answer:* 4
Rationale: Pillows should not be used to elevate the head or shoulders of a child in a body cast because the pillows will thrust the child's chest against the cast and cause discomfort and respiratory difficulty. Neurovascular checks are a critical component of care to ensure that the cast is not causing circulatory compromise. The nurse should observe for nonverbal signs of pain and should ask the older child if pain is experienced. A ride on a stretcher to the playroom or around the hospital provides changes of position and scenery.
Test-Taking Strategy: Use the process of elimination and note the key word "avoids." Visualize this type of cast to direct you to option 4. Review care to the child with a spica cast if you had difficulty with this question.
Level of Cognitive Ability: Application
Client Needs: Physiological Integrity
Integrated Concept/Process: Nursing Process/Implementation
Content Area: Child Health
Reference: Wong D, Hockenberry-Eaton M: *Wong's essentials of pediatric nursing,* ed 6, St Louis, 2001, Mosby, p. 1214.

10. *Answer:* 3
Rationale: Buck's skin traction is a type of skin traction used in fractures of the femur and in hip and knee contractures. It pulls the hip and leg into extension. Countertraction is applied by the child's body. Options 1, 2, and 4 describe skeletal traction.
Test-Taking Strategy: Use the process of elimination. Noting the key word "skin" in the question will assist in directing you to option 3. Review the purpose of Buck's traction if you had difficulty with this question.
Level of Cognitive Ability: Comprehension
Client Needs: Physiological Integrity
Integrated Concept/Process: Nursing Process/Planning
Content Area: Child Health
Reference: Wong D, Hockenberry-Eaton M: *Wong's essentials of pediatric nursing,* ed 6, St Louis, 2001, Mosby, p. 1217.

11. *Answer:* 4
Rationale: The neurovascular check for tissue perfusion is performed on the toes or fingers distal to an injury or cast and includes peripheral pulse, color, capillary refill time, warmth, and motion and sensation. Options 1, 2, and 3 may be components of care but are not the priority in this situation.
Test-Taking Strategy: Use the process of elimination and note the key word "priority." Option 4 is the only option that addresses a neurovascular check. Review the components of a neurovascular check if you had difficulty with this question.
Level of Cognitive Ability: Application
Client Needs: Physiological Integrity
Integrated Concept/Process: Nursing Process/Data Collection
Content Area: Child Health
Reference: Wong D, Hockenberry-Eaton M: *Wong's essentials of pediatric nursing,* ed 6, St Louis, 2001, Mosby, p. 1217.

12. *Answer:* 2
Rationale: When checking capillary refill, the nurse would expect to note that a compressed nail bed will return to its original color in less than 3 seconds. Options 1, 3, and 4 are unnecessary actions.
Test-Taking Strategy: Knowledge regarding a normal finding when checking the capillary refill is required to answer this question. Review this data collection technique if you had difficulty with this question.
Level of Cognitive Ability: Application
Client Needs: Physiological Integrity
Integrated Concept/Process: Nursing Process/Implementation
Content Area: Child Health
Reference: Wong D, Hockenberry-Eaton M: *Wong's essentials of pediatric nursing,* ed 6, St Louis, 2001, Mosby, p. 183.

13. *Answer:* 4
Rationale: Reduced sensation to touch or complaints of numbness or tingling at a site distal to a fracture may indicate poor tissue perfusion. This finding should be reported to the RN. Options 1, 2, and 3 are inappropriate and would delay the required and immediate interventions.
Test-Taking Strategy: Use the process of elimination and recall the signs of circulatory compromise. Noting the child's complaint will assist in directing you to option 4. Review the complications associated with a cast if you had difficulty with this question.
Level of Cognitive Ability: Application
Client Needs: Physiological Integrity
Integrated Concept/Process: Nursing Process/Implementation
Content Area: Child Health
Reference: Wong D, Hockenberry-Eaton M: *Wong's essentials of pediatric nursing,* ed 6, St Louis, 2001, Mosby, p. 1211.

14. *Answer:* 2
Rationale: Bed linens should not be placed on the traction ropes because of the risk of disrupting the traction apparatus. Options 1, 3, and 4 are appropriate measures when caring for a child in skeletal traction.
Test-Taking Strategy: Note the key word "avoids." Use the process of elimination and knowledge regarding the care to the child in traction to assist in directing you to option 2. Review these nursing measures if you had difficulty with this question.
Level of Cognitive Ability: Application
Client Needs: Physiological Integrity
Integrated Concept/Process: Nursing Process/Implementation
Content Area: Child Health
Reference: Wong D, Hockenberry-Eaton M: *Wong's essentials of pediatric nursing,* ed 6, St Louis, 2001, Mosby, p. 1217.

15. *Answer:* 4
Rationale: Synthetic casts dry quickly (in less than 30 minutes) and are lighter than plaster casts. Synthetic casts allow for greater mobility than a plaster cast. However, synthetic casts are not as strong as plaster casts and are more expensive.
Test-Taking Strategy: Use the process of elimination and note the key word "synthetic." Recalling the differences between a plaster and a synthetic cast will assist in directing you to option 4. Review these differences if you had difficulty with this question.
Level of Cognitive Ability: Application
Client Needs: Health Promotion and Maintenance
Integrated Concept/Process: Nursing Process/Implementation
Content Area: Child Health
Reference: Wong D, Hockenberry-Eaton M: *Wong's essentials of pediatric nursing,* ed 6, St Louis, 2001, Mosby, p. 1214.

REFERENCES

Burroughs A, Leifer G: *Maternity nursing,* ed 8, Philadelphia, 2002, WB Saunders.

McKinney E et al: *Maternal-child nursing,* Philadelphia, 2000, WB Saunders.

Murray S, McKinney E, Gorrie T: *Foundations of maternal-newborn nursing,* ed 3, Philadelphia, 2002, WB Saunders.

Schulte E, Price D, Gwin J: *Thompson's pediatric nursing,* ed 8, Philadelphia, 2001, WB Saunders.

Wong D: *Whaley and Wong's nursing care of infants and children,* ed 6, St Louis, 1999, Mosby.

Wong D, Hockenberry-Eaton M: *Wong's essentials of pediatric nursing,* ed 6, St Louis, 2001, Mosby.

Hematological and Oncological Disorders

I. SICKLE CELL DISEASE (SCD)

A. Description
   1. A group of diseases collectively termed hemoglobinopathies, in which hemoglobin (hemoglobin A [HgbA]) is partly or completely replaced by abnormal sickle hemoglobin (HgbS)
   2. Caused by the inheritance of a gene for a structurally abnormal portion of the hemoglobin (Hgb) chain
   3. HgbS is sensitive to changes in the oxygen content of the red blood cell (RBC)
   4. Insufficient oxygen causes the cells to assume a sickle shape, and the cells become rigid and clumped together, obstructing capillary blood flow
   5. Situations that precipitate sickling include fever and emotional or physical stress; any condition that increases the body's need for oxygen or alters the transport of oxygen can result in sickle cell crisis
   6. Risk factors include having parents heterozygous for HgbS or being African-American
   7. The sickling response is reversible under conditions of adequate oxygenation and hydration; after repeated sickling, the cell becomes permanently sickled
   8. The clinical manifestations are primarily the result of obstruction caused by sickled RBCs and increased RBC destruction
   9. Sickle cell crises are acute exacerbations of the disease that vary markedly in severity and frequency; these include vasoocclusive crisis, splenic sequestration, and aplastic crisis
   10. Care focuses on the prevention (preventing exposure to infection and maintaining normal hydration) and treatment (oxygen, hydration, pain management, and bed rest) of the crisis

B. Data collection
   1. Vasoocclusive crisis
      a. Most common type of crisis; caused by stasis of blood with clumping of the cells in the microcirculation, ischemia, and infarction
      b. Signs include fever, pain, and tissue engorgement
   2. Splenic sequestration
      a. Life-threatening crisis caused by the pooling of blood in the spleen
      b. Signs include profound anemia, hypovolemia, and shock
   3. Aplastic crisis
      a. Caused by the diminished production and increased destruction of RBCs, triggered by viral infection or the depletion of folic acid
      b. Signs include profound anemia and pallor

C. Implementation
   1. Administer oxygen as prescribed; blood transfusions may be prescribed to increase tissue perfusion
   2. Administer analgesics as prescribed (around the clock); administration of meperidine (Demerol) is avoided because of the risk of seizures
   3. Maintain adequate hydration and blood flow with intravenous (IV) normal saline as prescribed and with oral fluids
   4. Assist the child to assume a comfortable position so that the child keeps the extremities extended to promote venous return; elevate the head of the bed no more than 30 degrees, avoid putting strain on painful joints, and do not raise the knee gatch of the bed

5. Encourage consumption of a high-calorie, high-protein diet with folic acid supplementation
6. Administer antibiotics as prescribed to prevent infection
7. Monitor for signs of increasing anemia and shock (mental status changes, pallor, vital sign changes)
8. Instruct the child and parents about the early signs and symptoms of crisis and the measures to prevent crisis
9. Inform the parents of the **hereditary** aspects of the disorder

II. IRON DEFICIENCY ANEMIA

A. Description
1. Iron stores are depleted, resulting in a decreased supply of iron for the manufacture of hemoglobin in RBCs
2. Commonly results from blood loss, increased metabolic demands, syndromes of gastrointestinal (GI) malabsorption, and dietary inadequacy

B. Data collection
1. Pallor
2. Weakness and fatigue
3. Irritability

C. Implementation
1. Increase the oral intake of iron
2. Instruct the child and parents in food choices that are high in iron (Box 35-1)
3. Administer iron supplements as prescribed
4. Teach the child and parents that liquid iron preparation stains the teeth and should be taken through a straw
5. Instruct the child and parents about the side effects of iron supplements (black stools, constipation, and foul aftertaste)

III. APLASTIC ANEMIA

A. Description
1. A deficiency of circulating erythrocytes resulting from the arrested development of RBCs within the bone marrow

BOX 35-1

Iron-Rich Foods

Liver
Meats
Egg yolks
Dark, green leafy vegetables
Breads and cereals
Kidney beans
Raisins

2. There are several possible causes, including chronic exposure to myelotoxic agents, viruses, infection, autoimmune disorders, and allergic states
3. The definitive diagnosis is determined by bone marrow aspiration (demonstrates conversion of red bone marrow to fatty, red bone marrow)
4. Therapeutic management includes blood transfusions, splenectomy, corticosteroids, immunosuppressive therapy, bone marrow transplant (treatment of choice if a suitable donor exists), and the administration of antilymphocyte globulin (ALG) or antithymocyte globulin (ATG) to suppress the autoimmune response

B. Data collection
1. Pancytopenia (a deficiency of erythrocytes, leukocytes, and thrombocytes)
2. Petechiae, purpura, bleeding, pallor, weakness, tachycardia, and fatigue

C. Implementation
1. Blood transfusions may be prescribed; transfusions are discontinued as soon as the bone marrow begins to produce RBCs
2. Administer corticosteroids and immunosuppressive therapy as prescribed
3. Prepare the child for splenectomy; prescribed for the child with an enlarged spleen that is destroying normal RBCs or suppressing their development
4. Prepare the child for bone marrow transplant if planned
5. Administer ALG or ATG as prescribed and monitor for allergic reactions (fever, skin rash)
6. Advise the parents to obtain a Medic-Alert bracelet for the child

IV. HEMOPHILIA

A. Description
1. An X-linked recessive trait
2. Hemophilia A (classic hemophilia) results from a deficiency of factor VIII
3. Hemophilia B (Christmas disease) results from a deficiency of factor IX
4. Males inherit hemophilia from their mothers, and females inherit the carrier status from their fathers
5. Some females who are carriers have an increased tendency to bleed, and, although it is rare, females can have hemophilia if their fathers have the disorder and their mothers are carriers of the genetic disorder
6. The primary treatment is replacement of the missing clotting factor; products used are

factor VIII concentrate and desmopressin acetate (DDAVP)

B. Data collection
  1. Abnormal bleeding in response to trauma or surgery
  2. Joint bleeding causing pain, tenderness, swelling, and limited range of motion
  3. Tendency to bruise easily
  4. Prolonged partial thromboplastin time (PTT)
  5. Normal bleeding time, prothrombin time (PT), and platelet count

C. Implementation
  1. Factor VIII concentrate or DDAVP may be prescribed
  2. Monitor for bleeding and maintain bleeding precautions
  3. Monitor for joint pain; immobilize the affected extremity if joint pain occurs
  4. Monitor neurological status (child is at risk for intracranial hemorrhage)
  5. Monitor urine for hematuria
  6. Control bleeding by immobilization, elevation, and the application of ice; additionally, apply pressure (15 minutes) for superficial bleeding
  7. Instruct the child and parents about the signs of internal bleeding
  8. Instruct the parents how to control the bleeding
  9. Instruct the parents regarding activities for the child, emphasizing the avoidance of contact sports
  10. Instruct the parents to obtain a Medic-Alert bracelet for the child

V. β-THALASSEMIA MAJOR

A. Description
  1. An autosomal recessive disorder
  2. Also called Cooley's anemia and includes a group of disorders characterized by the reduced production of one of the globin chains in the synthesis of hemoglobin
  3. The incidence is highest in individuals of Mediterranean descent
  4. Treatment is supportive, and the goal of therapy is to maintain normal hemoglobin levels by the administration of blood transfusions
  5. Bone marrow transplantation may be offered as an alternative therapy

B. Data collection
  1. Severe anemia
  2. Pallor
  3. Failure to thrive
  4. Hepatosplenomegaly
  5. Microcytic, hypochromic RBCs

C. Implementation
  1. Instruct in the administration of folic acid (vitamin B_9) as prescribed, which stimulates the production of blood cells
  2. Blood transfusions may be prescribed; monitor for transfusion reactions
  3. Monitor for iron overload and administer chelation therapy with deferoxamine (Desferal) as prescribed to treat iron overload and to prevent organ damage from the elevated levels of iron caused by the multiple transfusion therapy
  4. Provide genetic counseling

VI. LEUKEMIA (Table 35-1)

A. Description
  1. Malignant exacerbation in the number of leukocytes, usually at an immature stage, in the bone marrow
  2. Affects the bone marrow, causing anemia from decreased erythrocytes, infection from neutropenia, and bleeding from decreased platelet production
  3. The cause is unknown and appears to involve gene damage of cells, leading to the transformation of cells from a normal state to a malignant state
  4. Risk factors include genetic, viral, immunological, and environmental factors, and exposure to radiation, chemicals, and medications
  5. Acute lymphocytic leukemia (ALL) is the most frequent type of cancer in children; peak onset is age 2 to 6 years
  6. Is more common in boys than girls after age 1 year
  7. Treatment involves the use of chemotherapeutic agents with or without cranial radiation
  8. Bone marrow transplantation (BMT) may also be performed to treat some children with leukemia

B. Data collection
  1. Infiltration of the bone marrow causes fever, pallor, fatigue, anorexia, hemorrhage (usually

TABLE 35-1

Classification of Leukemia

Acute Lymphocytic Leukemia (ALL)	Acute Myelogenous Leukemia (AML)
Mostly lymphoblasts present in bone marrow	Mostly myeloblasts present in bone marrow
Age of onset is less than 15 years	Age of onset is between 15 and 39 years

petechiae), and bone and joint pain; pathological fractures can occur as a result of bone marrow invasion with leukemic cells

2. Signs of infection as a result of neutropenia
3. Hepatosplenomegaly, lymphadenopathy
4. Normal, elevated, or a low white blood cell (WBC) count
5. Decreased hemoglobin and hematocrit levels
6. Decreased platelet count
7. Positive bone marrow biopsy identifying leukemic blast (immature) phase cells
8. Signs of increased intracranial pressure, such as severe headache, vomiting, papilledema, irritability, lethargy, and eventually coma, as a result of central nervous system involvement
9. Signs of cranial nerve (cranial nerve VII, or the facial nerve, is most commonly affected) or spinal nerve involvement; clinical manifestations relate to the area involved
10. Clinical manifestations that indicate the invasion of leukemic cells to the kidneys, testes, prostate, ovaries, gastrointestinal (GI) tract, and lungs

C. Infection (Box 35-2)
   1. A major cause of death in the immunosuppressed child
   2. Can occur through autocontamination or cross-contamination
   3. Most common sites of infection are the skin (any break in the skin is a potential site of infection), respiratory tract, and GI tract

D. Bleeding (Box 35-3)
   1. Children with platelet counts below 20,000/mm^3 may need a platelet transfusion
   2. For children with severe blood loss, packed red blood cells may be prescribed

E. Fatigue and nutrition
   1. Assist the child in selecting a well-balanced diet
   2. Provide small meals that require little chewing
   3. Assist the child in self-care and mobility activities
   4. Allow adequate rest periods during care
   5. Do not perform activities unless they are essential

F. Chemotherapy
   1. Monitor for severe bone marrow suppression; during the period of greatest bone marrow

BOX 35-2

Protecting the Child from Infection

Initiate protective isolation procedures
Maintain the child in a private room and a room with high-efficiency particulate air (HEPA) filtration or laminar air flow system if possible
Be sure that the child's room is cleaned daily
Maintain frequent and thorough handwashing
Use strict aseptic technique for all nursing procedures
Limit the number of caregivers entering the child's room, and ensure that anyone entering the child's room is wearing a mask
Keep supplies for the child separate from supplies for other children
Reduce exposure to environmental organisms by eliminating raw fruits and vegetables and fresh flowers, and by not leaving standing water in the child's room
Assist the child with daily bathing, using antimicrobial soap
Assist the child to perform oral hygiene frequently
Assess for signs and symptoms of infection
Monitor temperature, pulse, and blood pressure
Change wound dressings daily and inspect wounds for redness, swelling, or drainage
Assess urine for color and cloudiness
Assess the skin and oral mucous membranes for signs of infection
Check lung sounds
Encourage the child to cough and deep breathe
Monitor the white blood cell and neutrophil count
Notify the physician if signs of infection are present and prepare to obtain specimens for culture of open lesions, urine, and sputum
Initiate a bowel program to prevent constipation and rectal trauma
Avoid invasive procedures such as injections, rectal temperatures, and urinary catheterization
Administer antibiotic, antifungal, and antiviral medication as prescribed
Administer granulocyte colony-stimulating factor (GCSF) as prescribed
Instruct the parents to keep the child away from crowds and those with infections
Instruct the parents that the child should not receive immunization with a live virus
Keep any child with chickenpox or any child who has been exposed to the virus away from the child with leukemia
Instruct the parents to inform the teacher that they should be notified immediately if a case of chickenpox occurs in another child at school

BOX 35-3

Protecting the Child from Bleeding

Examine the child for signs and symptoms of bleeding
Handle the child gently
Measure abdominal girth; an increase can indicate internal hemorrhage
Instruct the child to use a soft toothbrush and to avoid dental floss
Provide soft foods that are cool to warm in temperature
Avoid injections, if possible, to prevent trauma to the skin and bleeding
Apply firm and gentle pressure to a needle-stick site for at least 10 minutes
Pad side rails and sharp corners of the bed and furniture
Discourage the child from engaging in activities involving the use of sharp objects
Instruct the child to avoid constrictive or tight clothing
Use caution when taking the blood pressure to prevent skin injury
Instruct the child to avoid blowing the nose
Avoid rectal suppositories, enemas, and rectal thermometers
Examine all body fluids and excrement for the presence of blood
Count the number of pads or tampons used if the female adolescent is menstruating
Instruct the child in the signs and symptoms of bleeding
Instruct the parents to avoid administering nonsteroidal antiinflammatory drugs (NSAIDs) and products that contain aspirin to the child

suppression (the nadir), blood counts will be extremely low

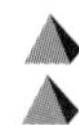

2. Monitor for infection and bleeding
3. Protect the child from life-threatening infections
4. Monitor for nausea, vomiting, and diarrhea
5. Administer antiemetics as prescribed
6. Monitor for signs of dehydration
7. Monitor for signs of hemorrhagic cystitis
8. Monitor for signs of peripheral neuropathy
9. Assess oral mucous membranes for mucositis; administer frequent mouth rinses (normal saline with or without sodium bicarbonate solution) to promote healing if mucositis occurs
10. Instruct the parents in signs and symptoms to monitor for after chemotherapy and when to notify the physician
11. Inform the parents that hair loss may occur from chemotherapy (hair will regrow in 3 to 6 months and may be a slightly different color or texture)
12. Instruct the parents about the care of a central venous access device as necessary
13. Listen to the child and family, and encourage them to verbalize their feelings and express their concerns
14. Introduce the family to other families of children with cancer
15. Consult social services and chaplains as necessary

VII. HODGKIN'S DISEASE (Box 35-4)

A. Description
1. A malignancy of the lymph nodes that originates in a single lymph node or a single chain of nodes
2. It predictably metastasizes to nonnodal or extralymphatic sites, especially the spleen, liver, bone marrow, lungs, and mediastinum
3. Characterized by the presence of Reed-Sternberg cells in the lymph nodes
4. Possible causes include viral infections and previous exposure to alkalating chemical agents
5. The prognosis is dependent on the stage of disease; the prognosis is excellent in children with localized disease
6. The primary treatment modalities are radiation and chemotherapy; each may be used alone or in combination, depending on the clinical staging of the disease
7. BMT may be a consideration in treating Hodgkin's disease

B. Data collection
1. Painless enlargement of lymph nodes

BOX 35-4

Staging of Hodgkin's Disease

STAGE I
Involvement of a single lymph node region or a extralymphatic organ or site

STAGE II
Involvement of two or more lymph node regions on the same side of the diaphragm or localized involvement of an extralymphatic organ or site

STAGE III
Involvement of lymph node regions on both sides of the diaphragm or localized involvement of an extralymphatic organ or site or spleen or both

STAGE IV
Diffuse or disseminated involvement of one or more extralymphatic organs with or without associated lymph node involvement

2. Enlarged, firm, nontender, movable nodes in the supraclavicular area; in children, the "sentinel" node located near the left clavicle may be the first enlarged node
3. Nonproductive cough as a result of mediastinal lymphadenopathy
4. Abdominal pain as a result of enlarged retroperitoneal nodes
5. Advanced lymph node and extralymphatic involvement may cause systemic symptoms such as low-grade and/or intermittent fever, anorexia, nausea, weight loss, night sweats, and pruritus
6. Positive biopsy of lymph node (presence of Reed-Sternberg cell) and a positive bone marrow biopsy
7. Computed tomography (CT) scan of the liver, spleen, and bone marrow to detect metastasis

C. Implementation
1. For stages 1 and 2 without mediastinal node involvement, the treatment of choice is extensive external radiation of the involved lymph node regions
2. With more extensive disease, radiation along with multiagent chemotherapy is utilized
3. Monitor for drug-induced pancytopenia, which increases the risk for infection, bleeding, and anemia
4. Monitor for signs of infection and bleeding
5. Protect the child from infection
6. Provide a safe, hazard-free environment
7. Monitor for side effects related to chemotherapy or radiation; the most common complication of radiation to the neck area is hypothyroidism
8. Monitor for nausea and vomiting and administer antiemetics as prescribed
9. Monitor for skin irritation and breakdown as a result of radiation therapy

VIII. NEPHROBLASTOMA (WILMS' TUMOR)

A. Description
1. A tumor of the kidney that may present unilaterally and localized or bilaterally, sometimes with metastasis to other organs
2. The peak incidence is at 3 years of age
3. Its occurrence is associated with a genetic inheritance and with several congenital anomalies
4. Therapeutic management includes a combined treatment of surgery (partial to total nephrectomy) and chemotherapy with or without radiation, depending on the clinical stage and histological pattern

B. Data collection
1. Swelling or mass within the abdomen (mass is characteristically firm, nontender, confined to one side, and deep within the flank)
2. Abdominal pain
3. Urinary retention and/or hematuria
4. Anemia (secondary to hemorrhage within the tumor)
5. Pallor, anorexia, lethargy (occurs as a result of anemia)
6. Hypertension (caused by secretion of excess amounts of renin by the tumor)
7. Weight loss and fever
8. Symptoms of lung involvement, such as dyspnea, shortness of breath, and pain in the chest if metastasis has occurred

C. Preoperative implementation
1. Monitor vital signs, particularly blood pressure
2. Place a sign at bedside: "Do Not Palpate Abdomen"
3. Avoid palpation of the abdomen
4. Measure abdominal girth

D. Postoperative implementation
1. Monitor temperature and blood pressure closely
2. Monitor for signs of hemorrhage and infection
3. Maintain I&O and urine output closely
4. Monitor for abdominal distention, bowel sounds, and for other signs of GI activity, because of the risk for intestinal obstruction

IX. NEUROBLASTOMA

A. Description
1. An embryonal tumor found in children that arises from the neural crest
2. The primary site is in the abdomen because the tumor arises from the adrenal gland or from the retroperitoneal sympathetic chain; other sites may be within the head, neck, chest, or pelvis
3. Most presenting signs are caused by the tumor compressing on adjacent normal tissue and organs
4. Diagnostic evaluation is aimed at locating the primary site of the tumor
5. The prognosis is poor because of the frequency of invasiveness of the tumor and because in most cases, a diagnosis is not made until after metastasis has occurred
6. Therapeutic management
   a. Surgery to remove as much of the tumor as possible and to obtain biopsies; in stages I and II, complete surgical removal of the tumor is the treatment of choice

   b. Surgery is usually limited to biopsy in stages III and IV because of the extensive metastasis
   c. Radiation is commonly used with stage III disease and provides palliation for metastatic lesions in bones, lungs, liver, or brain
   d. Chemotherapy is the mainstay of treatment for extensive local or disseminated disease

B. Data collection
   1. Firm, nontender, irregular mass in the abdomen that crosses the midline
   2. Urinary frequency or retention from compression of the kidney, ureter, or bladder
   3. Lymphadenopathy, especially in the cervical and supraclavicular area
   4. Bone pain if skeletal involvement occurs
   5. Supraorbital ecchymosis, periorbital edema, and exophthalmos as a result of invasion of retrobulbar soft tissue
   6. Pallor, weakness, irritability, anorexia, weight loss
   7. Signs of respiratory impairment (thoracic lesion)
   8. Signs of neurological impairment (intracranial lesion)
   9. Paralysis from compression of the spinal cord

C. Preoperative implementation
   1. Monitor for signs and symptoms related to the location of the tumor
   2. Provide emotional support to the child and parents

D. Postoperative implementation
   1. Monitor for postoperative complications related to the location (organ) of the surgery
   2. Monitor for complications related to chemotherapy or radiation if prescribed
   3. Provide support to the parents and encourage them to express their feelings; many parents suffer from guilt for not having recognized signs in the child earlier
   4. Refer the parents to appropriate community services

X. OSTEOGENIC SARCOMA

A. Description
   1. The most common bone cancer in children
   2. Usually found in the metaphysis of long bones, especially in the lower extremities, with most tumors occurring in the femur
   3. Peak age of incidence is between 10 and 25 years
   4. Symptoms in its earliest stage are almost always attributed to extremity injury or normal growing pains
   5. Treatment may include surgical resection by limb salvage to remove affected tissue or amputation
   6. Chemotherapy plays a vital role in treatment and may be used both before and after surgery

B. Data collection
   1. Localized pain at the affected site (may be severe or dull) that may be attributed to trauma or the vague complaint of "growing pains"; pain is often relieved by a flexed position
   2. Palpable mass
   3. Limping if weight-bearing limb is affected
   4. Progressive limited range of motion and the child curtails physical activity
   5. Child may be unable to hold heavy objects
   6. Pathological fractures at the tumor site

C. Implementation
   1. Prepare the child and family for prescribed treatment modalities, which may include surgical resection by limb salvage to remove affected tissue, amputation, and chemotherapy
   2. Provide honesty and support for the child and family
   3. Prepare for prosthetic fitting as necessary
   4. Assist the child in dealing with problems of self-image

XI. EWING'S SARCOMA

A. Description
   1. A tumor that invades the soft tissue around the bone, especially the femur, vertebrae, ribs, and pelvic bones
   2. Peak incidence is age 7 to12 years

B. Data collection
   1. Pain
   2. Soft tissue swelling around the affected bone
   3. Neurological symptoms if a vertebral tumor is present
   4. Respiratory symptoms if a rib tumor is present
   5. Anorexia, fever, malaise, fatigue, and weight loss if metastatic disease is present

C. Implementation: prepare the child and family for treatments that may include chemotherapy, radiation, or excision of the tumor

XII. BRAIN TUMORS

A. Description
   1. An infratentorial (below the tentorium cerebelli) tumor is located in the posterior third of the brain (primarily in the cerebellum or brainstem) and accounts for the frequency of

symptoms resulting from increased intracranial pressure (ICP)

2. A supratentorial tumor is located within the anterior two thirds of the brain, mainly the cerebrum
3. The signs and symptoms of the brain tumor depend on its anatomical location and size, and to some extent the age of the child
4. Therapeutic management includes surgery, radiation, and chemotherapy; the treatment of choice is total removal of the tumor without residual neurological damage

B. Data collection
1. Headache that is worse on awakening and improves during the day
2. Vomiting that is unrelated to feeding or eating
3. Ataxia
4. Seizures
5. Behavioral changes
6. Clumsiness; awkward gait or difficulty walking
7. Diplopia
8. Facial weakness

C. Preoperative implementation
1. Perform neurological assessments
2. Institute safety measures
3. Assess weight loss and nutritional status
4. Initiate seizure precautions
5. The child's head will be shaved (provide a favorite cap or hat for the child)
6. Prepare the child as much as possible; tell the child that he or she will wake up with a large head dressing

D. Postoperative implementation
1. Assess neurological and motor function and level of consciousness (LOC)
2. Monitor temperature closely, which may be elevated because of hypothalamus or brainstem involvement during surgery; maintain a cooling blanket by the bedside
3. Monitor for signs of respiratory infection
4. Monitor for signs of meningitis (opisthotonos, Kernig and Brudzinski signs)
5. Monitor for signs of increased intracranial pressure (ICP) or hemorrhage (check the back of the head dressing for posterior pooling of blood)
6. Assess pupillary response; sluggish, dilated, or unequal pupils are reported immediately because they may indicate increased ICP and potential brainstem herniation
7. Monitor for colorless drainage on the dressing or from the ears or nose, which indicates cerebrospinal fluid (CSF) and should be reported immediately
8. Check the physician's order for positioning, including the degree of neck flexion
   a. If a large tumor was removed, the child is not placed on the operative side because the brain may suddenly shift to that cavity
   b. In an infratentorial procedure, the child is usually positioned flat and on either side
   c. In a supratentorial procedure, the head is usually elevated above the heart level to facilitate CSF drainage and to decrease excessive blood flow to the brain to prevent hemorrhage
   d. Never place the child in Trendelenburg position because it increases ICP and the risk of hemorrhage
9. Monitor IV fluids carefully
10. Promote measures that prevent vomiting (vomiting increases ICP and the risk for incisional rupture)
11. Provide a quiet environment
12. Administer analgesics as prescribed
13. Provide emotional support to the child and parents, and promote maximum functioning in the child

PRACTICE QUESTIONS

1. A pediatric nursing instructor asks a nursing student to describe the cause of the clinical manifestations that occur in sickle cell disease. Which of the following is the appropriate response by the nursing student?
   1. "Sickled cells increase the blood flow through the body and cause a great deal of pain."
   2. "The sickled cells mix with the unsickled cells and cause the immune system to become depressed."
   3. "Bone marrow depression occurs because of the development of sickled cells."
   4. "Sickled cells are unable to flow easily through the microvasculature and their clumping obstructs blood flow."
2. A child with sickle cell disease is admitted to the hospital for treatment of vasoocclusive pain crisis. The oxygen saturation level is 92%. The nurse prepares to administer care for the child. Which of the following would not be a component of the plan of care?
   1. Monitoring IV fluids for rehydration
   2. Administering meperidine (Demerol) for pain management
   3. Administering oxygen
   4. Increasing fluid intake
3. A nurse instructs the mother of a child with sickle cell disease regarding the precipitating factors related to pain crisis. The nurse provides instructions knowing that which of the following is not a precipitating factor?

1. Infection
2. Trauma
3. Fluid overload
4. Stress

4. Oral iron supplements are prescribed for the 6-year-old child with iron deficiency anemia. The nurse instructs the mother to administer the iron with which of the following best food items?
   1. Water
   2. Milk
   3. Apple juice
   4. Orange juice
5. A nurse caring for a child with aplastic anemia reviews the laboratory results and notes a white blood cell (WBC) count of 6000/μL and a platelet count of 27,000/mm^3. Which of the following nursing interventions will the nurse suggest to incorporate into the plan of care?
   1. Maintain strict isolation precautions
   2. Encourage naps
   3. Encourage a diet high in iron
   4. Encourage quiet play activities
6. A nurse reinforces instructions regarding home care to the parents of a 3-year-old child hospitalized with hemophilia. Which statement by a parent indicates a need for further instructions?
   1. "I will supervise my child closely."
   2. "I will pad corners of the furniture."
   3. "I will remove household items that can easily fall over."
   4. "I will avoid immunizations being administered and dental hygiene treatments for my child."
7. A nurse is reinforcing home care instructions to the mother of a 10-year-old child with hemophilia. Which of the following activities would the nurse suggest that the child could safely participate with peers?
   1. Basketball
   2. Swimming
   3. Soccer
   4. Field hockey
8. A nursing student is presenting a clinical conference and discusses the etiology related to β-thalassemia. The student informs the group that the child at greatest risk of developing this disorder is:
   1. A child whose intake of iron is extremely poor
   2. A breastfed child by a mother with chronic anemia
   3. A child of Mediterranean descent
   4. A child of Mexican descent
9. A nurse reinforces instructions to the parents of a child with leukemia regarding measures related to monitoring for infection. Which statement by the parents indicates a need for further instructions?
   1. "I need to use proper handwashing techniques."
   2. "I need to take a rectal temperature daily on my child."
   3. "I need to inspect my child's skin daily for redness."
   4. "I need to inspect my child's mouth daily for lesions."
10. A 6-year-old child with leukemia is hospitalized and is receiving chemotherapy. Laboratory results indicate that the child is neutropenic and protective isolation procedures are initiated. The grandmother of the child visits and brings a fresh bouquet of flowers picked from her garden and asks the nurse for a vase for the flowers. Which of the following would be the most appropriate response to the grandmother?
    1. "I have a vase in the utility room and I will get it for you."
    2. "The flowers from your garden are beautiful, but should not be placed in the child's room at this time."
    3. "I will get the vase and wash it well before you put the flowers in it."
    4. "When you bring the flowers into the room, place them on the bed side stand as far away from the child as possible."
11. A nurse is reviewing the health record of a 10-year-old child suspected of having Hodgkin's disease. Which of the following would the nurse expect to note documented in the record that is most characteristic of this disease?
    1. Painful, enlarged inguinal lymph nodes
    2. Fever and malaise
    3. Painless, firm, and movable adenopathy in the cervical area
    4. Anorexia and weight loss
12. A 4-year-old child is hospitalized with a suspected diagnosis of Wilms' tumor. The nurse assists in developing a plan of care and suggests to include avoiding which of the following?
    1. Palpating the abdomen for a mass
    2. Checking the urine for the presence of hematuria
    3. Monitoring the temperature for the presence of fever
    4. Monitoring the blood pressure for the presence of hypertension
13. A student nurse is conducting a clinical conference and is discussing osteogenic sarcoma. Which of the following would not be a component of the information provided by the student during this conference?
    1. The symptoms of the disease in the early stage are almost always attributed to normal growing pains
    2. The femur is the most common site of this sarcoma

3. Limping, if a weight-bearing limb is affected, is a clinical manifestation
4. The child does not experience pain at the primary tumor site

14. A 13-year-old child is diagnosed with a Ewing's sarcoma of the femur. After a course of chemotherapy, it has been decided that leg amputation is necessary. After the amputation, the child becomes very frightened because of aching and cramping felt in the missing limb. Which of the following would be the most appropriate nursing statement to assist in alleviating the child's fear?
1. "This aching and cramping are normal and temporary and will subside."
2. "This normally occurs after the surgery and we will teach you ways to deal with it."
3. "The pain medication that I give you will take these feelings away."
4. "This pain is not real pain and relaxation exercises will help it go away."

15. A nurse is monitoring for bleeding in a child after surgery for removal of a brain tumor. The nurse checks the head dressing for the presence of blood and notes a colorless drainage on the back of the dressing. Which of the following would be the most appropriate nursing intervention?
1. Circle the area of drainage and continue to monitor
2. Reinforce the dressing
3. Notify the registered nurse (RN)
4. Document the findings and continue to monitor

ANSWERS

1. *Answer:* 4
Rationale: All of the clinical manifestations of sickle cell disease are a result of the sickled cells being unable to flow easily through the microvasculature, and their clumping obstructs blood flow. With reoxygenation, most of the sickled red blood cells resume their normal shape. Options 1, 2, and 3 are inaccurate.
Test-Taking Strategy: Use the process of elimination. Recalling that sickled cells clump will assist in directing you to the correct option. Review the pathophysiology associated with sickle cell disease if you had difficulty with this question.
Level of Cognitive Ability: Comprehension
Client Needs: Physiological Integrity
Integrated Concept/Process: Teaching/Learning
Content Area: Child Health
Reference: Schulte E, Price D, Gwin J: *Thompson's pediatric nursing,* ed 8, Philadelphia, 2001, WB Saunders, p. 132.

2. *Answer:* 2
Rationale: Management of severe pain that occurs with vasoocclusive crisis includes the use of strong narcotic analgesics such as morphine sulfate and hydromorphone hydrochloride (Dilaudid). Meperidine is contraindicated because of its side effects and increased risk of seizures. Oxygen is administered when hypoxia is present and the oxygen saturation level is less than 95%. Increased fluid intake both orally and by IV are important components of care.
Test-Taking Strategy: Use the process of elimination. Note the key word "not" in the stem of the question. Noting that the oxygen saturation level is 92% will assist in eliminating option 3. Eliminate options 1 and 4 knowing that hydration is necessary and because these options are similar. Review care to the client with sickle cell disease if you had difficulty with this question.
Level of Cognitive Ability: Application
Client Needs: Physiological Integrity
Integrated Concept/Process: Nursing Process/Planning
Content Area: Child Health
Reference: Schulte E, Price D, Gwin J: *Thompson's pediatric nursing,* ed 8, Philadelphia, 2001, WB Saunders, p. 133.

3. *Answer:* 3
Rationale: Pain crisis may be precipitated by infection, dehydration, hypoxia, trauma, or general stress. The mother of a child with sickle cell disease should encourage fluid intake of 1.5 to 2 times the daily requirement to prevent dehydration.
Test-Taking Strategy: Use the process of elimination. Note the key word "not." Recalling that fluids is a main component of treatment in sickle cell disease to prevent dehydration and pain crisis will direct you to option 3. Review the precipitating factors of pain crisis if you had difficulty with this question.
Level of Cognitive Ability: Comprehension
Client Needs: Health Promotion and Maintenance
Integrated Concept/Process: Teaching/Learning
Content Area: Child Health
Reference: Schulte E, Price D, Gwin J: *Thompson's pediatric nursing,* ed 8, Philadelphia, 2001, WB Saunders, p. 132.

4. *Answer:* 4
Rationale: Vitamin C increases the absorption of iron by the body. The mother should be instructed to administer the medication with a citrus fruit or juice high in vitamin C.
Test-Taking Strategy: Use the process of elimination. Recalling that vitamin C increases the absorption of iron will assist in eliminating options 1 and 2. From the remaining options, select option 4 because this food item contains the highest amount of vitamin C. Review the procedure for administering oral iron if you had difficulty with this question.
Level of Cognitive Ability: Application
Client Needs: Health Promotion and Maintenance
Integrated Concept/Process: Teaching/Learning

Content Area: Child Health
Reference: Schulte E, Price D, Gwin J: *Thompson's pediatric nursing,* ed 8, Philadelphia, 2001, WB Saunders, p. 130.

5. *Answer:* 4
Rationale: Precautionary measures to prevent bleeding should be taken when a child has a low platelet count. These include no injections, no rectal temperatures, use of a soft toothbrush, and abstinence from contact sports or activities that could cause an injury. Strict isolation would be required if the WBC count was low. Options 2 and 3 are unrelated to the risk of bleeding.
Test-Taking Strategy: Use the process of elimination. Note that the WBC count is normal and that the platelet count is low. Recall that a low platelet count places the client at risk for bleeding. This will assist in eliminating options 1, 2, and 3. Review normal WBC and platelet counts if you had difficulty with this question.
Level of Cognitive Ability: Comprehension
Client Needs: Physiological Integrity
Integrated Concept/Process: Nursing Process/Planning
Content Area: Child Health
Reference: Chernecky C, Berger B: *Laboratory tests and diagnostic procedures,* ed 3, Philadelphia, 2001, WB Saunders, p. 827.

6. *Answer:* 4
Rationale: The nurse needs to stress the importance of immunizations, dental hygiene, and routine well-child care. Options 1, 2, and 3 are appropriate statements. The parents are also provided instructions regarding measures to take in the event of blunt trauma, especially trauma involving the joints, and are instructed to apply prolonged pressure to superficial wounds until the bleeding has stopped.
Test-Taking Strategy: Use the process of elimination and note the key words "need for further instructions." Recalling that bleeding is a concern in this disorder will assist in eliminating options 1, 2, and 3 because they include measures of protection and safety for the child. Review home care measures for the child with hemophilia if you had difficulty with this question.
Level of Cognitive Ability: Application
Client Needs: Health Promotion and Maintenance
Integrated Concept/Process: Teaching/Learning
Content Area: Child Health
Reference: Schulte E, Price D, Gwin J: *Thompson's pediatric nursing,* ed 8, Philadelphia, 2001, WB Saunders, p. 235.

7. *Answer:* 2
Rationale: Children with hemophilia need to avoid contact sports and need to take precautions, such as wearing elbow and knee pads and helmets when participating in other sports. The safest activity that will prevent injury is swimming.
Test-Taking Strategy: Use the process of elimination. Note the key word "safely." Recalling that bleeding is a major concern in this condition will assist in directing you to option 2. Also, note that the activities in options 1, 3, and 4 present the potential for injury. Review home care instructions for the child with hemophilia if you had difficulty with this question.
Level of Cognitive Ability: Application
Client Needs: Health Promotion and Maintenance
Integrated Concept/Process: Teaching/Learning
Content Area: Child Health
Reference: Schulte E, Price D, Gwin J: *Thompson's pediatric nursing,* ed 8, Philadelphia, 2001, WB Saunders, p. 236.

8. *Answer:* 3
Rationale: β-Thalassemia is an autosomal recessive disorder. This disorder is found primarily in individuals of Mediterranean descent. The disease has also been reported in Asians and Africans.
Test-Taking Strategy: Knowledge regarding the etiology associated with this disorder is required to answer this question. Review this disorder if you had difficulty with this question.
Level of Cognitive Ability: Comprehension
Client Needs: Physiological Integrity
Integrated Concept/Process: Teaching/Learning
Content Area: Child Health
Reference: Wong D, Hockenberry-Eaton M: *Wong's essentials of pediatric nursing,* ed 6, St Louis, 2001, Mosby, p. 994.

9. *Answer:* 2
Rationale: The risk of injury to fragile mucous membranes is so great in the child with leukemia that only oral, axillary, or tympanic temperatures should be taken. Rectal abscesses can easily occur to damaged rectal tissue. No rectal temperatures should be taken. Additionally oral temperatures should be avoided if the child has oral ulcers. Options 1, 3, and 4 are appropriate teaching measures.
Test-Taking Strategy: Use the process of elimination and note the key word "need for further instructions." Options 1 and 3 can be easily eliminated first. From the remaining options, note the word "rectal" in option 2. Recalling that rectal temperatures should be avoided will direct you to this option. Review home care instructions related to infection in the leukemic child if you had difficulty with this question.
Level of Cognitive Ability: Application
Client Needs: Health Promotion and Maintenance
Integrated Concept/Process: Teaching/Learning
Content Area: Child Health
Reference: Schulte E, Price D, Gwin J: *Thompson's pediatric nursing,* ed 8, Philadelphia, 2001, WB Saunders, p. 233.

10. *Answer:* 2
Rationale: For the hospitalized neutropenic child, flowers or plants should not be kept in the room because standing water and damp soil harbor *Aspergillus* and *Pseudomonas,* to which these children are very susceptible. Additionally fruits and vegetables not peeled before being eaten harbor molds and should be avoided until the white blood cell count rises.
Test-Taking Strategy: Use the process of elimination and knowledge regarding protective isolation procedures for a neutropenic child. Note that options 1 and 3 are similar and should be eliminated first. From the remaining options, select option 2 because this nursing response maintains the procedure required. Review protective isolation procedures for the neutropenic child if you had difficulty with this question.
Level of Cognitive Ability: Application
Client Needs: Safe, Effective Care Environment
Integrated Concept/Process: Communication and Documentation
Content Area: Child Health
Reference: Schulte E, Price D, Gwin J: *Thompson's pediatric nursing,* ed 8, Philadelphia, 2001, WB Saunders, p. 231.

11. *Answer:* 3
Rationale: Clinical manifestations specifically associated with Hodgkin's disease include painless, firm, and movable adenopathy in the cervical and supraclavicular area. Hepatosplenomegaly is also noted. Although anorexia, weight loss, fever, and malaise are associated with Hodgkin's disease, these manifestations are seen in many disorders.
Test-Taking Strategy: Use the process of elimination. Note the key words "most characteristic." Eliminate options 2 and 4 first because these symptoms are general and vague. Recalling that painless adenopathy is associated with Hodgkin's disease will direct you to option 3. Review the clinical manifestations related to Hodgkin's disease if you had difficulty with this question.
Level of Cognitive Ability: Comprehension
Client Needs: Physiological Integrity
Integrated Concept/Process: Nursing Process/Data Collection
Content Area: Child Health
Reference: Schulte E, Price D, Gwin J: *Thompson's pediatric nursing,* ed 8, Philadelphia, 2001, WB Saunders, p. 338.

12. *Answer:* 1
Rationale: A Wilms' tumor is a tumor of the kidney. If Wilms' tumor is suspected, the mass should not be palpated. Excessive manipulation can cause seeding of the tumor and the spread of cancerous cells. Fever, hematuria, and hypertension are clinical manifestations associated with Wilms' tumor.
Test-Taking Strategy: Use the process of elimination and note the key word "avoiding." Knowledge that this tumor is located in the kidney will assist in eliminating options 2, 3, and 4 because of the relationship of these options to renal function. Review nursing interventions for the child with Wilms' tumor if you had difficulty with this question.
Level of Cognitive Ability: Application
Client Needs: Physiological Integrity
Integrated Concept/Process: Nursing Process/Planning
Content Area: Child Health
Reference: Schulte E, Price D, Gwin J: *Thompson's pediatric nursing,* ed 8, Philadelphia, 2001, WB Saunders, p. 196.

13. *Answer:* 4
Rationale: A clinical manifestation of osteogenic sarcoma is progressive, insidious, intermittent pain at the tumor site. By the time these children receive medical attention, they may be in considerable pain from the tumor. Options 1, 2, and 3 are accurate regarding osteogenic sarcoma.
Test-Taking Strategy: Use the process of elimination. Note the key word "not." Knowledge that osteogenic sarcoma is a malignant tumor of the bone will direct you to option 4. Review the clinical manifestations associated with osteogenic sarcoma if you had difficulty with this question.
Level of Cognitive Ability: Comprehension
Client Needs: Physiological Integrity
Integrated Concept/Process: Teaching/Learning
Content Area: Child Health
Reference: Wong D, Hockenberry-Eaton M: *Wong's essentials of pediatric nursing,* ed 6, St Louis, 2001, Mosby, p. 1235.

14. *Answer:* 1
Rationale: After amputation, phantom limb pain is a temporary condition that some children may experience. This sensation of aching or cramping in the missing limb is most distressing to the child. The child needs to be reassured that the condition is normal and only temporary.
Test-Taking Strategy: Use the process of elimination and therapeutic communication techniques to answer this question. Note that the issue of the question relates to alleviating the child's fear. Option 1 is the only option that will alleviate fear. Options 2, 3, and 4 infer that this pain may be permanent. Review care to the child after amputation if you had difficulty with this question.
Level of Cognitive Ability: Application
Client Needs: Psychosocial Integrity
Integrated Concept/Process: Communication and Documentation
Content Area: Child Health
Reference: Wong D, Hockenberry-Eaton M: *Wong's essentials of pediatric nursing,* ed 6, St Louis, 2001, Mosby, p. 1221.

15. *Answer:* 3
Rationale: Colorless drainage on the dressing would indicate the presence of cerebrospinal fluid and should be reported to the RN immediately. The RN would then contact the physician. Options 1, 2, and 4 delay required immediate interventions.
Test-Taking Strategy: Use the process of elimination. Note the key words "colorless drainage." This should quickly alert you to the possibility of the presence of cerebrospinal fluid. Therefore, eliminate options 1, 2, and 4. Review care to the child with a brain tumor if you had difficulty with this question.
Level of Cognitive Ability: Application
Client Needs: Physiological Integrity
Integrated Concept/Process: Nursing Process/Implementation
Content Area: Child Health
Reference: Schulte E, Price D, Gwin J: *Thompson's pediatric nursing,* ed 8, Philadelphia, 2001, WB Saunders, p. 280.

REFERENCES

Burroughs A, Leifer G: *Maternity nursing,* ed 8, Philadelphia, 2002, WB Saunders.

Chernecky C, Berger B: *Laboratory tests and diagnostic procedures,* ed 3, Philadelphia, 2001, WB Saunders.

McKinney E et al: *Maternal-child nursing,* Philadelphia, 2000, WB Saunders.

Murray S, McKinney E, Gorrie T: *Foundations of maternal- newborn nursing,* ed 3, Philadelphia, 2002, WB Saunders.

Schulte E, Price D, Gwin J: *Thompson's pediatric nursing,* ed 8, Philadelphia, 2001, WB Saunders.

Wong D: *Whaley & Wong's nursing care of infants and children,* ed 6, St Louis, 1999, Mosby.

Wong D, Hockenberry-Eaton M: *Wong's essentials of pediatric nursing,* ed 6, St Louis, 2001, Mosby.

Communicable Diseases and Acquired Immunodeficiency Syndrome

I. RUBEOLA (MEASLES)

A. Description
1. Agent: virus
2. Incubation period: 10 to 20 days
3. Communicable period: from 4 days before to 5 days after the rash appears; mainly during prodromal (catarrhal) stage
4. Source: respiratory tract secretions, blood, or urine of infected person
5. Transmission: airborne or direct contact with infectious droplets

B. Data collection
1. Fever
2. Malaise
3. Coryza and cough
4. Rash appears as red, discrete maculopapules that blanch easily with pressure and gradually turn a brownish color (lasts 6 to 7 days); rash begins behind the ears and spreads downward to the feet
5. Koplik spots: small, red spots with a bluish white center and a red base; located on the mucosa and last 3 days

C. Implementation
1. Respiratory precautions if the child is hospitalized
2. Restrict to quiet activities and bed rest
3. Use a cool mist vaporizer for cough and coryza
4. Dim lights if photophobia is present
5. Administer antipyretics for fever

II. ROSEOLA (EXANTHEMA SUBITUM)

A. Description
1. Agent: Human herpesvirus type 6 (HHV-6)
2. Incubation period: 5 to 15 days
3. Communicable period: unknown but thought to extend from the febrile stage to the time the rash first appears
4. Source: unknown
5. Transmission: unknown

B. Data collection
1. Fever for 3 to 5 days followed by a rash (rose-pink maculas that blanch with pressure)
2. The rash appears 2 to 3 days after the onset of fever and lasts 1 to 2 days

C. Implementation: supportive

III. RUBELLA (GERMAN MEASLES)

A. Description
1. Agent: rubella virus
2. Incubation period: 14 to 21 days
3. Communicable period: 7 days before to approximately 5 days after the rash appears
4. Source: nasopharyngeal secretions; virus is also present in blood, stool, and urine
5. Transmission
   a. Airborne or direct contact with infectious droplets
   b. Indirectly via articles freshly contaminated with nasopharyngeal secretions, feces, or urine
   c. Transplacental

B. Data collection
1. Low-grade fever
2. Malaise
3. Pinkish red maculopapular rash that begins on the face and spreads to the entire body
4. Petechiae spots may occur on the soft palate

C. Implementation
1. Supportive treatment
2. Isolate the infected child from pregnant women

IV. MUMPS

A. Description
1. Agent: paramyxovirus
2. Incubation period: 14 to 21 days
3. Communicable period: immediately before and after the swelling begins
4. Source: saliva of infected person and possibly urine
5. Transmission
   a. Direct contact with infected person
   b. Droplet spread from infected person

B. Data collection
1. Fever
2. Headache and malaise
3. Anorexia
4. Earache aggravated by chewing, followed by parotid glandular swelling

C. Implementation
1. Respiratory precautions
2. Bed rest until the parotid glandular swelling subsides
3. Avoid foods that require chewing
4. Apply hot or cold compresses as prescribed to the neck
5. To relieve orchitis, apply warmth and local support with tight-fitting underpants

V. CHICKENPOX (VARICELLA)

A. Description
1. Agent: varicella zoster virus (VZV)
2. Incubation period: 13 to 17 days
3. Communicable period: 1 to 2 days before the onset of the rash to 6 days after the first crop of vesicles, when crusts have formed
4. Source: respiratory tract secretions of infected person; skin lesions
5. Transmission: direct contact, droplet (airborne) spread, and contaminated objects

B. Data collection
1. Slight fever, malaise, and anorexia followed by a macular rash that first appears on the trunk and scalp and moves to the extremities
2. Lesions become pustules, begin to dry, and develop a crust
3. Lesions may appear on the mucous membranes of the mouth, genital area, and rectal area

C. Implementation
1. In the hospital setting, strict isolation
2. In the home setting, isolate the infected child until the vesicles have dried; isolate high-risk children from the infected child

VI. PERTUSSIS (WHOOPING COUGH)

A. Description
1. Agent: *Bordetella pertussis*
2. Incubation period: 5 to 21 days (usually 10 days)
3. Communicable period: greatest during the catarrhal stage
4. Source: discharge from the respiratory tract of the infected person
5. Transmission: direct contact or droplet spread from infected person; indirect contact with freshly contaminated articles

B. Data collection: symptoms of respiratory infection followed by increased severity of cough

C. Implementation
1. Isolation during the catarrhal stage; if the child is hospitalized, institute respiratory precautions
2. Administer antimicrobial therapy as prescribed
3. Administer pertussis-immune globulin as prescribed
4. Reduce environmental factors that promote paroxysms of cough, such as dust, smoke, and sudden changes in temperature
5. Encourage fluid intake
6. Provide high humidity with the use of a humidifier or tent

VII. DIPHTHERIA

A. Description
1. Agent: *Corynebacterium diphtheriae*
2. Incubation period: 2 to 5 days
3. Communicable period: variable; until virulent bacilli are no longer present (three negative cultures), usually 2 weeks but as long as 4 weeks
4. Source: discharge from the mucous membrane of the nose and nasopharynx, skin, and other lesions of the infected person
5. Transmission: direct contact with infected person, carrier, or contaminated articles

B. Data collection
1. Low-grade fever, malaise, sore throat
2. Foul-smelling, mucopurulent nasal discharge
3. Gray membrane on the tonsils and pharynx
4. Lymphadenitis (neck edema)

C. Implementation
1. Strict isolation of the hospitalized child
2. Administer antitoxin as prescribed (preceded by a skin or conjunctival test to rule out sensitivity to horse serum)
3. Bed rest
4. Administer antibiotics as prescribed

VIII. POLIOMYELITIS

A. Description
1. Agent: enteroviruses
2. Incubation period: 7 to 14 days
3. Communicable period: not exactly known; the virus is present in the throat and feces shortly after infection and persists for approximately 1 week in the throat and 4 to 6 weeks in the feces
4. Source: oropharyngeal secretions and feces of the infected person
5. Transmission: direct contact with infected person; fecal-oral and oropharyngeal routes

B. Data collection
1. Fever, malaise, anorexia, nausea, headache, sore throat
2. Abdominal pain followed by soreness and stiffness of the trunk, neck, and limbs that progresses to flaccid paralysis

C. Implementation
1. Enteric precautions
2. Supportive treatment
3. Bed rest
4. Monitor for respiratory paralysis
5. Physical therapy

IX. SCARLET FEVER

A. Description
1. Agent: group A, β-hemolytic streptococci
2. Incubation period: 1 to 7 days
3. Communicable period: during the incubation period and clinical illness, approximately 10 days; during the first 2 weeks of the carrier stage, although may persist for months
4. Source: nasopharyngeal secretions of infected person and carriers
5. Transmission: direct contact with infected person or droplet spread; indirectly by contact with contaminated articles, ingestion of contaminated milk, or other foods

B. Data collection
1. Abrupt high fever, vomiting, headache, malaise, abdominal pain
2. A red, fine papular rash in the axilla, groin, and neck that spreads to cover the entire body
3. The rash blanches with pressure except in areas of deep creases and folds of the joints (Pastia's sign)
4. The tongue is coated and papillae become red and swollen (white strawberry tongue); by the fourth to fifth day the white coat sloughs off leaving prominent papillae (red strawberry tongue)
5. Tonsils are edematous and covered with a gray-white exudate
6. Pharynx is edematous and beefy-red in color

C. Implementation
1. Respiratory precautions until 24 hours after the initiation of treatment
2. Supportive therapy
3. Bed rest
4. Encourage fluid intake
5. Administer antibiotics as prescribed

X. ERYTHEMA INFECTIOSUM (FIFTH DISEASE)

A. Description
1. Agent: human parvovirus B19 (HPV)
2. Incubation period: 4 to 14 days; may be as long as 20 days
3. Communicable period: uncertain but before the onset of symptoms in most children
4. Source: infected person
5. Transmission: unknown; possibly respiratory secretions and blood

B. Data collection
1. Fever, myalgia, lethargy, nausea, vomiting, abdominal pain
2. Stages of the rash
   a. Erythema of the face (slapped face appearance) chiefly on the cheeks; disappears by 1 to 4 days
   b. Approximately 1 day after the rash appears on the face, maculopapular red spots appear, symmetrically distributed in the extremities; rash progresses from proximal to distal surfaces and may last a week or more
   c. Rash subsides but may reappear if the skin becomes irritated or traumatized by such factors as the sun, heat, cold, or friction

C. Implementation
1. Respiratory isolation in the hospitalized child
2. Pregnant women should not be in contact with or care for the infected person
3. Supportive
4. Administer antipyretics, analgesics, and anti-inflammatory medications as prescribed

XI. INFECTIOUS MONONUCLEOSIS

A. Description
1. Agent: Epstein-Barr (EB) virus
2. Incubation period: 4 to 6 weeks
3. Communicable period: unknown; the virus is shed before the onset of the disease until 6 months or longer after recovery
4. Source: oral secretions
5. Transmission: direct intimate contact, infected blood

B. Data collection
   1. Fever, sore throat, malaise, headache, fatigue, nausea, abdominal pain
   2. Lymphadenopathy and hepatosplenomegaly
C. Implementation
   1. Supportive
   2. Monitor for signs of splenic rupture, which includes abdominal pain, left upper quadrant pain, or left shoulder pain

XII. ROCKY MOUNTAIN SPOTTED FEVER

A. Description
   1. Agent: *Rickettsia rickettsii*
   2. Incubation period: 2 to 14 days
   3. Source: tick; mammal source: wild rodents, dogs
   4. Transmission: bite of infected tick
B. Data collection
   1. Fever, malaise, anorexia, vomiting, headache, myalgia
   2. Maculopapular or petechial rash primarily on the extremities (ankles and wrists) but may spread to other areas, characteristically on the palms and soles
C. Implementation
   1. Vigorous supportive care
   2. Administer antibiotics as prescribed
   3. Teaching regarding protection from tick bites

XIII. ENTEROBIASIS (PINWORM)

A. Description
   1. Agent: *Enterobius vermicularis*
   2. Source
      a. Universally present in temperate climatic zones
      b. Eggs are ingested or inhaled (eggs float in the air), hatch in the upper intestine, mature in 2 to 8 weeks, and migrate to the cecal area; females then mate, migrate out the anus, and lay eggs
   3. Transmission
      a. Favored in crowded conditions
      b. Ingestion or inhalation of eggs
      c. Hands to mouth or fecal-oral route
      d. Contaminated items (pinworm eggs persist in the environment for 2 to 3 weeks)
B. Data collection: intense perianal itching, irritability, restlessness, poor sleep, bed-wetting, distractibility, short attention span; in females, the worm may migrate to the vagina and urethra and cause infection
C. Implementation
   1. Identify the worms
      a. Use of a flashlight to inspect the anal area 2 to 3 hours after the child is asleep
      b. Tape test: transparent, sticky tape is used to obtain a specimen from the child's perianal area; specimen is collected in the morning as soon as the child awakens and before a bowel movement or a bath
   2. Enteric precautions
   3. Antihelmintic medications (all household members are treated); course of medication is repeated in 2 weeks after the first course to prevent reinfection
   4. Teach home care measures to prevent reinfection

XIV. IMMUNIZATIONS

A. Immunization schedule (Box 36-1)
B. General contraindications to immunizations
   1. Severe febrile illness
   2. Live virus vaccines are generally not administered to anyone with an altered immune system
   3. Allergic reaction to a previously administered vaccine or a substance in the vaccine
C. Hepatitis B vaccine
   1. Protects against hepatitis B
   2. The first dose of hepatitis B is administered between the ages of birth and 2 months, the second dose is administered between the ages of 1 and 4 months, and the third dose is administered between the ages of 6 and 18 months
   3. All children 0 through 18 years old need three doses of hepatitis B vaccine if they haven't already received them
   4. Contraindication: anaphylactic reaction to common baker's yeast
D. DTaP (diphtheria, tetanus, acellular pertussis) and Td
   1. Protects against diphtheria, tetanus, and pertussis

BOX 36-1

Recommended Immunization Schedule for Healthy Infants and Children

Birth	Hepatitis B
1 month	Hepatitis B
2 months	IPV, DTaP, Hib
4 months	DTaP, Hib, IPV
6 months	DTaP, Hib, hepatitis B, IPV
12 - 15 months	Hib, MMR
12 - 18 months	DtaP, varicella zoster
4 - 6 years	DTaP, IPV, MMR
11 - 12 years	MMR (if not administered at 4-6 years)
11 - 16 years	Td

2. DTaP is administered at 2 months, 4 months, 6 months, between 15 and 18 months old, and between 4 and 6 years old
3. The fourth dose of DTaP can be given at 12 months of age if 6 months have elapsed since the previous dose and if the child might not return for follow-up care by 18 months of age
4. Td (tetanus, diphtheria booster) is given at 11 to 12 years of age if at least 5 years have passed since the last dose of DTaP/DPT (DPT = diphtheria, tetanus, pertussis)
5. Contraindication: encephalopathy within 7 days of administration of previous dose of DPT

E. Hib (*Haemophilus influenzae* type b) vaccine
1. Protects against *H. influenzae* type b
2. Hib is administered at 2 months, 4 months, 6 months, and between 12 and 15 months of age
3. Depending on the brand of Hib vaccine used for the first and second doses, a dose at 6 months of age may not be needed
4. Contraindication: nonidentified

F. IPV (inactivated poliovirus vaccine)
1. Protects against polio
2. IPV is administered at 2 months, 4 months, 6 months, and between 4 and 6 years of age
3. The third dose of IPV is administered between 6 and 18 months of age
4. Contraindication: Anaphylactic reaction to neomycin or streptomycin

G. MMR (measles, mumps, rubella)
1. Protects against measles, mumps, and rubella (German measles)
2. The first dose of MMR is administered between 12 and 15 months of age; the second dose is administered at 4 to 6 years of age (if the second dose was not given by 4 to 6 years of age, it should be given at the next visit)
3. MMR contains minute amounts of neomycin; measles and mumps vaccine, which are grown on chick embryo tissue cultures, are not believed to contain significant amounts of egg cross-reacting proteins
4. Contraindications
   a. Pregnancy
   b. Known altered immunodeficiency
   c. Allergic to contents of immunization (before the administration of MMR vaccine, assess for a known history of allergy to neomycin or related antibiotics)
   d. Presence of recently acquired passive immunity through blood transfusions, immunoglobulin, or maternal antibodies (MMR should be postponed for a minimum of 3 months after passive immunization with immunoglobulins or blood transfusions, except washed blood cells, which do not interfere with the immune response)

H. Varicella zoster vaccine
1. Protects against chickenpox
2. Varicella zoster vaccine is administered between 12 and 18 months of age
3. Susceptible children 13 years of age and older (who have not had chickenpox or have not been previously vaccinated) need two doses given 4 to 8 weeks apart
4. Contraindications
   a. Pregnancy
   b. Immunocompromised individuals
   c. Children receiving corticosteroids

I. OPV (oral poliovirus vaccine)
1. No longer recommended for routine vaccination
2. Not administered to anyone with an altered immune system or to any household contacts of an immunosuppressed child (the virus multiplies in the gastrointestinal tract and is excreted in the stool)

XV. ACQUIRED IMMUNODEFICIENCY SYNDROME (AIDS)

A. Description
1. A disorder caused by the human immunodeficiency virus (HIV) and is characterized by a generalized dysfunction of the immune system
2. Both the cellular immunity and the humoral immunity are compromised
3. Horizontal transmission of HIV occurs through intimate sexual contact or parenteral exposure to blood or body fluids containing visible blood
4. Vertical (perinatal) transmission occurs when an HIV-infected pregnant woman passes the infection to her infant
5. The most common opportunistic infection of children infected with HIV is *Pneumocystis carinii* pneumonia (PCP); it occurs most frequently between the ages of 3 and 6 months, when HIV status may be indeterminate
6. The goals of therapy include slowing the growth of the virus, preventing and treating opportunistic infections, and providing nutritional support and symptomatic treatment

B. Data collection
1. During neonatal period
   a. Lymphadenopathy
   b. Hepatosplenomegaly
   c. *P. carinii* pneumonia (PCP)

d. Progressive encephalopathy
e. Microcephaly
2. Infants
a. Failure to thrive
b. Diarrhea
c. Developmental delays
d. Oral candidiasis
e. Hepatosplenomegaly
f. Chronic cough and lymphoid interstitial pneumonia (LIP)
g. Chronic otitis media
3. Children/adolescents
a. Malaise and fatigue
b. Night sweats
c. Weight loss
d. Diarrhea
e. Fever
f. **Regression** of developmental milestones
g. Generalized lymphadenopathy
h. Nephropathy
i. PCP and LIP
j. Encephalopathy

C. Diagnostic tests
1. Enzyme-linked immunosorbent assay (ELISA)
a. ELISA determines the response of antibodies to the HIV virus
b. Useful in children older than 18 months
2. Western blot
a. Confirms the presence of HIV antibodies
b. Useful in children older than 18 months
c. A positive HIV antibody test in children younger than 18 months indicates only that the mother is infected; other diagnostic tests will be used, including the virus culture, polymerase chain reaction (PCR) for detection of proviral DNA, and p24 antigen detection, which is HIV-specific
3. p24 antigen
a. Used to detect HIV antigen in children younger than 18 months
b. Test can be useful at any age
c. Only a positive result is significant
d. Two or more positive results are diagnostic for HIV infection
4. CD4+: used to assess a child's immune status, risk for disease progression, and the need for PCP prophylaxis after 1 year of age

D. Prophylaxis
1. Provide prophylaxis as prescribed against PCP during the first year of life to the infant born to an HIV-infected woman; after 1 year of age, the need for prophylaxis is determined by the presence of severe immunosuppression or a history of PCP
2. Provide continued prophylaxis through 12 months of age for children diagnosed with HIV
3. For HIV-infected children older than 12 months, continued prophylaxis is based on CD4+ counts and whether PCP has previously occurred

E. Parent instructions regarding care to the child
1. Frequent handwashing
2. Assess for fever, malaise, fatigue, weight loss, vomiting and diarrhea, altered activity level, and oral lesions, and notify the physician if these occur
3. The signs and symptoms of opportunistic infections
4. The administration of antiretroviral medications as prescribed
5. The child should avoid exposure to other illnesses
6. Keep immunizations up-to-date
7. Keep the child home when sick
8. Do not kiss the child on the mouth
9. Monitor weight
10. Provide a high-calorie and high-protein diet
11. Do not share eating utensils
12. Wash eating utensils in the dishwasher
13. Cover unused food and formula and refrigerate
14. Discard unused refrigerated formula and food after 24 hours
15. Wear gloves for care, especially when in contact with body fluids and changing diapers
16. Change diapers frequently, away from food areas
17. Fold soiled disposable diapers inward and tab, and dispose in a tightly covered plastic-lined container
18. Dispose of trash daily
19. Cover sandboxes when not in use to create a barrier to germs
20. Clean up spills with bleach solution (10:1 ratio of water to bleach)

F. Immunizations
1. Immunization against common childhood illnesses is recommended for all children exposed to and infected with HIV
2. The varicella (chickenpox) vaccine is avoided
3. Oral polio virus (OPV) is not recommended for routine vaccination for any child
4. Pneumococcal and influenza vaccines are recommended
5. Measles, mumps, rubella (MMR) vaccine is administered if the child is not severely immunocompromised (the child receiving IV gamma globulin prophylaxis may not respond to the MMR vaccine)

PRACTICE QUESTIONS

1. A child with rubeola (measles) is being admitted to the hospital. In preparing for the admission of the child, the nurse plans to place the child of which precautions?
   1. Contact
   2. Enteric
   3. Respiratory
   4. Protective
2. Several children have contracted rubeola (measles) in a local school. The school nurse conducts a teaching session to the mothers of the school children. Which statement made by a mother indicates a need for further teaching regarding this communicable disease?
   1. "Respiratory symptoms such as a profuse runny nose, cough, and fever occur before the development of a rash."
   2. "Small, blue, white spots with a red base may appear in the mouth."
   3. "The rash usually begins behind the ears and spreads downward toward the feet."
   4. "The communicable period ranges from 10 days before the onset of symptoms to 15 days after the rash appears."
3. A mother of a 15-month-old child brings the child to the clinic and reports that the child has a fever and has developed a rash on the neck and trunk of the body. Roseola is diagnosed. The mother is concerned that her other children will contract the disease. The nurse provides which of the following instructions to the mother regarding the prevention of transmission of the disease?
   1. The disease is transmitted through the urine and feces so the other children should use a separate bathroom
   2. Disease transmission is unknown
   3. The disease is transmitted through the respiratory tract so the child should be isolated from the other children as much as possible
   4. The disease is transmitted by contact with body fluids so any items contaminated with body fluids need to be discarded in a separate receptacle
4. A nurse provides instructions to the mother of a child with mumps regarding respiratory precautions. The mother asks the nurse about the length of time required for the respiratory precautions. The nurse most appropriately responds that:
   1. "Respiratory precautions are necessary for the entire time of illness."
   2. "Respiratory precautions are necessary until the swelling is gone."
   3. "Respiratory precautions are indicated during the period of communicability."
   4. "Respiratory precautions are indicated for 18 days after the onset of parotid swelling."
5. A mother brings her 6-year-old child to the clinic because the child has developed a rash on the trunk and on the scalp. The mother reports that the child has had a low-grade temperature, has not felt like eating, and has been generally tired. The child is diagnosed with chickenpox. The mother inquires about the communicable period associated with chickenpox. The nurse plans to base the response on which of the following?
   1. The communicable period is unknown
   2. The communicable period is 1 to 2 days before the onset of the rash to 6 days after the onset of lesions and the crusting of lesions
   3. The communicable period is 10 days before the onset of symptoms to 15 days after the rash appears
   4. The communicable period ranges from 2 weeks or less up to several months
6. A nurse assists in preparing home care instructions to the parents of a child hospitalized with pertussis. The child is in the convalescent stage and is being prepared for discharge. Which of the following will not be included in the instructions?
   1. Maintain respiratory precautions and a quiet environment for at least 2 weeks
   2. Coughing spells may be triggered by dust or smoke
   3. Encourage fluid intake
   4. Good handwashing techniques must be instituted to prevent spreading the disease to others
7. A 6-month-old infant receives a DTaP (diphtheria, tetanus, and acellular pertussis) immunization at the well-baby clinic. The mother returns home and calls the clinic to report that the infant has developed swelling and redness at the site of injection. The nurse tells the mother to:
   1. Apply a warm pack to the injection site
   2. Bring the infant back to the clinic
   3. Apply an ice pack to the injection site
   4. Monitor the infant for a fever
8. A child is diagnosed with scarlet fever. The nurse collects data on the child knowing that which of the following is not a clinical manifestation associated with this disease?
   1. Pastia's sign
   2. White strawberry tongue
   3. Edematous and beefy, red-colored pharynx
   4. Koplik spots
9. A nurse provides home care instructions to the parents of a child with infectious mononucleosis. The nurse tells the parents to:
   1. Maintain the child on bed rest for 2 weeks
   2. Maintain respiratory precautions for 1 week
   3. Notify the physician if the child develops a fever
   4. Notify the physician if the child develops abdominal pain or left shoulder pain

10. The mother of a preschooler who attends day care calls the clinic nurse and tells the nurse that the child is constantly itching the perianal area and that the area is irritated. The nurse suspects the possibility of pinworm (enterobiasis) infection. The nurse instructs the mother to obtain a tape test rectal specimen. The nurse instructs the mother to obtain the specimen:
    1. When the child is put to bed
    2. After toileting
    3. After bathing
    4. In the morning when the child awakens
11. A nursing student is assigned to administer immunizations to children in a clinic. The nursing instructor asks the student about the contraindications to receiving an immunization. The student responds correctly by telling the instructor that a contraindication for receiving an immunization is if a child has:
    1. A cold
    2. Otitis media
    3. Mild diarrhea
    4. A severe febrile illness
12. A clinic nurse prepares to administer an MMR (measles, mumps and rubella) vaccine to a 5-year-old child. The nurse administers this vaccine:
    1. Intramuscularly in the anterolateral aspect of the thigh
    2. Intramuscularly in the deltoid muscle
    3. Subcutaneously in the outer aspect of the upper arm
    4. Subcutaneously in the gluteal muscle
13. A child is scheduled to receive an MMR (measles, mumps, rubella) vaccine. The nurse preparing to administer the vaccine reviews the child's record and questions the order if which of the following is documented in the child's record?
    1. A local reaction at the site of injection of a previous MMR vaccine
    2. A history of an anaphylactoid reaction to neomycin
    3. A history of frequent respiratory infections
    4. Recent recovery from a cold
14. An infant with a human immunodeficiency virus (HIV)-infected mother is seen in the clinic on a monthly basis and is being monitored for symptoms indicative of HIV. The nurse collects data on the infant knowing that the most common opportunistic infection of children infected with HIV is:
    1. Gastroenteritis
    2. Meningitis
    3. *Pneumocystis carinii* pneumonia (PCP)
    4. Lymphoid interstitial pneumonia (LIP)
15. A child with human immunodeficiency virus (HIV) is receiving zidovudine (AZT, Retrovir). The nurse monitors which laboratory study to determine if the child is experiencing an adverse reaction from the medication?
    1. Sedimentation rate
    2. Complete blood count (CBC)
    3. Calcium level
    4. Potassium level

ANSWERS

1. *Answer:* 3
Rationale: Rubeola is transmitted via airborne particles or direct contact with infectious droplets. Respiratory precautions are required and a mask is worn by those in contact with the child. Gowns and gloves are not indicated. Articles that are contaminated should be bagged and labeled. Options 1, 2, and 4 are not indicated in rubeola.
Test-Taking Strategy: Use the process of elimination. Recalling that rubeola is transmitted via the airborne route will easily direct you to option 3. Review the route of transmission and therapeutic management of rubeola if you had difficulty with this question.
Level of Cognitive Ability: Application
Client Needs: Safe, Effective Care Environment
Integrated Concept/Process: Nursing Process/Planning
Content Area: Child Health
Reference: Schulte E, Price D, Gwin J: *Thompson's pediatric nursing*, ed 8, Philadelphia, 2001, WB Saunders, p. 244.

2. *Answer:* 4
Rationale: The communicable period for rubeola ranges from 4 days before to 5 days after the rash appears, mainly during the prodromal (catarrhal) stage. Options 1, 2, and 3 are accurate descriptions of rubeola. The small blue-white spots found in this communicable disease are called Koplik spots. Option 4, the incorrect option, describes the incubation period for rubella, not rubeola.
Test-Taking Strategy: Use the process of elimination. Note the key words "need for further teaching" in the stem of the question. Recalling that the communicable period for rubeola ranges from 4 days before to 5 days after the rash appears will direct you to option 4. Review the clinical manifestations associated with rubeola if you had difficulty with this question.
Level of Cognitive Ability: Comprehension
Client Needs: Health Promotion and Maintenance
Integrated Concept/Process: Teaching/Learning
Content Area: Child Health

Reference: Schulte E, Price D, Gwin J: *Thompson's pediatric nursing,* ed 8, Philadelphia, 2001, WB Saunders, p. 244.

3. *Answer:* 2
Rationale: The method of transmission of roseola is unknown. Options 1, 3, and 4 are not accurate transmission routes of roseola.
Test-Taking Strategy: Use the process of elimination. Eliminate options 1 and 4 first because they are similar. From the remaining options, recall that the method of transmission of roseola is unknown. Review the characteristics of roseola if you had difficulty with this question.
Level of Cognitive Ability: Application
Client Needs: Health Promotion and Maintenance
Integrated Concept/Process: Teaching/Learning
Content Area: Child Health
Reference: Schulte E, Price D, Gwin J: *Thompson's pediatric nursing,* ed 8, Philadelphia, 2001, WB Saunders, p. 242.

4. *Answer:* 3
Rationale: Mumps is transmitted via direct contact or droplet spread from an infected person and possibly by contact with the urine. Respiratory precautions are indicated during the period of communicability.
Test-Taking Strategy: Use the process of elimination. Options 1 and 2 can be eliminated first because they are similar. From the remaining options, select option 3, because it is the global option, and addresses communicability. Also, the time frame indicated in option 4 seems rather lengthy. Review the infectious period related to mumps if you had difficulty with this question.
Level of Cognitive Ability: Application
Client Needs: Safe, Effective Care Environment
Integrated Concept/Process: Teaching/Learning
Content Area: Child Health
Reference: Schulte E, Price D, Gwin J: *Thompson's pediatric nursing,* ed 8, Philadelphia, 2001, WB Saunders, p. 245.

5. *Answer:* 2
Rationale: The communicable period for chickenpox is 1 to 2 days before the onset of the rash to 6 days after the onset of lesions and the crusting of lesions. In roseola, the communicable period is unknown. Option 3 describes rubella. Option 4 describes diphtheria.
Test-Taking Strategy: Use the process of elimination. Option 1 can be easily eliminated. Eliminate options 3 and 4 next because the time frames in these two options seem rather lengthy and are similar. If you had difficulty with this question, review the communicable period for chickenpox.
Level of Cognitive Ability: Comprehension
Client Needs: Safe, Effective Care Environment
Integrated Concept/Process: Nursing Process/Planning
Content Area: Child Health
Reference: Schulte E, Price D, Gwin J: *Thompson's pediatric nursing,* ed 8, Philadelphia, 2001, WB Saunders, p. 241.

6. *Answer:* 1
Rationale: Pertussis is transmitted by direct contact or respiratory droplets from coughing. The communicable period occurs primarily during the catarrhal stage. Respiratory precautions are not required during the convalescent phase. Options 2, 3, and 4 are components of home care instructions.
Test-Taking Strategy: Use the process of elimination. Note the key words "convalescent" in the question and "not" in the stem of the question. Options 3 and 4 can be eliminated because they are general interventions associated with convalescence. Knowing that coughing spells are associated with pertussis will assist in directing you to option 1. Additionally, 2 weeks of respiratory precautions is not required. If you had difficulty with this question, review home care instructions for the child with pertussis.
Level of Cognitive Ability: Application
Client Needs: Health Promotion and Maintenance
Integrated Concept/Process: Nursing Process/Planning
Content Area: Child Health
Reference: Schulte E, Price D, Gwin J: *Thompson's pediatric nursing,* ed 8, Philadelphia, 2001, WB Saunders, p. 245.

7. *Answer:* 3
Rationale: Occasionally, tenderness, redness, or swelling may occur at the site of the injection. This can be relieved with ice packs for the first 24 hours followed by warm compresses if the inflammation persists. It is not necessary to bring the infant back to the clinic. Option 4 may be an appropriate intervention but is not specific to the issue of the question.
Test-Taking Strategy: Use the process of elimination. Option 4 can be eliminated first because it does not relate specifically to the issue of the question. Eliminate option 2 next as an unnecessary intervention. From the remaining options, general principles related to the effects of heat and cold will direct you to option 3. Review interventions following immunizations and injections if you had difficulty with this question.
Level of Cognitive Ability: Application
Client Needs: Health Promotion and Maintenance
Integrated Concept/Process: Nursing Process/Implementation
Content Area: Child Health
Reference: Schulte E, Price D, Gwin J: *Thompson's pediatric nursing,* ed 8, Philadelphia, 2001, WB Saunders, p. 119.

8. *Answer:* 4
Rationale: Pastia's sign describes a rash seen in scarlet fever that will blanch with pressure except in areas of deep creases and the folds of joints. The tongue is initially coated with a white furry covering with red projecting papillae (white strawberry tongue). By the fourth to fifth day, the white strawberry tongue sloughs off, leaving a red swollen tongue (strawberry tongue). The pharynx is edematous and beefy red in color. Koplik spots are associated with rubeola.
Test-Taking Strategy: Use the process of elimination noting the key word "not" in the stem of the question. Recalling that Koplik spots are associated with rubeola will assist in answering this question. Review the clinical manifestations associated with scarlet fever if you had difficulty with this question.
Level of Cognitive Ability: Comprehension
Client Needs: Physiological Integrity
Integrated Concept/Process: Nursing Process/Data Collection
Content Area: Child Health
Reference: Wong D, Hockenberry-Eaton M: *Wong's essentials of pediatric nursing,* ed 6, St Louis, 2001, Mosby, p. 464.

9. *Answer:* 4
Rationale: The parents need to be instructed to notify the physician if abdominal pain, especially in the left upper quadrant, or left shoulder pain occurs because this may indicate splenic rupture. Children with enlarged spleens are also instructed to avoid contact sports until splenomegaly resolves. Bed rest is not necessary and children usually self-limit their activity. Respiratory precautions are not required, although transmission can occur via direct intimate contact or contact with infected blood. Fever is treated with acetaminophen (Tylenol).
Test-Taking Strategy: Use the process of elimination and knowledge regarding the organs affected in mononucleosis. Options 1 and 2 can be eliminated first because they are unnecessary interventions in this infection. From the remaining options, recalling that splenic rupture is a concern will direct you to option 4. Review the complications associated with mononucleosis if you had difficulty with this question.
Level of Cognitive Ability: Application
Client Needs: Health Promotion and Maintenance
Integrated Concept/Process: Teaching/Learning
Content Area: Child Health
Reference: Schulte E, Price D, Gwin J: *Thompson's pediatric nursing*, ed 8, Philadelphia, 2001, WB Saunders, p. 323.

10. *Answer:* 4
Rationale: Diagnosis is confirmed by direct visualization of the worms. Parents can view the sleeping child's anus with a flashlight. The worm is white, thin, about 1/2 inch long, and moves. A simple technique, the tape test, is used to capture worms and eggs. Transparent tape is lightly touched to the anus and then applied to a slide for examination. The best specimens are obtained as the child awakens, before toileting or bathing.
Test-Taking Strategy: Use the process of elimination. Thinking about the test and the purpose of the test (to obtain a specimen that contains worms and eggs) will direct you to option 4. Review the procedure for this test if you are unfamiliar with it.
Level of Cognitive Ability: Application
Client Needs: Physiological Integrity
Integrated Concept/Process: Nursing Process/Implementation
Content Area: Child Health
Reference: Schulte E, Price D, Gwin J: *Thompson's pediatric nursing*, ed 8, Philadelphia, 2001, WB Saunders, p. 192.

11. *Answer:* 4
Rationale: A severe febrile illness is a reason to delay immunization, but only until the child has recovered from the acute stage of the illness. Minor illnesses such as a cold, otitis media, or mild diarrhea are not contraindications to immunization.
Test-Taking Strategy: Use the process of elimination focusing on the issue of the question, a contraindication to receiving an immunization. Reviewing each option carefully will easily direct you to option 4. If you had difficulty with this question, review the contraindications associated with immunizations.
Level of Cognitive Ability: Application
Client Needs: Physiological Integrity
Integrated Concept/Process: Nursing Process/Implementation
Content Area: Child Health
Reference: Schulte E, Price D, Gwin J: *Thompson's pediatric nursing*, ed 8, Philadelphia, 2001, WB Saunders, p. 387.

12. *Answer:* 3
Rationale: MMR is administered subcutaneously in the outer aspect of the upper arm. The gluteal muscle is most often used for intramuscular injections. MMR is not administered by the intramuscular route.
Test-Taking Strategy: Use the process of elimination. Knowledge that MMR is administered subcutaneously will assist in eliminating options 1 and 2. From the remaining options, recalling that the gluteal muscle is most often used for intramuscular injections will assist in directing you to option 3. Review the procedures related to the administration of MMR if you had difficulty with this question.
Level of Cognitive Ability: Application
Client Needs: Physiological Integrity
Integrated Concept/Process: Nursing Process/Implementation
Content Area: Child Health
Reference: Schulte E, Price D, Gwin J: *Thompson's pediatric nursing*, ed 8, Philadelphia, 2001, WB Saunders, p. 386.

13. *Answer:* 2
Rationale: MMR contains minute amounts of neomycin. A history of an anaphylactoid reaction to neomycin is considered a contraindication to the MMR vaccine. The general contraindication to all immunizations is a severe febrile illness. The presence of minor illnesses such as a common cold is not a contraindication. Additionally, a history of frequent respiratory infections is not a contraindication to receiving a vaccine. A local reaction to an immunization is treated with ice packs for the first 24 hours after injection followed by warm compresses if the inflammation persists.
Test-Taking Strategy: Use the process of elimination. Recalling that a general contraindication to all immunizations is a severe febrile illness will assist in eliminating options 3 and 4. From the remaining options, note that option 1 identifies a local reaction. This will direct you to option 2, the systemic reaction, and a potential life-threatening condition. Review the contraindications to receiving immunizations if you had difficulty with this question.
Level of Cognitive Ability: Application
Client Needs: Safe, Effective Care Environment
Integrated Concept/Process: Nursing Process/Implementation
Content Area: Child Health
Reference: Schulte E, Price D, Gwin J: *Thompson's pediatric nursing*, ed 8, Philadelphia, 2001, WB Saunders, p. 386.

14. *Answer:* 3
Rationale: The most common opportunistic infection of children infected with HIV is PCP. It occurs most frequently between the ages of 3 and 6 months, when HIV status may be indeterminate. LIP is a form of chronic pneumonitis and is also characteristic of HIV infection; however, it is not the most common opportunistic infection. Although gastrointestinal disturbances and neurological abnormalities may occur in the child with HIV infection, options 1 and 2 are not specific opportunistic infections noted in the HIV infected infant or child.

Test-Taking Strategy: Use the process of elimination and note the key words "most common opportunistic infection." This focus will direct you to option 3. Review the common manifestations associated with HIV, if you had difficulty with this question.
Level of Cognitive Ability: Application
Client Needs: Physiological Integrity
Integrated Concept/Process: Nursing Process/Data Collection
Content Area: Child Health
Reference: Wong D: *Whaley and Wong's nursing care of infants and children*, ed 6, St Louis, 1999, Mosby, p. 1695.

15. ***Answer:*** 2
Rationale: Zidovudine effectively interferes with HIV replication but can cause bone marrow suppression. Anemia occurs most commonly after 4 to 6 weeks of therapy. Hematology studies need to be monitored for anemia and granulocytopenia. Renal and liver function tests should also be monitored. Options 1, 3, and 4 are not associated with the use of zidovudine.
Test-Taking Strategy: Use the process of elimination. Recalling that anemia is a concern with the administration of this medication will direct you to option 2. Review the adverse effects related to this medication if you had difficulty with this question.
Level of Cognitive Ability: Application
Client Needs: Physiological Integrity
Integrated Concept/Process: Nursing Process/Data Collection
Content Area: Child Health
Reference: Hodgson B, Kizior R: *Saunders nursing drug handbook 2002*, Philadelphia, 2002, WB Saunders, pp. 1168.

REFERENCES

Advisory Committee on Immunization Practices: *When do children and teens need vaccinations?* St. Paul, 2000, Immunization Action Coalition: Item P4050.

Advisory Committee on Immunization Practices: *Summary of rules for childhood immunization*, St Paul, 2000, Immunization Action Coalition: Item P2010.

Burroughs A, Leifer G: *Maternity nursing*, ed 8, Philadelphia, 2002, WB Saunders.

Hodgson B, Kizior R: *Saunders nursing drug handbook 2002*, Philadelphia, 2002, WB Saunders.

McKinney E et al: *Maternal-child nursing*, Philadelphia, 2002, WB Saunders.

Murray S, McKinney E, Gorrie T: *Foundations of maternal-newborn nursing*, ed 3, Philadelphia, 2002, WB Saunders.

Schulte E, Price D, Gwin J: *Thompson's pediatric nursing*, ed 8, Philadelphia, 2001, WB Saunders.

Web site: http://www2.cdc.gov/mmwr/.

Web site: http://www.immunize.org

Wong D: *Whaley and Wong's nursing care of infants and children*, ed 6, St Louis, 1999, Mosby.

Pediatric Medication Administration

I. MEDICATIONS AND THE PEDIATRIC CLIENT (Figure 37-1)

A. Pediatric clients are smaller than an adult and their medications have to be adapted to their size and age

B. Neonates and premature infants have immature body systems

C. The absorption, distribution, metabolism, and excretion of medications differ substantially, and the pediatric client will react more quickly to medication than an adult

D. Medication reactions are not as predictable in a pediatric client as they are in an adult

II. ADMINISTERING ORAL MEDICATION

A. Most oral pediatric medications are in liquid or suspension form because children usually are not able to swallow a tablet

B. Solutions may be measured using an oral syringe; if an oral syringe is not available, hypodermic syringes without the needle can be used for dosage measurement

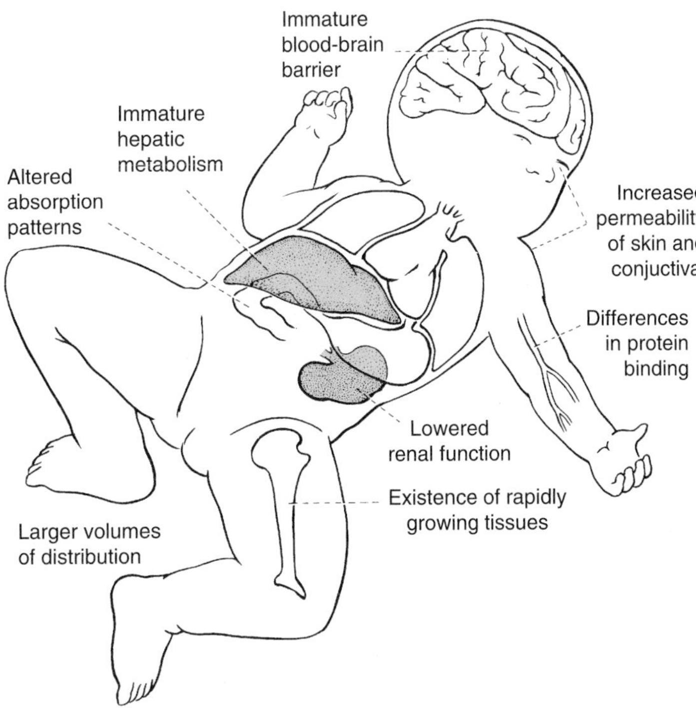

FIG. 37-1 Some of the multiple factors that modify drug disposition in the newborn infant. (Modified from Hirata T, Smith D, editors: *Introduction to clinical pediatrics*, ed 2, Philadelphia, 1977, WB Saunders.)

C. When volumes are extremely small, oral liquids are measured using a calibrated medication dropper

D. Be alert to liquid medications prepared as suspensions because a medication in suspension settles to the bottom of the bottle between uses, and thorough mixing is required before pouring the medication

E. Suspensions must be administered immediately after measurement to prevent settling and administering an incomplete dosage

F. Administer oral medications with the child sitting in an upright position with the head elevated to prevent aspiration if the child cries or resists

G. Never pinch the child's nostrils when administering medication

H. Do not place medication in a bottle

I. Draw the required dose of an unpleasant medication into a small syringe and place the syringe into the side and toward the back of the infant's mouth; administer the medication slowly, allowing the infant to swallow

J. Place the small child sideways on the lap; the child's closest arm should be placed under the adult's arm and behind the adult's back; cradle the child's head and hold the child's hand and administer the medication slowly using a plastic spoon or small plastic cup

K. Mix liquid medications with less than an ounce of fluid to disguise the taste if necessary

L. Check the child's mouth if a tablet or capsule has been administered to ensure that it has been swallowed; if swallowing is a problem, some tablets can be crushed and given in small amounts of foods

M. Crush tablets if necessary and mix with 1 teaspoon of pureed fruit or flavored syrup; enteric-coated and time-released tablets or capsules cannot be crushed

III. ADMINISTERING PARENTERAL MEDICATIONS (Figure 37-2)

A. Subcutaneous (SC) and intramuscular (IM) medications

1. Medications most often given via the subcutaneous route are insulin and most immunizations

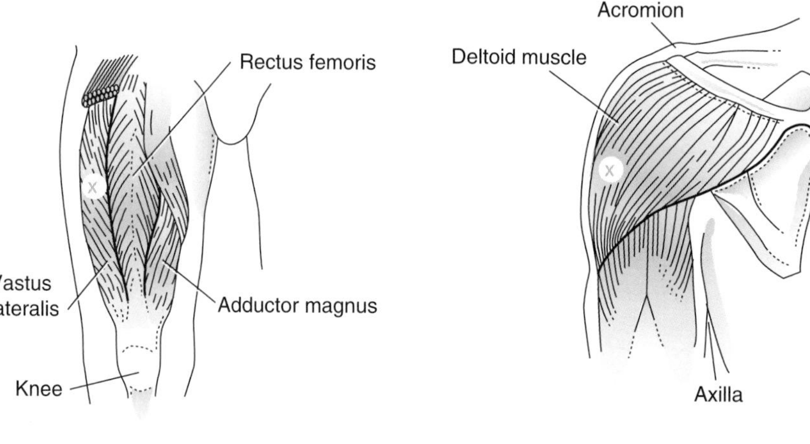

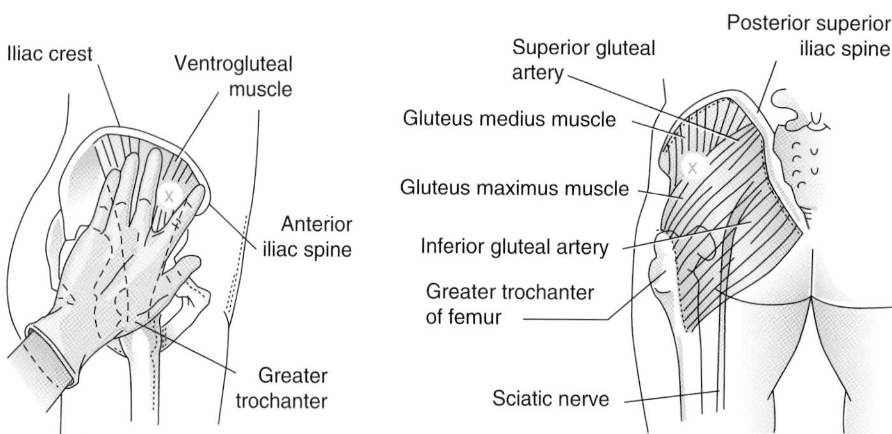

FIG. 37-2 Injection sites. (From Schulte E, Price D, Gwin J: *Thompson's pediatric nursing*, ed 8, Philadelphia, 2001, WB Saunders.)

2. Any site with sufficient subcutaneous tissue may be used for SC injections; common sites include the central third of the lateral aspect of the upper arm, the abdomen, and the center third of the anterior thigh
3. The safe use of all injection sites is based on normal muscle development and the size of the child
4. The preferred site for IM injections in infants is the vastus lateralis; it is the largest muscle mass in infants and small children and has few major nerves and blood vessels
5. After age 3 years, the ventrogluteal site may be used for intramuscular injections
6. The dorsogluteal site should not be used in any child who has not been walking for at least 2 years, and it is generally avoided in children under 6 years of age
7. The deltoid is also avoided in children under 6 years, and it should be used only for very small amounts of medication
8. Usually not more than 0.5 mL (infant) to 2.0 mL (child) is injected per IM or SC site, and the site of injection is rotated if frequent injections are necessary
9. The usual needle length and gauge for pediatric clients is ½ to 1 inch long and 22 to 25 gauge
10. Needle length can also be estimated by grasping the muscle for injection between the thumb and forefinger; half the distance would be the needle length
11. Pediatric dosages for SC and IM administration are calculated to the nearest hundredth and measured using a tuberculin (TB) syringe
12. Place an adhesive bandage or decorated bandage over the puncture site, particularly for toddlers and preschoolers

B. Monitoring intravenous (IV) medications
   1. When a child is receiving an IV medication, the IV site needs to be monitored for signs of infiltration and inflammation
   2. Signs of inflammation include redness, heat, swelling, and tenderness
   3. Signs of infiltration include swelling, coldness, pain, and lack of blood return
   4. Signs of infiltration or inflammation need to be reported

IV. CALCULATION OF MEDICATION DOSAGE BY BODY WEIGHT

A. Conversion of body weight
   1. Pounds (lb) to kilograms (kg)
      a. 1 kg = 2.2 lb
      b. To convert from lb to kg, divide by 2.2
      c. The answer, in kg, will be smaller than the lb you are converting since you are dividing
      d. Answers are expressed to the nearest tenth
   2. Kilograms (kg) to pounds (lb)
      a. 1 kg = 2.2 lb
      b. To convert from kg to lb, multiply by 2.2
      c. The answer, in lb, will be larger than the kg you are converting since you are multiplying
      d. Express weight to the nearest tenth

B. Calculating daily dosages
   1. Dosages are expressed in terms of mg/kg/day, or mg/lb/day
   2. The total daily dosage is usually administered in divided (more than one) doses per day
   3. Express the child's body weight in kg or lb to correlate with the dosage specifications
   4. Calculate the total daily dosage
   5. Divide the total daily dosage by the number of doses to be administered in one day

V. CALCULATION OF BODY SURFACE AREA (BSA) (Figure 37-3)

A. The body surface area is determined by comparing body weight and height with averages or norms on a graph called a nomogram

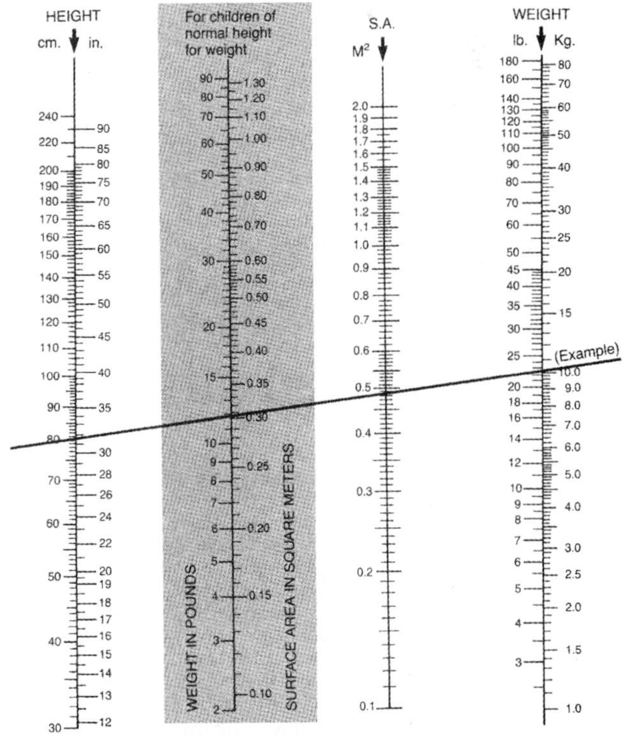

FIG. 37-3 Nomogram. (From Schulte E, Price D, Gwin J: *Thompson's pediatric nursing*, ed 8, Philadelphia, 2001, WB Saunders.)

B. Not all children are the same size at the same age; therefore the nomogram chart is used to determine the BSA of a child
C. Look at the nomogram chart (Fig. 37-3) and note that the height is on the left hand side of the chart and the weight is on the right hand side
D. Place a ruler on the chart
E. Line up the left side of the ruler on the height and the right side of the ruler on the weight; read the BSA where the point of the straight edge of the ruler intersects with the surface area (SA) column; this gives the estimated surface area in square meters (m^2)

EXAMPLE: Use the nomogram and calculate the BSA for a child whose height is 58 inches and weight is 12 kg.

ANSWER: 0.66 m^2

VI. CALCULATION BASED ON BODY SURFACE AREA (BSA)

A. When dosage recommendations for children specify milligrams or units per square meter (m^2), calculating the dosage is simple multiplication

EXAMPLE: The dosage recommendation is 4 mg per m^2. The child has a BSA of 1.1 m^2. What is the dose to be administered?

ANSWER: 1.1×4 mg = 4.4 mg

B. When dosages are specified only for adults, a formula is used to calculate a child's dose from the adult dosage
C. The average adult body surface area is approximately 1.7 m^2

EXAMPLE: A physician has prescribed an antibiotic for a child. The average adult dose is 250 mg. The child has a BSA of 0.41 square meter (m^2). What is the dose for the child?

ANSWER: 60.29 or 60.3 mg

$$\frac{\text{BSA of Child}}{1.7\ \text{m}^2} \times \text{adult dose} = \text{child's dose}$$

$$\frac{0.41}{1.7} \times 250\ \text{mg} = 60.29 \text{ or } 60.3\ \text{mg}$$

PRACTICE QUESTIONS

1. Penicillin V (Veetids), 250 mg PO every 8 hours, is prescribed for a child with a respiratory infection. The child's weight is 45 pounds. The safe pediatric dose is 25 to 50 mg/kg/day. The nurse determines that:
   1. The dose is too low
   2. The dose is too high
   3. The dose is within the safe dosage range
   4. There is not enough information to determine the safe dose
2. A physician has prescribed phenobarbital sodium (Luminal Sodium), 25 mg PO BID, for a child with febrile seizures. The medication label reads: phenobarbital sodium, 20 mg per 5 mL. The nurse has determined that the dose prescribed is a safe dose for the child. The nurse administers how many milliliters per dose to the child?
   1. 1. 2 mL
   2. 4.5 mL
   3. 6.25 mL
   4. 7.0 mL
3. Cloxacillin (Tegopen), 100 mg PO every 8 hours, is prescribed for a child with an elevated temperature who is suspected of having a respiratory tract infection. The child weighs 17 lb. The safe pediatric dose is 50 mg/kg/day. The nurse determines that:
   1. The dose is too low
   2. The dose is too high
   3. The dose is within the safe dosage range
   4. There is not enough information to determine the safe dose
4. Sulfisoxazole (Gantrisin), 1.0 g PO four times a day, is prescribed for an adolescent with a urinary tract infection. The medication label reads: 500-mg tablets. The nurse has determined that the dose prescribed is safe. The nurse administers how many tablets per dose to the adolescent?
   1. 0.5 tablet
   2. 1 tablet
   3. 2 tablets
   4. 3 tablets
5. Diphenhydramine hydrochloride (Benadryl), 25 mg PO every 6 hours, is prescribed for a child with an allergic reaction. The child weighs 25 kg. The safe pediatric dose is 5 mg/kg/day. The nurse determines that:
   1. The dose is too low
   2. The dose is too high
   3. The dose is within the safe dosage range
   4. There is not enough information to determine the safe dose
6. Penicillin G procaine (Wycillin), 1,000,000 units (U) IM, is prescribed for the child with an infection. The medication label reads: 1,200,000 U per 2 mL. The nurse has determined that the dose prescribed is safe. The nurse administers how many milliliters per dose to the child?
   1. 0.8 mL
   2. 1.2 mL
   3. 1.44 mL
   4. 1.66 mL
7. Morphine sulfate, 2.5 mg is prescribed for a child with cancer. The safe pediatric dose is 0.05 to 0.1

mg/kg/dose. The child weighs 50 kg. The nurse determines that:
1. The dose is too low
2. The dose is too high
3. The dose is within the safe dosage range
4. There is not enough information to determine the safe dosage range

8. Morphine sulfate, 2.5 mg subcutaneously, is prescribed for a child postoperatively. The medication label reads: 1/15 grains (gr) per mL. The nurse has determined that the dose is safe. The nurse administers how many mL to the child?
1. 0.62 mL
2. 0.82 mL
3. 1.35 mL
4. 1.62 mL

9. A physician's order reads: ampicillin (Omnipen), 125 mg IM every 6 hours. The medication label reads: 1 gram (g) and reconstitute with 7.4 mL of bacteriostatic water. The nurse draws up how many mL to administer one dose?
1. 0.54 mL
2. 0.92 mL
3. 1.1 mL
4. 7.4 mL

10. A pediatric client with ventricular septal defect repair is placed on a maintenance dosage of digoxin (Lanoxin) elixir. The safe dosage is 0.07 mg/kg/day, and the client's weight is 7.2 kg. The physician orders the digoxin to be given BID. The nurse prepares how much digoxin to administer to the client at each dose?
1. 0.25 mg
2. 0.37 mg
3. 0.50 mg
4. 2.50 mg

ANSWERS

1. *Answer:* 3
Rationale: Convert pounds to kilograms by dividing by 2.2
Pounds to kilograms: 45 lb divided by 2.2 lb/kg = 20.45 kg
Dosage parameters: 25 mg/kg/day × 20.45 kg = 511.25 mg/day
50 mg/kg/day × 20.45 kg = 1022.50 mg/day
Dose frequency: 250 mg × 3 doses (every 8 hours) = 750 mg/day
Dose is within the safe dosage range.
Test-Taking Strategy: Use the process of elimination. Identify the key components of the question and what the question is asking. In this case, the question asks for the safe dosage range for medication. Change pounds to kilograms. Calculate the dosage parameters using the safe dose range identified in the question and the child's weight in kg. Remember to determine the total daily dosage before selecting an option. Review pediatric medication calculations if you had difficulty with this question.
Level of Cognitive Ability: Comprehension
Client Needs: Safe, Effective Care Environment
Integrated Concept/Process: Nursing Process/Planning
Content Area: Child Health
Reference: Kee J, Marshall S: *Clinical calculations: with applications to general and specialty areas*, ed 4, Philadelphia, 2000, WB Saunders, p. 219.

2. *Answer:* 3
Rationale: Use the medication calculation formula.
Formula:

$$\frac{\text{Desired}}{\text{Available}} \times \text{Volume} = \frac{25 \text{ mg}}{20 \text{ mg}} = 5\text{mL} = 6.25 \text{ mL per dose}$$

Test-Taking Strategy: Use the process of elimination. Identify the key components of the question and what the question is asking. In this case, the question asks for the milliliters per dose. Use the formula to determine the correct dosage. Review pediatric medication calculations if you had difficulty with this question.
Level of Cognitive Ability: Application
Client Needs: Safe, Effective Care Environment
Integrated Concept/Process: Nursing Process/Implementation
Content Area: Child Health
Reference: DeWit S: *Fundamental concepts and skills for nursing*, Philadelphia, 2001, WB Saunders, p. 642.

3. *Answer:* 3
Rationale: Convert pounds to kilograms by dividing by 2.2
Pounds to kilograms: 17 lb divided by 2.2 lb/kg = 7.72 kg
Safe dose parameter: 50 mg/kg/day × 7.72 kg = 386 mg/day
Dosage frequency: 100 mg × 3 doses (every 8 hours) = 300 mg/day
Dose is within the safe dosage range.
Test-Taking Strategy: Use the process of elimination. Identify the key components of the question and what the question is asking. In this case, the question asks for the safe dose of the medication. Change pounds to kilograms. Calculate the dosage using the safe dose identified in the question and the child's weight in kilograms. Remember to determine the total daily dosage before selecting an option. Review pediatric medication calculations if you had difficulty with this question.
Level of Cognitive Ability: Comprehension
Client Needs: Safe, Effective Care Environment
Integrated Concept/Process: Nursing Process/Planning
Content Area: Child Health
Reference: Kee J, Marshall S: *Clinical calculations: with applications to general and specialty areas*, ed 4, Philadelphia, 2000, WB Saunders, p. 219.

4. *Answer:* 3
Rationale: Change 1 g to mg knowing that 1000 mg = 1 g. When converting from g to mg (larger to smaller) move the decimal point 3 places to the right. Therefore 1.0 g = 1000 mg. Then, use the medication calculation formula.
Formula:

$$\frac{\text{Desired}}{\text{Available}} \times \text{tablet} = \frac{1000 \text{ mg}}{500 \text{ mg}} = 1 \text{ tablet} = 2 \text{ tablets}$$

Test-Taking Strategy: Use the process of elimination. Identify the key components of the question and what the question is asking. In this case, the question asks for tablets per dose. Change grams to milligrams first. Then, use the formula to determine the correct dosage. Review pediatric medication calculations if you had difficulty with this question.
Level of Cognitive Ability: Application
Client Needs: Safe, Effective Care Environment
Integrated Concept/Process: Nursing Process/Implementation
Content Area: Child Health
Reference: DeWit S: *Fundamental concepts and skills for nursing,* Philadelphia, 2001, WB Saunders, p. 642.

5. *Answer:* 3
Rationale: Safe dose parameter: 5 mg/kg/day × 25 kg = 125 mg/day
Dosage frequency: 25 mg × 4 doses (every 6 hours) = 100 mg/day
Dose is within the safe dosage range.
Test-Taking Strategy: Use the process of elimination. Identify the key components of the question and what the question is asking. In this case, the question asks for the safe dose of the medication. Calculate the dosage parameters using the safe dose identified in the question and the child's weight in kilograms. Remember to determine the total daily dosage before selecting an option. Review pediatric medication calculations if you had difficulty with this question.
Level of Cognitive Ability: Comprehension
Client Needs: Safe, Effective Care Environment
Integrated Concept/Process: Nursing Process/Planning
Content Area: Child Health
Reference: Kee J, Marshall S: *Clinical calculations: with applications to general and specialty areas,* ed 4, Philadelphia, 2000, WB Saunders, p. 219.

6. *Answer:* 4
Rationale: Use the medication calculation formula.
Formula:

$$\frac{\text{Desired}}{\text{Available}} \times \text{Volume} = \frac{1{,}000{,}000}{1{,}200{,}000} = 2 \text{ mL} = 1.66 \text{ mL per dose}$$

Test-Taking Strategy: Use the process of elimination. Identify the key components of the question and what the question is asking. In this case, the question asks for the mL per dose. Use the formula to determine the correct dose. Review pediatric medication calculations if you had difficulty with this question.
Level of Cognitive Ability: Application
Client Needs: Safe, Effective Care Environment
Integrated Concept/Process: Nursing Process/Implementation
Content Area: Child Health
Reference: DeWit S: *Fundamental concepts and skills for nursing,* Philadelphia, 2001, WB Saunders, p. 642.

7. *Answer:* 3
Rationale:
Dosage parameters: 0.05 mg/kg/dose × 50 kg = 2.5 mg/dose
0.1 mg/kg/dose × 50 kg = 5 mg/dose
Dose is within the safe dosage range.
Test-Taking Strategy: Use the process of elimination. Identify the key components of the question and what the question is asking. In this case, the question asks for the safe dosage range of the medication. Calculate the dosage parameters, using the safe dosage range identified in the question and the child's weight in kilograms. Review pediatric medication calculations if you had difficulty with this question.
Level of Cognitive Ability: Comprehension
Client Needs: Safe, Effective Care Environment
Integrated Concept/Process: Nursing Process/Planning
Content Area: Child Health
Reference: Kee J, Marshall S: *Clinical calculations: With applications to general and specialty areas,* ed 4, Philadelphia, 2000, WB Saunders, p. 219.

8. *Answer:* 1
Rationale: Convert gr to mg then use the medication calculation formula.

1 gr = 60 mg
1/15 gr × 60 mg = 4 mg

Formula:

$$\frac{\text{Desired}}{\text{Available}} \times \text{Volume} = \frac{2.5 \text{ mg}}{4 \text{ mg}} = 1 \text{ mL} = 0.62 \text{ mL}$$

Test-Taking Strategy: Use the process of elimination. Identify the key components of the question and what the question is asking. In this case, the question asks for the milliliters per dose. Begin by converting grains to milligrams. Then, use the formula to determine the correct dose. Review pediatric medication calculations if you had difficulty with this question.
Level of Cognitive Ability: Application
Client Needs: Safe, Effective Care Environment
Integrated Concept/Process: Nursing Process/Implementation
Content Area: Child Health
Reference: DeWit S: *Fundamental concepts and skills for nursing,* Philadelphia, 2001, WB Saunders, p. 642.

9. *Answer:* 2
Rationale: Convert 1 g to milligrams. In the metric system, to convert larger to smaller multiply by 1000 or move the decimal 3 places to the right. Then, use the medication calculation formula.
1 g = 1000 mg
Formula:

$$\frac{\text{Desired}}{\text{Available}} \times \text{Volume} = \text{mL per dose}$$

$$\frac{125 \text{ mg}}{1000 \text{ mg}} \times 7.4 \text{ mL} = 0.925 \text{ mL} = 0.92 \text{ mL per dose}$$

Test-Taking Strategy: Use the process of elimination. Identify the key components of the question and what the question is asking. In this case, the question asks for the milliliters per

dose. Convert grams to milligrams first. Next, use the formula to determine the correct dosage knowing that 1000 mg = 7.4 mL. Review pediatric medication calculations if you had difficulty with this question.
Level of Cognitive Ability: Application
Client Needs: Safe, Effective Care Environment
Integrated Concept/Process: Nursing Process/Planning
Content Area: Fundamental Skills
Reference: Kee J, Marshall S: *Clinical calculations: with applications to general and specialty areas*, ed 4, Philadelphia, 2000, WB Saunders, p. 78.

10. ***Answer:*** **1**
Rationale: Calculate the dosage by weight first; therefore 0.07 mg/day × 7.2 kg = 0.50 mg/day. Next, note that the physician orders digoxin BID; therefore 2 doses in 24 hours will be administered. 0.50 mg/day divided by 2 doses = 0.25 mg for each dose
Test-Taking Strategy: Use the process of elimination. Identify the key components of the question and what the question is asking. Read the question carefully noting the key words "BID" and "each dose." Calculate the dosage by weight first and then determine the mg per each dose. Review pediatric medication calculations if you had difficulty with this question.
Level of Cognitive Ability: Application
Client Needs: Safe, Effective Care Environment
Integrated Concept/Process: Nursing Process/Implementation
Content Area: Child Health
Reference: Kee J, Marshall S: *Clinical calculations: with applications to general and specialty areas*, ed 4, Philadelphia, 2000, WB Saunders, p. 78.

REFERENCES

DeWit S: *Fundamental concepts and skills for nursing*, Philadelphia, 2001, WB Saunders.

Hodgson B, Kizior R: *Saunders nursing drug handbook 2002*, Philadelphia, 2002, WB Saunders.

Kee J, Marshall S: *Clinical calculations: with applications to general and specialty areas*, ed 4, Philadelphia, 2000, WB Saunders.

Schulte E, Price D, Gwin J: *Thompson's pediatric nursing, ed 8*, Philadelphia, 2001, WB Saunders.

Wong D: *Whaley & Wong's nursing care of infants and children*, ed 6, St Louis, 1999, Mosby.

Wong D, Hockenberry-Eaton M: *Wong's essentials of pediatric nursing*, ed 6, St Louis, 2001, Mosby.

UNIT VIII

The Adult Client with an Integumentary Disorder

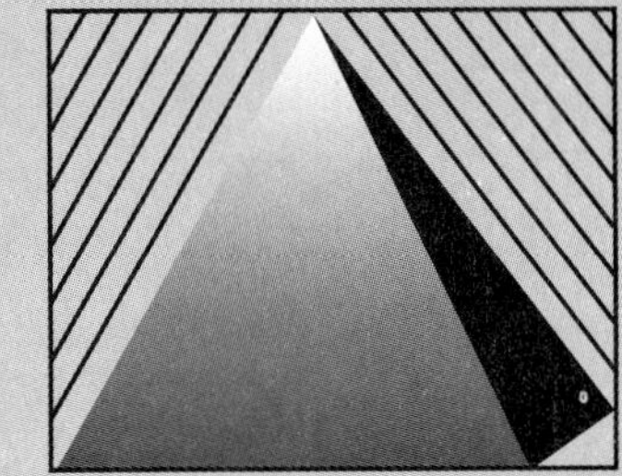

PYRAMID TERMS

Burns Cell destruction of the layers of the skin and the resultant depletion of fluid and electrolytes.

Chemical Burns Caused by tissue contact with strong acids, alkalis, or organic compounds. Systemic toxicity from cutaneous absorption can occur.

Decubitus Localized area of skin breakdown that occurs as a result of poor circulation to the area; also called pressure ulcer.

Deep Full-Thickness Burn Involves injury to the muscle and bone. Injured area appears black. Edema is absent.

Electrical Burn Caused by heat generated by an electrical energy as it passes through the body. Results in internal tissue damage.

Full-Thickness Burn Injured area appears deep red, black, white, or brown. Injured surface appears dry. Tissue disruption is noted, with fat exposed. Skin is edematous.

Herpes Zoster (Shingles) An acute viral infection of the nerve structure caused by varicella-zoster. Herpes zoster is contagious to individuals who have not had chickenpox.

Kaposi's Sarcoma Small, purplish brown lesions that are the most common malignancy associated with acquired immunodeficiency syndrome.

Lyme Disease An infection acquired from a tick bite. Ticks live in wooded areas and survive by attaching to a host.

Partial-Thickness Superficial Burn A mottled red base and broken epidermis; a wet, shiny, weeping surface is present. Large blisters cover an extensive area. Skin is edematous and painful.

Skin Cancer A malignant lesion of the skin that may or may not metastasize. Causes include chronic friction and irritation to a skin area and exposure to ultraviolet rays. Diagnosis is confirmed by a skin biopsy that is positive for cancer cells.

Smoke Inhalation Injury Results from the inhalation of superheated air, steam, toxic fumes, or smoke, and leads to respiratory insufficiency.

Superficial-Thickness Burn Mild to severe erythema is noted, and the skin blanches with pressure.

Thermal Burn Caused by exposure to flames, hot liquids, steam, or hot objects.

PYRAMID TO SUCCESS

The Pyramid to Success focuses on the concept that the integumentary system provides the first line of defense against infections. Focus on the protective measures necessary to prevent infection. Pyramid points address the risk factors related to the development of integumentary disorders, the preventive measures related to skin cancer, and the content related to Kaposi's sarcoma, and Lyme disease. Focus on the emergency measures related to a client with a burn, fluid resuscitation, monitoring for complications, and skin grafting. Psychosocial issues relate to the body image disturbances that can occur as a result of the integumentary disorder. The Integrated Concepts and Processes addressed in this unit include Clinical Problem-Solving Process (Nursing Process), Caring, Communication and Documentation, Cultural Awareness, Self-Care, and Teaching/Learning.

CLIENT NEEDS

Safe, Effective Care Environment

Asepsis
Confidentiality related to the disorder
Establishing priorities
Handling infectious materials
Informed consent for treatments and procedures
Standard (universal) precautions

Health Promotion and Maintenance

Disease prevention measures
Health promotion programs
Reinforcing instructions to the client regarding care to integumentary disorder

Psychosocial Integrity

Adapting to role changes
Unexpected body image changes
Use of support systems
Using coping mechanisms

Physiological Integrity

Basic care and comfort
Adequate nutrition for healing
Comfort interventions
Monitoring laboratory values
Fluid and electrolyte imbalances
Monitoring for complications
Providing emergency care

REFERENCES

Black J, Hawks J, Keene A: *Medical-surgical nursing: clinical management for positive outcomes*, ed 6, Philadelphia, 2001, WB Saunders.
DeWit S: *Fundamental concepts and skills for nursing*, Philadelphia, 2001, WB Saunders.
National Council of State Boards of Nursing, editors: *Test plan for the National Council Licensure Examination for Practical/Vocational Nurses*, Chicago, 2001, Author.
Potter P, Perry A: *Fundamentals of nursing*, ed 5, St Louis, 2001, Mosby.

Integumentary System

I. ANATOMY AND PHYSIOLOGY

A. The skin is the largest sensory organ of the body

B. Functions

1. First line of defense against infections
2. Protects underlying tissues and organs
3. Receives stimuli from the external environment
4. Maintains normal body temperature
5. Excretes salts, water, and organic wastes
6. Protects the body from dehydration
7. Synthesizes vitamin D_3, which converts to calcitriol, for normal calcium metabolism
8. Stores nutrients
9. Protects the internal organs from injury
10. Detects touch, pressure, pain, and temperature and relays that information to the nervous system

C. Layers

1. Epidermis
2. Dermis
3. Subcutaneous fat

D. Accessory structures

1. Nails
2. Hair
3. Glands
   a. Sebaceous
   b. Sweat

E. Normal bacterial flora

1. A pH of 4.2 to 5.6 halts the growth of bacteria
2. Organisms are shed with normal exfoliation
3. Normal bacterial flora
   a. Gram-positive and gram-negative staphylococcus
   b. *Pseudomonas*
   c. *Streptococcus*

II. RISK FACTORS

A. Exposure to chemical and environmental pollutants

B. Exposure to radiation

C. Exposure to the sun

D. Lack of personal hygiene habits

E. Use of cosmetics and harsh soaps

F. Medications, such as long-term corticosteroids and/or anticoagulant therapy

G. Nutritional deficiencies

H. Moderate to severe emotional stress

I. Injured areas with potential entry points for infection

J. Changes associated with developmental stages and aging

III. PSYCHOSOCIAL IMPACT

A. Change in body image

B. Fear of rejection

C. Social isolation (from embarrassment about changes in skin appearance)

D. Decreased self-esteem

E. Restrictions in physical activity

F. Pain

G. Disruption or loss of employment

H. Cost of medications, if prescribed

I. Cost of hospitalizations and follow-up care, including dressing supplies

IV. DIAGNOSTIC TESTS

A. Skin biopsy

1. Description: obtaining a small piece of skin tissue for histopathological study
2. Implementation preprocedure

a. Obtain informed consent
b. Cleanse site as prescribed
3. Implementation postprocedure
a. Place the specimen when obtained by physician in the appropriate container as directed and send to the pathology laboratory for analysis
b. Use aseptic technique for biopsy site dressings
c. Check the biopsy site for bleeding and infection

B. Skin cultures
1. Description
a. Noninvasive procedure
b. A small skin culture sample is obtained, using a sterile applicator
c. Sample is sent to laboratory to identify an existing organism
2. Implementation: ensure that skin culture samples are obtained before beginning antibiotic therapy
3. Implementation postprocedure: send the skin culture sample to the laboratory

C. Wood's light examination
1. Description: the skin is viewed under ultraviolet light through a special glass (Wood's glass) to identify superficial infections of the skin
2. Implementation preprocedure: darken room before the examination
3. Implementation postprocedure: assist the client while adjustment from a darkened room occurs

D. Skin testing
1. Description
a. The administration of an allergen to the skin's surface or into the dermis
b. Administered by patch, scratch, or intradermal techniques
2. Implementation preprocedure
a. The client is instructed to discontinue systemic corticosteroids or antihistamine therapy for 48 hours before test
b. Obtain informed consent
c. Resuscitation equipment needs to be available if a scratch test is performed, because it may induce an anaphylactic reaction
3. Implementation postprocedure
a. Instruct the client to keep the skin-testing patch area dry
b. Instruct the client to avoid activities that may produce sweating if a patch test was performed
c. Record the site, date, and time of the test and the date and the time for follow-up site reading
d. Inspect the site for erythema, papules, vesicles, edema, and induration
e. Provide the client with a list of potential allergens, if identified

V. SKIN DISORDERS

A. Contact dermatitis
1. Description: an inflammatory response of the skin that produces skin changes after contact with a specific antigen
2. Data collection
a. Pruritus and burning
b. Edema
c. Erythema at the point of contact
d. Vesicles with drainage
3. Implementation
a. Elevation of the extremity to reduce edema
b. Application of cool, wet dressings and tepid baths as prescribed
c. Maintain a cool environment
d. Prevent scratching and rubbing of the affected area
e. Assist with skin testing as prescribed to determine allergen(s)
f. Instruct the client to avoid contact with the allergen when determined
g. Instruct the client to avoid harsh soaps
h. Instruct the client to avoid using heating pads or blankets
i. Prescribed medications may include antibiotics for infection, antipruritics or antihistamines for itching, or corticosteroids for inflammation

B. Poison ivy, poison oak, and poison sumac
1. Description: a dermatitis that develops from contact with urushiol from poison ivy, oak, or sumac plants
2. Data collection
a. Papulovesicular lesions
b. Severe itching
3. Implementation
a. Cleanse the skin of plant oils
b. Application of cool, wet dressings with Burow's solution, as prescribed, to relieve the itching
c. Prescribed treatments may include the application of lotions or topical corticosteroids, and/or oral corticosteroids

C. **Lyme disease**
1. Description
a. An infection caused by *Borrelia burgdorferi* acquired from a tick bite
b. Ticks lives in wooded areas and survive by attaching to a host
2. Data collection (Table 38-1)

TABLE 38-1

Stages of Lyme Disease

First Stage	Second Stage	Third Stage
Symptoms can occur several days to months after the bite A small red pimple develops that spreads into a ring-shaped rash Rash may be large or small or may not occur at all Flulike symptoms occur, such as headaches, stiff neck, muscle aches, and fatigue	Occurs several weeks after the tick bite Joint pain Neurological complications Symptoms of heart disease	Large joints become involved Arthritis progresses

3. Implementation
   a. Gently remove the tick with tweezers or fingers, wash the skin with antiseptic, and dispose of tick by flushing it down the toilet
   b. Obtain a blood test 4 to 6 weeks after a bite to detect the presence of the disease (testing before this time is not reliable)
   c. Instruct the client in the administration of antibiotics, as prescribed, if the disease is confirmed
   d. Instruct the client to avoid areas that contain ticks, such as wooded grassy areas, especially in the summer
   e. Instruct the client to wear tight-fitting clothing while outside and to spray the body with tick repellent before going outside
   f. Instruct the client to examine the body when returning inside
   g. Lymerix, a vaccine for **Lyme disease**, is available and may be recommended for high-risk individuals

D. Erysipelas and cellulitis
1. Description
   a. Erysipelas is an acute, superficial, rapidly spreading inflammation of the dermis and lymphatics caused by beta-hemolytic streptococcus group A that enters the tissue via an abrasion, bite, trauma, or wound
   b. Cellulitis is a skin infection into the deeper dermis and subcutaneous fat, and the causative organism is usually *Streptococcus pyogenes*
2. Data collection
   a. Pain and itching
   b. Swelling, redness, and warmth
   c. Presence of nodules
3. Implementation
   a. Promote rest
   b. Apply warm compresses as prescribed to promote circulation and to decrease discomfort, erythema, and edema
   c. Antibiotics may be prescribed for infection (begin administration after a culture of the area)

E. Psoriasis
1. Description
   a. A chronic, noninfectious skin inflammation involving keratin synthesis that results in psoriatic patches
   b. Possible causes of the disorder include stress, trauma, infection, and changes in climate
   c. The disorder may also be exacerbated by the use of certain medications
   d. Koebner's phenomenon is the development of psoriatic lesions at a site of injury, such as a scratched or sunburned area
2. Data collection
   a. Pruritus
   b. Shedding, silvery white, scaling plaques; usually affects the scalp, knees, shins, elbows, and sacral regions
   c. A yellow discoloration, pitting, and a thickening of the nails
   d. Joint inflammation
3. Implementation
   a. Administer and instruct the client regarding daily soaks and tepid, wet compresses as prescribed to the affected areas
   b. Assist the client to remove the scales during the soak
   c. Apply corticosteroids and cover the areas with warm moist dressings or occlusive dressings as prescribed to decrease infection
   d. Use plastic wrap or plastic bags as the occlusive dressing, and apply rubber gloves on the client's hands
   e. Use a bed cradle to keep covers off the client's skin
   f. Instruct the client not to scratch the affected areas
   g. Monitor for and instruct the client to recognize the signs and symptoms of infection

h. Administer antipsoriatics as prescribed, anticipating the use of anthralin (Anthra-Derm (coal tar), followed by exposure to ultraviolet light (tar preparations suppress miotic activity and produce an antiinflammatory effect)
i. Prepare the client for photochemotherapy (psoralens and ultraviolet A [PUVA] light therapy) as prescribed anticipating the administration of a photosensitizing medication 2 hours before the ultraviolet light
j. Prepare to administer keratolytics and antimicrobials as prescribed
k. Instruct the client to wear light cotton clothing over affected areas
l. Instruct the client to avoid over-the-counter medications
m. Instruct the client regarding prescribed treatments and medications
n. Assist the client to identify ways to reduce stress

F. **Skin cancer** (Box 38-1)
1. Description
a. A malignant lesion of the skin, which may or may not metastasize
b. Causes include chronic friction and irritation to a skin area and exposure to ultraviolet rays
c. Diagnosis is confirmed by a skin biopsy that is positive for cancer cells
2. Types
a. Basal cell: the most common form, arising from the basal cells contained in the epidermis
b. Squamous cell: the second most common **skin cancer** in Caucasians; it is a tumor of the epidermal keratinocytes and can infiltrate surrounding structures, metastasize to lymph nodes, and be subsequently fatal
c. Malignant melanoma: cancer of the melanocytes that can metastasize to the brain, lungs, bone, liver, and skin and is ultimately fatal
3. Data collection
a. Change in color, size, or shape of a preexisting lesion

BOX 38-1

Appearance of Skin Cancer Lesions

A waxy nodule
An irregular, circular, bordered lesion with hues of tan, black, or blue
A small, red, nodular lesion
An oozing, bleeding, crusting lesion

b. Pruritus
c. Local soreness
4. Implementation
a. Instruct clients regarding preventive measures
b. Instruct clients to monitor for lesions that do not heal or that change characteristics
c. Instruct clients to have moles or lesions removed that are subject to chronic irritation
d. Instruct clients to avoid contact with chemical irritants
e. Instruct clients to use sun-screening lotions and layered clothing when outdoors
f. Assist with surgical excision of the lesion as prescribed

G. **Kaposi's sarcoma**
1. Description: small, purplish brown lesions that are the most common malignancy associated with acquired immunodeficiency syndrome
2. Data collection
a. Purplish, reddish-brown lesions on the skin
b. Raised, oblong, tender, or nontender and slow-growing skin tumors
c. Organ involvement includes the lymph nodes, airways or lungs, or any part of gastrointestinal (GI) tract from the mouth to the anus
3. Implementation
a. Maintain body fluid precautions
b. Provide protective isolation if the immune system is depressed
c. Prepare the client for radiation as prescribed
d. Prepare the client for chemotherapy as prescribed
e. Immunotherapy may be prescribed to stabilize the immune system

H. **Herpes zoster (shingles)**
1. Description
a. An acute viral infection of the dorsal nerve root ganglion, caused by varicella-zoster virus
b. Can be caused by the reactivation of the varicella-zoster virus or exposure to varicella-zoster or can occur during any immunocompromised state
c. Diagnosis is determined by visual examination, skin cultures and skin stains that identify the organism, and by an antinuclear antibody (ANA) blood test that will produce a positive result
d. A culture provides the definitive diagnosis
e. **Herpes zoster** is contagious to individuals who have not had chickenpox

2. Data collection
   a. Unilaterally clustered skin vesicles along peripheral sensory nerves on the trunk, thorax, or face
   b. Fever
   c. Burning and neuralgia
   d. Pruritus
   e. Paresthesia
3. Implementation
   a. Isolate the client, because exudate from the lesions contain the virus
   b. Maintain strict wound and skin precautions
   c. Monitor vital signs
   d. Monitor for signs and symptoms of infection
   e. Keep blisters intact if formed
   f. Assist the client with acetic acid compresses and tepid baths as prescribed
   g. A nerve block using lidocaine (Xylocaine) may be performed
   h. Medications may include antiviral agents, analgesics, antianxiety agents, antipruritics, and corticosteroids
   i. Use an air mattress and a bed cradle on the client's bed
   j. Prevent the client from scratching and rubbing the affected area
   k. Instruct the client to wear light-weight, loose cotton clothing and to avoid wool and synthetic clothing

I. Paronychia
1. Description
   a. An infection of the tissue around the nail bed
   b. The disorder most commonly occurs in middle-aged women and in clients with diabetes mellitus
2. Data collection
   a. Redness and swelling around the nail bed
   b. Soreness at the nail bed
3. Implementation
   a. Monitor temperature
   b. Monitor for infection around the nails
   c. Assist the client with warm soaks as prescribed
   d. Prepare to assist with incision and drainage of the infected area if prescribed
   e. Antibiotic or fungicidal ointments may be prescribed

J. Impetigo
1. Description: a bacterial infection of the skin caused by *Streptococcus* or *Staphylococcus* or both
2. Data collection
   a. Skin lesions that appear as vesicles
   b. Lesions progress to crusted pustules
3. Implementation
   a. Allow the lesions to dry by air exposure
   b. Assist the client with cleansing with hexachlorophene soap as prescribed
   c. Assist with compresses as prescribed to remove crusts and to allow for healing
   d. Apply and instruct the client in the use of antibiotic ointments as prescribed
   e. Apply and instruct the client in the use of emollients as prescribed to prevent the skin from cracking
   f. Instruct the client in the methods to prevent the spread of the disease
   g. Instruct the client to use separate towels, linens, and dishes

K. Boils
1. Description
   a. A deep bacterial inflammation of a hair follicle caused by staphylococcus
   b. Commonly occur on the face, neck, arms, legs, and groin
2. Data collection
   a. Redness on skin
   b. Tender and painful furuncle
   c. Skin swelling at the site
   d. A yellow or white center at the furuncle
3. Implementation
   a. Instruct the client in good hand washing technique to prevent the spread of infection
   b. Apply hot, moist compresses until drainage occurs
   c. Assist the physician in incision and drainage, which relieves the pain and allows the escape of purulent drainage
   d. Instruct the client in the use of separate bath linens
   e. Instruct the client in daily cleanliness
   f. Instruct the client in the administration of antibiotics if prescribed

L. Frostbite
1. Description
   a. Damage to tissues and blood vessels as a result of prolonged exposure to cold
   b. Fingers, toes, nose, and ears are often affected
2. Data collection
   a. Numbness
   b. Paresthesia
   c. Pallor
   d. Severe pain, swelling, erythema, and blistering occur once the client is in a warm environment
   e. Necrosis and gangrene may develop in severe cases

3. Implementation
   a. Handle the tissues gently
   b. Rewarm the affected part with tepid water about 105° F as prescribed
   c. Do not massage the area because this may result in further tissue damage
   d. Do not open blisters
   e. Apply bulky dressings as prescribed to permit drainage and provide protection

M. Scabies
1. Description
   a. A parasitic skin disorder caused by an infestation of the *Sarcoptes scabiei* (itch mite)
   b. Is endemic among schoolchildren and institutionalized populations
   c. Risk factors include contact with an infected person or contaminated article
   d. There is a 1-month delay between the initial infestation and the onset of pruritis in the host
   e. Sites can include are the hands, feet, finger webs, nipples, umbilicus, penis, soles, and palms
2. Data collection
   a. Threadlike, brownish, linear burrows up to 1 cm long
   b. Secondary lesions consist of vesicles, crusts, reddish-brown nodules, and excoriations
   c. Intense pruritis that worsens at night
3. Implementation
   a. Administer antihistamines or topical corticosteroids to relieve itching as prescribed
   b. Apply topical antiscabies creams or lotions such as lindane (Kwell, Scabene), crotamiton (Eurax), or permethrin 5% (Elimite) as prescribed
   c. Lindane (Kwell, Scabene) should not be used in children younger than age 2 because of the risk of neurotoxicity and seizures
   d. Instruct the client to apply the antiscabies preparation thinly to the entire skin from the neck down (face and scalp are not affected in scabies) and to leave on for 12 to 24 hours, as prescribed
   e. Instruct the client to apply antiscabies creams to dry skin because moist skin increases absorption and the potential for side effects
   f. After treatment with antiscabies preparations, instruct the client to remove the medication by washing with soap and water

N. Acne vulgaris
1. Description
   a. A common, self-limiting, multifactorial disorder
   b. Requires active treatment for control until it spontaneously resolves
   c. The types of lesions are comedones (open and closed), pustules, papules, and nodules
   d. The exact cause is unknown
   e. There is no evidence that consumption of foods such as chocolate, nuts, or fatty foods affect acne
   f. Exacerbations coincide with the menstrual cycle from hormonal activity
   g. Heat, humidity, and excessive perspiration have a role in increased acne
2. Data collection
   a. Closed comedone: whiteheads and noninflamed lesions that develop as a follicle and enlarge with the retention of horny cells
   b. Open comedones: blackheads that result from continuing accumulation of horny cells and sebum that dilates the follicles
   c. Pustules and papules result as the inflammatory process progresses
   d. Nodules result from total disintegration of a comedome and subsequent collapse of the follicle; deep scarring can result from nodules
3. Implementation
   a. Instruct the client in the administration (provide written instructions) of topical or oral antibiotics as prescribed
   b. Instruct the client in the use of isotretinoin (Accutane) if prescribed to inhibit sebum production and reduce sebaceous gland size
   c. Instruct the client about the adverse effects of isotretinoin (Accutane), which include cheilitis (lip inflammation), skin dryness, elevated triglycerides, and eye discomfort
   d. Instruct the client to stop taking vitamin A supplements during treatment with isotretinoin (Accutane)
   e. Inform the client that improvement may not be apparent for 4 to 6 weeks
   f. Instruct the client in appropriate skin-cleansing methods, with emphasis on not scrubbing the face and using only the agreed-upon topical agents
   g. Instruct the client not to squeeze, prick, or pick at lesions
   h. Instruct the client to use products labeled noncomedogenic and cosmetics that are water-based and to avoid contact with excessively oil-based products
   i. Instruct the client on the importance of follow-up treatment

O. **Decubitus**
1. Description
   a. An impairment of skin integrity
   b. Localized areas of necrosis of the skin and subcutaneous tissue due to pressure
   c. Prevention of skin breakdown is a major role of the nurse, particularly in caring for the bedridden or immobile client
2. Risk factors
   a. Malnutrition
   b. Incontinence
   c. Immobility
   d. Decreased sensory perception
   e. Skin shearing
3. Data collection (Table 38-2)
4. Implementation
   a. Institute measures to prevent **decubiti**
   b. Monitor the nutritional status of the client
   c. Provide adequate nutritional intake to promote tissue integrity
   d. Monitor for an alteration in skin integrity
   e. Relieve or remove pressure on the skin
   f. Turn and reposition the immobile client every 2 hours, or more frequently if necessary
   g. Ambulate the client
   h. Provide active and passive exercises every 8 hours
   i. Keep the skin clean and dry and the sheets wrinkle-free
   j. Apply moisture barrier as prescribed to protect the skin
   k. Use assistive devices to prevent pressure, such as an alternating air pressure mattress or sheepskin padding
   l. Apply medications or dressings to the wound as prescribed

VI. BURN INJURIES

A. Description: cell destruction of the layers of the skin and the resultant depletion of fluid and electrolytes

B. **Burn** size
1. Small **burns**: the body's response to injury is localized to the injured area
2. Large or extensive **burns**
   a. Consists of 25% or more of the total body surface area (TBSA)
   b. The body's response to the injury is systemic
   c. Affects all of the major systems of the body

C. Estimating the extent of injury (Table 38-3)

D. **Burn** depth
1. **Superficial thickness**
   a. Mild to severe erythema
   b. Skin blanches with pressure
   c. Painful and tingling
   d. Pain is eased by cooling
   e. Discomfort lasts about 48 hours
   f. Healing occurs in about 3 to 7 days
   g. Skin grafts are not required
2. **Partial thickness**
   a. Large blisters covering an extensive area
   b. Edema
   c. Mottled red base and broken epidermis, with a wet, shiny, and weeping surface
   d. Painful; injured area is sensitive to cold air
   e. Superficial **partial thickness** heals in 14 to 21 days
   f. Deep **partial thickness** heals in 21 to 28 days
   g. Grafts may be used if the healing process is prolonged
3. **Full thickness**
   a. Deep red, black, white, or brown area

TABLE 38-2

Stages of Decubiti

Stage 1	Stage 2	Stage 3	Stage 4
A reddened area that returns to normal skin color after 15 to 20 minutes of pressure relief, such as turning the client to another position The skin is intact Area is red and does does not blanche with external pressure	Area in which the top layer of skin is missing The ulcer usually is shallow with a pink to red base; a white or yellow eschar may be present	Deep ulcers that extend into the dermis and subcutaneous tissues White, gray, or yellow eschar usually is present at the bottom of the ulcer, and the ulcer crater may have a lip or edge Purulent drainage is common	Deep ulcers that extend into muscle and bone Brown or black eschar Purulent drainage is common

TABLE 38-3

Methods to Estimate Extent of Burn Injury

Rule of Nines/Adult		Lund and Browder Method
Head and neck	9%	Modifies percentages for body segments according to age
Anterior trunk	18%	
Posterior trunk	18%	Provides a more accurate estimate of the burn size
Arms (9%)	18%	
Legs (18%)	36%	Uses a diagram of the body divided into sections, with the representative % of the TBSA for ages greater than 1 year
Perineum	1%	Should be reevaluated after initial wound debridement

b. Injured surface appears dry
c. Edema
d. Tissue disruption with fat exposed
e. Little pain
f. Spontaneous healing will not occur; healing takes weeks to months
g. Requires removal of eschar and split- or full-thickness skin grafting
h. Scarring and wound contractures are likely to develop without preventive measures

4. **Deep-full thickness**
   a. Involves injury to the muscle and bone
   b. Injured area appears black
   c. Edema is absent
   d. Pain is absent
   e. No blisters
   f. Eschar is hard and inelastic
   g. Healing time takes weeks to months
   h. Grafts are required

E. **Burn** location
1. **Burns** of the head, neck, and chest are associated with pulmonary complications
2. **Burns** of the face are associated with corneal abrasion
3. **Burns** of the ear are associated with auricular chondritis
4. Hands and joints require intensive therapy to prevent disability
5. The perineal area is prone to autocontamination by urine and feces
6. Circumferential **burns** of the extremities can produce a tourniquet-like effect and lead to vascular compromise
7. Circumferential thorax **burns** lead to inadequate chest wall expansion and pulmonary insufficiency

VII. TYPES OF BURNS

A. Thermal **burns**: caused by exposure to flames, hot liquids, steam, or hot objects

B. Chemical **burns**
1. Caused by tissue contact with strong acids, alkalis, or organic compounds
2. Systemic toxicity from cutaneous absorption can occur

C. Electrical **burns**
1. Caused by heat generated by an electrical energy as it passes through the body
2. Results in internal tissue damage
3. Cutaneous **burns** cause muscle and soft tissue damage that may be extensive, particularly in high-voltage electrical injuries
4. The voltage, type of current, contact site, and duration of contact are important to identify
5. Alternating current is more dangerous than direct current because it is associated with cardiopulmonary arrest, ventricular fibrillation, tetanic muscle contractions, and long bone or vertebral fractures

D. Radiation **burns**: caused by exposure to a radioactive source

VIII. INHALATION INJURIES

A. **Smoke inhalation injury**
1. Description: results from the inhalation of superheated air, steam, toxic fumes, or smoke, and leads to respiratory insufficiency
2. Data collection
   a. Facial **burns**
   b. Erythema
   c. Swelling of oropharynx and nasopharynx
   d. Singed nasal hairs
   e. Tachycardia
   f. Flaring nostrils, stridor, wheezing, and dyspnea
   g. Hoarse voice
   h. Sooty sputum and cough

B. Carbon monoxide poisoning
1. Carbon monoxide is a colorless, odorless, and tasteless gas that has an affinity for hemoglobin 200 times greater than that of oxygen

2. Oxygen molecules are displaced and carbon monoxide reversibly binds to hemoglobin to form carboxyhemoglobin
3. Tissue hypoxia occurs

C. Direct thermal heat injury
1. Description
a. Can occur to the lower airways by the inhalation of steam or explosive gases or the aspiration of scalding liquids
b. Can occur to the upper airways, which appear erythematous and edematous, with mucosal blisters and ulcerations
c. Mucosal edema can lead to upper airway obstruction, especially during the first 24 to 48 hours
d. All clients with head or neck **burns** should be monitored closely for the development of airway obstruction and are immediately considered for endotracheal intubation if obstruction occurs
2. Data collection
a. Erythema and edema of the upper airways
b. Mucosal blisters and ulcerations

IX. MANAGEMENT OF THE BURN INJURY

A. Emergent phase
1. Description
a. Begins at the time of injury and ends with the restoration of capillary permeability, usually at 48 to 72 hours after the injury; includes resuscitative phase
b. The primary goal is to prevent hypovolemic shock and preserve vital organ functioning
2. Prehospital care
a. Begins at the scene of accident and ends when emergency care is obtained
b. Remove the victim from the source of the **burn**
c. Assess airway, breathing, and circulation
d. Assess for associated trauma
e. Conserve body heat
f. Cover **burns** with sterile or clean cloths
g. Remove constricting jewelry and clothing
h. Transport
3. Emergency department care: continuation of care administered at the scene of the injury
4. Major **burns**
a. A patent airway is established and 100% oxygen is administered as prescribed if the **burn** occurred in an enclosed area
b. Prepare for the administration of IV fluids to maintain fluid balance
c. Monitor vital signs closely
d. Insert a Foley catheter as prescribed and maintain urine output at 30 to 50 mL per hour
e. Maintain NPO status
f. Prepare for insertion of a nasogastric tube as prescribed to prevent paralytic ileus, to prevent vomiting, and to reduce the risk of aspiration
g. Administer tetanus prophylaxis as prescribed
h. Pain medication will be administered by the IV route
i. Prepare the client for an escharotomy or fasciotomy as prescribed
5. Minor **burns**
a. Administer oral analgesics as prescribed
b. Administer tetanus prophylaxis as prescribed
c. Assist with wound care, which may include cleansing, debriding loose tissue, and removing any damaging agents, followed by application of topical antimicrobial cream and a sterile dressing

B. Resuscitation phase
1. Description
a. Begins with the initiation of fluids and ends when capillary integrity returns to near-normal levels, and the large fluid shifts have decreased
b. The amount of fluid administered is based on the client's weight and extent of injury
c. Most fluid replacement formulas are calculated from the time of injury and not from the time of arrival at the hospital
d. The goal is to prevent shock by maintaining adequate circulating blood volume and maintaining vital organ perfusion
2. Fluid resuscitation
a. Successful fluid resuscitation is evaluated by stable vital signs, an adequate urine output, palpable peripheral pulses, and a clear sensorium
b. Urinary output is the most common and most sensitive noninvasive assessment parameter for cardiac output and tissue perfusion
3. Implementation
a. Monitor temperature and for signs of infection
b. Monitor daily weights, expecting a weight gain of 15 to 20 lb in the first 72 hours
c. Monitor gastric output and pH levels and for gastric discomfort and bleeding indicating a stress ulcer
d. Administer antacids, H_2-receptor antagonists and mucosal barrier fortifier, sucralfate (Carafate), as prescribed
e. Auscultate bowel sounds for ileus and monitor for abdominal distention and GI dysfunction

f. Monitor stools for occult blood
g. Monitor pulses and capillary refill of the affected extremities and assess perfusion of the distal extremity with a circumferential **burn**
h. Place the client on an air-fluidized bed and use a bed cradle to keep sheets off the client's skin

4. Pain management
   a. Medicate the client before painful procedures
   b. Avoid IM or SC routes because absorption through the soft tissue is unreliable when hypovolemia and large fluid shifts are occurring
   c. Avoid oral route owing to the possibility of GI dysfunction
5. Nutrition
   a. Essential to promote wound healing and prevent infection
   b. Maintain NPO status until the bowel sounds are heard, then advance to clear liquids as prescribed
   c. Nutrition may be provided via enteral tube feeding, peripheral parenteral nutrition, or central parenteral nutrition
6. Escharotomy
   a. A lengthwise incision is made through the **burn** eschar to relieve constriction and pressure and improve circulation
   b. Performed at the bedside without anesthesia because nerve endings have been destroyed by the **burn** injury
   c. After the escharotomy, monitor pulses, color, movement, and sensation of affected extremity and control any bleeding with pressure
   d. Apply topical antimicrobial agents and dressings to the area as prescribed after the procedure
7. Fasciotomy
   a. An incision is made extending through the subcutaneous tissue and fascia
   b. The procedure is performed if adequate tissue perfusion does not return after an escharotomy
   c. Performed in the operating room with the client under general anesthesia
   d. Postprocedure care similar to escharotomy

C. Wound care
   1. Description: cleansing, debridement, and dressing of the **burn** wounds
   2. Hydrotherapy
      a. Wounds are cleansed by immersion, showering, or spraying
      b. Hydrotherapy is generally not used for clients who are hemodynamically unstable or those with new skin grafts
   3. Debridement (Table 38-4)
      a. Removal of eschar to prevent bacterial proliferation under the eschar and to promote wound healing
      b. Debridement may be mechanical, enzymatic, or surgical

D. Wound closure (Table 38-5)
   1. Description
      a. Prevents infection and loss of fluid
      b. Promotes healing and prevents contractures
      c. Performed on the fifth to twenty-first day depending on the extent of the **burn**
   2. Temporary wound coverings (Boxes 38-2 and 38-3)
   3. Autografting
      a. Permanent wound coverage
      b. Surgical removal of a thin layer of the client's own unburned skin and application of the client's skin to the excised **burn** wound
      c. Performed in the operating room under anesthesia

TABLE 38-4

Debridement

Mechanical	Enzymatic	Surgical
Use of scissors and forceps to lift and trim away loose eschar Wet to dry or wet to wet dressing changes A painful procedure	Application of prepared proteolytic and fibrinolytic topical enzymes that digest necrotic tissue and facilitate eschar removal Requires a moist environment to be effective and is applied directly to the burn wound Pain and bleeding are major problems	Excision of eschar and coverage of wound *Tangential:* Very thin layers of eschar are shaved until viable tissue is reached *Fascial:* Used for very deep burns and removes burn tissue and underlying fat down to the fascia

TABLE 38-5

Open Method Versus Closed Method of Wound Care

Method	Advantages	Disadvantages
OPEN Antimicrobial cream is applied, and wound is left open to the air without a dressing Antimicrobial cream is applied every 12 hours	Visualization of the wound Easier mobility and joint range of motion Simplicity in wound care	Increased chance of hypothermia from exposure
CLOSED Gauze dressings are carefully wrapped from the distal to the proximal area of the extremity to ensure circulation is not compromised No two burn surfaces should be allowed to touch; touching promotes webbing of digits, contractures, and poor cosmetic outcome Dressings are changed every 8 to 12 hours	Decreases evaporative fluid and heat loss Aids in debridement	Mobility limitations Prevents effective range of motion exercises Wound assessment is limited

BOX 38-2

Types of Skin Grafts

SPLIT THICKNESS
Graft of half of the epidermis; applied in sheets or postage stamplike pieces

FULL THICKNESS
Graft consisting of epidermis and dermis; commonly used for reconstructive surgery months or years after the initial injury

PEDICLE FLAP
Commonly used for reconstructive surgery months or years after the initial injury

CULTURED EPITHELIUM
Use of the client's unburned skin
Keratinocytes are isolated and epithelial cells are cultured in a laboratory; these cells are then attached to the burn wound

BOX 38-3

Temporary Wound Coverings

BIOLOGICAL
Amnion
Amniotic membranes from human placenta
Dressing is changed every 48 hours with amnion
Allograft (Homograft)
Donated human cadaver skin is harvested within 24 hours after death
Monitor for wound exudate and signs of infection
Rejection can occur within 24 hours
Xenograft (Heterograft)
Porcine skin is harvested after slaughter and preserved for storage
Rejection can occur within 24 to 72 hours
Xenograft over granulation tissue is replaced every 2 to 5 days until the wound heals naturally or until closure with autograft is complete

BIOSYNTHETIC AND SYNTHETIC
Visual inspection of wound is possible as dressings are transparent or translucent
Monitor for wound exudate and signs of infection

d. Monitor for bleeding after the graft because bleeding beneath an autograft can prevent adherence
e. Autografts are immobilized after surgery for 3 to 7 days to allow time to adhere and attach to the wound bed
f. Position for immobilization and elevation of the graft site to prevent movement and shearing of the graft

4. Care to the graft site
   a. Elevate and immobilize the graft site
   b. Keep the site free from pressure
   c. Avoid weight bearing
   d. Monitor for foul-smelling drainage, increased temperature, increased white blood cell (WBC) count, hematoma, and fluid accumulation
5. Care to the donor site
   a. The fine-mesh gauze dressing is allowed to dry
   b. Cover with nonadherent dressing and absorbent gauze as prescribed
   c. Nonadherent dressing will separate as healing occurs
   d. The gauze can be gently lifted and trimmed away as new epithelium forms below it
   e. Keep site dry, open to air, and free from pressure

f. Prevent the client from scratching the donor site
g. Apply lubricating lotions to soften the area and reduce itching after the donor site is healed
h. Donor site can be reused once healing has occurred

E. Physical therapy
1. An individualized program of splinting, positioning, exercises, ambulation, activities of daily living, and physical therapy is implemented early in the acute phase of recovery to maximize functional and cosmetic outcomes
2. Apply splints as prescribed to maintain proper joint position and prevent contractures; do not apply pressure to skin areas with splints because it could lead to further tissue and nerve damage
3. Scarring is controlled by elastic wraps and bandages that apply continuous pressure to the healing skin during the period when the skin is vulnerable to shearing
4. Antiburn scar support garments are worn 23 hours a day until the **burn** scar tissue has matured, which takes 18 months to 2 years

F. Rehabilitative phase (Box 38-4)
1. Description
a. Final phase of **burn** care
b. Overlaps the acute-care phase and goes well beyond hospitalization
c. Goals of this phase are designed so that the client can gain independence and achieve maximal function
2. Goals
a. Promoting wound healing
b. Minimizing deformities
c. Increasing strength and function
d. Providing emotional support

PRACTICE QUESTIONS

1. Which of the following individuals would be at the greatest risk for development of an integumentary disorder?
   1. An elderly woman
   2. An adolescent
   3. An outdoor construction worker
   4. A physical education teacher

BOX 38-4

Surgical Options for Contractures and Scarring

Split-thickness and full-thickness skin grafts
Skin flaps
Z-plasties
Tissue expansion

2. A client scheduled for a skin biopsy asks the nurse how painful the procedure is. The most appropriate response by the nurse is:
   1. "There is no pain associated with this procedure."
   2. "There is some pain, but the physician will prescribe an analgesic after the procedure."
   3. "The local anesthetic may cause a burning or stinging sensation."
   4. "A preoperative medication will be given so you will be sleeping and will not feel any pain."
3. A nurse has reinforced discharge instructions to a client who had a skin biopsy. Which statement by the client indicates a need for further instruction?
   1. "I will call the physician if I see any drainage from the wound."
   2. "I will return in 7 days to have the sutures removed."
   3. "I will use the antibiotic ointment as prescribed."
   4. "I will remove the dressing when I get home and wash the site with tap water."
4. A nurse prepares to assist the physician to examine the client's skin with a Wood's light. Which of the following would be included in the plan for this procedure?
   1. Obtain an informed consent
   2. Darken the room for the examination
   3. Shave the skin and scrub with Betadine solution
   4. Prepare a local anesthetic
5. A nurse is checking for the presence of cyanosis in a dark-skinned client. Which body area would provide the best information?
   1. Back of the hands
   2. Earlobes
   3. Palms of the hands
   4. Sacrum
6. A nurse reinforces instructions to a client who is to return to the physician's office in 1 week for a patch test. The patch test will be done to identify the allergen causing the dermatitis. Which of the following instructions is most appropriate to provide to the client?
   1. Remain NPO before the test
   2. Shower using an antibacterial soap on the morning of the test
   3. Discontinue the prescribed antihistamine 2 days before the test
   4. Consume fluids only on the day of the test
7. A nurse reinforces discharge instructions to a client after patch testing. Which statement by the client indicates the need for further instruction?
   1. "I will return to the clinic in 2 days for the initial reading."
   2. "If the patch comes off I need to reapply it."
   3. "I need to avoid activities that will cause me to sweat."
   4. "I need to keep the test sites dry at all times."

8. A nurse reinforces instructions to a client who has complained of chronic dry skin and episodes of pruritus. Which of the following, if stated by the client, indicates a need for further instructions?
   1. "I should drink 8 to 10 glasses of water a day."
   2. "I need to avoid using astringents on my skin."
   3. "I should limit myself to one shower a day and apply emollient to my skin after the shower."
   4. "I should use a dehumidifier especially during the winter months."
9. The nurse prepares to assist in instructing a client about Lyme disease. Which of the following information would the nurse include in the instructions?
   1. It is contagious by skin contact with an infected individual
   2. It is caused by the inhalation of spores from bird droppings
   3. It is caused by contamination from cat feces
   4. It is caused by a tick carried by deer
10. After diagnostic evaluation, it has been determined that the client has Lyme disease, stage II. The nurse understands that which of the following is most indicative of this stage?
    1. Erythematous rash
    2. Neurological deficits
    3. Arthralgias
    4. Joint enlargements
11. The client arrives at the health care clinic and tells the nurse that he was just bitten by a tick and would like to be tested for Lyme disease. The client tells the nurse that he removed the tick and flushed it down the toilet. Which of the following nursing actions is most appropriate?
    1. Tell the client that a blood test is needed immediately
    2. Inform the client that there is not a test available for Lyme disease
    3. Inform the client the he will need to return in 4 to 6 weeks to be tested because testing before this time is not reliable
    4. Tell the client that testing is not necessary unless arthralgia develops
12. A client calls the emergency room and tells the nurse that he has been cleaning a wooded area in the back yard and has discovered that he came directly in contact with poison ivy shrubs. The client tells the nurse that he cannot see anything on the skin and asks the nurse what to do. Which of the following is the most appropriate nursing response?
    1. "Come to the emergency room."
    2. "It is not necessary to do anything if you cannot see anything on your skin."
    3. "Take a shower immediately lathering and rinsing several times."
    4. "Apply calamine lotion immediately to the exposed skin areas."
13. A client with acquired immunodeficiency syndrome (AIDS) is diagnosed with cutaneous Kaposi's sarcoma. Based on this diagnosis, the nurse understands that this has been determined by which of the following?
    1. Appearance of reddish-blue lesions noted on the skin
    2. Swelling in the lower extremities
    3. Punch biopsy of the cutaneous lesions
    4. Swelling in the genitalia area
14. Which of the following individuals is least likely at risk for the development of Kaposi's sarcoma?
    1. A man with a history of same sex partners
    2. A renal transplant recipient
    3. A client receiving antineoplastic medications
    4. An individual working in an environment where exposure to asbestos exists
15. A nurse prepares to give a bath and change the bed linens on a client with cutaneous Kaposi's sarcoma lesions. The lesions are open and draining a scant amount of serous fluid. Which of the following would the nurse use during the bathing of this client?
    1. Gown, gloves, and a mask
    2. Gown and gloves
    3. Gloves
    4. Gown and gloves to change the bed linens and gloves only for the bath
16. A client is being admitted to the hospital for treatment of acute cellulitis of the lower left leg. The client asks the nurse to explain what cellulitis means. The nurse bases the response on the understanding that the characteristics of cellulitis include:
    1. A skin infection into the deep dermis and subcutaneous fat
    2. An acute superficial infection
    3. An inflammation of the lymphatics
    4. A superficial infection caused by staphylococcus
17. A nurse prepares to care for a client with acute cellulitis of the lower leg. Which of the following would the nurse anticipate to be prescribed for the client?
    1. Warm compresses to the affected area
    2. Cold compresses to the affected area
    3. Intermittent heat lamp treatments four times daily
    4. Alternating hot to cold compresses continuously
18. The nurse is caring for a client with a diagnosis of psoriasis. The nurse reviews the health record knowing that which of the following characteristics is not associated with this skin disorder?
    1. A discoloration and pitting of the nails
    2. Silvery, white, scaly patches on the scalp, elbows, knees, and sacral regions
    3. Complaints of pruritus
    4. Red, purplish scaly lesions

19. Ultraviolet A (PUVA) light therapy is prescribed as a component of the treatment plan for a client with psoriasis. Which of the following would not be a component of the plan of care related to this light treatment?
   1. Eye goggles need to be worn to prevent exposure to UVL
   2. The face needs to be shielded with a loosely applied covering
   3. The client will stand in a light treatment chamber for 30 minutes
   4. Only the area requiring treatment should be exposed to the UVL
20. A nurse notes that the physician has documented a diagnosis of herpes zoster in the client's chart. Based on an understanding of the cause of this disorder, the nurse would determine that this diagnosis was made after which diagnostic test?
   1. Skin biopsy
   2. Wood's light examination
   3. Culture of the lesion
   4. Patch test
21. A nurse is assigned to care for a client with herpes zoster. Which of the following characteristics would the nurse expect to note when assessing the lesions of this infection?
   1. A generalized body rash
   2. Small blue-white spots with a red base
   3. A fiery red edematous rash on the cheeks
   4. Clustered skin vesicles
22. A nurse employed in a long-term care facility is planning the clinical assignments for the day. Which of the following staff members would not be assigned to the client with a diagnosis of herpes zoster?
   1. A staff member who never had mumps
   2. An experienced nursing assistant who never had chickenpox
   3. A staff member who never had roseola
   4. A nursing assistant who never had German measles
23. A client returns to the clinic for follow-up treatment after a skin biopsy of a suspicious lesion performed 1 week ago. The biopsy report indicates that the lesion is a melanoma. The nurse understands that which of the following describes the characteristic of this type of a lesion?
   1. Is highly metastatic
   2. Metastasis is rare
   3. Is characterized by local invasion
   4. Is encapsulated
24. A nurse is reviewing the health care record of a client with a lesion diagnosed as malignant melanoma. The nurse would most likely expect to note which of the following characteristics of this type of lesion documented in the client's record?
   1. A small papule with a dry, rough scale
   2. A firm nodular lesion topped with crust
   3. A pearly papule with a central crater and a waxy border
   4. An irregularly shaped lesion
25. A nurse reinforces discharge instructions after cryosurgery for treatment of a malignant skin lesion. Which of the following would the nurse plan to include in the instructions?
   1. To clean the site with hydrogen peroxide to prevent infection
   2. To apply ice to the site for comfort
   3. To apply alcohol soaked dressings twice a day
   4. To avoid showering for 7 to 10 days
26. A nurse reinforces instructions to a group of clients regarding measures that will assist in preventing skin cancer. Which of the following would not be a part of the instructions?
   1. Use sunscreen when participating in outdoor activities
   2. Examine the body monthly for any lesions that may be suspicious
   3. Wear a hat, opaque clothing, and sunglasses when in the sun
   4. Avoid sun exposure before 11:00 AM and after 3:00 PM
27. A nurse reviews a client's chart and notes that the physician has documented a diagnosis of paronychia. Based on this diagnosis, which of the following would the nurse expect to note during data collection?
   1. Swelling of the skin near the parotid gland
   2. Red, shiny skin around the nail bed
   3. White, silvery patches on the elbows
   4. White, taut skin in the popliteal area
28. A nurse reinforces instructions to a client diagnosed with impetigo. Which of the following would not be a component of the instructions?
   1. Continue with antibiotics as prescribed
   2. Separate washing of dishes from other household members
   3. Wash laundry with other household members' items
   4. To wash hands thoroughly and frequently throughout the day
29. A client arrives at the emergency room and has experienced frostbite to the right hand. Which of the following would the nurse note on data collection of the client's hand?
   1. A fiery, red skin with edema in the nail beds
   2. A pink, edematous hand
   3. Black fingertips surrounded by an erythematous rash
   4. A white color to the skin that is insensitive to touch

30. A nurse is assigned to assist in caring for a client with frostbite of the toes. Which of the following would the nurse anticipate to be prescribed for this condition?
    1. Rapid and continuous rewarming of the toes in a warm water bath until flushing of the skin occurs
    2. Rapid and continuous rewarming of the toes in hot water for 15 to 20 minutes
    3. Rapid and continuous rewarming of the toes when flushing occurs
    4. Rapid and continuous rewarming of the toes in cold water for 45 minutes
31. An evening nurse reviews the nursing documentation in the client's chart and notes that the day nurse has documented that the client has a stage II pressure ulcer (decubitus) in the sacral area. Which of the following would the nurse expect to note when checking the client's sacral area?
    1. Skin is intact
    2. Partial-thickness skin loss of the epidermis
    3. A deep craterlike appearance
    4. The presence of sinus tracts
32. Which of the following conditions would least likely be a risk factor for the development of skin breakdown?
    1. A client who is unable to move about and is confined to bed
    2. A client incontinent of urine and feces
    3. A client with chronic nutritional deficiencies
    4. A client with a lowered mental awareness status
33. A nurse inspects the oral cavity of a client with candidiasis (thrush). Which of the following would the nurse expect to note?
    1. The presence of numerous small, red, pinpoint lesions
    2. The presence of blisters
    3. The presence of white patches
    4. The presence of purple-colored patches
34. A nurse plans to instruct a client with candidiasis (thrush) of the oral cavity how to care for the disorder. Which of the following would not be a component of the instructions?
    1. To rinse the mouth four times daily with a commercial mouthwash
    2. To avoid spicy foods
    3. To avoid citrus juices and hot liquids
    4. To eat foods that are liquid or pureed
35. Isotretinoin (Accutane) is prescribed for a client with severe cystic acne. Which of the following, if stated by the client, would indicate a need for further instruction regarding this medication?
    1. "I need to continue to take my vitamin A supplements."
    2. "I need to use emollients and lip balms for my dry skin."
    3. "The medication may cause dryness and burning in my eyes."
    4. "I will need to return for a blood test to check my triglyceride level."
36. A nurse inspects the skin of a client suspected of having scabies. Which of the following findings would the nurse note if this disorder was present?
    1. The appearance of vesicles or pustules with a thick, honey-colored crust
    2. The presence of white patches scattered about the trunk
    3. Multiple straight or wavy threadlike lines beneath the skin
    4. Patchy hair loss and round red macules with scales
37. A nurse is told that an assigned client is suspected of having scabies. Which of the following precautions will the nurse institute during the care of the client?
    1. Wear a mask and gloves
    2. Wear gloves only
    3. Wear a gown and gloves
    4. Avoid touching the client's clothes
38. An adult client was burned as a result of an explosion. The burn initially affected the client's entire face (anterior half of the head), upper half of the anterior torso, and caused circumferential burns to the lower half of both of the arms. The client's clothes caught on fire and the client ran, causing subsequent burn injuries to the posterior surface of the head and the upper half of the posterior torso. Using the Rule of Nines, the extent of the total burn injury would be which of the following?
    1. 31.5%
    2. 36%
    3. 40.5%
    4. 45%
39. A nurse is caring for a client who has just been admitted to the nursing unit after suffering flame burns to the face and chest. The nurse notes a hoarse cough and that the client is expectorating sputum with black flecks. The client's eyelashes and eyebrows are singed and the eyelids are swollen. The client becomes restless and the color becomes dusky. The nurse interprets these data to indicate which of the following?
    1. The client is afraid and is having a panic attack because of the unfamiliar surroundings
    2. Pain is present from the burn injury
    3. The client is hypotensive
    4. The burn has probably caused laryngeal edema, which has occluded the airway
40. Which of the following would be the anticipated therapeutic outcome of an escharotomy procedure performed for a circumferential arm burn?

1. Brisk bleeding from the site
2. Formation of granulation tissue
3. Decreasing edema formation
4. Return of distal pulses

41. A client is undergoing radiation therapy to treat lung cancer. After treatment, the nurse notes that the chest and neck are red, and the client is complaining of pain at the radiation site. The nurse interprets this data as
    1. A superficial injury to tissue from the radiation
    2. An allergic reaction to the radiation
    3. A cutaneous reaction to products formed by the lysis of the neoplastic cells
    4. An ischemic injury, much like decubitus formation

42. A nurse is caring for a client with circumferential burns of the both legs. Which of the following leg positions is most appropriate for this type of a burn?
    1. In a dependent position
    2. Flat without elevation
    3. Elevation above the level of the heart
    4. Elevation of the knee gatch on the bed

43. A nurse is caring for a burn client in protective isolation. Which of the following is not a component of protective isolation techniques?
    1. Using sterile sheets and linens
    2. Strict handwashing
    3. Wearing gloves and a gown only when caring for the client
    4. Wearing protective garb including a mask, cap, shoe covers, gloves, scrub clothes, and plastic aprons

44. A nurse is caring for a client after an autograft and grafting to a burn wound on the right knee. Which of the following would the nurse anticipate to be prescribed for the client?
    1. Immobilization for 3 to 7 days
    2. Placing the affected leg flat
    3. Placing the affected leg in a dependent position
    4. Immobilization for 24 hours

45. A nurse reinforces discharge instructions regarding skin care to a client after grafting to burn injuries sustained to the left chest and left arm. Which of the following would not be a component of the discharge instructions?
    1. Bathe using a mild soap and rinsing thoroughly
    2. Avoid the use of lanolin products to the newly healed skin area
    3. Avoid direct sunlight to the newly healed skin area
    4. Never wear warm clothing over the newly healed skin area

ANSWERS

1. *Answer:* 3

Rationale: Prolonged exposure to the sun, unusual cold, or other conditions can damage the skin. An elderly client may be at a higher risk than a younger individual because immobility and lack of nutrition would increase the elder person's risk. An adolescent may be prone to the development of acne, but this does not occur in all adolescents. The physical education teacher is at low or no risk of developing an integumentary problem.

Test-Taking Strategy: Use the process of elimination. Note the key words "greatest risk." Eliminate option 4 first. Eliminate options 1 and 2 next because not all elderly or adolescents are at risk for the development of integumentary disorders. If you had difficulty with this question, review the risk factors associated with integumentary disorders.

Level of Cognitive Ability: Comprehension

Client Needs: Health Promotion and Maintenance

Integrated Concept/Process: Nursing Process/Data Collection

Content Area: Adult Health/Integumentary

Reference: Black J, Hawks J, Keene A: *Medical-surgical nursing: clinical management for positive outcomes*, ed 6, Philadelphia, 2001, WB Saunders, p. 1305.

2. *Answer:* 3

Rationale: Depending on the size and location of the lesion, a biopsy is usually a quick and almost painless procedure. The most common source of pain is the initial local anesthetic, which can produce a burning or stinging sensation. Options 1, 2, and 4 are incorrect.

Test-Taking Strategy: Use the process of elimination. Eliminate option 1 first because of the word "no." Eliminate option 2 next because this option addresses postprocedure, which is not the issue of the client's question to the nurse. Eliminate option 4 because a preoperative medication that puts the client to sleep is not a part of the procedure for a skin biopsy. If you had difficulty with this question, review the procedure related to a skin biopsy.

Level of Cognitive Ability: Application

Client Needs: Psychosocial Integrity

Integrated Concept/Process: Nursing Process/Implementation

Content Area: Adult Health/Integumentary

Reference: Black J, Hawks J, Keene A: *Medical-surgical nursing: clinical management for positive outcomes*, ed 6, Philadelphia, 2001, WB Saunders, 1307.

3. *Answer:* 4

Rationale: After a skin biopsy, the nurse instructs the client to keep the dressing dry and in place for a minimum of 8 hours. After the dressing is removed, the site is cleaned once a day with tap water or saline to remove any dry blood or crusts. The physician may prescribe an antibiotic ointment to minimize local bacterial colonization. The nurse instructs the client to

report any redness or excessive drainage at the site. Sutures are usually removed 7 to 10 days after biopsy.
Test-Taking Strategy: Use the process of elimination and note the key words "indicates a need for further instruction." Eliminate option 3 first because the client verbalizes a physician's prescription. Eliminate options 1 and 2 next. A client needs to report signs of drainage and needs to return to the physician for follow-up care and suture removal. Consider the alteration in skin integrity that occurs with a skin biopsy. This should assist in directing you to the correct option. Review postprocedure instructions after a skin biopsy if you had difficulty with this question.
Level of Cognitive Ability: Comprehension
Client Needs: Health Promotion and Maintenance
Integrated Concept/Process: Teaching/Learning
Content Area: Adult Health/Integumentary
Reference: Black J, Hawks J, Keene A: *Medical-surgical nursing: clinical management for positive outcomes*, ed 6, Philadelphia, 2001, WB Saunders, p. 1307.

4. *Answer:* 2
Rationale: Examination of the skin under a Wood's light is always carried out in a darkened room. This is a noninvasive examination; therefore an informed consent is not required. A hand-held, long wavelength, ultraviolet light or Wood's light is used. The skin does not need to be shaved, nor is a local anesthetic necessary. Areas of blue-green or red fluorescence are associated with certain skin infections. The procedure is painless.
Test-Taking Strategy: Use the process of elimination. Recalling that this is a noninvasive procedure will assist in eliminating options 1, 3, and 4. Review this procedure if you had difficulty answering this question.
Level of Cognitive Ability: Application
Client Needs: Physiological Integrity
Integrated Concept/Process: Nursing Process/Planning
Content Area: Adult Health/Integumentary
Reference: Black J, Hawks J, Keene A: *Medical-surgical nursing: clinical management for positive outcomes*, ed 6, Philadelphia, 2001, WB Saunders, p. 1276.

5. *Answer:* 3
Rationale: In a dark-skinned client, the nurse examines the lips, tongue, nail beds, conjunctiva, and palms and soles at regular intervals for subtle color changes. In a client with cyanosis, the lips and tongue are gray; and the palms, soles, conjunctiva, and nail beds have a bluish tinge.
Test-Taking Strategy: Use the process of elimination. Focus on the key words "dark-skinned" and use the process of elimination. This will assist in directing you to option 3. Review this important assessment technique if you had difficulty with this question.
Level of Cognitive Ability: Comprehension
Client Needs: Physiological Integrity
Integrated Concept/Process: Nursing Process/Data Collection
Content Area: Adult Health/Integumentary
Reference: DeWit S: *Fundamental concepts and skills for nursing*, Philadelphia, 2001, WB Saunders, p. 374.

6. *Answer:* 3
Rationale: Client preparation for a patch test includes informing the client to discontinue the administration of systemic corticosteroids or antihistamines for at least 48 hours before the test. To prevent suppression of the inflammatory response to an allergen, these medications must be discontinued. Options 1, 2, and 4 are unnecessary.
Test-Taking Strategy: Use the process of elimination. Eliminate options 1 and 4 first. These options are similar and there is no need to restrict food or remain NPO before the procedure. A "patch" test does not require a body shower with an antibacterial soap. Also, note the relationship between "allergen" in the question and "antihistamine" in the option. Review this test if you had difficulty with this question.
Level of Cognitive Ability: Application
Client Needs: Health Promotion and Maintenance
Integrated Concept/Process: Nursing Process/Implementation
Content Area: Adult Health/Integumentary
Reference: DeWit S: *Fundamental concepts and skills for nursing*, Philadelphia, 2001, WB Saunders, p. 653.

7. *Answer:* 2
Rationale: The nurse instructs the client to keep the test sites dry at all times. The nurse also discourages excessive physical activity that will result in sweating. Reapplying the patch can interfere with an accurate interpretation of the allergic reactions. The nurse reinforces the necessity of removing loose or nonadherent test patches for reapplication at a later date. The initial reading is performed 2 days after application and the final reading is performed 2 to 5 days later.
Test-Taking Strategy: Use the process of elimination and note the key words "need for further instruction." Eliminate options 3 and 4 first because keeping the test site dry and avoiding sweating are similar. From the remaining options, recalling that follow-up care is important after any procedure will assist in directing you to option 2. If you had difficulty with this question, review the client teaching points after a patch test.
Level of Cognitive Ability: Comprehension
Client Needs: Health Promotion and Maintenance
Integrated Concept/Process: Teaching/Learning
Content Area: Adult Health/Integumentary
Reference: DeWit S: *Fundamental concepts and skills for nursing*, Philadelphia, 2001, WB Saunders, p. 653.

8. *Answer:* 4
Rationale: The client should avoid using a dehumidifier because this will further dry room air. Instead, they should use a room humidifier during the winter months or whenever the furnace is in use. The client should be taught to maintain a daily fluid intake of 3000 mL unless contraindicated, and should avoid alcohol and caffeine ingestion. They should avoid applying rubbing alcohol, astringents, or other drying agents to the skin. One bath or one shower per day for 15 to 20 minutes with warm water and a mild soap should be immediately followed by the application of an emollient to prevent evaporation of water from the hydrated epidermis.
Test-Taking Strategy: Use the process of elimination and note the key words "need for further instructions." Recalling that a dehumidifier is going to dry the air in the environment will

assist in directing you to option 4. If you had difficulty with this question, review client teaching points related to dry skin and pruritis.
Level of Cognitive Ability: Comprehension
Client Needs: Health Promotion and Maintenance
Integrated Concept/Process: Teaching/Learning
Content Area: Adult Health/Integumentary
Reference: Black J, Hawks J, Keene A: *Medical-surgical nursing: clinical management for positive outcomes*, ed 6, Philadelphia, 2001, WB Saunders, p. 1286.

9. *Answer:* 4
Rationale: Lyme disease is a multisystem infection that results from a bite by a tick carried by several species of deer. Persons bitten by the *Ixodes* ticks are infected with the spirochete *Borrelia burgdorferi*. Histoplasmosis is caused by the inhalation of spores from bat or bird droppings. Toxoplasmosis is caused from the ingestion of cysts from contaminated cat feces. Lyme disease cannot be transmitted from one person to another.
Test-Taking Strategy: Use the process of elimination. Recalling that this disease is caused by a bite will assist in eliminating the incorrect options. If you had difficulty with this question, review the cause of Lyme disease.
Level of Cognitive Ability: Application
Client Needs: Health Promotion and Maintenance
Integrated Concept/Process: Nursing Process/Implementation
Content Area: Adult Health/Integumentary
Reference: Black J, Hawks J, Keene A: *Medical-surgical nursing: clinical management for positive outcomes*, ed 6, Philadelphia, 2001, WB Saunders, p. 337.

10. *Answer:* 2
Rationale: Stage II of Lyme disease develops within 1 to 6 months in the majority of untreated individuals. The most serious problems include cardiac conduction defects and neurological disorders, such as Bell's palsy and paralysis. These problems are not usually permanent. Arthralgias and joint enlargements are noted in stage III. A rash appears in stage I.
Test-Taking Strategy: Use the process of elimination. Eliminate options 3 and 4 first because they are similar. Recalling that a rash appears initially after the tick bite will assist in eliminating option 1. If you had difficulty with this question, review the clinical manifestations associated with each stage of Lyme disease.
Level of Cognitive Ability: Comprehension
Client Needs: Physiological Integrity
Integrated Concept/Process: Nursing Process/Data Collection
Content Area: Adult Health/Integumentary
Reference: Black J, Hawks J, Keene A: *Medical-surgical nursing: clinical management for positive outcomes*, ed 6, Philadelphia, 2001, WB Saunders, p. 1829.

11. *Answer:* 3
Rationale: There is a blood test available to detect Lyme disease; however, it is not a reliable test if performed before 4 to 6 weeks after the tick bite. Options 1, 2, and 4 are incorrect.
Test-Taking Strategy: Use the process of elimination. Eliminate option 1 first because of the word "immediately." A blood test is available; therefore eliminate option 2. Eliminate option 4 because treatment should begin before the arthralgia develops. If you had difficulty with this question, review the method of diagnosing Lyme disease.
Level of Cognitive Ability: Application
Client Needs: Physiological Integrity
Integrated Concept/Process: Nursing Process/Implementation
Content Area: Adult Health/Integumentary
Reference: Ignatavicius D, Workman M: *Medical-surgical: critical thinking for collaborative care*, ed 4, Philadelphia, 2002, WB Saunders, p. 361.

12. *Answer:* 3
Rationale: When an individual comes in contact with a poison ivy plant, the sap from the plant forms an invisible film on the human skin. The client should be instructed to immediately shower and that the skin should be lathered several times and rinsed each time in running water. Calamine lotion is a treatment that is used if dermatitis develops. It is not necessary for the client to be seen in the emergency room at this time.
Test-Taking Strategy: Recall that dermatitis can develop from contact with an allergen. Also, recalling that contact with poison ivy results in an invisible film will assist in directing you to option 3. Review the immediate treatment for contact with poison ivy, if you had difficulty with this question.
Level of Cognitive Ability: Application
Client Needs: Health Promotion and Maintenance
Integrated Concept/Process: Nursing Process/Implementation
Content Area: Adult Health/Integumentary
Reference: *Mosby's medical, nursing, and allied health dictionary*, ed 6, St Louis, 2002, Mosby, p. 1363.

13. *Answer:* 3
Rationale: Kaposi's sarcoma lesions begin as red, dark blue, or purple macules on the lower legs that change into plaques. These large plaques ulcerate or open and drain. The lesions spread by metastasis through the upper body then to the face and oral mucosa. It can also spread to the lymphatic system, lungs, and gastrointestinal (GI) tract. Late disease results in swelling and pain in the lower extremities, penis, scrotum, or face. Diagnosis is made by punch biopsy of cutaneous lesions and biopsy of pulmonary and GI lesions.
Test-Taking Strategy: Use the process of elimination. Eliminate options 2 and 4 first. These symptoms occur late in the development of Kaposi's sarcoma. Note the key words "this has been determined." These words should assist in directing you to the option that will confirm the diagnosis, which will be the biopsy of the lesions. Review this skin disorder if you had difficulty with this question.
Level of Cognitive Ability: Comprehension
Client Needs: Physiological Integrity
Integrated Concept/Process: Nursing Process/Data Collection
Content Area: Adult Health/Integumentary
Reference: Ignatavicius D, Workman M: *Medical-surgical: critical thinking for collaborative care*, ed 4, Philadelphia, 2002, WB Saunders, p. 374.

14. *Answer:* 4
Rationale: Kaposi's sarcoma is a vascular malignancy that presents as a skin disorder. It is a common acquired immunodeficiency syndrome indicator. Malignancy is seen most frequently in men with a history of same sex partners.

Although the cause of Kaposi's sarcoma is not known, it is considered to be due to an alteration or failure in the immune system. The renal transplant recipient and the client receiving antineoplastic medications are at risk for immunosuppression. Exposure to asbestos is not related to the development of Kaposi's sarcoma.
Test-Taking Strategy: Use the process of elimination. Note the key words "least likely." You can easily eliminate option 1 first. Next, note the similarity between options 2 and 3. These clients are at risk for immunosuppression. With this in mind, these options can be eliminated leaving option 4 as the correct option. If you had difficulty with this question, review the risk factors associated with Kaposi's sarcoma.
Level of Cognitive Ability: Comprehension
Client Needs: Physiological Integrity
Integrated Concept/Process: Nursing Process/Data Collection
Content Area: Adult Health/Integumentary
Reference: Ignatavicius D, Workman M: *Medical-surgical: critical thinking for collaborative care,* ed 4, Philadelphia, 2002, WB Saunders, p. 383.

15. ***Answer:*** 2
Rationale: Gowns and gloves are required if the nurse anticipates contact with soiled items, such as wound drainage. Masks are not required unless droplet or airborne precautions are necessary.
Test-Taking Strategy: Use the process of elimination. Think about the method of transmission when answering a question of this type. Read the question noting the task that is presented and in this case, it is bathing and changing linens. Eliminate option 1 because the method of transmission is not respiratory in nature. Eliminate options 3 and 4 because neither provide adequate protection based on the method of transmission. If you had difficulty with this question, review standard precautions.
Level of Cognitive Ability: Application
Client Needs: Safe, Effective Care Environment
Integrated Concept/Process: Nursing Process/Implementation
Content Area: Adult Health/Integumentary
Reference: DeWit S: *Fundamental concepts and skills for nursing,* Philadelphia, 2001, WB Saunders, p. 216.

16. ***Answer:*** 1
Rationale: Cellulitis is a skin infection into deeper dermis and subcutaneous fat that results in deep red erythema without sharp borders and spreads widely through tissue spaces. The skin is erythematous, edematous, tender, and sometimes nodular. Erysipelas is an acute superficial rapidly spreading inflammation of the dermis and lymphatics.
Test-Taking Strategy: Knowledge regarding the characteristics of cellulitis is required to answer the question. If you had difficulty with this question, review the characteristics of cellulitis and erysipelas.
Level of Cognitive Ability: Application
Client Needs: Physiological Integrity
Integrated Concept/Process: Nursing Process/Planning
Content Area: Adult Health/Integumentary
Reference: DeWit S: *Fundamental concepts and skills for nursing,* Philadelphia, 2001, WB Saunders, p. 782.

17. ***Answer:*** 1
Rationale: Warm compresses may be used to decrease the discomfort, erythema, and edema. After tissue and blood cultures are obtained, antibiotics are initiated. Heat lamps can cause more disruption to already inflamed tissue. Continuous cold and hot compresses are not the best measures.
Test-Taking Strategy: Use the process of elimination noting that option 1 is different from the other options. Option 1 addresses "warm" compresses, whereas options 2, 3, and 4 address either cold or hot measures. If you had difficulty with this question, review the treatment associated with cellulitis.
Level of Cognitive Ability: Application
Client Needs: Physiological Integrity
Integrated Concept/Process: Nursing Process/Planning
Content Area: Adult Health/Integumentary
Reference: DeWit S: *Fundamental concepts and skills for nursing,* Philadelphia, 2001, WB Saunders, p. 782.

18. ***Answer:*** 4
Rationale: Psoriatic patches are covered with silvery, white scaly patches. Affected areas include the scalp, elbows, knees, shins, sacral area, and trunk. Thickening, pitting, and discoloration of the nails occur. Pruritus may occur. The lesions in psoriasis are not red, purplish scaly lesions.
Test-Taking Strategy: Knowledge regarding the clinical manifestations associated with psoriasis is required to answer the question. If you had difficulty with this question, review the manifestations associated with psoriasis.
Level of Cognitive Ability: Comprehension
Client Needs: Physiological Integrity
Integrated Concept/Process: Nursing Process/Data Collection
Content Area: Adult Health/Integumentary
Reference: Ignatavicius D, Workman M: *Medical-surgical: critical thinking for collaborative care,* ed 4, Philadelphia, 2002, WB Saunders, p. 403.

19. ***Answer:*** 3
Rationale: Safety precautions are required during ultraviolet A light therapy. Most light therapy treatments require the person to stand in a light treatment chamber for up to 15 minutes. It is best to expose only those areas requiring treatment to the light therapy. Protective wrap around goggles prevent exposure of the eyes to ultraviolet light. The face should be shielded with a loosely applied covering if it is unaffected. Direct contact with the light bulbs of the treatment unit should be avoided to prevent burning of the skin.
Test-Taking Strategy: Use the process of elimination and note the key word "not." Note that option 3 addresses a time frame of 30 minutes, which is an extensive time period for exposure to ultraviolet light. If you had difficulty with this question, review the procedure for ultraviolet light treatments.
Level of Cognitive Ability: Application
Client Needs: Safe, Effective Care Environment
Integrated Concept/Process: Nursing Process/Planning
Content Area: Adult Health/Integumentary
Reference: Ignatavicius D, Workman M: *Medical-surgical: critical thinking for collaborative care,* ed 4, Philadelphia, 2002, WB Saunders, p. 1543.

20. ***Answer:*** 3
Rationale: Herpes zoster is caused by a reactivation of the varicella zoster virus, the cause of the virus for chickenpox. A viral culture of the lesion provides the definitive diagnosis. In a Wood's light examination, the skin is viewed under ultraviolet light to identify superficial infections of the skin. A patch test is a skin test that involves the administration of an allergen to the skin's surface to identify specific allergies. A biopsy will determine tissue type.
Test-Taking Strategy: Use the process of elimination and focus on the diagnosis. Recall that herpes zoster is caused by a virus. This will assist in eliminating options 2 and 4. From the remaining options, remember that a biopsy will determine tissue type, whereas a culture will identify an organism. Review this skin disorder if you had difficulty with this question.
Level of Cognitive Ability: Comprehension
Client Needs: Physiological Integrity
Integrated Concept/Process: Nursing Process/Data Collection
Content Area: Adult Health/Integumentary
Reference: Ignatavicius D, Workman M: *Medical-surgical: critical thinking for collaborative care,* ed 4, Philadelphia, 2002, WB Saunders, p. 1534.

21. ***Answer:*** 4
Rationale: The primary lesion of herpes zoster is a vesicle. The classic presentation is grouped vesicles on an erythematous base along a dermatome. Because they follow nerve pathways, the lesions do not cross the body's midline. Options 1, 2, and 3 are incorrect descriptions.
Test-Taking Strategy: Use the process of elimination. Remembering that these lesions occur as grouped vesicles along a nerve pathway will assist in answering the question. If you had difficulty with this question, review the characteristics of herpes zoster lesions.
Level of Cognitive Ability: Comprehension
Client Needs: Physiological Integrity
Integrated Concept/Process: Nursing Process/Data Collection
Content Area: Adult Health/Integumentary
Reference: Ignatavicius D, Workman M: *Medical-surgical: critical thinking for collaborative care,* ed 4, Philadelphia, 2002, WB Saunders, p. 1536.

22. ***Answer:*** 2
Rationale: Herpes zoster is caused by a reactivation of the varicella zoster virus, the causative virus for chickenpox. Individuals who have not been exposed to the varicella zoster virus are susceptible to chickenpox. Options 1, 3, and 4 are not associated with the herpes zoster virus.
Test-Taking Strategy: Use the process of elimination. Recalling that herpes zoster is caused by a reactivation of the varicella zoster virus, the causative virus for chickenpox, will assist in answering the question. Review the relationship between herpes zoster and chickenpox if you had difficulty with this question.
Level of Cognitive Ability: Application
Client Needs: Safe, Effective Care Environment
Integrated Concept/Process: Nursing Process/Planning
Content Area: Adult Health/Integumentary
Reference: Ignatavicius D, Workman M: *Medical-surgical: critical thinking for collaborative care,* ed 4, Philadelphia, 2002, WB Saunders, p. 1535.

23. ***Answer:*** 1
Rationale: Melanomas are pigmented malignant lesions originating in the melanin-producing cells of the epidermis. This skin cancer is highly metastatic, and a person's survival depends on early diagnosis and treatment. Basal cell carcinomas arise in the basal cell layer of the epidermis. Early malignant basal cell lesions often go unnoticed and although metastasis is rare, underlying tissue destruction can progress to include vital structures. Squamous cell carcinomas are malignant neoplasms of the epidermis. They are characterized by local invasion and the potential for metastasis.
Test-Taking Strategy: Knowledge regarding the various types of skin cancers and recalling that melanomas are highly metastatic will assist in directing you to the correct option. If you had difficulty with this question, review the characteristics of skin cancers.
Level of Cognitive Ability: Comprehension
Client Needs: Physiological Integrity
Integrated Concept/Process: Nursing Process/Data Collection
Content Area: Adult Health/Integumentary
Reference: Ignatavicius D, Workman M: *Medical-surgical: critical thinking for collaborative care,* ed 4, Philadelphia, 2002, WB Saunders, p. 1546.

24. ***Answer:*** 4
Rationale: A melanoma is an irregularly shaped pigmented papule or plaque with a red, white, or blue-toned color. Basal cell carcinoma appears as a pearly papule with a central crater and rolled waxy border. Squamous cell carcinoma is a firm nodular lesion topped with a crust or a central area of ulceration. Actinic keratosis, a premalignant lesion, appears as a small macule or papule with dry, rough, adherent yellow or brown scale.
Test-Taking Strategy: Use the process of elimination. Remembering that irregularly shaped lesions are a cause for concern will assist you in answering the question. If you had difficulty with this question, review the characteristics of malignant skin lesions.
Level of Cognitive Ability: Comprehension
Client Needs: Physiological Integrity
Integrated Concept/Process: Nursing Process/Data Collection
Content Area: Adult Health/Integumentary
Reference: Ignatavicius D, Workman M: *Medical-surgical: critical thinking for collaborative care,* ed 4, Philadelphia, 2002, WB Saunders, p. 1546.

25. ***Answer:*** 1
Rationale: Cryosurgery involves the local application of liquid nitrogen to isolated lesions and causes cell death and tissue destruction. The nurse prepares the client for swelling and increased tenderness of the treated area when the skin thaws. Tissue freezing is followed in 1 to 2 days by hemorrhagic blister formation. The nurse instructs the client to clean the treatment site with hydrogen peroxide to prevent secondary infection. A topical antibiotic may also be prescribed. Application of a warm damp wash cloth intermittently to the

site will provide relief from any discomfort. Alcohol-soaked dressings will cause irritation. It is not necessary to avoid showering.
Test-Taking Strategy: Use the process of elimination. Eliminate option 4 first because there is no reason for the client to avoid showers. Eliminate option 3 (alcohol-soaked dressing) next. From the remaining options, note that option 1 addresses the prevention of infection. If you had difficulty with this question, review client instructions after cryosurgery.
Level of Cognitive Ability: Application
Client Needs: Health Promotion and Maintenance
Integrated Concept/Process: Nursing Process/Planning
Content Area: Adult Health/Integumentary
Reference: Ignatavicius D, Workman M: *Medical-surgical: critical thinking for collaborative care,* ed 4, Philadelphia, 2002, WB Saunders, p. 1547.

26. *Answer:* 4
Rationale: The client should be instructed to avoid sun exposure between the hours of 11:00 AM and 3:00 PM. Sunscreen, a hat, opaque clothing, and sunglasses should be worn for outdoor activities. The client should be instructed to examine the body monthly for the appearance of any possible cancerous or any precancerous lesions.
Test-Taking Strategy: Use the process of elimination. Note the key word "not." Careful reading of the question will easily direct you to option 4. Review client teaching in the prevention of skin cancer if you had difficulty with this question.
Level of Cognitive Ability: Application
Client Needs: Health Promotion and Maintenance
Integrated Concept/Process: Self-Care
Content Area: Adult Health/Integumentary
Reference: Ignatavicius D, Workman M: *Medical-surgical: critical thinking for collaborative care,* ed 4, Philadelphia, 2002, WB Saunders, p. 1548.

27. *Answer:* 2
Rationale: Paronychia or infection around the nail is characterized by red, shiny skin often associated with painful swelling. These infections frequently result from trauma, picking at the nail, or disorders such as dermatitis. Often these become secondarily infected with bacteria or fungus, which later involves the nail. Options 1, 3, and 4 are incorrect descriptions of this disorder.
Test-Taking Strategy: Use the process of elimination. If you knew that this disorder related to an infection of the nail you would easily be directed to the correct option. If you had difficulty with this question, review the definition of this disorder.
Level of Cognitive Ability: Comprehension
Client Needs: Physiological Integrity
Integrated Concept/Process: Nursing Process/Data Collection
Content Area: Adult Health/Integumentary
Reference: Ignatavicius D, Workman M: *Medical-surgical: critical thinking for collaborative care,* ed 4, Philadelphia, 2002, WB Saunders, p. 1510.

28. *Answer:* 3
Rationale: Thorough handwashing, separating laundry, and separating washing of the client's dishes are required because this infection is contagious as long as skin lesions are present. Antibiotics are administered and should be continued as prescribed.
Test-Taking Strategy: Note the key word "not." Recalling that this infection is contagious will direct you to option 3. If you had difficulty with this question, review client instructions related to home care and the prevention of transmission of the infection.
Level of Cognitive Ability: Application
Client Needs: Health Promotion and Maintenance
Integrated Concept/Process: Teaching/Learning
Content Area: Adult Health/Integumentary
Reference: DeWit S: *Fundamental concepts and skills for nursing,* Philadelphia, 2001, WB Saunders, p. 388.

29. *Answer:* 4
Rationale: Findings in frostbite include a white or blue color and the skin will be hard, cold, and insensitive to touch. As thawing occurs, flushing of the skin, the development of blisters or blebs, or tissue edema appears. Gangrene can develop in 9 to 15 days.
Test-Taking Strategy: Use the process of elimination and focus on the diagnosis, frostbite. The words "insensitive to touch" should assist in directing you to the correct option. If you had difficulty with this question, review the characteristics associated with frostbite.
Level of Cognitive Ability: Comprehension
Client Needs: Physiological Integrity
Integrated Concept/Process: Nursing Process/Data Collection
Content Area: Adult Health/Integumentary
Reference: DeWit S: *Fundamental concepts and skills for nursing,* Philadelphia, 2001, WB Saunders, p. 342.

30. *Answer:* 1
Rationale: Frostbite is ideally treated with rapid and continuous rewarming of the tissue in a water bath for 15 to 20 minutes or until flushing of the skin occurs. Hot or cold water is not used in the treatment of frostbite.
Test-Taking Strategy: Use the process of elimination. Eliminate options 2 and 4 first avoiding options that address "hot" or "cold." Eliminate option 3 because interventions would begin immediately. If you had difficulty with this question, review the interventions associated with frostbite.
Level of Cognitive Ability: Application
Client Needs: Physiological Integrity
Integrated Concept/Process: Nursing Process/Planning
Content Area: Adult Health/Integumentary
Reference: DeWit S: *Fundamental concepts and skills for nursing,* Philadelphia, 2001, WB Saunders, p. 342.

31. *Answer:* 2
Rationale: In a stage II pressure ulcer, the skin is not intact. There is partial-thickness skin loss of the epidermis or dermis. The ulcer is superficial and may look like an abrasion, blister, or shallow crater. The skin is intact in stage I. A deep craterlike appearance occurs in stage III, and sinus tracts develop in stage IV.
Test-Taking Strategy: Use the process of elimination and knowledge of the characteristics associated with each stage of pressure ulcers. If you had difficulty with this question, review

the characteristics associated with each stage of pressure ulcers.
Level of Cognitive Ability: Comprehension
Client Needs: Physiological Integrity
Integrated Concept/Process: Nursing Process/Data Collection
Content Area: Adult Health/Integumentary
Reference: DeWit S: *Fundamental concepts and skills for nursing,* Philadelphia, 2001, WB Saunders, p. 289.

32. *Answer:* 4
Rationale: Bed or chair confinement, inability to move, loss of bowel or bladder control, poor nutrition, absent or inconsistent care giving, and a lowered mental awareness can all contribute to the development of skin breakdown. The least likely risk as presented in the options is the lowered mental awareness status. Options 1, 2, and 3 identify physiological conditions, which are the risk priorities.
Test-Taking Strategy: Note the key words "least likely." Use Maslow's Hierarchy of Needs theory. Remember that physiological needs are the priority. This will assist you in eliminating options 1, 2, and 3. Review the risk factors associated with skin breakdown if you had difficulty with this question.
Level of Cognitive Ability: Comprehension
Client Needs: Physiological Integrity
Integrated Concept/Process: Nursing Process/Data Collection
Content Area: Adult Health/Integumentary
Reference: DeWit S: *Fundamental concepts and skills for nursing,* Philadelphia, 2001, WB Saunders, p. 290.

33. *Answer:* 3
Rationale: Candidiasis (thrush) is noted as white patches on the tongue, palate, and buccal mucosa. The lesions adhere firmly to the tissues. The lesions are often referred to as milk curds because of their appearance. Clients often describe the lesions as dry and hot.
Test-Taking Strategy: Remembering that candidiasis (thrush) presents as white patches will assist in answering the question. If you had difficulty with this question, review the characteristics associated with this disorder.
Level of Cognitive Ability: Comprehension
Client Needs: Physiological Integrity
Integrated Concept/Process: Nursing Process/Data Collection
Content Area: Adult Health/Integumentary
Reference: Ignatavicius D, Workman M: *Medical-surgical: critical thinking for collaborative care,* ed 4, Philadelphia, 2002, WB Saunders, p. 1536.

34. *Answer:* 1
Rationale: Clients cannot tolerate commercial mouthwashes because the high alcohol concentration in these products can cause pain and discomfort to the lesions. A solution of warm water, half strength peroxide, or mouthwash formulas without alcohol are better tolerated and may promote healing. A change in the diet to liquid or pureed food often eases the discomfort of eating. The client should avoid spicy foods, citrus juice, and hot liquids.
Test-Taking Strategy: Note the key word "not" and use the process of elimination. Recalling that commercial mouthwashes contain alcohol will direct you to option 1. Review the client teaching points related to candidiasis (thrush) if you had difficulty with this question.
Level of Cognitive Ability: Application
Client Needs: Health Promotion and Maintenance
Integrated Concept/Process: Self-Care
Content Area: Adult Health/Integumentary
Reference: Ignatavicius D, Workman M: *Medical-surgical: critical thinking for collaborative care,* ed 4, Philadelphia, 2002, WB Saunders, p. 1536.

35. *Answer:* 1
Rationale: In severe cystic acne, isotretinoin may be prescribed to inhibit inflammation. Adverse effects include elevated triglycerides, skin dryness, eye discomfort such as dryness and burning, and cheilitis (lip inflammation). Close medical follow-up monitoring is required, and dry skin and cheilitis can be decreased by the use of emollients and lip balms. Vitamin A supplements are stopped during this treatment.
Test-Taking Strategy: Use the process of elimination and note the key words "need for further instruction." Recalling that isotretinoin is a metabolite of vitamin A will direct you to option 1. If you had difficulty with this question review the action, side effects, and adverse effects of this medication.
Level of Cognitive Ability: Comprehension
Client Needs: Health Promotion and Maintenance
Integrated Concept/Process: Nursing Process/Evaluation
Content Area: Adult Health/Integumentary
Reference: Schulte E, Price D, Gwin J: *Thompson's pediatric nursing,* ed 8, Philadelphia, 2001, WB Saunders, p. 340.

36. *Answer:* 3
Rationale: Scabies can be identified by the multiple straight or wavy threadlike lines noted beneath the skin. The skin lesions are caused by the female, which burrows beneath the skin and lays its eggs. The eggs hatch in a few days and the baby mites find their way to the skin surface where they mate and complete the life cycle. Options 1, 2, and 4 are not characteristics of scabies.
Test-Taking Strategy: Recalling that scabies burrows beneath the skin surface will assist in the process of elimination and provide direction in selecting the correct option. If you had difficulty with this question, review the characteristics associated with scabies.
Level of Cognitive Ability: Comprehension
Client Needs: Physiological Integrity
Integrated Concept/Process: Nursing Process/Data Collection
Content Area: Adult Health/Integumentary
Reference: Ignatavicius D, Workman M: *Medical-surgical: critical thinking for collaborative care,* ed 4, Philadelphia, 2002, WB Saunders, p. 1540.

37. *Answer:* 3
Rationale: The Centers for Disease Control and Prevention recommend the wearing of gowns and gloves for close contact with a person infested with scabies. Masks are not necessary. Transmission via clothing and other inanimate objects is uncommon. Scabies is usually transmitted from person to person by direct skin contact. All contacts that the client has had should be treated at the same time.

Test-Taking Strategy: Consider the mode of transmission of scabies and use the process of elimination. Since scabies is transmitted by direct skin contact, eliminate options 1, 2, and 4. If you had difficulty with question, review standard precautions and the transmission mode of scabies.
Level of Cognitive Ability: Application
Client Needs: Safe, Effective Care Environment
Integrated Concept/Process: Nursing Process/Implementation
Content Area: Adult Health/Integumentary
Reference: Ignatavicius D, Workman M: *Medical-surgical: critical thinking for collaborative care,* ed 4, Philadelphia, 2002, WB Saunders, p. 1540.

38. *Answer:* 2
Rationale: According to the Rule of Nines, with the initial burn, the anterior half of head equals 4.5%, the upper half of the anterior torso equals 9%, and the lower half of both arms equals 9%. The subsequent burn included the posterior half of head equaling 4.5% and the upper half of posterior torso equaling 9%. This totals 36%.
Test-Taking Strategy: Knowledge regarding the Rule of Nines is required to answer this question. Remember: 9 (head), 18 (arms), 36 (thorax), 36 (legs), 1 (perineum), equaling 99. If you had difficulty with this question, review the Rule of Nines.
Level of Cognitive Ability: Comprehension
Client Needs: Physiological Integrity
Integrated Concept/Process: Nursing Process/Data Collection
Content Area: Adult Health/Integumentary
Reference: DeWit S: *Fundamental concepts and skills for nursing,* Philadelphia, 2001, WB Saunders, p. 317.

39. *Answer:* 4
Rationale: The client exhibits several warning signs of an inhalation injury, namely, a history of a flame burn to the face, hoarseness, cough, carbonaceous sputum, singed facial hair, facial edema, and then color change. Additionally, one of the cardinal signs of hypoxia is restlessness and anxiety.
Test-Taking Strategy: Use the ABCs to answer the question. The only option that addresses airway is option 4. If you had difficulty with this question, review the clinical manifestations associated with burns to the face.
Level of Cognitive Ability: Analysis
Client Needs: Physiological Integrity
Integrated Concept/Process: Nursing Process/Data Collection
Content Area: Adult Health/Integumentary
Reference: Ignatavicius D, Workman M: *Medical-surgical: critical thinking for collaborative care,* ed 4, Philadelphia, 2002, WB Saunders, p. 1566.

40. *Answer:* 4
Rationale: Escharotomies are performed to alleviate the compartment syndrome that can occur when edema forms under nondistensible eschar in a circumferential burn. Escharotomies are performed through avascular eschar to subcutaneous fat. Although bleeding may occur from the site, it is considered a complication rather than an anticipated therapeutic outcome. Formation of granulation tissue is not the intent of an escharotomy. Escharotomy will not affect the formation of edema.
Test-Taking Strategy: Note the issue of the question, a therapeutic outcome. Use the ABCs (airway, breathing, circulation) to answer the question. The only option that addresses circulation is option 4. If you had difficulty with this question, review the purpose of an escharotomy.
Level of Cognitive Ability: Analysis
Client Needs: Physiological Integrity
Integrated Concept/Process: Nursing Process/Evaluation
Content Area: Adult Health/Integumentary
Reference: Ignatavicius D, Workman M: *Medical-surgical: critical thinking for collaborative care,* ed 4, Philadelphia, 2002, WB Saunders, p. 1572.

41. *Answer:* 1
Rationale: Superficial injury from radiation causes erythema and pain, hyperpigmentation, dry desquamation, or moist desquamation. Options 2, 3, and 4 are not associated with the description presented in the question.
Test-Taking Strategy: Use the process of elimination. Focus on the description in the question and note the word "superficial" in the correct option. If you had difficulty with this question, review the effects of radiation burns.
Level of Cognitive Ability: Comprehension
Client Needs: Physiological Integrity
Integrated Concept/Process: Nursing Process/Data Collection
Content Area: Adult Health/Integumentary
Reference: Ignatavicius D, Workman M: *Medical-surgical: critical thinking for collaborative care,* ed 4, Philadelphia, 2002, WB Saunders, p. 1575.

42. *Answer:* 3
Rationale: Circumferential burns of the extremities may compromise circulation. Elevating injured extremities above the level of the heart and active exercise help to reduce dependent edema formation. Options 1, 2, and 4 are incorrect.
Test-Taking Strategy: Use the process of elimination remembering that when an injury occurs such as a burn, edema develops. Option 3 addresses a position that will reduce edema. If you had difficulty with this question, review care to the client experiencing this type of a burn injury.
Level of Cognitive Ability: Application
Client Needs: Physiological Integrity
Integrated Concept/Process: Nursing Process/Implementation
Content Area: Adult Health/Integumentary
Reference: Ignatavicius D, Workman M: *Medical-surgical: critical thinking for collaborative care,* ed 4, Philadelphia, 2002, WB Saunders, p. 1558.

43. *Answer:* 3
Rationale: Thorough handwashing should be done before and after each contact with the burn-injured client. Sterile sheets and linens are used. Protective garb including gloves, cap, masks, shoe covers, scrub clothes, and plastic aprons need to be worn when caring for the client.
Test-Taking Strategy: Use the process of elimination and note the key word "not. " Option 2 can be easily eliminated first. From the remaining options, select option 3 because this is the least thorough technique to prevent infection. Also, note the absolute word "only" in option 3. If you had difficulty

with this question, review protective isolation techniques when caring for a burn client.
Level of Cognitive Ability: Application
Client Needs: Safe, Effective Care Environment
Integrated Concept/Process: Nursing Process/Implementation
Content Area: Adult Health/Integumentary
Reference: Ignatavicius D, Workman M: *Medical-surgical: critical thinking for collaborative care,* ed 4, Philadelphia, 2002, WB Saunders, p. 1561.

44. *Answer:* 1
Rationale: Autografts placed over joints or on the lower extremities are often elevated and immobilized after surgery for 3 to 7 days. This period of immobilization allows the autograft time to adhere and attach to the wound bed.
Test-Taking Strategy: Use the process of elimination. Eliminate options 2 and 3 first because they are similar. Note that the autograft was placed over a joint. This should direct you to select the option that identifies the longer period of immobilization. If you had difficulty with this question, review care to an autograft placed over a joint.
Level of Cognitive Ability: Application
Client Needs: Physiological Integrity
Integrated Concept/Process: Nursing Process/Planning
Content Area: Adult Health/Integumentary
Reference: Ignatavicius D, Workman M: *Medical-surgical: critical thinking for collaborative care,* ed 4, Philadelphia, 2002, WB Saunders, p. 1578.

45. *Answer:* 4
Rationale: Newly healed skin is more sensitive to the cold and the client should be instructed to wear warm clothing. The client should wash using a mild soap, rinsing thoroughly, and patting the skin dry using a clean towel. Newly healed skin sunburns easily and direct sunlight needs to be avoided. Products that contain perfume, alcohol, or lanolin should be avoided because they tend to irritate newly healed skin.
Test-Taking Strategy: Use the process of elimination and note the key word "not." Read each option carefully noting that the correct option uses the absolute word "never." If you had difficulty with this question, review home care instructions regarding skin care.
Level of Cognitive Ability: Application
Client Needs: Health Promotion and Maintenance
Integrated Concept/Process: Self-Care
Content Area: Adult Health/Integumentary
Reference: Ignatavicius D, Workman M: *Medical-surgical: critical thinking for collaborative care,* ed 4, Philadelphia, 2002, WB Saunders, p. 1579.

REFERENCES

Black J, Hawks J, Keene A: *Medical-surgical nursing: clinical management for positive outcomes,* ed 6, Philadelphia, 2001, WB Saunders.

DeWit S: *Fundamental concepts and skills for nursing,* Philadelphia, 2001, WB Saunders.

Ignatavicius D, Workman M: *Medical-surgical: Critical thinking for collaborative care,* ed 4, Philadelphia, 2002, WB Saunders.

Mosby's medical, nursing, and allied health dictionary, ed 6, St Louis, 2002, Mosby.

Shulte E, Price D, Gwin J: *Thompson's pediatric nursing,* ed 8, Philadelphia, 2001, WB Saunders.

Integumentary Medications

I. EMOLLIENTS AND LOTIONS

A. Emollients (Box 39-1)
   1. Oily or fatty substances that soften and soothe irritated skin by allowing the skin to retain water
   2. Available as creams or ointments
   3. Used for dry, scaly, itchy, inflammatory conditions

B. Lotions (Box 39-2)
   1. Liquid suspensions or dispersions
   2. Require shaking before application
   3. Although lotions are predominantly water, they have a drying effect on the skin when the water evaporates
   4. Used as a wash for the skin, as soaks, or as wet dressings on ulcers or **burns**
   5. Used for subacute inflammatory lesions after the severe exudate phase has ceased
   6. Medicated lotions are often used as antiinflammatory agents because they provide a drying, protective, and cooling effect

BOX 39-1

Emollients

Cold cream
Glycerin
Lanolin
Petrolatum
Zinc ointment

BOX 39-2

Lotions

Aluminum acetate solution (Burow's solution)
Calamine lotion (Caladryl lotion)
Potassium permanganate solution
Zinc stearate

II. RUBS AND LINIMENTS (Box 39-3)

A. Used for the temporary relief of muscular aches, rheumatism, arthritis, sprains, and neuralgia

B. Over-the-counter (OTC) products contain combinations of antiseptics, local anesthetics, analgesics, and counter irritants

C. Some products contain salicylates and, if used over a large area of the skin, may cause salicylate side effects such as tinnitus, nausea, or vomiting

D. A heating pad is not used with these products, as irritation or burning of the skin may occur

III. ANTIINFECTIVE AGENTS

A. Description
   1. Includes antiseptics and antibacterial, antifungal, antiviral, and antiparasitic medications
   2. Topical antibiotics are safe and effective in certain conditions; extensive use may encourage the emergence of resistant bacteria

BOX 39-3

Rubs and Liniments

Aspercreme
Ben-Gay
Deep-Down Rub
Hot cream/balm/stick
Myoflex

B. Antiseptics
1. Sodium hypochlorite (Dakin solution)
   a. A chloride solution that loosens, dissolves, and deodorizes necrotic tissue and blood clots
   b. It kills most common bacteria, including spores, amebas, fungi, protozoa, viruses, and yeast
   c. It is used for irrigating and cleaning necrotic or purulent wounds
   d. Loses its potency during storage, so fresh solution is prepared frequently
   e. It should not be in contact with healing or normal tissue
2. Chlorhexidine gluconate (Hibiclens)
   a. Effective for cleaning wounds caused by staphylococci and other gram-positive bacteria
   b. Used for irrigating and cleansing wounds, but not for packing wounds because it may cause contact dermatitis
3. Acetic acid
   a. Effective for irrigating, cleansing, and packing wounds infected by *Pseudomonas aeruginosa*
   b. Healthy skin surrounding the wound must be protected with a petroleum barrier because it excoriates the skin
4. Hydrogen peroxide
   a. As a 3% solution, it has effervescent action that releases gas and breaks up necrotic tissue
   b. It is used to irrigate and clean necrotic tissue and pus from open wounds
   c. It is not used to pack wounds because it decomposes too rapidly
   d. When epithelial tissue begins to form, hydrogen peroxide is discontinued because it inhibits tissue formation
5. Hexachlorophene (pHisoHex, Septisol)
   a. A combination of hexachlorophene and alcohol
   b. Hexachlorophene is a bacteriostatic agent with activity against staphylococci and other gram-positive bacteria
   c. Hexachlorophene is heavily absorbed through broken skin and can cause neurotoxicity; it should not be used on wounds
   d. The alcohol component dries and irritates tissue, is not a very effective germicide, and forms a film that can actually promote infection
   e. All hexachlorophene products are well rinsed from the skin after their use to prevent systemic absorption

BOX 39-4

Antibacterials, Antifungals, Antiparasitics

ANTIBACTERIALS
Bacitracin
Mity-Mycin
Mupirocin (Bactroban)
Mycitracin triple antibiotic
Neomycin
Neo-Polycin ointment
Polymyxin B
Triple antibiotic

ANTIFUNGALS
Acyclovir (Zovirax)

ANTIPARASITICS
Crotamiton (Eurax)
Lindane (Kwell)
Permethrin 5% (Elimite)

C. Antibacterials (Box 39-4)
1. Description: used for superficial skin infections
2. Mupirocin (Bactroban)
   a. Topical antibacterial active against *Staphylococcus aureus*, beta-hemolytic streptococci, or *Streptococcus pyogenes*
   b. Applied three times daily; if improvement is not observed within 3 to 5 days, it is discontinued

D. Antifungals
1. May cause erythema, stinging, blistering, peeling, pruritis, urticaria, and general skin irritation
2. Client is reevaluated if no results are obtained after 4 weeks of treatment

E. Antiviral: Acyclovir (Zovirax)
1. Inhibits DNA replication in the virus
2. Used for **herpes** simplex types 1 and 2, varicella zoster, Epstein-Barr virus, and cytomegalovirus
3. Can cause mild pain and transient burning and stinging
4. Applied completely over the lesion every 3 hours six times daily for 1 week
5. Rubber gloves are used to apply the ointment, to prevent the spread of infection

F. Antiparasitics
1. Used to treat scabies (mites) and pediculosis (lice)
2. May be harmful during pregnancy and in young children
3. May irritate the skin, eyes, and mucous membranes
4. May cause allergic reactions

IV. ANTIPRURITICS (Box 39-5)

A. Used to allay itching
B. Applied as wet dressings, pastes, lotions, creams, or ointments
C. Persons with dry skin should be instructed to bathe less frequently

V. KERATOLYTICS (Box 39-6)

A. Description
   1. Preparations that dissolve keratin
   2. Soften scales and loosen the horny layer of the skin, resulting in minimal peeling or extensive desquamation
   3. Used to treat superficial fungal infections, dermatitis, psoriasis, and localized dermatitis
B. Salicylic acid
   1. Used to treat seborrheic dermatitis, acne, and psoriasis, and to thin and remove calluses
   2. Can be absorbed systematically and can cause salicylism, characterized by dizziness and tinnitus; is not applied to large surface areas or open wounds
C. Podophyllum resin
   1. Used for various types of **skin cancer**
   2. Causes lesions to slough off, leaving a superficial ulcer and moderate dermatitis
   3. After the therapy is discontinued, the lesions are treated with a mild antiseptic ointment; healing usually occurs within a few days
D. Cantharidin (Cantharone)
   1. Used in treating warts
   2. Has an exfoliation effect only on the epidermal cells
   3. May cause tingling, itching, and burning
   4. Site may be very tender for 2 to 6 days
E. Masoprocol (Actinex)
   1. Has antiproliferative activity against keratinocytes and is used to treat keratosis
   2. Occlusive dressings are not to be used
   3. Transient burning may be experienced after administration

VI. STIMULANTS AND IRRITANTS (Box 39-7)

A. Description: produce a mild irritation to the surface of the skin, causing hyperemia and inflammation that promote the healing process
B. Coal tar
   1. Used in treating psoriasis, seborrheic dermatitis, and atopic dermatitis
   2. Has an unpleasant odor and frequently stains the skin and hair
   3. Can cause phototoxicity
C. Compound benzoin tincture
   1. Protects the skin when the client has bed sores, ulcers, cracked nipples, or fissures of any orifice
   2. Causes a mild irritation that produces increased blood flow and healing

VII. PROTECTIVES (Box 39-8)

A. Description
   1. Preparations that provide a film on the skin to protect it from irritations such as light, moisture, air, and dust
   2. Promote natural healing without the usual formation of dry crust over the wound
   3. Allow exudate to collect beneath the dressing, forming an artificial blister

BOX 39-5
Antipruritics

Calamine or phenol
Corn starch or oatmeal baths
Solutions of potassium permanganate, aluminum subacetate, boric acid, or normal saline

BOX 39-6
Keratolytics

Cantharidin (Cantharone)
Masoprocol (Actinex)
Podophyllum resin (Pod-Ben-25)
Podofilox (Condylox)
Resorcinol (Fostex Medicated Bar, Meted-2, Sebulex)
Salicylic acid (Wart-Off, Freezone, Compound W)

BOX 39-7
Stimulants and Irritants

Coal tar
Compound benzoin tincture

BOX 39-8
Protectives

DuoDerm
Ensure-It (Deseret)
Mediskin and Silver
Op-Site
Polyskin
Tegaderm
Tegasorb
Uniflex
Vigilon
Zinc oxide paste (Unna's boot)

4. Designed to be left in place for up to 7 days or until leakage occurs around the dressing
5. Uniflex, PolySkin, and Ensure-It; may be used to cover central and peripheral intravenous (IV) sites
6. Op-Site, Tegasorb, Mediskin and Silver, and Vigilon may be used for skin **burns**

B. Sunscreens
1. Act by absorbing ultraviolet rays
2. The best sunscreens contain PABA (para-aminobenzoic acid)
3. Most effective when applied about 30 minutes to 1 hour before exposure to the sun; should be reapplied after swimming or sweating
4. Can cause contact dermatitis and photosensitivity reactions

C. Nonadherent dressings
1. Woven or nonwoven dressings that may be impregnated with saline, petrolatum, or antimicrobials
2. Nonadherent dressings include Adaptic, Exu-Dry, Sofsorb, Telfa, Vaseline gauze, and Xeroform

VIII. GROWTH FACTORS

A. Description
1. Used to promote wound healing
2. Stimulate cells to divide and migrate, which results in wound healing, formation of granulation tissue, and new epidermis

B. Procuren solution
1. Promotes healing by actively stimulating growth and granulation tissue, capillaries, and epithelium
2. Applied to the wound and covered with petrolatum-impregnated gauze
3. The material is left in place for 12 hours and then washed off; during the remaining 12 hours of the day, the wound is covered with sulfadiazine (Silvadene)

IX. ENZYMES

A. Description
1. Used to promote healing of wounds and to debride skin ulcers
2. Reduce inflammation resulting from trauma and infection
3. Dissolve fibrin clots, which helps reduce the size of surface hematomas
4. To be effective, must be in contact with affected tissue in adequate concentrations for a sufficient length of time
5. Wound may need to be surgically debrided before application; if not administered to a clean, debrided wound, healing may be delayed

B. Enzymes that promote wound healing (Box 39-9)
1. Papain (Panafil, Panafil White)
   a. Does not injure or affect health tissue or cells
   b. Enzyme must be in immediate contact with the purulent wound material
   c. Wounds are cleansed with prescribed irrigating solution between applications
   d. Hydrogen peroxide cannot be used to irrigate the wound because it inactivates the papain
   e. Light dressings and cellophane wrap may be used over the wound to prevent soiling of clothing
   f. Dressings are changed frequently to prevent contamination and to remove necrotic debris
2. Hyaluronidase (Wydase)
   a. Facilitates the absorption of fluid administered by subcutaneous hypodermoclysis
   b. Can be injected subcutaneously into an infiltrated IV site when a potent vasoconstrictor such as norepinephrine (Levophed) or metaraminol (Aramine) has infiltrated
   c. It reduces the sloughing of tissue likely to occur secondarily to infiltration

C. Enzymes to remove exudates (Box 39-10)
1. Description
   a. Alter the thick, purulent drainage to a thin, liquid material that can be easily wiped or irrigated off the wound
   b. Enzyme contact with the wound is necessary to promote wound healing
   c. Wound needs to be cleansed, and crosshatching of eschar on **burns** is performed before application

BOX 39-9

Enzymes That Promote Wound Healing

Hyaluronidase (Wydase)
Papain (Panafil) (Panafil White)

BOX 39-10

Enzymes to Remove Exudates

Collagenase (Santyl)
Dextranomer (Debrisan)
Fibrinolysin and desoxyribonuclease (Elase)
Sutilains (Travase)

2. Sutilains (Travase)
   a. Used to remove nonviable or necrotic tissue and purulent enzymes from **burns**, ulcers, traumatic injury, and peripheral vascular disease wounds
   b. Inactive on viable tissue
3. Collagenase (Santyl)
   a. Used as a topical debriding agent
   b. Provides effective debridement of the collagen tissue at the wound edges where necrotic tissue is anchored
   c. Encourages the formation of granulation tissue at the wound edges and quicker epithelialization of wounds
   d. Apply with a tongue depressor directly into deep wounds
   e. Before application, cleanse wound of debris by gently rubbing with a gauze pad with sterile water or Dakin solution, followed by sterile normal saline
   f. Remove all excess ointment each time dressing is changed
   g. Apply only to injured area; causes erythema in healthy tissues
   h. Protect healthy tissue by applying zinc oxide paste
   i. Discontinued when necrotic tissue is gone
4. Fibrinolysin and desoxyribonuclease (Elase)
   a. Used to debride wounds, including **burns**, **decubitus** ulcers, and inflamed or infected lesions
   b. Clean wound with sterile water, pat dry; flush away necrotic debris with normal saline; then, apply a thin layer and cover with petrolatum gauze

D. Dextranomer (Debrisan)
1. Not a debriding agent but is a cleansing agent that actually absorbs peptides and proteins
2. Effective in wet wounds only
3. It is not packed tightly into the wound because maceration of surrounding tissue may occur from contact with the agent

X. CORTICOSTEROIDS

A. Have antiinflammatory, antipruritic, and vasoconstrictive actions

B. Contraindications
1. Clients demonstrating previous sensitivity to corticosteroids
2. Those with current systemic fungal, viral, or bacterial infections
3. Those with current complications related to corticosteroid therapy

C. Local adverse effects
1. Hypopigmentation
2. Acneiform eruptions
3. Contact dermatitis
4. Burning, dryness, irritation, itching
5. Overgrowth of bacteria, fungi, and viruses
6. Skin atrophy

D. Systemic adverse effects
1. Occur rarely
2. Adrenal suppression
3. Cushing's syndrome
4. Striae, skin atrophy
5. Ocular effects (glaucoma and cataracts)

E. Topical corticosteroids
1. Monitor plasma cortisol levels if prolonged therapy is necessary
2. Wash area just before application to increase medication penetration
3. Apply sparingly in a light film, rubbing gently
4. May apply to skin alone or with a dry occlusive dressing if prescribed by the physician
5. Instruct the client to report burning, irritation, or signs of infection to the physician

XI. ACNE PRODUCTS (Box 39-11)

A. Description
1. Mild acne can be treated with bar soaps, soapfree cakes, liquid cleansers, lotions, gels, and creams

BOX 39-11

Acne Products

CLEANSERS
Acnomel
Brasivol
Clearasil Medicated Astringent
Fostex
pHisoDerm
Stri-Dex

DRYING AGENTS
Acnomel
Dry and Clear
Ionax
Listerex

MISCELLANEOUS
Adapalene (Differin)
Alpha-Hydroxy Acids
Antibiotics
Azelaic acid (Azelex)
Bensulfoid cream (benzoyl peroxide and sulfur)
Benzamycin gel (benzoyl peroxide and sulfur)
Benzoyl peroxide wash, gel
Isotretinoin (Accutane)
Rosorcinol (as an ingredient in other preparations)
Salicylic acid (as an ingredient in other preparations)
Trentinoin (Retin-A)

2. For moderate acne, topical antiinflammatory medication such as benzoyl peroxide, tretinoin (Retin-A), isotretinoin (Accutane), azelaic acid (Azelex), and adapalene (Differin) may be prescribed; antibiotics may also be prescribed
3. Side effects can include excessive redness, extreme dryness of the skin leading to blistering and crusting, temporary pigmentation changes, and peeling of the skin
4. All products are kept away from the eyes, inside the nose, mucous membranes, and hair

B. Benzoyl peroxide: a keratolytic agent that is bacteriostatic and may decrease the production of irritant free fatty acids in the follicle

C. Tretinoin (Retin-A) and adapalene (Differin): acids of vitamin A that are used to treat acne vulgaris; may also be used to treat **skin cancer** and aging of the skin

D. Tretinoin (Retin-A)
1. Decreases cohesiveness of the epithelial cells, increasing cell mitosis and turnover; potentially irritating, particularly when used correctly
2. Within 48 hours of use, the skin generally becomes red and begins to peel
3. Temporary hyperpigmentation and hypopigmentation can occur
4. Client should avoid sun exposure because photosensitivity may occur
5. Applied liberally to the skin; the hands are washed thoroughly immediately after applying
6. Therapeutic results should be seen after 2 to 3 weeks but may not be optimal until after 6 weeks
7. Client may use cosmetics, but the skin needs to be cleaned thoroughly before applying the cosmetics

E. Isotretinoin (Accutane)
1. A metabolite of vitamin A
2. Used to treat severe cystic acne, and its use is reserved for persons who have not responded to other therapies, including systemic antibiotics
3. Can cause xerosis and facial desquamation, palmoplantar desquamation, pruritus, brittle nails, and hair loss
4. Is administered with meals two times daily for a 15- to 20-week course; if another course of therapy is needed, an 8-week lapse of time should occur
5. Photosensitivity may occur, so the client needs to be instructed to decrease sun exposure
6. Alcohol consumption should be eliminated during therapy because alcohol may potentiate serum triglyceride elevation

F. Local antibiotics
1. Used to treat acne; include clindamycin (Cleocin T), erythromycin, tetracycline (Topicycline), and meclocycline (Meclan)
2. Therapeutic response generally requires 6 to 12 weeks of therapy
3. Side effects include acute contact dermatitis, transient stinging or burning, staining of the skin, erythema, and skin tenderness

XII. POISON IVY TREATMENT (Box 39-12)

XIII. BURN PRODUCTS (Box 39-13)

A. Nitrofurazone (Furacin)
1. Applied topically to the **burn** as a solution, ointment, or cream
2. Has a broad spectrum of antibacterial activity
3. Used in **burns** when bacterial resistance to other agents is a problem
4. Topical: apply 1/16 inch film directly to **burn**
5. Side effects: contact dermatitis, rash
6. Less common side effects: pruritus, local edema

B. Mafenide (Sulfamylon)
1. A water-soluble cream that is bacteriostatic for both gram-negative and gram-positive organisms
2. Is used to treat **burns** to reduce the bacteria present in avascular tissues
3. Diffuses through the devascularized areas of the skin; may precipitate metabolic acidosis (usually compensated by hyperventilation)
4. Apply 1/16 inch film directly to the **burn**

BOX 39-12
Poison Ivy Treatment Products

Calamine
Calomox
IV-Chex
Ivy-Rid
Rhuli cream/spray/gel

BOX 39-13
Burn Products

Mafenide (Sulfamylon)
Nitrofurazone (Furacin)
Silver nitrate
Silver sulfadiazine (Flint SSD, Silvadene)

5. Side effects can include local pain, rash
6. Systemic effects include bone marrow depression, hemolytic anemia, metabolic acidosis
7. Keep **burn** covered with mafenide at all times
8. Notify physician if hyperventilation occurs; if acidosis develops, mafenide is washed off the skin

C. Silver sulfadiazine (Flint SSD, Silvadene)
1. Has a broad spectrum of activity against gram-negative bacteria, gram-positive bacteria, and yeast
2. Released slowly from the cream, which is selectively toxic to bacteria
3. Used primarily to prevent sepsis in clients with **burns**
4. Is not a carbonic anhydrase inhibitor and therefore does not cause acidosis
5. Rash and itching do occur from topical application
6. Apply 1/16 inch film (keep **burn** covered at all times with silver sulfadiazine)
7. Side effects include rash, itching
8. Systemic effects include leukopenia, interstitial nephritis
9. Monitor complete blood cell (CBC) count, particularly the white blood cells (WBC) frequently; if leukopenia develops, the physician will discontinue the medication

D. Silver nitrate
1. An antiseptic solution active against gram-negative bacteria
2. Dressings are applied to the **burn**, which are then kept moist with silver nitrate, which stains anything that it comes in contact with; this discoloration is not usually permanent
3. Used on extensive **burns** that may precipitate fluid and electrolyte imbalances
4. Apply to dressing; do not apply to wounds, cuts, or broken skin

PRACTICE QUESTIONS

1. A camp nurse asks the children preparing to swim in the lake if they have applied sunscreen. The nurse tells the children that sunscreen is most effective when applied:
   1. 1 hour before exposure to the sun
   2. Immediately before exposure to the sun
   3. 15 minutes before exposure to the sun
   4. Immediately after swimming
2. The nurse is assigned to care for a client with a burn injury to the lower legs. Nitrofurazone (Furacin) is prescribed to be applied to the sites of injury. The nurse plans to:
   1. Apply saline-soaked dressings over the medication
   2. Apply 1 inch film directly to the burn sites
   3. Apply 1/16 inch film directly to the burn sites
   4. Apply ½ inch film directly to the burn sites after cleansing the wounds
3. Mafenide (Sulfamylon) is prescribed for the client with a burn injury. When applying the medication, the client complains of local discomfort and burning. The most appropriate nursing action is to:
   1. Discontinue the medication
   2. Call the physician
   3. Apply a thinner film than prescribed to the burn site
   4. Inform the client that this is normal
4. A burn client is receiving treatments of topical mafenide (Sulfamylon) to the site of injury. The nurse would suspect that a systemic effect has occurred if which of the following is noted in the client?
   1. Local pain at the burn site
   2. Local rash at the burn site
   3. Hyperventilation
   4. Elevated blood pressure
5. Sodium hypochlorite (Dakin solution) is prescribed for a client with a leg wound containing purulent drainage. The nurse is assisting in developing a plan of care for the client. Which of the following would not be a component of the treatment plan with the use of this solution?
   1. Avoid contact with normal skin tissue
   2. Rinse off immediately after irrigation
   3. Soak sterile dressing with solution and pack into the wound
   4. Prepare solution before use
6. Tretinoin (Retin-A) is prescribed for a client with acne. The client calls the physician's office and tells the nurse that the skin has become very red and is beginning to peel. The nurse most appropriately responds by telling the client:
   1. To come to the clinic immediately
   2. To discontinue the medication
   3. To notify the physician
   4. That this is a normal occurrence with the use of this medication
7. A nurse provides instructions to a client regarding the use of tretinoin (Retin-A). Which of the following would not be a component of the instructions regarding the use of this medication?
   1. Wash hands thoroughly after applying the medication
   2. Optimal results will be seen after 6 weeks
   3. Apply a thin layer to the skin
   4. Cleanse the skin thoroughly before applying the medication
8. Isotretinoin (Accutane) is prescribed for a client to treat severe cystic acne. The nurse tells the client that the length of the usual prescribed course of treatment is:

1. 1 month
2. 8 weeks
3. 15 to 20 weeks
4. 1 year

9. Isotretinoin (Accutane) is prescribed for a client with severe acne. Before the administration of this medication, the nurse would expect that which laboratory test will be prescribed?
   1. Complete blood count
   2. White blood cell count
   3. Triglyceride level
   4. Platelet count
10. A client with severe acne is seen at the physician's office. The physician prescribes isotretinoin (Accutane). The nurse reviews the client's health record and would notify the physician if the client is presently taking which of the following medications?
   1. Digoxin (Lanoxin)
   2. Phenytoin (Dilantin)
   3. Vitamin A
   4. Furosemide (Lasix)
11. Fibrinolysin and desoxyribonuclease (Elase) dry powder are prescribed to treat a skin ulcer. The nurse assists in developing a plan of care for the client. Which of the following nursing interventions would not be a component of the plan regarding this treatment?
   1. Clean the wound with a sterile solution before applying
   2. Prepare a solution just before use
   3. Apply a thick layer of medication and cover with a dry, sterile dressing
   4. Apply a thin layer of medication and cover with a petrolatum gauze
12. Minoxidil solution (Rogaine) is prescribed for the client to treat hair loss. The nurse instructs the client regarding the medication knowing that the usual dosage for this medication is:
   1. 0.5 mL applied two times daily
   2. 1 mL applied at bedtime
   3. 1 mL applied two times a day
   4. 1 mL applied four times a day
13. A nurse employed in a physician's office is collecting data from a client. The nurse notes that the client is taking azelaic acid (Azelex). Because of the medication prescription, the nurse suspects that the client is being treated for:
   1. Herpes simplex
   2. Acne
   3. Eczema
   4. Hair loss
14. Collagenase (Santyl) is prescribed for a client with a severe burn to the hand. The nurse provides instructions to the client regarding the use of the medication. Which statement by the client indicates an accurate understanding of the use of this medication?
   1. "I will apply the ointment once a day and leave it open to the air."
   2. "I will apply the ointment once a day and cover it with a sterile dressing."
   3. "I will apply the ointment twice a day and leave it open to the air."
   4. "I will apply the ointment at bedtime and in the morning and cover it with a sterile dressing."
15. Minoxidil (Rogaine) is prescribed for a client to treat hair loss. The client asks the nurse if the hair will continue to grow when the medication is stopped. The most appropriate nursing response is:
   1. "The hair will continue to grow."
   2. "Newly gained hair is lost in 3 to 4 months."
   3. "It depends on how long you have been taking the minoxidil."
   4. "I'm not sure, you need to ask your physician."
16. Coal tar has been prescribed for a client with a diagnosis of psoriasis. The nurse is asked to describe the treatment to the client. Which of the following will not be a component of the description of this treatment provided to the client?
   1. The medication has an unpleasant odor
   2. The medication can stain the skin and hair
   3. The medication can cause systemic effects
   4. The medication can cause phototoxicity
17. A client is diagnosed with herpes simplex. The physician tells the nurse that a topical medication for treatment will be prescribed. The nurse expects that which of the following medications will be prescribed?
   1. Triple antibiotic
   2. Acyclovir (Zovirax)
   3. Mupirocin (Bactroban)
   4. Masoprocol (Actinex)
18. Salicylic acid is prescribed for a client with a diagnosis of psoriasis. The nurse suspects the presence of systemic toxicity from this medication if which of the following occurs in the client?
   1. Decreased respirations
   2. Diarrhea
   3. Constipation
   4. Tinnitus
19. A hospitalized client with severe seborrheic dermatitis is receiving treatments of topical glucocorticoid applications followed by the application of an occlusive dressing. The nurse monitors for which systemic effect that can occur from this treatment?
   1. Adrenal suppression
   2. Adrenal hyperactivity
   3. Local infection
   4. Thinning of the skin
20. A nurse is applying a topical glucocorticoid to a client with eczema. The nurse monitors for systemic

absorption of the medication if the medication was being applied to which of the following body areas?
1. Back
2. Axilla
3. Palms of the hands
4. Soles of the feet

21. A topical glucocorticoid is prescribed for a client with dermatitis. The nurse provides instructions to the client regarding the use of the medication. Which of the following, if stated by the client, would indicate a need for further instruction?
1. "I need to apply the medication in a thin film."
2. "I should gently rub the medication into the skin."
3. "I should place a bandage over the site after applying the medication."
4. "The medication will help to relieve the inflammation and itching."

22. Lindane (Kwell) is prescribed for the treatment of scabies. The nurse would question the order if the medication were prescribed for which of the following clients?
1. A 42-year-old woman
2. An elderly client
3. A 6-year-old child
4. A 52-year-old man with hypertension

23. A client is seen in the clinic for complaints of skin itchiness that has been persistent over the past several weeks. After an assessment, it has been determined that the client has scabies. Lindane (Kwell) is prescribed and the nurse is asked to provide instructions to the client regarding the use of the medication. The nurse tells the client to:
1. Leave the cream on for 8 to 12 hours and then remove by washing
2. Apply a thick layer of cream to the entire body
3. Apply the cream as prescribed for 2 days in a row
4. Apply to the entire body and scalp, excluding the face

24. An outbreak of pediculosis capitus has occurred at the local school. The nurse is assisting in providing instructions to the mothers of the children attending the school regarding the application of permethrin 5% (Elimite). The nurse tells the mothers to:
1. Apply at bedtime and rinse off in the morning
2. Apply before washing the hair
3. Avoid saturating the hair and scalp when applying
4. Allow to remain on the hair 10 minutes and then rinse with water

25. A female client tells a nurse that her skin is very dry and irritated. Which of the following products would the nurse suggest that the client apply to the dry skin?
1. A glycerin emollient
2. Aspercreme
3. Myoflex
4. Acetic acid solution

ANSWERS

1. *Answer:* 1

Rationale: Sunscreens are most effective when applied about 30 minutes to 1 hour before exposure to the sun so that they can penetrate the skin. All sunscreens should be reapplied after swimming or sweating.

Test-Taking Strategy: Use the process of elimination. Knowledge that sunscreens need to penetrate the skin will assist in eliminating options 2 and 3. From the remaining options, noting the key words "most effective" will direct you to option 1. Review protective skin measures if you had difficulty with this question.

Level of Cognitive Ability: Application

Client Needs: Health Promotion and Maintenance

Integrated Concept/Process: Nursing Process/Implementation

Content Area: Pharmacology

Reference: Lehne R: *Pharmacology for nursing care,* ed 4, Philadelphia, 2001, WB Saunders, p. 1160.

2. *Answer:* 3

Rationale: Furacin is applied topically to the burn and has a broad spectrum of antibiotic activity. It is used in a burn injury when bacterial resistance to other agents is a real or potential problem. A film of $\frac{1}{16}$ inch is applied directly to the burn. Saline-soaked dressings are not used.

Test-Taking Strategy: Use the process of elimination. Option 1 can be eliminated because infection is a major concern with the burn client and a wet dressing can more easily harbor bacteria. Recalling that a very thin film is required will direct you to option 3 from the remaining options. Review the use of this medication for burn therapy if you had difficulty with this question.

Level of Cognitive Ability: Application

Client Needs: Physiological Integrity

Integrated Concept/Process: Nursing Process/Planning

Content Area: Pharmacology

Reference: Ignatavicius D, Workman M: *Medical-surgical: critical thinking for collaborative care,* ed 4, Philadelphia, 2002, WB Saunders, p. 1581.

3. *Answer:* 4

Rationale: Mafenide is bacteriostatic for both gram-negative and gram-positive organisms and is used to treat burn injuries to reduce bacteria present in avascular tissues. The client should be informed that the medication will cause local discomfort and burning.

Test-Taking Strategy: Use the process of elimination. Eliminate options 1 and 3 because it is not within the scope of nursing practice to alter or discontinue a medication. From the remaining options, recalling that this is a normal expected

occurrence will direct you to option 4. If you had difficulty with this question, review this medication.
Level of Cognitive Ability: Application
Client Needs: Physiological Integrity
Integrated Concept/Process: Nursing Process/Implementation
Content Area: Pharmacology
Reference: Ignatavicius D, Workman M: *Medical-surgical: critical thinking for collaborative care*, ed 4, Philadelphia, 2002, WB Saunders, p. 1581.

4. *Answer:* 3
Rationale: Mafenide can suppress renal excretion of acid and cause acidosis evidenced by hyperventilation. Clients receiving this treatment should be monitored for acid-base status, and if the acidosis becomes severe, the medication is discontinued for 1 to 2 days. Options 1 and 2 describe local rather than systemic effects. An elevated blood pressure may be expected in the client with pain.
Test-Taking Strategy: Use the process of elimination. Note the key words "systemic effect." Options 1 and 2 can be eliminated because these are local rather than systemic effects. From the remaining options, recall that the client in pain would likely have an elevated blood pressure. This should direct you to option 3. Review the systemic effects of this medication if you had difficulty with this question.
Level of Cognitive Ability: Comprehension
Client Needs: Physiological Integrity
Integrated Concept/Process: Nursing Process/Data Collection
Content Area: Pharmacology
Reference: Hodgson B, Kizior R: *Saunders nursing drug handbook 2002*, Philadelphia, 2002, WB Saunders, p. 673.

5. *Answer:* 3
Rationale: Dakin solution is a chloride solution that is used for irrigating and cleaning necrotic or purulent wounds. It can be used for packing necrotic wounds. It cannot be used to pack purulent wounds because the solution is inactivated by copious pus. It should not come in contact with healing or normal tissue, and it should be rinsed off immediately if used for irrigation. Solutions are unstable and must be prepared fresh for each use.
Test-Taking Strategy: Use the process of elimination. Note the key words "purulent drainage" and "not." Eliminate options 1 and 2 first because they are similar and indicate avoiding healthy tissue. It makes sense to prepare the solution before use; therefore eliminate option 4. If you are unfamiliar with the use of this solution, review this content.
Level of Cognitive Ability: Application
Client Needs: Physiological Integrity
Integrated Concept/Process: Nursing Process/Planning
Content Area: Pharmacology
Reference: Karch A: *Focus on nursing pharmacology*, Philadelphia, 2000, Lippincott, p. 744.

6. *Answer:* 4
Rationale: Tretinoin decreases cohesiveness of the epithelial cells, increasing cell mitosis and turnover. It is potentially irritating particularly when used correctly. Within 48 hours of use, the skin generally becomes red and begins to peel.
Test-Taking Strategy: Use the process of elimination. Options 1 and 3 can be eliminated first because they are similar. Eliminate option 2 next because it is not within the scope of nursing practice to advise a client to discontinue a medication. Review the effects of this medication if you had difficulty with this question.
Level of Cognitive Ability: Application
Client Needs: Physiological Integrity
Integrated Concept/Process: Nursing Process/Implementation
Content Area: Pharmacology
Reference: Hodgson B, Kizior R: *Saunders nursing drug handbook 2002*, Philadelphia, 2002, WB Saunders, p. 1112.

7. *Answer:* 3
Rationale: Tretinoin is applied liberally to the skin. The hands are washed thoroughly immediately after applying. Therapeutic results should be seen after 2 to 3 weeks but may not be optimal until after 6 weeks. The skin needs to be cleansed thoroughly before applying the medication.
Test-Taking Strategy: Use the process of elimination and note the key word "not." Eliminate options 1 and 4 first using the principles of asepsis. From the remaining options, knowledge regarding the use of the medication will assist in directing you to option 3. Review this medication if you had difficulty with this question.
Level of Cognitive Ability: Application
Client Needs: Health Promotion and Maintenance
Integrated Concept/Process: Teaching/Learning
Content Area: Pharmacology
Reference: Hodgson B, Kizior R: *Saunders nursing drug handbook 2002*, Philadelphia, 2002, WB Saunders, p. 1112.

8. *Answer:* 3
Rationale: Isotretinoin is administered two times daily for 15 to 20 weeks. If needed, a second course may be given, but not until 2 months have elapsed after completing the first course.
Test-Taking Strategy: Knowledge regarding the use of this medication is required to answer this question. Review this medication if you had difficulty with this question.
Level of Cognitive Ability: Application
Client Needs: Health Promotion and Maintenance
Integrated Concept/Process: Nursing Process/Implementation
Content Area: Pharmacology
Reference: Hodgson B, Kizior R: *Saunders nursing drug handbook 2002*, Philadelphia, 2002, WB Saunders, p. 605.

9. *Answer:* 3
Rationale: Isotretinoin can elevate triglyceride levels. Blood triglyceride content should be measured before treatment and periodically thereafter until the effect of the medication on the triglycerides have been evaluated.
Test-Taking Strategy: Use the process of elimination. Eliminate options 1 and 2 first because a complete blood count will also measure the white blood cell count. From the remaining options, it is necessary to know that the medication can affect the triglyceride level in the client. Review this medication if you had difficulty with this question.
Level of Cognitive Ability: Comprehension
Client Needs: Physiological Integrity

Integrated Concept/Process: Nursing Process/Planning
Content Area: Pharmacology
Reference: Hodgson B, Kizior R: *Saunders nursing drug handbook 2002*, Philadelphia, 2002, WB Saunders, p. 605.

10. *Answer:* 3
Rationale: Vitamin A, a derivative of isotretinoin, can produce generalized intensification of isotretinoin toxicity. Because of the potential for increased toxicity, vitamin A supplements should be discontinued before isotretinoin therapy.
Test-Taking Strategy: Use the process of elimination. Recalling that isotretinoin is a derivative of vitamin A will easily direct you to the correct option. If you are unfamiliar with this medication, review the contraindications associated with its use.
Level of Cognitive Ability: Application
Client Needs: Safe, Effective Care Environment
Integrated Concept/Process: Nursing Process/Implementation
Content Area: Pharmacology
Reference: Hodgson B, Kizior R: *Saunders nursing drug handbook 2002*, Philadelphia, 2002, WB Saunders, p. 605.

11. *Answer:* 3
Rationale: The wound should be cleansed with a sterile solution and gently patted dry. A thin layer of Elase is applied and covered with a petrolatum gauze. If a dry powder is used, the solution should be prepared just before use.
Test-Taking Strategy: Use the process of elimination and note the word "not." Noting the word "thick" in option 3 should assist in directing you to this option. Review the method of application of this medication if you had difficulty with this question.
Level of Cognitive Ability: Application
Client Needs: Physiological Integrity
Integrated Concept/Process: Nursing Process/Planning
Content Area: Pharmacology
Reference: Ignatavicius D, Workman M: *Medical-surgical: critical thinking for collaborative care*, ed 4, Philadelphia, 2002, WB Saunders, p. 1577.

12. *Answer:* 3
Rationale: Minoxidil solution is used for topical treatment of baldness. The usual dosage is 1 mL applied two times a day.
Test-Taking Strategy: Knowledge regarding the usual dosage for minoxidil solution is required to answer this question. Review this medication if you had difficulty with this question.
Level of Cognitive Ability: Application
Client Needs: Physiological Integrity
Integrated Concept/Process: Teaching/Learning
Content Area: Pharmacology
Reference: Lehne R: *Pharmacology for nursing care*, ed 4, Philadelphia, 2001, WB Saunders, p. 464.

13. *Answer:* 2
Rationale: Azelaic acid is a topical medication used to treat mild to moderate acne. It appears to work by suppressing the growth of *Propionibacterium acnes* and by decreasing proliferation of keratinocytes.
Test-Taking Strategy: Knowledge regarding the use of azelaic acid is required to answer this question. Review this medication if you had difficulty with this question.
Level of Cognitive Ability: Comprehension
Client Needs: Physiological Integrity
Integrated Concept/Process: Nursing Process/Data Collection
Content Area: Pharmacology
Reference: Lehne R: *Pharmacology for nursing care*, ed 4, Philadelphia, 2001, WB Saunders, p. 1155.

14. *Answer:* 2
Rationale: Collagenase is used to promote debridement of dermal lesions and severe burns. It is applied once daily and covered with a sterile dressing.
Test-Taking Strategy: Note the key words "indicates an accurate understanding." Knowledge regarding the use of this medication will direct you to option 2. Review this medication if you had difficulty with this question.
Level of Cognitive Ability: Comprehension
Client Needs: Health Promotion and Maintenance
Integrated Concept/Process: Teaching/Learning
Content Area: Pharmacology
Reference: Ignatavicius D, Workman M: *Medical-surgical: critical thinking for collaborative care*, ed 4, Philadelphia, 2002, WB Saunders, p. 1577.

15. *Answer:* 2
Rationale: Hair regrowth is most likely when baldness has developed recently and has been limited to a small area. Upon discontinuation of the medication, newly gained hair is lost in 3 to 4 months, and the natural progression of hair loss resumes.
Test-Taking Strategy: Use the process of elimination. Option 4 can be easily eliminated because it is nontherapeutic and places the client's question on hold. From the remaining options, knowledge regarding the clinical response and effects of this medication will direct you to option 2. Review this medication if you had difficulty with this question.
Level of Cognitive Ability: Application
Client Needs: Psychosocial Integrity
Integrated Concept/Process: Nursing Process/Implementation
Content Area: Pharmacology
Reference: Lehne R: *Pharmacology for nursing care*, ed 4, Philadelphia, 2001, WB Saunders, p. 1159.

16. *Answer:* 3
Rationale: Coal tar is used to treat psoriasis and other chronic disorders of the skin. It suppresses DNA synthesis, mitotic activity, and cell proliferation. It has an unpleasant odor, can frequently stain the skin and hair, and can cause phototoxicity. Systemic toxicity does not occur.
Test-Taking Strategy: Use the process of elimination and note the key word "not." The name of the medication will assist in eliminating options 1 and 2. From the remaining options, it is necessary to know that the medication does not cause systemic effects. Review this treatment if you had difficulty with this question.
Level of Cognitive Ability: Application
Client Needs: Physiological Integrity
Integrated Concept/Process: Teaching/Learning
Content Area: Pharmacology
Reference: Lehne R: *Pharmacology for nursing care*, ed 4, Philadelphia, 2001, WB Saunders, p. 1157.

17. *Answer:* 2
Rationale: Acyclovir is a topical antiviral agent that inhibits DNA replication in the virus. It has activity against herpes simplex types 1 and 2, varicella-zoster, Epstein-Barr, and cytomegalovirus. Triple antibiotic would not be effective in treating herpesvirus. Mupirocin is a topical antibacterial active against impetigo caused by staphylococcus or streptococcus. Masoprocol is a keratolytic.
Test-Taking Strategy: Use the process of elimination. Recalling that herpes simplex is a virus will direct you to the option that identifies an antiviral medication. Review this medication if you had difficulty with this question.
Level of Cognitive Ability: Comprehension
Client Needs: Physiological Integrity
Integrated Concept/Process: Nursing Process/Planning
Content Area: Pharmacology
Reference: Lehne R: *Pharmacology for nursing care,* ed 4, Philadelphia, 2001, WB Saunders, p. 1013.

18. *Answer:* 4
Rationale: Salicylic acid is readily absorbed through the skin and systemic toxicity (salicylism) can result. Symptoms include tinnitus, hyperpnea, dizziness, and psychological disturbances. Constipation and diarrhea are not associated with salicylism.
Test-Taking Strategy: Use the process of elimination. Noting the name of the medication will assist in directing you to the correct option if you can recall the toxic effects that occur with acetyl "salicylic" acid (aspirin). If you are unfamiliar with the toxic effects of salicylic acid, review this content.
Level of Cognitive Ability: Comprehension
Client Needs: Physiological Integrity
Integrated Concept/Process: Nursing Process/Data Collection
Content Area: Pharmacology
Reference: Lehne R: *Pharmacology for nursing care,* ed 4, Philadelphia, 2001, WB Saunders, p. 1153.

19. *Answer:* 1
Rationale: Topical glucocorticoids can be absorbed in sufficient amounts to produce systemic toxicity. Principal concerns are growth retardation (in children) and adrenal suppression in all age groups. Options 3 and 4 identify local rather than systemic reactions.
Test-Taking Strategy: Use the process of elimination. Options 3 and 4 can be eliminated first because they are local reactions. From the remaining options, recalling the concerns related to systemic toxicity is required to answer the question. Review these systemic effects if you had difficulty with this question.
Level of Cognitive Ability: Application
Client Needs: Physiological Integrity
Integrated Concept/Process: Nursing Process/Data Collection
Content Area: Pharmacology
Reference: Lehne R: *Pharmacology for nursing care,* ed 4, Philadelphia, 2001, WB Saunders, p. 660.

20. *Answer:* 2
Rationale: Topical glucocorticoids can be absorbed into the systemic circulation. Absorption is higher from regions where the skin is especially permeable (scalp, axilla, face, eyelids, neck, perineum, genitalia) and lower from regions where penetrability is poor (back, palms, soles).
Test-Taking Strategy: Focus on the issue of the question "systemic absorption." Eliminate options 3 and 4 because these body areas are similar in terms of skin substance. From the remaining options, think about permeability of the skin area. This will direct you to option 2. Review this medication if you had difficulty with this question.
Level of Cognitive Ability: Application
Client Needs: Physiological Integrity
Integrated Concept/Process: Nursing Process/Data Collection
Content Area: Pharmacology
Reference: Lehne R: *Pharmacology for nursing care,* ed 4, Philadelphia, 2001, WB Saunders, p. 660.

21. *Answer:* 3
Rationale: Clients should be advised not to use occlusive dressings (bandages or plastic wraps) to cover the affected site after the application of the topical glucocorticoid, unless the physician specifically prescribes wound coverage. Options 1, 2, and 4 are accurate statements related to the use of this medication.
Test-Taking Strategy: Use the process of elimination and note the key words "need for further instruction." Eliminate option 4 knowing that this is the action for glucocorticoids. The words "thin" in option 1 and "gently" in option 2 should assist you in eliminating these options. If you had difficulty with this question, review this medication.
Level of Cognitive Ability: Comprehension
Client Needs: Health Promotion and Maintenance
Integrated Concept/Process: Teaching/Learning
Content Area: Pharmacology
Reference: Lehne R: *Pharmacology for nursing care,* ed 4, Philadelphia, 2001, WB Saunders, p. 787.

22. *Answer:* 3
Rationale: Lindane can penetrate the intact skin and can cause convulsions if absorbed in sufficient quantities. Clients at highest risk for convulsions are premature infants, children, and clients with preexisting seizure disorders. Lindane should not be used on pediatric clients unless safer medications have failed to control the infection.
Test-Taking Strategy: Knowledge regarding the contraindications associated with the use of lindane is required to answer this question. If you are unfamiliar with these contraindications, review this content.
Level of Cognitive Ability: Comprehension
Client Needs: Safe, Effective Care Environment
Integrated Concept/Process: Nursing Process/Implementation
Content Area: Pharmacology
Reference: Lehne R: *Pharmacology for nursing care,* ed 4, Philadelphia, 2001, WB Saunders, p. 1099.

23. *Answer:* 1
Rationale: Lindane is applied in a thin layer to the entire body below the head. No more than 30 g (1 oz) should be used. The medication is removed by washing 8 to 12 hours later. Usually, only one application is required.

Test-Taking Strategy: Knowledge regarding the use of lindane is required to answer this question. If you are unfamiliar with the use of this medication, review this procedure.
Level of Cognitive Ability: Application
Client Needs: Health Promotion and Maintenance
Integrated Concept/Process: Nursing Process/Implementation
Content Area: Pharmacology
Reference: Lehne R: *Pharmacology for nursing care,* ed 4, Philadelphia, 2001, WB Saunders, p. 1098.

24. *Answer:* 4
Rationale: The instructions for the use of permethrin include wash, rinse, and towel dry the hair; apply sufficient volume to saturate the hair and scalp; allow to remain on the hair 10 minutes and then rinse with water. Options 1, 2, and 3 are incorrect instructions.
Test-Taking Strategy: Note that both options 1 and 4 address a time frame for allowing the medication to remain on the hair. Recognizing this may provide you with the clue that one of these options is correct. From this point, it is necessary to know the procedure for this treatment. If you are unfamiliar with this treatment, review this content.
Level of Cognitive Ability: Application
Client Needs: Health Promotion and Maintenance
Integrated Concept/Process: Nursing Process/Implementation
Content Area: Pharmacology
Reference: Lehne R: *Pharmacology for nursing care,* ed 4, Philadelphia, 2001, WB Saunders, p. 1098.

25. *Answer:* 1
Rationale: Glycerin is an emollient that is used for dry, cracked, and irritated skin. Aspercreme and Myoflex are used to treat muscular aches. Acetic acid solution is used for irrigating, cleansing, and packing wounds infected by *Pseudomonas aeruginosa.*
Test-Taking Strategy: Use the process of elimination. Note the key words "skin is very dry and irritated." These key words and knowledge of the products indicated in the options will assist in directing you to option 1. Review these products if you had difficulty with this question.
Level of Cognitive Ability: Application
Client Needs: Health Promotion and Maintenance
Integrated Concept/Process: Self-Care
Content Area: Pharmacology
Reference: Ignatavicius D, Workman M: *Medical-surgical: critical thinking for collaborative care,* ed 4, Philadelphia, 2002, WB Saunders, p. 1515.

REFERENCES

Black J, Hawks J, Keene A: *Medical-surgical nursing: clinical management for positive outcomes,* ed 6, Philadelphia, 2001, WB Saunders.

DeWit S: *Fundamental concepts and skills for nursing,* Philadelphia, 2001, WB Saunders.

Hodgson B, Kizior R: *Saunders nursing drug handbook 2002,* Philadelphia, 2002, WB Saunders.

Ignatavicius D, Workman M: *Medical-surgical: critical thinking for collaborative care,* ed 4, Philadelphia, 2002, WB Saunders.

Karch A: *Focus on nursing pharmacology,* Philadelphia, 2000, Lippincott.

Lehne R: *Pharmacology for nursing care,* ed 4, Philadelphia, 2001, WB Saunders.

Potter P, Perry A: *Fundamentals of nursing,* ed 5, St Louis, 2001, Mosby.

UNIT IX

The Adult Client with an Oncological Disorder

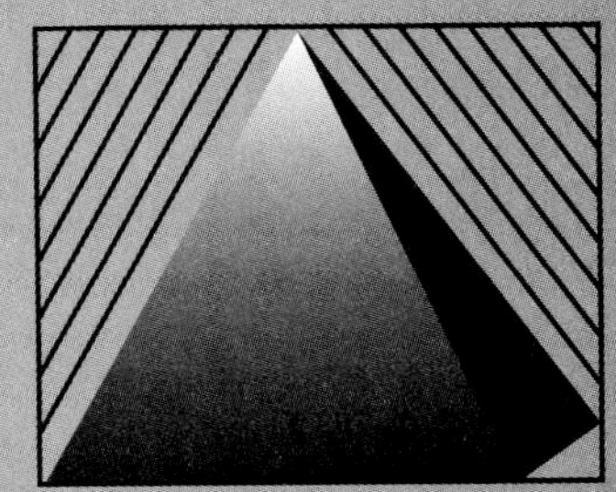

PYRAMID TERMS

Benign Usually refers to growths that are encapsulated, remain localized, and are slow growing.

Cancer A neoplastic disorder that can involve all body organs. Cells lose their normal growth-controlling mechanism, and the growth of cells is uncontrolled.

Carcinogen A physical, chemical, or biological stressor that causes neoplastic changes in normal cells.

Carcinoma In Situ A lesion with all the histological characteristics of malignancies except invasion.

Carcinomas Originate from epithelial cells, solid tumors, the skin, gastrointestinal (GI) tract, lungs, uterus, breast, and other organs.

Hospice A concept of care for terminally ill clients that includes intensive caring rather than intensive care. The family and client are the focus of nursing care, and the goal is to relieve pain and facilitate the optimal quality of life.

Lymphomas Originate from lymphoid tissue.

Leukemias or Myelomas Originate from blood-forming organs.

Malignant Refers to growths that are not encapsulated, metastasize, and grow; a cancerous lesion having the characteristics of disorderly, uncontrolled, and chaotic proliferation of cells.

Metastasis The transfer of disease from one organ or part to another not directly connected with it. Secondary malignant lesions, originating from the primary tumor, are located in anatomically distant places.

Nadir The period when an antineoplastic medication has its most profound effects on the bone marrow.

Neoplasia A new growth, which may be benign or malignant.

Sarcomas Originate from muscle, bone, fat, or the lymph system or from connective tissues.

Staging A method of classifying malignancies based on the presence and extent of the tumor within the body.

Tumor Markers Specific bodily substances that seem to indicate tumor progression or regression.

Undifferentiated Cells Cells that have lost the capacity for specialized functions.

PYRAMID TO SUCCESS

Pyramid points focus on treatment modalities related to an oncological disorder, such as pain management, internal and external radiation, chemotherapy, and on oncological disorders as skin cancer, leukemia, breast cancer, and lung cancer. Specific focus is on the nursing care related to these treatment modalities and disorders, and to client adaptation and the impact of the treatment or disorder. Specifically, focus on the complications related to chemotherapy and the nursing measures required in monitoring for these complications, and in preventing life-threatening conditions such as infection and bleeding. Specific laboratory values include the white blood cell count (WBC) and the platelet count. The Integrated Concepts and Processes addressed in this unit include Clinical Problem-Solving Process (Nursing Process), Caring, Communication and Documentation, Cultural Awareness, Self-Care, and Teaching/Learning.

CLIENT NEEDS

Safe, Effective Care Environment

Advance directives
Advocacy related to client's decisions
Asepsis
Client rights
Confidentiality regarding diagnosis
Establishing priorities
Handling hazardous and infectious materials related to radiation and chemotherapy
Informed consent for treatments and procedures
Oncology-related consultations and referrals
Standard (universal) and protective precautions

Health Promotion and Maintenance

Client lifestyle choices
Expected body image changes related to chemotherapy and treatments
Health promotion programs regarding risks for cancer
Health screening measures for cancer
Instructions regarding monthly self-breast or self-testicular examinations
Prevention of disease related to infection

Psychosocial Integrity

Ability to cope, adapt, and/or problem solve during illness or stressful events
Assisting in mobilizing appropriate support and resource systems
Assisting the client and family to cope with alteration in body image
End-of-life issues
Grief and loss related to death and the dying process
Promoting a positive environment to maintain optimal quality of life
Religious, spiritual, and cultural preferences

Physiological Integrity

Providing basic care and comfort
Promoting nutrition
Managing pain
Diagnostic tests and laboratory values such as WBC and platelet counts
Monitoring for the expected and unexpected responses to radiation and chemotherapy
Protecting the client from the life-threatening side effects of treatments

REFERENCES

Black J, Hawks J, Keene A: *Medical-surgical nursing: Clinical management for positive outcomes,* ed 6, Philadelphia, 2001, WB Saunders.
Chernecky C, Berger B: *Laboratory tests and diagnostic procedures,* ed 3, Philadelphia, 2001, WB Saunders.
Clark J, Queener S, Karb V: *Pharmacologic basis of nursing practice,* ed 6, St Louis, 2000, Mosby.
DeWit S: *Fundamental concepts and skills for nursing,* Philadelphia, 2001, WB Saunders.
Hill S, Howlett H: *Success in practical nursing: personal and vocational issues,* ed 4, Philadelphia, 2001, WB Saunders.
National Council of State Boards of Nursing: *Test plan for the National Council Licensure Examination for Practical/Vocational Nurses,* Chicago, 2001, Author.
Potter P, Perry A: *Fundamentals of nursing,* ed 5, St Louis, 2001, Mosby.
Perry A, Potter P: *Clinical nursing skills and techniques,* ed 5, St Louis, 2002, Mosby.
Wilson J: *Infection control in clinical practice,* ed 2, St Louis, 2002, Balliere Tindall.

Oncological Disorders

I. CANCER

A. Description
   1. A neoplastic disorder that can involve all body organs
   2. Cells lose their normal growth-controlling mechanism and the growth of cells is uncontrolled

B. **Metastasis:** can occur through the lymphatics, the bloodstream, seeding, or transfer and spread from one site to another

C. **Staging:** a method used to describe the tumor and includes the extent of the tumor, the extent to which malignancy has increased in size, the involvement of regional nodes, and metastatic development

D. Risk factors (Box 40-1)

E. Prevention
   1. Avoid obesity
   2. Decrease fat intake
   3. Increase total fiber in diet
   4. Decrease alcohol consumption
   5. Avoid salt-cured/nitrate-cured foods
   6. Avoid exposure to **carcinogens**
   7. Obtain adequate rest and exercise to decrease stress

BOX 40-1

Risk Factors

Chemical carcinogens
Radiation carcinogens such as sunlight or x-rays
Viral factors
Genetic factors
Demographic/geographic factors
Dietary factors such as obesity, use of alcohol, high-fat and low-fiber diets
Psychological factors such as stress

F. Early detection (Box 40-2)
   1. Mammography
   2. Papanicolaou (Pap) test
   3. Stools for occult blood
   4. Sigmoidoscopy
   5. Breast self-examination
   6. Testicular self-examination
   7. Skin inspection

II. BREAST SELF-EXAMINATION (BSE)

A. Performing BSE
   1. Perform 7 to 10 days after menses
   2. Postmenopausal or clients who have had a hysterectomy should select a specific day of the month and perform BSE monthly on that day

B. Procedure
   1. Before a mirror
      a. Inspect with arms at the side
      b. Raise arms overhead to inspect for changes in size or contour, dimpling, or changes in the nipple
      c. Inspect by resting the palms on the hips and pressing down firmly to flex chest muscles

BOX 40-2

Warning Signs of Cancer

Change in bowel or bladder habits
Any sore that does not heal
Unusual bleeding or discharge
Thickening or lump in breast or elsewhere
Indigestion
Obvious change of wart or mole
Nagging cough or hoarseness

2. Lying down
   a. Place a pillow under the right breast
   b. Use the pads of the middle three fingers of the left hand, press firmly, and feel for lumps or changes using a rubbing, circular pattern to cover all breast tissue
   c. Gently squeeze the nipple, looking for discharge
   d. Perform BSE on the left breast using the same method
3. In the shower
   a. With fingers flat, move gently over every part of each breast
   b. Check for lumps or thickening

III. TESTICULAR SELF-EXAMINATION (TSE)

A. Select a day of the month and perform the examination on the same day each month
B. Perform after a warm bath or shower
C. Hold the scrotum in one hand
D. Examine each testicle separately by gently rolling it between the thumb and fingers of the other hand
E. Check for hard lumps or knots

IV. DIAGNOSTIC TESTS

A. Tomography
   1. Description
      a. X-ray films showing details of structures otherwise hidden by overlying radiopaque bone
      b. Allows views of tissues at various planes as if slices have been made through the tissue
   2. Implementation: no special preparation is required
B. Computed tomography (CT scan)
   1. Description
      a. X-ray technique that produces cross-sectional body images at progressive depths
      b. Can differentiate normal tissues from abnormal masses and accurately identify their size and location
      c. An oral or IV contrast agent may be administered to increase the sensitivity of the CT scan
   2. Implementation
      a. Obtain informed consent if a dye is injected
      b. Assess the client for allergies to the dye
      c. Clients should be told that they will lie on a table and the x-ray machine will move around them
      d. Client should be told that the test is painless unless an IV contrast dye is used, which may cause a burning sensation on injection
      e. Inform the client that the dye may cause nausea, vomiting, flushing, itching, and a bitter taste in the mouth
      f. Client should be told that the x-ray machine can be very noisy
C. Ultrasound
   1. Description
      a. Uses high-frequency sound waves to visualize organs and masses
      b. A noninvasive method of identifying and following the growth of neoplasms without radiation exposure
   2. Implementation
      a. Test preparation may include cleansing the bowel with enemas if the abdominal area is to be tested, and having the client drink 6 to 8 glasses of water without voiding before the test
      b. Inform the client that he or she will not be allowed to void until after the test
      c. Inform the client that the test is painless and that only a slight pressure may be felt
      d. Inform the client that lubricant gel is applied to the area but is easily wiped off after the test
D. Magnetic resonance imaging (MRI) (Refer to Chapter 54 for information regarding this diagnostic test)
E. Radioisotope scans
   1. Description
      a. Radioisotopes are used to locate tumors and lesions within the brain, kidneys, liver, lungs, pericardium, and bones
      b. When the radioisotope enters the client's body, the fate of the radioisotope can be followed or traced by the scanning machine
      c. Abnormal tissue appears different on the scan because the isotope is metabolized differently by this tissue
      d. A scan of the organ will reveal a high uptake of the radioisotope at the site of a tumor, and the area in which the concentration of the radioisotope is unusually high is called a hot spot
      e. The area of less concentration of a radioactive isotope is called a cold spot
   2. Implementation
      a. The client receives a tracer dose of the appropriate radioisotope, either orally or by injection
      b. Before the scanning procedure can be performed, the radioisotope must be assimi-

lated by the organ under study; the length of time for organ assimilation of the radioisotope will vary
   c. During the procedure the client is asked to lie still and breathe normally while the scanner measures the radioactivity concentrated in the organ under study and records its findings
   d. Sedation before this procedure may be prescribed for the restless, agitated, or anxious client

F. Lymphangiogram
1. Description
   a. Examines the lymphatic system, the primary site of **metastasis** for tumors with good lymphatic drainage
   b. The test is performed by injecting dye into the interdigital webs of the feet
   c. The dye is picked up by the lymphatic system; the dye may take several hours to infuse into the lymphatics of the abdomen
   d. X-ray studies are then obtained
2. Implementation
   a. Obtain an informed consent
   b. Assess the client for allergies
   c. Note that the test cannot be performed for 48 hours after another contrast study
   d. Inform the client that the test is fairly long and uncomfortable
   e. Instruct the client to drink plenty of fluids after the test
   f. Inform the client that the dye may continue to discolor the urine for several days
   g. Inform the client that he or she must return the next day for follow-up x-ray studies

G. Biopsy
1. Description
   a. Surgical incision of a small piece of tissue for microscopic examination
   b. Used to either rule out or confirm a diagnosis of malignancy
   c. A total biopsy excises the entire tumor for examination
   d. An excisional biopsy excises only a part of the tumor
   e. After excision, a frozen section or a permanent paraffin section is done to examine the specimen
   f. The advantage of the frozen section is the speed with which the section can be prepared and the diagnosis made, because only minutes are required for this test
   g. Permanent paraffin section takes about 24 hours; however, it provides clearer details than does the frozen section
2. Implementation
   a. The procedure is usually performed in an outpatient surgical setting
   b. Prepare the client for the surgery following the physician's instructions
   c. Obtain an informed consent

H. Blood studies
1. Routine tests do not test for specific types of **cancer** but indicate the presence of any number of problems
2. Other blood tests, such as **tumor markers** and biochemical tests, identify the extent of a particular type of **cancer**
3. These specific tests are not used to make the diagnosis of **cancer** but only to check its progression

V. PAIN CONTROL

A. Causes of pain
1. Bone destruction
2. Obstruction of an organ
3. Compression of peripheral nerves
4. Infiltration/distention of tissue
5. Inflammation/necrosis
6. Psychological, such as fear or anxiety

B. Implementation
1. Collaborate with other members of the health care team to develop a pain management program
2. Administer oral preparations if possible and if they provide adequate relief of pain
3. Mild and moderate pain may be treated with salicylates, acetaminophen (Tylenol), and nonsteroidal antiinflammatory drugs (NSAIDs)
4. Severe pain is treated with narcotics, such as codeine sulfate, meperidine (Demerol), morphine sulfate, and hydromorphone hydrochloride (Dilaudid)
5. Continuous IV and subcutaneous infusions of narcotics provide superior pain control
6. Monitor for side effects and effectiveness of medications
7. Provide nonpharmacological techniques of pain control such as relaxation, guided imagery, biofeedback, and diversion
8. Do not undermedicate the **cancer** client who is in pain

VI. SURGERY

A. Description: used to diagnose, stage, and treat **cancer**

B. Curative surgery
1. For **cancer** that is localized to the organ of origin and regional lymph nodes

2. **Cancers** that recur locally can be excised, resulting in occasional cure or remission or both
3. Metastatic lesions that appear in the lungs, liver, or brain can be removed to attempt a surgical cure
4. Excision of a metastatic lesion is considered if no other evidence of disease exists and the metastatic lesion appeared after a relatively long disease-free period

C. Palliative surgery
1. Performed if the risk/benefit ratio is favorable and if it can benefit the client and improve quality of life
2. Reduces pain, relieves airway obstruction, relieves obstructions in the gastrointestinal (GI) and urinary tract
3. Performed to relieve pressure on the brain and spinal cord
4. Performed to prevent hemorrhage
5. Performed to remove infected and ulcerated tumors and drain abscesses

D. Reconstructive surgery: performed to improve the quality of life by restoring maximal function and appearance

E. Preventive surgery
1. Performed in clients with multiple high-risk factors
2. Performed in certain conditions that may increase the risk of **cancer**, such as polyps or ulcerative colitis

VII. CHEMOTHERAPY (REFER TO CHAPTER 41 FOR INFORMATION REGARDING CHEMOTHERAPY)

VIII. RADIATION THERAPY

A. Description
1. Destroys **cancer** cells with minimal exposure of normal cells to the damaging effects of radiation; the cells damaged either die or become unable to divide
2. Effective on tissues directly within the path of the radiation beam
3. Side effects include skin changes and irritation, alopecia, fatigue, and altered taste sensation; also, the effects vary according to the site of treatment
4. Teletherapy and brachytherapy are the types of radiation therapy most commonly used to treat **cancer**

B. Teletherapy (Box 40-3)
1. Also called beam radiation; the actual radiation source is external to client

BOX 40-3

Teletherapy: Client Education

Wash area with water or mild soap and water, using the hand rather than a washcloth; rinse the soap thoroughly, and pat dry with a soft towel or cloth
Do not remove the radiation markings from the skin
Use no powders, ointments, lotions, or creams on the area unless prescribed
Wear soft clothing over the area, avoiding belts, buckels, straps, or any clothing that binds or rubs the skin
Avoid sun and heat exposure
Monitor for moist desquamation (weeping of the skin)
If moist desquamation occurs, cleanse the area with warm water and pat dry, apply antibiotic ointment or corticosteroid cream as prescribed, and expose the site to air

2. The client does not emit radiation and does not pose a hazard to anyone else

C. Brachytherapy
1. The radiation source comes into direct, continuous contact with tumor tissues for a specific time
2. The radiation source is within the client; for a period of time, the client emits radiation and can pose a hazard to others
3. Includes either an unsealed source or a sealed source of radiation
4. Unsealed radiation source
   a. Administered via the oral or IV route or as an instillation into body cavities
   b. The source is not completely confined to one body area, and it enters body fluids and is eventually eliminated via various excreta, which are radioactive and harmful to others; most of the source is eliminated from the body within 48 hours; then neither the client nor the excreta are radioactive or harmful
5. Sealed radiation sources (Box 40-4 and Box 40-5)
   a. A sealed, temporary or permanent radiation source (solid implant) implanted within the tumor target tissues
   b. The client emits radiation while the implant is in place, but the excreta are not radioactive
6. Removal of sealed radiation sources
   a. The client is no longer radioactive
   b. Inform the client that sexual partners cannot "catch" **cancer**
   c. Inform the female client that she may resume sexual intercourse after 7 to 10 days, if the implant was cervical or vaginal
   d. Provide a Betadine douche if prescribed, if the implant was placed in the cervix

BOX 40-4

Care of the Client with a Sealed Radiation Source

Place the client in a private room with a private bath
Place a caution sign on the client's door
Organize nursing tasks to minimize exposure to the radiation source
Nursing assignments to a client with a radiation implant should be rotated
Limit time to one-half hour per care provider per shift
Wear a dosimeter film badge to measure radiation exposure
Wear a lead shield to reduce the transmission of radiation
A nurse should never care for more than one client with a radiation implant at one time
Do not allow a pregnant nurse to care for the client
Do not allow children under the age of 16 or a pregnant woman to visit the client
Limit visitors to one-half hour per day; visitors should be at least 6 feet from the source
Save bed linens and dressings until the source is removed; then dispose of in the usual manner
Other equipment can be removed from the room at any time

BOX 40-5

A Dislodged Radiation Source

Do not touch a dislodged radiation source with bare hands
If the radiation source dislodges, use long-handled forceps to place the source in the lead container kept in the client's room, and call the physician
If unable to locate the radiation source, bar visitors and notify the physician

e. Administer a Fleet enema if prescribed
f. Advise the client who had a cervical or vaginal implant to notify the physician if nausea, vomiting, diarrhea, frequent urination, vaginal or rectal bleeding, hematuria, foul-smelling vaginal discharge, abdominal pain or distention, or a fever occurs

IX. BONE MARROW TRANSPLANTATION

A. Description
1. Used in the treatment of **leukemia** for clients who have closely matched donors and who are experiencing temporary remission with chemotherapy
2. The goal of treatment is to rid the client of all leukemic or other **malignant** cells through treatment with high doses of chemotherapy and whole-body irradiation
3. Since these treatments are lethal to bone marrow, without the replacement of bone marrow function through transplantation, the client would die of infection or hemorrhage

B. Transplantation: bone marrow is administered through the client's central IV line in a manner similar to a blood transfusion

C. Posttransplantation period
1. The client remains without any natural immunity until the donor marrow begins to proliferate and engraftment (transfused bone marrow cells move to the marrow-forming sites of the recipient's bones) occurs
2. Infection and severe thrombocytopenia are major concerns until engraftment occurs
3. Major complications include failure to engraft and graft-versus-host disease (GVHD)

X. SKIN CANCER (REFER TO CHAPTER 38 FOR INFORMATION REGARDING SKIN CANCER)

XI. LEUKEMIA (Box 40-6)

A. Description
1. **Malignant** exacerbation in the number of leukocytes, usually at an immature stage, in the bone marrow
2. May be acute, with a sudden onset and short duration, or chronic, with a slow onset and persistent symptoms over a period of years
3. Affects the bone marrow, causing anemia, leukopenia, the production of immature cells, thrombocytopenia, and a decline in immunity
4. The cause is unknown and appears to involve gene damage of cells, leading to the transfor-

BOX 40-6

Classification of Leukemia

ACUTE LYMPHOCYTIC LEUKEMIA (ALL)
Mostly lymphoblasts present in bone marrow
Age of onset is less than 15 years

ACUTE MYELOGENOUS LEUKEMIA (AML)
Mostly myeloblasts present in bone marrow
Age of onset is between 15 and 39 years

CHRONIC MYELOGENOUS LEUKEMIA (CML)
Mostly granulocytes present in bone marrow
Age of onset after 50 years of age

CHRONIC LYMPHOCYTIC LEUKEMIA (CLL)
Mostly lymphocytes present in bone marrow
Age of onset is after 50 years of age

mation of cells from a normal state to a **malignant** state
5. Risk factors include genetic, viral, immunological, and environmental factors and exposure to radiation, chemicals, and medications

B. Data collection
1. Anorexia, fatigue, weakness, and weight loss
2. Signs of bleeding
3. Petechiae
4. Prolonged bleeding after minor abrasions or lacerations
5. Elevated temperature
6. Lymphadenopathy and splenomegaly
7. Normal, elevated, or reduced white blood cell (WBC) count
8. Decreased hemoglobin and hematocrit levels
9. Decreased platelet count
10. Positive bone marrow biopsy identifying leukemic blast phase cells

C. Infection
1. A major cause of death in the immunosuppressed client
2. Can occur through autocontamination or cross-contamination
3. Common sites of infection are the skin, respiratory tract, and GI tract
4. Initiate protective isolation procedures
5. Perform frequent and thorough handwashing
6. Ensure that anyone entering the client's room is wearing a mask
7. Use strict aseptic technique for all procedures
8. Keep supplies for the client separate from supplies for other clients
9. Limit the number of caregivers entering the client's room
10. Maintain the client in a private room
11. Place the client in a room with high-efficiency particulate air (HEPA) filtration or a laminar airflow system if possible
12. Reduce exposure to environmental organisms by eliminating raw fruits and vegetables and fresh flowers and by not leaving standing water in the client's room
13. Be sure that the client's room is cleaned daily
14. Assist the client with daily bathing, using an antimicrobial soap
15. Assist the client to perform oral hygiene frequently
16. Initiate a bowel program for constipation and to prevent rectal trauma
17. Avoid invasive procedures such as injections, rectal temperatures, and urinary catheterization
18. Monitor for signs and symptoms of infection
19. Change wound dressings daily, and inspect wounds for redness, swelling, or drainage
20. Monitor urine for color and cloudiness
21. Monitor skin and oral mucous membranes for signs of infection
22. Encourage the client to cough and deep breathe
23. Monitor temperature, pulse, and blood pressure
24. Monitor WBC and neutrophil count
25. The physician is notified if signs of infection are present; prepare to obtain specimens for culture of open lesions, urine, and sputum
26. Antibiotic, antifungal, and antiviral medication may be prescribed
27. Instruct the client to avoid crowds and those with infections
28. Instruct the client that neither they nor their household contacts should receive immunization with a live virus

D. Bleeding
1. During the period of greatest bone marrow suppression (the **nadir**), the platelet count may be extremely low, less than $10,000/mm^3$
2. The client is at risk for bleeding when the platelet count falls below $50,000/mm^3$, and spontaneous bleeding frequently occurs when the platelet count is lower than $20,000/mm^3$
3. Clients with platelet counts below $20,000/mm^3$ may need a platelet transfusion
4. For clients with severe blood loss, packed red blood cells (RBCs) may be prescribed
5. Monitor laboratory values
6. Monitor the client for signs and symptoms of bleeding
7. Handle the client gently
8. Measure abdominal girth; an increase in girth can indicate internal hemorrhage
9. Instruct the client to use a soft toothbrush and avoid dental floss
10. Instruct the client to use only an electric razor for shaving
11. Provide soft foods that are cool to warm
12. Avoid injections if possible to prevent trauma to the skin and bleeding
13. Apply firm and gentle pressure to a needlestick site for at least 10 minutes
14. Pad side rails and sharp corners of the bed and furniture
15. Discourage the client from engaging in activities involving sharp objects
16. Instruct the client to avoid constrictive or tight clothing
17. Use caution when taking blood pressures to prevent skin injury

18. Instruct the client to avoid blowing the nose
19. Avoid rectal suppositories, enemas, and thermometers
20. Examine all body fluids and excrement for the presence of blood
21. If the female client is menstruating, count the number of pads or tampons used
22. Instruct client to avoid NSAIDs and products that contain aspirin

E. Fatigue and nutrition
1. Assist the client in selecting a well-balanced diet
2. Provide small meals that require little chewing
3. Assist the client in self-care and mobility activities
4. Allow adequate rest periods during care
5. Do not perform activities unless they are essential

F. Chemotherapy (refer to Chapter 41 for information regarding chemotherapy and the client with leukemia)

XII. HODGKIN'S DISEASE

A. Description
1. A malignancy of the lymph nodes that originates in a single lymph node or a single chain of nodes
2. **Metastasis** occurs to other adjacent lymph structures and eventually invades nonlymphoid tissue
3. Usually involves lymph nodes, tonsils, spleen, and bone marrow and is characterized by the presence of Reed-Sternberg cells in the lymph nodes
4. Possible causes include viral infections and previous exposure to alkalating chemical agents
5. Prognosis is dependent on the stage of the disease

B. Data collection
1. Persistent fever
2. Night sweats
3. Loss of appetite and significant weight loss
4. Fatigue and weakness
5. Pruritus
6. Anemia and thrombocytopenia
7. Enlarged lymph nodes, spleen, and liver
8. Positive biopsy of lymph nodes with cervical nodes most often affected first
9. Presence of Reed-Sternberg cells
10. Positive CT scan of liver and spleen

C. Implementation
1. For the early stages without mediastinal node involvement, the treatment of choice is extensive external radiation of involved lymph node regions
2. With more extensive disease, radiation along with multiagent chemotherapy is used
3. Monitor for side effects related to chemotherapy or radiation
4. Discuss the possibility of sterility with the male client receiving radiation and inform the client of options related to sperm banks

XIII. MULTIPLE MYELOMA

A. Description
1. A **malignant** proliferation of plasma cells and tumors within the bone
2. Causes destruction to bone tissue, decreased production of immunoglobulin and antibodies, and increased levels of uric acid and calcium, which can lead to renal failure
3. The cause is unknown

B. Data collection
1. Bone (skeletal) pain, especially in the pelvis, spine, and ribs
2. Weakness and fatigue
3. Signs of respiratory infection
4. Anemia
5. Elevated temperature
6. Elevated calcium and uric acid levels
7. Decreased platelet count
8. Bone fractures
9. Spinal cord compression and paraplegia
10. Renal failure

C. Implementation
1. Encourage fluids up to 3 to 4 liters a day to maintain an adequate output 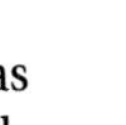
2. Monitor IV fluids and administer diuretics as prescribed to increase renal excretion of calcium
3. Encourage ambulation to prevent renal problems and to slow down bone resorption 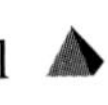 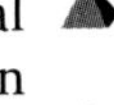
4. Provide skeletal support during moving, turning, and ambulating to prevent pathological fractures 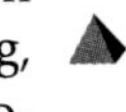
5. Provide a hazard-free environment 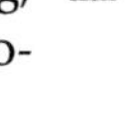 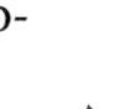
6. Monitor for signs of bleeding, infection, and skeletal fractures 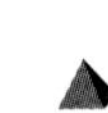
7. Administer analgesics as prescribed to control pain and antibiotics as prescribed for infection
8. Chemotherapy will be prescribed

XIV. TESTICULAR CANCER

A. Description
1. Arises from germinal epithelium from the sperm-producing germ cells or from

nongerminal epithelium from other structures in the testicles
2. Most often occurs between the ages of 20 and 40 years
3. **Metastasis** occurs to the lung, liver, bone, and adrenal glands

B. Prevention: routine testicular self-examination

C. Data collection
1. Painless testicular swelling
2. Dragging sensation in scrotum
3. Abdominal masses
4. Palpable lymphadenopathy
5. Gynecomastia
6. Infertility
7. Late signs include back or bone pain and respiratory symptoms

D. Implementation
1. Chemotherapy will be prescribed
2. Prepare the client for radiation therapy as prescribed
3. Prepare the client for unilateral orchiectomy if prescribed for diagnosis and primary surgical management
4. Prepare the client for radical retroperitoneal lymph node dissection if prescribed to stage the disease and reduce tumor volume so that chemotherapy and radiation therapy are more effective
5. Discuss reproduction, sexuality, and fertility information and options with the client
6. Identify with the client reproductive options such as sperm storage, donor insemination, and adoption

E. Postoperative implementation
1. Monitor vital signs
2. Monitor for signs of bleeding
3. Monitor for signs of wound infection
4. Monitor I&O
5. The physician is notified if chills, fever, increasing pain or tenderness at the incision site, or drainage of the incision occurs
6. Instruct the client that he may resume normal activities except for lifting objects heavier than 20 pounds or stair climbing
7. Instruct the client to perform monthly testicular self-examination on the remaining testis

XV. CERVICAL CANCER

A. Description
1. Preinvasive **cancer** is limited to the cervix
2. Invasive **cancer** is in the cervix and other pelvic structures
3. **Metastasis** is usually confined to the pelvis, but distant **metastasis** occurs through lymphatic spread
4. Premalignant changes are described on a continuum from dysplasia, which is the earliest premalignancy change, to **carcinoma in situ** (CIS), the most advanced premalignant change (Box 40-7)

B. Precipitating factors
1. Low socioeconomic groups
2. Early first marriage
3. Early and frequent intercourse
4. Multiple sex partners
5. High parity
6. Poor hygiene

C. Data collection
1. Painless postmenstrual and postcoital vaginal bleeding
2. Foul-smelling or serosanguineous vaginal discharge
3. Pelvic, lower back, leg, or groin pain
4. Anorexia and weight loss
5. Leakage of urine and feces from the vagina
6. Dysuria and hematuria
7. Cytological changes on Papanicolaou test

D. Implementation (Box 40-8)

E. Laser therapy
1. Used when all boundaries of the lesion are visible during colposcopic examination
2. Energy from the beam is absorbed by fluid in the tissues, causing them to vaporize
3. Minimal bleeding is associated with the procedure
4. Slight vaginal discharge is expected after the procedure, and healing occurs in 6 to 12 weeks

BOX 40-7

Preinvasive Cancers: Cervical Intraepithelial Neoplasia (CIN)

CIN I: mild dysplasia
CIN II: moderate dysplasia
CIN III: severe dysplasia to cancer in situ (CIS)

BOX 40-8

Treatment for Cervical Cancer

NONSURGICAL
External radiation
Internal radiation implants (intracavitary)
Chemotherapy
Laser therapy
Cryosurgery

SURGICAL
Conization
Hysterectomy
Pelvic exenteration

F. Cryosurgery
  1. Freezing of the tissues by a probe with subsequent necrosis
  2. No anesthesia is required, although cramping may occur during the procedure
  3. A heavy watery discharge will occur for several weeks after the procedure
  4. Instruct the client to avoid intercourse and the use of tampons while the discharge is present

G. Conization
  1. A cone-shaped area of cervix is removed
  2. Performed in women who desire further pregnancies
  3. Long-term follow-up care is needed as new lesions can develop
  4. The risks of the procedure include hemorrhage, uterine perforation, incompetent cervix, cervical stenosis, and preterm labor in future pregnancies

H. Hysterectomy
  1. Description
    a. For microinvasive **cancer** if childbearing is not desired
    b. A vaginal approach is most commonly performed
    c. A radical hysterectomy and bilateral lymph node dissection may be performed for **cancer** that has spread beyond the cervix but not to the pelvic wall
  2. Postoperative implementation
    a. Monitor vital signs
    b. Assist with coughing and deep-breathing exercises
    c. Assist with range of motion (ROM) exercises and provide early ambulation
    d. Apply antiembolism stockings as prescribed
    e. Monitor input and output (I&O) and hydration status
    f. Monitor bowel sounds
    g. Monitor vaginal bleeding; note that more than one saturated pad per hour may indicate excessive bleeding
    h. Assess incision site for signs of infection
    i. Monitor Foley catheter drainage
    j. Administer pain medication as prescribed
    k. Instruct the client to limit stair climbing for 1 month and to avoid tub baths and sitting for long periods
    l. Avoid strenuous activity or lifting anything weighing more than 20 pounds
    m. Instruct the client to avoid sexual intercourse for 3 to 6 weeks
    n. Instruct the client in the signs associated with complications

I. Pelvic exenteration (Box 40-9)

BOX 40-9

Types of Pelvic Exenteration

ANTERIOR
Removal of uterus, ovaries, fallopian tubes, vagina, bladder, urethra, and pelvic lymph nodes

POSTERIOR
Removal of uterus, ovaries, fallopian tubes, descending colon, rectum, and anal canal

TOTAL
Combination of anterior and posterior

  1. Description
    a. A radical surgical procedure performed for recurrent **cancer** if there is no evidence of tumor outside the pelvis and no lymph node involvement
    b. When the bladder is removed, an ileal conduit will be created and located on the right side of the abdomen to divert urine
    c. A colostomy may need to be created and will be located on the left side of the abdomen for the passage of feces
  2. Postoperative implementation
    a. Nursing care measures are similar to postoperative care after hysterectomy
    b. Monitor the incision site for vaginal bleeding and infection
    c. Administer perineal irrigations with half-strength normal saline (NS) and hydrogen peroxide as prescribed
    d. Provide sitz baths as prescribed
    e. Instruct the client that the perineal opening, if present, may drain for several months
    f. Instruct the client in the care of the ileal conduit and colostomy
    g. Provide sexual counseling, as vaginal intercourse is not possible after anterior and total pelvic exenteration

XVI. OVARIAN CANCER

A. Description
  1. Grows rapidly, spreads fast, and is often bilateral
  2. **Metastasis** occurs by direct spread to the organs in the pelvis, by distal spread through lymphatic drainage, or by peritoneal seeding
  3. Prognosis is usually poor because the tumor is usually detected late
  4. An exploratory laparotomy is performed to diagnose and stage the tumor

B. Data collection

1. Abdominal discomfort or swelling
2. GI disturbances
3. Dysfunctional vaginal bleeding
4. Abdominal mass

C. Implementation
1. External radiation is used if the tumor has invaded other organs
2. Postoperative chemotherapy is used for all stages of ovarian **cancer**
3. Intraperitoneal chemotherapy, which involves the instillation of chemotherapy into the abdominal cavity
4. Immunotherapy, which alters the immunological response of the ovary and promotes tumor resistance
5. Total abdominal hysterectomy and bilateral salpingo-oophorectomy

XVII. ENDOMETRIAL CANCER

A. Description
1. A slow-growing tumor associated with menopausal years
2. **Metastasis** occurs through the lymphatic system to the ovaries and pelvis via the blood to the lungs, liver, and bone or intraabdominally to the peritoneal cavity

B. Precipitating factors
1. History of uterine polyps
2. Nulliparity
3. Polycystic ovary disease
4. Estrogen stimulation
5. Late menopause
6. Family history

C. Data collection
1. Postmenopausal bleeding
2. Watery, serosanguineous discharge
3. Low back, pelvic, or abdominal pain
4. Enlarged uterus in advanced stages

D. Nonsurgical implementation
1. External radiation or internal radiation used alone or in combination with surgery, depending on the stage of **cancer**
2. Chemotherapy to treat advanced and recurrent disease
3. Progestational therapy with medroxyprogesterone (Depo-Provera) or megestrol acetate (Megace) for estrogen-dependent tumors
4. Tamoxifen (Nolvadex), an antiestrogen, may also be prescribed

E. Surgical implementation: total abdominal hysterectomy and bilateral salpingo-oophorectomy

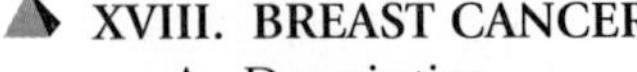

XVIII. BREAST CANCER

A. Description
1. Classified as invasive when it penetrates the tissue surrounding the mammary duct and grows in an irregular pattern
2. **Metastasis** occurs via lymph nodes
3. Common sites of metastatic disease are the bone, lungs, brain, and liver
4. Diagnosis is made by breast biopsy through a needle aspiration or by surgical removal of the tumor with microscopic examination made for **malignant** cells

B. Precipitating factors
1. Family history
2. Early menarche and late menopause
3. Previous **cancer** of breast, uterus, or ovaries
4. Nulliparity
5. Obesity
6. High-dose radiation exposure to the chest

C. Data collection
1. Mass usually felt in the upper outer quadrant or beneath the nipple
2. A fixed, irregular, nonencapsulated mass
3. A painless mass except in the very late stages
4. Nipple retraction or elevation
5. Asymmetry, with affected breast being higher
6. Bloody or clear nipple discharge
7. Skin dimpling, retraction, or ulceration
8. Skin edema or peau d'orange
9. Axillary lymphadenopathy
10. Lymphedema of affected arm
11. Symptoms of bone or lung **metastasis**
12. Presence of lesion on mammography

D. Prevention: monthly breast self-examination (BSE)

E. Nonsurgical implementation
1. Chemotherapy
2. Radiation therapy
3. Hormonal manipulation via the use of estrogen in postmenopausal women or tamoxifen (Nolvadex) for estrogen receptor-positive tumors

F. Surgical implementation
1. Surgical breast procedures (Box 40-10)
2. Oophorectomy for estrogen receptive-positive tumors
3. Ablative therapy with adrenalectomy or chemical ablation therapy

G. Postoperative implementation
1. Monitor vital signs
2. Position semi-Fowler's on the back or unaffected side with the affected arm above the level of the heart to promote drainage and prevent lymphedema
3. Turn the client only to the back and unaffected side
4. Encourage coughing and deep breathing

BOX 40-10

Surgical Breast Procedures

LUMPECTOMY
Excision and removal of the tumor
Lymph node dissection may also be performed

SIMPLE MASTECTOMY
Breast tissue and the nipple are removed
Lymph nodes are left intact

PARTIAL MASTECTOMY
The tumor is removed along with a small amount of surrounding tissue

MODIFIED RADICAL MASTECTOMY
Breast tissue, nipple, and lymph nodes are removed
Muscles are left intact

HALSTED RADICAL MASTECTOMY
Breast tissue, nipple, underlying muscles, and lymph nodes are removed

BOX 40-11

Client Instructions after Mastectomy

Avoid overuse of the arm during the first few months
To prevent lymphedema, keep the affected arm elevated
Provide incision care with lanolin to soften and prevent wound contracture
Encourage use of Reach for Recovery volunteers
Encourage the client to perform BSE on the remaining breast
Protect the affected hand and arm
Avoid strong sunlight to the affected arm
Do not let the affected arm hang dependent
Do not carry a pocketbook or anything heavy over the affected arm
Avoid trauma, cuts, bruises, or burns to the affected side
Avoid wearing constricted clothing or jewelry on the affected side
Wear gloves when gardening
Use thick oven mitts when cooking
Use a thimble when sewing
Apply lanolin hand cream several times daily
Use cream cuticle remover
Call the physician if signs of inflammation occur in the affected arm
Wear a Medic-Alert bracelet stating lymphedema arm

5. If a Hemovac or a Jackson-Pratt drain is in place, maintain suction and record the amount of drainage and drainage characteristics
6. Monitor operative sites for swelling or the presence of fluid collection under the skin flaps
7. Monitor for signs of infection
8. Place a sign above the bed stating "No IVs, No IMs, No BPs, venipunctures"
9. Provide the use of a pressure sleeve as prescribed if edema is severe
10. Administer diuretics as prescribed for severe lymphedema
11. Provide a low-salt diet as prescribed for severe lymphedema
12. Monitor the site for restriction of dressing, impaired sensation, color changes of skin
13. Assist with exercises as prescribed to decrease lymphedema and muscle weakness
14. See Box 40-11 for client instructions following mastectomy

XIX. GASTRIC CANCER

A. Description
   1. An abnormal **malignant** growth in the stomach
   2. Risk factors include a diet high in complex carbohydrates, grains, and salt, and low in fresh, green leafy vegetables and fresh fruit; smoking; alcohol; foods containing nitrates; and a history of gastric ulcers
   3. Complications include hemorrhage, obstruction, and **metastasis**
   4. The goal of treatment is to remove the tumor and provide a nutritional program

B. Data collection
   1. Fatigue
   2. Anorexia and weight loss
   3. Nausea and vomiting
   4. Indigestion and epigastric discomfort
   5. A sensation of pressure in the stomach
   6. Dysphagia
   7. Palpable mass

C. Implementation
   1. Monitor vital signs
   2. Monitor hemoglobin and hematocrit levels
   3. Monitor weight
   4. Monitor nutritional status
   5. Encourage small, bland, easily digestible meals with vitamin and mineral supplements
   6. Administer pain medication as prescribed
   7. Prepare the client for chemotherapy or radiation therapy as prescribed
   8. Prepare the client for surgical resection of the tumor as prescribed (Box 40-12)

D. Postoperative implementation (Refer to Chapter 44 for information regarding postoperative care)

BOX 40-12

Surgical Implementation for Gastric Cancer

SUBTOTAL GASTRECTOMY

Billroth I

Also called gastroduodenostomy

Partial gastrectomy, and remaining segment is anastomosed to the duodenum

Billroth II

Also called gastrojejunostomy

Partial gastrectomy, with remaining segment anastomosed to the jejunum

TOTAL GASTRECTOMY

Also called esophagojejunostomy

Removal of the stomach with attachment of the esophagus to the jejunum or duodenum

XX. INTESTINAL TUMORS

A. Description
   1. **Malignant** lesions that develop in the cells lining the bowel wall or as polyps in the colon or rectum
   2. Complications include bowel perforation with peritonitis, abscess and/or fistula formation, frank hemorrhage, and complete intestinal obstruction
   3. Metastasis occurs via the circulatory or lymphatic system, or by direct extension to other areas in the colon or other organs

B. Data collection
   1. Blood in stools
   2. Anorexia, vomiting, and weight loss
   3. Malaise and anemia
   4. Abnormal stools
      a. Ascending colon tumor: diarrhea
      b. Descending colon tumor: constipation or some diarrhea, or flat, ribbonlike stool due to a partial obstruction
      c. Rectal tumor: alternating constipation and diarrhea
   5. Guarding or abdominal distention
   6. Abdominal mass (a late sign)
   7. Cachexia (a late sign)

C. Implementation
   1. Monitor for signs of complications, which include bowel perforation with peritonitis, abscess and/or fistula formation, frank hemorrhage, and complete intestinal obstruction
   2. Monitor for signs of intestinal perforation including low blood pressure, rapid and weak pulse, distended abdomen, and elevated temperature
   3. Monitor for signs of intestinal obstruction, which may include vomiting (may be fecal contents), pain, constipation, and abdominal distention
   4. Note that an early sign of intestinal obstruction includes increased peristaltic activity, which produces an increase in bowel sounds; as the obstruction progresses, hypoactive sounds are heard
   5. Prepare for radiation before surgery to facilitate surgical resection and after surgery to decrease the risk of recurrence or to reduce pain, hemorrhage, bowel obstruction, or **metastasis**
   6. Postoperative chemotherapy is used to assist in the control of symptoms and spread of the disease

D. Surgical implementation: bowel resection and creation of colostomy of ileostomy (Refer to Chapter 44 for information regarding the preoperative and postoperative care related to surgery)

XXI. LUNG CANCER

A. Description
   1. **Malignant** tumor of the lung that may be primary or metastatic
   2. The lungs are a common target for **metastasis** from other organs
   3. Bronchiogenic carcinoma spreads through direct extension and lymphatic dissemination
   4. The four major types of lung **cancer** include small cell (oat cell), epidermal (squamous cell), adenocarcinoma, and large cell anaplastic carcinoma
   5. Diagnosis is made by a chest x-ray study, which will show a lesion or mass, and bronchoscopy and sputum studies, which will demonstrate a positive cytology for **cancer** cells

B. Causes
   1. Cigarette smoking
   2. Exposure to environmental pollutants
   3. Exposure to occupational pollutants

C. Data collection
   1. Cough and hemoptysis
   2. Dyspnea
   3. Hoarseness
   4. Chest pain
   5. Anorexia and weight loss
   6. Weakness

D. Implementation
   1. Monitor vital signs
   2. Monitor breathing patterns and for signs of respiratory impairment
   3. Administer analgesics as prescribed for pain management

4. Position the client upright for ease in breathing
5. Administer oxygen as prescribed and humidification to moisten and loosen secretions
6. Monitor pulse oximetry
7. Provide respiratory treatments as prescribed
8. Administer bronchodilators and corticosteroids as prescribed to decrease bronchospasm, inflammation, and edema
9. Provide a high-protein, high-calorie diet
10. Provide activity as tolerated, rest periods, and active and passive ROM exercises
11. Monitor for bleeding, infection, and electrolyte imbalance

E. Nonsurgical implementation
1. Radiation therapy for localized intrathoracic lung **cancers**
2. Chemotherapy to promote tumor regression
3. Immunotherapy directed at enhancing an effective response, which favorably affects the course of disease
4. Nonspecific immune therapy with bacille Calmette-Guérin (BCG) vaccine as prescribed

F. Surgical implementation
1. Laser therapy: to relieve endobronchial obstruction
2. Thoracotomy with pneumonectomy: surgical removal of a lung for bronchiogenic carcinoma
3. Thoracotomy with lobectomy: surgical removal of one lobe of the lung for tumors confined to a single lobe
4. Thoracotomy with segmental resection: surgical removal of lobe segment for clients unable to tolerate lobectomy or pneumonectomy

G. Preoperative and postoperative implementation (Refer to Chapter 46 for care to the client undergoing thoracic surgery)

XXII. LARYNGEAL CANCER

A. Description
1. A **malignant** tumor of the larynx
2. Laryngeal **cancer** presents as **malignant** ulcerations with underlying filtration
3. **Metastasis** to the lung is common
4. Diagnosis is made by laryngoscopy and biopsy showing a positive cytology for **cancer** cells

B. Causes
1. Cigarette smoking
2. Alcohol abuse
3. Exposure to environmental pollutants
4. Exposure to radiation
5. Voice strain

C. Data collection
1. Persistent hoarseness
2. Persistent sore throat
3. Painless neck mass
4. A feeling of a lump in the throat
5. Burning sensation in the throat
6. Dysphagia
7. Change in voice quality
8. Dyspnea
9. Hemoptysis
10. Weakness and weight loss
11. Foul breath

D. Implementation
1. Place client in Fowler's position to promote optimal air exchange
2. Monitor respiratory status
3. Monitor for signs of aspiration of food and fluid
4. Provide activity as tolerated
5. Provide a high-calorie, high-vitamin, high-protein diet
6. Provide nutritional support as prescribed
7. Administer oxygen as prescribed
8. Provide respiratory treatments as prescribed
9. Administer analgesic as prescribed

E. Nonsurgical implementation
1. Radiation therapy if the **cancer** is limited to a small area in one vocal cord
2. Chemotherapy, which may be done in combination with radiation and surgery

F. Surgical implementation
1. Small tumor excision or total laryngectomy: performed for infiltrate tumors that involve vocal cord paralysis and for tumors that do not respond to radiation therapy
2. Radical neck dissection: performed when lymph node involvement is present and involves a laryngectomy and tracheostomy

G. Preoperative and postoperative implementation (Refer to Chapter 46 for care to the client undergoing surgery)

XXIII. CANCER OF THE PROSTATE

A. Description
1. A slow-growing **cancer** of the prostrate gland, which is usually an androgen-dependent type adenocarcinoma
2. The risk increases in the male with each decade after age 50
3. **Metastasis** occurs via direct invasion of surrounding tissues, spread through the bloodstream and lymphatics, and via **metastasis** to the bony pelvis and spine
4. Bone **metastasis** is a concern

B. Data collection
   1. Asymptomatic in early stages
   2. Hard, pea-sized nodule palpated on rectal examination
   3. Hematuria
   4. Late symptoms include weight loss, urinary obstruction, and pain radiating from the lumbosacral area down the leg
   5. Prostate-specific antigen (PSA) test does not necessarily indicate malignancy and is used routinely to monitor the client's response to therapy
   6. Elevated serum acid phosphatase level indicates spread

C. Nonsurgical implementation
   1. Prepare the client for hormone manipulation therapy as prescribed
   2. Administer hormones as prescribed to slow the rate of growth of the tumor
   3. Prepare the client for radiation (internal or external), which may be prescribed alone or in conjunction with surgery and may be prescribed before or after surgery to reduce the lesion and limit **metastasis**
   4. Prepare the client for the administration of chemotherapy in hormone-resistant tumors

D. Surgical implementation
   1. Prepare the client for orchiectomy if prescribed, which will limit the production of testosterone
   2. Prepare the client for transurethral resection of the prostate (TURP) or prostatectomy if prescribed (Refer to Chapter 50 for information regarding preoperative and postoperative care following TURP and prostatectomy)

XXIV. BLADDER CANCER

A. Description
   1. Papillomatous growths in the bladder urothelium that undergo **malignant** changes and may infiltrate the bladder wall
   2. Predisposing factors include cigarette smoking, exposure to industrial chemicals, and exposure to radiation
   3. Common sites of **metastasis** include the liver, bones, and lungs
   4. As the tumor progresses, it can extend into the rectum, vagina, other pelvic soft tissues, and retroperitoneal structures

B. Data collection
   1. Gross painless hematuria
   2. Frequency, urgency, dysuria
   3. Clot-induced obstruction
   4. Bladder biopsy confirms diagnosis

C. Radiation
   1. Most bladder **cancers** are poorly radiosensitive and require high doses of radiation
   2. Radiation therapy is more acceptable for advanced disease that cannot be eradicated by surgery
   3. Palliative radiation may be used to relieve pain, bowel obstruction, and control potential hemorrhage and leg edema secondary to venous or lymphatic obstruction
   4. Intracavitary radiation may be prescribed, which protects adjacent tissue
   5. External radiation combined with chemotherapy or surgery may be prescribed because the external radiation alone may be ineffective
   6. Complications of radiation
      a. Abacterial cystitis
      b. Proctitis
      c. Fistula formation
      d. Ileitis or colitis
      e. Bladder ulceration and hemorrhage

D. Chemotherapy
   1. Intravesical instillation
      a. An alkalating chemotherapeutic agent is instilled in the bladder
      b. Treat the urine as a biohazard and dispose of properly
      c. For 6 hours after intravesical chemotherapy, disinfect the toilet with household bleach after voiding
   2. Systemic chemotherapy: used to treat inoperable or late tumors
   3. Complications of chemotherapy
      a. Bladder irritation
      b. Hemorrhagic cystitis

E. Surgical implementation
   1. Transurethral resection of bladder tumor: Performed for very early tumors for cure or for inoperable tumors for palliation
   2. Partial cystectomy
      a. The removal of up to half of the bladder
      b. Done in early tumors and for clients who cannot tolerate a radical cystectomy
      c. During the initial postoperative period, bladder capacity is markedly reduced to about 60 mL; however, as the bladder tissue expands, the capacity increases to 200 to 400 mL
      d. Maintenance of a continuous output of urine after surgery is critical to prevent bladder distention and stress on the suture line
      e. A urethral and suprapubic catheter may be in place, and the suprapubic catheter may be left in place for 2 weeks until healing occurs
   3. Cystectomy and urinary diversion

a. Removal of the bladder and urethra in women and the bladder, urethra, and usually prostate and seminal vesicles in men
b. When the bladder and the urethra are removed, permanent urinary diversion is required
c. The surgery may be performed in two stages if the tumor is extensive, with the creation of the urinary diversion first and the cystectomy several weeks later
d. If a radical cystectomy is performed, lower extremity lymphedema may occur as a result of lymph node dissection, and impotence may occur in the male client

4. Ileal conduit
   a. Also called ureteroileostomy or Bricker procedure
   b. Ureters are implanted into a segment of the ileum with the formation of an abdominal stoma
   c. The urine flows into the conduit and is continually propelled out through the stoma by peristalsis
   d. The client is required to wear an appliance over the stoma to collect the urine
   e. Complications include obstruction, pyelonephritis, leakage at the anastomosis site, stenosis, hydronephrosis, calculi, skin irritation and ulceration, and stomal defects
5. Kock pouch or Indiana pouch
   a. Kock pouch: a continent internal ileal reservoir created from a segment of the ileum and ascending colon; the ureters are implanted into the side of the reservoir, and a special nipple valve is constructed to attach the reservoir to the skin
   b. Indiana pouch: a continent reservoir is created from the ascending colon and terminal ileum, making a pouch larger than the Kock pouch
   c. Postoperatively, the client will have a 24 to 26 Foley catheter in place to drain urine continuously until the pouch has healed
   d. The catheter is irrigated gently with normal saline to prevent obstruction from mucus or clots as prescribed
   e. After removal of the catheter, the client is instructed how to self-catheterize and drain the reservoir at 4- to 6-hour intervals
6. Creation of a neobladder
   a. Similar to the creation of an internal reservoir except that instead of emptying through an abdominal stoma, it empties through a pelvic outlet into the urethra
   b. The client empties the neobladder by relaxing the external sphincter and creating abdominal pressure or by intermittent self-catheterization
7. Percutaneous nephrostomy or pyelostomy
   a. Used when the **cancer** is inoperable, to prevent obstruction
   b. Involves a percutaneous or surgical insertion of a nephrostomy tube into the kidney for drainage
   c. Nursing implementation involves stabilizing the tube to prevent dislodgement and monitoring output
8. Ureterostomy
   a. May be performed as a palliative procedure if the ureters are obstructed by the tumor
   b. The ureters are attached to the surface of the abdomen, where the urine flows directly into a drainage appliance without a conduit
   c. Potential problems include infection, skin irritation, and obstruction to urinary flow as a result of strictures at the opening
9. Vesicostomy
   a. The bladder is sutured to the abdomen, and a stoma is created in the bladder wall
   b. The bladder empties through the stoma

F. Preoperative implementation
1. Administer bowel preparation as prescribed, which may include clear liquid diet, laxatives and enemas, and antibiotics to lower the bacterial count in the bowel ▲
2. Assist the surgeon and enterostomal nurse in selecting an appropriate skin site for creation of the abdominal stoma
3. Encourage the client to talk about his or her feelings related to the stoma creation

G. Postoperative implementation
1. Monitor vital signs
2. Monitor incision site
3. Assess stoma (should be red and moist) every hour for the first 24 hours (Box 40-13) ▲
4. Note edema in the stoma, which may be present in the immediate postoperative period ▲
5. If the stoma appears dark and dusky, the physician is notified immediately because this indicates necrosis ▲
6. Monitor for prolapse or retraction of the stoma
7. Monitor for return of bowel function
8. Monitor for peristalsis, which will return in 3 to 4 days
9. Maintain NPO status as prescribed until bowel sounds return
10. Monitor urine flow, which is continuous (30 to 60 mL per hour) after surgery ▲

BOX 40-13

Urinary Stoma Care

Instruct the client to change the appliance in the morning when urinary production is slowest
Collect equipment, remove collection bag, use water or commercial solvent to loosen adhesive
Hold a rolled gauze pad against the stoma to collect and absorb urine during the procedure
Cleanse the skin around stoma and under the drainage bag with mild, nonresidue soap and water
Inspect the skin for excoriation and instruct the client to prevent urine from coming in contact with the skin
After the skin is dry, apply skin adhesive around the appliance
Instruct the client to cut the stoma opening of the skin barrier just large enough to fit over the stoma (no more that 3 mm larger than the stoma)
Instruct the client that the stoma will begin to shrink requiring a smaller stoma opening on the skin barrier
Apply skin barrier before attaching the pouch or faceplate
Place the appliance over the stoma and secure in place
Encourage self-care; teach the client to use a mirror
Instruct the client that the pouch may be drained by a bedside bag or leg bag, especially at night
Instruct the client to empty the urinary collection bag when it is one-third to one-half full to prevent pulling of the appliance and leakage
Instruct the client to check the appliance seal if perspiring occurs
Instruct the client to leave the urinary pouch in place as long as it is not leaking, and change every 5 to 7 days
During appliance changes, leave the skin open to air as long as possible
Use a nonkaraya gum product because urine erodes karaya gum
To control odor, instruct the client to drink adequate fluids, to wash appliance thoroughly with soap and lukewarm water, to soak collection pouch in dilute white vinegar for 20 to 30 minutes, or to place a special deodorant tablet into the pouch while it is being worn
Instruct the client who takes baths to keep the level of the water below the stoma and avoid oily soaps
If the client plans to shower, instruct the client to direct the flow of water away from the stoma

BOX 40-14

Self-Irrigation and Catheterization of Stoma

IRRIGATION

Instruct the client to wash hands and use clean technique
Instruct the client to use a catheter and syringe and to instill 60 mL of normal saline or water into the reservoir and to gently aspirate or allow to drain
Instruct the client to irrigate until the drainage remains free of mucus but to be cautious not to overirrigate

CATHETERIZATION

Instruct the client to wash hands and use a clean technique
Initially, the client is taught to insert a catheter every 2 to 3 hours to drain the reservoir; during each week thereafter, the interval is increased by 1 hour until the catheterization is done every 4 to 6 hours
Lubricate the catheter well with water-soluble lubricant and instruct the client never to force the catheter into the reservoir
If resistance is met, instruct the client to pause, rotate the catheter, and apply gentle pressure to insert
Instruct the client to notify the physician if unable to insert catheter
When urine has stopped, instruct the client to take several deep breaths and move the catheter in and out 2 to 3 inches to ensure that the pouch is empty
Instruct the client to withdraw the catheter slowly and to pinch the catheter when withdrawn so that it does not leak urine
Instruct the client to carry catheterization supplies with him/her

11. The physician is notified if the urine output is less than 30 mL per hour or if there is no urine output for more than 15 minutes ▲
12. Ureteral stents or catheters may be in place for 2 to 3 weeks or until healing occurs
13. Maintain stability with catheters to prevent dislodgement ▲
14. Monitor for hematuria ▲
15. Monitor for signs of peritonitis ▲
16. Monitor for bladder distention after a partial cystectomy
17. Monitor for shock, hemorrhage, thrombophlebitis, and lower extremity lymphedema after a radical cystectomy
18. Monitor the urinary drainage pouch for leaks and check skin integrity
19. Monitor pH of the urine (do not place the dipstick in the stoma) because strongly alkali urine can cause skin irritation and facilitate crystal formation
20. Instruct the client regarding the potential for urinary tract infection (UTI) or the development of calculi
21. Instruct the client to assess skin for irritation, to monitor urinary drainage pouch for any leakage, and self-catheterization procedure (Box 40-14) ▲
22. Encourage the client to express feelings about changes in body image, embarrassment, and sexual dysfunction

PRACTICE QUESTIONS

1. A nurse is instructing a client to perform a testicular self examination (TSE). Which instruction would the nurse provide to the client?
   1. Examine the testicles while lying down
   2. The best time for the examination is after a shower
   3. Gently feel the testicle with one finger to feel for a growth
   4. Testicular examinations should be done at least every 6 months
2. A nurse is assisting in conducting a health promotion program at a local school. Which of the following will not be identified as a risk factor associated with cancer?
   1. Viral factors
   2. Stress
   3. Low-fat and high-fiber diets
   4. Exposure to radiation
3. A client with cancer is receiving chemotherapy and develops thrombocytopenia. Which goal should be given the highest priority in the nursing plan of care?
   1. Ambulate the client three times a day
   2. Monitor the client's temperature
   3. Monitor the client for bleeding
   4. Monitor the client for pathological fractures
4. A nurse inspects the oral cavity of a client with cancer and notes white patches on the mucous membranes. The nurse determines that this occurrence:
   1. Is common
   2. Is characteristic of a thrush infection
   3. Is indicative that oral hygiene needs to be improved
   4. Suggests that the client is anemic
5. A nurse is monitoring the laboratory results of a client preparing to receive chemotherapy. The nurse determines that the white blood cell count (WBC) is normal if which of the following results were present?
   1. 3000 to $6000/mm^3$
   2. 4000 to $9000/mm^3$
   3. 7000 to $15,000/mm^3$
   4. 2000 to $5000/mm^3$
6. A nurse is instructing a group of female clients about breast self-examination (BSE). The nurse would instruct the clients to perform the examination:
   1. At the onset on menstruation
   2. 1 week after menstruation begins
   3. Every month during ovulation
   4. Weekly at the same time of day
7. A nurse instructs the client in breast self-examination (BSE). The nurse instructs the client to lie down and to examine the left breast. The nurse instructs the client that while examining the left breast, to place a pillow:
   1. Under the right shoulder
   2. Under the left shoulder
   3. Under the small of the back
   4. Under the right scapula
8. A nurse is teaching breast self-examination (BSE) to a client who had a hysterectomy. The nurse tells the client to perform the BSE:
   1. 7 to 10 days after menses
   2. Just before the menses begins
   3. At ovulation time
   4. At a specific day of the month and on that same day every month thereafter
9. A client suspected of having an abdominal tumor is scheduled for a computed tomography (CT) scan with dye injection. The nurse tells the client which of the following about the test?
   1. The test may be painful
   2. The dye injected may cause a warm, flushing sensation
   3. Fluids will be restricted after the test
   4. The test takes approximately 2 hours
10. A 32-year-old female client has a history of fibrocystic disorder of the breasts. The nurse gathering data from the client asks whether the breast lumps are more noticeable:
    1. In the spring months
    2. In the autumn
    3. After menses
    4. Before menses
11. A client has undergone mastectomy. The nurse interprets that the client is making the best adjustment to the loss of the breast if which of the following behaviors is observed?
    1. Participating in the care of the surgical drain
    2. Reading postoperative care booklet
    3. Refusing to look at wound
    4. Asking for pain medication when needed
12. A client is preparing for discharge 10 days after radical vulvectomy. The nurse plans to tell the client that which of the following activities is acceptable after discharge because it will not precipitate complications?
    1. Sexual activity
    2. Walking
    3. Sitting for lengthy periods
    4. Driving a car
13. A client has undergone vaginal hysterectomy. The nurse avoids which of the following in the care of this client?
    1. Removal of antiembolism stockings twice daily
    2. Assisting with range of motion leg exercises
    3. Elevating the knee gatch on the bed
    4. Checking placement of pneumatic compression boots
14. A client suspected of an ovarian tumor is scheduled for a pelvic ultrasound. The nurse plans to tell the

client that preparation for the ultrasound includes which of the following?
1. NPO before the procedure
2. A light breakfast only
3. Drinking six to eight glasses of water without voiding before the test
4. Wearing comfortable clothing and shoes for the procedure

15. A client is diagnosed as having a bowel tumor. Several diagnostic tests are prescribed. The nurse understands that which of the following tests will confirm the diagnosis of malignancy?
1. Magnetic resonance imaging (MRI)
2. Computed tomography (CT) scan
3. Abdominal ultrasound
4. Biopsy of the tumor

16. A client is diagnosed with multiple myeloma and the client asks the nurse about the diagnosis. The nurse bases the response on which of the following characteristics of the disorder?
1. Malignant exacerbation in the number of leukocytes
2. Altered red blood cell production
3. Altered production of lymph nodes
4. Malignant proliferation of plasma cells and tumors within the bone

17. A nurse is reviewing the laboratory results of a client diagnosed with multiple myeloma. Which of the following would the nurse expect to specifically note with this diagnosis?
1. Decreased number of plasma cells in the bone marrow
2. Increased white blood cells
3. Increased calcium level
4. Decreased blood urea nitrogen (BUN)

18. A nurse is assisting in developing a plan of care for the client with multiple myeloma. A priority nursing intervention would include which of the following?
1. Coughing and deep breathing
2. Encouraging fluids
3. Monitoring the red blood cell count
4. Providing frequent oral care

19. A nurse is assigned to care for a client with Hodgkin's disease. The nurse plans care knowing that which of the following is not a characteristic of this disease?
1. Presence of Reed-Sternberg cells
2. Involvement of lymph nodes, spleen, and liver
3. Occurs most often in older adults
4. Prognosis depends on the stage of the disease

20. A nurse is assisting in conducting a health promotion program regarding testicular cancer to community members. The nurse tells the members that which of the following is not a sign of testicular cancer?
1. Painless testicular swelling
2. Heavy sensation in the scrotum
3. Alopecia
4. Back pain

21. A nurse is reviewing the laboratory results of a client with leukemia who received a regimen of chemotherapy. Which laboratory value would the nurse specifically note as a result of the massive cell destruction that occurs with the chemotherapy?
1. Anemia
2. Decreased platelets
3. Decreased leukocyte count
4. Increased uric acid level

22. A nurse is preparing a client with a bowel tumor for surgery. The physician has informed the client that the surgery is palliative in the treatment of the tumor. The nurse understands that this type of surgery is performed to:
1. Restore maximal function and appearance
2. Eliminate high-risk factors
3. Reduce pain
4. Cure the client

23. A client is receiving external radiation to the neck for cancer of the larynx. The nurse plans care knowing that the most likely side effect to be expected is:
1. Constipation
2. Dyspnea
3. Sore throat
4. Diarrhea

24. A nurse inspects the skin of a client receiving external radiation therapy and documents a finding noted as moist desquamation. The nurse understands that the most appropriate description of moist desquamation is which of the following?
1. Reddened skin
2. A rash
3. Weeping of the skin
4. Dermatitis

25. A nurse is providing instructions to a client receiving external radiation therapy. Which of the following would not be a component of the instructions?
1. Avoid exposure to sunlight
2. Wash the skin with a mild soap and pat dry
3. Apply pressure on the radiated area to prevent bleeding
4. Eat a high-protein diet

26. A nurse is caring for a client with an internal radiation implant. When caring for the client, the nurse should observe which of the following principles?
1. Limit the time with the client to 1 hour per shift
2. Do not allow pregnant women into the client's room
3. Individuals under 16 years old may be allowed to go in the room as long as they are 6 feet away from the client
4. Remove dosimeter badge when entering the client's room

27. A client was hospitalized for a cervical radiation implant for the treatment of cervical cancer. The implant is removed, the client is to be discharged, and the nurse reinforces discharge instructions. Which statement by the client indicates the need for further discharge instructions?
    1. "Cream may be used to relieve dryness or itching."
    2. "Foul-smelling vaginal discharge is a sign of an infection."
    3. "Sexual intercourse may be resumed after 7 to 10 days."
    4. "Some vaginal bleeding is expected for 1 to 3 months."
28. A cervical radiation implant is placed in the client for treatment of cervical cancer. What activity order would the nurse most likely expect to note in the physician's orders?
    1. Out of bed in a chair only
    2. Ambulate to the bathroom only
    3. Bed rest
    4. Out of bed ad lib
29. A nurse teaches skin care to the client receiving external radiation therapy. Which of the following statements, if made by the client, would indicate the need for further instruction?
    1. "I will handle the area gently."
    2. "I will avoid the use of deodorants."
    3. "I will limit sun exposure to one hour daily."
    4. "I will wear loose fitting clothing."
30. A client is hospitalized for insertion of a internal cervical radiation implant. While giving care, the nurse finds the radiation implant in the bed. The initial action by the nurse is to:
    1. Call the physician
    2. Pick up the implant with gloved hands and flush down the toilet
    3. Reinsert the implant into the vagina immediately
    4. Pick up the implant with long-handled forceps and place in a lead container
31. A nurse is assisting in developing a plan of care for a client experiencing hematological toxicity as a result of chemotherapy. Which of the following would be included in the plan of care?
    1. Restricting all visitors
    2. Restricting fluid intake
    3. Inserting an indwelling urinary catheter to prevent skin breakdown
    4. Restricting fresh fruits and vegetables in the diet
32. A nurse is reviewing the laboratory results of a client receiving chemotherapy. The platelet count is 10,000/mm^3. Based on this laboratory value, the priority nursing action is to monitor which of the following?
    1. Level of consciousness
    2. Temperature
    3. Bowel sounds
    4. Skin turgor
33. A nurse is caring for a client who is 4 days postoperative after a pelvic exenteration. The physician has changed the client's diet from NPO to clear liquids. The nurse checks which of the following before administering the clear liquids?
    1. Ability to ambulate
    2. Urine specific gravity
    3. Incision appearance
    4. Bowel sounds
34. A client is admitted to the hospital with a diagnosis of suspected Hodgkin's disease. Which of the following assessment signs would the nurse most likely expect to note documented in the client's record?
    1. Weakness
    2. Fatigue
    3. Weight gain
    4. Enlarged lymph nodes
35. When reviewing the health care record of a client with ovarian cancer, the nurse recognizes which symptom as typical of the disease?
    1. Hypermenorrhea
    2. Abdominal distention
    3. Diarrhea
    4. Abnormal bleeding
36. A nurse is reviewing the complications of conization with a client who has microinvasive cervical cancer. Which of the following complications is not associated with this procedure?
    1. Infection
    2. Infertility
    3. Ovarian perforation
    4. Hemorrhage
37. A nurse is caring for a client dying of ovarian cancer. During care, the client states, "If I can just live long enough to attend my daughter's graduation, I'll be ready to die." Which phase of coping is this client experiencing?
    1. Denial
    2. Bargaining
    3. Depression
    4. Anger
38. A nurse is caring for a client after a modified radical mastectomy. Which of the following findings would indicate that the client is experiencing a complication related to the surgery?
    1. Sanguineous drainage in the drainage tube
    2. Pain at the incisional site
    3. Complaints of decreased sensation near the operative site
    4. Arm edema on the operative side
39. A nurse is reviewing the health record of a client with laryngeal cancer. The nurse would expect to

note which most common risk factor for this type of cancer in the record?
1. Use of chewing tobacco
2. Cigarette smoking
3. Urban living
4. Alcohol abuse

40. A female client who has been receiving radiation therapy for bladder cancer tells the nurse that it feels as if she is voiding through the vagina. The nurse interprets that the client may be experiencing:
1. Extreme stress due to the diagnosis of cancer
2. Altered perineal sensation as a side effect of radiation therapy
3. The development of a vesicovaginal fistula
4. Rupture of the bladder

41. A client with leukemia is receiving busulfan (Myleran). Allopurinol (Zyloprim) is prescribed for the client. The nurse understands that the purpose of the allopurinol (Zyloprim) is to:
1. Prevent gouty arthritis
2. Prevent hyperuricemia
3. Prevent stomatitis
4. Prevent diarrhea

42. A client receiving chemotherapy is experiencing stomatitis. The nurse advises the client to use which of the following as the best substance to rinse the mouth?
1. Hydrogen peroxide mixture
2. Weak salt and bicarbonate mouth rinse
3. Lemon-flavored mouthwash
4. Alcohol-based mouthwash

43. A nurse is assisting in conducting a health promotion program and the topic of the discussion relates to the risk factors of gastric cancer. Which of the following is not associated with the incidence of this type of cancer?
1. History of gastric polyps
2. History of pernicious anemia
3. A diet of smoked, highly salted and spiced food
4. High meat and carbohydrate consumption

44. A nurse is reviewing the preoperative orders of a client with a colon tumor who is scheduled for abdominal perineal resection. The nurse notes that the physician has prescribed neomycin sulfate (Mycifradin Sulfate) for the client. The nurse determines that this medication has been prescribed:
1. Because the client has an infection
2. To prevent an infection
3. To decrease the bacteria in the bowel
4. Because the client is allergic to penicillin

45. A nurse is caring for a client after a radical neck dissection and creation of a tracheostomy performed for laryngeal cancer. The nurse is reinforcing discharge instructions to the client. Which of the following would not be a component of the instructions regarding care to the stoma?
1. Apply a thin layer of petrolatum to the skin around the stoma to prevent cracking
2. Protect the stoma from water
3. Use an air conditioner to provide cool air to assist in breathing
4. Keep powders and sprays away from the stoma site

46. A nurse is caring for a client with cancer of the prostate after a prostatectomy. The nurse reinforces discharge instructions and plans to include which of the following?
1. Notify the physician if small blood clots are noticed during urination
2. Driving in a car may be resumed in 1 week
3. Restrict fluid intake to prevent incontinence
4. Avoid lifting objects heavier than 20 pounds for at least 6 weeks

47. A nurse is assisting in providing a teaching session to a community group regarding the risks and causes of bladder cancer. Which of the following is not associated with this type of cancer?
1. It most often occurs in women
2. It is generally seen in clients older than age 40
3. Environmental health hazards have been attributed as a cause
4. Using cigarettes, artificial sweeteners, and coffee drinking can increase the risk

48. A nurse is reviewing the history of a client with bladder cancer. The nurse would expect to note which most common symptom of this type of cancer documented in the record?
1. Frequency of urination
2. Urgency on urination
3. Hematuria
4. Dysuria

49. A nurse is inspecting the stoma of a client after a ureterostomy. Which of the following would the nurse expect to note?
1. A pale stoma
2. A red and moist stoma
3. A dry stoma
4. A dark-colored stoma

50. A nurse is caring for a client after a radical mastectomy. Which of the following nursing interventions would assist in preventing lymphedema of the affected arm?
1. Placing cool compresses on the affected arm
2. Elevating the affected arm on a pillow above heart level
3. Maintaining an IV site below the antecubital area on the affected side
4. Avoiding arm exercises in the immediate postoperative period

ANSWERS

1. *Answer:* 2

Rationale: The TSE is recommended monthly after a warm bath or shower when the scrotal skin is relaxed. The client should stand to examine the testicles. Using both hands, with fingers under the scrotum and thumbs on top, the client should gently roll the testicles feeling for any lumps.
Test-Taking Strategy: Use the process of elimination. Eliminate option 4 first because of the words "6 months." Next eliminate option 3 because of the word "one." From the remaining options, eliminate option 1 by trying to visualize the process of the self-examination. If you had difficulty with this question, review this self-examination.
Level of Cognitive Ability: Application
Client Needs: Health Promotion and Maintenance
Integrated Concept/Process: Self-Care
Content Area: Adult Health/Oncology
Reference: DeWit S: *Fundamental concepts and skills for nursing,* Philadelphia, 2001, WB Saunders, p. 388.

2. *Answer:* 3

Rationale: Viruses may be one of multiple agents acting to initiate carcinogenesis and have been associated with several types of cancer. Increased stress has been associated with causing the growth and proliferation of cancer cells. Two forms of radiation, ultraviolet and ionizing, can lead to cancer. High-fiber diets may reduce the risk of colon cancer. A diet high in fat may increase the risk of developing some cancers.
Test-Taking Strategy: Note the key word "not." Read each option carefully using the process of elimination. Recalling the risk factors related to cancer will direct you to option 3. Review these risk factors if you had difficulty with this question.
Level of Cognitive Ability: Comprehension
Client Needs: Health Promotion and Maintenance
Integrated Concept/Process: Teaching/Learning
Content Area: Adult Health/Oncology
Reference: DeWit S: *Fundamental concepts and skills for nursing,* Philadelphia, 2001, WB Saunders, p. 390.

3. *Answer:* 3

Rationale: Thrombocytopenia indicates a decrease in the number of platelets in the circulating blood. A major concern is monitoring for and preventing bleeding. Option 2 relates to monitoring for infection, particularly if leukopenia is present. Options 1 and 4, although important in the plan of care, are not directly related to thrombocytopenia.
Test-Taking Strategy: Use the process of elimination and note the key word "thrombocytopenia." Recalling that this condition places the client at risk of bleeding will assist in eliminating options 1, 2, and 4. If you are unfamiliar with the nursing interventions related to this disorder, review this content.
Level of Cognitive Ability: Application
Client Needs: Physiological Integrity
Integrated Concept/Process: Nursing Process/Planning
Content Area: Adult Health/Oncology
Reference: DeWit S: *Fundamental concepts and skills for nursing,* Philadelphia, 2001, WB Saunders, p. 866.

4. *Answer:* 2

Rationale: Candidiasis is a fungal infection caused by *Candida albicans*. When it occurs in the mouth, it is called thrush and appears as white plaques. Although it can occur in an immunocompromised client, it is not considered to be common. Options 3 and 4 are not accurate regarding this infection.
Test-Taking Strategy: Use the process of elimination. Options 1 and 3 can be eliminated first. Recalling that the anemic client is more likely to exhibit pallor will assist in eliminating option 4 and will direct you to option 2. If you are unfamiliar with the manifestations associated with thrush, review this content.
Level of Cognitive Ability: Comprehension
Client Needs: Physiological Integrity
Integrated Concept/Process: Nursing Process/Data Collection
Content Area: Adult Health/Oncology
Reference: Ignatavicius D, Workman M: *Medical-surgical: critical thinking for collaborative care,* ed 4, Philadelphia, 2002, WB Saunders, p. 1759.

5. *Answer:* 2

Rationale: The normal WBC count ranges from 4,500 to 11,000/mm^3. Option 1 indicates a low value. Options 3 and 4 indicate elevated values.
Test-Taking Strategy: Recalling the normal WBC count is required to answer this question. Learn this value if you are unfamiliar with it.
Level of Cognitive Ability: Comprehension
Client Needs: Physiological Integrity
Integrated Concept/Process: Nursing Process/Data Collection
Content Area: Adult Health/Oncology
Reference: DeWit S: *Fundamental concepts and skills for nursing,* Philadelphia, 2001, WB Saunders, p. 209.

6. *Answer:* 2

Rationale: The BSE should be performed monthly several days after the menstrual period. It is not recommended to perform the examination weekly. At the onset of menstruation and during ovulation, hormonal changes occur that may alter breast tissue.
Test-Taking Strategy: Use the process of elimination. Option 4 can be eliminated first because of the word "weekly." Eliminate options 1 and 3 next because of the similarity in regard to the hormonal changes that occur during these times. If you are unfamiliar with the procedure for performing BSE, review this self-examination.
Level of Cognitive Ability: Application
Client Needs: Health Promotion and Maintenance
Integrated Concept/Process: Self-Care
Content Area: Adult Health/Oncology
Reference: DeWit S: *Fundamental concepts and skills for nursing,* Philadelphia, 2001, WB Saunders, p. 388.

7. *Answer:* 2

Rationale: The nurse would instruct the client to lie down and place a towel or pillow under the shoulder on the side of the breast to be examined. If the left breast it to be examined, the pillow would be placed under the left shoulder. Options 3 and 4 are incorrect.

Test-Taking Strategy: Attempt to visualize this procedure to select the correct option. Remember to examine the left, the pillow is placed under the left; to examine the right, the pillow is placed under the right. If you are unfamiliar with the procedure for performing BSE, review this self-examination.
Level of Cognitive Ability: Application
Client Needs: Health Promotion and Maintenance
Integrated Concept/Process: Self-Care
Content Area: Adult Health/Oncology
Reference: DeWit S: *Fundamental concepts and skills for nursing,* Philadelphia, 2001, WB Saunders, p. 388.

8. *Answer:* 4
Rationale: If the client has had a hysterectomy or is no longer menstruating, the BSE should be performed on the same day every month. Options 1 and 2 are inappropriate because the client who had a hysterectomy would not be menstruating. It is best not to perform the BSE at ovulation time because of the hormonal changes that occur.
Test-Taking Strategy: Use the process of elimination and note the key word "hysterectomy." Options 1 and 2 can be easily eliminated. Eliminate option 3 because of the hormonal changes that occur at this time. If you are unfamiliar with the procedure for performing BSE, review this self-examination.
Level of Cognitive Ability: Application
Client Needs: Health Promotion and Maintenance
Integrated Concept/Process: Self-Care
Content Area: Adult Health/Oncology
Reference: DeWit S: *Fundamental concepts and skills for nursing,* Philadelphia, 2001, WB Saunders, p. 389.

9. *Answer:* 2
Rationale: The CT scan causes no pain and can last for 15 to 60 minutes. The dye may cause a warm flushing sensation when injected. Fluids are encouraged after the procedure. If an iodine dye is used, the client should be asked about allergies to seafood or iodine.
Test-Taking Strategy: Use the process of elimination and note the key words "dye injection." Noting the relationship between these key words and option 2 will assist in answering the question. Review this diagnostic test if you had difficulty with this question.
Level of Cognitive Ability: Comprehension
Client Needs: Physiological Integrity
Integrated Concept/Process: Nursing Process/Implementation
Content Area: Adult Health/Oncology
Reference: DeWit S: *Fundamental concepts and skills for nursing,* Philadelphia, 2001, WB Saunders, p. 409.

10. *Answer:* 4
Rationale: The nurse asks the client with fibrocystic breast disorder about worsening of symptoms (breast lumps, painful breasts, and possible nipple discharge) before the onset of menses. This is associated with cyclical hormone changes. Options 1, 2, and 3 do not provide significant data regarding this disorder.
Test-Taking Strategy: The key words are "more noticeable." This implies that there is a predictable variation in symptoms. Use knowledge of the effects of various hormones in the body to analyze the options and choose correctly. Review fibrocystic disorder, if you had difficulty with this question.
Level of Cognitive Ability: Application
Client Needs: Physiological Integrity
Integrated Concept/Process: Nursing Process/Data Collection
Content Area: Adult Health/Oncology
Reference: Ignatavicius D, Workman M: *Medical-surgical: critical thinking for collaborative care,* ed 4, Philadelphia, 2002, WB Saunders, p. 1734.

11. *Answer:* 1
Rationale: The client demonstrates the best adjustment by participating in own care. This would include care of surgical drains that would be in place for a short time after discharge. Asking for pain medication is also an action-oriented option, but it does not relate to acceptance of the loss of the breast. Reading the postoperative care booklet is useful, but is not the best of the options presented. Refusing to look at the wound indicates a lack of adjustment to the loss.
Test-Taking Strategy: Note the key words "best adjustment." This tells you that more than one or all of the options may be partially or totally correct. Use prioritizing skills noting that option 1 is the most action-oriented behavior. Review the psychosocial needs of the client after mastectomy if you had difficulty with this question.
Level of Cognitive Ability: Analysis
Client Needs: Psychosocial Integrity
Integrated Concept/Process: Nursing Process/Evaluation
Content Area: Adult Health/Oncology
Reference: Ignatavicius D, Workman M: *Medical-surgical: critical thinking for collaborative care,* ed 4, Philadelphia, 2002, WB Saunders, p. 1744.

12. *Answer:* 2
Rationale: The client should resume activity slowly, and walking is a beneficial activity. The client should be instructed to rest when fatigue occurs. Activities to be avoided include driving, heavy housework, wearing tight clothing, crossing the legs, and prolonged standing or sitting. Sexual activity is prohibited for 4 to 6 weeks after surgery.
Test-Taking Strategy: Use the process of elimination and note the key words "not precipitate complications." With this in mind, evaluate each of the options in terms of the stress or harm it could cause to the perineal area. This will direct you to option 2. Review home care measures after vulvectomy if you had difficulty with this question.
Level of Cognitive Ability: Application
Client Needs: Physiological Integrity
Integrated Concept/Process: Nursing Process/Planning
Content Area: Adult Health/Oncology
Reference: Ignatavicius D, Workman M: *Medical-surgical: critical thinking for collaborative care,* ed 4, Philadelphia, 2002, WB Saunders, p. 1779.

13. *Answer:* 3
Rationale: The client is at risk of deep vein thrombosis or thrombophlebitis after this surgery, as for any other major surgery. For this reason, the nurse implements measures that will prevent this complication. Range of motion exercises, antiembolism stockings, and pneumatic compression boots

are all helpful. The nurse should avoid using the knee gatch in the bed, which inhibits venous return, thus placing the client more at risk for deep vein thrombosis or thrombophlebitis.
Test-Taking Strategy: Use the process of elimination and note the key word "avoids." Recalling the complications after this type of surgery and the interventions that will prevent these complications will direct you to option 3. Review these postoperative nursing interventions if you had difficulty with this question.
Level of Cognitive Ability: Application
Client Needs: Physiological Integrity
Integrated Concept/Process: Nursing Process/Implementation
Content Area: Adult Health/Oncology
Reference: Ignatavicius D, Workman M: *Medical-surgical: critical thinking for collaborative care,* ed 4, Philadelphia, 2002, WB Saunders, p. 763.

14. ***Answer:*** 3
Rationale: A pelvic ultrasound requires the ingestion of large volumes of water just before the procedure. A full bladder is necessary so that this organ will be visualized as such and not mistaken as a possible pelvic growth. An abdominal ultrasound may require that the client abstain from food or fluid for several hours before the procedure. Option 4 is unrelated to this specific procedure.
Test-Taking Strategy: Use the process of elimination. Noting the key word "pelvic" will assist in directing you to option 3. Review preparation for a pelvic ultrasound if you had difficulty with this question.
Level of Cognitive Ability: Application
Client Needs: Physiological Integrity
Integrated Concept/Process: Nursing Process/Implementation
Content Area: Adult Health/Oncology
Reference: Ignatavicius D, Workman M: *Medical-surgical: critical thinking for collaborative care,* ed 4, Philadelphia, 2002, WB Saunders, p. 1176.

15. ***Answer:*** 4
Rationale: A biopsy is done to determine whether a tumor is malignant or benign. An MRI, CT scan, and ultrasound will visualize the presence of a mass but will not confirm a diagnosis of malignancy.
Test-Taking Strategy: Use the process of elimination and note the key word "confirm." This key word will direct you to option 4. Review the purpose of the tests if you had difficulty with this question.
Level of Cognitive Ability: Comprehension
Client Needs: Physiological Integrity
Integrated Concept/Process: Nursing Process/Data Collection
Content Area: Adult Health/Oncology
Reference: DeWit S: *Fundamental concepts and skills for nursing,* Philadelphia, 2001, WB Saunders, p. 37.

16. ***Answer:*** 4
Rationale: Multiple myeloma is a neoplastic condition characterized by abnormal malignant proliferation of plasma cells and the accumulation of mature plasma cells in the bone marrow. Option 1 describes the leukemic process. Options 2 and 3 are not characteristics of multiple myeloma.
Test-Taking Strategy: Use the process of elimination and knowledge regarding the pathophysiology associated with this disorder to answer the question. Focusing on the name of the diagnosis will assist in directing you to option 4. Review this information if you are unfamiliar with this oncological disorder.
Level of Cognitive Ability: Comprehension
Client Needs: Physiological Integrity
Integrated Concept/Process: Nursing Process/Planning
Content Area: Adult Health/Oncology
Reference: Black J, Hawks J, Keene A: *Medical-surgical nursing: clinical management for positive outcomes,* ed 6, Philadelphia, 2001, WB Saunders, p. 2120.

17. ***Answer:*** 3
Rationale: Findings indicative of multiple myeloma are an increased number of plasma cells in the bone marrow, anemia, hypercalcemia as a result of the release of calcium from the deteriorating bone tissue, and an elevated BUN. An increased white blood cell count may or may not be present and is not specifically related to multiple myeloma.
Test-Taking Strategy: Knowledge regarding the pathophysiology associated with this disorder and the effects it produces on the body is required to answer the question. Review this information if you are unfamiliar with this oncological disorder.
Level of Cognitive Ability: Comprehension
Client Needs: Physiological Integrity
Integrated Concept/Process: Nursing Process/Data Collection
Content Area: Adult Health/Oncology
Reference: Black J, Hawks J, Keene A: *Medical-surgical nursing: clinical management for positive outcomes,* ed 6, Philadelphia, 2001, WB Saunders, p. 2120.

18. ***Answer:*** 2
Rationale: Hypercalcemia secondary to bone destruction is a priority concern in the client with multiple myeloma. The nurse should encourage fluids in adequate amounts to maintain an output of 1.5 to 2.0 liters per day. Clients require about 3 liters of fluid per day. The fluid is needed not only to dilute the calcium, but also to prevent protein from precipitating in the renal tubules. Options 1, 3, and 4 may be a component of the plan of care, but are not the priority in this client.
Test-Taking Strategy: Knowledge regarding the clinical manifestations that occur in multiple myeloma is required to answer the question. Recalling that encouraging fluids is specific to the care of a client with this disorder will direct you to option 2. Review the specific manifestations of this disorder if you had difficulty with this question.
Level of Cognitive Ability: Application
Client Needs: Physiological Integrity
Integrated Concept/Process: Nursing Process/Planning
Content Area: Adult Health/Oncology
Reference: Black J, Hawks J, Keene A: *Medical-surgical nursing: clinical management for positive outcomes,* ed 6, Philadelphia, 2001, WB Saunders, p. 2121.

19. ***Answer:*** 3
Rationale: Hodgkin's disease is a disorder of young adults and primarily occurs between the ages of 20 and 40 years. Options 1, 2, and 4 are characteristics of this disease.

Test-Taking Strategy: Use the process of elimination and note the key word "not." Recalling that Hodgkin's disease occurs in the young adult will direct you to option 3. Review the characteristics of this disorder if you had difficulty with this question.
Level of Cognitive Ability: Comprehension
Client Needs: Physiological Integrity
Integrated Concept/Process: Nursing Process/Planning
Content Area: Adult Health/Oncology
Reference: Black J, Hawks J, Keene A: *Medical-surgical nursing: clinical management for positive outcomes*, ed 6, Philadelphia, 2001, WB Saunders, p. 2173.

20. *Answer:* 3
Rationale: Alopecia is not a finding in testicular cancer; however, it may occur as a result of radiation or chemotherapy. Options 1, 2, and 4 are findings in testicular cancer. Back pain may indicate metastasis to the retroperitoneal lymph nodes.
Test-Taking Strategy: Note the key word "not." Use the process of elimination, remembering that alopecia occurs as a result of chemotherapy rather than from the disease. Review the manifestations associated with testicular cancer if you had difficulty with this question
Level of Cognitive Ability: Application
Client Needs: Health Promotion and Maintenance
Integrated Concept/Process: Teaching/Learning
Content Area: Adult Health/Oncology
Reference: Black J, Hawks J, Keene A: *Medical-surgical nursing: clinical management for positive outcomes*, ed 6, Philadelphia, 2001, WB Saunders, p. 964.

21. *Answer:* 4
Rationale: Hyperuricemia is especially common after treatment for leukemias and lymphomas, because the therapy results in massive cell kill. Although options 1, 2, and 3 may also be noted, an increased uric acid level is specifically related to cell destruction.
Test-Taking Strategy: Note the key word "specifically note" and "massive cell destruction." Recalling the cell response to destruction will assist in directing you to option 4. Review this concept if you had difficulty with this question.
Level of Cognitive Ability: Comprehension
Client Needs: Physiological Integrity
Integrated Concept/Process: Nursing Process/Data Collection
Content Area: Adult Health/Oncology
Reference: Ignatavicius D, Workman M: *Medical-surgical: critical thinking for collaborative care*, ed 4, Philadelphia, 2002, WB Saunders, p. 1633.

22. *Answer:* 3
Rationale: Palliative surgery that can benefit the client with cancer and improve quality of life includes procedures that reduce pain, relieve airway obstructions, relieve obstruction in the gastrointestinal and urinary tracts, relieve pressure on the brain and spinal cord, and prevent hemorrhage. Options 1, 2, and 4 do not describe palliative surgery.
Test-Taking Strategy: Note the key word "palliative." Knowledge of the definition of this word will assist in directing you to option 3. Review the various types of surgery if you had difficulty with this question.
Level of Cognitive Ability: Comprehension
Client Needs: Physiological Integrity
Integrated Concept/Process: Nursing Process/Planning
Content Area: Adult Health/Oncology
Reference: Ignatavicius D, Workman M: *Medical-surgical: critical thinking for collaborative care*, ed 4, Philadelphia, 2002, WB Saunders, p. 426.

23. *Answer:* 3
Rationale: In general, only the area in the treatment field is affected by the radiation. Skin reactions, fatigue, nausea, and anorexia may occur with radiation to any site, whereas other side effects occur only when specific areas are involved in treatment. A client receiving radiation to the larynx is most likely to experience a sore throat. Options 1 and 4 may occur with radiation to the gastrointestinal (GI) tract. Dyspnea may occur with lung involvement.
Test-Taking Strategy: Use the process of elimination. Eliminate options 1 and 4 first because they are similar and GI related. Consider the anatomical location of the radiation therapy to assist in directing you to option 3. Review the effects of radiation therapy if you had difficulty with this question.
Level of Cognitive Ability: Application
Client Needs: Physiological Integrity
Integrated Concept/Process: Nursing Process/Planning
Content Area: Adult Health/Oncology
Reference: Ignatavicius D, Workman M: *Medical-surgical: critical thinking for collaborative care*, ed 4, Philadelphia, 2002, WB Saunders, p. 427.

24. *Answer:* 3
Rationale: Moist desquamation occurs when the basal cells of the skin are destroyed. The dermal level is exposed, which results in the leakage of serum. Reddened skin, a rash, and dermatitis may occur with external radiation but is not described as a moist desquamation.
Test-Taking Strategy: Use the process of elimination. Noting the key word "moist" will direct you to option 3. Options 1, 2, and 4 are eliminated because they are similar and describe a dry rather than a moist skin alteration. Review the signs associated with a moist desquamation if you had difficulty with this question.
Level of Cognitive Ability: Comprehension
Client Needs: Physiological Integrity
Integrated Concept/Process: Nursing Process/Data Collection
Content Area: Adult Health/Oncology
Reference: Ignatavicius D, Workman M: *Medical-surgical: critical thinking for collaborative care*, ed 4, Philadelphia, 2002, WB Saunders, p. 1563.

25. *Answer:* 3
Rationale: The client should avoid pressure on the radiated area and should wear loose-fitting clothing. Options 1, 2, and 4 are accurate instructions regarding radiation therapy.
Test-Taking Strategy: Use the process of elimination and note the key word "not." The word "pressure" in option 3 should be an indication that this is an inappropriate measure. Review client teaching points related to skin care and radiation therapy if you had difficulty with this question.
Level of Cognitive Ability: Application
Client Needs: Health Promotion and Maintenance

Integrated Concept/Process: Nursing Process/Implementation
Content Area: Adult Health/Oncology
Reference: Ignatavicius D, Workman M: *Medical-surgical: critical thinking for collaborative care*, ed 4, Philadelphia, 2002, WB Saunders, p. 1563.

26. *Answer:* 2
Rationale: The time that the nurse spends in a room of a client with an internal radiation implant is 30 minutes per 8-hour shift. The dosimeter badge must be worn when in the client's room. Children younger than 16 years old and pregnant women are not allowed in the client's room.
Test-Taking Strategy: Use the process of elimination. Option 4 can be eliminated first. Knowledge of the time frame related to exposure to the client will assist in eliminating option 1. From the remaining options, select option 2 because of the possible risks associated with exposure to the mother and fetus. Review these principles if you had difficulty with this question.
Level of Cognitive Ability: Application
Client Needs: Safe, Effective Care Environment
Integrated Concept/Process: Nursing Process/Implementation
Content Area: Adult Health/Oncology
Reference: Ignatavicius D, Workman M: *Medical-surgical: critical thinking for collaborative care*, ed 4, Philadelphia, 2002, WB Saunders, p. 428.

27. *Answer:* 2
Rationale: Foul-smelling vaginal discharge is expected and will occur for some time after removal of a radiation implant from the cervix. Options 1, 3, and 4 are accurate discharge instructions.
Test-Taking Strategy: Note the key words "need for further discharge instructions." Recalling that foul-smelling vaginal discharge is expected will direct you to option 2. Review these points if you had difficulty with this question.
Level of Cognitive Ability: Comprehension
Client Needs: Health Promotion and Maintenance
Integrated Concept/Process: Teaching/Learning
Content Area: Adult Health/Oncology
Reference: Ignatavicius D, Workman M: *Medical-surgical: critical thinking for collaborative care*, ed 4, Philadelphia, 2002, WB Saunders, p. 1774.

28. *Answer:* 3
Rationale: The client with a cervical radiation implant should be maintained on bed rest in the dorsal position to prevent movement of the radiation source. The head of the bed is elevated to a maximum of 10 to 15 degrees for comfort. Avoid turning the client on the side. If the client needs to be turned, a pillow is placed between the knees and, with the body in straight alignment, the client is log rolled.
Test-Taking Strategy: Consider the anatomical location of the implant and the risk of dislodgement to answer the question. Additionally, note that options 1, 2, and 4 are similar. If you had difficulty with this question, review care to the client with a radiation implant.
Level of Cognitive Ability: Comprehension
Client Needs: Safe, Effective Care Environment
Integrated Concept/Process: Nursing Process/Planning
Content Area: Adult Health/Oncology
Reference: Ignatavicius D, Workman M: *Medical-surgical: critical thinking for collaborative care*, ed 4, Philadelphia, 2002, WB Saunders, p. 1774.

29. *Answer:* 3
Rationale: The client needs to be instructed to avoid exposure to the sun. Options 1, 2, and 4 are accurate measures in the care of a client receiving external radiation therapy.
Test-Taking Strategy: Use the process of elimination. Note the key words "need for further instruction." Eliminate option 1 because of the word "gently" and option 4 because of the word "loose." From the remaining options, recalling that sun exposure is to be avoided will assist in answering the question. Review skin care measures for the client receiving external radiation if you had difficulty with this question.
Level of Cognitive Ability: Comprehension
Client Needs: Health Promotion and Maintenance
Integrated Concept/Process: Teaching/Learning
Content Area: Adult Health/Oncology
Reference: Ignatavicius D, Workman M: *Medical-surgical: critical thinking for collaborative care*, ed 4, Philadelphia, 2002, WB Saunders, p. 1547.

30. *Answer:* 4
Rationale: A lead container and long-handled forceps should be kept in the client's room at all times during internal radiation therapy. If the implant becomes dislodged, the nurse should pick up the implant with long-handled forceps and place it in the lead container. Options 1, 2, and 3 are inaccurate interventions.
Test-Taking Strategy: Use the process of elimination. Note the key word "initial." Option 3 is not an appropriate action. Eliminate option 2 next because the implant would not be discarded. Although the physician would be notified, the initial action is option 4. Review the measures related to a dislodged implant if you had difficulty with this question.
Level of Cognitive Ability: Application
Client Needs: Safe, Effective Care Environment
Integrated Concept/Process: Nursing Process/Implementation
Content Area: Adult Health/Oncology
Reference: Ignatavicius D, Workman M: *Medical-surgical: critical thinking for collaborative care*, ed 4, Philadelphia, 2002, WB Saunders, p. 1774.

31. *Answer:* 4
Rationale: In a client experiencing hematological toxicity, a low-bacteria diet is implemented. This includes avoiding fresh fruits and vegetables and thorough cooking of all foods. Not all visitors are restricted, but the client is protected from people with known infections. Fluids should be encouraged. Invasive measures such as an indwelling urinary catheter should be avoided to prevent infections.
Test-Taking Strategy: Use the process of elimination. Eliminate option 1 because of the word "all." Next, eliminate option 2 because it is not reasonable to restrict fluids in a client receiving chemotherapy who is already at risk for fluid and electrolyte imbalances. Eliminate option 3 because of the risk of infection that exists with this measure. Review interventions

for the client with hematological toxicity if you had difficulty with this question.
Level of Cognitive Ability: Application
Client Needs: Safe, Effective Care Environment
Integrated Concept/Process: Nursing Process/Planning
Content Area: Adult Health/Oncology
Reference: Ignatavicius D, Workman M: *Medical-surgical: critical thinking for collaborative care,* ed 4, Philadelphia, 2002, WB Saunders, p. 437.

32. *Answer:* 1
Rationale: A high risk of hemorrhage exists when the platelet count is less than 20,000/mm^3. Fatal central nervous system (CNS) hemorrhage or massive gastrointestinal (GI) hemorrhage can occur when the platelet count is less than 10,000/mm^3. The client should be monitored for changes in level of consciousness, which may be an early indication of an intracranial hemorrhage. Option 2 is a priority when the WBC count is low and the client is at risk for an infection. Although options 3 and 4 are important, they are not the priority in this situation.
Test-Taking Strategy: Use the process of elimination and note the key word "priority." Recalling the normal platelet count and determining that a low count places the client at risk for bleeding will assist in eliminating options 2, 3, and 4. Review the normal platelet count and the nursing interventions for a client with a low count if you had difficulty with this question.
Level of Cognitive Ability: Analysis
Client Needs: Physiological Integrity
Integrated Concept/Process: Nursing Process/Implementation
Content Area: Adult Health/Oncology
Reference: Ignatavicius D, Workman M: *Medical-surgical: critical thinking for collaborative care,* ed 4, Philadelphia, 2002, WB Saunders, p. 831.

33. *Answer:* 4
Rationale: The client is kept NPO until peristalsis returns, usually in 4 to 6 days after surgery. When signs of bowel function return, clear fluids are given to the client. If no distention occurs, the diet is advanced as tolerated. It is most important to monitor for bowel sounds before feeding the client. Options 1, 2, and 3 are unrelated to the issue of the question.
Test-Taking Strategy: Use the process of elimination. Note the key words "priority" and "NPO to clear liquids." Option 4 is the only option that relates to GI function, which is the issue of the question. Review care to the client after abdominal surgery if you had difficulty with this question.
Level of Cognitive Ability: Application
Client Needs: Physiological Integrity
Integrated Concept/Process: Nursing Process/Implementation
Content Area: Adult Health/Oncology
Reference: Ignatavicius D, Workman M: *Medical-surgical: critical thinking for collaborative care,* ed 4, Philadelphia, 2002, WB Saunders, p. 1775.

34. *Answer:* 4
Rationale: Hodgkin's disease is a chronic progressive neoplastic disorder of lymphoid tissue characterized by the painless enlargement of lymph nodes with progression to extralymphatic sites, such as the spleen and liver. Weight loss is most likely to be noted. Fatigue and weakness may occur, but are not significantly related to the disease.
Test-Taking Strategy: Use the process of elimination. Option 3 can be easily eliminated first because in such a disorder, weight loss is most likely to occur. Options 1 and 2 are similar and rather vague symptoms that can occur in many disorders. Also, recalling that Hodgkin's disease affects the lymph nodes will easily direct you to option 4. Review the manifestations associated with Hodgkin's disease if you had difficulty with this question.
Level of Cognitive Ability: Comprehension
Client Needs: Physiological Integrity
Integrated Concept/Process: Nursing Process/Data Collection
Content Area: Adult Health/Oncology
Reference: Ignatavicius D, Workman M: *Medical-surgical: critical thinking for collaborative care,* ed 4, Philadelphia, 2002, WB Saunders, p. 859.

35. *Answer:* 2
Rationale: Clinical manifestations of ovarian cancer include abdominal distention, urinary frequency and urgency, pain from pressure caused by the growing tumor and the effects of urinary or bowel obstruction, and constipation. Abnormal bleeding, often resulting in hypermenorrhea, is associated with uterine cancer.
Test-Taking Strategy: Use the process of elimination. Eliminate options 1 and 4 first because they are similar. From the remaining options, consider the anatomical location of the diagnosis. This will assist in directing you to option 2. Review the manifestations associated with ovarian cancer if you had difficulty with this question.
Level of Cognitive Ability: Comprehension
Client Needs: Physiological Integrity
Integrated Concept/Process: Nursing Process/Data Collection
Content Area: Adult Health/Oncology
Reference: Ignatavicius D, Workman M: *Medical-surgical: critical thinking for collaborative care,* ed 4, Philadelphia, 2002, WB Saunders, p. 1776.

36. *Answer:* 3
Rationale: Conization is generally not performed on women who desire to bear children because it can lead to incompetence of the cervix or infertility. Other complications of the procedure include hemorrhage, infection, and less frequently cervical stenosis.
Test-Taking Strategy: Use the process of elimination. Note the key word "not" and the words "cervical cancer." Select option 3 because this option addresses an "ovarian" condition not a cervical one. Review the complications associated with this procedure if you had difficulty with this question.
Level of Cognitive Ability: Comprehension
Client Needs: Physiological Integrity
Integrated Concept/Process: Nursing Process/Implementation
Content Area: Adult Health/Oncology
Reference: Ignatavicius D, Workman M: *Medical-surgical: critical thinking for collaborative care,* ed 4, Philadelphia, 2002, WB Saunders, p. 1774.

37. *Answer:* 2
Rationale: Denial, bargaining, anger, depression, and acceptance are recognized stages that a person facing a life-threatening illness experiences. The client's statement is indicative of bargaining. Denial is expressed as shock and disbelief and may be the first response to hearing bad news. Depression may be manifested by hopelessness, weeping openly, or remaining quiet or withdrawn. Anger may also be a first response to upsetting news and the predominant theme is "why me?" or the blaming of others.
Test-Taking Strategy: Focus on the client's statement as identified in the question to assist in selecting the correct option. From this point, you should be able to eliminate options 1, 3, and 4. Review these stages if you had difficulty with this question.
Level of Cognitive Ability: Analysis
Client Needs: Psychosocial Integrity
Integrated Concept/Process: Nursing Process/Data Collection
Content Area: Adult Health/Oncology
Reference: DeWit S: *Fundamental concepts and skills for nursing,* Philadelphia, 2001, WB Saunders, p. 189.

38. *Answer:* 4
Rationale: Arm edema on the operative side (lymphedema) is a complication after mastectomy and can occur immediately after surgery, or months or even years after surgery. Options 1, 2, and 3 are expected occurrences after mastectomy and are not indicative of a complication.
Test-Taking Strategy: Use the process of elimination considering the normal expected occurrences after a mastectomy. If you had difficulty with this question, review the complications after mastectomy.
Level of Cognitive Ability: Comprehension
Client Needs: Physiological Integrity
Integrated Concept/Process: Nursing Process/Data Collection
Content Area: Adult Health/Oncology
Reference: Black J, Hawks J, Keene A: *Medical-surgical nursing: clinical management for positive outcomes,* ed 6, Philadelphia, 2001, WB Saunders, p. 1025.

39. *Answer:* 2
Rationale: The most common risk factor associated with laryngeal cancer is cigarette smoking. Approximately three fourths of those diagnosed with this form of cancer smoke either now or in the past. Alcohol abuse may have a synergistic effect with cigarette smoking. Air pollution is also a contributing cause, as well as chronic laryngitis and voice abuse.
Test-Taking Strategy: Use the process of elimination and note the key words "most common." Begin to answer this question by eliminating options 3 and 4. Because cancer of the upper and lower airway is most often related to tobacco, these are the options that are most likely correct. From the remaining options, recalling that cigarettes are the most harmful guides you to choose this option over the chewing tobacco. Review these risk factors if you had difficulty with this question.
Level of Cognitive Ability: Comprehension
Client Needs: Health Promotion and Maintenance
Integrated Concept/Process: Nursing Process/Data Collection
Content Area: Adult Health/Oncology
Reference: Black J, Hawks J, Keene A: *Medical-surgical nursing: clinical management for positive outcomes,* ed 6, Philadelphia, 2001, WB Saunders, p. 1661.

40. *Answer:* 3
Rationale: A vesicovaginal fistula is a genital fistula that occurs between the bladder and the vagina. The fistula is an abnormal opening between these two body parts and if this occurs, the client may experience drainage of urine through the vagina. The client's complaint is not associated with options 1, 2, and 4.
Test-Taking Strategy: Use the process of elimination. Noting the key words "voiding through the vagina" should direct you to option 3. Review the symptoms associated with vesicovaginal fistula if you had difficulty with this question.
Level of Cognitive Ability: Comprehension
Client Needs: Physiological Integrity
Integrated Concept/Process: Nursing Process/Data Collection
Content Area: Adult Health/Oncology
Reference: Black J, Hawks J, Keene A: *Medical-surgical nursing: clinical management for positive outcomes,* ed 6, Philadelphia, 2001, WB Saunders, p. 1003.

41. *Answer:* 2
Rationale: Allopurinol decreases uric acid production and reduces uric acid concentrations in both serum and urine. In the client receiving chemotherapy, uric acid levels elevate as a result of the massive cell destruction that occurs from the chemotherapy. This medication prevents or treats hyperuricemia secondary to chemotherapy. Although the medication is used to treat gout, it is not the purpose in this client situation. This medication is not used to prevent stomatitis or diarrhea.
Test-Taking Strategy: Use the process of elimination. Recalling that hyperuricemia occurs as a result of chemotherapy will assist in directing you to option 2. If you had difficulty with this question or are unfamiliar with the action of this medication, review this content.
Level of Cognitive Ability: Comprehension
Client Needs: Physiological Integrity
Integrated Concept/Process: Nursing Process/Planning
Content Area: Adult Health/Oncology
Reference: Hodgson B, Kizior R: *Saunders nursing drug handbook 2002*, Philadelphia, 2002, WB Saunders, p. 26.

42. *Answer:* 2
Rationale: An acidic environment in the mouth is favorable for bacterial growth. Therefore the client is advised to rinse the mouth at least before every meal and at bedtime with a weak salt and sodium bicarbonate mouth rinse. This lessens the growth of bacteria and limits plaque formation. The other substances are irritating to oral tissue, which is already at risk. If hydrogen peroxide must be used, it should be a very weak solution, because it dries the mucous membranes.
Test-Taking Strategy: Use the process of elimination. Options 3 and 4 can be eliminated first because of the irritating effects of these solutions. From the remaining options, note the word "weak" in the correct option. Review the treatment measures for stomatitis if you had difficulty with this question.
Level of Cognitive Ability: Application

Client Needs: Physiological Integrity
Integrated Concept/Process: Nursing Process/Implementation
Content Area: Adult Health/Oncology
Reference: Black J, Hawks J, Keene A: *Medical-surgical nursing: clinical management for positive outcomes*, ed 6, Philadelphia, 2001, WB Saunders, p. 684.

43. *Answer:* 4
Rationale: High meat and carbohydrate consumption plays a role in the development of cancer of the pancreas. Options 1, 2, and 3 are risk factors related to gastric cancer.
Test-Taking Strategy: Use the process of elimination. Note that the question asks about the risk factors associated with gastric cancer and note the key word "not." Eliminate options 1 and 2 because they are directly related to gastric disorders. Eliminate option 3 knowing that spicy foods cause gastric irritation. Review the risk factors associated with gastric cancer if you had difficulty with this question.
Level of Cognitive Ability: Comprehension
Client Needs: Health Promotion and Maintenance
Integrated Concept/Process: Teaching/Learning
Content Area: Adult Health/Oncology
Reference: Black J, Hawks J, Keene A: *Medical-surgical nursing: clinical management for positive outcomes*, ed 6, Philadelphia, 2001, WB Saunders, p. 1201.

44. *Answer:* 3
Rationale: To reduce the risk of contamination at the time of surgery, the bowel is emptied and cleansed. Laxatives and enemas are given to empty the bowel. Intestinal antiinfectives such as neomycin are administered to decrease the bacteria in the bowel.
Test-Taking Strategy: Use the process of elimination. Eliminate options 1 and 4 first because there is no reference made to this information in the question. Recalling the concepts related to the flora of the intestinal tract will assist in directing you to option 3 as the primary purpose of this medication. Review this preoperative intervention if you had difficulty with this question.
Level of Cognitive Ability: Comprehension
Client Needs: Physiological Integrity
Integrated Concept/Process: Nursing Process/Planning
Content Area: Adult Health/Oncology
Reference: Black J, Hawks J, Keene A: *Medical-surgical nursing: clinical management for positive outcomes*, ed 6, Philadelphia, 2001, WB Saunders, p. 784.

45. *Answer:* 3
Rationale: Air conditioners need to be avoided to protect from excessive coldness. A humidifier in the home should be used if excessive dryness is a problem. Options 1, 2, and 4 are appropriate interventions regarding stoma care after radical neck dissection and creation of a tracheotomy.
Test-Taking Strategy: Use the process of elimination. Noting the key word "not" will assist in eliminating options 2 and 4. From the remaining options, recalling that a humidifier rather than an air conditioner is recommended will assist in selecting the correct option. If you had difficulty with this question, review discharge instructions after radical neck dissection.
Level of Cognitive Ability: Application
Client Needs: Health Promotion and Maintenance
Integrated Concept/Process: Teaching/Learning
Content Area: Adult Health/Oncology
Reference: Black J, Hawks J, Keene A: *Medical-surgical nursing: clinical management for positive outcomes*, ed 6, Philadelphia, 2001, WB Saunders, p. 688.

46. *Answer:* 4
Rationale: Small pieces of tissue or blood clots can be passed during urination for up to 2 weeks after surgery. Driving a car and sitting for long periods of time are restricted for at least 3 weeks. A daily fluid intake of 2 to 2.5 liters per day should be maintained to limit clot formation and prevent infection. Option 4 is an accurate discharge instruction after prostatectomy.
Test-Taking Strategy: Use the process of elimination. Option 3 can be easily eliminated first. Eliminate option 2 next, because 1 week is a rather short period. Recalling that blood clots are expected after this type of surgery will assist in directing you to option 4. Review client teaching points after prostatectomy if you had difficulty with this question.
Level of Cognitive Ability: Application
Client Needs: Health Promotion and Maintenance
Integrated Concept/Process: Nursing Process/Implementation
Content Area: Adult Health/Oncology
Reference: Black J, Hawks J, Keene A: *Medical-surgical nursing: clinical management for positive outcomes*, ed 6, Philadelphia, 2001, WB Saunders, p. 960.

47. *Answer:* 1
Rationale: The incidence of bladder cancer is three times greater in men than in women and affects Caucasians twice as often as African-Americans. Options 2, 3, and 4 are associated with the incidence of bladder cancer.
Test-Taking Strategy: Use the process of elimination and note the key word "not." Basic information regarding the risks associated with cancer will assist in eliminating options 3 and 4. From the remaining options, knowledge regarding the risk factors associated with bladder cancer will direct you to option 1. If you had difficulty with this question, review these risks.
Level of Cognitive Ability: Comprehension
Client Needs: Health Promotion and Maintenance
Integrated Concept/Process: Teaching/Learning
Content Area: Adult Health/Oncology
Reference: Black J, Hawks J, Keene A: *Medical-surgical nursing: clinical management for positive outcomes*, ed 6, Philadelphia, 2001, WB Saunders, p. 809.

48. *Answer:* 3
Rationale: The most common symptom in clients with cancer of the bladder is hematuria. The client may also experience irritative voiding symptoms such as frequency, urgency, and dysuria and these symptoms are often associated with cancer in situ.
Test-Taking Strategy: Use the process of elimination and note the key words "most common." Options 1, 2, and 4 are symptoms that are also associated with bladder infection. Review the clinical manifestations associated with bladder cancer if you had difficulty with this question.

Level of Cognitive Ability: Comprehension
Client Needs: Physiological Integrity
Integrated Concept/Process: Nursing Process/Data Collection
Content Area: Adult Health/Oncology
Reference: Black J, Hawks J, Keene A: *Medical-surgical nursing: clinical management for positive outcomes,* ed 6, Philadelphia, 2001, WB Saunders, p. 810.

49. ***Answer:*** 2
Rationale: After ureterostomy, the stoma should be red and moist. A pale stoma may indicate an inadequate amount of vascular supply. A dry stoma may indicate body fluid deficit. Any sign of darkness or duskiness in the stoma may mean loss of vascular supply and must be corrected immediately or necrosis can develop.
Test-Taking Strategy: Use the process of elimination. You should easily be able to eliminate options 1 and 4. From the remaining options, note the key word moist in option 2. This should indicate that this is an expected and positive finding. If you had difficulty with this question, review expected and unexpected findings after ureterostomy.
Level of Cognitive Ability: Comprehension
Client Needs: Physiological Integrity
Integrated Concept/Process: Nursing Process/Data Collection
Content Area: Adult Health/Oncology
Reference: Black J, Hawks J, Keene A: *Medical-surgical nursing: clinical management for positive outcomes,* ed 6, Philadelphia, 2001, WB Saunders, p. 813.

50. ***Answer:*** 2
Rationale: After mastectomy, the arm should be elevated above the level of the heart. Arm exercises should be encouraged. No blood pressure readings, injections, IV lines, or blood draws should be performed on the affected arm. Cool compresses are not a suggested measure to prevent lymphedema from occurring.
Test-Taking Strategy: Note the key words "assist in preventing." Use the process of elimination and note the relationship between the words lymph "edema" in the question and "elevating" in the correct option. Review these measures if you had difficulty with this question.
Level of Cognitive Ability: Application
Client Needs: Physiological Integrity
Integrated Concept/Process: Nursing Process/Implementation
Content Area: Adult Health/Oncology
Reference: Black J, Hawks J, Keene A: *Medical-surgical nursing: clinical management for positive outcomes,* ed 6, Philadelphia, 2001, WB Saunders, p. 1025.

REFERENCES

Black J, Hawks J, Keene A: *Medical-surgical nursing: clinical management for positive outcomes,* ed 6, Philadelphia, 2001, WB Saunders.

Chernecky C, Berger B: *Laboratory tests and diagnostic procedures,* ed 3, Philadelphia, 2001, WB Saunders.

Clark J, Queener S, Karb V: *Pharmacologic basis of nursing practice,* ed 6, St Louis, 2000, Mosby.

DeWit S: *Fundamental concepts and skills for nursing,* Philadelphia, 2001, WB Saunders.

Hodgson B, Kizior R: *Saunders nursing drug handbook 2002,* Philadelphia, 2002, WB Saunders.

Ignatavicius D, Workman M: *Medical-surgical: critical thinking for collaborative care,* ed 4, Philadelphia, 2002, WB Saunders.

Potter P, Perry A: *Fundamentals of nursing,* ed 5, St Louis, 2001, Mosby.

Perry A, Potter P: *Clinical nursing skills and techniques,* ed 5, St Louis, 2002, Mosby.

41 Antineoplastic Medications

I. GENERAL CONSIDERATIONS

A. Description
1. Kill or inhibit the reproduction of neoplastic cells
2. The effect of antineoplastic medications may not be limited to neoplastic cells; normal cells are also affected by the medication
3. Cell cycle phase-specific medications affect cells only during a certain phase of the reproductive cycle
4. Cell cycle phase-nonspecific medications affect cells in any phase of the reproductive cycle
5. Usually several medications are used in combination to increase the therapeutic response
6. Antineoplastic medications may be combined with other treatments such as surgery and radiation
7. The routes of antineoplastic medication administration can vary; the intravenous (IV) route is the preferred route
8. Side effects result from the effects of the antineoplastic medication on normal cells

B. Side effects
1. Mucositis
2. Alopecia
3. Anorexia, nausea, and vomiting
4. Diarrhea
5. Anemia
6. Low white blood cell (WBC) count (neutropenia)
7. Thrombocytopenia
8. Infertility

C. Implementation
1. Physiological integrity
   a. Monitor complete blood count (CBC), WBC count, platelet count, and electrolytes
   b. Initiate bleeding precautions if thrombocytopenia occurs
   c. When the platelet count is less than 50,000 cells/μL, any small trauma can lead to episodes of prolonged bleeding; when less than 20,000 cells/μL, spontaneous and uncontrollable bleeding can occur
   d. Monitor for petechiae, ecchymosis, bleeding of the gums, and nosebleeds because the decreased platelet count can precipitate bleeding tendencies
   e. Avoid intramuscular (IM) injections and venipunctures as much as possible to prevent bleeding
   f. Initiate neutropenic precautions if the WBC count decreases
   g. Monitor for fever, sore throat, unusual bleeding, or signs and symptoms of infection
   h. Inform the client that loss of appetite may also be due to a bitter taste in the mouth from the medications
   i. Monitor for nausea and vomiting and provide a high-calorie diet with protein supplements
   j. Antiemetics are administered several hours before chemotherapy and for 12 to 48 hours afterward, as prescribed, because antineoplastic medications stimulate the vomiting centers
   k. Encourage hydration; IV fluids will be administered before and during therapy
   l. Promote a fluid intake of at least 2000 mL a day to maintain adequate renal function
   m. Administer allopurinol (Zyloprim) as prescribed to reduce the serum uric acid that occurs from the rapid destruction of cells by the antineoplastic medication

2. Safe, effective care environment
   a. IV chemotherapy is prepared in an air-vented space
   b. Antineoplastic medications are administered in short, high-dose, intermittent courses, as prescribed, to maximize antineoplastic effects while allowing normal cells to recover
   c. Gloves, gown, and a mask are worn when handling IV medications
   d. Monitor for phlebitis with IV administration, as these medications irritate the veins
   e. Monitor for extravasation (leakage of medication into surrounding skin and subcutaneous tissue), which causes tissue necrosis, and the physician is notified if this occurs; heat or ice is applied depending on the medication, and an antidote may be injected into the site
   f. Discard IV equipment in designated containers
3. Psychosocial integrity
   a. Instruct the client in the potential for hair loss and that varying degrees of hair loss may occur after the first or second treatment
   b. Discuss the purchase of a wig before treatment starts
   c. Inform the client that new hair growth will occur several months after the final treatment
   d. Instruct the client about the need for contraception, as these medications have teratogenic effects
   e. Discuss the potential effect of infertility, which may be irreversible
   f. Encourage pretreatment counseling
4. Health promotion and maintenance
   a. If diarrhea is a problem, instruct the client to avoid hot foods and high-fiber foods, which increase peristalsis
   b. Instruct the client to inspect the oral mucosa for erythema and ulcers, to rinse mouth after meals, and to provide good oral hygiene
   c. Instruct the client to use saline or sodium bicarbonate mouth rinses for mouth sores
   d. Instruct the client in the use of antifungal medications for mouth sores, if prescribed for the development of a superinfection
   e. Instruct the client to avoid crowds and persons with infections and to report signs of infection such as fever, chills, or sore throat
   f. Instruct individuals with colds or infections to wear a mask when visiting or to avoid visiting the client
   g. Instruct the client to use a soft toothbrush and an electric razor to minimize the risk of bleeding 
   h. Instruct the client to avoid aspirin-containing products to minimize the risk of bleeding
   i. Instruct the client to avoid alcohol to minimize the risk of toxicity
   j. Instruct the client to consult the physician before receiving vaccinations

D. Anaphylactic reactions
1. Precautions
   a. Obtain an allergy history
   b. A test dose may be administered when prescribed by the physician
   c. Stay with the client during the administration of medication
   d. Monitor vital signs
   e. Have emergency equipment and medications readily available
   f. An IV line is needed for the administration of emergency medications if needed
2. Signs of anaphylactic reaction
   a. Dyspnea
   b. Chest tightness or pain
   c. Pruritis/urticaria
   d. Tachycardia
   e. Dizziness
   f. Anxiety/agitation
   g. Flushed appearance
   h. Inability to speak
   i. Nausea and abdominal pain
   j. Hypotension
   k. Decreased sensorium
   l. Cyanosis
3. Implementation for anaphylactic reaction
   a. Stop the medication
   b. Maintain airway
   c. The physician is notified
   d. An IV access is maintained with 0.9% normal saline
   e. Place the client in supine position with the legs elevated if not contraindicated
   f. Monitor vital signs
   g. Emergency medications may be prescribed

II. ALKALATING MEDICATIONS (Box 41-1)

A. Description
1. Affects the synthesis of DNA by causing cross-linking of DNA to inhibit cell reproduction
2. Cell cycle phase-nonspecific medications

B. Side effects
1. Anorexia, nausea, and vomiting
2. Stomatitis
3. Skin rash

BOX 41-1

Alkalating Medications

NITROGEN MUSTARDS
Chlorambucil (Leukeran)
Cyclophosphamide (Cytoxan)
Estramustine phosphate sodium (Emcyt)
Ifosfamide (Ifex)
Mechlorethamine HCl (Mustargen)
Melphalan (Alkeran)

NITROSOUREAS
Busulfan (Myleran)
Carmustine (BCNU)
Chlorozotozin (DCNU)
Lomustine (CCNU)
Semustine (Methyl CCNU)
Streptozocin (Zanosar)

ALKYLATING-LIKE MEDICATIONS
Altretamine (Hexalen)
Carboplatin (Paraplatin)
Cisplatin (Platinol)
Dacarbazine (DTIC)
Thiotepa

4. Pain during IV administration
5. Busulfan (Myleran) may cause hyperuricemia
6. Chlorambucil (Leukeran) and mechlorethamine HCl (Mustargen) may cause gonadal suppression and hyperuricemia
7. Cisplatin (Platinol) may cause ototoxicity, tinnitus, hypokalemia, hypocalcemia, hypomagnesemia, and nephrotoxicity
8. Cyclophosphamide (Cytoxan) may cause alopecia, gonadal suppression, hemorrhagic cystitis, and hematuria

C. Implementation
1. Monitor vital signs and the temperature for signs of infection
2. Monitor CBC, WBC, platelet, uric acid, and electrolyte counts
3. The medication is withheld if the platelet count is less than 75,000 cells/(L or the WBC count is less than 4,000 cells/(L, and notify the physician
4. Pulmonary function test results are monitored
5. Chest radiographs and renal and liver function studies are monitored
6. The client is hydrated with IV and/or oral fluids before the antineoplastic medication is administered as prescribed
7. An antiemetic is administered 30 to 60 minutes before the antineoplastic medication if prescribed
8. As prescribed, IV site pain is reduced by altering IV rates, diluting the medication, or warming the injection site to distend vein and increase blood flow
9. Monitor IV site for irritation and phlebitis
10. When the client is receiving cisplatin (Platinol), monitor the client for dizziness, tinnitus, hearing loss, incoordination, and numbness or tingling of extremities
11. Monitor for signs of hemorrhagic cystitis, such as hematuria or dysuria, during cyclophosphamide (Cytoxan) or ifosfamide (Ifex) therapy, and encourage the client to drink increased fluids (2 to 3 liters per day)
12. Instruct the client that cyclophosphamide (Cytoxan), when prescribed orally, is administered without food
13. Instruct the client to follow a diet low in purines to alkalize urine and lower uric acid blood levels
14. Instruct the client how to avoid infection
15. Instruct the client to report signs of infection or bleeding
16. Instruct the client about good oral hygiene and the use of a soft toothbrush

III. ANTITUMOR ANTIBIOTIC MEDICATIONS (Box 41-2)

A. Description
1. Interferes with DNA and ribonucleic acid synthesis
2. Cell cycle phase-nonspecific medications

B. Side effects
1. Nausea and vomiting
2. Fever
3. Bone marrow depression
4. Skin rash
5. Alopecia
6. Stomatitis
7. Gonadal suppression
8. Hyperuricemia
9. Vesication (blistering of tissue at IV site)
10. Plicamycin (Mithracin) affects bleeding time

BOX 41-2

Antitumor Antibiotic Medications

Bleomycin sulfate (Blenoxane)
Dactinomycin (Actinomycin D)
Daunorubicin (Cerubidine)
Doxorubicin (Adriamycin)
Idarubicin (Idamycin)
Mitomycin (Mutamycin)
Mitoxantrone (Novantrone)
Plicamycin (Mithracin)

11. Daunorubicin (Cerubidine) may cause congestive heart failure (CHF) and dysrhythmias
12. Doxorubicin (Adriamycin) and idarubicin (Idamycin) may cause cardiotoxicity, cardiomyopathy, and electrocardiogram (ECG) changes
13. Pulmonary toxicity can occur with bleomycin sulfate (Blenoxane)

C. Implementation
1. Monitor vital signs and temperature for signs of infection
2. Monitor CBC, WBC, platelets, uric acid, bleeding time, and electrolyte counts
3. The medication is withheld if the platelets are less than 75,000 cells/μL or the WBC count is less than 4000 cells/μL, and the physician is notified
4. Pulmonary function test results are monitored
5. The ECG is monitored for changes
6. Monitor lung sounds for rales
7. Monitor for signs of CHF, including dyspnea, crackles, peripheral edema, and weight gain
8. Chest radiographs and renal and liver function studies are monitored
9. The client is hydrated with IV and/or oral fluids before the antineoplastic medication
10. An antiemetic is administered 30 to 60 minutes before the antineoplastic medication
11. As prescribed, IV site pain is reduced by altering IV rates, diluting the medication, or warming the injection site to distend the vein and increase blood flow
12. Monitor IV site for irritation, phlebitis, and vesication
13. Monitor for myocardial toxicity, dyspnea, dysrhythmias, hypotension, and weight gain when doxorubicin (Adriamycin) or idarubicin (Idamycin) is administered
14. Monitor the pulmonary status when bleomycin (Blenoxane) is administered
15. Aspirin, anticoagulants, and thrombolytic agents are avoided when plicamycin (Mithracin) is administered

IV. ANTIMETABOLITE MEDICATIONS (Box 41-3)

A. Description
1. Halt the synthesis of cell protein
2. Replace normal proteins required for DNA synthesis
3. Cell cycle phase-specific and affect the S phase

B. Side effects
1. Anorexia, nausea, and vomiting
2. Diarrhea
3. Alopecia
4. Stomatitis
5. Depression of bone marrow
6. Cytarabine HCl (ara-C, Cytosar-U) may cause alopecia, stomatitis, hyperuricemia, and hepatotoxicity
7. 5-Fluorouracil (5-FU, Adrucil) may cause alopecia, stomatitis, diarrhea, phototoxicity reactions, and cerebellar dysfunction
8. 6-Mercaptopurine (Purinethol) may cause hyperuricemia and hepatotoxicity
9. Methotrexate (Folex) may cause alopecia, stomatitis, hyperuricemia, photosensitivity, hepatotoxicity, hematological, GI, and skin toxicity

C. Implementation
1. Monitor vital signs and temperature for signs of infection
2. Monitor the CBC, WBC, uric acid, and platelet count
3. The medication is withheld if the WBC count is less than 4000 cells/μL or the platelet count is less than 75,000 cells/μL, and the physician is notified
4. Monitor renal function studies
5. Monitor for cerebellar dysfunction
6. Monitor for photosensitivity
7. Antiemetics are administered 30 to 60 minutes before the antineoplastic medication as prescribed

BOX 41-3

Antimetabolite Medications

FOLIC ACID ANTAGONIST
Methotrexate (Folex)

PYRIMIDINE ANALOGS
Cytarabine HCl (Ara-C; Cytosar-U)
Floxuridine (FUDR)
5-Fluorouracil (5-FU; Adrucil)
Procarbazine HCl (Matulane)

PURINE ANALOGS
6-Mercaptopurine (Purinethol)
Thioguanine

MISCELLANEOUS RIBONUCLEOTIDE REDUCTASE INHIBITORS
Hydroxyurea (Hydrea)
Trimetrexate glucuronate (NeuTrexin)

ANTIMICROTUBULE
Pentostatin (Nipent)

OTHER ANTIMETABOLITE MEDICATIONS
5-Azacytidine
Cladribine (Leustatin)
Fludarabine (Fludara)
Hexamethylmelamine
Vidarabine (Vira-A)

8. Monitor the IV site for extravasation
9. Encourage fluid intake of 2 to 3 liters a day
10. Encourage good oral hygiene
11. Instruct the client how to avoid infections and bleeding
12. When the client is receiving 5-fluorouracil (5-FU, Adrucil), monitor for signs of cerebellar dysfunction, such as dizziness, weakness, and ataxia, and for stomatitis and diarrhea, which may necessitate medication discontinuation
13. When the client is receiving methotrexate (Folex) in large doses, leucovorin (folinic acid or citrovorum factor) may be prescribed to prevent fatal toxicity (known as leucovorin rescue)
14. When the client is receiving 5-fluorouracil (5-FU; Adrucil) or methotrexate (Folex), instruct the client to use sunscreen and wear protective clothing to prevent photosensitivity reactions

V. VINCA (PLANT) ALKALOIDS (Box 41-4)

A. Description
1. Prevent mitosis, causing cell death
2. Mitotic inhibitor that prevents cell division
3. Cell cycle phase-specific and act on the M phase

B. Side effects
1. Leukopenia
2. Neurotoxicity with vincristine sulfate (Oncovin), manifested as numbness and tingling in the fingers and toes
3. Ptosis
4. Hoarseness
5. Motor instability
6. Anorexia, nausea, and vomiting
7. Constipation
8. Peripheral neuropathy
9. Alopecia
10. Stomatitis
11. Hyperuricemia
12. Phlebitis at IV site

BOX 41-4

Plant (Vinca) Alkaloids

Etoposide (VePesid)
Paclitaxel (Taxol)
Docetaxel (Taxotere)
Teniposide (Vumon)
Vinblastine sulfate (Velban)
Vincristine sulfate (Oncovin)
Vindesine (Eldisine)
Vinorelbine (Navelbine)

C. Implementation
1. Monitor vital signs
2. Monitor WBC, CBC, uric acid, and platelet counts
3. Monitor for hoarseness
4. Check the eyes for ptosis
5. Monitor motor stability and initiate safety precautions as necessary
6. Monitor for neurotoxicity with vincristine sulfate (Oncovin) manifested as numbness and tingling in the fingers and toes

VI. HORMONAL MEDICATIONS AND ENZYMES (Box 41-5)

A. Description
1. Suppress the immune system and block normal hormones in hormone-sensitive tumors
2. Change the hormonal balance and slow the growth rates of certain tumors

B. Side effects
1. Anorexia, nausea, and vomiting
2. Leukopenia
3. Impaired pancreatic function with asparaginase (Elspar)
4. Gynecomastia
5. Breast swelling
6. Hot flashes
7. Weight gain
8. Hemorrhagic cystitis, hypouricemia, and hypercholesterolemia, with mitotane (Lysodren)
9. Hypertension
10. Thromboembolitic disorders
11. Edema
12. Sex characteristic alterations
13. Electrolyte imbalances

BOX 41-5

Hormonal Medications and Enzymes

ANDROGENS
Testolactone (Teslac)
Fluoxymesterone (Halotestin)

HORMONAL ANTAGONISTS, ENZYMES
Aminoglutethimide (Cytadren)
Asparaginase (Elspar)
Diethylstilbestrol (DES; Stilphostrol)
Flutamide (Eulexin)
Goserelin acetate (Zoladex)
Leuprolide acetate (Lupron)
Megestrol acetate (Megace)
Mitotane (Lysodren)
Tamoxifen citrate (Nolvadex)

14. Tamoxifen citrate (Nolvadex) may cause edema, hypercalcemia, and elevated cholesterol and triglyceride levels
15. Tamoxifen citrate (Nolvadex) decreases the effects of estrogen
16. Diethylstilbestrol (DES; Stilphostrol) may cause impotence and gynecomastia in men
17. Diethylstilbestrol (DES; Stilphostrol) may alter effects of insulin, oral anticoagulants, and oral hypoglycemic agents

C. Implementation
1. Monitor vital signs
2. Ask the client about the medications currently taking
3. Monitor serum calcium levels with androgens
4. Monitor for signs of alterations in sexual characteristics
5. Monitor pancreatic function with asparaginase (Elspar)
6. Encourage an oral intake of 2 to 3 liters of fluids per day
7. Monitor uric acid and cholesterol levels
8. Monitor for signs of hemorrhagic cystitis

VII. IMMUNOTHERAPY: BIOLOGICAL RESPONSE MODIFIERS

A. Description
1. Stimulate the immune system to recognize **cancer** cells and take action to eliminate or destroy them
2. Interleukins: help different immune system cells to recognize and destroy abnormal body cells
3. Interferons: slow down tumor cell division, stimulate proliferation and activation of natural killer cells, and help **cancer** cells resume a more normal appearance and revert to their previous characteristics

B. Colony-stimulating factors (CSF): induce more rapid bone marrow recovery after suppression by chemotherapy (Box 41-6)

BOX 41-6

Colony-Stimulating Factors (CSF)

GRANULOCYTE/MACROPHAGE COLONY-STIMULATING FACTOR (GM-CSF)
Sargramostim (Leukine, Prokine)

GRANULOCYTE COLONY-STIMULATING FACTOR (G-CSF)
Filgrastim (Neupogen)

ERYTHROPOIETIN (EPO)
Epoetin alfa (Epogen)

PRACTICE QUESTIONS

1. A client with breast cancer is being treated with cyclophosphamide (Cytoxan). The nurse plans care knowing that this medication is:
   1. Cell cycle phase-specific
   2. Cell cycle phase-nonspecific
   3. A hormonal medication
   4. An antimetabolite
2. A client with bladder cancer is receiving cisplatin (Platinol) and vincristine (Oncovin). The nurse plans care knowing that the purpose of administering both of these medications is to:
   1. Prevent gastrointestinal side effects
   2. Prevent alopecia
   3. Decrease the destruction of cells
   4. Decrease medication resistance and reduce medication toxicity
3. A nurse is instructed to initiate bleeding precautions on a client receiving an antineoplastic medication intravenously. The nurse reviews the laboratory results and would expect to note which of the following?
   1. A white blood cell (WBC) of 5000/μL
   2. A platelet count of 70,000 cells/μL
   3. A clotting time of 10 minutes
   4. An ammonia level of 20 μg/dL
4. A nurse is caring for a client who is receiving an intravenous (IV) infusion of an antineoplastic medication. During the infusion, the client complains of pain at the insertion site. On inspection of the site, the nurse notes redness and swelling and that the infusion of the medication has slowed in rate. The most appropriate nursing action is to:
   1. Elevate the extremity of the IV site and slow the infusion
   2. Apply ice and maintain the infusion rate as prescribed
   3. Administer pain medication to reduce the discomfort
   4. Notify the registered nurse
5. A client with leukemia is receiving busulfan (Myleran). Allopurinol (Zyloprim) is prescribed for the client. The nurse administers the allopurinol knowing that its purpose is to prevent:
   1. Gouty arthritis
   2. Hyperuricemia
   3. Stomatitis
   4. Diarrhea
6. A nurse is reinforcing medication instructions to a client with breast cancer who will be taking cyclophosphamide (Cytoxan). Which of the following would the nurse include in the instructions?
   1. Take the medication with food
   2. Increase fluid intake to 2000 to 3000 mL daily

3. Decrease sodium intake while taking the medication
4. Increase potassium intake while taking the medication

7. A nurse is assigned to care for a client with non-Hodgkin's lymphoma who is receiving daunorubicin (Cerubidine). Which of the following signs would indicate to the nurse that the client is experiencing a toxic effect related to the medication?
   1. Nausea and vomiting
   2. Fever
   3. Dyspnea
   4. Diarrhea

8. A nurse assigned to care for a client with testicular cancer who is receiving plicamycin (Mithracin) is preparing to administer the prescribed daily medications to the client. The nurse would question which of the following medications if noted on the client's medication record?
   1. Warfarin (Coumadin)
   2. Allopurinol (Zyloprim)
   3. Acetaminophen (Tylenol)
   4. Ondansetron (Zofran)

9. A client with squamous cell carcinoma of the larynx is receiving IV bleomycin sulfate (Blenoxane). The nurse anticipates that which of the following diagnostic studies will be prescribed for this client?
   1. Pulmonary function studies
   2. Electrocardiogram
   3. Cervical x-ray studies
   4. Echocardiogram

10. Cytarabine HCl (Cytosar-U) is prescribed for the client with acute lymphocytic leukemia. The nurse plans care knowing that this is a:
   1. Cell cycle phase-nonspecific medication
   2. Hormone medication
   3. Cell cycle phase-specific medication
   4. A medication that affects cells in any phase of the reproductive cell cycle

11. The nurse is assisting in preparing a teaching plan for the client receiving an antineoplastic medication. The nurse suggests including which of the following in the plan of care?
   1. Take aspirin (acetylsalicylic acid, ASA) as needed for headache
   2. Drink beverages containing alcohol in moderate amounts
   3. Consult with the physician before receiving immunizations
   4. Be sure to receive the flu and pneumonia vaccine

12. The client with lung cancer is receiving a high dose of methotrexate (Folex). Leucovorin (citrovorum factor, folic acid) is also prescribed. The nurse who is assisting in planning care for the client understands that the purpose of administering the leucovorin is to:
   1. Preserve normal cells
   2. Promote DNA synthesis
   3. Promote medication excretion
   4. Promote the synthesis of nucleic acids

13. The client with ovarian cancer is being treated with vincristine (Oncovin). The nurse caring for the client monitors for which side effect specific to this medication?
   1. Diarrhea
   2. Numbness and tingling in the fingers and toes
   3. Chest pain
   4. Hair loss

14. Asparaginase (Elspar), an antineoplastic agent, is prescribed for a client. The nurse assigned to care for the client collects data from the client. The nurse would report which of the following conditions contraindicated with the administration of asparaginase?
   1. Myocardial infarction
   2. Chronic obstructive pulmonary disease
   3. Diabetes mellitus
   4. Pancreatitis

15. Tamoxifen (Nolvadex) is prescribed for the client with metastatic breast carcinoma. The nurse assists in planning care knowing that the primary action of this medication is to:
   1. Increase DNA and RNA synthesis
   2. Compete with estradiol for binding to estrogen in tissues containing high concentrations of receptors
   3. Increase estrogen concentration and estrogen response
   4. Promote the biosynthesis of nucleic acids

16. The client with metastatic breast cancer is receiving tamoxifen (Nolvadex). The nurse assigned to care for the client monitors for signs of which of the following during therapy with this medication?
   1. Leukocytosis
   2. Weight loss
   3. Hypercalcemia
   4. Hypotension

17. Megestrol acetate (Megace), an antineoplastic medication, is prescribed for a client with metastatic endometrial carcinoma. The nurse assigned to the client collects data regarding the client's medical history. The nurse would report which of the following conditions that requires caution with the administration of megestrol acetate?
   1. Asthma
   2. Myocardial infarction
   3. Thrombophlebitis
   4. Gout

18. A female client with carcinoma of the breast is admitted to the hospital for treatment with intravenous vincristine (Oncovin). The client tells the nurse that she has been told by her friends that she

is going to lose all of her hair. The most appropriate nursing response is which of the following?
1. "You will not lose your hair."
2. "Your friends are correct."
3. "Hair loss may occur, but it will grow back just as it is now."
4. "Hair loss may occur, and it will grow back, but it may have a different color or texture."

19. A nurse is assisting in preparing instructions for a client who developed stomatitis after administration of a course of antineoplastic medications. Which of the following instructions does the nurse most appropriately suggest to include in the plan of care?
1. To rinse the mouth with diluted baking soda or saline
2. To avoid foods and fluids for the next 24 hours
3. To swab the mouth daily with lemon and glycerin swabs
4. To brush the teeth and use waxed dental floss three times a day

20. A client with acute myelocytic leukemia is being treated with busulfan (Myleran). The nurse monitors for signs of which of the following that specifically occurs from the administration of this medication?
1. Hyperglycemia
2. Renal failure
3. Hyperkalemia
4. Congestive heart failure

ANSWERS

1. *Answer:* 2
Rationale: Cyclophosphamide is an antineoplastic medication of the alkalating classification. Medications in this classification are cell cycle phase nonspecific and affect all phases of the reproductive cell cycle. Cell phase-specific medications affect cells only during a certain phase of the reproductive cycle.
Test-Taking Strategy: Knowledge regarding the classification of this medication and the specific action of alkalating agents is required to answer the question. If you had difficulty with this question, review the action of alkalating medications.
Level of Cognitive Ability: Comprehension
Client Needs: Physiological Integrity
Integrated Concept/Process: Nursing Process/Planning
Content Area: Pharmacology
Reference: Hodgson B, Kizior R: *Saunders nursing drug handbook 2002*, Philadelphia, 2002, WB Saunders, p. 288.

2. *Answer:* 4
Rationale: Cisplatin is an alkalating-like medication and vincristine is a vinca alkaloid. Alkalating medications are cell cycle phase nonspecific. Vinca alkaloids are cell cycle phase specific. Combinations of medications are used to enhance tumoricidal effects. Use of combination medications decrease medication resistance, increase destruction of cancer cells, and reduce medication toxicity.
Test-Taking Strategy: Use the process of elimination and knowledge regarding the rationale of combination medication therapy to answer the question. Eliminate options 1 and 2 first. It may be possible, with some specific interventions, to reduce gastrointestinal effects and alopecia, but it is unlikely that these occurrences can be prevented. Review the purpose of combination therapy if you had difficulty with this question.
Level of Cognitive Ability: Comprehension
Client Needs: Physiological Integrity
Integrated Concept/Process: Nursing Process/Planning
Content Area: Pharmacology
Reference: Hodgson B, Kizior R: *Saunders nursing drug handbook 2002*, Philadelphia, 2002, WB Saunders, p. 243.

3. *Answer:* 2
Rationale: Bleeding precautions need to be initiated when the platelet count drops. Bleeding precautions include avoiding all trauma such as rectal temperatures or injections. The normal platelet count is 150,000 to 450,000 cells/μL. The normal WBC is 5000 to 10,000/μL. When the WBC count falls, neutropenic precautions need to be implemented. The normal clotting time is 8 to 15 minutes. The normal ammonia value is 15 to 45 μg/dL.
Test-Taking Strategy: Use the process of elimination and knowledge regarding normal laboratory values. Options 1, 3, and 4 identify normal laboratory values. Remember, correlate a low platelet count with the need for bleeding precautions and a low WBC count with the need for neutropenic precaution. Review these normal laboratory values if you had difficulty with this question.
Level of Cognitive Ability: Analysis
Client Needs: Safe, Effective Care Environment
Integrated Concept/Process: Nursing Process/Data Collection
Content Area: Pharmacology
Reference: Hodgson B, Kizior R: *Saunders nursing drug handbook 2002*, Philadelphia, 2002, WB Saunders, p. 48.

4. *Answer:* 4
Rationale: When antineoplastic medications are administered by IV, great care must be taken to prevent the medication from escaping into the tissues surrounding the injection site, because pain, tissue damage, and necrosis can result. The nurse monitors for signs of extravasation, such as redness or swelling at the insertion site and a decreased infusion rate. If extravasation occurs, the registered nurse needs to be notified who will then contact the physician.
Test-Taking Strategy: Use the process of elimination and focus on the data in the question. Eliminate options 1 and 2 first.

The nurse would not slow the IV rate and the nurse would not be able to maintain the prescribed rate in this situation. Administering pain medication to reduce discomfort at an IV site is not an appropriate action. Further investigation of the cause of the discomfort is required. This leaves option 4 as the correct nursing action. Review care to the client receiving IV chemotherapy if you had difficulty with this question.
Level of Cognitive Ability: Application
Client Needs: Physiological Integrity
Integrated Concept/Process: Nursing Process/Implementation
Content Area: Pharmacology
Reference: Hodgson B, Kizior R: *Saunders nursing drug handbook 2002*, Philadelphia, 2002, WB Saunders, p. 52.

5. *Answer:* 2
Rationale: Busulfan is as alkalating medication used in the treatment of acute myelocytic leukemia and in the palliative treatment of chronic myelogenous leukemia. Hyperuricemia can result from the use of this medication because it may produce uric acid nephropathy, renal stones, and acute renal failure. Allopurinol, an antigout medication, is used with chemotherapy to prevent or treat hyperuricemia. Allopurinol is not used to prevent diarrhea.
Test-Taking Strategy: Knowledge regarding the side effects associated with busulfan and the purpose of administering allopurinol during the administration of antineoplastic medication is required to answer this question. Review both of these medications if you had difficulty with this question.
Level of Cognitive Ability: Application
Client Needs: Physiological Integrity
Integrated Concept/Process: Nursing Process/Implementation
Content Area: Pharmacology
Reference: Hodgson B, Kizior R: *Saunders nursing drug handbook 2002*, Philadelphia, 2002, WB Saunders, p. 144.

6. *Answer:* 2
Rationale: Hemorrhagic cystitis is a toxic effect that can occur with the use of cyclophosphamide. The client needs to be instructed to drink copious amounts of fluid during administration of this medication. Clients should also monitor urine output for hematuria. The medication should be taken on an empty stomach unless gastrointestinal upset occurs. Hyperkalemia can result from the use of the medication; therefore the client would not be encouraged to increase potassium intake. The client would not be instructed to alter their sodium intake.
Test-Taking Strategy: Use the process of elimination. If you correlated cyclophosphamide with hemorrhagic cystitis, then, by the process of elimination, option 2 would be selected. If you had difficulty with this question, review the toxic effects associated with this medication.
Level of Cognitive Ability: Comprehension
Client Needs: Health Promotion and Maintenance
Integrated Concept/Process: Teaching/Learning
Content Area: Pharmacology
Reference: Hodgson B, Kizior R: *Saunders nursing drug handbook 2002*, Philadelphia, 2002, WB Saunders, p. 288.

7. *Answer:* 3
Rationale: Cardiotoxicity and/or cardiomyopathy manifested as congestive heart failure (CHF) is a toxic effect of daunorubicin; as is bone marrow depression. Nausea and vomiting is a frequent side effect associated with the medication that begins a few hours after administration and lasts 24 to 48 hours. Fever is a frequent side effect and diarrhea can occur occasionally.
Test-Taking Strategy: Use the process of elimination, keeping in mind that the question is asking for a toxic effect. This concept should direct you to the option addressing a sign of CHF. Additionally, the correct option presents the most serious concern. If you had difficulty with this question, review the toxic effects associated with daunorubicin.
Level of Cognitive Ability: Analysis
Client Needs: Physiological Integrity
Integrated Concept/Process: Nursing Process/Data Collection
Content Area: Pharmacology
Reference: Hodgson B, Kizior R: *Saunders nursing drug handbook 2002*, Philadelphia, 2002, WB Saunders, p. 308.

8. *Answer:* 1
Rationale: Plicamycin is an antitumor antibiotic. Because plicamycin affects bleeding time, the use of aspirin, anticoagulants, and thrombolytic agents should be avoided. Warfarin is an anticoagulant and the risk of hemorrhage is increased if administered during plicamycin therapy. Allopurinol, an antigout medication, may be used with chemotherapy to prevent or treat hyperuricemia secondary to blood dyscrasias caused by cancer chemotherapy. Acetaminophen may be used to treat mild discomfort. Ondansetron is an antiemetic used to prevent or treat nausea and vomiting during chemotherapy.
Test-Taking Strategy: Knowledge regarding classification of the medications identified in the options is needed to answer the question. If you are unfamiliar with these medications, review these classifications and purposes for use.
Level of Cognitive Ability: Comprehension
Client Needs: Physiological Integrity
Integrated Concept/Process: Nursing Process/Implementation
Content Area: Pharmacology
Reference: Hodgson B, Kizior R: *Saunders nursing drug handbook 2002*, Philadelphia, 2002, WB Saunders, p. 895.

9. *Answer:* 1
Rationale: Bleomycin sulfate is an antineoplastic medication that can cause interstitial pneumonitis, which can progress to pulmonary fibrosis. Pulmonary function studies, along with hematological, hepatic, and renal function tests, need to be monitored. The nurse needs to monitor for dyspnea, which may indicate pulmonary toxicity. The medication will be discontinued immediately if pulmonary toxicity occurs.
Test-Taking Strategy: Use the process of elimination. Eliminate options 2 and 4 first because they are both cardiac related and therefore similar. From the remaining options, select option 1 because it relates to airway. If you had difficulty with this question, review the toxic effects of this medication.
Level of Cognitive Ability: Analysis
Client Needs: Physiological Integrity

Integrated Concept/Process: Nursing Process/Planning
Content Area: Pharmacology
Reference: Hodgson B, Kizior R: *Saunders nursing drug handbook 2002*, Philadelphia, 2002, WB Saunders, p. 131.

10. ***Answer:*** 3
Rationale: Cytarabine is an antimetabolite. Antimetabolites are classified as cell cycle specific. Alkalating medications affect all phases of the cell reproductive cycle. Hormone medications suppress the immune system and block normal hormones in hormone-sensitive tumors.
Test-Taking Strategy: Use the process of elimination. Eliminate options 1 and 4 first because they are similar. From the remaining options, recalling that this medication is an antimetabolite is required to answer the question. Review the action of this medication if you had difficulty with this question.
Level of Cognitive Ability: Application
Client Needs: Physiological Integrity
Integrated Concept/Process: Nursing Process/Planning
Content Area: Pharmacology
Reference: Hodgson B, Kizior R: *Saunders nursing drug handbook 2002*, Philadelphia, 2002, WB Saunders, p. 294.

11. ***Answer:*** 3
Rationale: Because antineoplastic medications lower the body's resistance, clients must be informed not to receive immunizations or vaccines without a physician's approval. Aspirin and aspirin-containing products need to be avoided to minimize the risk of bleeding. Alcohol needs to be avoided to minimize the risk of toxicity.
Test-Taking Strategy: Use general guidelines related to medication administration. Also, remembering that antineoplastic medications lower the body's resistance will direct you to option 3. Review client teaching points regarding these medications if you had difficulty with this question.
Level of Cognitive Ability: Application
Client Needs: Health Promotion and Maintenance
Integrated Concept/Process: Nursing Process/Planning
Content Area: Pharmacology
Reference: Hodgson B, Kizior R: *Saunders nursing drug handbook 2002*, Philadelphia, 2002, WB Saunders, p. 48.

12. ***Answer:*** 1
Rationale: High concentrations of methotrexate cause harm and damage to normal cells. To save normal cells, leucovorin is given. This is known as leucovorin rescue. Options 2, 3, and 4 do not identify the purpose for administering leucovorin.
Test-Taking Strategy: Use the process of elimination. Eliminate options 2 and 4 first because they are similar. Nucleic acids include RNA and DNA. Eliminate option 3 because increased fluids and diuretics are usually administered to promote medication excretion. If you had difficulty with this question, review leucovorin rescue.
Level of Cognitive Ability: Comprehension
Client Needs: Physiological Integrity
Integrated Concept/Process: Nursing Process/Planning
Content Area: Pharmacology
Reference: Hodgson B, Kizior R: *Saunders nursing drug handbook 2002*, Philadelphia, 2002, WB Saunders, p. 708.

13. ***Answer:*** 2
Rationale: A side effect specific to vincristine is peripheral neuropathy, which occurs in nearly every client. This can be manifested as numbness and tingling in the fingers and toes. Constipation rather than diarrhea is most likely to occur with this medication, although diarrhea may occur occasionally. Hair loss occurs with nearly all of the antineoplastic medications. Chest pain is unrelated to this medication.
Test-Taking Strategy: Use the process of elimination. Eliminate options 1 and 4 first because these side effects are associated with many of the antineoplastic agents. Note that the question asks for the side effect "specific" to this medication. Correlate peripheral neuropathy with vincristine. Review the side effects of vincristine if you had difficulty with this question.
Level of Cognitive Ability: Application
Client Needs: Physiological Integrity
Integrated Concept/Process: Nursing Process/Data Collection
Content Area: Pharmacology
Reference: Hodgson B, Kizior R: *Saunders nursing drug handbook 2002*, Philadelphia, 2002, WB Saunders, p. 1149.

14. ***Answer:*** 4
Rationale: Asparaginase is contraindicated if hypersensitivity exists and in cases of pancreatitis or if the client has a history of pancreatitis. The medication impairs pancreatic function, and pancreatic function tests should be performed before therapy begins and when a week or more has elapsed between the administration of the doses. The client needs to be monitored for signs of pancreatitis, which include nausea, vomiting, and abdominal pain.
Test-Taking Strategy: Knowledge regarding the contraindications associated with asparaginase is required to answer this question. Review this medication if you had difficulty answering this question.
Level of Cognitive Ability: Application
Client Needs: Physiological Integrity
Integrated Concept/Process: Nursing Process/Implementation
Content Area: Pharmacology
Reference: Hodgson B, Kizior R: *Saunders nursing drug handbook 2002*, Philadelphia, 2002, WB Saunders, p. 80.

15. ***Answer:*** 2
Rationale: Tamoxifen is an antineoplastic medication that competes with estradiol for binding to estrogen in tissues containing high concentrations of receptors. It is used in the treatment of metastatic breast carcinoma in women and men. It is also effective in delaying the recurrence of cancer after mastectomy. It reduces DNA synthesis and estrogen response.
Test-Taking Strategy: Use the process of elimination. Eliminate options 1 and 4 first because they are similar. Nucleic acids include DNA and RNA. From this point, select option 2 because it is unlikely that treatment of metastatic breast carcinoma would focus on increasing estrogen concentration and estrogen response. If you had difficulty with this question, review the action of this medication.
Level of Cognitive Ability: Application
Client Needs: Physiological Integrity
Integrated Concept/Process: Nursing Process/Planning
Content Area: Pharmacology

Reference: Hodgson B, Kizior R: *Saunders nursing drug handbook 2002*, Philadelphia, 2002, WB Saunders, p. 1143.

16. *Answer:* 3
Rationale: Tamoxifen may increase calcium, cholesterol, and triglyceride levels. The nurse should assess for hypercalcemia while the client is taking this medication. Signs of hypercalcemia include increased urine volume, excessive thirst, nausea, vomiting, constipation, hypotonicity of muscles, and deep bone or flank pain. Leukopenia, weight gain, and hypertension are most likely to occur.
Test-Taking Strategy: Knowledge regarding the side effects associated with this medication is required to answer this question. Review this medication if you had difficulty answering this question.
Level of Cognitive Ability: Analysis
Client Needs: Physiological Integrity
Integrated Concept/Process: Nursing Process/Data Collection
Content Area: Pharmacology
Reference: Hodgson B, Kizior R: *Saunders nursing drug handbook 2002*, Philadelphia, 2002, WB Saunders, p. 1143.

17. *Answer:* 3
Rationale: Megestrol acetate suppresses the release of luteinizing hormone from the anterior pituitary by inhibiting pituitary function and regressing tumor size. It is used with caution if the client has a history of thrombophlebitis.
Test-Taking Strategy: Knowledge regarding the cautions associated with administration of this medication is required to answer the question. Review this medication if you had difficulty answering this question.
Level of Cognitive Ability: Application
Client Needs: Physiological Integrity
Integrated Concept/Process: Nursing Process/Implementation
Content Area: Pharmacology
Reference: Hodgson B, Kizior R: *Saunders nursing drug handbook 2002*, Philadelphia, 2002, WB Saunders, p. 687.

18. *Answer:* 4
Rationale: Alopecia, hair loss, can occur after administration of many antineoplastic medications. Alopecia is reversible, but new hair growth may have a different color and texture.
Test-Taking Strategy: Use knowledge regarding side effects of antineoplastic medications and therapeutic communication techniques to answer this question. Option 1 is incorrect and option 2 is a nontherapeutic response. Recalling that new hair growth may have a different color and texture will assist in directing you to option 4. Review content related to hair loss and antineoplastic medications if you had difficulty with this question.
Level of Cognitive Ability: Application
Client Needs: Psychosocial Integrity
Integrated Concept/Process: Communication and Documentation
Content Area: Pharmacology
Reference: Hodgson B, Kizior R: *Saunders nursing drug handbook 2002*, Philadelphia, 2002, WB Saunders, p. 48.

19. *Answer:* 1
Rationale: Stomatitis, ulceration in the mouth, can occur as a result of the administration of antineoplastic medications. The client should be instructed to examine the mouth daily and to report any signs of ulceration. If stomatitis occurs, the client should be instructed to rinse the mouth with diluted baking soda or saline. Food and fluid are important and should not be restricted. The client should avoid tooth brushing and flossing when stomatitis is severe. Lemon and glycerin swabs may cause pain and further irritation.
Test-Taking Strategy: Use the process of elimination. Recalling that stomatitis involves ulcerations in the mucous membrane of the mouth will assist in eliminating the incorrect options. Eliminate option 2 first because foods and fluids would not be restricted in a client who received antineoplastic medication. Eliminate option 3 because lemon can be irritating to ulcerated lesions. Eliminate option 4 because a toothbrush and floss will also irritate ulcerations and may cause bleeding. If you had difficulty with this question, review the client teaching points related to stomatitis.
Level of Cognitive Ability: Application
Client Needs: Physiological Integrity
Integrated Concept/Process: Nursing Process/Planning
Content Area: Pharmacology
Reference: Hodgson B, Kizior R: *Saunders nursing drug handbook 2002*, Philadelphia, 2002, WB Saunders, p. 48.

20. *Answer:* 2
Rationale: Busulfan can cause an increase in the uric acid level. Hyperuricemia can produce uric acid nephropathy, renal stones, and acute renal failure. Options 1, 3, and 4 are unrelated to the administration of this medication.
Test-Taking Strategy: Knowledge regarding the adverse effects of this medication is required to answer this question. If you had difficulty with this question, review the effects of busulfan.
Level of Cognitive Ability: Application
Client Needs: Physiological Integrity
Integrated Concept/Process: Nursing Process/Data Collection
Content Area: Pharmacology
Reference: Hodgson B, Kizior R: *Saunders nursing drug handbook 2002*, Philadelphia, 2002, WB Saunders, p. 144.

REFERENCES

Clark J, Queener S, Karb V: *Pharmacologic basis of nursing practice*, ed 6, St Louis, 2000, Mosby.

Hodgson B, Kizior R: *Saunders nursing drug handbook 2002*, Philadelphia, 2002, WB Saunders.

Ignatavicius D, Workman M: *Medical-surgical: critical thinking for collaborative care*, ed 4, Philadelphia, 2002, WB Saunders.

Karch A: *Focus on nursing pharmacology*, Philadelphia, 2000, Lipincott.

Lehne R: *Pharmacology for nursing care*, ed 4, Philadelphia, 2001, WB Saunders.

UNIT X

The Adult Client with an Endocrine Disorder

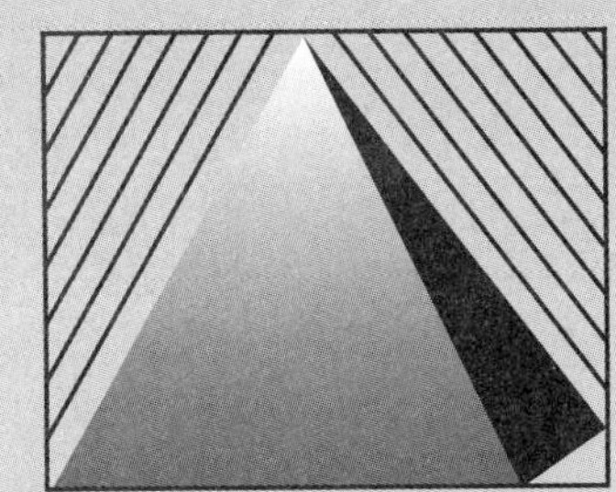

PYRAMID TERMS

Addisonian Crisis A life-threatening disorder caused by adrenal hormone insufficiency. It is precipitated by infection, trauma, stress, or surgery. Death can occur from shock, vascular collapse, or hyperkalemia.

Addison's Disease Hyposecretion of adrenal cortex hormones (glucocorticoids and mineralocorticoids) from the adrenal gland, resulting in deficiency of the steroid hormones. The condition is fatal if left untreated.

Adrenalectomy The surgical removal of an adrenal gland. Lifelong steroid replacement is necessary with a bilateral adrenalectomy. Temporary steroid replacement, up to 2 years, is necessary for a unilateral adrenalectomy.

Chvostek's Sign A spasm of the facial muscles elicited by tapping the facial nerve in the region of the parotid gland. It is noted in hypocalcemia.

Cushing's Syndrome A condition resulting from the hypersecretion of glucocorticoids from the adrenal cortex.

Dawn Phenomenon Results from a nocturnal release of growth hormone, which may cause blood glucose elevations at about 3 AM. Treatment includes administering an evening dose of intermediate-acting insulin at 10 PM.

Diabetic Ketoacidosis (DKA) A complication of diabetes mellitus that develops when a severe insulin deficiency occurs. DKA is a life-threatening condition. Hyperglycemia that progresses to ketoacidosis occurs; seen in clients with type 1 diabetes mellitus, undiagnosed diabetics, and persons who stop prescribed treatment for diabetes. It develops over several hours to days.

Diabetes Insipidus The hyposecretion of antidiuretic hormone (ADH) and a deficiency of vasopressin. Results in failure of tubular reabsorption of water in the kidneys.

Diabetes Mellitus A chronic and potentially disabling disease characterized by elevated blood glucose levels. A chronic disorder of glucose intolerance and impaired carbohydrate, protein, and lipid metabolism because of a deficiency of insulin. A deficiency of insulin results in hyperglycemia.

Graves' Disease (Hyperthyroidism) Known as thyrotoxicosis. A hyperthyroid state resulting from a hypersecretion of thyroid hormone.

Hyperglycemia Elevated blood glucose level.

Hyperosmolar Hyperglycemia Nonketotic Syndrome (HHNS) Extreme hyperglycemia without acidosis. Usually occurs in patients with non-insulin-dependent diabetes when diabetes is uncontrolled or undiagnosed, or during stress or infection. The major difference between HHNS and DKA is the lack of ketone production with HHNS. Onset is usually slow, taking from hours to days.

Hypoglycemia (Insulin Reaction) Described as a blood glucose level below 50 to 60 mg/dL. Occurs as a result of too much insulin, not enough food, or excessive activity.

Hypophysectomy The removal of the pituitary gland.

Myxedema (Hypothyroidism) A hypothyroid state resulting from a hyposecretion of thyroid hormone. The condition occurs in adulthood.

Myxedema Coma A rare but serious disorder that results from a persistent low thyroid production. It can be precipitated by acute illness, rapid withdrawal of thyroid medication, anesthesia and surgery, hypothermia, and the use of sedatives and narcotics.

Somogyi's Phenomenon A rebound phenomenon that occurs during the initial period of serum glucose control. It develops at peak insulin times and during the night. Normal or elevated blood glucose levels are present at bedtime, a decrease occurs at about 2 to 3 AM to hypoglycemic levels, and a subsequent increase occurs as a result of the production of counterregulatory hormones. Treatment includes decreasing the evening (predinner or bedtime) dose of intermediate-acting insulin, or increasing the bedtime snack.

Thyroidectomy Removal of the thyroid gland. Performed in conditions in which persistent hyperthyroidism exists.

Thyroid Storm An acute and fatal thyroid condition that occurs from manipulation of the thyroid gland during surgery and the release of thyroid hormone into the bloodstream. It can also occur from severe infection and stress.

Trousseau's Sign A sign found in hypocalcemia in which carpal spasm can be elicited by compressing the upper arm and causing ischemia to the nerves distally.

PYRAMID TO SUCCESS

The endocrine system is made up of organs or glands that secrete hormones and release them directly into the circulation. The endocrine system can be easily understood if you remember that basically one of two situations can occur: hyposecretion or hypersecretion of hormones from the organ or gland. When an excess of the hormone occurs, treatment is aimed at blocking the hormone release through medication or surgery. When a deficit of the hormone exists, treatment is aimed at replacement therapy. Pyramid points focus on diabetes mellitus—the prevention and treatment of complications and insulin therapy, hypoglycemic and hyperglycemic reactions, and diabetic ketoacidosis—Addison's disease and addisonian crisis, Cushing's syndrome, thyroid disorders, thyroid storm, and care to the client after thyroidectomy or adrenalectomy. The Integrated Concepts and Processes addressed in this unit include the Clinical Problem-Solving Process (Nursing Process), Caring, Communication and Documentation, Cultural Awareness, Self-Care, and Teaching/Learning.

CLIENT NEEDS

Safe, Effective Care Environment

Accident prevention in the client with altered mental status
Advocacy related to the client's decisions
Asepsis
Confidentiality related to the client's condition
Establishing priorities
Handling hazardous and infectious materials
Informed consent related to diagnostic tests and procedures

Health Promotion and Maintenance

Addressing lifestyle choices
Describing expected body image changes
Disease prevention related to potential complications
Health screening related to diabetes
Reinforcing instructions regarding the prescribed treatment plan
Reinforcing instructions regarding the effect of diet therapy, exercise, and administration of insulin to the diabetic client

Psychosocial Integrity

Coping mechanisms related to the endocrine disturbance
Role changes and support systems
Sensory or perceptual alterations related to the disorder
Unexpected body image disturbances

Physiological Integrity

Basic care and comfort measures
Expected effects of medication administration
Identifying potential complications
Laboratory values of diagnostic tests
Providing care in emergencies

REFERENCES

Black J, Hawks J, Keene A: *Medical-surgical nursing: clinical management for positive outcomes*, ed 6, Philadelphia, 2001, WB Saunders.
Chernecky C, Berger B: *Laboratory tests and diagnostic procedures*, ed 3, Philadelphia, 2001, WB Saunders.
Clark J, Queener S, Karb V: *Pharmacologic basis of nursing practice*, ed 6, St Louis, 2000, Mosby.
DeWit S: *Fundamental concepts and skills for nursing*, Philadelphia, 2001, WB Saunders.
Hill S, Howlett H: *Success in practical nursing: personal and vocational issues*, ed 4, Philadelphia, 2001, WB Saunders.
National Council of State Boards of Nursing. *Test plan for the National Council Licensure Examination for Practical/Vocational Nurses*, Chicago, 2001, Author.
Potter P, Perry A: *Fundamentals of nursing*, ed 5, St Louis, 2001, Mosby.
Perry A, Potter P: *Clinical nursing skills and techniques*, ed 5, St Louis, 2002, Mosby.
Wilson J: *Infection control in clinical practice*, ed 2, St Louis, 2002, Balliere Tindall.

Endocrine System

I. ANATOMY AND PHYSIOLOGY OF ENDOCRINE GLANDS (Box 42-1)
   A. Functions
      1. Maintenance and regulation of vital functions
      2. Response to stress and injury
      3. Growth and development
      4. Energy metabolism
      5. Reproduction
      6. Fluid, electrolyte, and acid-base balance
   B. Pituitary gland (Box 42-2)
      1. The master gland
      2. Located at the base of the brain
      3. Influenced by the hypothalamus
      4. Directly affects the function of other endocrine glands
      5. Promotes growth of body tissue
      6. Influences water absorption by the kidney
      7. Controls sexual development and function
   C. Adrenal gland
      1. Rests on each kidney
      2. Regulates sodium and electrolyte balance
      3. Affects carbohydrate, fat, and protein metabolism
      4. Influences the development of sexual characteristics

BOX 42-1

Endocrine Glands

Pituitary
Adrenal
Thyroid
Parathyroid
Pancreas
Ovaries
Testes

BOX 42-2

Pituitary Gland

ANTERIOR LOBE PRODUCTION
ACTH (adrenocorticotropic hormone)
TSH (thyroid-stimulating hormone)
STH (somatotropic growth-stimulating hormone)
FSH (follicle-stimulating hormone)
LH (luteinizing hormone)
PRL (prolactin)
GH (growth hormone)
MSH (melanocyte-stimulating hormone)

POSTERIOR LOBE PRODUCTION
ADH (vasopressin, antidiuretic hormone)
Oxytocin

      5. Sustains the "flight-or-fight" response
      6. Adrenal cortex
         a. The outer shell of the adrenal gland
         b. Synthesizes glucocorticoids and mineralocorticoids and secretes small amounts of sex hormones (androgens, estrogens)
      7. Adrenal medulla
         a. The inner core of the adrenal gland
         b. Works as part of the sympathetic nervous system
         c. Produces epinephrine and norepinephrine
   D. Thyroid gland
      1. Located in the anterior part of the neck
      2. Controls the rate of body metabolism and growth
      3. Produces thyroxine (T_4), triiodothyronine (T_3), and thyrocalcitonin
   E. Parathyroid gland
      1. Located near the thyroid
      2. Controls calcium and phosphorus metabolism
      3. Produces parathyroid hormone (PTH)

F. Pancreas
   1. Located posterior to the liver
   2. Influences carbohydrate metabolism
   3. Indirectly influences fat and protein metabolism
   4. Produces insulin and glucagon

G. Ovaries and testes
   1. Ovaries
      a. Located in the pelvic cavity
      b. Produces estrogen and progesterone
   2. Testes
      a. Located in the scrotum
      b. Controls the development of the secondary sex characteristics
      c. Produces testosterone

II. DIAGNOSTIC TESTS

A. Stimulation/suppression tests
   1. Stimulation testing
      a. In the client with a suspected underactivity of an endocrine gland, a stimulus may be provided to determine whether the gland is capable of normal hormone production
      b. Measured amounts of selected hormones are administered to stimulate the target gland to maximal production
      c. Hormone levels are measured
      d. Failure of the hormone to rise with stimulation indicates hypofunction
   2. Suppression tests
      a. Used when hormone levels are high or in the upper range of normal
      b. Failure of hormone production to be suppressed during standardized testing indicates hyperfunction

B. Radioactive iodine (RAI) uptake
   1. A thyroid function test that measures absorption of the iodine isotope to determine how the thyroid gland is functioning
   2. The amount of radioactivity is measured 2, 6, and 24 hours after ingestion of the capsule
   3. Normal value is 5% to 35% in 24 hours
   4. Elevated values are indicative of **hyperthyroidism**, **thyrotoxicosis**, decreased iodine intake, or increased iodine excretion
   5. Decreased values indicate a low T_4, the use of antithyroid medications, thyroiditis, myxedema, or **hypothyroidism**

C. T_3 and T_4 resin uptake test
   1. Blood tests for the diagnosis of thyroid disorders
   2. T_3 and T_4 regulate thyroid-stimulating hormone
   3. Normal values
      a. T_3: 80 to 230 ng/dL
      b. T_4: 5.0 to 12.0 μg/dL
      c. Thyroxine, free (FT_4): 0.8 to 2.4 ng/dL
   4. The T_3 is elevated in **hyperthyroidism**, decreases with the aging process, and may be decreased in **hypothyroidism**
   5. The T_4 is elevated in **hyperthyroidism** and decreased in **hypothyroidism**

D. Thyroid-stimulating hormone (TSH)
   1. Blood test used to differentiate the diagnosis of primary **hypothyroidism**
   2. Normal value is: 0.2 to 5.4 μU/mL
   3. Elevated values indicate primary **hypothyroidism**
   4. Decreased values indicate **hyperthyroidism** or secondary **hypothyroidism**

E. Thyroid scan
   1. Performed to identify nodules or growths in the thyroid gland
   2. A radioisotope of iodine or technetium is administered before scanning the thyroid gland
   3. Reassure the client that the level of radioactive medication is not dangerous to self or others
   4. Determine whether the client has received radiographic contrast agents within the last 3 months, because these may invalidate scan
   5. Check with the physician regarding discontinuing medications containing iodine for 14 days before the test and the need to discontinue thyroid medication 4 to 6 weeks before the test
   6. Instruct the client to maintain a NPO status after midnight on the day before the test; if iodine is used, the client will fast for an additional 45 minutes after ingestion of the oral isotope and the scan will be performed in 24 hours
   7. If technetium is used, it is administered by the intravenous (IV) route 30 minutes before the scan

F. Needle aspiration of thyroid tissue
   1. Aspiration of thyroid tissue for cytological examination
   2. No client preparation is necessary
   3. Light pressure is applied to the aspiration site after the procedure

G. Glucose tolerance test (GTT)
   1. Aids in the diagnosis of **diabetes mellitus**
   2. If the glucose levels peak at higher than normal at 1 and 2 hours after injection or ingestion of glucose and are slower than normal to return to fasting levels, then **diabetes mellitus** is confirmed
   3. Client preparation

a. Eat a high-carbohydrate (200- to 300-g) diet for 3 days before the test
b. Avoid alcohol, coffee, and smoking for 36 hours before testing
c. Fast for 10 to 16 hours before the test
d. Avoid strenuous exercise for 8 hours before and after the test
e. Withhold morning insulin or oral hypoglycemic medication (client with **diabetes mellitus**)
f. The test will take 3 to 5 hours, requires intravenous or oral administration of glucose, and multiple blood samples

H. Glycosylated hemoglobin
1. Description
a. Glycosylated hemoglobin is blood glucose bound to hemoglobin
b. HbA_{1c} (glycosylated hemoglobin A) is a reflection of how well blood glucose levels have been controlled for up to the previous 4 months
c. **Hyperglycemia** in a client with **diabetes mellitus** is usually a cause of an increase in HbA_{1c}
2. Values
a. Values are expressed as a percentage of total hemoglobin
b. Diabetic with good control: 7.5% or less
c. Diabetic with fair control: 7.6% to 8.9%
d. Diabetic with poor control: 9% or greater
3. Nursing consideration: fasting is not required

III. DISORDERS OF PITUITARY GLAND (Box 42-3)

A. Hypopituitarism
1. Description: hyposecretion of growth hormone (GH) by the anterior pituitary gland
2. Data collection
a. Retarded physical growth
b. Premature aging
c. Low intellectual development
d. Poor development of secondary sex characteristics

BOX 42-3

Pituitary Disorders

ANTERIOR PITUITARY
Hypopituitarism
Hyperpituitarism

POSTERIOR PITUITARY
Diabetes insipidus
SIADH (syndrome of inappropriate antidiuretic hormone)

3. Implementation
a. Provide emotional support to client and family
b. Encourage the client and family to express feelings related to altered body image
c. Prepare to administer human growth hormone (hGH)

B. Hyperpituitarism
1. Description
a. The hypersecretion of GH by the anterior pituitary gland that results in giantism or acromegaly
b. Giantism occurs in childhood before the closure of the epiphyses of the long bones
c. Acromegaly occurs in middle age, after the closure of the epiphyses of the long bones
2. Data collection
a. Large hands and feet
b. Thickening and protrusion of the jaw
c. Arthritic changes
d. Visual disturbances
e. Diaphoresis
f. Oily, rough skin
g. Organomegaly
h. Hypertension
i. Dysphagia
j. Deepening of the voice
3. Implementation
a. Provide emotional support to the client and family and encourage client and family to express feelings related to altered body image
b. Provide frequent skin care
c. Provide pharmacological and nonpharmacological interventions for joint pain
d. Prepare the client for radiation of the pituitary gland if prescribed
e. Prepare the client for **hypophysectomy** if planned

C. **Hypophysectomy**
1. Description
a. Removal of the pituitary gland
b. Complications include increased intracranial pressure, bleeding, rhinorrhea, and meningitis
2. Postoperative implementation
a. Initiate postoperative care similar to craniotomy care
b. Monitor vital signs
c. Monitor level of consciousness and neurological status
d. Monitor for increased intracranial pressure (ICP) 
e. Monitor for bleeding
f. Elevate the head of the bed
g. Monitor for adrenal insufficiency 

h. Administer corticosteroids as prescribed on time
i. Monitor fluids and electrolytes values
j. Monitor for temporary **diabetes insipidus** resulting from antidiuretic hormone (ADH) disturbances
k. Avoid water intoxication
l. Instruct the client to avoid sneezing, coughing, and blowing the nose
m. Instruct the client in the administration of prescribed medications

D. **Diabetes insipidus**
1. Description
a. The hyposecretion of ADH and a deficiency of vasopressin
b. Results in failure of tubular reabsorption of water in the kidneys
2. Data collection
a. Polyuria of 4 to 24 L per day
b. Polydipsia
c. Dehydration
d. Decreased skin turgor, dry mucous membranes
e. Inability to concentrate urine; a low urinary specific gravity of 1.006 or less
f. Fatigue, muscle pain, and weakness
g. Headache
h. Postural hypotension
i. Tachycardia
3. Implementation
a. Monitor vital signs and neurological and cardiovascular status
b. Monitor electrolyte values
c. Prepare to administer vasopressin tannate (Pitressin Tannate) or DDAVP (desmopressin acetate) as prescribed
d. Monitor input and output (I&O), weights, specific gravity of urine
e. Instruct the client to avoid foods or liquids with a diuretic-type action
f. Maintain the intake of adequate fluids
g. Instruct the client in the administration of medications as prescribed
h. Instruct the client to wear a Medic-Alert bracelet

E. **Syndrome of inappropriate antidiuretic hormone (SIADH) secretion**
1. Description
a. A disorder of the posterior pituitary gland in which a continued release of the ADH occurs
b. Results in water intoxication
2. Data collection
a. Changes in level of consciousness (LOC)
b. Mental status changes
c. Weight gain
d. Hypertension
e. Signs of fluid volume overload
f. Tachycardia
g. Anorexia, nausea, and vomiting
h. Hyponatremia
3. Implementation
a. Monitor vital signs
b. Monitor neurological and cardiac status
c. Protect the client from injury
d. Monitor I&O
e. Obtain daily weights
f. Restrict water intake as prescribed
g. Monitor fluid and electrolyte balance
h. Administer diuretics and monitor IV fluids as prescribed

IV. DISORDERS OF ADRENAL GLANDS (Box 42-4)

A. **Addison's disease**
1. Description
a. Hyposecretion of adrenal cortex hormones (glucocorticoids and mineralocorticoids)
b. The condition is fatal if left untreated
2. Data collection
a. Weakness
b. Gastrointestinal (GI) disturbances and weight loss
c. Emotional disturbances
d. Bronze pigmentation to the skin
e. Electrolyte imbalances such as hyponatremia and hyperkalemia
f. Hypotension
g. **Hypoglycemia**
h. Elevated blood urea nitrogen (BUN)
3. Implementation
a. Monitor vital signs
b. Monitor weight and I&O
c. Maintain fluid and electrolyte balance
d. Monitor for infection
e. Instruct the client in a high-protein, high-carbohydrate diet
f. Instruct the client in the avoidance of stress
g. Instruct the client to avoid individuals with an infection

BOX 42-4

Disorders of Adrenal Glands

ADRENAL CORTEX
Addison's disease
Cushing's syndrome
Aldosteronism (Conn's syndrome)

ADRENAL MEDULLA
Pheochromocytoma

h. Instruct the client in the need for lifelong corticosteroids
i. Instruct the client to avoid over-the-counter medications
j. Instruct the client to avoid strenuous exercise
k. Instruct the client to wear a Medic-Alert bracelet
l. Observe for **addisonian crisis** secondary to stress, infection, trauma, or surgery

B. **Addisonian crisis**
1. Description
a. A life-threatening disorder caused by acute adrenal insufficiency
b. It is precipitated by infection, trauma, stress, or surgery
c. Can cause hyponatremia, hyperkalemia, **hypoglycemia**, and shock
2. Data collection
a. Severe headache
b. Severe abdominal, leg, and lower back pain
c. Generalized weakness
d. Irritability and confusion
e. Severe hypotension
f. Signs of shock
3. Implementation
a. Monitor vital signs
b. Monitor neurological status, noting irritability and confusion
c. Monitor I&O
d. Monitor IV fluids as prescribed to restore electrolyte balance
e. Administer adrenocorticosteroids as prescribed on time
f. Protect the client from infection
g. Maintain bed rest and provide a quiet environment

C. **Cushing's syndrome**
1. Description
a. A condition resulting from the hypersecretion of glucocorticoids from the adrenal cortex
b. Can result from the prolonged administration of corticosteroids
2. Data collection
a. Obesity with thin extremities
b. Moonface
c. Buffalo hump
d. Fragile skin that easily bruises
e. Hirsutism (masculine characteristics in female)
f. Mood swings
g. Muscular weakness
h. Signs of infection
i. Signs of osteoporosis
j. Hypertension
k. Hypokalemia
l. **Hyperglycemia** and glycosuria
m. Elevated white blood cell (WBC) count
n. Sodium and water retention
3. Implementation
a. Monitor I&O and weight
b. Monitor for urinary glucose
c. Provide good skin care
d. Allow the client to discuss feelings related to body appearance
e. High-protein, low-calorie diet with potassium supplements
f. Prepare the client for **adrenalectomy** if prescribed
g. Prepare the client for radiation if prescribed
h. Administer hormone replacement therapy as prescribed
i. Administer steroids as prescribed if **adrenalectomy** was performed
j. Instruct the client in the administration of medications as prescribed
k. Instruct the client to avoid infection, stress, and accidents
l. Instruct the client in measures for adequate nutrition and rest

D. Aldosteronism (Conn's syndrome)
1. Description
a. A hypersecretion of aldosterone from the adrenal cortex of the adrenal gland
b. Caused by an adrenal lesion that is usually benign
2. Data collection
a. Generalized weakness
b. Increased thirst, nocturia, and polyuria
c. Weight gain and edema
d. Headache
e. Hypertension
f. Positive **Chvostek's sign**
g. Hypokalemia and hypernatremia
3. Implementation
a. Monitor vital signs
b. Monitor I&O and weight
c. Monitor muscular strength
d. Monitor electrolytes
e. Maintain sodium restriction as prescribed
f. Administer antihypertensives and potassium supplements as prescribed
g. Prepare the client for surgical removal of the tumor if prescribed

E. Pheochromocytoma
1. Description
a. A catecholamine-producing tumor, usually found in the adrenal gland but also may be found in the abdomen
b. It causes hypersecretion of the hormones of the adrenal medulla and the secretion of

excessive amounts of epinephrine and nor-epinephrine
c. It is typically a benign tumor but can be malignant
d. Surgical excision of adrenal gland is the primary treatment
2. Data collection
a. Hypertension and headaches
b. Hypermetabolism
c. Diaphoresis, palpitations, and tachycardia
d. Apprehension
e. Emotional instability
f. **Hyperglycemia** and glycosuria
g. Pain in the chest or abdomen with nausea and vomiting
h. Weight loss
3. Implementation
a. Monitor vital signs
b. Monitor cardiovascular, neurological, and renal status
c. Monitor for hypertensive attacks as hypertension can precipitate a cerebrovascular accident or sudden blindness
d. Keep phentolamine (Regitine) at the bedside for treatment of a hypertensive crisis
e. Prepare to administer medication as prescribed to control the blood pressure
f. Be alert to stimuli that can precipitate a hypertensive crisis such as increased abdominal pressure, micturition, and vigorous abdominal palpation
g. Avoid preoperative use of opiates because they can precipitate a hypertensive crisis
h. Monitor urine for glucose and acetone
i. Promote rest and nonstressful environment
j. Provide a diet high in calories, vitamins, and minerals
k. Prohibit caffeine-containing beverages and food

F. **Adrenalectomy**
1. Description
a. The surgical removal of an adrenal gland
b. Lifelong steroid replacement is necessary with a bilateral **adrenalectomy**
c. Temporary steroid replacement, up to 2 years, is necessary for a unilateral **adrenalectomy**
d. Catecholamine levels drop as a result of surgery, which can result in cardiovascular collapse, hypotension, and shock; the client needs to be monitored closely
e. Hemorrhage can also occur as a result of the high vascularity of the adrenal glands
2. Preoperative implementation
a. Prepare the client for the surgical procedure
b. Monitor electrolytes and correct electrolyte imbalances
c. Monitor for cardiac irregularities
d. Monitor for **hyperglycemia**
e. Protect the client from infections
f. Administer steroids as prescribed
3. Postoperative implementation
a. Monitor vital signs
b. Monitor I&O and if urinary output is less that 30 mL per hour notify physician because this may be indicative of impending shock and renal failure
c. Monitor daily weights
d. Monitor electrolytes
e. Monitor for signs of shock and hemorrhage particularly during first 24 to 48 hours
f. Check the dressing
g. Monitor for paralytic ileus as manifested by abdominal distention and pain, nausea, vomiting, and diminished or absent bowel sounds because paralytic ileus can develop from internal bleeding
h. Monitor IV fluids as prescribed to maintain blood volume
i. Administer pain medication as prescribed, remembering that meperidine (Demerol) can cause hypotension
j. Administer steroid replacement as prescribed
k. Instruct the client in the importance of steroid therapy after surgery

V. DISORDERS OF THE THYROID GLAND (Box 42-5)

A. **Hypothyroidism (Myxedema)**
1. Description
a. A hypothyroid state resulting from a hyposecretion of thyroid hormone
b. Occurs during adulthood
2. Data collection
a. Slowed rate of body metabolism
b. Lethargy and fatigue
c. Intolerance to cold
d. Weight gain
e. Dry skin and hair
f. Loss of body hair

BOX 42-5

Disorders of the Thyroid Gland

Hypothyroidism (myxedema)
Hyperthyroidism (Graves' disease)

g. Bradycardia
h. Constipation
i. Generalized puffiness and nonpitting edema
j. Forgetfulness and loss of memory
k. Menstrual disturbances
l. Cardiac disorders

3. Implementation
   a. Monitor vital signs
   b. Monitor for cardiac complications
   c. Administer thyroid replacement medication as prescribed
   d. Instruct the client in low-calorie, low-cholesterol, low-saturated fat diet
   e. Monitor the client for anorexia and constipation
   f. Provide roughage and fluids to prevent constipation
   g. Provide a warm environment for the client
   h. Avoid sedatives and narcotics because of intolerance
   i. Monitor for overdose of thyroid medications characterized by tachycardia, restlessness, nervousness, and insomnia

B. **Myxedema coma**
1. Description
   a. A rare but serious disorder that results from persistent low thyroid production
   b. It can be precipitated by acute illness, rapid withdrawal of thyroid medication, anesthesia and surgery, hypothermia, and the use of sedatives and narcotics
2. Data collection
   a. Hypotension
   b. Hypothermia
   c. Bradycardia
   d. Mental depression
   e. Mood swings
   f. Hyponatremia
   g. **Hypoglycemia**
   h. Coma
3. Implementation
   a. Maintain a patent airway
   b. Monitor vital signs and LOC
   c. Monitor the client's temperature frequently
   d. Monitor IV fluids as prescribed
   e. Monitor electrolytes and glucose level
   f. Keep the client warm
   g. Monitor for changes in mental status
   h. Administer corticosteroids as prescribed
   i. Avoid the use of sedatives and hypnotics

C. **Hyperthyroidism (Graves' disease)**
1. Description
   a. A hyperthyroid state resulting from a hypersecretion of thyroid hormone
   b. Also known as thyrotoxicosis
2. Data collection
   a. Increased rate of body metabolism
   b. Enlarged thyroid gland (goiter)
   c. Cardiac dysrhythmias such as tachycardia and palpitations
   d. Protruding eyeballs (exophthalmos)
   e. Hypertension
   f. Heat intolerance
   g. Diaphoresis
   h. Weight loss
   i. Smooth soft skin and hair
   j. Nervousness and fine tremors of hands
   k. Personality changes
   l. Irritability and agitation
   m. Mood swings
3. Implementation
   a. Provide adequate rest
   b. Administer sedatives as prescribed
   c. Provide a cool and quiet environment
   d. Obtain daily weights
   e. Provide a high-calorie diet
   f. Avoid stimulants
   g. Provide psychosocial support
   h. Administer antithyroid medications as prescribed to block thyroid synthesis
   i. Administer iodine preparations as prescribed, which inhibit the release of thyroid hormone
   j. Administer propranolol (Inderal) for tachycardia as prescribed
   k. Prepare the client for radioiodine therapy as prescribed to destroy thyroid cells
   l. Prepare the client for **thyroidectomy** if prescribed

D. **Thyroid storm**
1. Description
   a. An acute and fatal thyroid condition that occurs from manipulation of the thyroid gland during surgery and the release of thyroid hormone into the bloodstream
   b. It can also occur from severe infection and stress
2. Data collection
   a. Fever
   b. Diaphoresis
   c. Dehydration
   d. Tachycardia
   e. Congestive heart failure and pulmonary edema
   f. Nausea, vomiting, and diarrhea
   g. Jaundice
   h. Tremors
   i. Irritability, agitation, and restlessness
   j. Delirium and coma
3. Implementation
   a. Monitor vital signs

b. Decrease temperature avoiding the use of salicylates because they increase free thyroid hormone levels
c. Avoid palpating the thyroid gland
d. Monitor I&O
e. Monitor fluid and electrolyte balance
f. Monitor for dehydration and overhydration
g. Monitor pulmonary and cardiac status
h. Administer iodine preparations, which inhibit the release of thyroid hormone, as prescribed
i. Administer propranolol (Inderal) for tachycardia and to reverse toxic manifestations of **thyroid storm** as prescribed
j. Administer glucocorticoids as prescribed to allay stress effects
k. Administer cardiac medications as prescribed to decrease heart activity

E. **Thyroidectomy**

1. Description
   a. Removal of the thyroid gland
   b. Performed in conditions where persistent hyperthyroidism exists
2. Preoperative implementation
   a. Obtain vital signs
   b. Obtain weight
   c. Monitor electrolyte levels
   d. Monitor for **hyperglycemia** and glycosuria
   e. Monitor level of consciousness
   f. Monitor for signs of **thyroid storm**
   g. Administer antithyroid medications as prescribed to deplete iodine and hormones
   h. Administer iodine as prescribed to decrease vascularity of the thyroid gland

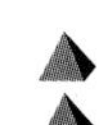

3. Postoperative implementation
   a. Monitor for respiratory distress
   b. Have tracheotomy set, oxygen, and suction at the bedside
   c. Maintain semi-Fowler's position
   d. Monitor for signs of bleeding
   e. Check the dressing anteriorly and at the back of the neck
   f. Limit talking and assess the level of hoarseness
   g. Monitor for laryngeal nerve damage as evidenced by respiratory obstruction, dysphonia, high-pitched voice, stridor, dysphagia, and restlessness
   h. Monitor for signs of tetany, which can be due to trauma to the parathyroid gland
   i. Prepare for the administration of calcium gluconate as prescribed for tetany (Box 42-6)

BOX 42-6

Signs of Tetany

Positive Chvostek's sign
Positive Trousseau's sign
Numbness of extremities and spasm of glottis
Irritability
Wheezing and dyspnea
Visual disturbances
Muscle and abdominal cramps

VI. DISORDERS OF THE PARATHYROID GLAND

A. Hypoparathyroidism

1. Description
   a. A condition caused by hyposecretion of parathyroid hormone by the parathyroid gland
   b. Can occur after **thyroidectomy** from removal of parathyroid tissue
2. Data collection
   a. Hypocalcemia and hyperphosphatemia
   b. Numbness and tingling in the face
   c. Muscle cramps and cramps in the abdomen or in the extremities
   d. Positive **Trousseau's sign** or **Chvostek's sign**
   e. Signs of overt tetany such as bronchospasm, laryngospasm, carpopedal spasm, dysphagia, photophobia, cardiac dysrhythmias, seizures
   f. Hypotension
   g. Anxiety, irritability, depression
3. Implementation
   a. Monitor vital signs
   b. Monitor for signs of hypocalcemia and tetany
   c. Initiate seizure precautions
   d. Place a tracheotomy set, oxygen, and suctioning at the bedside
   e. Prepare for the administration of IV calcium gluconate or calcium chloride for hypocalcemia
   f. Provide a high-calcium and low-phosphorus diet
   g. Instruct the client in the administration of calcium supplements as prescribed
   h. Instruct the client in the administration of vitamin D supplements as prescribed; vitamin D enhances the absorption of calcium from the GI tract
   i. Instruct the client in the administration of phosphate binders as prescribed to promote the excretion of phosphate through the GI tract

j. Instruct the client to wear a Medic-Alert bracelet

B. Hyperparathyroidism
1. Description: A condition caused by hypersecretion of parathyroid hormone by the parathyroid gland
2. Data collection
a. Hypercalcemia and hypophosphatemia
b. Fatigue and muscle weakness
c. Skeletal pain and tenderness
d. Bone deformities that result in pathological fractures
e. Anorexia, nausea, vomiting, epigastric pain
f. Weight loss
g. Constipation
h. Hypertension
i. Cardiac dysrhythmias
j. Renal stones
3. Implementation
a. Monitor vital signs, particularly the blood pressure (BP)
b. Monitor for cardiac dysrhythmias
c. Monitor I&O and for signs of renal stones
d. Monitor for skeletal pain; move client slowly and carefully
e. Encourage fluids
f. Administer furosemide (Lasix) as prescribed to lower calcium levels
g. Monitor IV normal saline, prescribed to lower calcium levels
h. Administer phosphates as prescribed, which interfere with calcium absorption
i. Administer calcitonin (Calcimar) as prescribed to decrease skeletal calcium release and increase renal clearance of calcium
j. Administer calcium chelators as prescribed to lower calcium levels
k. Monitor calcium and phosphorus levels
l. Notify the physician immediately if a precipitous drop in the calcium level occurs; assess for tingling and numbness in the muscles and signs of hypocalcemia
m. Prepare the client for parathyroidectomy as prescribed

C. Parathyroidectomy
1. Description: removal of one or more of the parathyroid glands
2. Implementation preoperative
a. Monitor electrolytes, calcium, phosphate, and magnesium levels
b. Ensure that calcium levels are decreased to near normal
c. Inform the client that talking may be painful for the first day or two after surgery
3. Postoperative implementation
a. Monitor for respiratory distress
b. Place a tracheotomy set, oxygen, and suctioning at the bedside
c. Monitor vital signs
d. Place the client in semi-Fowler's position
e. Monitor the neck dressing for bleeding; 1 to 5 mL serosanguineous drainage is expected
f. Monitor for hypocalcemic crisis as evidenced by tingling and twitching in the extremities and face
g. Monitor for positive **Trousseau's sign** and **Chvostek's sign,** which signal the potential of tetany
h. Monitor for laryngeal nerve damage
i. Monitor for changes in voice pattern and hoarseness
j. Instruct the client in the administration of calcium and vitamin D as prescribed

VII. DISORDERS OF THE PANCREAS

A. **Diabetes mellitus** (Box 42-7)
1. Description
a. A chronic disorder of impaired glucose intolerance and carbohydrate, protein, and lipid metabolism; caused by a deficiency of insulin
b. A deficiency of insulin results in **hyperglycemia**
c. Macrovascular complications include coronary disease, cardiomyopathy, hypertension, cerebrovascular disease, peripheral vascular disease, and infection
d. Microvascular complications include retinopathy, nephropathy, and neuropathy
2. Data collection
a. Polyuria
b. Polydipsia
c. Polyphagia
d. **Hyperglycemia**
e. Weight loss
f. Blurred vision
g. Slow wound healing
h. Vaginal infections
i. Weakness and paresthesias
j. Signs of inadequate circulation to the feet

BOX 42-7

Major Types of Diabetes Mellitus

Type 1: insulin-dependent diabetes mellitus
Type 2: non-insulin-dependent diabetes mellitus

3. Diet
   a. The total number of calories is individualized on the basis of the client's current or desired weight and the presence of other existing health problems
   b. As prescribed by the physician, the client may be advised to follow the food exchange from the American Diabetic Association diet or the dietary guidelines for Americans (Food Guide Pyramid) issued by the U.S. Departments of Agriculture and Health and Human Services
   c. Incorporate diet into individual client needs, lifestyle, and cultural and socioeconomic patterns
4. Exercise
   a. Lowers blood glucose level
   b. Reduces cardiovascular risks
   c. Improves circulation and muscle tone
   d. Decreases total cholesterol and triglyceride levels
   e. Encourages weight loss
   f. Instruct the client in dietary adjustments when exercising; dietary adjustments are individualized
   g. Instruct the client to monitor blood glucose before exercising; if the client plans to participate in extended periods of exercise, blood glucose levels should be checked before, during, and after the exercise period
   h. Initially, the client who requires insulin should be instructed to eat a 15-g carbohydrate snack (a fruit exchange) or a snack of complex carbohydrate with a protein before engaging in moderate exercise, to prevent **hypoglycemia**
   i. If the client requires extra food during exercise to prevent **hypoglycemia**, it need not be deducted from the regular meal plan
   j. If the blood glucose level is greater than 250 mg/dL and urinary ketones are present, the client is instructed not to exercise until the blood glucose is closer to normal and urinary ketones are negative
5. Oral hypoglycemic medications
   a. Prescribed for clients with **diabetes mellitus** type 2
   b. Assess the client's knowledge of **diabetes mellitus** and the use of oral antidiabetic agents
   c. Assess vital signs and blood glucose levels
   d. Find out about the medications that the client is currently taking
   e. Aspirin, alcohol, sulfonamides, oral contraceptives, and monoamine oxidase inhibitors (MAOIs) increase the hypoglycemic effect
   f. Glucocorticoids, thiazide diuretics, and estrogen increase blood glucose levels
   g. Instruct the client how to recognize symptoms of **hypoglycemia** and **hyperglycemia**
   h. Instruct the client to avoid over-the-counter medications unless prescribed by the physician
   i. Instruct the client not to ingest alcohol with sulfonylureas
   j. Inform the client that insulin may be needed during stress, surgery, or infection
   k. Instruct the client of the necessity to comply with the prescribed medication regimen
   l. Advise the client to wear a Medic-Alert bracelet
6. Insulin
   a. Used in the treatment of type 1 **diabetes mellitus** and in type 2 **diabetes mellitus** when diet and weight control therapy have failed to maintain satisfactory blood glucose levels
   b. Regular insulin is used in the emergency treatment of **diabetic ketoacidosis**
   c. Aspirin, alcohol, oral anticoagulants, oral hypoglycemics, beta-blockers, tricyclic antidepressants, tetracycline, and MAOIs increase the hypoglycemic effect of insulin
   d. Glucocorticoids, thiazide diuretics, thyroid agents, oral contraceptives, and estrogen increase blood glucose levels
   e. Illness, infection, and stress increase the need for insulin, and insulin should not be withheld during illness, infection, or stress because **hyperglycemia** and ketoacidosis can result
   f. Instruct the client to recognize symptoms of **hypoglycemia** and **hyperglycemia**
   g. The peak action time of insulin is very important because of the possibility of hypoglycemic reactions occurring during that time

B. Complications of insulin therapy
1. Local allergic reactions
   a. Redness, swelling, tenderness, and induration or a wheal at the site of injection 1 to 2 hours after administration
   b. Usually occurs during the early stages of insulin therapy
   c. Instruct the client to avoid the use of alcohol to cleanse the skin before injection
   d. The physician may prescribe an antihistamine to be taken 1 hour before injection
2. Insulin lipodystrophy
   a. Lipoatrophy is loss of subcutaneous fat and appears as slight dimpling or more serious pitting of subcutaneous fat; the use of

human insulin helps to prevent this complication
   b. Liperhypertrophy is the development of fibrofatty masses at the injection site and is caused by repeated use of an injection site
   c. Instruct the client to avoid injecting insulin into affected sites
   d. Instruct the client about the importance of rotating insulin injection sites
3. Insulin resistance
   a. The client taking insulin develops immune antibodies that bind the insulin, thereby decreasing the insulin available for use in the body
   b. Treatment consists of administering a purer insulin preparation; occasionally prednisone is prescribed to block the production of antibodies
4. **Dawn phenomenon**
   a. Results from a nocturnal release of growth hormone, which may cause the blood glucose to begin to rise at about 3:00 AM
   b. Treatment includes administering an evening dose of intermediate-acting insulin at 10:00 PM
5. **Somogyi's phenomenon**
   a. A rebound phenomenon that occurs during the initial period of blood glucose control; develops at peak insulin times and during the night
   b. Normal or elevated blood glucose levels are present at bedtime, a decrease occurs at about 2:00 to 3:00 AM to hypoglycemic levels, and a subsequent increase occurs as a result of the production of counterregulatory hormones
   c. Treatment includes decreasing the evening (predinner or bedtime) dose of intermediate-acting insulin, or increasing the bedtime snack
6. **Insulin waning**
   a. A progressive rise in the blood glucose level from bedtime to morning
   b. Treatment includes increasing the evening (predinner or bedtime) dose of intermediate- or long-acting insulin, or instituting a dose of insulin before the evening meal if one is not already prescribed

C. Insulin administration
1. Subcutaneous injections and mixing insulin: refer to Chapter 43
2. Insulin pens
   a. A device that uses a small, prefilled insulin cartridge that is loaded into a penlike holder; a disposable needle is attached to the device for injection
   b. The client inserts the needle for injection, and the insulin is delivered by dialing in a dose or pushing a button for every 1- to 2-unit increment administered
3. Jet injectors
   a. A device that delivers insulin through the skin under pressure in an extremely fine stream
   b. Insulin administered by this device usually absorbs faster
   c. Can cause bruising at the site of insulin delivery
4. Insulin pumps
   a. Continuous subcutaneous insulin infusion is administered by an externally worn device that contains a syringe attached to a long, thin, narrow-lumened tube with a needle or Teflon catheter attached to the end
   b. The client inserts the needle or Teflon catheter into the subcutaneous tissue (usually on the abdomen) and secures it with tape or a transparent dressing; the pump is worn either on a belt or in a pocket; the needle or Teflon catheter is changed at least every 3 days
   c. A continuous basal rate of insulin infuses, and on the basis of the blood glucose level, the anticipated food intake, and the activity level, the client delivers a bolus of insulin before each meal
   d. The pump uses Regular insulin (buffered to prevent the precipitation of insulin crystals within the catheter); some physicians may prescribe the use of Lispro insulin
5. Implantable insulin delivery
   a. An insulin pump is implanted in the peritoneal cavity, where insulin can be absorbed in a more physiological manner
   b. Not widely used because mechanical problems associated with the pump, the catheter, and the insulin delivery exist
6. Inhalant insulin delivery
   a. Regular insulin is administered in an inhaler during inspiration
   b. A less effective method of administration; absorption across the nasal mucosa is rapid; however, only a small amount of insulin is actually absorbed
7. Pancreas transplants
   a. The goal of pancreatic transplantation is to halt or reverse the complications of **diabetes mellitus**
   b. The pancreas is transplanted into the peritoneal cavity; the exocrine secretions drain into the urinary bladder

c. Performed on a limited number of clients (mostly clients receiving kidney transplantations simultaneously)
d. Immunosuppressive therapy is prescribed to prevent and treat rejection

D. Self-monitoring of blood glucose
1. Provides the client with the current blood glucose level and information to maintain good glycemic control
2. Requires a finger prick to obtain a drop of blood for testing
3. Must be used with caution in clients with diabetic retinopathy and neuropathy
4. Instruct the client in the proper procedure for obtaining the blood glucose level
5. Inform the client that the procedure must be carried out precisely to obtain accurate results
6. Stress the importance of following the manufacturer's instructions
7. Stress the importance of handwashing before and after performing the procedure to prevent infection
8. Instruct the client to calibrate the monitor as instructed by the manufacturer
9. Instruct the client to check the expiration date on the test strips
10. Instruct the client that if the blood glucose results do not seem reasonable, to reread the instructions, reassess technique, check the expiration date of the test strips, and perform the procedure again to verify results

E. Urine testing
1. A less reliable indicator as compared with blood glucose monitoring
2. Instruct the client in the procedure for testing urine for glucose and ketones
3. Teach the client that the second voided urine specimen is most accurate
4. The presence of ketones may indicate impending **ketoacidosis**
5. Urine ketone testing should be performed during illness and whenever the client with type 1 **diabetes mellitus** has glycosuria or persistently elevated blood glucose levels (greater than 240 mg/dL for two consecutive testing periods)

VIII. ACUTE COMPLICATIONS OF DIABETES MELLITUS

A. **Hypoglycemia**
1. Description
a. Occurs when the blood glucose level falls to less than 50 to 60 mg/dL
b. Caused by too much insulin or oral hypoglycemic agents, too little food, or excessive activity
2. Data collection (Table 42-1)
a. Mild **hypoglycemia:** a capillary blood glucose level of 40 to 60 mg/dL
b. Moderate **hypoglycemia:** a capillary blood glucose level of 20 to 40 mg/dL
c. Severe **hypoglycemia:** the client is unconscious or experiencing seizures
3. Implementation
a. Give 10 to 15 g of a fast-acting simple carbohydrate (Box 42-8)

BOX 42-8

Simple Carbohydrates to Treat Hypoglycemia

Three or four commercially prepared glucose tablets
4 to 6 ounces of fruit juice or regular soda
6 to 10 Life Savers or hard candy
2 to 3 teaspoons of sugar or honey

TABLE 42-1

Signs and Symptoms of Hypoglycemia

Mild	Moderate	Severe
Sweating	Inability to concentrate	Disoriented behavior
Tremor	Headache	Difficulty arousing from sleep
Tachycardia	Light-headedness	Loss of consciousness
Palpitations	Confusion	Seizures
Nervousness	Memory lapses	
Hunger	Numbness of the lips and tongue	
	Slurred speech	
	Impaired coordination	
	Emotional changes	
	Irrational or combative behavior	
	Double vision	
	Drowsiness	

b. Retest the blood glucose level in 15 minutes, and retreat if it is less than 70 to 75 mg/dL
c. If symptoms persist for more than 15 minutes after the initial treatment, the treatment is repeated even if testing of blood glucose is not possible
d. Once symptoms resolve, a snack containing protein and carbohydrate, such as milk or cheese and crackers, is recommended unless the client plans to eat a regular meal or snack within 30 to 60 minutes

4. Implementation for severe **hypoglycemia**
   a. If the client is unconscious and cannot swallow, an injection of glucagon is administered either subcutaneously or intramuscularly
   b. After the injection of glucagon, it may take up to 20 minutes for the client to regain consciousness
   c. A simple carbohydrate followed by a snack should be given to prevent recurrence of **hypoglycemia**
   d. In the hospital or emergency department, the client may be treated with an IV injection of 25 to 50 mL of 50% dextrose in water
   e. The client needs to be instructed to always carry some form of fast-acting simple carbohydrate with him or her
   f. If the client has a hypoglycemic reaction and does not have any of the recommended emergency foods available, any available food should be eaten; high-fat foods slow the absorption of glucose, and the hypoglycemic symptoms may not resolve quickly
   g. Family members need to be instructed on the administration of glucagon
   h. The client is instructed that if a severe hypoglycemic reaction occurs, the physician needs to be notified

B. **Diabetic ketoacidosis (DKA)**
1. Description
   a. A life-threatening complication of **diabetes mellitus** that develops when a severe insulin deficiency occurs
   b. The main clinical manifestations include **hyperglycemia**, dehydration and electrolyte loss, and acidosis
   c. The major causes include a decreased or missed dose of insulin, illness or infection, and undiagnosed and untreated **diabetes mellitus**
   d. It develops over a period of several hours to days
2. Data collection (Box 42-9)
   a. Blood glucose levels may vary from 300 to 800 mg/dL
   b. Low serum bicarbonate and a low pH
   c. Sodium and potassium levels may be low, normal, or high depending on the amount of water loss and dehydration status
3. Implementation
   a. Restore circulating volume and protect against cerebral, coronary, or renal hypoperfusion
   b. Treat dehydration with rapid IV infusions of 0.9% or 0.45% saline as prescribed; dextrose is added to IV fluids, such as D5NS (dextrose 5% in normal saline) or 5% dextrose and 0.45% saline, when the blood glucose level reaches 250 to 300 mg/dL
   c. Treat **hyperglycemia** with IV Regular insulin administration as prescribed
   d. Correct electrolyte imbalance (potassium level may be elevated as a result of dehydration and acidosis)
   e. Monitor potassium level closely because when the client receives treatment for the dehydration and acidosis, the serum potassium will decrease and potassium replacement may be required
4. Insulin IV administration
   a. Regular insulin only is used for IV administration 
   b. A dose of 5 to 10 units of Regular insulin by IV bolus may be prescribed before a continuous infusion is begun
   c. The IV dose of Regular insulin for continuous infusion is mixed in 0.9% or 0.45% saline as prescribed
   d. The insulin solution is flushed through the entire IV infusion set and the first 50 mL of solution is discarded before connecting and

BOX 42-9

Signs and Symptoms of Diabetic Ketoacidosis

Polyuria
Polydipsia
Blurred vision
Weakness
Headache
Hypotension
Weak, rapid pulse
Anorexia, nausea, vomiting, and abdominal pain
Acetone breath (a fruity odor)
Kussmaul respirations
Mental status changes

administering it to the client; insulin molecules adhere to the glass and plastic of IV infusion sets
e. The insulin infusion is always placed on an IV infusion controller
f. Monitor vital signs and for signs of fluid overload
g. Monitor potassium levels, glucose levels, urinary output, and for signs of increased intracranial pressure
h. If the blood glucose level falls too far, too fast before the brain has time to equilibrate, water is pulled from the blood to the cerebrospinal fluid and the brain, causing cerebral edema and increased intracranial pressure
i. The potassium level will fall rapidly within the first hour of treatment as the dehydration and the acidosis are treated
j. Potassium is administered IV as prescribed when the potassium reaches normal level to prevent hypokalemia; ensure adequate renal function before administering potassium

5. Client education (Box 42-10)

C. **Hyperglycemia hyperosmolar nonketotic syndrome (HHNS)**

1. Description
a. Extreme **hyperglycemia** without ketosis and acidosis
b. Occurs most often in individuals with type 2 **diabetes mellitus**
c. The major difference between **HHNS** and **DKA** is that ketosis and acidosis do not occur with **HHNS**
d. Onset is usually slow and takes hours to days to develop
2. Data collection
a. Blood glucose level is from 600 to 1200 mg/dL
b. Hypotension
c. Dehydration
d. Tachycardia
e. Mental status changes
f. Neurological deficits
g. Seizures
3. Implementation
a. Similar to the treatment for **DKA**
b. Includes fluid replacement, correction of electrolyte imbalances, and insulin administration
c. Insulin plays a less critical role in the treatment of **HHNS** than it does for the treatment of **DKA** because insulin is not needed for reversal of acidosis in **HHNS**

BOX 42-10

Client Education: Guidelines During Illness

Take insulin or oral hypoglycemic medications as prescribed
Test blood glucose and test the urine for ketones every 3 to 4 hours
If the usual meal plan cannot be followed, substitute soft foods six to eight times a day
If vomiting, diarrhea, or fever occurs, consume liquids every 1/2 to 1 hour to prevent dehydration and to provide calories
Notify the physician if vomiting, diarrhea, or fever persists, if blood glucose levels are greater than 250 to 300 mg/dL, when ketonuria is present for more than 24 hours, when unable to take food or fluids for a period of 4 hours, or when illness persists for more than 2 days

IX. CHRONIC COMPLICATIONS OF DIABETES MELLITUS

A. Diabetic retinopathy
1. Description
a. A chronic and progressive noninflammatory impairment of the retinal circulation that eventually causes hemorrhage
b. Permanent vision changes and blindness can occur
c. The client has difficulty with carrying out the daily tasks of blood glucose testing and insulin injections
2. Data collection
a. A change in vision caused by ruptured vessels
b. Blurred vision resulting from macular edema
c. Sudden loss of vision as a result of retinal detachment
d. Cataracts resulting from lens opacity
3. Implementation
a. Maintain safety
b. Early prevention by the control of hypertension and blood glucose levels
c. Photocoagulation (laser therapy) to remove hemorrhagic tissue to decrease scarring
d. Vitrectomy to remove vitreous hemorrhages and thus decrease tension on the retina, preventing detachment
e. Cataract removal with lens implant

B. Diabetic nephropathy
1. Description: a progressive decrease in kidney function
2. Data collection
a. Microalbuminuria
b. Thirst

c. Fatigue
d. Anemia
e. Weight loss
f. Signs of malnutrition
g. Frequent urinary tract infections
h. Signs of a neurogenic bladder

3. Implementation
   a. Early prevention by the control of hypertension and blood glucose levels
   b. Assess vital signs
   c. Monitor I&O
   d. Monitor BUN and creatinine levels, and for albuminuria
   e. Restrict dietary protein, sodium, and potassium as prescribed
   f. Avoid nephrotoxic medications
   g. Prepare the client for dialysis procedures as prescribed
   h. Prepare the client for kidney transplants as prescribed
   i. Prepare the client for pancreas transplants as prescribed

C. Diabetic neuropathy
1. Description
   a. General deterioration of the nervous system
   b. Complications include foot injuries resulting from trauma and the development of ulcers, frequently requiring amputation
2. Data collection
   a. Paresthesias
   b. Decreased or absent reflexes
   c. Decreased sensation to vibration or light touch
   d. Pain, aching, and burning in the lower extremities
   e. Poor peripheral pulses
   f. Skin breakdown and signs of infection
   g. Dizziness and postural hypotension
   h. Nausea and vomiting
   i. Diarrhea or constipation
   j. Incontinence
   k. Dyspareunia
   l. Impotence
   m. Hypoglycemic unawareness
3. Implementation
   a. Early prevention by the control of hypertension and blood glucose levels
   b. Careful foot care to prevent trauma (Box 42-11)
   c. Apply topical medication for temporary relief of neuralgia, if prescribed
   d. Administer medications as prescribed for pain relief
   e. Initiate bladder-training programs
   f. Instruct in the use of estrogen-containing lubricants for women with dysparunia
   g. Prepare the male client with impotence for penile injections or implantable devices as prescribed
   h. Prepare for surgical decompression for compression lesions related to the cranial nerves as prescribed

BOX 42-11

Preventive Foot Care Instructions

Meticulous skin care and proper foot care
Inspect feet daily and monitor feet for redness, swelling, or break in skin integrity
Notify the physician if redness or a break in the skin occurs
Avoid thermal injuries from hot water, heating pads, and baths
Wash feet with warm (not hot) water and dry thoroughly (avoid foot soaks)
Do not soak feet
Do not treat corns, blisters, or ingrown toenails
Do not cross legs or wear tight garments that may constrict blood flow
Apply moisturizing lotion to the feet but not between the toes
Prevent moisture from accumulating between the toes
Wear loose socks and well-fitting (not tight) shoes, and instruct the client not to go barefoot
Change into clean cotton socks daily
Wear socks to keep the feet warm
Do not wear the same pair of shoes two days in a row
Do not wear open-toed shoes or shoes with a strap that goes between the toes
Check shoes for cracks or tears in the lining and for foreign objects before putting them on
Break in new shoes gradually
Cut toenails straight across and smooth nails with an emery board
Do not smoke

X. OPERATIVE CARE FOR THE DIABETIC CLIENT

A. Preoperative care
1. Check with physician regarding withholding oral hypoglycemic medications or insulin
2. Some long-acting oral hypoglycemic medications are discontinued 24 to 48 hours before surgery
3. Insulin dose may be adjusted or withheld if IV insulin administration is planned during surgery
4. Monitor blood glucose level
5. Administer IV fluids as prescribed

B. Postoperative care
   1. IV glucose and insulin infusions may be prescribed until the client can tolerate oral feedings
   2. Supplemental short-acting insulin may be prescribed on the basis of blood glucose results
   3. Monitor blood glucose levels frequently if the client is receiving total parenteral nutrition
   4. When the client is tolerating food, ensure that the client receives an adequate amount of carbohydrates daily to prevent **hypoglycemia** and ketosis

PRACTICE QUESTIONS

1. A nurse is caring for a client after hypophysectomy. The nurse notices clear nasal drainage from the client's nostril. The initial nursing action would be to:
   1. Continue to observe drainage
   2. Test the drainage for glucose
   3. Lower the head of the bed
   4. Obtain a culture of the drainage
2. After several diagnostic tests, a client is diagnosed with diabetes insipidus. The nurse understands that which symptom is indicative of this disorder?
   1. Diarrhea
   2. Polydipsia
   3. Weight gain
   4. Fatigue
3. A nurse caring for a client with Addison's disease would expect to note which of the following?
   1. Obesity
   2. Edema
   3. Hypotension
   4. Hirsutism
4. A client with Cushing's syndrome verbalizes concern to the nurse regarding the appearance of the buffalo hump that has developed. Which of the following statements by the nurse is most appropriate?
   1. "This is permanent, but looks are deceiving and not that important."
   2. "Don't be concerned, this problem can be covered with clothing."
   3. "Try not to worry about it, there are other things to be concerned about."
   4. "Usually these physical changes slowly improve after treatment."
5. A nurse assists in developing a plan of care for a client with Graves' disease. Which of the following would the nurse include in the plan of care?
   1. Provide three small meals a day
   2. Provide the client with extra blankets
   3. Provide a high-fiber diet
   4. Provide a restful environment
6. A nurse is caring for a client after thyroidectomy. The nurse notes that calcium gluconate is prescribed for the client. The nurse determines that this medication has been prescribed to:
   1. Treat thyroid storm
   2. Prevent cardiac irritability
   3. Stimulate the release of parathyroid hormone
   4. Treat hypocalcemic tetany
7. A nurse is collecting data on the client after a thyroidectomy. The nurse notes that the client has developed hoarseness and a weak voice. Which of the following nursing actions is appropriate?
   1. Notify the physician immediately
   2. Reassure the client that this is usually a temporary condition
   3. Check for signs of bleeding
   4. Administer calcium gluconate
8. A client is admitted to the emergency room and a diagnosis of myxedema coma is made. Which nursing action would the nurse prepare to carry out initially?
   1. Warm the client
   2. Administer fluids
   3. Maintain a patent airway
   4. Administer thyroid hormone
9. A client is taking NPH insulin daily every morning. The nurse instructs the client that the most likely time for a hypoglycemic reaction to occur is:
   1. 2 to 4 hours after administration
   2. 4 to 12 hours after administration
   3. 12 to 16 hours after administration
   4. 18 to 24 hours after administration
10. A nurse is assisting in preparing a teaching plan for the client with diabetes mellitus regarding proper foot care. Which of the following instructions should be included in the plan?
    1. Soak feet in hot water
    2. Apply a lanolin lotion to dry feet
    3. Always have a podiatrist cut your toenails; never cut them yourself
    4. Avoid using soap on the feet
11. A nurse provides dietary instructions to a client with diabetes mellitus regarding the prescribed diabetic diet. Which statement, if made by the client, indicates a need for further teaching?
    1. "I need to drink diet soft drinks."
    2. "I'll eat a balanced meal plan."
    3. "I need to buy special dietetic foods."
    4. "I'll snack on fruit instead of cake."
12. An external insulin pump is prescribed for a client with diabetes mellitus. The client asks the nurse about the functioning of the pump. The nurse plans to base the response on the information that the pump:
    1. Gives a small continuous dose of Regular insulin subcutaneously and the client can bolus self with an additional dosage from the pump before each meal

2. Is timed to release programmed doses of Regular or NPH insulin into the bloodstream at specific intervals
3. Is surgically attached to the pancreas and infuses Regular insulin into the pancreas, which in turn releases the insulin into the bloodstream
4. Continuously infuses small amounts of NPH insulin into the bloodstream while regularly monitoring blood glucose levels

13. A client newly diagnosed with diabetes mellitus has been stabilized with daily insulin injections. The nurse assists in preparing a discharge teaching plan regarding the insulin and includes which of the following concepts?
 1. Increase the amount of insulin before unusual exercise
 2. Acetone in the urine will signify a need for less insulin
 3. Always keep insulin vials refrigerated
 4. Systematically rotate insulin injection sites

14. A nurse reinforces teaching with a client with diabetes mellitus about differentiating between hypoglycemia and ketoacidosis. The client demonstrates an understanding of the teaching by stating that glucose will be taken if which of the following symptoms develop?
 1. Fruity breath odor
 2. Shakiness
 3. Blurred vision
 4. Polyuria

15. A client with diabetes mellitus demonstrates acute anxiety when admitted to the hospital for the treatment of hyperglycemia. The most appropriate intervention to decrease the client's anxiety would be to:
 1. Administer a sedative
 2. Make sure the client knows all the correct medical terms to understand what is happening
 3. Ignore the signs and symptoms of anxiety so that they will soon disappear
 4. Convey empathy, trust, and respect toward the client

16. A nurse reinforces instructions to a client newly diagnosed with type 1 diabetes mellitus. The nurse evaluates accurate understanding of measures to prevent diabetic ketoacidosis (DKA) when the client says:
 1. "I will stop taking my insulin if I'm too sick to eat."
 2. "I will decrease my insulin dose during times of illness."
 3. "I will notify my physician if my blood glucose level is greater than 250 mg/dL."
 4. "I will adjust my insulin dose according to the level of glucose in my urine."

17. A physician prescribes levothyroxine (Synthroid) orally 0.15 mg per day for a client with hypothyroidism. The nurse prepares to administer this medication:
 1. Three times a day in equal doses of 0.5 mg each to ensure consistent serum drug levels
 2. In the morning to prevent sleeplessness
 3. Only when the client complains of fatigue and cold intolerance
 4. At various times of the day to prevent tolerance from occurring

18. A nurse is monitoring a client receiving chlorpropamide (Diabinese). The nurse understands that which of the following is not a therapeutic outcome for this client?
 1. A decrease in polyuria
 2. A blood glucose of 110 mg/dL
 3. A decrease in polyphagia
 4. A glycosylated hemoglobin of 18%

19. A nurse is monitoring a client newly diagnosed with diabetes mellitus for sign of complications. Which of the following, if exhibited in the client, would indicate hyperglycemia and warrant physician notification?
 1. Hypertension
 2. Diaphoresis
 3. Polyuria
 4. Increased pulse rate

20. A nurse is reinforcing instructions with a client with diabetes mellitus recovering from diabetic ketoacidosis (DKA) in measures to prevent a recurrence. The nurse tells the client to:
 1. Eat 6 small meals per day
 2. Receive appropriate follow-up health care
 3. Monitor blood glucose levels frequently
 4. Test urine for ketone levels

21. A nurse is collecting data from a client with type 2 diabetes mellitus. Which statement by the client indicates an understanding of the medication regimen?
 1. "I am taking oral insulin instead of shots."
 2. "The medication that I am taking helps release the insulin I already make."
 3. "By taking these medications I am able to eat more."
 4. "When I become ill I need to increase the number of pills I take."

22. A client with type 1 diabetes mellitus is having trouble remembering the type, duration, and onset of action of insulin and the client's family members have not been supportive. The nurse's best statement to the client would be:
 1. "You can't always depend on your family to help."
 2. "Let me go over the types of insulin with you again."
 3. "It's not really necessary for you to remember this."
 4. "What is it you don't understand?"

23. A nurse is doing discharge teaching with a client who has Cushing's syndrome. Which of the following statements by the client indicates that the

instructions related to dietary management were understood?
1. "I am fortunate that I do not need to follow any special diet."
2. "I will need to limit the amount of protein in my diet."
3. "I am fortunate that I can eat all the salty foods I enjoy."
4. "I can eat foods that have a lot of potassium in them."

24. A client with type 1 diabetes mellitus calls the nurse to report recurrent episodes of hypoglycemia. Which statement by the client indicates an inadequate understanding of NPH insulin and exercise?
1. "The best time for me to exercise is late afternoon."
2. "The best time for me to exercise is after lunch."
3. "The best time for me to exercise is after breakfast."
4. "The best time for me to exercise is before bedtime."

25. A nurse is collecting data from an elderly client who is being admitted to the hospital for a diagnostic workup for primary hyperparathyroidism. The nurse understands that which client complaint would be characteristic of this disorder?
1. Diarrhea
2. Polyuria
3. Polyphagia
4. Weight gain

26. A nurse is caring for a postoperative parathyroidectomy client. Which client complaint would indicate that a serious life-threatening complication may be developing requiring immediate notification of the physician?
1. Difficulty voiding
2. Abdominal cramps
3. Laryngeal stridor
4. Mild to moderate incisional pain

27. A nurse is preparing to discharge a client who has had a parathyroidectomy. The nurse teaches the client about the prescribed oral calcium supplements and tells the client to:
1. Store the calcium in the refrigerator to maintain potency
2. Check the pulse daily, and not to take the calcium if it is below 60 beats per minute
3. Take the calcium with food or after a meal
4. Avoid sunlight because it can cause skin color change

28. A nurse notes that a client with type 1 diabetes mellitus has lipodystrophy on both upper thighs. The nurse would most appropriately inquire if the client:
1. Cleanses the skin with alcohol before each injection
2. Rotates sites for injection
3. Aspirates for blood before injection into the subcutaneous tissue
4. Administers the insulin at a 45-degree angle

29. A nurse is caring for a client with type 1 diabetes mellitus. Which of the following client complaints would alert the nurse of a possible hypoglycemic reaction?
1. Hot, dry skin
2. Muscle cramps
3. Anorexia
4. Tremors

30. A male client with type 1 diabetes mellitus tells the nurse that he might lose his job because he has been having frequent hypoglycemic reactions. When these reactions occur, his boss thinks that he is drunk and that he has been drinking on the job. Which action by the nurse would best assist this client to meet his needs?
1. Contact the local employment office to help him find another job
2. Ask the client if he indeed has been drinking at work
3. Examine factors that may be causing frequent hypoglycemic episodes
4. Ask the client what he does to treat his hypoglycemia

31. A nurse needs to maintain food and fluid intake to minimize the risk of dehydration in an elderly client with diabetes mellitus who has gastroenteritis. An appropriate nursing intervention to perform is to:
1. Offer water only until the client is able to tolerate solid foods
2. Withhold all fluids until vomiting has ceased for at least 4 hours
3. Encourage the client to take 8 to 12 ounces of fluid every hour while awake
4. Maintain a clear liquid diet for at least 5 days before advancing the diet to allow inflammation of the bowel to dissipate

32. A client who is currently taking levothyroxine (Synthroid) complains of cold intolerance, constipation, dry skin, weight gain, and puffy eyes. Based on these findings, the nurse would anticipate which of the following physician prescriptions?
1. Increase levothyroxine dosage after checking the T_4 level
2. Decrease levothyroxine dosage after checking the T_4 level
3. Discontinue the levothyroxine because the client is having an adverse reaction
4. No change in medication dosage because these are common side effects that will diminish with time

33. A nurse is caring for a client with diabetes insipidus receiving vasopressin tannate (Pitressin tannate).

The nurse understands that which of the following is not a therapeutic effect of this medication?
1. Increased gastrointestinal tract smooth muscle tone and contractions
2. Decreased urine output
3. Increased rebasorption of water by the renal tubules
4. Vasodilation of vascular vessels

34. A client is diagnosed with pheochromocytoma. The nurse assisting in preparing a nursing care plan for the client understands that pheochromocytoma is a condition that:
1. Causes profound hypotension
2. Causes the release of excessive amounts of catecholamines
3. Is not a curable condition and is treated symptomatically
4. Is manifested by severe hypoglycemia

35. A nurse is collecting data on a client admitted to the hospital with a diagnosis of pheochromocytoma. The nurse observes for the major symptom associated with pheochromocytoma when the nurse:
1. Tests the client's urine for glucose
2. Takes the client's weight
3. Palpates the skin for its temperature
4. Takes the client's blood pressure

36. A nurse is caring for a client with pheochromocytoma. The client is scheduled for an adrenalectomy. In the preoperative period, the priority nursing action would be to monitor:
1. Vital signs
2. Urine for glucose and acetone
3. Intake and output
4. Blood urea nitrogen (BUN) laboratory values

37. A nurse is caring for a client with pheochromocytoma. The client asks for a snack and something warm to drink. The most appropriate choice for this client to meet nutritional needs would be which of the following?
1. Graham crackers and warm milk
2. Toast with peanut butter and cocoa
3. Crackers with cheese and tea
4. Vanilla wafers and coffee with cream and sugar

38. A nurse is caring for a client with pheochromocytoma. Which of the following data would indicate a potential complication associated with this disorder?
1. A urinary output of 50 mL per hour
2. Rales heard on auscultation
3. A blood urea nitrogen (BUN) of 20 mg/dL
4. A coagulation time of 5 minutes

39. A client with pheochromocytoma is scheduled for surgery and says to the nurse, "I'm not sure that surgery is the best thing to do?" The most appropriate response by the nurse is which of the following?
1. "You have concerns about the surgical treatment for your condition?"
2. "There is no reason to worry. Your doctor is a wonderful surgeon."
3. "You are very ill. Your physician has made the correct decision."
4. "I think you are making the right decision to have the surgery."

40. A nurse is caring for a client after thyroidectomy and is monitoring for signs of thyroid storm. The nurse understands that which of the following is a manifestation associated with this disorder?
1. Low-grade temperature
2. Bradycardia
3. Hypotension
4. Constipation

ANSWERS

1. *Answer:* 2

Rationale: After hypophysectomy, the client should be monitored for rhinorrhea, which could indicate a cerebrospinal fluid (CSF) leak. If this occurs, the drainage should be collected and tested for the presence of CSF. The head of the bed should not be lowered to prevent increased intracranial pressure. Clear nasal drainage would not indicate the need for a culture. Continuing to observe the drainage without taking action could result in a serious complication.

Test-Taking Strategy: Note the key word "initial." This indicates that an action is required. Option 3 can be easily eliminated. Option 4 can be eliminated because the drainage is clear. Because an action is required, eliminate option 1. Review the complications after hypophysectomy if you had difficulty with this question.

Level of Cognitive Ability: Application

Client Needs: Physiological Integrity

Integrated Concept/Process: Nursing Process/Implementation

Content Area: Adult Health/Endocrine

Reference: Ignatavicius D, Workman M: *Medical-surgical: critical thinking for collaborative care,* ed 4, Philadelphia, 2002, WB Saunders, p. 1407.

2. *Answer:* 2
Rationale: Polydipsia and polyuria are classic symptoms of diabetes insipidus. The urine is pale in color and the specific gravity is low. Anorexia and weight loss occur.
Test-Taking Strategy: Use the process of elimination. Eliminate option 4 first because this symptom is rather vague and occurs in many conditions. Knowledge of the manifestations of diabetes insipidus will assist in eliminating options 1 and 3. If you had difficulty with this question, review the clinical manifestations associated with diabetes insipidus.
Level of Cognitive Ability: Comprehension
Client Needs: Physiological Integrity
Integrated Concept/Process: Nursing Process/Data Collection
Content Area: Adult Health/Endocrine
Reference: Ignatavicius D, Workman M: *Medical-surgical: critical thinking for collaborative care,* ed 4, Philadelphia, 2002, WB Saunders, p. 1409.

3. *Answer:* 3
Rationale: Common manifestations of Addison's disease include postural hypotension from fluid loss, syncope, muscle weakness, anorexia, nausea and vomiting, abdominal cramps, weight loss, depression, and irritability.
Test-Taking Strategy: Knowledge regarding the clinical manifestations associated with Addison's disease is required to answer this question. If you had difficulty with this question, review this endocrine disorder.
Level of Cognitive Ability: Comprehension
Client Needs: Physiological Integrity
Integrated Concept/Process: Nursing Process/Data Collection
Content Area: Adult Health/Endocrine
Reference: Ignatavicius D, Workman M: *Medical-surgical: critical thinking for collaborative care,* ed 4, Philadelphia, 2002, WB Saunders, p. 403.

4. *Answer:* 4
Rationale: The client with Cushing's syndrome should be reassured that most physical changes resolve with treatment. Options 1, 2, and 3 are not therapeutic responses.
Test-Taking Strategy: Use knowledge regarding the physical changes that occur in Cushing's syndrome and therapeutic communication techniques to answer this question. Options 1, 2, and 3 are not therapeutic responses to a client. Review this disorder and therapeutic communication techniques if you had difficulty with this question.
Level of Cognitive Ability: Application
Client Needs: Psychosocial Integrity
Integrated Concept/Process: Communication and Documentation
Content Area: Adult Health/Endocrine
Reference: Ignatavicius D, Workman M: *Medical-surgical: critical thinking for collaborative care,* ed 4, Philadelphia, 2002, WB Saunders, p. 1416.

5. *Answer:* 4
Rationale: Because of the hypermetabolic state, the client with Graves' disease needs to be provided with an environment that is restful both physically and mentally. Six full meals a day that are well balanced and high in calories are required because of the accelerated metabolic rate. Foods that increase peristalsis such as high fiber foods need to be avoided. These clients suffer from heat intolerance and require a cool environment.
Test-Taking Strategy: The key concept to bear in mind when answering this question is that clients with Graves' disease experience an accelerated metabolic rate. This concept should assist in eliminating options 1, 2, and 3. Review care to the client with Graves' disease if you had difficulty with this question.
Level of Cognitive Ability: Application
Client Needs: Physiological Integrity
Integrated Concept/Process: Nursing Process/Planning
Content Area: Adult Health/Endocrine
Reference: Ignatavicius D, Workman M: *Medical-surgical: critical thinking for collaborative care,* ed 4, Philadelphia, 2002, WB Saunders, p. 1425.

6. *Answer:* 4
Rationale: Hypocalcemia can develop after thyroidectomy if the parathyroid glands are accidentally removed during surgery. Manifestations develop 1 to 7 days after surgery. If the client develops numbness and tingling around the mouth, fingertips, or toes; muscle spasms; or twitching, the physician is notified immediately. Calcium gluconate should be kept at the bedside.
Test-Taking Strategy: Noting the name of the medication (calcium gluconate) should easily direct you to option 4. Calcium would be given if hypocalcemic tetany occurs. Review this medication if you had difficulty with this question.
Level of Cognitive Ability: Analysis
Client Needs: Physiological Integrity
Integrated Concept/Process: Nursing Process/Planning
Content Area: Pharmacology
Reference: Ignatavicius D, Workman M: *Medical-surgical: critical thinking for collaborative care,* ed 4, Philadelphia, 2002, WB Saunders, p. 1429.

7. *Answer:* 2
Rationale: Weakness and hoarseness of the voice can occur as a result of trauma of the laryngeal nerve. If this develops, the client should be reassured that the problem will subside in a few days. Unnecessary talking should be discouraged. It is not necessary to notify the physician. These signs do not indicate bleeding or the need to administer calcium gluconate.
Test-Taking Strategy: Use the process of elimination. Options 3 and 4 can easily be eliminated because they are unrelated to the signs presented in the question. None of the information given requires physician notification. Review the expected findings after thyroidectomy if you had difficulty with this question.
Level of Cognitive Ability: Application
Client Needs: Physiological Integrity
Integrated Concept/Process: Nursing Process/Implementation
Content Area: Adult Health/Endocrine
Reference: Ignatavicius D, Workman M: *Medical-surgical: critical thinking for collaborative care,* ed 4, Philadelphia, 2002, WB Saunders, p. 1429.

8. *Answer:* 3
Rationale: The initial nursing action would be to maintain a patent airway. Oxygen would be administered followed by fluid replacement, keeping the client warm, monitoring vital signs, and administering thyroid hormones.
Test-Taking Strategy: Note the key words "carry out initially." All of the options are appropriate interventions, but use of the ABCs—airway, breathing, and circulation—will direct you to option 3. Review care to the client with myxedema coma if you had difficulty with this question.
Level of Cognitive Ability: Application
Client Needs: Physiological Integrity
Integrated Concept/Process: Nursing Process/Implementation
Content Area: Adult Health/Endocrine
Reference: Ignatavicius D, Workman M: *Medical-surgical: critical thinking for collaborative care,* ed 4, Philadelphia, 2002, WB Saunders, p. 1434.

9. *Answer:* 2
Rationale: NPH is an intermediate-acting insulin. The onset of action is 3 to 4 hours, it peaks in 4 to 12 hours, and its duration of action is 16 to 20 hours. Hypoglycemic reactions most likely occur during peak time.
Test-Taking Strategy: Knowledge regarding the onset, peak, and duration of action for NPH insulin is required to answer this question. Review the characteristics of NPH insulin if you had difficulty with this question.
Level of Cognitive Ability: Application
Client Needs: Health Promotion and Maintenance
Integrated Concept/Process: Teaching/Learning
Content Area: Pharmacology
Reference: Lehne R: *Pharmacology for nursing care,* ed 4, Philadelphia, 2001, WB Saunders, p. 619.

10. *Answer:* 2
Rationale: The client should be instructed not to soak the feet and to avoid hot water to prevent burns. The client may cut toe nails straight and even with the toe itself, and would consult a podiatrist if the toenails were thick, hard to cut, or if vision were poor. The client should be instructed to wash the feet daily using a mild soap.
Test-Taking Strategy: Use the process of elimination. Eliminate option 3 first because of the word "always" and option 1 because of the word "hot." From the remaining options, recalling the concern related to skin infection will assist in eliminating option 4. Review diabetic foot care instructions if you had difficulty with this question.
Level of Cognitive Ability: Application
Client Needs: Health Promotion and Maintenance
Integrated Concept/Process: Nursing Process/Planning
Content Area: Adult Health/Endocrine
Reference: Ignatavicius D, Workman M: *Medical-surgical: critical thinking for collaborative care,* ed 4, Philadelphia, 2002, WB Saunders, p. 1474.

11. *Answer:* 3
Rationale: It is important to emphasize to the client and family that they are not eating a diabetic diet but rather a balanced meal plan. Adherence to nutrition principles is an important component of diabetic management, and an individualized meal plan should be developed for the client. It is not necessary for the client to purchase special dietetic foods.
Test-Taking Strategy: Note the key words "indicates a need for further teaching." Basic principles related to the diabetic diet will direct you to option 3. Review these principles if you had difficulty with this question.
Level of Cognitive Ability: Comprehension
Client Needs: Health Promotion and Maintenance
Integrated Concept/Process: Teaching/Learning
Content Area: Adult Health/Endocrine
Reference: Ignatavicius D, Workman M: *Medical-surgical: critical thinking for collaborative care,* ed 4, Philadelphia, 2002, WB Saunders, p. 1477.

12. *Answer:* 1
Rationale: An insulin pump provides a small continuous dose of Regular insulin subcutaneously throughout the day and night, and the client can bolus self with an additional dosage from the pump before each meal as needed. Regular insulin is used in an insulin pump. An external pump is not surgically attached to the pancreas.
Test-Taking Strategy: Use the process of elimination. Recalling that Regular insulin is used in an insulin pump will assist in eliminating options 2 and 4. Careful reading of the question noting the word "external" will assist in eliminating option 3. Review the use of the insulin pump if you are unfamiliar with it.
Level of Cognitive Ability: Application
Client Needs: Physiological Integrity
Integrated Concept/Process: Nursing Process/Planning
Content Area: Adult Health/Endocrine
Reference: Ignatavicius D, Workman M: *Medical-surgical: critical thinking for collaborative care,* ed 4, Philadelphia, 2002, WB Saunders, p. 1461.

13. *Answer:* 4
Rationale: Insulin dosages should not be adjusted or increased before unusual exercise. If acetone is found in the urine, it may indicate the need for additional insulin. To minimize the discomfort associated with insulin injections, insulin should be administered at room temperature. Injection sites should be systematically rotated from one area to another. The client should be instructed to give injections in one area, about an inch apart, until the whole area has been used and then change to another site. This prevents dramatic changes in daily insulin absorption.
Test-Taking Strategy: Use the process of elimination. Eliminate option 3 first because of the word "always." Knowledge regarding insulin administration and the significance of acetone in the urine will assist in eliminating options 1 and 2. If you had difficulty with this question, review insulin management.
Level of Cognitive Ability: Application
Client Needs: Health Promotion and Maintenance
Integrated Concept/Process: Nursing Process/Planning
Content Area: Pharmacology
Reference: Ignatavicius D, Workman M: *Medical-surgical: critical thinking for collaborative care,* ed 4, Philadelphia, 2002, WB Saunders, p. 1462.

14. *Answer:* 2
Rationale: Shakiness is a sign of hypoglycemia and would indicate the need for food, or glucose. A fruity breath odor, blurred vision, and polyuria are signs of hyperglycemia.
Test-Taking Strategy: Knowledge regarding the signs and symptoms of hypoglycemia and hyperglycemia are required to answer this question. If you are unfamiliar with these signs, be sure to learn them.
Level of Cognitive Ability: Comprehension
Client Needs: Health Promotion and Maintenance
Integrated Concept/Process: Teaching/Learning
Content Area: Adult Health/Endocrine
Reference: Ignatavicius D, Workman M: *Medical-surgical: critical thinking for collaborative care*, ed 4, Philadelphia, 2002, WB Saunders, p. 1480.

15. *Answer:* 4
Rationale: The most appropriate intervention is to address the client's feelings related to the anxiety. Administering a sedative is not the most appropriate intervention. The nurse should not ignore the client's anxious feelings. A client will not relate to medical terms, particularly when anxiety exists.
Test-Taking Strategy: Use therapeutic communication techniques to answer the question. Remember that client's feelings come first. Keeping this in mind will easily direct you to option 4. Review these techniques if you had difficulty with this question.
Level of Cognitive Ability: Application
Client Needs: Psychosocial Integrity
Integrated Concept/Process: Caring
Content Area: Adult Health/Endocrine
Reference: Potter P, Perry A: *Fundamentals of nursing*, ed 5, St Louis, 2001, Mosby, p. 459.

16. *Answer:* 3
Rationale: During illness, the client should monitor blood glucose levels and notify the physician if the level is greater than 250 mg/dL. Insulin should never be stopped. In fact, insulin may need to be increased during times of illness. Doses should not be adjusted without the physician's advice.
Test-Taking Strategy: Use the process of elimination. Note that options 1, 2, and 4 all relate to adjustment of insulin doses. Therefore eliminate these options. Review diabetic management during illness if you had difficulty with this question.
Level of Cognitive Ability: Comprehension
Client Needs: Health Promotion and Maintenance
Integrated Concept/Process: Self-Care
Content Area: Adult Health/Endocrine
Reference: Ignatavicius D, Workman M: *Medical-surgical: critical thinking for collaborative care*, ed 4, Philadelphia, 2002, WB Saunders, p. 1462.

17. *Answer:* 2
Rationale: Levothyroxine is a synthetic thyroid hormone that increases cellular metabolism. It should be given in the morning in a single dose to prevent sleeplessness and at the same time each day to maintain a consistent drug level.
Test-Taking Strategy: Use the process of elimination. Options 1 and 3 can be eliminated because the nurse cannot change or alter a physician's order. From the remaining options, use principles related to medication administration to direct you to option 2. Review this medication if you had difficulty with this question.
Level of Cognitive Ability: Application
Client Needs: Physiological Integrity
Integrated Concept/Process: Nursing Process/Implementation
Content Area: Adult Health/Endocrine
Reference: Lehne R: *Pharmacology for nursing care*, ed 4, Philadelphia, 2001, WB Saunders, p. 640.

18. *Answer:* 4
Rationale: Chlorpropamide is an oral hypoglycemic agent administered to decrease serum glucose and the signs and symptoms of hyperglycemia. Therefore a decrease in both polyuria and polyphagia would indicate a therapeutic response. Laboratory values are also used to assess a client's response to treatment. A blood glucose of 110 mg/dL is within normal limits. However, a glycosylated hemoglobin of 18% indicates poor glycemic control.
Test-Taking Strategy: Note the key words "not a therapeutic outcome." Recalling that chlorpropamide is an oral hypoglycemic agent tells you to look for an option that would indicate hyperglycemia (lack of response to the medication). Options 1 and 3 are similar and are eliminated first. Next, eliminate option 2 because it is a normal blood glucose level. Review this medication if you had difficulty with this question.
Level of Cognitive Ability: Analysis
Client Needs: Physiological Integrity
Integrated Concept/Process: Nursing Process/Evaluation
Content Area: Adult Health/Endocrine
Reference: Lehne R: *Pharmacology for nursing care*, ed 4, Philadelphia, 2001, WB Saunders, p. 624.

19. *Answer:* 3
Rationale: The classic symptoms of hyperglycemia include polydipsia, polyuria, and polyphagia. Options 1, 2, and 4 are not signs of hyperglycemia.
Test-Taking Strategy: Focus on the issue, hyperglycemia. Remember the 3 Ps: polyuria, polydipsia, and polyphagia. Review the signs of hyperglycemia if you had difficulty with this question.
Level of Cognitive Ability: Comprehension
Client Needs: Physiological Integrity
Integrated Concept/Process: Nursing Process/Data Collection
Content Area: Adult Health/Endocrine
Reference: DeWit S: *Fundamental concepts and skills for nursing*, Philadelphia, 2001, WB Saunders, p. 552.

20. *Answer:* 3
Rationale: Client education after DKA should emphasize the need for home glucose monitoring two to four times a day. It is also important to instruct the client to notify the health care provider when illness occurs. The presence of urinary ketones indicates that DKA has already occurred. The client should eat well-balanced meals with snacks as prescribed.
Test-Taking Strategy: Focus on the issue of preventing DKA. Recall that the treatment of DKA focuses on maintenance of an appropriate blood glucose level. Option 1 is not an accurate component of diabetic care. Option 2 will not prevent

DKA, and option 4 does not prevent DKA but actually confirms the diagnosis. Review this complication of diabetes mellitus if you had difficulty with this question.
Level of Cognitive Ability: Application
Client Needs: Health Promotion and Maintenance
Integrated Concept/Process: Teaching/Learning
Content Area: Adult Health/Endocrine
Reference: Ignatavicius D, Workman M: *Medical-surgical: critical thinking for collaborative care,* ed 4, Philadelphia, 2002, WB Saunders, p. 1482.

21. *Answer:* 2
Rationale: Clients with type 2 diabetes mellitus have decreased or impaired insulin secretion. Oral hypoglycemic agents are given to these clients to facilitate glucose utilization. Insulin injections may be given during times of stress-induced hyperglycemia. Oral insulin is not available or effective because of the breakdown of the insulin by digestion.
Test-Taking Strategy: Focus on the issue, type 2 diabetes mellitus. Eliminate option 1 because there is no "oral insulin." Next, eliminate options 3 and 4 because they are not accepted treatment for diabetes mellitus. Review the treatment for diabetes mellitus if you had difficulty with this question.
Level of Cognitive Ability: Comprehension
Client Needs: Health Promotion and Maintenance
Integrated Concept/Process: Nursing Process/Evaluation
Content Area: Adult Health/Endocrine
Reference: DeWit S: *Fundamental concepts and skills for nursing,* Philadelphia, 2001, WB Saunders, p. 493.

22. *Answer:* 2
Rationale: Reinforcement of knowledge and behaviors is vital to the success of the client's self-care. Option 1 may devalue a client's family. Option 3 places the issue on "hold," and option 4 requests an explanation by the client. Option 2 clarifies previous information.
Test-Taking Strategy: Focus on the data in the question. Use therapeutic communication techniques to answer the question. This will direct you to option 2. Review these techniques if you had difficulty with this question.
Level of Cognitive Ability: Application
Client Needs: Psychosocial Integrity
Integrated Concept/Process: Communication and Documentation
Content Area: Adult Health/Endocrine
Reference: Potter P, Perry A: *Fundamentals of nursing,* ed 5, St Louis, 2001, Mosby, p. 459.

23. *Answer:* 4
Rationale: A diet low in calories, carbohydrates, and sodium but ample in protein and potassium content is encouraged for a client with Cushing's syndrome. Such a diet promotes weight loss, reduction of edema and hypertension, control of hypokalemia, and rebuilding of wasted tissue.
Test-Taking Strategy: Note the key words "instructions related to dietary management were understood." Eliminate option 1 because it indicates that no dietary change is necessary. Eliminate option 2 next because protein is usually limited only with renal disorders. Excess sodium is not healthy in general, so eliminate option 3. Review dietary management of Cushing's syndrome if you had difficulty with this question.
Level of Cognitive Ability: Comprehension
Client Needs: Health Promotion and Maintenance
Integrated Concept/Process: Self-Care
Content Area: Adult Health/Endocrine
Reference: Ignatavicius D, Workman M: *Medical-surgical: critical thinking for collaborative care,* ed 4, Philadelphia, 2002, WB Saunders, p. 1405.

24. *Answer:* 1
Rationale: A hypoglycemic reaction may occur in response to increased exercise. Clients should avoid exercise during the peak time of insulin. NPH insulin peaks at 4 to 12 hours; therefore late afternoon exercise will occur during the peak of the medication.
Test-Taking Strategy: Use the process of elimination and note the key words "inadequate understanding." Recalling the peak time of insulin will direct you to option 1. Review the measures to prevent hypoglycemia if you had difficulty with this question.
Level of Cognitive Ability: Comprehension
Client Needs: Health Promotion and Maintenance
Integrated Concept/Process: Nursing Process/Evaluation
Content Area: Adult Health/Endocrine
Reference: Ignatavicius D, Workman M: *Medical-surgical: critical thinking for collaborative care,* ed 4, Philadelphia, 2002, WB Saunders, p. 1478.

25. *Answer:* 2
Rationale: Hypercalcemia is the hallmark of hyperparathyroidism. Elevated serum calcium levels produce osmotic diuresis (polyuria). This diuresis lead to dehydration and the client would lose weight. Both options 1 and 3 are gastrointestinal (GI) symptoms but are not associated with the common GI symptoms typical of hyperparathyroidsim (nausea, vomiting, anorexia, constipation)
Test-Taking Strategy: Use the process of elimination. Note that options 1, 3, and 4 are similar and are all GI symptoms. Review the characteristics of hyperparathyroidism if you had difficulty with this question.
Level of Cognitive Ability: Analysis
Client Needs: Physiological Integrity
Integrated Concept/Process: Nursing Process/Data Collection
Content Area: Adult Health/Endocrine
Reference: DeWit S: *Fundamental concepts and skills for nursing,* Philadelphia, 2001, WB Saunders, p. 448.

26. *Answer:* 3
Rationale: During the postoperative period, the nurse carefully observes the client for signs of hemorrhage, which cause swelling and compression of adjacent tissue. Laryngeal stridor is a harsh, high-pitched sound heard on inspiration and expiration caused by compression of the trachea leading to respiratory distress. It is an acute emergency situation that requires immediate attention to avoid complete obstruction of the airway.
Test-Taking Strategy: Consider the anatomical location of the surgical procedure and use the ABCs—airway, breathing, and circulation—to select the correct option. Options 1, 2, and 4

are usual postoperative problems that are not life-threatening. Option 3 addresses airway. Review care to the client after parathyroidectomy if you had difficulty with this question.
Level of Cognitive Ability: Analysis
Client Needs: Physiological Integrity
Integrated Concept/Process: Nursing Process/Data Collection
Content Area: Adult Health/Endocrine
Reference: Ignatavicius D, Workman M: *Medical-surgical: critical thinking for collaborative care,* ed 4, Philadelphia, 2002, WB Saunders, p. 1438.

27. *Answer:* 3
Rationale: Oral calcium supplements need to be taken with food to enhance its absorption as well as decrease gastrointestinal irritation. All of the other options are unrelated to oral calcium therapy.
Test-Taking Strategy: Knowledge regarding administration of calcium is required to answer this question. Eliminate those options that seem unusual. Checking the pulse is usually done for patients using cardiac medications. Avoidance of sunlight and refrigeration of tablets are required for some medications, but is not a common intervention. Review this medication if you had difficulty with this question.
Level of Cognitive Ability: Application
Client Needs: Health Promotion and Maintenance
Integrated Concept/Process: Teaching/Learning
Content Area: Adult Health/Endocrine
Reference: Hodgson B, Kizior R: *Saunders nursing drug handbook 2002,* Philadelphia, 2002, WB Saunders, p. 153.

28. *Answer:* 2
Rationale: Lipodystrophy (hypertrophy of subcutaneous tissue at the injection site) occurs in some diabetic clients when the same injection sites are used for prolonged periods. Thus clients are instructed to adhere to a rotating injection site plan to avoid tissue changes. Cleansing with alcohol, aspiration, and angle of insulin administration does not produce tissue damage.
Test-Taking Strategy: Recalling the definition of lipodystrophy will direct you to the correct option. If you are unfamiliar with this complication of insulin therapy, review this component of diabetic teaching.
Level of Cognitive Ability: Application
Client Needs: Physiological Integrity
Integrated Concept/Process: Nursing Process/Data Collection
Content Area: Adult Health/Endocrine
Reference: Ignatavicius D, Workman M: *Medical-surgical: critical thinking for collaborative care,* ed 4, Philadelphia, 2002, WB Saunders, p. 1459.

29. *Answer:* 4
Rationale: Decreased blood glucose levels produce automatic nervous system symptoms, which are classically manifested as nervousness, irritability, and tremors. Option 1 is more likely to occur with hyperglycemia. Options 2 and 3 are unrelated to the signs of hypoglycemia.
Test-Taking Strategy: Focus on the issue, a hypoglycemic reaction. Recalling the signs associated with this reaction will direct you to option 4. Review this complication if you had difficulty with this question.
Level of Cognitive Ability: Comprehension
Client Needs: Physiological Integrity
Integrated Concept/Process: Nursing Process/Data Collection
Content Area: Adult Health/Endocrine
Reference: Ignatavicius D, Workman M: *Medical-surgical: critical thinking for collaborative care,* ed 4, Philadelphia, 2002, WB Saunders, p. 1479.

30. *Answer:* 3
Rationale: Hypoglycemic reactions present adrenergic symptoms of tremor, shakiness, and nervousness, which are similar to alcohol intoxication. The best action to deal with this client's psychosocial need is to identify and then eliminate those factors that precipitate these types of reactions. Option 1 presumes that the problem is unavoidable and thus the client is at fault. Option 2 is nontherapeutic because it presumes that the client may be drinking, and option 4 avoids the psychosocial aspects of the client's problem.
Test-Taking Strategy: Use the process of elimination. Note the relationship between the issue, hypoglycemic reactions and option 3. Review the psychosocial issues related to the complications of diabetes mellitus if you had difficulty with this question.
Level of Cognitive Ability: Application
Client Needs: Psychosocial Integrity
Integrated Concept/Process: Nursing Process/Implementation
Content Area: Adult Health/Endocrine
Reference: Ignatavicius D, Workman M: *Medical-surgical: critical thinking for collaborative care,* ed 4, Philadelphia, 2002, WB Saunders, p. 1479.

31. *Answer:* 3
Rationale: Fluids containing both glucose and electrolytes should be offered to the client every hour. Small amounts of fluid may be tolerated even when vomiting is present. Water alone is insufficient. Withholding all fluids is inappropriate. A clear liquid diet for 5 days is inappropriate.
Test-Taking Strategy: Use the process of elimination. Eliminate options 1 and 2 because of the words "only" and "all." The time frame in option 4 seems unreasonable; therefore select option 3. Review care to the diabetic client during illness if you had difficulty with this question.
Level of Cognitive Ability: Application
Client Needs: Physiological Integrity
Integrated Concept/Process: Nursing Process/Implementation
Content Area: Adult Health/Endocrine
Reference: Black J, Hawks J, Keene A: *Medical-surgical nursing: clinical management for positive outcomes,* ed 6, Philadelphia, 2001, WB Saunders, p. 1190.

32. *Answer:* 1
Rationale: Manifestations of hypothyroidism include cold intolerance, constipation, loss of initiative, thick dry skin, a notably puffy appearance of the skin around the eyes, slowed intellectual function including retarded speech and apathy, and a low metabolic rate. Levothyroxine is used to correct hypothyroidism. In this situation, the dosage is subtherapeutic and needs to be increased.
Test-Taking Strategy: Note the key words "currently taking levothyroxine." Recalling that the signs presented in the ques-

tion relate to the manifestations associated with hypothyroidism will direct you to option 1. Review this medication and the signs of hypothyroidism if you had difficulty with this question.
Level of Cognitive Ability: Analysis
Client Needs: Physiological Integrity
Integrated Concept/Process: Nursing Process/Planning
Content Area: Adult Health/Endocrine
Reference: Black J, Hawks J, Keene A:*Medical-surgical nursing: clinical management for positive outcomes,* ed 6, Philadelphia, 2001, WB Saunders, p. 1097.

33. *Answer:* 4
Rationale: Vasopressin, an antidiuretic hormone, causes vasoconstriction with reduced blood flow in coronary, peripheral, cerebral, and pulmonary vessels. Options 1, 2, and 3 are therapeutic effects of the medication.
Test-Taking Strategy: Note the key word "not" in the stem of the question. Eliminate options 2 and 3 first because they are similar. From the remaining options, recalling the pathophysiology related to diabetes insipidus will direct you to option 4. If you had difficulty with this question, review this disorder.
Level of Cognitive Ability: Comprehension
Client Needs: Physiological Integrity
Integrated Concept/Process: Nursing Process/Evaluation
Content Area: Adult Health/Endocrine
Reference: Hodgson B, Kizior R: *Saunders nursing drug handbook 2002,* Philadelphia, 2002, WB Saunders, p. 1139.

34. *Answer:* 2
Rationale: Pheochromocytoma is a catecholamine-producing tumor and causes secretion of excessive amounts of epinephrine and norepinephrine. Hypertension is the principal manifestation and the client has episodes of a high blood pressure accompanied by pounding headaches. The excessive release of catecholamine also results in excessive conversion of glycogen into glucose in the liver. Consequently, hyperglycemia and glucosuria occur during attacks. Pheochromocytoma is curable. The primary treatment is surgical removal of one or both of the adrenal glands depending on whether the tumor is unilateral or bilateral.
Test-Taking Strategy: Knowledge regarding the pathophysiology associated with pheochromocytoma is required to answer this question. Review this disorder if you had difficulty with this question.
Level of Cognitive Ability: Comprehension
Client Needs: Physiological Integrity
Integrated Concept/Process: Nursing Process/Planning
Content Area: Adult Health/Endocrine
Reference: Black J, Hawks J, Keene A: *Medical-surgical nursing: clinical management for positive outcomes,* ed 6, Philadelphia, 2001, WB Saunders, p. 1135.

35. *Answer:* 4
Rationale: Hypertension is the major symptom associated with pheochromocytoma. The blood pressure status is monitored by taking the client's blood pressure. Glycosuria, weight loss, and diaphoresis are also clinical manifestations of pheochromocytoma, but hypertension is the major symptom.
Test-Taking Strategy: Note the key words "major symptom." Use the principles associated with prioritizing and the ABCs—airway, breathing, and circulation. A method of assessing circulation is to take the blood pressure. Review the manifestations of this disorder if you had difficulty with this question.
Level of Cognitive Ability: Application
Client Needs: Physiological Integrity
Integrated Concept/Process: Nursing Process/Data Collection
Content Area: Adult Health/Endocrine
Reference: Black J, Hawks J, Keene A: *Medical-surgical nursing: clinical management for positive outcomes,* ed 6, Philadelphia, 2001, WB Saunders, p. 1135.

36. *Answer:* 1
Rationale: Hypertension is the hallmark of pheochromocytoma. Severe hypertension can precipitate a cerebrovascular accident or sudden blindness. Although all of the options are accurate nursing interventions for the client with pheochromocytoma, the priority nursing action is to monitor the vital signs, particularly the blood pressure.
Test-Taking Strategy: Note the key words "priority nursing action." Use the ABCs—airway, breathing, and circulation. Monitoring vital signs is the nursing action that would assess airway, breathing, and circulation. Also, note that options 2, 3, and 4 all refer to the assessment of the renal system. Review care to the client with pheochromocytoma if you had difficulty with this question.
Level of Cognitive Ability: Application
Client Needs: Physiological Integrity
Integrated Concept/Process: Nursing Process/Implementation
Content Area: Adult Health/Endocrine
Reference: Black J, Hawks J, Keene A: *Medical-surgical nursing: clinical management for positive outcomes,* ed 6, Philadelphia, 2001, WB Saunders, p. 1135.

37. *Answer:* 1
Rationale: The client with pheochromocytoma needs to be provided with a diet high in vitamins, minerals, and calories. Of particular importance is that food or beverages that contain caffeine such as chocolate, coffee, tea, or colas are prohibited.
Test-Taking Strategy: Use the process of elimination. Eliminate options 2, 3, and 4 because they are similar and contain food items that contain caffeine. Review dietary measures for the client with pheochromocytoma if you had difficulty with this question.
Level of Cognitive Ability: Application
Client Needs: Physiological Integrity
Integrated Concept/Process: Nursing Process/Implementation
Content Area: Adult Health/Endocrine
Reference: Black J, Hawks J, Keene A: *Medical-surgical nursing: clinical management for positive outcomes,* ed 6, Philadelphia, 2001, WB Saunders, p. 1137.

38. *Answer:* 2
Rationale: The complications associated with pheochromocytoma include hypertensive retinopathy and nephropathy, myocarditis, congestive heart failure (CHF), increased platelet aggregation, and cerebrovascular accident (CVA). Death can

occur from shock, CVA, renal failure, dysrhythmias, or dissecting aortic aneurysm. Rales heard on auscultation are indicative of CHF. A urinary output of 50 mL per hour is an appropriate output; the nurse would become concerned if the output was below 30 mL per hour. A BUN of 20 mg/dL is a normal finding. A coagulation time of 5 minutes is normal.
Test-Taking Strategy: Use the ABCs—airway, breathing, and circulation. Rales heard on auscultation in the lungs is associated with airway. Additionally, if you knew the normal hourly expectations associated with urinary output and the normal laboratory values for coagulation time and for the BUN, by the process of elimination, you will determine that option 2 is the correct option. Review the complications associated with pheochromocytoma if you had difficulty with this question.
Level of Cognitive Ability: Comprehension
Client Needs: Physiological Integrity
Integrated Concept/Process: Nursing Process/Data Collection
Content Area: Adult Health/Endocrine
Reference: Black J, Hawks J, Keene A: *Medical-surgical nursing: clinical management for positive outcomes,* ed 6, Philadelphia, 2001, WB Saunders, p. 1135.

39. ***Answer:*** 1
Rationale: Paraphrasing is restating the client's messages in the nurse's own words. Option 1 addresses the therapeutic communication technique of paraphrasing. The client is reaching out for understanding. In option 2, the nurse is offering a false reassurance and this type of response will block communication. Option 3 also represents a communication block in that it reflects a lack of the client's right to an opinion. In option 4, the nurse is expressing approval, which can be harmful to a nurse-client relationship.
Test-Taking Strategy: Use therapeutic communication techniques and always address the client's concerns and feelings. Option 1 is the only therapeutic option. Review these techniques if you had difficulty with this question.
Level of Cognitive Ability: Application
Client Needs: Psychosocial Integrity
Integrated Concept/Process: Communication and Documentation
Content Area: Adult Health/Endocrine
Reference: Potter P, Perry A: *Fundamentals of nursing,* ed 5, St Louis, 2001, Mosby, p. 460.

40. ***Answer:*** 3
Rationale: Clinical manifestations associated with thyroid storm include a fever as high as 106° F, severe tachycardia, profuse diarrhea, extreme vasodilation, hypotension, atrial fibrillation, hyperreflexia, abdominal pain, diarrhea, and dehydration. In this disorder, the client's condition can progress rapidly to coma and cardiovascular collapse.
Test-Taking Strategy: Knowledge regarding the manifestations associated with thyroid storm is required to answer the question. This condition is a rare but potentially fatal hypermetabolic state. If you are unfamiliar with this disorder, review this content.
Level of Cognitive Ability: Comprehension
Client Needs: Physiological Integrity
Integrated Concept/Process: Nursing Process/Data Collection
Content Area: Adult Health/Endocrine
Reference: Black J, Hawks J, Keene A: *Medical-surgical nursing: clinical management for positive outcomes,* ed 6, Philadelphia, 2001, WB Saunders, p. 1429.

REFERENCES

Black J, Hawks J, Keene A: *Medical-surgical nursing: clinical management for positive outcomes,* ed 6, Philadelphia, 2001, WB Saunders.

Chernecky C, Berger B: *Laboratory tests and diagnostic procedures,* ed 3, Philadelphia, 2001, WB Saunders.

Clark J, Queener S, Karb V: *Pharmacologic basis of nursing practice,* ed 6, St Louis, 2000, Mosby.

DeWit S: *Fundamental concepts and skills for nursing,* Philadelphia, 2001, WB Saunders.

Hodgson B, Kizior R: *Saunders nursing drug handbook 2002,* Philadelphia, 2002, WB Saunders.

Ignatavicius D, Workman M: *Medical-surgical: critical thinking for collaborative care,* ed 4, Philadelphia, 2002, WB Saunders.

Potter P, Perry A: *Fundamentals of nursing,* ed 5, St Louis, 2001, Mosby.

Perry A, Potter P: *Clinical nursing skills and techniques,* ed 5, St Louis, 2002, Mosby.

43 Endocrine Medications

I. PITUITARY MEDICATIONS

A. Description

1. Anterior pituitary gland: secretes growth hormone (GH), thyroid-stimulating hormone (TSH), adrenocorticotropic hormone (ACTH), and gonadotropins (follicle-stimulating hormone, or FSH, and luteinizing hormone, or LH)
2. Posterior pituitary gland: secretes antidiuretic hormones (ADH, vasopressin) and oxytocin

B. Growth hormones and related medications

1. Uses and side effects (Table 43-1)
2. Implementation
   a. Assess child's physical growth and compare growth with standards
   b. Recommend annual bone age determinations for children receiving growth hormones
   c. Monitor blood and urine glucose levels
   d. Teach the client and family about the importance of follow-up care regarding blood and urine glucose testing

II. ANTIDIURETIC HORMONES (Box 43-1)

A. Description

1. Enhance reabsorption of water in the kidneys, promoting an antidiuretic effect and regulating fluid balance
2. Used in **diabetes insipidus**

B. Side effects

1. Flushing
2. Headache
3. Nausea and abdominal cramps
4. Water intoxication
5. Hypertension with water intoxication
6. Nasal congestion with nasal administration

BOX 43-1

Antidiuretic Hormones

Desmopressin acetate (DDAVP, Stimate)
Lypressin (Diapid)
Vasopressin (Pitressin)

TABLE 43-1

Growth Hormone and Related Medications

Medication(s)	Use	Side Effects
Somatrem (Protropin)	Growth failure	Development of antibodies to GH
Somatropin (Humatrope)	Growth failure	Headache, muscle pain, weakness
		Mild hyperglycemia, allergic reaction (rash, swelling), pain at injection site
Sermorelin (Geref)	Growth failure	Pain, swelling, redness at injection site; facial flushing,nausea, vomiting, headache, altered taste, chest tightness
	Diagnose pituitary function	
Bromocriptine (Parlodel)	Acromegaly	Nausea, headache, dizziness
Octreotide (Sandostatin)	Acromegaly	Diarrhea, nausea, abdominal discomfort, increased glucose

C. Implementation
1. Monitor weight
2. Monitor intake and output (I&O) and urine osmolality
3. Monitor electrolytes
4. Restrict fluid intake as prescribed to prevent water intoxication
5. Monitor for signs of water intoxication, such as drowsiness, listlessness, and headache
6. Instruct the client how to use the intranasal medication
7. Instruct the client to report signs of water intoxication or symptoms of headache or shortness of breath

III. THYROID HORMONES (Box 43-2)

A. Description
1. Control the metabolic rate of tissues and accelerate heat production and oxygen consumption
2. To replace hormonal deficit in the treatment of **hypothyroidism, myxedema,** or cretinism
3. Enhance the action of oral anticoagulants, sympathomimetics, and antidepressants, and decrease the action of insulin, oral hypoglycemics, and digitalis preparations
4. Phenytoin (Dilantin) and aspirin can enhance the action of thyroid hormone

B. Side effects
1. Nausea and vomiting
2. Cramps and diarrhea
3. Weight loss
4. Nervousness and tremors
5. Headache
6. Hypertension
7. Tachycardia and dysrhythmias
8. Sweating and heat intolerance
9. Insomnia
10. Toxicity: **hyperthyroidism**

C. Implementation
1. Check the client for history of medications currently being taking
2. Monitor vital signs
3. Monitor weight
4. Monitor triiodothyronine (T_3), thyroxine (T_4), and TSH levels
5. Instruct the client to take the medication at the same time each day, preferably in the morning without food
6. Instruct the client in how to monitor pulse rate
7. Advise the client to report symptoms of **hyperthyroidism,** such as tachycardia, chest pain, palpitations, and excessive sweating
8. Instruct the client to avoid foods that can inhibit thyroid secretion, such as strawberries, peaches, pears, cabbage, turnips, spinach, kale, brussels sprouts, cauliflower, radishes, and peas
9. Advise the client to avoid over-the counter-medications
10. Instruct the client to wear a Medic-Alert bracelet

BOX 43-2

Thyroid Hormones

Levothyroxine (Synthroid, Levothroid, Levoxyl)
Liothyronine (Cytomel)
Liotrix (Thyrolar)
Thyroglobulin (Proloid)
Thyroid (Thyrar)

IV. ANTITHYROID MEDICATIONS (Box 43-3)

A. Description
1. Inhibit the synthesis of thyroid hormone
2. Used for **hyperthyroidism** or **Graves' disease**

B. Side effects
1. Nausea and vomiting
2. Diarrhea
3. Hypersensitivity
4. Agranulocytosis
5. Toxicity: **hypothyroidism**
6. Iodism: characterized by vomiting, abdominal pain, metallic taste in the mouth, rash, and sore salivary glands

C. Implementation
1. Monitor vital signs
2. Monitor T_3, T_4, and TSH levels
3. Monitor weight
4. Instruct the client to take medication with meals to avoid gastrointestinal (GI) upset
5. Instruct the client how to monitor the pulse rate
6. Inform the client of side effects and when to notify the physician
7. Advise the client to contact the physician if a fever or sore throat develops

BOX 43-3

Antithyroid Medications

Iodine solution (Lugol solution, potassium iodide solution)
Methimazole (Tapazole)
Propylthiouracil (PTU)

8. Instruct the client in the signs of **hypothyroidism**
9. Instruct the client regarding the importance of medication compliance and that abruptly stopping the medication could cause thyroid crisis (**thyroid storm**)
10. Instruct the client to monitor for signs and symptoms of thyroid crisis (fever, flushed skin, confusion and behavioral changes, tachycardia, dysrhythmias, and signs of heart failure)
11. Instruct the client to monitor for signs of iodism
12. Advise the client to consult the physician before eating iodized salt and iodine-rich foods
13. Instruct the client to avoid acetylsalicylic acid (aspirin) and medications containing iodine

V. PARATHYROID MEDICATIONS (Box 43-4)

A. Description
1. Parathyroid hormone regulates serum calcium levels
2. Low serum levels of calcium stimulate parathyroid hormone release
3. Hyperparathyroidism results in a high serum calcium level and bone demineralization, and medication is used to lower the serum calcium level
4. Hypoparathyroidism results in a low serum calcium level, which increases neuromuscular excitability, and the treatment includes calcium and vitamin D supplements
5. Parathyroid and antihypercalcemic agents may cause hypermagnesemia
6. Calcium salts administered with digoxin (Lanoxin) increases the risk of digoxin toxicity
7. Oral calcium salts reduce the absorption of tetracycline hydrochloride

B. Implementation
1. Monitor electrolyte and calcium levels
2. Monitor for signs and symptoms of hypocalcemia and hypercalcemia
3. Monitor for symptoms of tetany in the client with hypocalcemia
4. Instruct the client in the signs and symptoms of hypercalcemia and hypocalcemia
5. Instruct the client to check over-the-counter medication labels for the possibility of calcium content
6. Instruct the client receiving oral calcium to maintain an adequate intake of vitamin D, because vitamin D enhances the absorption of calcium

BOX 43-4

Medications to Treat Calcium Disorders

CALCIUM SUPPLEMENTS
Calcium carbonate (BioCal, Caltrate 600, Rolaids, Tums)
Calcium carbonate, oyster-shell derived (Os-Cal 500, Oysco, Oyst-Cal)
Calcium citrate (Citracal)
Calcium glubionate (Calcionate, Neo-Calglucon)
Calcium gluconate
Calcium lactate
Dibasic calcium phosphate
Tribasic calcium phosphate (Posture)

VITAMIN D SUPPLEMENTS
Calcifediol (Calderol)
Calcitriol (Calcijex, Rocaltrol)
Dihydrotachysterol (DHT, Hytakerol)
Ergocalciferol (Calciferol, Drisdol)

CALCIUM REGULATORS
Alendronate (Fosamax)
Calcitonin human (Cibacalcin)
Calcitonin salmon (Calcimar, Miacalcin)
Etidronate (Didronel)
Pamidronate (Aredia)
Risedronate(Actonel)
Tiludronate (Skelid)

ANTIHYPERCALCEMICS
Edetate disodium (Disotate, Endrate)
Gallium nitrate (Ganite)

VI. ADRENOCORTICOTROPIC HORMONES (Box 43-5)

A. Description
1. Stimulate the adrenal cortex to secrete cortisol
2. Produce an antiinflammatory effect
3. Used to diagnose adrenocortical disorders (Box 43-6)
4. Used to treat acute multiple sclerosis

B. Side effects
1. Nausea and vomiting

BOX 43-5

Medications for Adrenal Replacement Therapy

Betamethasone (Celestone)
Cortisone (Cortone)
Fludrocortisone (Florinef)
Hydrocortisone (Cortef)
Triamcinolone (Aristocort, Kenacort)
Dexamethasone (Decadron)
Methylprednisolone (Depo-Medrol, Solu-Medrol)
Prednisolone (Delta-Cortef, Prelone)
Prednisone (Orasone, Deltasone, Meticorten)

BOX 43-6

Medications Used in Diagnosing Adrenal Gland Dysfunction

Corticotropin (Acthar)
Corticotropin repository (Acthar gel)
Cosyntropin (Cortrosyn)

2. Increased appetite
3. Mood swings
4. Petechiae
5. Water and sodium retention
6. Hypokalemia
7. Hypocalcemia

C. Implementation
1. Monitor vital signs
2. Monitor I&O, weight, and for edema
3. Monitor for signs of infection
4. Monitor electrolyte and calcium levels
5. Avoid administering to the client with adrenocortical hyperfunction
6. Instruct the client to decrease salt intake
7. Instruct the client to report side effects such as muscle weakness, edema, petechiae, ecchymosis, decrease in growth, decreased wound healing, and menstrual irregularities
8. Monitor for adverse effects when the medication is discontinued; dose should be tapered and not stopped abruptly, because adrenal hypofunction may result
9. Advise the client to wear a Medic-Alert bracelet

VII. CORTICOSTEROIDS (GLUCOCORTICOIDS) (Box 43-5)

A. Description
1. Produce metabolic effects
2. Alter the normal immune response and suppress inflammation
3. Promote sodium and water retention and potassium excretion
4. Produce antiinflammatory, antiallergic, and antistress effects
5. May be used as a replacement for adrenocorticoid insufficiency

B. Side effects
1. **Hyperglycemia**
2. Hypokalemia
3. Sodium and water retention
4. Edema
5. Cause muscle wasting, osteoporosis, growth retardation in children, peptic ulcer, increased serum glucose levels, hypertension, convulsions, mood swings, cataracts, glaucoma, fragile skin, hirsutism, altered fat distribution
6. Mask the signs and symptoms of infection

C. Contraindications and cautions
1. Contraindicated in hypersensitivity, psychosis, and fungal infections
2. Use with caution in **diabetes mellitus**
3. Dexamethasone (Decadron) decreases the effects of oral anticoagulants and oral antidiabetic agents
4. Increase the potency of medications taken concurrently, such as aspirin and nonsteroidal antiinflammatory drugs (NSAIDs), thus increasing the risk of GI bleeding and ulceration
5. Use of potassium-wasting diuretics increases potassium loss, resulting in hypokalemia
6. Barbiturates, phenytoin (Dilantin), and rifampin (Rifadin) decrease the effect of prednisone
7. The action of dexamethasone (Decadron) is decreased by the use of phenytoin (Dilantin), theophylline, rifampin (Rifadin), barbiturates, and antacids
8. NSAIDs, aspirin, and estrogen increase the effect of dexamethasone (Decadron)
9. Should be used with extreme caution in clients with infections because they mask the signs and symptoms of an infection
10. Advise the client to wear a Medic-Alert bracelet

D. Implementation
1. Monitor vital signs
2. Monitor serum electrolytes and blood glucose level
3. Monitor for hypokalemia and **hyperglycemia**
4. Monitor I&O, weight, and for edema
5. Monitor for hypertension
6. Check the client's medical history for glaucoma, cataracts, peptic ulcer, mental health disorders, or **diabetes mellitus**
7. Monitor the older client for signs and symptoms of increased osteoporosis
8. Monitor for changes in muscle strength
9. Prepare a schedule for the client on short-term, tapered doses
10. Instruct the client to take at mealtime or with food
11. Advise the client to eat foods high in potassium
12. Instruct the client to avoid individuals with respiratory infections
13. Advise the client to inform all health care providers of taking the medication

14. Instruct the client to report signs and symptoms of a medication overdose or **Cushing's syndrome,** including a moon face, puffy eyelids, edema in the feet, increased bruising, dizziness, bleeding, and menstrual irregularities
15. Note that the client may need additional doses during periods of stress such as surgery
16. Instruct the client not to stop the medication abruptly, as abrupt withdrawal can result in severe adrenal insufficiency
17. Advise the client to consult with the physician before receiving vaccinations
18. Advise the client to wear a Medic-Alert bracelet

E. Mineralocorticoids
1. Description
a. Steroid hormones that enhance the reabsorption of sodium and chloride and promote the excretion of potassium and hydrogen from the renal tubules, thereby helping to maintain fluid and electrolyte balance
b. Used for replacement therapy in primary and secondary adrenal insufficiency in **Addison's disease**
2. Medication: fludrocortisone (Florinef)
3. Side effects
a. Sodium and water retention
b. Hypokalemia
c. Hypocalcemia
d. Increased susceptibility to infection
e. Delayed wound healing
f. GI distress
g. Diarrhea or constipation
h. Increased appetite
i. Weight gain
j. Insomnia
k. Mood swings
l. Abdominal distention
4. Implementation
a. Monitor vital signs
b. Monitor weight
c. Monitor electrolytes and calcium level
d. Instruct the client to take medication with food or milk
e. Instruct the client to consume a high potassium diet
f. Instruct the client not to stop the medication abruptly
g. Instruct the client to notify the physician if signs of infection, muscle aches, sudden weight gain, or headaches occur
h. Instruct the client to avoid exposure to disease or trauma
i. Instruct the client not to take aspirin or any other medication without consulting the physician
j. Instruct the client to wear a Medic-Alert bracelet

VIII. ANDROGENS (Box 43-7)

A. Description
1. Used to either replace deficient hormones or treat hormone-sensitive disorders
2. Can cause bleeding if the client is taking oral anticoagulants (increase the effect of anticoagulants)
3. Cause decreased serum glucose concentration, thereby reducing insulin requirements in the client with **diabetes mellitus**
4. Hepatotoxic medications are avoided with the use of androgens because of the risk of additive damage to the liver
5. Usually avoided in men with known prostatic or breast carcinoma because androgens often stimulate growth of these tumors

B. Side effects
1. Masculine secondary sexual characteristics (body hair growth, lowered voice, muscle growth)
2. Bladder irritation and urinary tract infections
3. Breast tenderness
4. Gynecomastia
5. Priapism
6. Menstrual irregularities
7. Virilism
8. Edema
9. Nausea, vomiting, or diarrhea
10. Acne
11. Changes in libido
12. Hepatotoxicity

C. Implementation
1. Monitor vital signs
2. Monitor for edema, weight gain, and skin changes

BOX 43-7

Androgens

Fluoxymesterone (Android-F Halotestin)
Methyltestosterone (Android, Testred, Virilon)
Testosterone (Andro, Histerone, Testaqua)
Testosterone (Androderm, Testoderm)
Testosterone (Testopel pellets)
Testosterone cypionate (Andronate, Depotest)
Testosterone enanthate (Delatest, Delatestryl, Everone)
Testosterone propionate (Testex)

3. Monitor mental status and neurological function
4. Monitor for signs of liver dysfunction, including right upper quadrant abdominal pain, malaise, fever, jaundice, pruritus
5. Monitor for the development of secondary sexual characteristics
6. Instruct the client to take with meals or a snack
7. Instruct the client to notify the physician if priapism develops
8. Instruct the client to notify the physician if fluid retention occurs
9. Instruct women to use a nonhormonal contraceptive while on therapy

IX. ESTROGENS AND PROGESTINS

A. Description
1. Estrogens are steroids that stimulate female reproductive tissue
2. Progestins are steroids that specifically stimulate the uterine lining
3. Estrogen and progestin preparations may be used to stimulate the endogenous hormones to restore hormonal balance or to treat hormone-sensitive tumors (suppress tumor growth) (Boxes 43-8 and 43-9)

B. Contraindications and cautions
1. Estrogens
   a. Contraindicated in clients with breast cancer, endometrial hyperplasia, or endometrial cancer
   b. Increase the risk of toxicity when used with hepatotoxic medications
2. Progestins: contraindicated in clients with thromboembolitic disorders and avoided in clients with breast tumors or hepatic disease

C. Side effects
1. Breast tenderness
2. Nausea, vomiting, and diarrhea

BOX 43-8

Estrogens

Chlorotrianisene (Tace)
Dienestrol (Dienestrol)
Diethylstibesterol (DES)
Estradiol (Estrace, Climara, Estraderm, FemPatch, Vivelle)
Estradiol cypionate (Depo-Estradiol)
Estradiol valerate (Delestrogen)
Estrogens, congugated (Premarin)
Estrogens, esterified (Estratab)
Estrone (Aquest, Estragyn 5)
Estropipate (Ogen, Ortho-Est)
Ethinyl Estradiol (Estinyl)

BOX 43-9

Progestins

Hydroxyprogesterone (Hylutin)
Levonorgestrel (Norplant)
Medroxyprogesterone (Cycrin, Provera)
Medroxyprogesterone (Depo-Provera)
Medroxyprogesterone and conjugated estrogens (Premphase, Prempro)
Megestrol (Megace)
Norethindrone acetate (Aygestin)
Progesterone (Prometrium)
Progesterone (Gesterol, Crinone, Progestasert)

3. Malaise, depression, excessive irritability
4. Weight gain
5. Edema and fluid retention
6. Atherosclerosis
7. Hypertension
8. Migraine headaches and vomiting (estrogen)

D. Implementation
1. Monitor vital signs
2. Monitor for hypertension
3. Monitor for edema and weight gain
4. Advise the client not to smoke
5. Advise the client to undergo routine breast and pelvic examinations

X. ORAL CONTRACEPTIVES

A. Description
1. These medications contain a combination of estrogen and a progestin or a progestin alone
2. Estrogen-progestin combinations suppress ovulation and change the cervical mucus, making it difficult for sperm to enter
3. Medications that contain only progestins are less effective than the combined medications
4. Usually taken for 21 consecutive days and stopped for 7 days; then, the administration cycle is repeated
5. Provide reversible prevention of pregnancy
6. Useful in controlling irregular or excessive menstrual cycles
7. Risk factors associated with the development of complications related to the use of oral contraceptives include smoking, obesity, and hypertension
8. Contraindicated in women with hypertension and thrombolytic disease
9. Avoided with the use of hepatotoxic medications
10. Interfere with the activity of bromocriptine (Parlodel) and anticoagulants and increase the toxicity of tricyclic antidepressants
11. May alter blood glucose levels

B. Side effects
   1. Breakthrough bleeding
   2. Excessive cervical mucus formation
   3. Breast tenderness

C. Implementation
   1. Monitor vital signs and weight
   2. Instruct the client in the administration of the medication (it may take up to 1 week for full contraceptive effect to occur when the medication is begun)
   3. Instruct the client with **diabetes mellitus** to monitor blood glucose levels carefully
   4. Instruct the client to report signs of thromboembolitic complications
   5. Instruct the client to notify the physician if vaginal bleeding or menstrual irregularities occur or if pregnancy is suspected
   6. Inform the client that many medications interfere with the effectiveness of birth control pills
   7. Instruct the client to perform breast self-examination monthly and about the importance of yearly physical examinations
   8. If the client decides to discontinue the oral contraceptive to become pregnant, recommend that the client use an alternative form of birth control for 2 months after discontinuation to ensure more complete excretion of hormonal agents before conception

XI. FERTILITY MEDICATIONS (Box 43-10)

A. Description
   1. Act to stimulate follicle development and ovulation in functioning ovaries and are combined with human chorionic gonadotropin (hCG) to maintain the follicles once ovulation has occurred
   2. Contraindicated in the presence of primary ovarian, thyroid, or adrenal dysfunction, ovarian cysts, pregnancy, and idiopathic uterine bleeding
   3. Used with caution in clients with thromboembolitic or respiratory diseases

BOX 43-10

Fertility Medications

Bromocriptine (Parlodel)
Chorionic gonagotropin (A.P.L., Profasi)
Clomiphene (Clomid)
Follitropin alfa (Gonal-F)
Follitropin beta (Follistin)
Menotropins (Humegon, Pergonal)
Urofollitropin (Metrodin, Fertinex)

B. Side effects
   1. Risk of multiple births and birth defects
   2. Ovarian overstimulation (abdominal pain, distention, ascites, pleural effusion)
   3. Headache
   4. Fluid retention and bloating
   5. Nausea
   6. Uterine bleeding
   7. Ovarian enlargement
   8. Gynecomastia
   9. Febrile reactions

C. Implementation
   1. Instruct the client regarding administration of the medication
   2. Provide a calendar of treatment days and instructions on when intercourse should occur to increase therapeutic effectiveness of the medication
   3. Provide information about the risks and hazards of multiple births
   4. Instruct the client to notify the physician if signs of ovarian stimulation occur
   5. Inform the client about the need for regular follow-up evaluation

XII. MEDICATIONS FOR PENILE ERECTION DYSFUNCTION

A. Description
   1. Alprostadil (Caverject, MUSE) is a prostaglandin that relaxes smooth muscle and promotes blood flow into the corpus cavernosum
   2. Sildenafil (Viagara) may be classified as a cardiovascular agent and selectively inhibits receptors and increases nitrous oxide levels, allowing blood flow into the corpus cavernosum
   3. Contraindicated in the presence of any anatomical obstruction or condition that might predispose to priapism and in clients with penile implants
   4. Caution should be used in clients with bleeding disorders
   5. Sildenafil (Viagara) is used cautiously in clients with coronary artery disease, active peptic ulcer, or retinitis pigmentosa
   6. Sildenafil (Viagara) cannot be administered to clients taking any organic nitrates 

B. Side effects
   1. Alprostadil (Caverject, MUSE): pain at the injection site, infection, priapism, fibrosis, rash
   2. Sildenafil (Viagara): headache, flushing, dyspepsia, urinary tract infection, diarrhea, dizziness, rash

C. Implementation
1. Obtain a health and medication history
2. Instruct the client regarding administration of the medication; Alprostadil (Caverject, MUSE) is injected, and Sildenafil (Viagara) is taken orally
3. Inform the client of the side effects necessitating the need to notify the physician

XIII. MEDICATIONS FOR DIABETES MELLITUS

A. Insulin and oral hypoglycemic medications
1. Description
a. Insulin increases glucose transport into cells and promotes conversion of glucose to glycogen, decreasing serum glucose levels
b. Oral hypoglycemic agents stimulate the pancreas to produce more insulin and increase the sensitivity of peripheral receptors to insulin, thereby decreasing serum glucose levels
2. Contraindications and concerns
a. Insulin is contraindicated in clients with hypersensitivity
b. Oral hypoglycemic agents are contraindicated in type 1 **diabetes mellitus** and in those individuals allergic to sulfonylureas
c. Sulfonylureas can affect cardiac function and oxygen consumption and lead to cardiac dysrhythmias
d. Use of hypoglycemic medications with beta-adrenergic blocking agents mask signs and symptoms of **hypoglycemia**
e. Anticoagulants, chloramphenicol (Chloromycetin), clofibrate (Atromid-S), salicylates, propranolol (Inderal), monoamine oxidase inhibitors (MAOIs), pentamidine (Pentam 300), and sulfonamides may cause **hypoglycemia**
f. Corticosteroids, sympathomimetics, thiazide diuretics, phenytoin (Dilantin), thyroid preparations, oral contraceptives, and estrogen compounds may cause **hyperglycemia**
g. Side effects of the sulfonylureas include gastrointestinal symptoms and dermatological reactions; **hypoglycemia** can occur when an excessive dose is administered or when meals are omitted or delayed, food intake is decreased, or activity is increased
h. Chlorpropamide (Diabenese) can cause a disulfiram (Antabuse) type of reaction when alcohol is ingested

B. Oral hypoglycemic medications
1. Prescribed for clients with type 2 **diabetes mellitus**
2. Sulfonylureas
a. Classified as first- and second-generation sulfonylureas (Box 43-11)
b. Stimulate the beta cells to produce more insulin
3. Nonsulfonylureas (Box 43-11)
a. Affect the hepatic and GI production of glucose
b. May be used in combination with a sulfonylurea
4. Implementation
a. Assess the client's knowledge of **diabetes mellitus** and the use of oral antidiabetic agents
b. Obtain a medication history regarding the medications that the client is currently taking
c. Monitor vital signs and blood glucose levels
d. Instruct the client to recognize symptoms of **hypoglycemia** and **hyperglycemia**
e. Instruct the client to avoid over-the-counter medications unless prescribed by the physician

BOX 43-11

First- and Second-Generation Sulfonylureas and Nonsulfonylureas

FIRST-GENERATION SULFONYLUREA

Short-Acting
Tolbutamide (Orinase)
Intermediate-Acting
Acetohexamide (Dymelor)
Tolazamide (Tolinase)
Long-Acting
Chlorpropamide (Diabenese)

SECOND-GENERATIONSULFONYLUREAS

Glipizide (Glucotrol, Glucotrol XL)
Glyburide (DiaBeta, Micronase, Glynase)
Glimepiride (Amaryl)

NONSULFONYLUREAS

Biguanide
Metformin (Glucophage)
Alpha Glucosidase Inhibitor
Acarbose (Precose)
Miglitol (Glyset)
Thiozolidinediones
Troglitazone (Rezulin)
Pioglitazone (Actos)
Rosiglitazone (Avandia)
Meglitinide
Rapaglinide (Prandin)

f. Instruct the client not to ingest alcohol with sulfonylureas
g. Inform the client that insulin may be needed during stress, surgery, or infection
h. Instruct the client in the necessity of compliance with prescribed medication
i. Advise the client to wear a Medic-Alert bracelet

C. Insulin (Table 43-2)
1. Primarily acts in the liver, muscle, and adipose tissue by attaching to receptors on cellular membranes and facilitating the passage of glucose, potassium, and magnesium
2. Prescribed for clients with type 1 **diabetes mellitus**
3. Storing insulin
   a. Exposure to extremes in temperature is avoided; insulin should not be frozen or kept in direct sunlight or a hot car
   b. Before injection, insulin should be at room temperature
   c. If a vial of insulin will be used up in a month, it may be kept at room temperature; otherwise, the vial should be refrigerated
4. Insulin injection sites
   a. The main areas for injections are the abdomen, arms (posterior surface), thighs (anterior surface), and hips
   b. Insulin injected into the abdomen may absorb more evenly and rapidly than at other sites
   c. Systematic rotation within one anatomical area is recommended to prevent lipodystrophy; client should be instructed not to use the same site more than once in a 2- to 3-week period
   d. Injections should be 1.5 inches apart within the anatomical area
   e. Heat, massage, and exercise of the injected area can increase absorption rates and may result in **hypoglycemia**
   f. Injection into scar tissue may delay absorption of insulin
5. Administering insulin
   a. To prevent dosage errors, be certain that there is a match of the insulin concentration noted on the vial with the calibration of units on the insulin syringe; the usual concentration of insulin is U 100 (100 units per mL)
   b. Most insulin syringes have a 27- to 29-gauge needle that is approximately 0.5 inch long
   c. Before use, roll, not shake (to avoid bubbles) the insulin bottle to ensure that the insulin and ingredients are mixed well; otherwise an inaccurate dose will be drawn
   d. Premixed insulins (NPH to Regular insulin) are available as 70/30 (most commonly used), 80/20, 60/40, 50/50
   e. A 3-week supply of insulin may be prepared and kept in the refrigerator; prefilled syringes should be kept flat or with the needle in an upright position to avoid clogging of the needle
   f. Inject air into the insulin bottle (a vacuum makes it difficult to draw up the insulin)
   g. It is recommended to draw up the Regular (shorter-acting) insulin first
   h. Regular Insulin may be mixed with any other type of insulin
   i. Insulin zinc suspensions may be mixed only with each other and Regular insulin, not with other types of insulin
   j. Administer a mixed dose of insulin within 5 to 15 minutes of preparation; after this time the Regular insulin binds with the NPH insulin and its action is reduced
   k. Aspiration is generally not recommended with self-injection of insulin
   l. Administer insulin at a 45- to 90-degree angle and at a 45- to 60-degree angle in thin persons
   m. REMEMBER: Regular insulin is the only type of insulin that can be administered intravenously

TABLE 43-2

Common Types of Insulin

Type	Onset	Peak	Duration
RAPID-ACTING			
Lispro (Humalog)	10-15 minutes	1 hour	3 hours
SHORT-ACTING			
Humulin Regular	0.5-1 hour	2-3 hours	4-6 hours
INTERMEDIATE-ACTING			
Humulin NPH	3-4 hours	4-12 hours	16-20 hours
Humulin Lente	3-4 hours	4-12 hours	16-20 hours
LONG-ACTING			
Humulin Ultralente	6-8 hours	12-16 hours	20-30 hours
PREMIXED			
70% NPH and 30% Regular	0.5-1 hour	2-12 hours	18-24 hours

D. Glucagon
1. A hormone secreted by the alpha cells of the islets of Langerhans in the pancreas
2. Increases blood glucose by stimulating glycogenolysis in the liver
3. Can be administered subcutaneously, intramuscularly, or intravenously
4. Used to treat insulin-induced **hypoglycemia** when the client is semiconscious or unconscious and is unable to ingest liquids
5. The blood glucose level begins to increase within 5 to 20 minutes after administration
6. Instruct the family in the procedure for administration
7. Refer to Chapter 42 for additional information regarding implementation for severe **hypoglycemia**

E. Diazoxide (Proglycem)
1. Increases blood glucose by inhibiting insulin release from the beta cells and stimulating the release of epinephrine from the adrenal medulla
2. Used to treat chronic **hypoglycemia** caused by hyperinsulinism resulting from islet cell cancer or hyperplasia
3. It is not used for **hypoglycemic** reactions from insulin

PRACTICE QUESTIONS

1. Somatrem (Protropin) is administered to a client with pituitary dwarfism. The expected therapeutic effect of this medication is to:
   1. Promote weight gain
   2. Stimulate linear growth
   3. Increase bone density
   4. Decrease the mobilization of fats
2. A nurse is monitoring a client receiving desmopressin (DDAVP). Which of the following, if noted in the client, would indicate an adverse reaction to the medication?
   1. Increased urination
   2. Weight loss
   3. Drowsiness
   4. Insomnia
3. A nurse reinforces instructions to a client taking levothyroxine (Synthroid). The nurse determines that the teaching was effective if the client states to take the medication:
   1. With food
   2. On an empty stomach
   3. At bed time
   4. At lunch time
4. Thyroid replacement therapy is prescribed for a client diagnosed with hypothyroidism. The client asks the nurse when the medication will no longer be needed. The most appropriate nursing response is which of the following?
   1. "You will need to ask your physician."
   2. "Most clients require medication therapy for about 1 year."
   3. "It depends on the results of the laboratory values."
   4. "The medication will need to be continued for life."
5. A nurse reinforces medication instructions to a client taking levothyroxine (Synthroid). The nurse instructs the client to notify the physician if which of the following occurs?
   1. Cold intolerance
   2. Tremors
   3. Excessively dry skin
   4. Fatigue
6. A nurse reviews the health record of a client seen in the physician's office and notes that the client is taking propylthiouracil (PTU) daily. The nurse suspects that the client has a history of:
   1. Cushing's syndrome
   2. Addison's disease
   3. Myxedema
   4. Graves' disease
7. A nurse is reinforcing instructions to a client regarding the administration of lypressin (Diapid). The nurse instructs the client that the medication will be taken by which of the following routes?
   1. Oral
   2. Subcutaneous
   3. Intranasal
   4. Intramuscular
8. A client is seen by the physician for complaints of fatigue, a lack of energy, constipation, and depression. After diagnostic studies, hypothyroidism is diagnosed. Levothyroxine (Synthroid) is prescribed. The nurse tells the client that the expected outcome of the medication is to:
   1. Increase energy levels
   2. Achieve normal thyroid hormone levels
   3. Increase blood glucose levels
   4. Alleviate depression
9. Propythiouracil (PTU) is prescribed for a client with hyperthyroidism. The nurse reinforces instructions to the client regarding the medication. The nurse informs the client to notify the physician if which of the following signs occur?
   1. Drowsiness
   2. Sore throat
   3. Polyuria
   4. Dry mouth
10. A client is scheduled for subtotal thyroidectomy. Iodine solution (Lugol solution) is prescribed. The nurse understands that the therapeutic effect of this medication is to:

1. Increase thyroid hormone production
2. Suppress thyroid hormone production
3. Replace thyroid hormone
4. Prevent the oxidation of iodide

11. A nurse reinforces instructions to the client taking fludrocortisone (Florinef). The nurse tells the client to notify the physician if which of the following occurs?
 1. Weight loss
 2. Nausea
 3. Swelling of the feet
 4. Fatigue

12. Calcium carbonate (Os-Cal) is prescribed for a client with hypocalcemia. The nurse most appropriately instructs the client to take the medication:
 1. With meals
 2. 2 hours after meals
 3. 1 hour before meals
 4. 1 hour before breakfast

13. Calcitriol (Rocaltrol) is prescribed for the client with hypocalcemia. The nurse provides dietary instructions to the client. Which of the following food items would the nurse instruct the client to avoid while taking this medication?
 1. Oysters
 2. Milk
 3. Whole grain cereals
 4. Sardines

14. A daily dose of prednisone (Deltasone) is prescribed for a client. A nurse provides instructions to the client regarding administration of the medication and tells the client that the best time to take this medication is:
 1. At bedtime
 2. At noon
 3. Early morning
 4. Anytime, at the same time, each day

15. A hospitalized client with diabetes mellitus received NPH insulin in the morning. When would the nurse expect the peak action of the insulin dose to occur?
 1. 2 to 4 hours after administration
 2. 4 to 12 hours after administration
 3. 12 to 16 hours after administration
 4. 18 to 24 hours after administration

16. A nurse is teaching the client how to mix Regular insulin and NPH insulin in the same syringe. Which of the following actions, if performed by the client, would indicate the need for further teaching?
 1. Injects air into NPH insulin vial first
 2. Injects the amount of air equal to the desired dose of insulin into the vial
 3. Withdraws the NPH insulin first
 4. Withdraws the Regular insulin first

17. A nurse is reinforcing home care instructions to a client recently diagnosed with diabetes mellitus. The client is taking NPH insulin daily and asks the nurse how to store the unopened vials of insulin. Which of the following instructions would the nurse provide to the client?
 1. Freeze the insulin
 2. Refrigerate the insulin
 3. Keep the insulin at room temperature
 4. Keep in a dark dry place

18. A client with diabetes mellitus is self-administering NPH insulin from a vial that is kept at room temperature. The client asks the nurse about the length of time an unrefrigerated vial of insulin will maintain its potency. The most appropriate response is which of the following?
 1. 2 weeks
 2. 1 month
 3. 2 months
 4. 6 months

19. Lispro insulin (Humalog), a rapid-acting form of insulin, is prescribed for a client. The nurse instructs the client to administer the insulin:
 1. Immediately before eating
 2. 30 minutes before eating
 3. 45 minutes before eating
 4. 60 minutes before eating

20. Tolbutamide (Orinase) is prescribed for the client with diabetes mellitus. The nurse instructs the client to avoid which of the following while taking this medication?
 1. Carbonated beverages
 2. Organ meats
 3. Alcohol
 4. Whole grain cereals

ANSWERS

1. *Answer:* 2

Rationale: Protropin is a growth stimulator used in the long-term treatment of growth failure resulting from growth hormone deficiency. It stimulates linear growth, increases the number and size of muscle cells, and red cell mass. It affects carbohydrate metabolism by antagonizing the action of insulin, increasing mobilization of fats, and increasing cellular protein synthesis.

Test-Taking Strategy: Use the client diagnosis in the question to assist in the process of elimination in answering the question. Note the relationship between "dwarfism" in the question and

"growth" in the correct option. Review the action of this medication if you had difficulty with this question.
Level of Cognitive Ability: Analysis
Client Needs: Physiological Integrity
Integrated Concept/Process: Nursing Process/Evaluation
Content Area: Pharmacology
Reference: Hodgson B, Kizior R: *Saunders nursing drug handbook 2002*, Philadelphia, 2002, WB Saunders, p. 1017.

2. *Answer:* 3
Rationale: Water intoxication or hyponatremia is an adverse reaction to DDAVP. Early signs include drowsiness, listlessness, and headache. Decreased urination, rapid weight gain, confusion, seizures, and coma may also occur in overhydration.
Test-Taking Strategy: Use the process of elimination. Knowledge that this medication is used in the treatment of diabetes insipidus will assist in eliminating options 1 and 2. Recalling the action of the medication will assist you in determining that water intoxication is an adverse reaction. This thought process will assist in directing you to option 3. Review the adverse reactions related to this medication if you had difficulty with this question.
Level of Cognitive Ability: Analysis
Client Needs: Physiological Integrity
Integrated Concept/Process: Nursing Process/Data Collection
Content Area: Pharmacology
Reference: Hodgson B, Kizior R: *Saunders nursing drug handbook 2002*, Philadelphia, 2002, WB Saunders, p. 317.

3. *Answer:* 2
Rationale: Oral doses of levothyroxine should be taken on an empty stomach to enhance absorption. The medication should be taken in the morning before breakfast.
Test-Taking Strategy: Use the process of elimination. Eliminate options 1 and 4 first because they are similar. From the remaining options, recalling the purpose of the medication and that it is administered in the morning will direct you to option 2. Review this medication if you had difficulty with this question.
Level of Cognitive Ability: Comprehension
Client Needs: Health Promotion and Maintenance
Integrated Concept/Process: Nursing Process/Evaluation
Content Area: Pharmacology
Reference: Hodgson B, Kizior R: *Saunders nursing drug handbook 2002*, Philadelphia, 2002, WB Saunders, p. 643.

4. *Answer:* 4
Rationale: For most hypothyroid clients, replacement therapy must be continued for life. Treatment provides symptomatic relief but does not produce a cure. The client should be told that although therapy will improve symptoms, these improvements do not constitute a reason to interrupt or discontinue the medication.
Test-Taking Strategy: Use the process of elimination. Recalling the physiology associated with hypothyroidism will direct you to option 4. If you are unfamiliar with this disorder and the medication therapy associated with it, review this content.
Level of Cognitive Ability: Application
Client Needs: Health Promotion and Maintenance
Integrated Concept/Process: Nursing Process/Implementation
Content Area: Pharmacology
Reference: Lehne R: *Pharmacology for nursing care*, ed 4, Philadelphia, 2001, WB Saunders, p. 640.

5. *Answer:* 2
Rationale: Excessive doses of levothyroxine can produce signs and symptoms of hyperthyroidism. These include tachycardia, angina, tremors, nervousness, insomnia, hyperthermia, heat intolerance, and sweating. The client should be instructed to notify the physician if these occur. Options 1, 3, and 4 are signs of hypothyroidism.
Test-Taking Strategy: Use the process of elimination recalling the symptoms associated with hypothyroidism, the purpose of administering levothyroxine, and the effects of the medication. Options 1, 3, and 4 are symptoms related to hypothyroidism. Review the adverse effects of the medication if you are unfamiliar with them.
Level of Cognitive Ability: Application
Client Needs: Health Promotion and Maintenance
Integrated Concept/Process: Nursing Process/Implementation
Content Area: Pharmacology
Reference: Lehne R: *Pharmacology for nursing care*, ed 4, Philadelphia, 2001, WB Saunders, p. 640.

6. *Answer:* 4
Rationale: PTU inhibits thyroid hormone synthesis and is used to treat hyperthyroidism or Graves' disease. Myxedema indicates hypothyroidism. Cushing's syndrome and Addison's disease are disorders related to adrenal function.
Test-Taking Strategy: Knowledge regarding the action of the medication and the treatment measures for Graves' disease are required to answer the question. If you are unfamiliar with either of these, review this content.
Level of Cognitive Ability: Analysis
Client Needs: Physiological Integrity
Integrated Concept/Process: Nursing Process/Data Collection
Content Area: Pharmacology
Reference: Lehne R: *Pharmacology for nursing care*, ed 4, Philadelphia, 2001, WB Saunders, p. 642.

7. *Answer:* 3
Rationale: Lypressin is administered by the intranasal route. It is used for diabetes insipidus. The usual adult dosage is 1 to 2 sprays into each nostril 4 times daily.
Test-Taking Strategy: Knowledge that lypressin is administered by the nasal route is required to answer the question. Review this medication if you had difficulty with this question.
Level of Cognitive Ability: Application
Client Needs: Health Promotion and Maintenance
Integrated Concept/Process: Nursing Process/Implementation
Content Area: Pharmacology
Reference: Lehne R: *Pharmacology for nursing care*, ed 4, Philadelphia, 2001, WB Saunders, p. 654.

8. *Answer:* 2
Rationale: Laboratory determination of the serum thyroid-stimulating hormone level (TSH) is an important means of evaluation of therapy with levothyroxine. Effective therapy will cause the elevated TSH levels to decrease. These levels will

begin their decline within hours of the onset of therapy and will continue to drop as plasma levels of thyroid hormone build up. If an adequate dosage is established, TSH levels will remain suppressed for the duration of the therapy.
Test-Taking Strategy: Note the key words "expected outcome." Relate the diagnosis hypo "thyroidism" with "thyroid" hormone levels in the correct option. If you had difficulty with this question, review the therapeutic effect of levothyroxine.
Level of Cognitive Ability: Application
Client Needs: Physiological Integrity
Integrated Concept/Process: Teaching/Learning
Content Area: Pharmacology
Reference: Lehne R: *Pharmacology for nursing care*, ed 4, Philadelphia, 2001, WB Saunders, p. 640.

9. ***Answer:*** 2
Rationale: An adverse effect of PTU is agranulocytosis. The client needs to be informed of the early signs of this adverse effect, which includes fever or sore throat. Drowsiness is an occasional side effect of the medication. Polyuria and dry mouth are unrelated to this medication.
Test-Taking Strategy: Use the process of elimination. Recalling that agranulocytosis is an adverse effect of PTU will direct you to option 2. Review this medication if you had difficulty with this question.
Level of Cognitive Ability: Application
Client Needs: Health Promotion and Maintenance
Integrated Concept/Process: Nursing Process/Implementation
Content Area: Pharmacology
Reference: Lehne R: *Pharmacology for nursing care*, ed 4, Philadelphia, 2001, WB Saunders, p. 642.

10. ***Answer:*** 2
Rationale: Lugol solution is administered to hyperthyroid individuals in preparation for thyroidectomy to suppress thyroid function. Initial effects develop within 24 hours; peak effects develop in 10 to 15 days. Options 1, 3, and 4 are incorrect.
Test-Taking Strategy: Use the process of elimination. Eliminate options 1 and 3 first because they are similar. From the remaining options, select option 2 because of its relationship to the issue of the question. If you had difficulty with this question, review the purpose of this medication.
Level of Cognitive Ability: Comprehension
Client Needs: Physiological Integrity
Integrated Concept/Process: Nursing Process/Evaluation
Content Area: Pharmacology
Reference: Lehne R: *Pharmacology for nursing care*, ed 4, Philadelphia, 2001, WB Saunders, p. 644.

11. ***Answer:*** 3
Rationale: Excessive doses of fludrocortisone cause retention of sodium and water and excessive excretion of potassium resulting in expansion of blood volume, hypertension, cardiac enlargement, edema, and hypokalemia. The client needs to be informed about the signs of sodium and water retention, such as unusual weight gain, or swelling of the feet or lower legs. If these signs occur, the physician needs to be notified.
Test-Taking Strategy: Use the process of elimination. Recalling that fludrocortisone can cause water retention will direct you to option 3. If you are unfamiliar with the adverse effects associated with this medication, review this content.
Level of Cognitive Ability: Application
Client Needs: Health Promotion and Maintenance
Integrated Concept/Process: Nursing Process/Implementation
Content Area: Pharmacology
Reference: Lehne R: *Pharmacology for nursing care*, ed 4, Philadelphia, 2001, WB Saunders, p. 664.

12. ***Answer:*** 1
Rationale: The client should be instructed to take oral calcium with or after meals to promote absorption. The client should take the medication with a full glass of water.
Test-Taking Strategy: Use the process of elimination. Eliminate options 3 and 4 first because they are similar. From the remaining options, it is necessary to know that this medication is taken with meals. Review this medication if you had difficulty with this question.
Level of Cognitive Ability: Application
Client Needs: Physiological Integrity
Integrated Concept/Process: Teaching/Learning
Content Area: Pharmacology
Reference: Lehne R: *Pharmacology for nursing care*, ed 4, Philadelphia, 2001, WB Saunders, p. 819.

13. ***Answer:*** 3
Rationale: The client taking an antihypocalcemic medication should be instructed to avoid eating foods that can suppress calcium absorption. These foods include Swiss chard, beets, bran, and whole-grain cereals.
Test-Taking Strategy: Use the process of elimination. Note that the client's diagnosis is "hypocalcemia" and note the key word "avoid." Eliminate options 1 and 4 first because they are similar. From the remaining options, recalling the food items that can suppress calcium absorption will direct you to option 3. Review these foods if you had difficulty with this question.
Level of Cognitive Ability: Application
Client Needs: Health Promotion and Maintenance
Integrated Concept/Process: Nursing Process/Implementation
Content Area: Pharmacology
Reference: Lehne R: *Pharmacology for nursing care*, ed 4, Philadelphia, 2001, WB Saunders, p. 808.

14. ***Answer:*** 3
Rationale: Glucocorticoids should be administered before 9 AM, and the client should be instructed to do so. Administration at this time helps minimize adrenal insufficiency and mimics the burst of glucocorticoids released naturally by the adrenals each morning.
Test-Taking Strategy: Knowledge regarding the administration of glucocorticoids is required to answer this question. If you had difficulty with this question, review these concepts.
Level of Cognitive Ability: Application
Client Needs: Health Promotion and Maintenance
Integrated Concept/Process: Nursing Process/Implementation
Content Area: Pharmacology
Reference: Lehne R: *Pharmacology for nursing care*, ed 4, Philadelphia, 2001, WB Saunders, p. 659.

15. *Answer:* 2
Rationale: NPH insulin is an intermediate-acting insulin. Its onset of action is 3 to 4 hours, it peaks in 4 to 12 hours, and its duration of action is 16 to 20 hours.
Test-Taking Strategy: Read the question carefully noting that the question is asking about NPH insulin. Recalling the onset of action, peak, and duration of action of NPH insulin will direct you to option 2. Review these points regarding both NPH and Regular insulin if you are unfamiliar with them.
Level of Cognitive Ability: Comprehension
Client Needs: Physiological Integrity
Integrated Concept/Process: Nursing Process/Planning
Content Area: Pharmacology
Reference: Lehne R: *Pharmacology for nursing care,* ed 4, Philadelphia, 2001, WB Saunders, p. 619.

16. *Answer:* 3
Rationale: When preparing a mixture of Regular insulin with another insulin preparation, the Regular insulin should be drawn into the syringe first. This sequence will avoid contaminating the vial of Regular insulin with insulin of another type. Options 1, 2, and 4 are correct.
Test-Taking Strategy: Use the process of elimination and note the key words "need for further teaching." Recalling the appropriate method of preparing insulin for injection will direct you to option 3. Review this procedure if you had difficulty with this question.
Level of Cognitive Ability: Comprehension
Client Needs: Health Promotion and Maintenance
Integrated Concept/Process: Teaching/Learning
Content Area: Pharmacology
Reference: Lehne R: *Pharmacology for nursing care,* ed 4, Philadelphia, 2001, WB Saunders, p. 617.

17. *Answer:* 2
Rationale: Unopened vials of insulin should be stored under refrigeration until needed. Vials should not be frozen. Open vials in use may be kept at room temperature and should be kept away from heat and direct light.
Test-Taking Strategy: Use the process of elimination and note the key word "store" in the question. Remembering that insulin should not be frozen will assist in eliminating option 1. Eliminate options 3 and 4 because they are similar. Review client teaching points related to insulin if you had difficulty with this question.
Level of Cognitive Ability: Application
Client Needs: Health Promotion and Maintenance
Integrated Concept/Process: Teaching/Learning
Content Area: Pharmacology
Reference: Lehne R: *Pharmacology for nursing care,* ed 4, Philadelphia, 2001, WB Saunders, p. 620.

18. *Answer:* 2
Rationale: An unrefrigerated insulin vial will maintain its potency for up to 1 month. Direct sunlight and heat must be avoided.
Test-Taking Strategy: Note the key word "unrefrigerated" to assist in directing you to the correct option. Review the concepts related to insulin stability if you had difficulty with this question.
Level of Cognitive Ability: Application
Client Needs: Health Promotion and Maintenance
Integrated Concept/Process: Nursing Process/Implementation
Content Area: Pharmacology
Reference: Lehne R: *Pharmacology for nursing care,* ed 4, Philadelphia, 2001, WB Saunders, p. 620.

19. *Answer:* 1
Rationale: The effect of Lispro insulin begins within 5 minutes of subcutaneous injection and persists for 2 to 4 hours. Lispro insulin acts more rapidly than Regular insulin but has a shorter duration of action. Because of its rapid onset, it can be administered immediately before eating. In contrast, Regular insulin is generally administered 30 to 60 minutes before meals.
Test-Taking Strategy: Use the process of elimination. Noting the key words "rapid acting" will assist in eliminating options 3 and 4.From the remaining options, remember that the question is asking about Lispro, not Regular insulin. Review this type of insulin if you had difficulty with this question.
Level of Cognitive Ability: Application
Client Needs: Health Promotion and Maintenance
Integrated Concept/Process: Teaching/Learning
Content Area: Pharmacology
Reference: Lehne R: *Pharmacology for nursing care,* ed 4, Philadelphia, 2001, WB Saunders, p. 618.

20. *Answer:* 3
Rationale: When alcohol is combined with tolbutamide, a disulfiram-like reaction may occur. This syndrome includes flushing, palpitations, and nausea. Also, alcohol can potentiate the hypoglycemic effects of tolbutamide. Clients must be warned about alcohol consumption while taking this medication.
Test-Taking Strategy: Use the process of elimination. Eliminate options 1, 2, and 4 because these food items are allowed in a diabetic diet. From the remaining options, remembering that alcohol can affect the action of many medications will assist in directing you to option 3. Review this medication if you had difficulty with this question.
Level of Cognitive Ability: Application
Client Needs: Health Promotion and Maintenance
Integrated Concept/Process: Teaching/Learning
Content Area: Pharmacology
Reference: Lehne R: *Pharmacology for nursing care,* ed 4, Philadelphia, 2001, WB Saunders, p. 625.

REFERENCES

Clark J, Queener S, Karb V: *Pharmacologic basis of nursing practice,* ed 6, St Louis, 2000, Mosby.
Hodgson B, Kizior R: *Saunders nursing drug handbook 2002,* Philadelphia, 2002, WB Saunders.
Ignatavicius D, Workman M: *Medical-surgical: critical thinking for collaborative care,* ed 4, Philadelphia, 2002, WB Saunders.
Karch A: *Focus on nursing pharmacology,* Philadelphia, 2000, Lippincott.
Lehne R: *Pharmacology for nursing care,* ed 4, Philadelphia, 2001, WB Saunders.

UNIT XI

The Adult Client with a Gastrointestinal Disorder

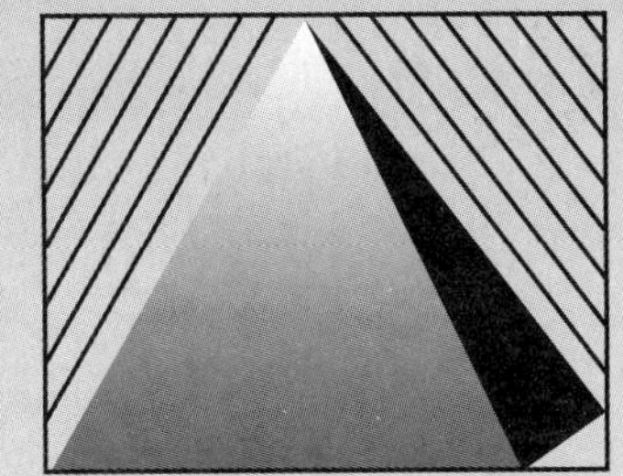

PYRAMID TERMS

Ascites Accumulation of fluid within the peritoneal cavity that results in venous congestion of the hepatic capillaries. This leads to plasma leaking directly from the liver surface and portal vein.

Asterixis Also termed liver flap. A course tremor characterized by rapid, nonrhythmic extensions and flexions in the wrist and fingers.

Billroth I Also called gastroduodenostomy; partial gastrectomy with the remaining segment anastomosed to the duodenum.

Billroth II Also called gastrojejunostomy; partial gastrectomy with the remaining segment anastomosed to the jejunum.

Cholecystectomy Removal of the gallbladder.

Cholecystitis An inflammation of the gallbladder that may occur as an acute or chronic process. Acute inflammation is associated with gallstones (cholelithiasis). Chronic cholecystitis results when inefficient bile emptying and gallbladder muscle wall disease cause a fibrotic and contracted gallbladder.

Choledochotomy Incision into the common bile duct to remove the stone.

Cirrhosis A chronic, progressive disease of the liver characterized by diffuse damage to cells with fibrosis and nodular regeneration. Repeated destruction of hepatic cells causes the formation of scar tissue.

Crohn's Disease An inflammatory disease that can occur anywhere in the gastrointestinal (GI) tract but most often affects the terminal ileum and leads to thickening and scarring, a narrowed lumen, fistulas, ulcerations, and abscesses. It is characterized by remissions and exacerbations.

Diverticulitis Inflammation of one or more diverticuli. Results when diverticulum perforates, with local abscess formation. A perforated diverticulum can progress to intraabdominal perforation with generalized peritonitis.

Diverticulosis Outpouching or herniations of the intestinal mucosa. They can occur in any part of the intestine but are most common in the sigmoid colon.

Dumping Syndrome Rapid emptying of the gastric contents into the small intestine. Occurs after gastric resection.

Esophageal Varices Dilated and tortuous veins in the submucosa of the esophagus. They are caused by portal hypertension, are often associated with liver cirrhosis, and are at high risk for rupture if portal circulation pressure rises.

Fetor Hepaticus The fruity, musty breath odor associated with chronic liver disease.

Gastrectomy Also called esophagojejunostomy; removal of the stomach with attachment of the esophagus to the jejunum or duodenum.

Gastric Resection Also called antrectomy; involves removal of the lower half of the stomach and usually includes a vagotomy.

Hepatitis An inflammation of the liver caused by a virus, bacteria, or exposure to medications or hepatotoxins.

Hiatal Hernia Also known as esophageal or diaphragmatic hernia. A portion of the stomach herniates through the diaphragm and into the thorax. It results from weakening of the muscles of the diaphragm and is aggravated by factors that increase abdominal pressure such as pregnancy, ascites, obesity, tumors, and heavy lifting.

Pancreatitis An acute or chronic inflammation of the pancreas, with associated escape of pancreatic enzymes into surrounding tissue. Acute pancreatitis occurs suddenly as one attack or can be recurrent, but resolves. Chronic pancreatitis is a continual inflammation and destruction of the pancreas, with scar tissue replacing pancreatic tissue.

Peristalsis Wavelike rhythmic contractions that propel material through the GI tract.

Pyloroplasty Enlarging the pylorus to prevent or decrease pyloric obstruction, thereby enhancing gastric emptying.

Ulcerative Colitis Ulcerative and inflammatory disease of the bowel that results in poor absorption of nutrients. Acute ulcerative colitis results in vascular congestion, hemorrhage, edema, and ulceration of the bowel mucosa. Chronic ulcerative colitis causes muscular hypertrophy, fat deposits, and fibrous tissue with bowel thickening, shortening, and narrowing.

Vagotomy Surgical division of the vagus nerve to eliminate the vagal impulses that stimulate hydrochloric acid secretion in the stomach.

PYRAMID TO SUCCESS

Pyramid points focus on diagnostic tests, nursing care related to the various gastric or intestinal tubes, gastric surgery, cirrhosis, hepatitis, pancreatitis, and colostomy care. Focus on preprocedure and postprocedure care of the client undergoing a GI diagnostic test. Remember that an informed consent is required for any invasive procedure. Focus on diet restrictions before and after the diagnostic test, and remember that the gag reflex or bowel sounds must return before allowing a client to consume food or fluids. Pyramid points include instructions to the client and family regarding the prevention of GI disorders and the complications associated with the disorder. Focus on teaching the client and family about diet and nutrition specific to the disorder, tube and wound care, preventing the transmission of infection, and care to a colostomy or ileostomy. Remember that body image disturbances can occur in clients with a GI disorder. Specific focus relates to the client with a diversion, such as an ileostomy or colostomy, to the social isolation issues that can occur, and coping strategies. The Integrated Concepts and Processes addressed in this unit include the Clinical Problem-Solving Process (Nursing Process), Caring, Communication and Documentation, Cultural Awareness, Self-Care, and Teaching/Learning.

CLIENT NEEDS

Safe, Effective Care Environment

Confidentiality issues related to GI disorder
Consultation related to nutritional status
Establishing priorities
Handling infectious drainage and secretions
Informed consent for treatments and surgical procedures
Preventing the transmission of disease
Referrals to home care and community services
Standard (universal) precautions

Health Promotion and Maintenance

Health screening related to GI disorders
Health promotion programs related to GI disorders
Teaching related to colostomy or ileostomy care
Teaching related to prescribed dietary and other treatment measures
Teaching related to preventing the transmission of disease

Psychosocial Integrity

Body image changes related to colostomy or ileostomy
Coping mechanisms
Support systems

Physiological Integrity

Care of GI tubes
Diagnostic tests related to GI system
Elimination
Fluid and electrolyte imbalances
Infectious diseases of the GI tract
Medication therapy specific to GI disorder
Monitoring for complications related to tests, procedures, and surgical interventions
Nonpharmacological and pharmacological comfort measures
Nutrition and oral hydration
Personal hygiene

REFERENCES

Black J, Hawks J, Keene A: *Medical-surgical nursing: clinical management for positive outcomes*, ed 6, Philadelphia, 2001, WB Saunders.
Chernecky C, Berger B: *Laboratory tests and diagnostic procedures*, ed 3, Philadelphia, 2001, WB Saunders.
Clark J, Queener S, Karb V: *Pharmacologic basis of nursing practice*, ed 6, St Louis, 2000, Mosby.
DeWit S: *Fundamental concepts and skills for nursing*, Philadelphia, 2001, WB Saunders.
Hill S, Howlett H: *Success in practical nursing: personal and vocational issues*, ed 4, Philadelphia, 2001, WB Saunders.
National Council of State Boards of Nursing: *Test plan for the National Council Licensure Examination for Practical/Vocational Nurses*, Chicago, 2001, Author.
Potter P, Perry A: *Fundamentals of nursing*, ed 5, St Louis, 2001, Mosby.
Perry A, Potter P: *Clinical nursing skills and techniques*, ed 5, St Louis, 2002, Mosby.
Wilson J: *Infection control in clinical practice*, ed 2, St Louis, 2002, Balliere Tindall.

44 Gastrointestinal System

I. ANATOMY AND PHYSIOLOGY

A. Functions of the gastrointestinal (GI) system
  1. Processes food substances
  2. Absorbs the products of digestion into the blood
  3. Excretes unabsorbed materials
  4. Provides an environment for microorganisms to synthesize nutrients such as vitamin K
  5. For risk factors associated with the GI system, see Box 44-1

B. Mouth
  1. Contains the lips, cheeks, palate, tongue, teeth (mastication), salivary glands (lubrication), muscles, and maxillary bones
  2. Saliva contains the amylase enzyme (ptyalin), which aids in digestion

BOX 44-1

Risk Factors Associated with the GI System

Family history of GI disorders
Chronic laxative use
Tobacco use
Chronic alcohol use
Chronic high stress levels
Allergic reactions to food or medications
Long-term GI conditions such as ulcerative colitis may predispose to colorectal cancer
Previous abdominal surgery or trauma may lead to adhesions
Neurological disorders can impair movement, particularly with chewing and swallowing
Cardiac, respiratory, and endocrine disorders may lead to constipation
Diabetes mellitus may predispose to oral candidal infections

C. Esophagus
  1. A collapsible muscular tube, about 10 inches long
  2. Carries food from the pharynx to the stomach

D. Stomach: contains the cardia, fundus, body, and pylorus
  1. Mucus glands
    a. Located in mucosa
    b. Prevent autodigestion by providing an alkaline-protective covering
  2. Cardiac opening: prevents reflux into the esophagus
  3. Pyloric sphincter: regulates the rate of stomach emptying into the small intestine
  4. Hydrochloric acid: kills microorganisms, breaks food into small particles, and provides a chemical environment that is required by the gastric enzymes
  5. Pepsin: the chief coenzyme of gastric juice that converts proteins into proteases and peptones
  6. Intrinsic factor: necessary for the absorption of vitamin B_{12}
  7. Gastrin: controls gastric acidity

E. Small intestine
  1. The small intestine terminates into the cecum
  2. Duodenum: contains the openings of the bile and pancreatic ducts
  3. Jejunum: approximately 8 feet long
  4. Ileum: approximately 12 feet long

F. Intestinal juice enzymes
  1. Amylase digests starch to maltose
  2. Maltase reduces maltose to monosaccharide glucose
  3. Lactase splits lactose into galactose and glucose
  4. Sucrase reduces sucrose to fructose and glucose

5. Nucleoses split nucleic acids to nucleotides
6. Enterokinase activates trypsinogen to trypsin

G. Large intestine
1. Approximately 5 feet long
2. Absorbs water and eliminates wastes
3. Microbial production of vitamins K, B_{12}, riboflavin, and thiamine
4. Colon
   a. Ascending
   b. Transverse
   c. Descending
   d. Sigmoid
   e. Rectum
5. Ileocecal valve: prevents contents of large intestine from entering ileum
6. Anal sphincters: guard the anal canal

H. Peritoneum
1. Lines the abdominal cavity
2. Forms the mesentery, which supports the intestines and blood supply

I. Liver
1. The largest gland in the body weighing 3 to 4 pounds
2. Contains Kupffer's cells, which remove bacteria in the portal venous blood
3. Removes excess glucose and amino acids from the portal blood
4. Synthesizes glucose, amino acids, and fats
5. Aids in the digestion of fats, carbohydrates, and proteins
6. Stores and filters blood (200 to 400 mL of blood stored)
7. Stores vitamin A, D, B_{12}, and iron
8. Secretes bile to emulsify fats (500 to 1000 mL of bile a day)
9. Hepatic ducts
   a. Deliver bile to the gallbladder via the cystic duct
   b. Deliver bile to the duodenum via the common bile duct
   c. The common bile duct opens into the duodenum with the pancreatic duct at the ampulla of Vater
   d. The sphincter prevents the reflux of intestinal contents into the common bile duct and pancreatic duct

J. Gallbladder
1. Stores and concentrates bile
2. Contracts to force bile into the duodenum during the digestion of fats
3. The cystic duct joins the hepatic duct to form the common bile duct
4. The sphincter of Oddi guards the entrance into the duodenum
5. The presence of fatty materials in the duodenum stimulates the liberation of cholecystokinin, which causes contraction of the gallbladder and relaxation of the sphincter of Oddi

K. Pancreas
1. Exocrine gland
   a. Secretes sodium bicarbonate to neutralize the acidity of the stomach contents as they enter the duodenum
   b. Pancreatic juices contain enzymes for digesting carbohydrates, fats, and proteins
2. Endocrine gland
   a. Insulin secretion is produced by the islets of Langerhans
   b. Insulin is secreted into the bloodstream
   c. Insulin is important for carbohydrate metabolism

II. DIAGNOSTIC PROCEDURES

A. Upper GI (barium swallow)
1. Description: an examination of the upper GI tract under fluoroscopy after the client drinks barium sulfate
2. Preprocedure: instruct the client to fast from foods and fluids overnight before the study
3. Postprocedure
   a. A laxative may be prescribed after the procedure
   b. Instruct client to drink six to eight glasses of water each day for 2 days to help pass the barium
   c. Monitor stools for the passage of barium (stools will appear chalky white)

B. Lower GI (barium enema)
1. Description
   a. A fluoroscopic and radiographic examination of the large intestine after rectal instillation of barium sulfate
   b. May be done with or without air
2. Preprocedure
   a. Laxatives on the day before and the morning of the test
   b. Liquid diet 1 day before and on the morning of the test
3. Postprocedure
   a. Increase fluid intake for 24 to 48 hours
   b. Administer mild laxatives to facilitate emptying of the barium
   c. Monitor stool for passage of barium
   d. Notify physician if a bowel movement does not occur within 2 days

C. Gastroscopy
1. Description: insertion of an endoscopic instrument through the esophagus into the stomach and upper portion of the small intestine to visualize the mucosal lining

2. Preprocedure
   a. Obtain informed consent
   b. Remove dentures
   c. Administer sedative as required
   d. Obtain baseline vital signs
   e. Maintain NPO status for 12 hours before procedure
3. Postprocedure
   a. Monitor vital signs, respiratory, cardiac, and neurological status
   b. Monitor for return of gag reflex
   c. Do not administer food or fluid until gag reflex returns
   d. Monitor for signs of bleeding as evidenced by hypotension, pallor, and tachycardia
   e. Monitor for perforation as evidenced by pain, tachypnea, and rales

D. Sigmoidoscopy
1. Description: endoscopic visualization of the sigmoid colon using a sigmoidoscope
2. Preprocedure
   a. Obtain informed consent
   b. A full liquid diet the evening before the test
   c. Laxatives the evening before the test and an enema or suppository 1 hour before the test
3. Postprocedure
   a. Assess for side effects related to sedative if administered
   b. Normal activities and diet may be resumed
   c. Notify physician if temperature is higher than 101° F or if breathing difficulty, stomach pain, or bright red rectal bleeding occurs

E. Colonoscopy
1. Description: a fiberoptic endoscopy study in which the lining of the large intestine is visually examined
2. Preprocedure
   a. Obtain informed consent
   b. Clear liquid diet for 48 hours before the test
   c. Bowel preparation with laxatives on the evening before the test and an enema on the day of the test
3. Postprocedure
   a. Monitor vital signs
   b. Monitor for side effects if sedation was administered
   c. A normal diet may be resumed
   d. Monitor for signs of colon perforation as evidenced by abdominal pain or distention, malaise, fever, purulent rectal drainage, or lower GI bleeding

F. Gastric analysis
1. Description: passage of a nasogastric (NG) tube into the stomach to aspirate gastric contents for analysis of acidity, appearance, and volume
2. Preprocedure
   a. Fast for 12 hours before the test
   b. Avoiding tobacco and chewing gum for 6 hours before the test
3. Postprocedure
   a. May resume normal activities
   b. Refrigerate gastric samples if not tested within 4 hours

G. Gallbladder series
1. Description: oral cholecystography to study the dye-filled gallbladder by radiographic film
2. Preprocedure
   a. A low-fat meal on the evening before the test and then fasting at midnight the day before the test
   b. Administer six 0.5-g iopanoic acid (Telepaque) tablets 12 hours before the test
   c. Tablets should be taken with a large amount of water at 5-minute intervals
   d. Instruct the client to go to the emergency department if a rash, itching or hives, or difficulty in breathing occurs after taking the tablets
3. Postprocedure
   a. Inform the client that dysuria is common because the dye is excreted in the urine
   b. A normal diet may be resumed; however, a fatty meal may enhance dye excretion

H. Liver biopsy
1. Description: a needle is inserted through the abdominal wall to the liver to obtain a tissue sample for biopsy and microscopic examination
2. Preprocedure
   a. Obtain informed consent
   b. Assess hematological laboratory results
   c. Administer sedative as prescribed
   d. NPO after midnight on the day before the test
   e. Note that the client is placed in the supine or left lateral position during the procedure
3. Postprocedure
   a. Assess vital signs frequently
   b. Assess biopsy site for bleeding
   c. Monitor for peritonitis
   d. Maintain bed rest for 24 hours
   e. Place client on the right side for 1 to 2 hours to decrease the risk of hemorrhage

I. Paracentesis
1. Description: transabdominal removal of fluid from the peritoneal cavity for the analysis of electrolytes, red blood cells, white blood cells (WBCs), bacterial and viral cultures, and cytology studies

2. Preprocedure
   a. Obtain informed consent
   b. Have the client void before the start of procedure to empty bladder and to move bladder out of the way of paracentesis needle
   c. Measure abdominal girth, weight, and baseline vital signs
   d. Note that the client is usually placed supine in Fowler's position
3. Postprocedure
   a. Monitor vital signs
   b. Maintain bed rest
   c. Apply a dry sterile dressing to the insertion site
   d. Monitor the insertion site for bleeding
   e. Measure abdominal girth and weight
   f. Monitor for hematuria resulting from bladder trauma
   g. Instruct the client to notify physician if the urine becomes bloody, pink, or red

J. Stool specimens
1. Description: examination of stool by dipstick for the presence of bleeding
2. Preprocedure: instruct client to avoid aspirin, nonsteroidal antiinflammatory drugs (NSAIDs), or red meat, poultry, and fish 3 days before the collection

K. Liver and pancreas laboratory studies (see Chapter 10)
1. Alkaline phosphatase: released during liver damage or biliary obstruction
2. Prothrombin time (PT): prolonged with liver damage
3. Serum ammonia: assesses the ability of the liver to deaminate protein by-products
4. Liver enzymes (transaminase studies): elevated with liver damage
5. Cholesterol: increase indicates **pancreatitis** or biliary obstruction
6. Bilirubin: increase indicates liver damage or biliary obstruction
7. Amylase and lipase: elevations indicate **pancreatitis**

III. DATA COLLECTION

A. Abdominal assessment
1. Inspect skin for color, abnormalities, contour, and tautness, and the abdomen for distention
2. Auscultate for bowel sounds
3. Percuss for air or solids
4. Palpate for tenderness

B. Bowel sounds
1. Auscultate bowel sounds before percussion and palpation
2. Normal bowel sounds occur 5 to 34 times a minute or every 5 to 15 seconds
3. Auscultate in all quadrants
4. Listen at least 5 minutes in each quadrant before assuming sounds are absent

IV. NASOGASTRIC, ESOPHAGEAL, AND INTESTINAL TUBES (REFER TO CHAPTER 18 FOR DESCRIPTIONS AND NURSING CARE RELATED TO GI TUBES)

V. HIATAL HERNIA

A. Description
1. Also known as esophageal or diaphragmatic hernia
2. A portion of the stomach herniates through the diaphragm and into the thorax
3. Results from weakening of the muscles of the diaphragm and is aggravated by factors that increase abdominal pressure such as pregnancy, **ascites**, obesity, tumors, and heavy lifting
4. Complications include ulceration, hemorrhage, regurgitation and aspiration of stomach contents, and incarceration of the stomach in the chest with possible necrosis, peritonitis, and mediastinitis

B. Data collection
1. Heartburn
2. Feeling of fullness
3. Discomfort or pain
4. Regurgitation or vomiting
5. Dysphagia
6. Bleeding

C. Implementation
1. Provide small frequent meals and minimize the amount of liquids
2. Elevate the head of the bed while eating and for 30 minutes after eating
3. Administer antacids after meals and at bedtime as prescribed to relieve heartburn and to increase lower esophageal sphincter pressure
4. Administer histamine H_2-receptor antagonists as prescribed to control esophageal reflux
5. Avoid anticholinergics, which delay stomach emptying
6. Instruct the client to avoid vigorous coughing
7. Instruct the client to avoid constrictive clothing around waist
8. Instruct the client to avoid sharp, forward bending
9. Instruct the client to avoid highly seasoned and fatty foods

10. Instruct the client to avoid alcohol, smoking, caffeine, chocolate, and carbonated and acidic beverages
11. Instruct the client to avoid nighttime snacking to ensure that the stomach is empty
12. Encourage weight reduction because obesity increases intraabdominal pressure

D. Surgical implementation
   1. Indicated when the risk of complications such as aspiration exists and damage from chronic reflux is severe
   2. Surgical approaches include reinforcement of the lower esophageal sphincter (LES) to restore sphincter competence and prevent reflux
   3. Achieved by a procedure that involves wrapping of a portion of the stomach fundus around the distal esophagus to anchor it and reinforce the LES

VI. ESOPHAGEAL VARICES

A. Description
   1. Dilated and tortuous veins in the submucosa of the esophagus
   2. They are caused by **portal hypertension**, are often associated with liver **cirrhosis,** and are at high risk for rupture if portal circulation pressure rises
   3. Bleeding varices is an emergency
   4. The goal of treatment is to control bleeding, prevent complications, and prevent the recurrence of a bleed

B. Data collection
   1. Hematemesis
   2. Melena
   3. Tarry stools
   4. **Ascites**
   5. Jaundice
   6. Hepatomegaly and splenomegaly
   7. Dilated abdominal veins
   8. Hemorrhoids
   9. Bleeding and shock

C. Implementation
   1. Monitor vital signs
   2. Elevate the head of the bed
   3. Monitor for orthostatic hypotension
   4. Monitor lung sounds and for the presence of respiratory distress
   5. Administer oxygen as prescribed to prevent tissue hypoxia
   6. Maintain NPO status
   7. Monitor level of consciousness (LOC)
   8. Monitor input and output (I&O)
   9. Administer intravenous (IV) fluids as prescribed to restore fluid volume and electrolyte imbalances
   10. Monitor hemoglobin, hematocrit, and coagulation factors
   11. Blood or clotting factors are administered as prescribed
   12. Assist in inserting a nasogastric tube or a balloon tamponade as prescribed
   13. Assist with the administration of saline irrigation to the vasoconstrictor vessels as prescribed
   14. Prepare to assist with administering vasopressin (Pitressin) as prescribed to induce vasoconstriction and reduce bleeding
   15. Prepare to assist with administering nitroglycerin with the vasopressin (Pitressin), which produces a reduction in portal pressure
   16. Instruct the client to avoid activities that will initiate vasovagal responses
   17. Prepare the client for endoscopic procedures or surgical procedures as prescribed

D. Endoscopic injection (sclerotherapy)
   1. Injection of a sclerosing agent into and around bleeding varices
   2. Complications include chest pain, pleural effusion, aspiration pneumonia, esophageal stricture, and perforation of the esophagus

E. Endoscopic variceal ligation
   1. Ligation of the varices with an elastic rubber band
   2. Sloughing, followed by superficial ulceration, occurs in the area of ligation within 3 to 7 days

F. Surgical shunt procedures
   1. Splenorenal: involves splenectomy with anastomosis of the splenic vein to the left renal vein
   2. Portacaval: shunting of the blood from the portal vein to the inferior vena cava
   3. Mesocaval: involves a side anastomosis of the superior mesenteric vein to the proximal end of the inferior vena cava
   4. Transjugular intrahepatic portal/systemic
      a. Uses the normal vascular anatomy of the liver to create a shunt with the use of a metallic stent
      b. The shunt is between the portal and systemic venous systems within the liver and is aimed at relieving **portal hypertension**

VII. PEPTIC ULCER DISEASE

A. Description
   1. An ulceration in the mucosal wall of stomach, pylorus, or duodenum in portions that are accessible to gastric secretions

2. Erosion may extend through the muscle to the peritoneum
3. The most common peptic ulcers are gastric ulcers and duodenal ulcers

B. Gastric ulcers
1. Description
   a. Involves ulceration of the mucosal lining that extends to the submucosal layer of the stomach
   b. Predisposing factors include stress; smoking; the use of steroids, NSAIDs, or alcohol; a history of gastritis or family history of gastric ulcers
   c. Complications include hemorrhage, perforation, and pyloric obstruction
2. Data collection
   a. Gnawing, sharp pain in or left of the midepigastric region 1 to 2 hours after eating
   b. Nausea and vomiting
   c. Hematemesis
3. Implementation
   a. Monitor vital signs
   b. Monitor for bleeding
   c. Administer small, frequent bland feedings during the active phase
   d. Administer histamine H_2-receptor antagonists as prescribed to decrease the secretion of gastric acid
   e. Administer antacids as prescribed to neutralize gastric secretions
   f. Administer anticholinergics as prescribed to reduce gastric motility
   g. Administer mucosal barrier protectants as prescribed 1 hour before each meal
   h. Administer prostaglandins as prescribed for their protective and antisecretory actions
   i. Instruct the client to avoid alcohol
   j. Instruct the client to avoid caffeine and chocolate
   k. Instruct the client to avoid smoking
   l. Instruct the client to avoid aspirin or NSAIDs
   m. Instruct the client to obtain adequate rest and reduce stress
4. Implementation during active bleeding
   a. Monitor vital signs
   b. Monitor for signs of dehydration, hypovolemic shock, sepsis, and respiratory insufficiency
   c. Monitor I&O
   d. Maintain NPO status and administer IV fluid replacement as prescribed
   e. Monitor hemoglobin and hematocrit
   f. Assist with administering blood transfusion as prescribed
   g. Assist with insertion of an NG tube for decompression and for access for lavage
   h. Assist with normal saline or tap water lavage at room temperature to reduce active bleeding
   i. Prepare to assist with administering vasopressin (Pitressin) by IV as prescribed to induce vasoconstriction and reduce bleeding
5. Estimating the amount of blood loss
   a. Less than 500 mL: pulse rate begins to rise
   b. 500 to 1000 mL: pulse increases to 100 to 110 beats per minute, blood pressure (BP) begins to decrease, urine output declines and signs of shock are present
   c. 1000 to 2000 mL: pulse increases beyond 110 to 120 beats per minute and BP continues to decrease
   d. More than 2000 mL: pulse increases beyond 120 beats per minute and BP and urine output decline significantly
6. Surgical implementation
   a. Total **gastrectomy:** also called esophagojejunostomy; removal of the stomach with attachment of the esophagus to the jejunum or duodenum
   b. **Vagotomy:** surgical division of the vagus nerve to eliminate the vagal impulses that stimulate hydrochloric acid secretion in the stomach
   c. **Gastric resection:** also called antrectomy; involves removal of the lower half of the stomach and usually includes a **vagotomy**
   d. **Billroth I:** also called gastroduodenostomy; partial **gastrectomy** with remaining segment anastomosed to duodenum
   e. **Billroth II:** also called gastrojejunostomy; partial **gastrectomy** with remaining segment anastomosed to jejunum
   f. **Pyloroplasty:** enlarges the pylorus to prevent or decrease pyloric obstruction, thereby enhancing gastric emptying
7. Postoperative implementation
   a. Monitor vital signs
   b. Position in Fowler's for comfort and to promote drainage
   c. Monitor I&O
   d. Administer fluids and electrolyte replacements IV as prescribed
   e. Assess bowel sounds
   f. Monitor nasogastric suction as prescribed
   g. Do not irrigate NG tube or remove NG tube
   h. Assist physician with NG irrigation or removal of NG tube
   i. Maintain NPO status as prescribed for 1 to 3 days until **peristalsis** returns

j. Progress diet from NPO to sips of clear water to bland six small meals a day as prescribed when bowel sounds return

k. Monitor for postoperative complications of hemorrhage, **dumping syndrome**, diarrhea, hypoglycemia, and vitamin B_{12} deficiency

VIII. DUODENAL ULCERS

A. Description
1. A break in the mucosa of the duodenum
2. Risk factors and causes include alcohol intake, smoking, stress, caffeine, the use of aspirin, corticosteroids and NSAIDs, and infection with *Helicobacter pylori*
3. The goals of treatment are to eliminate the cause, decrease gastric acidity, and prevent complications
4. Complications include bleeding, perforation, gastric outlet obstruction, and intractable disease

B. Data collection
1. Burning pain in the midepigastric area 2 to 4 hours after eating and during the night
2. Pain that is often relieved by eating
3. Melena

C. Implementation
1. Monitor vital signs
2. Perform abdominal assessment
3. Instruct the client in a bland diet with small, frequent meals
4. Provide for adequate rest
5. Encourage the cessation of smoking
6. Instruct the client to avoid alcohol intake, caffeine, the use of aspirin, corticosteroids, and NSAIDs
7. Administer antacids as prescribed to neutralize acid secretions
8. Administer histamine H_2-receptor antagonists as prescribed to block the secretion of acid

D. Surgical implementation: surgery is performed only if the ulcer is unresponsive to medications or if hemorrhage, obstruction, or perforation occurs

IX. DUMPING SYNDROME

A. Description
1. Rapid emptying of the gastric contents into the small intestine
2. Occurs after **gastric resection**

B. Data collection
1. Symptoms occurring 30 minutes after eating
2. Nausea and vomiting
3. Abdominal cramping
4. Feelings of fullness
5. Diarrhea
6. Palpitation
7. Tachycardia
8. Perspiration
9. Weakness and dizziness
10. Borborygmi

C. Implementation
1. Instruct the client to eat a high-protein, high-fat, low-carbohydrate diet
2. Instruct the client to eat small meals and to avoid fluids with meals
3. Instruct the client to avoid sugar and salt
4. Instruct the client to lie down after meals
5. Instruct the client to take antiperistaltic and antispasmodic medications as prescribed to delay gastric emptying

X. VITAMIN B_{12} DEFICIENCY

A. Description
1. Results from either an inadequate intake of vitamin B_{12} or a lack of absorption of ingested vitamin B_{12} from the intestinal tract
2. Pernicious anemia results from a deficiency of intrinsic factor, which is necessary for intestinal absorption of vitamin B_{12}

B. Data collection
1. Severe pallor
2. Fatigue
3. Weight loss
4. Smooth, beefy red tongue
5. Slight jaundice
6. Paresthesias of the hands and feet
7. Disturbances with gait and balance

C. Implementation
1. Increase dietary intake of food rich in vitamin B_{12} if the anemia is the result of a dietary deficiency (Box 44-2)
2. Administer vitamin B_{12} injections as prescribed on a weekly basis initially and then monthly for maintenance (lifelong) if the anemia is the result of a deficiency of the intrinsic factor

BOX 44-2

Foods Rich in Vitamin B_{12}

Liver
Organ meats
Dried beans
Nuts
Green leafy vegetables
Citrus fruits
Brewer's yeast

XI. GASTRIC CANCER

A. Description
1. An abnormal malignant growth in the abdomen
2. Risk factors include a diet high in complex carbohydrates, grains, salt, and animal fat, and low in fresh green leafy vegetables and fresh fruit; smoking; alcohol; and a history of gastric ulcers.
3. Complications include hemorrhage, obstruction, metastasis, and **dumping syndrome**
4. The goal of treatment is to remove the tumor and provide a nutritional program

B. Data collection
1. Anorexia
2. Nausea and vomiting
3. Indigestion and epigastric discomfort
4. A sensation of pressure
5. Dysphagia
6. Weight loss
7. Palpable mass
8. Fatigue
9. Anemia
10. **Ascites**

C. Implementation
1. Monitor vital signs
2. Monitor nutritional status
3. Encourage small bland, easily digestible meals with vitamin and mineral supplements
4. Monitor weight
5. Administer pain medication as prescribed
6. Monitor hemoglobin and hematocrit and administer blood transfusion as prescribed
7. Provide emotional support
8. Prepare the client for chemotherapy or radiation therapy as prescribed
9. Prepare the client for surgical resection of the tumor as prescribed (Box 44-3)

D. Postoperative implementation
1. Monitor vital signs
2. Place in Fowler's position for comfort and to promote drainage
3. Monitor I&O
4. Administer fluids and electrolyte replacements IV as prescribed
5. Monitor bowel sounds
6. Monitor nasogastric suction as prescribed
7. Do not irrigate or remove NG tube
8. Assist the physician with NG irrigation or removal of NG tube
9. Maintain NPO status as prescribed for 1 to 3 days until **peristalsis** returns
10. Progress the diet from NPO to sips of clear water to six small, bland meals a day, as prescribed, when bowel sounds return

BOX 44-3

Surgical Treatment for Gastric Cancer

Total gastrectomy
Vagotomy
Gastric resection
Billroth I
Billroth II
Pyloroplasty

11. Monitor for postoperative complications of hemorrhage, **dumping syndrome**, diarrhea, hypoglycemia, and Vitamin B_{12} deficiency

XII. ULCERATIVE COLITIS

A. Description
1. Ulcerative and inflammatory disease of the bowel that results in poor absorption of nutrients
2. Commonly begins in the rectum and spreads upward toward the cecum
3. The colon becomes edematous and may develop bleeding lesions and ulcers
4. The ulcers may lead to perforation
5. Scar tissue develops and causes loss of elasticity and loss of ability to absorb nutrients
6. Characterized by various periods of remissions and exacerbations
7. Acute **ulcerative colitis** results in vascular congestion, hemorrhage, edema, and ulceration of the bowel mucosa
8. Chronic **ulcerative colitis** causes muscular hypertrophy, fat deposits, and fibrous tissue with bowel thickening, shortening, and narrowing

B. Data collection
1. Anorexia
2. Weight loss
3. Malaise
4. Abdominal tenderness and cramping
5. Severe diarrhea that may contain blood and mucus 
6. Dehydration and electrolyte imbalances
7. Anemia
8. Vitamin K deficiency

C. Implementation 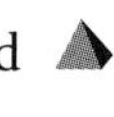
1. Maintain NPO status and administer IVs and electrolytes as prescribed during the acute phase
2. Total parenteral nutrition (TPN) may be prescribed during an acute phase
3. Restrict the client's activity to reduce intestinal activity
4. Monitor bowel sounds

5. Monitor for abdominal tenderness and cramping
6. Monitor stools noting color, consistency, and the presence or absence of blood
7. Monitor for perforation, peritonitis, and hemorrhage
8. After the acute phase, the diet progresses from clear liquids to low residue as tolerated
9. Instruct the client to consume a low-residue and high protein diet and to avoid foods as whole wheat grains, nuts, raw fruits, and vegetables
10. Instruct the client to avoid gas-forming foods and milk products
11. Instruct the client to thoroughly chew solid foods
12. Instruct the client to avoid caffeinated beverages, alcohol, and pepper
13. Encourage the client to stop smoking
14. Administer antidiarrheal medications as prescribed
15. Administer antimicrobial, corticosteroids, and immunosuppressants as prescribed to prevent infection and reduce inflammation

D. Surgical implementation
1. Total proctocolectomy with permanent ileostomy
   a. Involves removal of the colon, rectum, and anus with anal closure
   b. The end of the terminal ileum forms the stoma, which is located in the right lower quadrant
2. **Kock pouch** (ileostomy)
   a. An intraabdominal pouch is constructed from the terminal ileum
   b. The pouch is connected to the stoma with a nipplelike valve constructed from a portion of the ileum
   c. The stoma is flush with the skin
3. Ileoanal reservoir
   a. A two-stage procedure that involves the excision of the rectal mucosa, abdominal colectomy, construction of the reservoir to the anal canal, and a temporary loop ileostomy
   b. The ileostomy is closed in approximately 4 months after the capacity of the reservoir is increased
4. Preoperative colostomy/ileostomy
   a. Consult with enterostomal therapist to assist in identifying optimal placement of ostomy
   b. Instruct the client to eat a low-residue diet for a day or two before surgery as prescribed
   c. Administer intestinal antiseptics and antibiotics as prescribed to decrease bacterial content of the colon and to soften and decrease the bulk of the contents of colon 
   d. Administer laxatives and enemas as prescribed
5. Postoperative colostomy
   a. Place a petroleum gauze over the stoma as prescribed to keep it moist, followed by a dry sterile dressing if a pouch system is not in place
   b. Place a pouch system on the stoma as soon as possible
   c. Monitor the stoma for size, unusual bleeding, or necrotic tissue
   d. Monitor for color changes in the stoma
   e. Note that the normal stoma color is red or pink, indicating high vascularity
   f. Note that a pale pink stoma indicates low hemoglobin and hematocrit levels and a purple-black stoma indicates compromised circulation requiring physician notification
   g. Assess the functioning of the colostomy
   h. Expect that stool is liquid immediate postoperative but becomes more solid depending on the area of the colostomy; ascending colon—liquid stool; transverse colon—loose to semiformed; descending colon—close to normal
   i. Monitor the pouch system for proper fit and signs of leakage
   j. Empty pouch when one-third full
   k. Fecal matter should not be allowed to remain on skin
   l. Administer analgesics and antibiotics as prescribed
   m. Irrigate perineal wound if present as prescribed and monitor for signs of infection
   n. Instruct the client to avoid foods that cause excess gas formation and odor
   o. Instruct the client on stoma care and irrigations as prescribed (Box 44-4)
   p. Instruct the client that normal activities may be resumed when approved by the physician
6. Postoperative ileostomy
   a. Note that the healthy stoma is red
   b. Monitor for color change in the stoma to dark blue or black, and if it occurs, it should be reported to the physician
   c. Note that normal stool is liquid
   d. Monitor for dehydration and electrolyte imbalance
   e. Do not give suppositories through ileostomy

BOX 44-4

Colostomy Irrigation

DESCRIPTION

Instilling 500 to 1000 mL tepid H_2O through the stoma and allowing H_2O and stool to drain into collection bag

PROCEDURE

If ambulatory, position client sitting on toilet
If bed rest, position client on side
Hang irrigation bag so that bottom of bag is at the level of the client's shoulder or slightly higher
Insert irrigation tube carefully without force
Begin the flow of irrigation
Clamp tubing if cramping occurs, release tubing as cramping subsides
Avoid frequent irrigations with H_2O, which can lead to loss of fluids and electrolytes
Perform irrigation around the same time each day
Perform irrigation preferably 1 hour after a meal

XIII. CROHN'S DISEASE (REGIONAL ENTERITIS)

A. Description
   1. An inflammatory disease that can occur anywhere in the GI tract but most often affects the terminal ileum and leads to thickening and scarring, a narrowed lumen, fistulas, ulcerations, and abscesses
   2. It is characterized by remissions and exacerbations

B. Data collection
   1. Fever
   2. Cramplike pain after meals
   3. Diarrhea semisolid and may contain mucus, pus, and blood
   4. Abdominal distention
   5. Anorexia, nausea, and vomiting
   6. Weight loss
   7. Anemia

   8. Dehydration
   9. Electrolyte imbalances

C. Implementation: care is similar to the client with **ulcerative colitis**

XIV. INTESTINAL TUMORS

A. Description
   1. Malignant lesions that develop in the cells lining the bowel wall or develop as polyps in the colon or rectum
   2. Complications include bowel perforation with peritonitis, abscess and/or fistula formation, frank hemorrhage, and complete intestinal obstruction
   3. Metastasis occurs via the circulatory or lymphatic system or by direct extension to other areas in the colon or other organs

B. Data collection
   1. Blood in stools
   2. Abnormal stools
   3. Anorexia
   4. Vomiting
   5. Weight loss
   6. Malaise
   7. Anemia

   8. Ascending colon tumor: diarrhea
   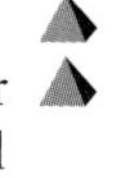
   9. Descending colon tumor: constipation or some diarrhea, or flat ribbon-like stool caused by a partial obstruction
   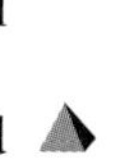
   10. Rectal tumor: alternating constipation and diarrhea
   11. Guarding or abdominal distention
   12. Abdominal mass (a late sign)
   13. Cachexia (a late sign)

C. Implementation
   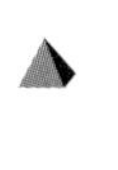
   1. Monitor for signs of complications, which include bowel perforation with peritonitis, abscess and/or fistula formation, frank hemorrhage, and complete intestinal obstruction
   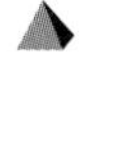
   2. Monitor for signs of intestinal perforation including low BP, rapid weak pulse, distended abdomen, and elevated temperature
   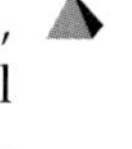
   3. Monitor for signs of intestinal obstruction, which may include vomiting (may be fecal contents), pain, constipation, and abdominal distention
   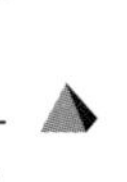
   4. Note that an early sign of intestinal obstruction includes increased peristaltic activity, which produces an increase in bowel sounds, and as the obstruction progresses, hypoactive sounds

D. Nonsurgical implementation
   1. Preoperative radiation to facilitate surgical resection and to decrease the risk of postoperative recurrence or to reduce pain, hemorrhage, bowel obstruction, or metastasis
   2. Postoperative chemotherapy used to assist in the control of symptoms and spread of the disease

E. Surgical implementation: bowel resection and creation of colostomy or ileostomy

XV. DIVERTICULOSIS AND DIVERTICULITIS

A. Description
   1. **Diverticulosis**
      a. Outpouching or herniations of the intestinal mucosa
      b. They can occur in any part of the intestine but are most common in the sigmoid colon

2. **Diverticulitis**
   a. Inflammation of one or more diverticuli
   b. Results when diverticulum perforates with local abscess formation
   c. A perforated diverticulum can progress to intraabdominal perforation with generalized peritonitis

B. Data collection
1. Left lower quadrant abdominal pain that increases with coughing, straining, or lifting
2. Elevated temperature
3. Nausea and vomiting
4. Flatulence
5. Cramplike pain
6. Abdominal distention and tenderness
7. Palpable, tender rectal mass
8. Blood in stools

C. Implementation
1. Provide bed rest during the acute phase
2. Maintain NPO status or provide clear liquids during the acute phase as prescribed
3. Introduce a fiber-containing diet gradually when the inflammation is resolved
4. Instruct the client to refrain from lifting, straining, coughing, or bending to avoid increased intraabdominal pressure
5. Administer antibiotics and pain medication as prescribed
6. Monitor for perforation, hemorrhage, fistulas, and abscesses
7. Instruct the client on the signs and symptoms of diverticular disease as fever, abdominal pain, and bloody stools
8. Instruct the client to eat soft, high-fiber foods such as whole grains
9. Instruct the client to eat fruits and vegetables with high fiber content and to avoid foods containing indigestible roughage or seeds
10. Instruct the client to avoid gas-forming foods, hot and cold liquids, and alcohol
11. Instruct the client to avoid enemas and laxatives other than bulk-forming products such as psyllium (Metamucil)

D. Surgical implementation
1. Colon resection with primary anastomosis
2. Temporary or permanent colostomy may be required for increased bowel inflammation

XVI. HEMORRHOIDS

A. Description
1. Dilated varicose veins of the anal canal
2. May be either internal, external, or prolapsed
3. Internal hemorrhoids lie above the anal sphincter and cannot be seen on inspection of the perianal area
4. External hemorrhoids lie below the anal sphincter and can be seen on inspection
5. Prolapsed hemorrhoids can become thrombosed or inflamed
6. Hemorrhoids are caused from **portal hypertension**, straining, irritation, increased venous or abdominal pressure

B. Data collection
1. Bright red rectal bleeding
2. Pain associated with thrombosis
3. Rectal itching
4. Mucus rectal discharge

C. Implementation
1. Apply cold packs to the anal rectal area followed by sitz baths as prescribed
2. Apply witch hazel soaks and topical anesthetics as prescribed
3. Encourage a high-fiber diet and fluids to promote bowel movements without straining
4. Administer stool softeners as prescribed

D. Endoscopic procedures
1. Sclerotherapy
2. Endoscopic ligation

E. Surgical procedures
1. Cryosurgery
2. Hemorrhoidectomy

F. Postoperative implementation
1. Assist the client to prone or side-lying position to prevent bleeding
2. Maintain ice packs over dressing as prescribed until the packing is removed by the physician
3. Monitor for urinary retention
4. Administer stool softeners as prescribed
5. Instruct the client to increase fluids and fiber foods
6. Instruct the client to limit sitting to short periods
7. Instruct the client in the use of sitz baths three to four times a day as prescribed

XVII. APPENDICITIS

A. Description
1. Inflammation of the appendix
2. When the appendix becomes inflamed or infected, rupture may occur within a matter of hours, leading to peritonitis and sepsis

B. Data collection
1. Pain in periumbilical area that descends to right lower quadrant
2. Abdominal pain that is most intense at McBurney's point
3. Rebound tenderness and abdominal rigidity
4. Low-grade fever
5. Elevated WBC count
6. Anorexia, nausea, and vomiting

7. Client in side-lying position with abdominal guarding and legs flexed
8. Constipation or diarrhea

C. Peritonitis: inflammation of the peritoneum
1. Increased fever and chills
2. Progressive abdominal distention and abdominal pain
3. Right guarding of abdomen
4. Tachycardia and tachypnea
5. Pallor
6. Restlessness

D. Appendectomy: surgical removal of the appendix
1. Preoperative implementation
   a. Maintain NPO status
   b. Administer IV fluids to prevent dehydration
   c. Monitor for changes in level of pain
   d. Monitor for signs of ruptured appendix and peritonitis
   e. Position right side-lying or low to semi-Fowler's position to promote comfort
   f. Monitor bowel sounds
   g. Apply ice packs to abdomen for 20 to 30 minutes every hour
   h. Administer antibiotics as prescribed
   i. Avoid application of heat to abdomen
   j. Avoid laxatives or enemas
2. Postoperative implementation
   a. Monitor temperature for signs of infection
   b. Assess incision for signs of infection as redness, swelling, and pain
   c. Maintain NPO status until bowel function has returned
   d. Advance diet gradually as tolerated when bowel sounds return
   e. If rupture of the appendix had occurred, expect a Penrose drain to be inserted, or incision may be left open to heal from the inside out
   f. Expect that drainage from Penrose drain may be profuse for the first 12 hours
   g. Position the client in right side-lying or low to semi-Fowler's position with legs flexed to facilitate drainage
   h. Change dressing as prescribed
   i. Record type and amount of drainage
   j. Perform wound irrigations if prescribed
   k. Maintain NG suction and patency of the NG tube if present
   l. Administer antibiotics and analgesics as prescribed

XVIII. CIRRHOSIS (Box 44-5)

A. Description

BOX 44-5

Types of Cirrhosis

LAENNEC'S CIRRHOSIS

Alcohol induced, nutritional, portal cirrhosis

Cellular necrosis causes eventual widespread scar tissue with fibrotic infiltration of the liver

POSTNECROTIC CIRRHOSIS

Occurs after massive liver necrosis

Results as a complication of acute viral hepatitis or exposure to hepatotoxins

Scar tissue causes destruction of liver lobules and entire lobes

BILIARY CIRRHOSIS

Develops from chronic biliary obstruction, bile stasis, and inflammation resulting in severe obstructive jaundice

CARDIAC CIRRHOSIS

Associated with severe right-sided congestive heart failure and results in an enlarged, edematous, congested liver

The liver becomes anoxic resulting in liver cell necrosis and fibrosis

1. A chronic progressive disease of the liver characterized by diffuse damage to cells with fibrosis and nodular regeneration
2. Repeated destruction of hepatic cells causes the formation of scar tissue

B. Complications
1. **Portal Hypertension:** a persistent increase in pressure within the portal vein that develops as a result of obstruction to flow
2. **Ascites**
   a. The accumulation of fluid within the peritoneal cavity that results in venous congestion of the hepatic capillaries
   b. This leads to plasma leaking directly from the liver surface and portal vein
3. Bleeding **esophageal varices:** fragile, thin-walled, distended esophageal veins that become irritated and rupture
4. Coagulation defects
   a. Decreased synthesis of bile fats in the liver prevents the absorption of fat-soluble vitamins
   b. Without vitamin K and clotting factors II, VII, IX, and X, the client is prone to bleeding
5. Jaundice: occurs because the liver is unable to metabolize bilirubin and because the edema, fibrosis, and scaring of the hepatic bile ducts interfere with normal bile and bilirubin secretion

6. Portal systemic encephalopathy: end-stage hepatic failure and **cirrhosis** characterized by altered LOC, neurological symptoms, impaired thinking, and neuromuscular disturbances
7. Hepatorenal syndrome
   a. Progressive renal failure associated with hepatic failure
   b. Characterized by a sudden decrease in urinary output, elevated blood urea nitrogen (BUN) and creatinine, decreased urine sodium excretion, and increased urine osmolarity

C. Data collection
1. Anorexia and weight loss
2. Early morning nausea and vomiting
3. Dyspepsia
4. Flatulence and changes in bowel habits
5. Emaciation
6. Fatigue
7. Jaundice
8. Abdominal pain or tenderness
9. **Ascites**
10. Peripheral edema
11. Dry skin and rashes
12. Petechiae or ecchymosis
13. Spider angiomas on the nose, cheeks, upper thorax, and shoulders
14. Hepatomegaly
15. Protruding umbilicus
16. Dilated abdominal veins
17. Presence of blood in vomitus
18. **Fetor hepaticus**: the fruity musty breath odor of chronic liver disease
19. Amenorrhea and testicular atrophy
20. Gynecomastia
21. Impotence
22. **Asterixis**, liver flap, a course tremor characterized by rapid nonrhythmic extension and flexions in the wrist and fingers
23. Delirium

D. Implementation
1. Elevate the head of bed to minimize shortness of breath
2. Provide a low-sodium diet initially restricting sodium to 200 to 500 mg and restricting protein to 50 to 60 g (to reduce excess protein breakdown by intestinal bacteria) daily as prescribed
3. Provide supplemental vitamins with thiamine, folate, and multivitamin as prescribed
4. TPN may be prescribed
5. Restrict fluid intake to 1500 mL daily as prescribed
6. Administer diuretics as prescribed
7. Monitor I&O
8. Monitor electrolyte balance
9. Weigh the client and measure abdominal girth daily
10. Monitor level of consciousness
11. Monitor for precoma state (tremors, delirium)
12. Monitor for **asterixis**
13. Maintain gastric intubation to assess bleeding
14. Maintain esophagogastric balloon tamponade to control bleeding varices if prescribed
15. Administer blood products as prescribed
16. Monitor coagulation laboratory results
17. Administer vitamin K if prescribed
18. Avoid hepatotoxin intake
19. Instruct the client to restrict alcohol
20. Administer low-sodium antacids as prescribed
21. Administer lactulose (Chronulac), which decreases the pH of the bowel, decreases production of ammonia by bacteria in the bowel, and facilitates excretion of ammonia
22. Administer neomycin (Mycifradin) as prescribed to inhibit protein synthesis in bacteria and decrease production of ammonia
23. Avoid medication such as narcotics, sedatives, and barbiturates
24. Prepare the client for paracentesis to remove abdominal fluid
25. Prepare the client for surgical shunting procedures if prescribed

XIX. CHOLECYSTITIS

A. Description
1. An inflammation of the gallbladder that may occur as an acute or chronic process
2. Acute inflammation is associated with gallstones (cholelithiasis)
3. Chronic **cholecystitis** results when inefficient bile emptying and gallbladder muscle wall disease cause a fibrotic and contracted gallbladder
4. A calculus **cholecystitis** occurs in the absence of gallstones and is due to bacterial invasion via the lymphatic or vascular systems

B. Data collection
1. Nausea and vomiting
2. Indigestion
3. Belching
4. Flatulence
5. Epigastric pain that radiates to the scapula 2 to 4 hours after eating fatty foods and may persist for 4 to 6 hours
6. Pain localized in right upper quadrant

7. Guarding, rigidity, and rebound tenderness
8. Mass palpated in the right upper quadrant
9. **Murphy's sign** (cannot take a deep breath when examiner's fingers are passed below hepatic margin)
10. Elevated temperature
11. Tachycardia
12. Signs of dehydration

C. Biliary obstruction
1. Jaundice
2. Dark orange and foamy urine
3. Steatorrhea and clay-colored feces
4. Pruritis

D. Implementation
1. Maintain NPO status during nausea and vomiting episodes
2. Maintain nasogastric decompression as prescribed for severe vomiting
3. Administer analgesics as prescribed to relieve pain and reduce spasm (Note: morphine or codeine may cause spasm of sphincter of Oddi and increase pain)
4. Administer antispasmodic (anticholinergics) as prescribed to relax smooth muscle
5. Administer antiemetics as prescribed for nausea and vomiting
6. Instruct the client with chronic **cholecystitis** to eat low-fat meals more frequently in small amounts
7. Instruct the client to avoid gas-forming foods
8. Prepare the client for nonsurgical and surgical procedures as prescribed

E. Nonsurgical implementation
1. Dissolution therapy
   a. To remove cholesterol stones
   b. Chenodeoxycholic acid (chenodiol) or ursodiol (Actigall) is administered PO to decrease size of stones or to dissolve small stones
   c. Direct contact with repeated injections and aspirations of a local choledotholytic agent via percutaneous catheter may be performed
2. Extracorporeal shock wave lithotripsy
   a. Shock waves are administered that disintegrate stones in the biliary system
   b. Oral dissolution follows

F. Surgical implementation
1. **Cholecystectomy:** removal of the gallbladder
2. **Choledochotomy:** incision into the common bile duct to remove the stone

G. Postoperative implementation
1. Monitor for respiratory complications secondary to pain at incision site
2. Encourage coughing and deep breathing
3. Encourage early ambulation
4. Instruct the client about splinting abdomen to prevent discomfort during coughing
5. Administer antiemetics as prescribed for nausea and vomiting
6. Administer analgesics as prescribed for pain relief
7. Maintain NPO status as prescribed for 24 to 48 hours
8. Maintain NG tube suction as prescribed
9. Advance the diet from clear liquids to solids when prescribed and as tolerated by the client
10. Maintain T tube (Box 44-6)

XX. PANCREATITIS

A. Description
1. An acute or chronic inflammation of the pancreas with associated escape of pancreatic enzymes into surrounding tissue
2. Acute **pancreatitis** occurs suddenly as one attack or can be recurrent, but resolves
3. Chronic **pancreatitis** is a continual inflammation and destruction of the pancreas, with scar tissue replacing pancreatic tissue
4. Precipitating factors include trauma, the use of alcohol, biliary tract disease, viral or bacterial disease, hyperlipidemia, hypercalcemia,

BOX 44-6

Care of a T Tube

DESCRIPTION

Surgically inserted to decompress biliary tree and maintain patency of the bile duct

IMPLEMENTATION

Place client in semi-Fowler's position to facilitate drainage

Monitor the amount, color, consistency, and odor of drainage

Monitor for inflammation and protect the skin from irritation

Keep the drainage system below the level of the gallbladder

Report sudden increases in bile output to the physician

Monitor for foul odor and purulent drainage and report to the physician

Avoid irrigation, aspiration, or clamping of the T tube without a physician's order

As prescribed, clamp tube before eating and observe for abdominal discomfort and distention, nausea, chills, or fever

Unclamp tube if nausea or vomiting occurs

cholelithiasis, hyperparathyroidism, ischemic vascular disease, and peptic ulcer disease

B. Acute
  1. Data collection
    a. Abdominal pain including a sudden onset, midepigastric or left upper quadrant location with radiation to the back
    b. Pain that is aggravated by a fatty meal, alcohol, or lying in a recumbent position
    c. Abdominal tenderness and guarding
    d. Nausea and vomiting
    e. Weight loss
    f. **Cullen's sign** (discoloration of the abdomen and periumbilical area)
    g. **Turner's sign** (bluish discoloration of the flanks)
    h. Absent or decreased bowel sounds
    i. Elevated temperature
    j. Hypotension
    k. Tachycardia
    l. Elevated WBC, glucose, bilirubin, alkaline phosphatase, and urinary amylase
    m. Elevated lipase and amylase
    n. Abnormally low calcium, sodium, and magnesium resulting from dehydration
  2. Implementation
    a. Maintain NPO status and maintain hydration with IV fluids
    b. Administer TPN for severe nutritional depletion
    c. Provide small, frequent high-carbohydrate, high-protein, and low-fat foods when prescribed and when tolerated by the client
    d. Administer supplemental preparations and vitamins and minerals to increase caloric intake if prescribed
    e. Maintain NG tube to decrease gastric distention and suppress pancreatic secretion
    f. Administer meperidine hydrochloride (Demerol) as prescribed for pain because it causes less incidence of spasm of the smooth muscle of the pancreatic ducts and sphincter of Oddi (Note: avoid morphine sulfate or codeine sulfate, which may cause spasms)
    g. Administer antacids as prescribed to neutralize gastric secretions
    h. Administer histamine-receptor-blocking medications as prescribed to decrease hydrochloric acid production so that pancreatic enzymes are not activated
    i. Administer anticholinergics as prescribed to decrease vagal stimulation, decrease GI motility, and inhibit pancreatic enzyme secretion
    j. Instruct the client in the importance of avoiding alcohol
    k. Instruct the client in the importance of follow-up visits with the physician
    l. Instruct the client to notify physician for acute abdominal pain, jaundice, clay-colored stools, and dark urine

C. Chronic
  1. Data collection
    a. Abdominal pain as continuous burning or gnawing, dullness with intense exacerbations
    b. Abdominal tenderness
    c. Left upper quadrant mass
    d. Steatorrhea and foul-smelling stools that may increase in volume as pancreatic insufficiency increases
    e. Weight loss
    f. Muscle wasting
    g. Jaundice
    h. Signs and symptoms of diabetes mellitus
  2. Implementation
    a. Administer meperidine hydrochloride (Demerol) as prescribed for pain because it causes less incidence of spasm of the smooth muscle of the pancreatic ducts and sphincter of Oddi (Note: avoid morphine sulfate or codeine sulfate, which may cause spasms)
    b. Maintain NPO status to avoid pain caused by eating
    c. TPN is administered for nutritional depletion as prescribed
    d. Provide small, frequent, high-carbohydrate, high-protein, low-fat diet when prescribed as tolerated by the client
    e. Provide supplemental preparations and vitamins and minerals to increase caloric intake
    f. Administer pancreatic enzymes as prescribed to aid in digestion and absorption of fat and protein
    g. Administer insulin or oral hypoglycemic medications as prescribed to control diabetes
    h. Instruct the client to avoid alcohol, caffeinated beverages, and rich fatty foods
    i. Instruct the client in the use of pancreatic enzyme medications
    j. Instruct the client in the treatment plan for glucose management
    k. Instruct the client to notify physician if increased steatorrhea occurs or if abdominal distention, cramping, and skin breakdown develop
    l. Instruct the client in the importance of follow-up visits

XXI. HEPATITIS

A. Description
  1. An inflammation of the liver caused by a virus, bacteria, or exposure to medications or hepatotoxins
  2. The goals of treatment include resting the inflamed liver to reduce metabolic demands and increasing the blood supply, thus promoting cellular regeneration and preventing complications

B. Types of viral hepatitis
  1. Hepatitis A (HAV), infectious hepatitis
  2. Hepatitis B (HBV), serum hepatitis
  3. Hepatitis C (HCV), non-A, non-B hepatitis or posttransfusion hepatitis
  4. Hepatitis D (HDV), delta agent hepatitis
  5. Hepatitis E (HEV), enterically transmitted or epidemic non-A, non-B hepatitis
  6. Hepatitis G (HGV), non-A, non-B, non-C hepatitis

C. Stages of viral hepatitis (Box 44-7)

D. Data collection
  1. Preicteric stage
    a. Flulike symptoms: malaise, fatigue
    b. Anorexia, nausea, vomiting, diarrhea
    c. Pain: headache, muscle aches, polyarthritis
    d. Serum bilirubin and enzyme levels are elevated
  2. Icteric stage
    a. Jaundice
    b. Pruritus
    c. Brown-colored urine
    d. Lighter-colored stools
    e. Decrease in preicteric phase symptoms
  3. Posticteric stage
    a. Energy levels increase
    b. Pain subsides
    c. GI symptoms are minimal to absent
    d. Serum bilirubin and enzyme levels return to normal

E. Laboratory assessment
  1. Alanine aminotransferase (ALT): Elevated to more than 1000 mU/mL and may rise to as high as 4000 mU/mL
  2. Aspartate aminotransferase (AST): May rise to 1000 to 2000 mU/mL
  3. Alkaline phosphatase levels
    a. May be normal or mildly elevated
    b. Normal adult blood value: 4.5 to 13 King-Armstrong units/dL
  4. Serum total bilirubin levels
    a. Elevated to greater than 2.5 mg/dL
    b. Normal: less than 1.5 mg/dL
    c. Elevated levels of bilirubin in the urine

BOX 44-7

Stages of Viral Hepatitis

PREICTERIC STAGE
The first stage of hepatitis preceding the appearance of jaundice

ICTERIC STAGE
The second stage of hepatitis, which includes the appearance of jaundice and associated symptoms such as elevated bilirubin levels, dark or tea-colored urine, and clay-colored stools

POSTICTERIC STAGE
The convalescent stage in which the jaundice decreases and the color of the urine and stool returns to normal

XXII. HEPATITIS A (HAV)

A. Description
  1. Formerly known as infectious hepatitis
  2. Commonly seen during the fall and early winter

B. Increased-risk individuals
  1. Commonly seen in young children
  2. Individuals in institutionalized settings
  3. Health care personnel

C. Transmission
  1. Fecal-oral route
  2. Person-to-person contact
  3. Parenteral
  4. Contaminated fruits, vegetables, or uncooked shellfish
  5. Contaminated water or milk
  6. Poorly washed utensils

D. Incubation period
  1. Incubation period is 2 to 6 weeks
  2. Infectious period is 2 to 3 weeks before and 1 week after developing jaundice

E. Testing
  1. Infection is established by the presence of hepatitis A virus (HAV) antibodies (anti-HAV) in the blood
  2. Immunoglobulin IgM and IgG are normally present in the blood, and increased levels indicate infection and inflammation
  3. Ongoing inflammation of the liver is evidenced by the presence of elevated IgM antibodies, which persist in the blood for 4 to 6 weeks
  4. Previous infection is indicated by the presence of elevated IgG antibodies

F. Complication: fulminant hepatitis
G. Prevention
1. Strict handwashing
2. Stool and needle precautions
3. Treatment of municipal water supplies
4. Serological screening of food handlers
5. Hepatitis A vaccine (Havrix)
6. Immune globulin (IG): for individuals exposed to HAV who have never received the hepatitis A vaccine; administer during the period of incubation and within 2 weeks of exposure
7. IG is recommended for household members and sexual contacts of individuals with hepatitis A
8. Preexposure prophylaxis with IG is recommended to individuals traveling to countries with poor or uncertain sanitation conditions

XXIII. HEPATITIS B (HBV)

A. Description
1. Is nonseasonal in nature
2. All age groups are affected
B. Increased-risk individuals
1. Drug addicts
2. Clients undergoing long-term hemodialysis
3. Health care personnel
C. Transmission
1. Blood or body fluid contact
2. Infected blood products
3. Infected saliva or semen
4. Contaminated needles
5. Sexual contact
6. Parenteral
7. Perinatal period
8. Blood or body fluids contact at birth
D. Incubation period: 6 to 24 weeks
E. Testing
1. Infection is established by the presence of hepatitis B antigen-antibody systems in the blood
2. Presence of hepatitis B surface antigens (HBsAG) is the serological marker to establish the diagnosis of hepatitis B
3. The client is considered infectious if these antigens are present in the blood
4. If the serological marker (HBsAG) is present after 6 months, it indicates a carrier state or chronic hepatitis
5. Normally the serological marker (HBsAG) level declines and disappears after the acute hepatitis B episode
6. The presence of antibodies to HBsAG (anti-HBS) indicates recovery and immunity to hepatitis B
7. Hepatitis B early antigen (HBeAG) is detected in the blood about 1 week after the appearance of HbsAG, and its presence determines the infective state of the client
F. Complications
1. Fulminant hepatitis
2. Chronic liver disease
3. **Cirrhosis**
4. Primary hepatocellular carcinoma

G. Prevention
1. Strict handwashing
2. Screening blood donors
3. Testing of all pregnant women
4. Needle precautions
5. Avoiding intimate sexual contact if hepatitis B surface antigen (HBsAG) is positive
6. Hepatitis B vaccine: Engerix-B, Recombivax HB
7. Hepatitis B Immune Globulin (HBIG): for individuals exposed to HBV, either through sexual contact or through the percutaneous or transmucosal route, who have never had hepatitis B and have never received hepatitis B vaccine

XXIV. HEPATITIS C (HCV)

A. Description
1. Occurs year round
2. Can occur in any age group
3. Is common among drug abusers and is the major cause of posttransfusion hepatitis
4. Risk factors are similar as those for HBV, as hepatitis C is also parenterally transmitted
B. Increased risk individuals
1. Parenteral drug users
2. Clients receiving frequent transfusions
3. Health care personnel
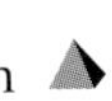
C. Transmission: same as HBV; primarily through blood
D. Incubation period: 5 to 10 weeks
E. Testing: Anti-HCV is the antibody to HCV and is most accurate in detecting chronic states of hepatitis C
F. Complications
1. Chronic liver disease
2. **Cirrhosis**
3. Primary hepatocellular carcinoma
G. Prevention
1. Strict handwashing
2. Needle precautions
3. Screening of blood donors

XXV. HEPATITIS D (HDV)

A. Description
1. Common in the Mediterranean and Middle Eastern areas

2. Seen with hepatitis B and may cause infection only in the presence of active HBV infection
3. Co-infection with the delta agent intensifies the acute symptoms of hepatitis B
4. Transmission and risk of infection are the same as for HBV, via contact with blood and blood products
5. Prevention of HBV infection with vaccine also prevents HDV infection, as HDV is dependent on HBV for replication

B. High-risk individuals
1. Drug users
2. Clients receiving hemodialysis
3. Clients receiving frequent blood transfusions

C. Transmission: same as HBV

D. Incubation period: 7 to 8 weeks

E. Testing: Serological hepatitis delta virus (HDV) determination is made by detection of the hepatitis D antigen (HDAg) early in the course of the infection and by detection of anti-HDV antibody in the later disease stages

F. Complications
1. Chronic liver disease
2. Fulminant hepatitis

G. Prevention: because hepatitis D must coexist with hepatitis B, the precautions that help prevent hepatitis B are also useful in preventing delta hepatitis

XXVI. HEPATITIS E (HEV)

A. Description
1. A water-borne virus
2. Prevalent in areas where sewage disposal is inadequate or where communal bathing in contaminated rivers is practiced
3. Risk of infection is the same as HAV
4. Presents as a mild disease except in infected women in the third trimester of pregnancy, with whom the mortality rate is high

B. Increased risk individuals
1. Travelers to countries that have a high incidence of hepatitis E, such as India, Burma (Myanmar), Afghanistan, Algeria, and Mexico
2. Eating or drinking food or water contaminated with the virus

C. Transmission: same as HAV

D. Incubation period: 2 to 9 weeks

E. Testing: specific serological tests for hepatitis E virus (HEV) include detection of IgM and IgG antibodies to hepatitis E (anti-HEV)

F. Complications
1. High mortality rate in pregnant women
2. Fetal demise

G. Prevention
1. Strict handwashing
2. Treatment of water supplies and sanitation measures

XXVII. HEPATITIS G (HGV)

A. Non-A, non-B, non-C hepatitis

B. Autoantibodies are absent

C. Risk factors are similar to those for hepatitis C

D. Hepatitis G (HGV) has been found in some blood donors, IV drug users, hemodialysis clients, and clients with hemophilia; however, HGV does not appear to cause significant liver disease

XXVIII. INSTRUCTIONS FOR HOME CARE FOR THE CLIENT AND FAMILY (Box 44-8)

PRACTICE QUESTIONS

1. A client presents to the emergency department with upper gastrointestinal (GI) bleeding and is in moderate distress. Which nursing action would be the first priority for this client?

BOX 44-8

Client and Family Education for Hepatitis

Strict and frequent handwashing
Do not share bathrooms unless the client strictly adheres to personal hygiene measures
Individual washcloths, towels, drinking and eating utensils, as well as toothbrushes and razors, must be labeled and identified
The client must not prepare food for other family members
The client should avoid alcohol and over-the-counter medications, particularly acetaminophen (Tylenol) and sedatives, because these medications are hepatotoxic
The client should increase activity gradually to prevent fatigue
The client should consume small, frequent, high-carbohydrate, low-fat foods
The client is not to donate blood
The client may maintain normal contact with people as long as proper personal hygiene is maintained
Close personal contact such as kissing should be discouraged until HBsAg test results are negative
The client is to avoid sexual activity until hepatitis B surface antigen (HBsAg) results are negative
The client needs to carry a Medic-Alert card noting the date of hepatitis onset
The client needs to inform other health professionals, such as medical or dental personnel, of the onset of hepatitis
The client needs to keep follow-up appointments with the health care provider

1. Thorough investigation of the precipitating events
2. Insertion of a nasogastric tube and hematest the emesis
3. Complete abdominal physical examination
4. Determination of vital signs

2. A nurse is caring for a client with possible cholelithiasis who is being prepared for a cholangiogram and provides instructions to the client about the procedure. Which client statement indicates that the client understands the purpose of this test?
   1. "They are going to look at my gallbladder and ducts."
   2. "This procedure will drain my gallbladder."
   3. "My gallbladder will be irrigated."
   4. "They will put medication in my gallbladder."

3. A nurse is caring for a client with acute pancreatitis and a history of alcoholism and is monitoring the client for complications. Which of the following information would be a sign of paralytic ileus?
   1. Firm, nontender mass palpable at the lower right costal margin
   2. Severe, constant pain with rapid onset
   3. Inability to pass flatus
   4. Loss of anal sphincter control

4. A nurse is caring for a client with a resolved intestinal obstruction who has a nasogastric tube in place. The client has tolerated the tube being clamped every 2 hours for 1 hour. The physician has now ordered the nasogastric tube to be discontinued. To determine if it is appropriate to discontinue the nasogastric tube, the nurse should check for:
   1. Proper nasogastric tube placement
   2. The client's serum electrolyte levels
   3. Presence of bowel sounds in all four quadrants
   4. The pH of the gastric aspirate

5. A nurse has administered approximately half of a high cleansing enema when the client complains of pain and cramping. Which of the following nursing actions is the most appropriate?
   1. Raise the enema bag so that the solution can be administered quickly
   2. Clamp the tubing for 30 seconds and restart the flow at a slower rate
   3. Reassure the client and continue the flow
   4. Discontinue the enema and notify the registered nurse

6. A nurse is preparing to administer a high cleansing enema. The nurse positions the client in the:
   1. Left lateral position with the right leg acutely flexed
   2. Right Sims' position
   3. Dorsal recumbent position
   4. Right lateral position with the left leg acutely flexed

7. A nurse has aspirated 40 mL of undigested formula from the client's nasogastric tube before administering an intermittent tube feeding. The nurse understands that before administering the tube feeding, the 40 mL of gastric aspirate should be:
   1. Discarded properly and recorded as output on the client's I&O record
   2. Poured into the nasogastric tube through a syringe with the plunger removed
   3. Mixed with the formula and poured into the nasogastric tube through a syringe without a plunger
   4. Diluted with water and injected into the nasogastric tube by putting pressure on the plunger

8. A nurse is participating in a health screening clinic, and is preparing teaching materials about colorectal cancer. The nurse would plan to include which most important risk factor for colorectal cancer in the material?
   1. Age over 20 years
   2. High-fiber, low-fat diet
   3. Distant relative with colorectal cancer
   4. Personal history of ulcerative colitis or gastrointestinal polyps

9. A hospitalized client with gastroesophageal reflux disease (GERD) is complaining of chest discomfort that feels like heartburn after a meal. After administering an ordered antacid, the nurse would encourage the client to lie in which of the following positions?
   1. Supine with the head of bed flat
   2. On the stomach with the head flat
   3. On the left side with the head of bed elevated 30 degrees
   4. On the right side with the head of bed elevated 30 degrees

10. A nurse is planning to teach a client with gastroesophageal reflux disease (GERD) about substances that will increase the lower esophageal sphincter (LES) pressure. The nurse tells the client to include which item in the diet?
    1. Fatty foods
    2. Nonfat milk
    3. Tea
    4. Coffee

11. A client has undergone esophagogastroduodenoscopy (EGD). The nurse places highest priority on which of the following items as part of the client's care plan?
    1. Checking for return of a gag reflex
    2. Giving warm gargles for a sore throat
    3. Monitoring the temperature
    4. Monitoring for complaints of heartburn

12. A nurse has taught a client about an upcoming endoscopic retrograde cholangiopancreatography (ERCP) procedure. The nurse evaluates that the client has not fully understood the information if the client makes which of the following statements?

1. "I know I must sign a consent form."
2. "I'm glad I don't have to lie still for this procedure."
3. "I'm glad some medication will be given IV to relax me."
4. "I hope the throat spray keeps me from gagging."

13. A client being seen in a physician's office has just been scheduled for a barium swallow the next day. The nurse writes down which of the following instructions for the client to follow before the test?
1. Remove all metal and jewelry before the test
2. Eat a regular supper and breakfast
3. Continue to take all oral medications as scheduled
4. Monitor own bowel movement pattern for constipation

14. A nurse is teaching the client about an upcoming colonoscopy procedure. The nurse would include in the instructions that the client will be placed in which of the following positions for the procedure?
1. Left Sims'
2. Right Sims'
3. Knee chest
4. Lithotomy

15. A nurse has given postprocedure instructions to a client who underwent colonoscopy. The nurse would evaluate that the client did not fully understand the directions if the client stated that:
1. Intake should be light at first, then progress to regular intake
2. It is normal to feel gassy or bloated after the procedure
3. The abdominal muscles may be tender from stretching during the procedure
4. It is all right to drive once the client has been home for an hour or so

16. A nurse is performing an abdominal examination. The initial assessment would be which of the following?
1. Auscultation
2. Inspection
3. Palpation
4. Percussion

17. A client is scheduled for an oral cholecystogram. The nurse would plan to obtain what type of diet for the evening meal before the test?
1. Low protein
2. High carbohydrate
3. Fat free
4. Liquid

18. Polyethylene glycol-electrolyte solution (GoLYTELY) is prescribed for a client scheduled for a colonoscopy. The client begins to experience diarrhea after administration of the solution. What action by the nurse is most appropriate?
1. Cancel the examination
2. Prepare to start an IV
3. Administer an enema
4. Explain that diarrhea is expected

19. A nasogastric tube has been inserted into a client and the physician prescribes that the tube be attached to intermittent suction. The nurse attaches the suction noting that the pressure should not exceed:
1. 10 mm Hg
2. 20 mm Hg
3. 25 mm Hg
4. 30 mm Hg

20. A nurse is caring for a client with a diagnosis of chronic gastritis. The nurse anticipates that this client is at risk for which of the following vitamin deficiencies?
1. Vitamin A
2. Vitamin B_{12}
3. Vitamin C
4. Vitamin E

21. A nurse is reviewing the medication record of a client with acute gastritis. Which of the following medications, if noted on the client's record, would the nurse question?
1. Digoxin (Lanoxin)
2. Indomethacin (Indocin)
3. Furosemide (Lasix)
4. Propranolol hydrochloride (Inderal)

22. A nurse is monitoring a client with a diagnosis of peptic ulcer. Which of the following findings would most likely indicate perforation of the ulcer?
1. Bradycardia
2. Numbness in the legs
3. Nausea and vomiting
4. A rigid, boardlike abdomen

23. A client with peptic ulcer disease is scheduled for a pyloroplasty and the client asks the nurse about the procedure. The nurse bases the response on which of the following?
1. A pyloroplasty involves cutting the vagus nerve
2. A pyloroplasty involves removing the distal portion of the stomach
3. A pyloroplasty involves removal of the ulcer and a large portion of the cells that produce hydrochloric acid
4. A pyloroplasty involves an incision and resuturing of the pylorus to relax the muscle and enlarge the opening from the stomach to the duodenum

24. A client with a peptic ulcer is scheduled for a vagotomy and the client asks the nurse about the purpose of this procedure. The nurse tells the client that a vagotomy:
1. Decreases food absorption in the stomach
2. Heals the gastric mucosa

3. Halts stress reactions
4. Reduces the stimulus to acid secretions

25. A nurse is caring for a client after a Billroth II procedure. On review of the postoperative orders, which of the following, if prescribed, would the nurse question and verify?
1. Irrigating the nasogastric (NG) tube
2. Coughing and deep breathing exercises
3. Leg exercises
4. Early ambulation

26. The nurse is providing discharge instructions to a client after gastrectomy. Which measure will the nurse instruct the client to follow to assist in preventing dumping syndrome?
1. Eat high-carbohydrate foods
2. Limit the fluids taken with meals
3. Ambulate after a meal
4. Sit in a high Fowler's position during meals

27. A nurse is monitoring a client for the early signs and symptoms of dumping syndrome. Which of the following symptoms will indicate this occurrence?
1. Abdominal cramping and pain
2. Bradycardia and indigestion
3. Sweating and pallor
4. Double vision and chest pain

28. A nurse is instructing the client who had a herniorrhaphy how to reduce postoperative swelling after the procedure. Which of the following would the nurse suggest to the client to prevent swelling?
1. Apply heat to the abdomen
2. Elevate the scrotum
3. Limit fluids
4. Maintain a low roughage diet

29. A nurse is reviewing the record of a client with Crohn's disease. Which of the following stool characteristics would the nurse expect to note documented in the record?
1. Bloody stools
2. Diarrhea
3. Constipation
4. Stool constantly oozing from the rectum

30. A nurse is performing a colostomy irrigation on a client. During the irrigation, the client begins to complain of abdominal cramps. Which of the following is the most appropriate nursing action?
1. Notify the registered nurse immediately
2. Increase the height of the irrigation
3. Stop the irrigation temporarily
4. Medicate for pain and resume irrigation

31. A nurse is teaching a client how to perform a colostomy irrigation. To enhance the effectiveness of the irrigation, what measure should the nurse instruct the client to do?
1. Increase fluid intake
2. Reduce the amount of irrigation solution
3. Massage the abdomen gently
4. Place heat on the abdomen

32. A nurse is reviewing the record of a client with a diagnosis of cirrhosis and notes that there is documentation of the presence of asterixis. To check for the presence of this sign, the nurse would do which of the following?
1. Ask the client to extend the arms
2. Check for the presence of Homan's sign
3. Instruct the client to lean forward
4. Measure the abdominal girth

33. A client with ascites is scheduled for a paracentesis. The nurse is assisting the physician in performing the procedure. Which of the following positions will the nurse assist the client to assume for this procedure?
1. Flat
2. Left side lying
3. Right side lying
4. Upright position

34. A nurse is reviewing the laboratory results of a client with cirrhosis and notes that the ammonia level is elevated. Which of the following diets would the nurse anticipate would most likely be prescribed for this client?
1. High carbohydrate
2. Moderate fat
3. High protein
4. Low protein

35. Lactulose (Chronulac) is prescribed for a client with a diagnosis of hepatic encephalopathy. Which finding indicates that the client is responding to this medication therapy as anticipated?
1. The fecal pH is acidic
2. The client experiences diarrhea
3. The client is able to tolerate a full diet
4. Vomiting occurs

36. An ultrasound of the gallbladder is scheduled for the client with a suspected diagnosis of cholecystitis. The nurse explains to the client that this test:
1. Requires the client to lie still for short intervals
2. Requires that the client be NPO
3. Is preceded by administration of oral tablets
4. Is uncomfortable

37. A nurse is providing preoperative teaching to a client scheduled for a cholecystectomy. Which of the following interventions would be of highest priority in the preoperative teaching plan?
1. Teaching coughing and deep breathing exercises
2. Teaching leg exercises
3. Instructions regarding fluid restrictions
4. Checking the client's understanding of the surgical procedure

38. A Penrose drain is in place on the first postoperative day after a cholecystectomy. Serosanguineous drainage is noted on the dressing covering the

drain. Which nursing intervention is most appropriate?
1. Notify the registered nurse immediately
2. Change the dressing
3. Circle the amount on the dressing with a pen
4. Continue to monitor the drainage

39. A client is admitted to the hospital for treatment of acute hepatitis B. Which activity order would the nurse expect to be prescribed?
1. Bed rest
2. Encourage ambulation
3. Out of bed in a chair
4. No activity restrictions

40. It had been determined that a client with hepatitis has contracted the infection from contaminated food. What type of hepatitis is this client most likely experiencing?
1. Hepatitis A
2. Hepatitis B
3. Hepatitis C
4. Hepatitis D

41. A nurse is reviewing the physician's orders written for a client admitted with acute pancreatitis. Which physician order would the nurse question if noted on the client's chart?
1. NPO status
2. Prepare to insert a nasogastric tube
3. An anticholinergic medication
4. Morphine sulfate for pain

42. A client with peptic ulcer states that stress frequently causes exacerbation of the disease. The nurse would interpret that which of the following items mentioned by the client is most likely responsible for the exacerbations?
1. Sleeping 8 to 10 hours a night
2. Eating 5 to 6 small meals per day
3. Ability to work at home periodically
4. Frequent need to work overtime on short notice

43. A client with peptic ulcer disease (PUD) needs dietary modification to reduce episodes of epigastric pain. The nurse would teach the client that which of the following items does not need to be limited or eliminated with this disease?
1. Wine
2. Baked chicken
3. Coffee
4. Fresh fruit

44. A nurse instructs the ileostomy client to do which of the following as part of essential care of the stoma?
1. Cleanse the peristomal skin meticulously
2. Take in high-fiber foods such as nuts
3. Massage the area below the stoma
4. Limit fluid intake to prevent diarrhea

45. A client with hiatal hernia chronically experiences heartburn after meals. The nurse would teach the client to avoid which of the following, which is contraindicated with hiatal hernia?
1. Taking in small, frequent, bland meals
2. Lying recumbent after meals
3. Raising the head of bed on 6-inch blocks
4. Taking histamine receptor-antagonist medication as prescribed

46. A nurse is monitoring for stoma prolapse in a client with a colostomy. The nurse would observe which of the following appearances in the stoma if prolapse occurred?
1. Sunken and hidden
2. Dark and bluish in color
3. Narrowed and flattened
4. Protruding and swollen

47. A client with a new colostomy is concerned about odor from stool in the ostomy drainage bag. The nurse teaches the client to include which of the following foods in the diet to reduce odor?
1. Yogurt
2. Broccoli
3. Cucumbers
4. Eggs

48. A nurse has given instructions to the client with an ileostomy about foods to eat to thicken the stool. The nurse would evaluate that the client did not fully understand the instructions if the client stated to eat which of the following foods to make the stool less watery?
1. Pasta
2. Boiled rice
3. Bran
4. Low-fat cheese

49. A nurse is doing preoperative teaching with the client who is about to undergo creation of a Kock pouch. The nurse interprets that the client has the best understanding of the nature of the surgery if the client makes which of the following statements?
1. "I will need to drain the pouch regularly with a catheter."
2. "I will need to wear a drainage bag for the rest of my life."
3. "The drainage from this type of ostomy will be formed."
4. "I will be able to pass stool by the rectum eventually."

50. The client with chronic pancreatitis needs information on dietary modification to manage the health problem. The nurse teaches the client to limit which of the following items in the diet?
1. Carbohydrate
2. Protein
3. Fat
4. Water-soluble vitamins

51. A client with acute pancreatitis is experiencing severe pain from the disorder. The nurse tells the

client to avoid which of the following positions that could aggravate the pain?
1. Sitting up
2. Lying flat
3. Leaning forward
4. Flexing the left leg

52. A nurse is evaluating the effect of dietary counseling on the client with cholecystitis. The nurse determines that the client understands the instructions given if the client stated that which of the following food items is acceptable in the diet?
1. Baked scrod
2. Sauces and gravies
3. Fried chicken
4. Fresh whipped cream

53. A client with cirrhosis is beginning to show signs of hepatic encephalopathy. The nurse would plan a dietary consult to limit the amount of which of the following ingredients in the client's diet?
1. Fat
2. Carbohydrate
3. Protein
4. Minerals

54. A client with Crohn's disease has an order to begin taking antispasmodic medication. The nurse should time the medication so that each dose is taken:
1. 30 minutes before meals
2. During meals
3. 60 minutes after meals
4. Upon arising and at bedtime

55. A client is admitted to the hospital with acute viral hepatitis. Which of the following signs or symptoms would the nurse expect to note based on this diagnosis?
1. Spider angiomas
2. Fatigue
3. Pale urine
4. Weight gain

56. A client with viral hepatitis who is discussing with the nurse the need to avoid alcohol states "I'm not sure I can do that." The nurse would respond by saying:
1. "Everything will be all right."
2. "I think you should talk more with the doctor about this."
3. "I don't believe that."
4. "I'm not sure that I understand. Would you please explain?"

57. Of the following infection control methods, which would be the priority to include in the plan of care to prevent hepatitis B in a client considered to be at high risk for exposure?
1. Correct handwashing technique
2. Hepatitis B vaccine
3. Proper personal hygiene
4. Use of immune globulin

58. A nurse provides home care instructions to a client with hepatitis B. Which statement by the client indicates the best understanding of how to prevent transmission of the disease?
1. "I should be vaccinated as soon as possible."
2. "I will never share a towel with anyone else."
3. "It is alright to kiss my wife."
4. "My wife should get the vaccine."

59. A client is admitted to the hospital with viral hepatitis and is complaining of a loss of appetite. To provide adequate nutrition, the nurse encourages the client to:
1. Eat a large supper when anorexia is most likely not as severe
2. Eat less often, preferably only 3 large meals daily
3. Drink a lot of fluids, especially carbonated beverages
4. Select foods high in fat

60. An African-American client has a diagnosis of acute viral hepatitis. Which of the following specific areas would the nurse inspect for jaundice in this client?
1. Flexor surfaces of the extremities
2. Hard palate of the mouth
3. Nail beds
4. Skin

61. A client with viral hepatitis states to the nurse, "I am so yellow." The nurse would most appropriately:
1. Assist the client in expressing feelings
2. Keep the client isolated from other clients and visitors
3. Provide information to the client about hepatitis
4. Restrict visitors until the jaundice subsides

62. A nurse provides instructions to a client after a liver biopsy. The nurse tells the client to:
1. Avoid alcohol for 8 hours
2. Save all stools to be checked for blood
3. Remain NPO for 24 hours
4. Lie on the right side for 2 hours

63. A sexually active 20-year-old client has developed viral hepatitis. Which of the following statements, if made by the client, would indicate a need for teaching?
1. "A condom should be used for sexual intercourse."
2. "I can never drink alcohol again."
3. "I won't go back to work right away."
4. "My close friends should get the vaccine."

64. A client is admitted to the hospital with severe jaundice and is having diagnostic testing. Since the client has no complaints of fatigue, the client is encouraged to ambulate in the hall to maintain muscle strength. The client paces around the room, but will not enter the hallway. Which of the following problems most likely is the reason for the client's reluctance to walk in the hall?
1. Fear of catching another disease
2. Not wanting to overexert and get overly tired

3. Feeling self-conscious about appearance
4. Unfamiliarity with the hospital

65. A client with viral hepatitis has no appetite and food makes the client nauseated. Which of the following nursing interventions would be most appropriate?
    1. Explain that high-fat diets are usually better tolerated
    2. Encourage foods low in calories
    3. Explain that the majority of calories need to be consumed in the evening hours
    4. Monitor for fluid and electrolyte imbalance

ANSWERS

1. *Answer:* 4

Rationale: The determination of vital signs indicates whether the client is in shock from blood loss and also provides a baseline blood pressure and pulse by which to monitor the progress of treatment. Signs and symptoms of shock include low blood pressure; rapid, weak pulse; increased thirst; cold, clammy skin; and restlessness. Vital signs should be monitored every 15 to 30 minutes, and the physician should be informed of any significant changes. The client may not be able to provide subjective data until the immediate physical needs are met. Although options 2 and 3 may be a component of care, they are not the first priority.
Test-Taking Strategy: Use the process of elimination and the ABCs—airway, breathing, and circulation. A client with acute upper GI bleeding is at risk for shock. Monitoring vital signs is the nursing action that will assess circulation, provide information about the client's circulating volume status, and alert the nurse to early stages of shock. Review care to the client with GI bleeding if you had difficulty with this question.
Level of Cognitive Ability: Application
Client Needs: Physiological Integrity
Integrated Concept/Process: Nursing Process/Implementation
Content Area: Adult Health/Gastrointestinal
Reference: DeWit S: *Fundamental concepts and skills for nursing,* Philadelphia, 2001, WB Saunders, p. 494.

2. *Answer:* 1

Rationale: A cholangiogram is for diagnostic purposes. It outlines both the gallbladder and the ducts, so gallstones that have moved into the ductal system can be detected. X-rays are used to visualize the biliary duct system after an IV injection of radiopaque dye. Options 2, 3, and 4 are incorrect.
Test-Taking Strategy: Use the process of elimination. Eliminate options 2, 3 and 4 because they are similar. Review this procedure if you had difficulty with this question.
Level of Cognitive Ability: Comprehension
Client Needs: Physiological Integrity
Integrated Concept/Process: Nursing Process/Evaluation
Content Area: Adult Health/Gastrointestinal
Reference: DeWit S: *Fundamental concepts and skills for nursing,* Philadelphia, 2001, WB Saunders, p. 409.

3. *Answer:* 3

Rationale: An inflammatory reaction such as acute pancreatitis can cause paralytic ileus, the most common form of nonmechanical obstruction. Inability to pass flatus is a clinical manifestation of paralytic ileus. Option 1 is the description of the physical finding of liver enlargement. The liver is usually enlarged in cases of cirrhosis or hepatitis. Although this client may have an enlarged liver, an enlarged liver is not a sign of paralytic ileus or intestinal obstruction. Pain is associated with paralytic ileus, but the pain usually presents as a more constant generalized discomfort. Pain that is severe, constant, and rapid in onset is more likely caused by strangulation of the bowel. Loss of sphincter control is not a sign of paralytic ileus.
Test-Taking Strategy: Use the process of elimination. Note the relationship between the words "paralytic ileus" and option 3. Review these clinical manifestations if you had difficulty with this question.
Level of Cognitive Ability: Comprehension
Client Needs: Physiological Integrity
Integrated Concept/Process: Nursing Process/Data Collection
Content Area: Adult Health/Gastrointestinal
Reference: DeWit S: *Fundamental concepts and skills for nursing,* Philadelphia, 2001, WB Saunders, p. 773.

4. *Answer:* 3

Rationale: Distention, vomiting, and abdominal pain are a few of the symptoms associated with intestinal obstruction, and a nasogastric tube may be used to empty the stomach and relieve distention and vomiting. Bowel sounds return to normal as the obstruction is relieved and normal bowel function is restored. Discontinuing the nasogastric tube before the return of normal bowel function may result in a return of the symptoms necessitating reinsertion of the nasogastric tube. Serum electrolyte levels, tube placement, and pH of gastric aspirate are important assessments for the client with a nasogastric tube in place, but would not assist in determining the readiness for removing the nasogastric tube.
Test-Taking Strategy: Use the process of elimination and focus on the issue, removing the nasogastric tube. Recalling the pathophysiology for intestinal obstruction and purpose of a nasogastric tube as a therapy will direct you to option 3. Review care to the client with an intestinal obstruction if you had difficulty with this question.
Level of Cognitive Ability: Comprehension
Client Needs: Physiological Integrity
Integrated Concept/Process: Nursing Process/Data Collection
Content Area: Adult Health/Gastrointestinal
Reference: DeWit S: *Fundamental concepts and skills for nursing,* Philadelphia, 2001, WB Saunders, p. 496.

5. *Answer:* 2
Rationale: Pain and cramping are usually due to intestinal spasm and will subside when the enema is stopped briefly. If the client complains of fullness or pain, the flow is stopped for 30 seconds and restarted at a slower rate. The higher the solution container is held above the rectum, the faster the flow and the greater the force in the rectum. There is no need to discontinue the enema and notify the registered nurse at this time.
Test-Taking Strategy: Use the process of elimination and knowledge of the procedure for enema administration to answer this question. Noting the client's symptoms will assist in directing you to the correct option. Review this procedure if you had difficulty with this question.
Level of Cognitive Ability: Application
Client Needs: Physiological Integrity
Integrated Concept/Process: Nursing Process/Implementation
Content Area: Adult Health/Gastrointestinal
Reference: DeWit S: *Fundamental concepts and skills for nursing*, Philadelphia, 2001, WB Saunders, p. 591.

6. *Answer:* 1
Rationale: The sigmoid and descending colon is located on the left side. Therefore, the left lateral position uses gravity to facilitate the flow of solution into the sigmoid and descending colon. Acute flexion of the right leg allows for adequate exposure of the anus. Options 2, 3, and 4 are incorrect positions.
Test-Taking Strategy: Use the process of elimination. Knowledge of anatomy of the rectum will assist in eliminating options 2 and 4. Attempt to visualize the remaining positions presented in options 1 and 3. This will assist in eliminating option 3. Review this procedure if you had difficulty with this question.
Level of Cognitive Ability: Application
Client Needs: Physiological Integrity
Integrated Concept/Process: Nursing Process/Implementation
Content Area: Adult Health/Gastrointestinal
Reference: DeWit S: *Fundamental concepts and skills for nursing*, Philadelphia, 2001, WB Saunders, p. 591.

7. *Answer:* 2
Rationale: After checking residual feeding contents, the gastric contents are reinstilled into the stomach by removing the syringe plunger and pouring the gastric contents via the syringe into the nasogastric tube. Removal of the contents could disturb the client's electrolyte balance and the contents are not discarded. Gastric contents are not mixed with formula.
Test-Taking Strategy: Use the process of elimination. Eliminate option 4 because of the word "pressure." Next eliminate option 3 because gastric contents are not mixed with formula. From the remaining options, recalling that gastric contents are not discarded will direct you to option 2. Review this procedure if you had difficulty with this question.
Level of Cognitive Ability: Comprehension
Client Needs: Physiological Integrity
Integrated Concept/Process: Nursing Process/Implementation
Content Area: Adult Health/Gastrointestinal
Reference: DeWit S: *Fundamental concepts and skills for nursing*, Philadelphia, 2001, WB Saunders, p. 504.

8. *Answer:* 4
Rationale: Common risk factors for colorectal cancer include age over 40; first-degree relative with colorectal cancer; high-fat, low-fiber diet; and history of bowel problems such as ulcerative colitis or familial polyposis.
Test-Taking Strategy: Use the process of elimination. Noting the key words "personal history" will direct you to option 4. Review these risk factors if you had difficulty with this question.
Level of Cognitive Ability: Application
Client Needs: Health Promotion and Maintenance
Integrated Concept/Process: Nursing Process/Planning
Content Area: Adult Health/Gastrointestinal
Reference: DeWit S: *Fundamental concepts and skills for nursing*, Philadelphia, 2001, WB Saunders, p. 585.

9. *Answer:* 3
Rationale: The discomfort of reflux is aggravated by positions that compress the abdomen and the stomach. These include lying flat either on the back or stomach after a meal, or lying on the right side. The left side-lying position with head of bed elevated is most likely to give relief to the client.
Test-Taking Strategy: Use the process of elimination. Evaluate each of the positions described in terms of their ability to put pressure on the stomach and cause reflux. Using knowledge of anatomy and these basic nursing positions, you should be able to eliminate each of the incorrect options. Review the measures to relieve reflux if you had difficulty with this question.
Level of Cognitive Ability: Application
Client Needs: Physiological Integrity
Integrated Concept/Process: Nursing Process/Implementation
Content Area: Adult Health/Gastrointestinal
Reference: DeWit S: *Fundamental concepts and skills for nursing*, Philadelphia, 2001, WB Saunders, p. 494.

10. *Answer:* 2
Rationale: Foods that increase the LES pressure will decrease reflux and lessen the symptoms of GERD. The food item that will increase the LES pressure is nonfat milk. The other items listed decrease the LES pressure, thus increasing reflux symptoms. Aggravating substances include chocolate, coffee, fatty foods, and alcohol.
Test-Taking Strategy: Use the process of elimination. Eliminate options 3 and 4 first because they are similar and both contain caffeine. From the remaining options, recalling the effects of fatty foods will direct you to option 2. Review these food items if you had difficulty with this question.
Level of Cognitive Ability: Application
Client Needs: Health Promotion and Maintenance
Integrated Concept/Process: Teaching/Learning
Content Area: Adult Health/Gastrointestinal
Reference: DeWit S: *Fundamental concepts and skills for nursing*, Philadelphia, 2001, WB Saunders, p. 494.

11. *Answer:* 1
Rationale: The nurse places highest priority on managing the client's airway. This includes assessing for return of the gag reflex. The client's vital signs are also monitored, and a sudden sharp increase in temperature could indicate perforation of

the gastrointestinal tract. This would be accompanied by other signs as well such as pain. Monitoring for sore throat and heartburn is also important; however, the client's airway still takes priority.
Test-Taking Strategy: Use the process of elimination. Note that the question contains the key words "highest priority." Use the ABCs—airway, breathing, and circulation. This will direct you to option 1. Review postprocedure care after EGD if you had difficulty with this question.
Level of Cognitive Ability: Application
Client Needs: Physiological Integrity
Integrated Concept/Process: Nursing Process/Data Collection
Content Area: Adult Health/Gastrointestinal
Reference: DeWit S: *Fundamental concepts and skills for nursing,* Philadelphia, 2001, WB Saunders, p. 409.

12. *Answer:* 2
Rationale: The client needs to lie still for ERCP, which takes about an hour to perform. The client also needs to sign a consent form. IV sedation is given to relax the client, and an anesthetic spray is used to help keep the client from gagging as the endoscope is passed.
Test-Taking Strategy: Use the process of elimination. Note the key words "has not fully understood." Invasive procedures require consent so option 1 can be eliminated. Noting the name of the procedure and considering the anatomical location will assist in eliminating options 3 and 4. Review this procedure if you had difficulty with this question.
Level of Cognitive Ability: Comprehension
Client Needs: Physiological Integrity
Integrated Concept/Process: Nursing Process/Evaluation
Content Area: Adult Health/Gastrointestinal
Reference: DeWit S: *Fundamental concepts and skills for nursing,* Philadelphia, 2001, WB Saunders, p. 409.

13. *Answer:* 1
Rationale: A barium swallow is an x-ray that uses a substance called barium for contrast to highlight abnormalities in the gastrointestinal (GI) tract. The client is told to remove all jewelry before the test, so that it won't interfere with x-ray visualization of the field. The client should fast for 8 to12 hours before the test, depending on physician instructions. Most oral medications are also withheld before the test, depending on the physician's instructions. It is important to monitor for constipation after the procedure, which can occur as a result of the presence of barium in the GI tract.
Test-Taking Strategy: Use the process of elimination. Note that the key words in the stem of the question are "barium swallow" and "before." This tells you that the correct option is an item that the client needs to comply with before the test is done. Eliminate option 4 first, because it is a part of aftercare. Eliminate option 3 next because of the word "all." Recalling that the procedure is a type of x-ray that involves barium for contrast and an NPO status will direct you to option 1. Review preprocedure instructions for this test if you had difficulty with this question.
Level of Cognitive Ability: Application
Client Needs: Physiological Integrity
Integrated Concept/Process: Nursing Process/Implementation
Content Area: Adult Health/Gastrointestinal
Reference: Ignatavicius D, Workman M: *Medical-surgical: critical thinking for collaborative care,* ed 4, Philadelphia, 2002, WB Saunders, p. 1172.

14. *Answer:* 1
Rationale: The client is placed in the left Sims' position for the procedure. This position takes the best advantage of the client's anatomy for ease in introducing the colonoscope. The other options are incorrect.
Test-Taking Strategy: Use concepts related to gastrointestinal anatomy to answer this question. The answer would be the same as would be used for giving the client an enema while lying down. When answering factual questions such as these, remember the guiding principles and attempt to visualize the procedure to help you select the correct option. Review this procedure if you had difficulty with this question.
Level of Cognitive Ability: Application
Client Needs: Physiological Integrity
Integrated Concept/Process: Nursing Process/Implementation
Content Area: Adult Health/Gastrointestinal
Reference: Ignatavicius D, Workman M: *Medical-surgical: critical thinking for collaborative care,* ed 4, Philadelphia, 2002, WB Saunders, p. 1176.

15. *Answer:* 4
Rationale: The client should not drive for several hours after this test because the client would have received sedative medications during the procedure. The client should resume intake slowly and progress as tolerated. The client may experience gas or abdominal tenderness for a short while after the procedure, and this is normal.
Test-Taking Strategy: Use the process of elimination. Note that the question contains the key words "did not fully understand." This tells you that the correct option is an incorrect statement on the part of the client. Use knowledge of events during the procedure to choose the correct option. Recalling that sedating medications are administered will direct you to option 4. Review postprocedure instructions if you had difficulty with this question.
Level of Cognitive Ability: Comprehension
Client Needs: Health Promotion and Maintenance
Integrated Concept/Process: Teaching/Learning
Content Area: Adult Health/Gastrointestinal
Reference: Ignatavicius D, Workman M: *Medical-surgical: critical thinking for collaborative care,* ed 4, Philadelphia, 2002, WB Saunders, p. 1176.

16. *Answer:* 2
Rationale: The appropriate technique for abdominal examination is inspection, auscultation, percussion, and palpation. Auscultation is performed after inspection and before percussion and palpation to ensure that the motility of the bowel and bowel sounds are not altered. The sequence of maneuvers is inspect, auscultate, percuss, and palpate.
Test-Taking Strategy: Use the process of elimination and think about the procedure. Remember that the sequence for abdominal examination differs from the usual systematic approach. Review this technique if you had difficulty with this question.
Level of Cognitive Ability: Application
Client Needs: Physiological Integrity

Integrated Concept/Process: Nursing Process/Data Collection
Content Area: Adult Health/Gastrointestinal
Reference: DeWit S: *Fundamental concepts and skills for nursing,* Philadelphia, 2001, WB Saunders, pp. 383, 385.

17. *Answer:* 3
Rationale: Normal dietary intake of fat should be maintained during the days preceding the test to empty bile from the gallbladder. A fat-free diet is ordered on the evening before the test. The fat-free supper prevents contraction of the gallbladder and allows accumulation of the contrast substance needed for x-ray visualization. Options 1, 2, and 4 are incorrect.
Test-Taking Strategy: Use the process of elimination. Recalling that an oral cholecystogram is an x-ray of the gallbladder will assist in directing you to the correct option. Think about the function of the gallbladder to assist in selecting the correct option. Review this test if you had difficulty with this question.
Level of Cognitive Ability: Application
Client Needs: Physiological Integrity
Integrated Concept/Process: Nursing Process/Planning
Content Area: Adult Health/Gastrointestinal
Reference: Ignatavicius D, Workman M: *Medical-surgical: critical thinking for collaborative care,* ed 4, Philadelphia, 2002, WB Saunders, p. 1173.

18. *Answer:* 4
Rationale: The solution GoLYTELY is a bowel evacuant used in preparation for colonoscopy to cleanse the bowel. It is expected to cause a mild diarrhea and will clear the bowel in 4 to 5 hours. Options 1, 2, and 3 are incorrect.
Test-Taking Strategy: Use the process of elimination. Options 1 and 2 are not within the scope of nursing practice and should be eliminated. Knowledge regarding the purpose of this medication will assist in eliminating option 3 and easily direct you to option 4. Review this medication if you had difficulty with this question.
Level of Cognitive Ability: Application
Client Needs: Physiological Integrity
Integrated Concept/Process: Nursing Process/Implementation
Content Area: Adult Health/Gastrointestinal
Reference: Hodgson B, Kizior R: *Saunders nursing drug handbook 2002,* Philadelphia, 2002, WB Saunders, p. 899.

19. *Answer:* 3
Rationale: When gastrointestinal (GI) tubes are attached to suction, it may be continuous or intermittent, with a pressure not exceeding 25 mm Hg. The specific pressure and the intervals are prescribed by the physician. Options 1, 2, and 4 are incorrect.
Test-Taking Strategy: Knowledge regarding the restrictions related to the amount of pressure with suction on a GI tube is required to answer this question. Review this procedure if you had difficulty with this question.
Level of Cognitive Ability: Comprehension
Client Needs: Physiological Integrity
Integrated Concept/Process: Nursing Process/Implementation
Content Area: Adult Health/Gastrointestinal
Reference: DeWit S: *Fundamental concepts and skills for nursing,* Philadelphia, 2001, WB Saunders, p.528.

20. *Answer:* 2
Rationale: Deterioration and atrophy of the lining of the stomach lead to the loss of function of the parietal cells. When the acid secretion decreases, the source of the intrinsic factor is lost, which results in the inability to absorb vitamin B_{12}. This leads to the development of pernicious anemia.
Test-Taking Strategy: Use the process of elimination. Knowledge regarding the pathophysiology related to the lining of the stomach is required to answer this question. If you are unfamiliar with vitamin B_{12} deficiency and its relationship to gastric disorders, review this content.
Level of Cognitive Ability: Comprehension
Client Needs: Physiological Integrity
Integrated Concept/Process: Nursing Process/Data Collection
Content Area: Adult Health/Gastrointestinal
Reference: deWit S: *Fundamental concepts and skills for nursing,* Philadelphia, 2001, WB Saunders, p.411.

21. *Answer:* 2
Rationale: Indomethacin is a nonsteroidal antiinflammatory drug (NSAID) that can cause ulceration of the esophagus, stomach, duodenum, and small intestine. It is contraindicated in a client with gastrointestinal disorders. Furosemide is a loop diuretic. Digoxin is an antidysrhythmic. Propranolol hydrochloride is a beta-adrenergic blocker. Furosemide, digoxin, and propranolol hydrochloride are not contraindicated in clients with gastric disorders.
Test-Taking Strategy: Knowledge regarding the side effects associated with the medications identified in the options is required to answer this question. If you are unfamiliar with these medications, review this content.
Level of Cognitive Ability: Comprehension
Client Needs: Safe, Effective Care Environment
Integrated Concept/Process: Nursing Process/Implementation
Content Area: Adult Health/Gastrointestinal
Reference: Hodgson B, Kizior R: *Saunders nursing drug handbook 2002,* Philadelphia, 2002, WB Saunders, p. 571.

22. *Answer:* 4
Rationale: Perforation is a surgical emergency. It is characterized by sudden, sharp, intolerable, severe pain beginning in the midepigastric area and spreading over the abdomen, which becomes rigid and boardlike. Nausea and vomiting may occur. Tachycardia may occur as hypovolemic shock develops. Numbness in the legs is not an associated finding.
Test-Taking Strategy: Use the process of elimination. Note the key words "most likely" in the stem of the question. Option 2 can be eliminated first. Eliminate option 1 next because tachycardia rather that bradycardia would develop if the client is bleeding. From the remaining options, focusing on the key words will assist in directing you to option 4. Review the signs of perforation if you had difficulty with this question.
Level of Cognitive Ability: Analysis
Client Needs: Physiological Integrity
Integrated Concept/Process: Nursing Process/Data Collection
Content Area: Adult Health/Gastrointestinal
Reference: Ignatavicius D, Workman M: *Medical-surgical: critical thinking for collaborative care,* ed 4, Philadelphia, 2002, WB Saunders, p. 1419.

23. *Answer:* 4
Rationale: Option 4 describes the procedure for a pyloroplasty. A vagotomy involves cutting the vagus nerve. A subtotal gastrectomy involves removing the distal portion of the stomach. A Billroth II procedure involves removal of the ulcer and a large portion of the cells that produce hydrochloric acid.
Test-Taking Strategy: Use the process of elimination. Note the relationship between the words "pyloroplasty" in the question and "pylorus" in the correct option. Review this procedure if you had difficulty with this question.
Level of Cognitive Ability: Comprehension
Client Needs: Physiological Integrity
Integrated Concept/Process: Nursing Process/Implementation
Content Area: Adult Health/Gastrointestinal
Reference: Ignatavicius D, Workman M: *Medical-surgical: critical thinking for collaborative care,* ed 4, Philadelphia, 2002, WB Saunders, p. 1230.

24. *Answer:* 4
Rationale: A vagotomy, or cutting of the vagus nerve, is done to eliminate parasympathetic stimulation of gastric secretion. Options 1, 2, and 3 are incorrect descriptions of a vagotomy.
Test-Taking Strategy: Knowledge regarding the procedure and purpose of a vagotomy is required to answer this question. If you are unfamiliar with this procedure, review this content.
Level of Cognitive Ability: Application
Client Needs: Physiological Integrity
Integrated Concept/Process: Nursing Process/Implementation
Content Area: Adult Health/Gastrointestinal
Reference: Ignatavicius D, Workman M: *Medical-surgical: critical thinking for collaborative care,* ed 4, Philadelphia, 2002, WB Saunders, p. 1229.

25. *Answer:* 1
Rationale: In a Billroth II resection, the proximal remnant of the stomach is anastomosed to the proximal jejunum. Patency of the NG tube is critical for preventing the retention of gastric secretions. The nurse, however, should never irrigate or reposition the gastric tube after gastric surgery unless specifically ordered by the physician. In this situation, the nurse should clarify the order. Options 2, 3, and 4 are appropriate postoperative interventions.
Test-Taking Strategy: Use the process of elimination. Eliminate options 2, 3, and 4 because they are general postoperative measures. Also, consider the anatomical location of the surgical procedure to assist in directing you to option 1. Review these postoperative measures if you had difficulty with this question.
Level of Cognitive Ability: Application
Client Needs: Safe, Effective Care Environment
Integrated Concept/Process: Nursing Process/Implementation
Content Area: Adult Health/Gastrointestinal
Reference: Ignatavicius D, Workman M: *Medical-surgical: critical thinking for collaborative care,* ed 4, Philadelphia, 2002, WB Saunders, p. 1230.

26. *Answer:* 2
Rationale: The client should be instructed to decrease the amount of fluid taken at meals. The client should also be instructed to avoid high-carbohydrate foods including fluids, such as fruit nectars; to assume a low-Fowler's position during meals; to lie down for 30 minutes after eating to delay gastric emptying, and to take antispasmodic medications as prescribed.
Test-Taking Strategy: Use the process of elimination. Eliminate options 3 and 4 first because these measures will promote gastric emptying. From the remaining options, select option 2 because this measure will delay gastric emptying. If you are unfamiliar with this syndrome, review these client teaching points.
Level of Cognitive Ability: Application
Client Needs: Health Promotion and Maintenance
Integrated Concept/Process: Teaching/Learning
Content Area: Adult Health/Gastrointestinal
Reference: Ignatavicius D, Workman M: *Medical-surgical: critical thinking for collaborative care,* ed 4, Philadelphia, 2002, WB Saunders, p. 1233.

27. *Answer:* 3
Rationale: Early manifestations occur 5 to 30 minutes after eating. Symptoms include vertigo, tachycardia, syncope, sweating, pallor, palpitations, and the desire to lie down.
Test-Taking Strategy: Knowledge regarding the early manifestations associated with dumping syndrome is required to answer this question. If you are unfamiliar with these manifestations, review this content.
Level of Cognitive Ability: Comprehension
Client Needs: Physiological Integrity
Integrated Concept/Process: Nursing Process/Data Collection
Content Area: Adult Health/Gastrointestinal
Reference: Ignatavicius D, Workman M: *Medical-surgical: critical thinking for collaborative care,* ed 4, Philadelphia, 2002, WB Saunders, p. 1233.

28. *Answer:* 2
Rationale: After herniorrhaphy, the client should be instructed to elevate the scrotum and apply ice packs while in bed to decrease pain and swelling. The client is also instructed to apply a scrotal support when out of bed. Options 1, 3, and 4 are incorrect.
Test-Taking Strategy: The issue of the question is to prevent swelling. Basic knowledge regarding the effects of heat and cold will assist in eliminating option 1. Options 3 and 4 can be eliminated next by focusing on the issue. Review postoperative care after herniorrhaphy if you had difficulty with this question.
Level of Cognitive Ability: Application
Client Needs: Health Promotion and Maintenance
Integrated Concept/Process: Self Care
Content Area: Adult Health/Gastrointestinal
Reference: Ignatavicius D, Workman M: *Medical-surgical: critical thinking for collaborative care,* ed 4, Philadelphia, 2002, WB Saunders, p. 1244

29. *Answer:* 2
Rationale: Crohn's disease is characterized by nonbloody diarrhea of usually not more than four to five stools daily. Over time, the diarrhea episodes do increase in frequency, duration, and severity. Options 3 and 4 are not characteristics of Crohn's disease.

Test-Taking Strategy: Use the process of elimination. Recalling the pathophysiology related to Crohn's disease will direct you to option 2. If you are unfamiliar with this disorder, review this content.
Level of Cognitive Ability: Comprehension
Client Needs: Physiological Integrity
Integrated Concept/Process: Nursing Process/Data Collection
Content Area: Adult Health/Gastrointestinal
Reference: Ignatavicius D, Workman M: *Medical-surgical: critical thinking for collaborative care,* ed 4, Philadelphia, 2002, WB Saunders, p. 1284.

30. *Answer:* 3
Rationale: If cramping occurs during colostomy irrigation, the irrigation flow is stopped temporarily and the client is allowed to rest. Cramping may occur from infusion that is too rapid or is causing too much pressure. Increasing the height of the irrigation will cause further discomfort. The registered nurse does not need to be notified immediately. Medicating the client for pain is not the most appropriate action.
Test-Taking Strategy: Use the process of elimination and focus on the issue of the question. Using the principles related to administering an enema will direct you to option 3. Review the procedure for colostomy irrigation if you had difficulty with this question.
Level of Cognitive Ability: Application
Client Needs: Physiological Integrity
Integrated Concept/Process: Nursing Process/Implementation
Content Area: Adult Health/Gastrointestinal
Reference: Ignatavicius D, Workman M: *Medical-surgical: critical thinking for collaborative care,* ed 4, Philadelphia, 2002, WB Saunders, p. 1250.

31. *Answer:* 3
Rationale: To enhance effectiveness of the irrigation, the client is instructed to change position, ambulate, massage the abdomen gently, and drink something warm. Options 1, 2, and 4 will not enhance the effectiveness of this procedure.
Test-Taking Strategy: Focus on the issue of the question, which is the measure that will enhance the effectiveness of the irrigation. This focus will assist in eliminating options 1, 2, and 4. Review this procedure if you had difficulty with this question.
Level of Cognitive Ability: Application
Client Needs: Health Promotion and Maintenance
Integrated Concept/Process: Self-Care
Content Area: Adult Health/Gastrointestinal
Reference: Ignatavicius D, Workman M: *Medical-surgical: critical thinking for collaborative care,* ed 4, Philadelphia, 2002, WB Saunders, p. 1252.

32. *Answer:* 1
Rationale: Asterixis is irregular flapping movements of the fingers and wrists when the hands and arms are outstretched, with the palms down, wrists bent up, and fingers spread. It is the most common sign that hepatic encephalopathy is developing.
Test-Taking Strategy: Use the process of elimination. Recalling the definition of asterixis will direct you to option 1. If you are unfamiliar with this assessment procedure, review this content.
Level of Cognitive Ability: Application
Client Needs: Physiological Integrity
Integrated Concept/Process: Nursing Process/Data Collection
Content Area: Adult Health/Gastrointestinal
Reference: Ignatavicius D, Workman M: *Medical-surgical: critical thinking for collaborative care,* ed 4, Philadelphia, 2002, WB Saunders, p. 1303.

33. *Answer:* 4
Rationale: An upright position allows the intestine to float posteriorly and helps prevent intestinal laceration during catheter insertion.
Test-Taking Strategy: Use the process of elimination. Attempt to visualize this procedure in selecting the correct option. Knowing that fluid will be aspirated from the abdominal cavity will assist in directing you to option 4. If you had difficulty with this question, review this procedure.
Level of Cognitive Ability: Application
Client Needs: Physiological Integrity
Integrated Concept/Process: Nursing Process/Implementation
Content Area: Adult Health/Gastrointestinal
Reference: Ignatavicius D, Workman M: *Medical-surgical: critical thinking for collaborative care,* ed 4, Philadelphia, 2002, WB Saunders, p. 1307.

34. *Answer:* 4
Rationale: Most of the ammonia in the body is found in the gastrointestinal tract. Protein provided by the diet is transported to the liver by the portal vein. The liver breaks down protein, which results in the formation of ammonia. A low-protein diet would be prescribed.
Test-Taking Strategy: Use the process of elimination. Noting that options 3 and 4 are opposite should provide you with the clue that one of these options is correct. Recalling the physiology of the liver will direct you to option 4. Review care of the client with cirrhosis if you had difficulty with this question.
Level of Cognitive Ability: Comprehension
Client Needs: Physiological Integrity
Integrated Concept/Process: Nursing Process/Planning
Content Area: Adult Health/Gastrointestinal
Reference: Ignatavicius D, Workman M: *Medical-surgical: critical thinking for collaborative care,* ed 4, Philadelphia, 2002, WB Saunders, p. 1303.

35. *Answer:* 1
Rationale: Lactulose is an osmotic laxative. The desired effect is two to three soft stools per day with an acid fecal pH. Lactulose creates an acid environment in the bowel, resulting in a decline of the colon's pH from 7 to 5. This causes ammonia to leave the circulatory system and move into the colon. Diarrhea may indicate excessive administration of the medication. Options 3 and 4 do not determine that a desired effect has occurred.
Test-Taking Strategy: Knowledge regarding the purpose and action of this medication is required to answer this question. Review this medication if you had difficulty with this question.
Level of Cognitive Ability: Analysis
Client Needs: Physiological Integrity
Integrated Concept/Process: Nursing Process/Evaluation

Content Area: Adult Health/Gastrointestinal
Reference: Ignatavicius D, Workman M: *Medical-surgical: critical thinking for collaborative care,* ed 4, Philadelphia, 2002, WB Saunders, p. 1312.

36. *Answer:* 1
Rationale: Ultrasound of the gallbladder is a noninvasive procedure and is frequently used for emergency diagnosis of acute cholecystitis. The client does not need to be NPO, but may be instructed to avoid carbonated beverages for 48 hours before the test to help decrease intestinal gas. It is a painless test that does not require administration of oral tablets as preparation.
Test-Taking Strategy: Focus on the issue, an ultrasound. Visualizing this procedure will direct you to option 1. Review this procedure if you had difficulty with this question.
Level of Cognitive Ability: Application
Client Needs: Physiological Integrity
Integrated Concept/Process: Nursing Process/Implementation
Content Area: Adult Health/Gastrointestinal
Reference: Ignatavicius D, Workman M: *Medical-surgical: critical thinking for collaborative care,* ed 4, Philadelphia, 2002, WB Saunders, p. 1176.

37. *Answer:* 1
Rationale: After cholecystectomy, breathing tends to be shallow because deep breathing is painful as a result of the location of the surgical procedure. Teaching the importance of performing coughing and deep breathing exercises is the priority.
Test-Taking Strategy: Use the process of elimination and recall the anatomical location of this surgical procedure. Use of the ABCs—airway, breathing, and circulation—will direct you to option 1. Review preoperative teaching for a cholecystectomy if you had difficulty with this question.
Level of Cognitive Ability: Application
Client Needs: Physiological Integrity
Integrated Concept/Process: Nursing Process/Implementation
Content Area: Adult Health/Gastrointestinal
Reference: Ignatavicius D, Workman M: *Medical-surgical: critical thinking for collaborative care,* ed 4, Philadelphia, 2002, WB Saunders, p. 1377.

38. *Answer:* 2
Rationale: Serosanguineous drainage with a small amount of bile is expected from the Penrose drain for the first 24 hours. Drainage then decreases and the drain is usually removed in 48 hours. The registered nurse does not need to be notified immediately. A sterile dressing covers the site and should be changed to prevent infection and skin excoriation..
Test-Taking Strategy: Use the process of elimination and note the key words "most appropriate." Eliminate options 3 and 4 first because they are similar. From the remaining options, recalling the expected findings after this surgical procedure will direct you to option 2. Review care to the client after cholecystectomy if you had difficulty with this question.
Level of Cognitive Ability: Application
Client Needs: Physiological Integrity
Integrated Concept/Process: Nursing Process/Implementation
Content Area: Adult Health/Gastrointestinal
Reference: Ignatavicius D, Workman M: *Medical-surgical: critical thinking for collaborative care,* ed 4, Philadelphia, 2002, WB Saunders, p. 1377.

39. *Answer:* 1
Rationale: Fatigue is a normal response to hepatic cellular damage. During the acute stage, rest is an essential intervention to reduce the liver's metabolic demands and increase its blood supply. Options 2, 3, and 4 are incorrect.
Test-Taking Strategy: Use the process of elimination. Note the key word "acute" in the question. Knowing that the liver will need to rest to heal will easily direct you to option 1. If you are unfamiliar with the care of a client with hepatitis, review this content.
Level of Cognitive Ability: Comprehension
Client Needs: Physiological Integrity
Integrated Concept/Process: Nursing Process/Implementation
Content Area: Adult Health/Gastrointestinal
Reference: Ignatavicius D, Workman M: *Medical-surgical: critical thinking for collaborative care,* ed 4, Philadelphia, 2002, WB Saunders, p. 494.

40. *Answer:* 1
Rationale: Hepatitis A is transmitted by the fecal-oral route via contaminated food or infected food handlers. Hepatitis B, C, and D are most commonly transmitted via infected blood or body fluids.
Test-Taking Strategy: Knowledge regarding the modes of transmission of the various types of hepatitis is required to answer this question. If you are unfamiliar with the modes of transmission of hepatitis, review this content.
Level of Cognitive Ability: Comprehension
Client Needs: Physiological Integrity
Integrated Concept/Process: Nursing Process/Data Collection
Content Area: Adult Health/Gastrointestinal
Reference: Ignatavicius D, Workman M: *Medical-surgical: critical thinking for collaborative care,* ed 4, Philadelphia, 2002, WB Saunders, p. 1315.

41. *Answer:* 4
Rationale: Meperidine (Demerol), rather than morphine sulfate, is the medication of choice because morphine sulfate can cause spasms in the sphincter of Oddi. Options 1, 2, and 3 are appropriate interventions for the client with acute pancreatitis.
Test-Taking Strategy: Use the process of elimination and note the key word "acute" in the question. Recalling treatment measures for acute pancreatitis and contraindications in the care of the client will direct you to option 4. Review these measures if you had difficulty with this question.
Level of Cognitive Ability: Analysis
Client Needs: Safe, Effective Care Environment
Integrated Concept/Process: Nursing Process/Implementation
Content Area: Adult Health/Gastrointestinal
Reference: Ignatavicius D, Workman M: *Medical-surgical: critical thinking for collaborative care,* ed 4, Philadelphia, 2002, WB Saunders, p. 1343.

42. *Answer:* 4
Rationale: Psychological or emotional stressors that exacerbate peptic ulcer disease may be found either at home or in

the workplace. The frequent need to work overtime on short notice is the option that is potentially most stressful, because it is the item that the client has least control over. An ability to work at home periodically is not necessarily stressful, because there is increased client control over timing of work and location. Adequate rest and proper dietary pattern (options 1 and 2) should alleviate symptoms, not worsen them.
Test-Taking Strategy: Use the process of elimination. Begin to answer this question by eliminating options 1 and 2 because they are healthy living habits. Recall that psychological stress may be worsened in situations where there is little client control. This will direct you to option 4. Review the causes of exacerbation of this disease if you had difficulty with this question.
Level of Cognitive Ability: Analysis
Client Needs: Physiological Integrity
Integrated Concept/Process: Nursing Process/Data Collection
Content Area: Adult Health/Gastrointestinal
Reference: Ignatavicius D, Workman M: *Medical-surgical: critical thinking for collaborative care,* ed 4, Philadelphia, 2002, WB Saunders, p. 1222.

43. *Answer:* 2
Rationale: Dietary modification for the client with PUD includes eliminating foods that are irritating to the client. Items that are generally eliminated or avoided are highly spiced foods, alcohol, caffeine, chocolate, and fresh fruits. Other foods may be taken according to the client's tolerance of that specific food.
Test-Taking Strategy: Use the process of elimination and focus on the client's diagnosis. Note the key words "does not need to be limited or eliminated." Recalling which types of foods and beverages are irritating to the gastrointestinal mucosa will direct you to option 2. Review the dietary measures for PUD if you had difficulty with this question.
Level of Cognitive Ability: Application
Client Needs: Health Promotion and Maintenance
Integrated Concept/Process: Teaching/Learning
Content Area: Adult Health/Gastrointestinal
Reference: Ignatavicius D, Workman M: *Medical-surgical: critical thinking for collaborative care,* ed 4, Philadelphia, 2002, WB Saunders, p. 1226.

44. *Answer:* 1
Rationale: The peristomal skin must receive meticulous cleansing because the ileostomy drainage has more enzymes and is more caustic to the skin than colostomy drainage. Foods, such as nuts and those with seeds, will pass through the ileostomy. The client should be taught that these foods will remain undigested. The area below the ileostomy may be massaged if needed if the ileostomy becomes blocked by high-fiber foods. Fluid intake should be at least six to eight glasses of water per day to prevent dehydration.
Test-Taking Strategy: Use the process of elimination. Note the key words "essential care" and "stoma." This tells you that the correct option will deal with the stoma directly. This focus will direct you to option 1. Review client teaching regarding ileostomy care if you had difficulty with this question.
Level of Cognitive Ability: Application
Client Needs: Health Promotion and Maintenance
Integrated Concept/Process: Self-Care
Content Area: Adult Health/Gastrointestinal
Reference: Ignatavicius D, Workman M: *Medical-surgical: critical thinking for collaborative care,* ed 4, Philadelphia, 2002, WB Saunders, p. 1282.

45. *Answer:* 2
Rationale: Hiatal hernia is due to a protrusion of a portion of the stomach above the diaphragm, where the esophagus usually is positioned. The client usually experiences pain because of reflux with ingestion of irritating foods, lying flat after meals or at night, and with consuming large or fatty meals. Relief is obtained with the intake of small, frequent, and bland meals; with use of histamine antagonists and antacids; and with elevation of the thorax after meals and during sleep.
Test-Taking Strategy: Use the process of elimination. Note the key word "contraindicated." This tells you that the correct answer will be the option that represents an aggravating factor for hiatal hernia discomfort. Visualize each option and think about the anatomical location of a hiatal hernia to direct you to option 2. Review these teaching points if you had difficulty with this question.
Level of Cognitive Ability: Application
Client Needs: Health Promotion and Maintenance
Integrated Concept/Process: Self-Care
Content Area: Adult Health/Gastrointestinal
Reference: Ignatavicius D, Workman M: *Medical-surgical: critical thinking for collaborative care,* ed 4, Philadelphia, 2002, WB Saunders, p. 1201.

46. *Answer:* 4
Rationale: A prolapsed stoma is one in which bowel protrudes through the stoma, with an elongated and swollen appearance. A stoma retraction is characterized by sinking of the stoma. Ischemia of the stoma would be associated with dusky or bluish color. A stoma with a narrowed opening, either at the level of the skin or fascia, is said to be stenosed.
Test-Taking Strategy: Use the process of elimination. Focusing on the key word "prolapse" will direct you to option 4. Review the different complications that can occur with ostomy formation if you had difficulty with this question.
Level of Cognitive Ability: Analysis
Client Needs: Physiological Integrity
Integrated Concept/Process: Nursing Process/Data Collection
Content Area: Adult Health/Gastrointestinal
Reference: Ignatavicius D, Workman M: *Medical-surgical: critical thinking for collaborative care,* ed 4, Philadelphia, 2002, WB Saunders, p. 1252

47. *Answer:* 1
Rationale: The client should be taught to include deodorizing foods in the diet, such as beet greens, parsley, buttermilk, and yogurt. Spinach also reduces odor, but is a gas-forming food as well. Broccoli, cucumbers, and eggs are gas-forming foods.
Test-Taking Strategy: Use the process of elimination. Recalling the effect of various foods on the gastrointestinal tract of the client with an ostomy will direct you to option 1. If this question was difficult, review the foods that cause odor or gas and those that have a deodorizing effect.
Level of Cognitive Ability: Application

Client Needs: Health Promotion and Maintenance
Integrated Concept/Process: Self-Care
Content Area: Adult Health/Gastrointestinal
Reference: Ignatavicius D, Workman M: *Medical-surgical: critical thinking for collaborative care*, ed 4, Philadelphia, 2002, WB Saunders, p. 1252.

48. *Answer:* 3
Rationale: Foods that help to thicken the stool of the client with an ileostomy include pasta, boiled rice, and low-fat cheese. Bran is high in dietary fiber, and thus will increase the output of watery stool by increasing propulsion through the bowel. Ileostomy output is liquid by nature. Addition or elimination of various foods can help to thicken or loosen this liquid drainage.
Test-Taking Strategy: Use the process of elimination and note the key words "did not fully understand." Recalling that high-fiber foods such as bran can aggravate watery stools will direct you to option 3. Review dietary measures for the client with an ileostomy if you had difficulty with this question.
Level of Cognitive Ability: Comprehension
Client Needs: Health Promotion and Maintenance
Integrated Concept/Process: Teaching/Learning
Content Area: Adult Health/Gastrointestinal
Reference: Ignatavicius D, Workman M: *Medical-surgical: critical thinking for collaborative care*, ed 4, Philadelphia, 2002, WB Saunders, p. 1252.

49. *Answer:* 1
Rationale: A Kock pouch is a continent ileostomy. As the ileostomy begins to function, the client drains it with a catheter every 3 to 4 hours, then decreasing to about three times a day or as needed when full. The client does not need to wear a drainage bag, but should wear an absorbent dressing to absorb mucus drainage from the stoma. Ileostomy drainage is liquid in nature. The client would be able to pass stool from the rectum only if an ileal-anal pouch or anastamosis was created.
Test-Taking Strategy: To answer this question accurately, it is necessary to understand the different surgical procedures that are performed with ileostomy, and their consequences on the bowel habits of the client. If this question was difficult, review this content.
Level of Cognitive Ability: Comprehension
Client Needs: Physiological Integrity
Integrated Concept/Process: Self-Care
Content Area: Adult Health/Gastrointestinal
Reference: Ignatavicius D, Workman M: *Medical-surgical: critical thinking for collaborative care*, ed 4, Philadelphia, 2002, WB Saunders, p. 1250.

50. *Answer:* 3
Rationale: The client should limit fat in the diet. The client should also take in small meals. This will also reduce the amount of carbohydrate and protein that the client must digest at any one time. The client does not need to limit water-soluble vitamins in the diet.
Test-Taking Strategy: Use the process of elimination. Recalling the pathophysiology related to pancreatic function will direct you to option 3. Review these dietary measures if you had difficulty with this question.
Level of Cognitive Ability: Application
Client Needs: Health Promotion and Maintenance
Integrated Concept/Process: Teaching/Learning
Content Area: Adult Health/Gastrointestinal
Reference: Ignatavicius D, Workman M: *Medical-surgical: critical thinking for collaborative care*, ed 4, Philadelphia, 2002, WB Saunders, p. 1163.

51. *Answer:* 2
Rationale: Positions such as sitting up, leaning forward and flexing the legs (especially the left leg) may alleviate some of the pain associated with pancreatitis. The pain is aggravated by lying supine or walking. This is because the pancreas is located retroperitoneally, and the edema and inflammation intensify the irritation of the posterior peritoneal wall with these positions.
Test-Taking Strategy: Use the process of elimination. Eliminate options 1 and 3 first because they are similar. From the remaining options, visualize the pancreas and the potential effects from stretching associated with the various positions listed. This will direct you to option 2. Review care to the client with pancreatitis if you had difficulty with this question.
Level of Cognitive Ability: Application
Client Needs: Physiological Integrity
Integrated Concept/Process: Nursing Process/Implementation
Content Area: Adult Health/Gastrointestinal
Reference: Ignatavicius D, Workman M: *Medical-surgical: critical thinking for collaborative care*, ed 4, Philadelphia, 2002, WB Saunders, p. 1344.

52. *Answer:* 1
Rationale: The client with cholecystitis should decrease overall intake of dietary fat. Foods that should be generally avoided to achieve this end include sauces and gravies, fatty meats, fried foods, products made with cream, and heavy desserts. The correct food item is baked scrod, which is low in fat.
Test-Taking Strategy: Use the process of elimination and recall that clients with cholecystitis should decrease fat intake. Also note that options 2, 3, and 4 are similar and are high in fat. Review dietary instructions for the client with cholecystitis if you had difficulty with this question.
Level of Cognitive Ability: Comprehension
Client Needs: Health Promotion and Maintenance
Integrated Concept/Process: Nursing Process/Evaluation
Content Area: Adult Health/Gastrointestinal
Reference: Ignatavicius D, Workman M: *Medical-surgical: critical thinking for collaborative care*, ed 4, Philadelphia, 2002, WB Saunders, p. 1332.

53. *Answer:* 3
Rationale: Ammonia is yielded as a product of protein metabolism. Clients with hepatic encephalopathy have high serum ammonia levels, which are responsible for the encephalopathy symptoms. Limiting protein intake will curb the elevation in serum ammonia and prevent further deterioration of the client's mental status.
Test-Taking Strategy: Use the process of elimination. Recalling the relationships among cirrhosis, encephalopathy, and protein intake will direct you to option 3. Review dietary meas-

ures for the client with cirrhosis if you had difficulty with this question.
Level of Cognitive Ability: Application
Client Needs: Health Promotion and Maintenance
Integrated Concept/Process: Nursing Process/Planning
Content Area: Adult Health/Gastrointestinal
Reference: Ignatavicius D, Workman M: *Medical-surgical: critical thinking for collaborative care,* ed 4, Philadelphia, 2002, WB Saunders, p. 1300.

54. *Answer:* 1
Rationale: To be effective in decreasing bowel motility, antispasmodic medications should be administered 30 minutes before mealtimes. The other options are incorrect.
Test-Taking Strategy: Use the process of elimination. By recalling that antispasmodics slow down gut motility, it can be reasoned that they should be taken before meals, an activity that normally stimulates increased gastrointestinal motility. Review the purpose of antispasmodic medications if you had difficulty with this question.
Level of Cognitive Ability: Application
Client Needs: Physiological Integrity
Integrated Concept/Process: Nursing Process/Implementation
Content Area: Adult Health/Gastrointestinal
Reference: Ignatavicius D, Workman M: *Medical-surgical: critical thinking for collaborative care,* ed 4, Philadelphia, 2002, WB Saunders, p. 431.

55. *Answer:* 2
Rationale: Common signs of acute viral hepatitis include weight loss, dark urine, and fatigue. The client is anorexic and finds food distasteful. The urine darkens because of excess bilirubin being excreted by the kidneys. Fatigue occurs during all phases of hepatitis. Spider angiomas, small, dilated blood vessels, are commonly seen in cirrhosis of the liver.
Test-Taking Strategy: Use the process of elimination. Recalling the function of the liver will direct you to option 2. Remember, lethargy is a classic symptom associated with hepatitis. If you had difficulty with this question, review the manifestations associated with hepatitis.
Level of Cognitive Ability: Analysis
Client Needs: Physiological Integrity
Integrated Concept/Process: Nursing Process/Data Collection
Content Area: Adult Health/Gastrointestinal
Reference: Ignatavicius D, Workman M: *Medical-surgical: critical thinking for collaborative care,* ed 4, Philadelphia, 2002, WB Saunders, p. 1314.

56. *Answer:* 4
Rationale: Clarifying the meaning of what has been said increases understanding for both the client and nurse. Providing false reassurance is inappropriate. Telling the client what to do implies that the nurse knows what is best and discourages independent thinking. Refusing to consider the client's ideas may cause the client to discontinue interaction with the nurse for fear of further rejection. Placing the client's feelings on hold by referring the client to the doctor for further information is a block to communication.
Test-Taking Strategy: Use therapeutic communication techniques. Remember to always focus on the client's feelings first. This will direct you to option 4. Review therapeutic communication techniques if you had difficulty with this question.
Level of Cognitive Ability: Application
Client Needs: Psychosocial Integrity
Integrated Concept/Process: Communication and Documentation
Content Area: Adult Health/Gastrointestinal
Reference: Potter P, Perry A: *Fundamentals of nursing,* ed 5, St Louis, 2001, Mosby, p. 459.

57. *Answer:* 2
Rationale: Immunization is the most effective method of preventing hepatitis B infection. Another general measure is handwashing. Immune globulin is used to prevent hepatitis A and is used for prophylaxis if traveling to endemic areas. Personal hygiene, such as handwashing after bowel movements and before eating, also helps prevent the transmission of hepatitis A.
Test-Taking Strategy: Use the process of elimination and note the key word "priority." Although two of the options are correct for preventing transmission of hepatitis B, the priority is immunization with hepatitis B vaccine. If you had difficulty with this question, review content associated with hepatitis.
Level of Cognitive Ability: Application
Client Needs: Safe, Effective Care Environment
Integrated Concept/Process: Nursing Process/Planning
Content Area: Adult Health/Gastrointestinal
Reference: Ignatavicius D, Workman M: *Medical-surgical: critical thinking for collaborative care,* ed 4, Philadelphia, 2002, WB Saunders, p. 1317.

58. *Answer:* 4
Rationale: Hepatitis B is transmitted through body fluids. The vaccine is recommended for both sexual and household contacts of clients with hepatitis B. Hepatitis B can be transmitted through intimate contact, such as kissing or sexual intercourse. The vaccine is used for prevention.
Test-Taking Strategy: Use the process of elimination. Eliminate option 2 because of the absolute word "never." Recalling the mode of transmission and the measures to prevent hepatitis will direct you to option 4. Review this content if you had difficulty with this question.
Level of Cognitive Ability: Comprehension
Client Needs: Health Promotion and Maintenance
Integrated Concept/Process: Teaching/Learning
Content Area: Adult Health/Gastrointestinal
Reference: Ignatavicius D, Workman M: *Medical-surgical: critical thinking for collaborative care,* ed 4, Philadelphia, 2002, WB Saunders, p.1317.

59. *Answer:* 3
Rationale: Although no special diet is required in the treatment of viral hepatitis, it is generally recommended that clients follow a low-fat diet since fat may be poorly tolerated because of decreased bile production. Small, frequent meals are preferable and may even prevent nausea. Frequently, the appetite is better in the morning so it is easier to eat a healthy breakfast. Carbonated beverages are used to counteract anorexia. An adequate fluid intake of 2500 to 3000 mL per day is also important.

Test-Taking Strategy: Use the process of elimination and focus on the issue, a lack of appetite. Eliminate option 4 because of the words "high in fat." Eliminate options 1 and 2 next because of the word "large." Review dietary measures for the client with hepatitis if you had difficulty with this question.
Level of Cognitive Ability: Application
Client Needs: Physiological Integrity
Integrated Concept/Process: Nursing Process/Implementation
Content Area: Adult Health/Gastrointestinal
Reference: Ignatavicius D, Workman M: *Medical-surgical: critical thinking for collaborative care,* ed 4, Philadelphia, 2002, WB Saunders, p. 1321.

60. *Answer:* 2
Rationale: Jaundice occurs in the skin and mucous membranes. In light-skinned persons, it is first seen in the sclera of the eyes and later in the skin. In dark-skinned persons, jaundice is observed in the inner canthus of the eyes and hard palate of the mouth. Pallor is detected in the nail beds, and flushing is detected in the flexor surfaces of the extremities.
Test-Taking Strategy: Use the process of elimination and focus on the client. Recalling that jaundice occurs in the skin and mucous membranes will direct you to option 2. Review data collection techniques for jaundice if you had difficulty with this question.
Level of Cognitive Ability: Application
Client Needs: Physiological Integrity
Integrated Concept/Process: Cultural Awareness
Content Area: Adult Health/Gastrointestinal
Reference: Ignatavicius D, Workman M: *Medical-surgical: critical thinking for collaborative care,* ed 4, Philadelphia, 2002, WB Saunders, p. 1314.

61. *Answer:* 1
Rationale: The client's feelings should be explored to discover how the client feels about the disease process and appearance so appropriate interventions can be planned. Options 2, 3, and 4 are inappropriate.
Test-Taking Strategy: Use the process of elimination and focus on the client's concern. Remembering to address the client's feelings will direct you to option 1. Review the psychosocial issues related to hepatitis if you had difficulty with this question.
Level of Cognitive Ability: Application
Client Needs: Psychosocial Integrity
Integrated Concept/Process: Nursing Process/Implementation
Content Area: Adult Health/Gastrointestinal
Reference: Ignatavicius D, Workman M: *Medical-surgical: critical thinking for collaborative care,* ed 4, Philadelphia, 2002, WB Saunders, p. 1317.

62. *Answer:* 4
Rationale: To splint the puncture site, the client is kept on the right side for a minimum of 2 hours. It is not necessary to remain NPO for 24 hours. Permission regarding the consumption of alcohol should be obtained from the physician. It is not necessary to save all stools.
Test-Taking Strategy: Use the process of elimination and focus on the issue, a liver biopsy. Recalling the anatomical location of this procedure will direct you to option 4. Review postprocedure instructions after a liver biopsy if you had difficulty with this question.
Level of Cognitive Ability: Application
Client Needs: Physiological Integrity
Integrated Concept/Process: Nursing Process/Implementation
Content Area: Adult Health/Gastrointestinal
Reference: Ignatavicius D, Workman M: *Medical-surgical: critical thinking for collaborative care,* ed 4, Philadelphia, 2002, WB Saunders, p. 426.

63. *Answer:* 2
Rationale: To prevent transmission of hepatitis, using a condom during sexual intercourse and vaccination of the partner or close friends are advised. Alcohol should be avoided for 1 year, as it is detoxified in the liver and may interfere with recovery. Rest is especially important until laboratory studies show that the liver function has returned to normal. The client's activity is increased gradually.
Test-Taking Strategy: Use the process of elimination and note the key words "need for teaching." Recalling the pathophysiology related to hepatitis and the key word "never" in option 2 will direct you to this option. Review client instructions regarding hepatitis if you had difficulty with this question.
Level of Cognitive Ability: Comprehension
Client Needs: Health Promotion and Maintenance
Integrated Concept/Process: Nursing Process/Evaluation
Content Area: Adult Health/Gastrointestinal
Reference: Ignatavicius D, Workman M: *Medical-surgical: critical thinking for collaborative care,* ed 4, Philadelphia, 2002, WB Saunders, p. 1317.

64. *Answer:* 3
Rationale: Clients with jaundice frequently have a body image disturbance because of a change in appearance. This can be manifested in negative verbal or nonverbal behavior. Options 1, 2, and 4 are unrelated to the data in the question.
Test-Taking Strategy: Use the process of elimination. Noting the key words "severe jaundice" will direct you to option 3. Review the psychosocial issues related to jaundice if you had difficulty with this question.
Level of Cognitive Ability: Comprehension
Client Needs: Psychosocial Integrity
Integrated Concept/Process: Nursing Process/Data Collection
Content Area: Adult Health/Gastrointestinal
Reference: Ignatavicius D, Workman M: *Medical-surgical: critical thinking for collaborative care,* ed 4, Philadelphia, 2002, WB Saunders, p. 1823.

65. *Answer:* 4
Rationale: If nausea persists, the client will need to be assessed for fluid and electrolyte imbalances. It is important to explain to the client that the majority of calories should be eaten in the morning hours, as nausea most often occurs in the afternoon and evening. Clients should select a diet high in calories because energy is required for healing. Changes in bilirubin interfere with fat absorption so low-fat diets are better tolerated.
Test-Taking Strategy: Use the process of elimination. Recalling the nutritional aspects of care for clients with viral hepatitis

will direct you to option 4. Review care to the client with viral hepatitis if you had difficulty answering this question.
Level of Cognitive Ability: Application
Client Needs: Physiological Integrity
Integrated Concept/Process: Nursing Process/Implementation
Content Area: Adult Health/Gastrointestinal
Reference: Ignatavicius D, Workman M: *Medical-surgical: critical thinking for collaborative care,* ed 4, Philadelphia, 2002, WB Saunders, p. 1321.

REFERENCES

Black J, Hawks J, Keene A: *Medical-surgical nursing: clinical management for positive outcomes,* ed 6, Philadelphia, 2001, WB Saunders.

Chernecky C, Berger B: *Laboratory tests and diagnostic procedures,* ed 3, Philadelphia, 2001, WB Saunders.

Clark J, Queener S, Karb V: *Pharmacologic basis of nursing practice,* ed 6, St Louis, 2000, Mosby.

DeWit S: *Fundamental concepts and skills for nursing,* Philadelphia, 2001, WB Saunders.

Hodgson B, Kizior R: *Saunders nursing drug handbook 2002,* Philadelphia, 2002, WB Saunders.

Ignatavicius D, Workman M: *Medical-surgical: critical thinking for collaborative care,* ed 4, Philadelphia, 2002, WB Saunders.

Potter P, Perry A: *Fundamentals of nursing,* ed 5, St Louis, 2001, Mosby.

Perry A, Potter P: *Clinical nursing skills and techniques,* ed 5, St Louis, 2002, Mosby.

45 Gastrointestinal Medications

I. ANTACIDS AND MUCOSAL PROTECTIVE MEDICATIONS (Box 45-1)

A. Description
1. React with gastric acid to produce neutral salts or salts of low acidity
2. Inactivate pepsin and enhance mucosal protection but do not coat the ulcer crater to protect it from the acid and pepsin
3. Used for peptic ulcer disease and gastroesophageal reflux disease (GERD)
4. Should be taken on a regular schedule
5. Are usually administered seven times a day, 1 and 3 hours after each meal and at bedtime
6. To provide maximum benefit, treatment should elevate the gastric pH above 5
7. Antacid tablets should be chewed thoroughly and followed with a glass of water or milk
8. Liquid preparations should be shaken before dispensing
9. Interactions with other medications can be minimized by allowing 1 hour between antacid administration and the administration of other medications
10. Can interfere with the action of sucralfate (Carafate), and to minimize this interaction, the medications should be administered 1 hour apart from each other

BOX 45-1

Antacids and Mucosal Protective Medications

Aluminum hydroxide gel (Amphogel, AlternaGEL)
Aluminum carbonate gel (Basaljel)
Bismuth subsalicylate (Pepto-Bismol)
Calcium carbonate (Tums)
Magnesium hydroxide (milk of magnesia, MOM)
Misoprostol (Cytotec)
Sulcralfate (Carafate)

B. Sucralfate (Carafate)
1. Creates a protective barrier against acid and pepsin
2. Administered orally; should be taken on an empty stomach
3. Administer at least 60 minutes apart from an antacid
4. May cause constipation
5. May impede absorption of warfarin sodium (Coumadin), phenytoin (Dilantin), theophylline, digoxin (Lanoxin), and some antibiotics and should be administered at least 2 hours apart from these medications

C. Misoprostol (Cytotec)
1. Used to prevent gastric ulcers caused by long-term therapy with nonsteroidal antiinflammatory drugs (NSAIDs)
2. Suppresses secretion of gastric acid
3. Promotes secretion of bicarbonate and cytoprotective mucus
4. Maintains submucosal blood flow by promoting vasodilation
5. Administered with meals
6. Causes diarrhea and abdominal pain
7. Contraindicated for use in pregnancy

D. Magnesium hydroxide
1. Rapid acting
2. Also referred to as milk of magnesia
3. Most prominent side effect is diarrhea
4. Usually administered in combination with aluminum hydroxide, an antacid that assists in preventing diarrhea
5. Contraindicated in clients with intestinal obstruction, appendicitis, or clients with undiagnosed abdominal pain

6. In clients with renal impairment, magnesium can accumulate to high levels, causing signs of toxicity

E. Aluminum hydroxide gel (Amphogel, Alterna GEL)
1. Slow acting
2. Contains significant amounts of sodium
3. Used with caution in clients with hypertension and heart failure
4. Most common side effect is constipation
5. Can reduce the effects of tetracyclines, warfarin sodium (Coumadin), and digoxin (Lanoxin)
6. Can reduce phosphate absorption and thereby cause hypophosphatemia

F. Calcium carbonate (Tums)
1. Rapid acting
2. Common side effect is constipation

G. Sodium bicarbonate
1. Rapid onset
2. Liberates carbon dioxide, increases intraabdominal pressure, and promotes flatulence
3. Used with caution in clients with hypertension and heart failure
4. Can cause systemic alkalosis in clients with renal impairment
5. Is useful for treating acidosis and elevating urinary pH to promote excretion of acidic medications after overdose

II. HISTAMINE H_2-RECEPTOR ANTAGONISTS (Box 45-2)

A. Description
1. Suppress secretions of gastric acid
2. Alleviate symptoms of heartburn and assist in preventing complications of peptic ulcer disease
3. Prevents stress ulcers and reduce the recurrence of all ulcers
4. Promotes healing in GERD
5. Contraindicated in hypersensitivity
6. Used with caution in clients with impaired renal or hepatic function

B. Cimetidine (Tagamet)
1. Can be administered orally, intramuscularly (IM), or intravenously (IV)
2. Food reduces the rate of absorption; if taken with meals, absorption will be slowed
3. Antacids can decrease the absorption of cimetidine
4. Cimetidine and antacids should be administered at least 1 hour apart from each other
5. Passes the blood-brain barrier, and central nervous system (CNS) side effects can occur
6. May cause mental confusion, agitation, psychosis, depression, anxiety, and disorientation
7. Dosage should be reduced in clients with renal impairment
8. IV administration can cause hypotension and dysrhythmias
9. If administered with warfarin sodium (Coumadin), phenytoin (Dilantin), theophylline or lidocaine, the dosages of these medications should be reduced

C. Ranitidine (Zantac)
1. Can be administered orally, IM, or IV
2. Side effects are uncommon
3. Unlike cimetidine, it does not penetrate the blood-brain-barrier
4. Zantac is not affected by food

D. Famotidine (Pepcid) and nizatidine (Axid)
1. Similar to Zantac and Tagamet
2. Do not need to be administered with food

E. Ranitidine bismuth citrate (Tritec)
1. Used to treat active duodenal ulcers associated with *Helicobacter pylori*
2. Administered with the antibiotic clarithromycin (Biaxin) (Box 45-3)

III. PROTON PUMP INHIBITORS (Box 45-4)

A. Suppress gastric acid secretion
B. Used with active ulcer disease, erosive esophagitis, and pathological hypersecretory conditions
C. Contraindicated in hypersensitivity
D. Common side effects include headache, diarrhea, abdominal pain, and nausea

BOX 45-2

Histamine H_2-Receptor Antagonists

Cimetidine (Tagamet)
Famotidine (Pepcid)
Nizatidine (Axid)
Ranitidine (Zantac)
Ranitidine bismuth citrate (Tritec)

BOX 45-3

Antimicrobials Effective Against *Helicobacter pylori*

Amoxicillin (Amoxil)
Clarithromycin (Biaxin)
Metronidazole (Flagyl)
Tetracycline (Achromycin)

BOX 45-4

Proton Pump Inhibitors

Omeprazole (Prilosec)
Lansoprazole (Prevacid)

IV. GASTROINTESTINAL STIMULANTS (Box 45-5)

A. Stimulates motility of the upper GI tract and increases rate of gastric emptying without stimulating gastric, biliary, or pancreatic secretions
B. Used for gastroesophageal reflux
C. May cause restlessness, drowsiness, extrapyramidal reactions, dizziness, insomnia, headache
D. Contraindicated in clients with sensitivity
E. Contraindicated in clients with mechanical obstruction, perforation, or GI hemorrhage
F. Can precipitate hypertensive crisis in clients with pheochromocytoma
G. Safety in pregnancy is not established
H. Reglan can cause Parkinson-like reactions, and if this occurs the medication is discontinued
I. Anticholinergics and narcotic analgesics antagonize the effects of metoclopramide (Reglan)
J. Alcohol, sedatives, cyclosporine (Sandimmune), and tranquilizers produce an additive effect

V. BILE ACID SEQUESTRANTS (Box 45-6)

A. Description
1. Used to treat pruritis associated with biliary disease
2. Acts by absorbing and combining with intestinal bile salts, which are then secreted in the feces, preventing intestinal reabsorption
3. May be used in the treatment of hypercholesterolemia in adults
4. Used cautiously in clients with bowel obstruction or severe constipation because of the adverse GI effects
5. Taste and palatability are often reasons for noncompliance and can be improved by the use of flavored products or mixing the medication with various juices
6. Stool softeners and other sources of fiber can be used to abate the GI side effects

B. Side effects
1. Constipation
2. Bloating
3. Flatulence
4. Nausea
5. Fecal impaction and intestinal obstruction
6. Exacerbation of hemorrhoids
7. Hypoprothrombinemia
8. Decreased vitamin absorption

VI. MEDICATIONS FOR CHOLELITHIASIS (Box 45-7)

A. Chenodiol (Chenix)
1. Decreases cholesterol production, lowering content of bile, thus facilitates dissolution of gallstones
2. Can cause diarrhea and possible hepatotoxicity
3. Baseline liver function studies should be performed
4. Client should be instructed to contact the physician if abdominal pain, sudden right upper quadrant pain, nausea, or vomiting occurs
5. Administer with food or milk
6. Avoid aluminum-containing antacids

B. Ursodiol (Actigall)
1. A naturally occurring bile salt
2. Suppresses hepatic synthesis and secretion of cholesterol and inhibits intestinal absorption of cholesterol
3. Requires months of therapy for dissolution of gallstone to occur
4. Ultrasound images are obtained within 6 month to determine effectiveness of therapy
5. Clients should be instructed to report nausea, vomiting, diarrhea, or rash to the physician
6. Administer with food or milk
7. Avoid aluminum-containing antacids

C. Monoctanoin (Moctanin)
1. Used when stones made of calcium are resistant to dissolution by oral chenodiol
2. Administered through a T tube, nasal biliary catheter, or percutaneous transhepatic catheter
3. Effective only when in contact with the stone
4. Major side effects include diarrhea, nausea, and abdominal pain

BOX 45-5

Gastrointestinal Stimulants

Bethanechol chloride (Urecholine, Duvoid)
Metoclopramide (Reglan)
Neostigmine methylsulfate (Prostigmin)

BOX 45-6

Bile Acid Sequestrants

Cholestyramine (Questran, Prevalite)
Colestipol (Colestid)

BOX 45-7

Medications for Cholelithiasis

Chenodiol (Chenix)
Monoctanoin (Moctanin)
Ursodiol (Actigall)

VII. MEDICATIONS TO TREAT HEPATIC ENCEPHALOPATHY (Box 45-8)

A. Lactulose (Cephulac)
   1. Reduces ammonia levels
   2. Improves protein tolerance in clients with advanced hepatic **cirrhosis**
   3. Lowers the colonic pH from 7 to 5; this acidification pulls ammonia into the bowel to be excreted in the feces, thus lowering the ammonia level
   4. Administered orally in the form of a syrup

B. Neomycin (Mycifradin)
   1. Reduces the number of colonic bacteria that normally convert urea and amino acids into ammonia
   2. Administered orally or via nasogastric (NG) tube
   3. Used with caution in clients with kidney impairment

VIII. PANCREATIC ENZYME REPLACEMENTS (Box 45-9)

A. Used to supplement or replace pancreatic enzymes
B. Taken with meals or a snack (food helps to buffer the stomach acid)
C. A high-fiber diet may increase the efficacy of the medication
D. Side effects include abdominal cramps or pain, nausea, and diarrhea
E. Products that contain calcium carbonate or magnesium hydroxide interfere with the action of the medication

IX. ANTIEMETICS (Box 45-10)

A. Medications used to control vomiting
B. The choice of the antiemetic is determined by the cause of the nausea and vomiting

BOX 45-8

Medications To Treat Hepatic Encephalopathy

Lactulose (Cephulac)
Neomycin (Mycifradin)

BOX 45-9

Pancreatic Enzyme Replacements

Pancreatin (Creon)
Pancrelipase (Cotazym, Pancrease, Viokase)

BOX 45-10

Commonly Administered Antiemetics

Diphenidol hydrochloride (Vontrol)
Dolasetron mesylate (Anzemet)
Dronabinol (Marinol)
Granisetron (Kytril)
Hydroxyzine hydrochloride (Atarax)
Hydroxyzine pamoate (Vistaril)
Meclizine hydrochloride (Antivert)
Metoclopramide (Reglan)
Ondansetron (Zofran)
Prochlorperazine (Compazine)
Promethazine hydrochloride (Phenergan)
Thiethylperazine malate (Torecon)
Trimethobenzamide hydrochloride (Tigan)

C. Monitor for drowsiness and protect the client from injury
D. Monitor vital signs and I&O
E. Limit odors in the client's room when the client is nauseated and/or vomiting
F. Limit oral intake to clear liquids when the client is nauseated and/or vomiting

X. LAXATIVES (Box 45-11)

A. Bulk-forming laxatives
   1. Description
      a. Absorb water into the feces and increase bulk to produce large and soft stools
      b. For short-term use
      c. Contraindicated in bowel obstruction
   2. Side effects
      a. GI disturbances
      b. Dehydration
      c. Electrolyte imbalance
      d. Dependency with chronic use

B. Stimulant cathartics
   1. Description: stimulate motility of large intestine
   2. Biscodyl (Dulcolax): do not administer within 60 minutes of an antacid or milk
   3. Cascara (castor oil): administer with juice; produces results in 2 to 6 hours

C. Saline cathartics
   1. Attract water into the large intestine to produce bulk
   2. Stimulate **peristalsis**
   3. Achieve results in 2 to 6 hours

D. Stool softeners
   1. Inhibit absorption of water so fecal mass remains large and soft
   2. Used to avoid straining

BOX 45-11

Laxatives

BULK-FORMING LAXATIVES
Methylcellulose (Citrucel)
Calcium polycarbophil (Fibercon)
Psyllium hydrophilic mucilloid (Metamucil, Fiberall, Konsyl, Serutan, Modane Bulk)

STIMULANT CATHARTICS
Bisacodyl (Dulcolax)
Cascara sagrada
Castor oil, emulsified (Neoloid)
Phenolphthalein (Ex-Lax)
Senna concentrate (Senexon, Senna-Gen)

OSMOTIC (SALINE) CATHARTICS
Glycerin suppositories (Senokot)
Lactulose (Chronulac)
Magnesium citrate (Citroma)
Magnesium hydroxide (milk of magnesia, MOM)
Magnesium sulfate (Epsom salt)
Potassium bitartrate and sodium bicarbonate (Coe-Two)
Sodium phosphates (Fleet Phospho-Soda)

STOOL SOFTENERS
Docusate calcium (Surfak)
Docusate sodium (Colace)
Docusate with casanthranol (Peri-Colace)

LUBRICANT
Mineral oil

E. Lubricants
   1. Act to soften the feces
   2. Ease the strain of passing stool
   3. Lessen irritation to hemorrhoids
   4. Mineral oil
      a. Can cause lipid pneumonia if accidentally aspirated
      b. Interferes with absorption of fat-soluble vitamins A, D, E, and K

XI. MEDICATIONS TO CONTROL DIARRHEA (Box 45-12)
   A. Opioids
      1. Decrease intestinal motility and **peristalsis**
      2. When poisons, infections, or bacterial toxins are the cause of the diarrhea, opioids worsen the condition by delaying the elimination of toxins
      3. Tincture of opium has an unpleasant taste and can be diluted with 15 to 30 mL of water for administration
   B. Other antidiarrheals: refer to Box 45-12

BOX 45-12

Medications to Control Diarrhea

OPIOIDS AND RELATED MEDICATIONS
Codeine phosphate; codeine sulfate
Difenoxin with atropine (Motofen)
Diphenoxylate hydrochloride with atropine (Lomotil)
Loperamide hydrochloride (Imodium)
Tincture of opium

ABSORBENT ANTIDIARRHEALS
Bismuth subsalicylate (Pepto-Bismol)
Kaolin and pectin (Kao-Spen, Kapectolin)
Somatostatin analog
Octreotide (Sandostatin)

XII. ANTISPASMODICS (Box 45-13)
   A. Description: relax smooth muscle of the GI tract
   B. Side effects
      1. Constipation or diarrhea
      2. Rash
      3. Euphoria
      4. Dizziness
      5. Drowsiness
      6. Headache
      7. Nausea
      8. Weakness

PRACTICE QUESTIONS

1. A client has been started on psyllium (Metamucil). The nurse would teach this client to take this medication with:
   1. Gelatin, applesauce, or pudding
   2. A full glass of liquid, followed by a second
   3. A multivitamin and mineral supplement
   4. A dose of antacid
2. A client with gastroparesis has been given a prescription for metoclopramide (Reglan) four times a day. The nurse teaches the client to take the medication:
   1. 30 minutes before meals and at bedtime
   2. With each meal and at bedtime
   3. 1 hour after each meal and at bedtime
   4. Every 6 hours spaced evenly around the clock
3. A nurse teaches a client taking metoclopramide (Reglan) to discontinue the medication immediately and call the physician if which of the following side effects occurs with long-term use?

BOX 45-13

Antispasmodics

Dicyclomine hydrochloride (Antispas)
Dicyclomine hydrochloride (Bentyl)

1. Anxiety or irritability
2. Dry mouth not minimized by the use of sugar-free hard candy
3. Excessive excitability
4. Uncontrolled rhythmic movements of the face or limbs

4. A client has just taken a dose of trimethobenzamide (Tigan). The nurse plans to monitor this client for relief of:
   1. Nausea and vomiting
   2. Abdominal pain
   3. Heartburn
   4. Constipation
5. A client has a PRN order for ondansetron (Zofran). The nurse would administer this medication to the postoperative client for relief of:
   1. Urinary retention
   2. Incisional pain
   3. Nausea and vomiting
   4. Paralytic ileus
6. A client has an order to take magnesium citrate to prevent constipation after a barium study of the upper gastrointestinal tract. The nurse plans to administer this medication:
   1. With a full glass of water
   2. With fruit juice only
   3. On ice
   4. At room temperature
7. A nurse is administering a dose of prochlorperazine (Compazine) to a client for nausea and vomiting. The nurse would monitor the client for which frequent side effect of this medication?
   1. Diarrhea
   2. Drooling
   3. Excessive lacrimation
   4. Blurred vision
8. A client has begun medication therapy with pancrelipase (Pancrease). The nurse would evaluate that the medication is having the optimal intended benefit if which of the following effects is observed?
   1. Reduction of steatorrhea
   2. Absence of abdominal pain
   3. Relief of heartburn
   4. Weight loss
9. A nurse is giving a client directions for proper use of aluminum hydroxide tablets (Alu-Caps). The nurse tells the client to:
   1. Chew the tablets thoroughly and follow with 4 ounces of water
   2. Swallow the tablets whole with a full glass of water
   3. Take the tablets at the same time as an antacid
   4. Take each dose of the tablets with a laxative to prevent constipation
10. A client with a history of duodenal ulcer is taking calcium carbonate chewable tablets. The nurse evaluates that the client is experiencing optimal effects of the medication if:
    1. Muscle twitching stops
    2. Heartburn is relieved
    3. Serum calcium levels rise
    4. Serum phosphorus levels decrease
11. A hospitalized client asks the nurse for sodium bicarbonate to relieve heartburn after a meal. The nurse determines that this client could not receive this medication if the client is currently being treated for which of the following conditions?
    1. Urinary calculi
    2. Chronic bronchitis
    3. Metabolic alkalosis
    4. Respiratory acidosis
12. An elderly client has recently been started on cimetidine (Tagamet). The nurse monitors the client for which most frequent central nervous system (CNS) side effects of this medication?
    1. Confusion
    2. Dizziness
    3. Tremors
    4. Hallucinations
13. A client with a gastric ulcer has an order for sucralfate (Carafate) 1 gram by mouth QID. The nurse schedules the medication for which of the following times?
    1. With meals and at bedtime
    2. 1 hour before meals and at bedtime
    3. Every 6 hours around the clock
    4. 1 hour after meals and at bedtime
14. A physician has written an order for ranitidine (Zantac) 300 mg once daily. The nurse schedules the medication for which of the following times?
    1. Before breakfast
    2. After lunch
    3. With supper
    4. At bedtime
15. A client has been taking omeprazole (Prilosec) for 4 weeks. The nurse would evaluate that the client is receiving the optimal intended effect of the medication if the client reports absence of which of the following symptoms?
    1. Constipation
    2. Heartburn
    3. Diarrhea
    4. Flatulence
16. A client is taking cascara sagrada and develops abdominal cramps. The nurse interprets that the client is most likely experiencing:
    1. A common side effect of this medication
    2. Partial bowel obstruction
    3. A case of influenza
    4. Peptic ulcer disease
17. A physician prescribes bisacodyl (Dulcolax) for a client in preparation for a diagnostic test and wants

the client to achieve a rapid effect from the medication. The nurse then tells the client to take the medication:
1. With a large meal
2. On an empty stomach
3. At bedtime with a snack
4. With two glasses of juice

18. A client who is advised to take senna (Senokot) for the treatment of constipation asks the nurse how this medication works. The nurse would incorporate which of the following when formulating a response?
1. It coats the bowel wall and makes it slippery
2. It adds fiber and bulk to the stool
3. It accumulates water and increases peristalsis
4. It stimulates the vagus nerve to improve bowel tone

19. A client has a PRN order for loperamide (Imodium). The nurse should plan to administer this medication if the client has:
1. Hematest-positive nasogastric tube drainage
2. Abdominal pain
3. Constipation
4. An episode of diarrhea

20. A nurse has given instructions to the client who just received a prescription for diphenoxylate with atropine (Lomotil). The nurse evaluates that the client understands the use of the medication and its properties if the client states to:
1. Stay within the prescribed dose because it can be habit-forming
2. Take the medication with a bulk-forming laxative
3. Expect increased salivation while taking the medication
4. Anticipate side effects related to central nervous system excitability

21. A client has received a dose of dimenhydrinate (Dramamine). The nurse determines that the medication has been effective if the client states relief of:
1. Headache
2. Chills
3. Nausea and vomiting
4. Buzzing sound in the ears

22. A nurse is preparing to administer a dose of hydroxyzine hydrochloride (Vistaril) to a client by the intramuscular route. The nurse tells the client to expect:
1. Pain at the injection site from the medication
2. Relief from nausea within 5 minutes
3. Excessive salivation as a side effect
4. Increased alertness lasting generally 4 hours

23. A physician tells a nurse that a client can be given droperidol (Inapsine) for the relief of postoperative nausea. The nurse expects that the physician will order the medication by which of the following routes?
1. Oral
2. Intramuscular
3. Subcutaneous
4. Intranasally

24. A client is receiving propantheline (Pro-Banthine) as adjunctive treatment for peptic ulcer disease. The nurse plans to administer this medication:
1. With meals
2. Just after meals
3. 30 minutes before meals
4. With antacids

25. A client is taking docusate sodium (Colace). The nurse monitors which of the following to determine whether the client is having therapeutic effect from this medication?
1. Abdominal pain
2. Hematest-negative stools
3. Reduction in steatorrhea
4. Regular bowel movements

ANSWERS

1. *Answer:* 2

Rationale: Metamucil is a bulk-forming laxative. It should be taken with a full glass of water or juice, followed by another glass of liquid. This will help prevent impaction of the medication in the stomach or small intestine. The other options are incorrect.

Test-Taking Strategy: Use the process of elimination. Option 4 can be eliminated first because most medications are not taken with antacids. Eliminate options 1 and 3 next because they have no physiological benefit for medication effect. Review the administration of this medication if you had difficulty with this question.

Level of Cognitive Ability: Application

Client Needs: Physiological Integrity

Integrated Concept/Process: Teaching/Learning

Content Area: Pharmacology

Reference: Hodgson B, Kizior R: *Saunders nursing drug handbook 2002*, Philadelphia, 2002, WB Saunders, p. 941.

2. *Answer:* 1

Rationale: The client should be taught to take this medication 30 minutes before meals and at bedtime. This allows the medication time to begin working before the client takes in food, which requires digestion and movement. The other options are incorrect.

Test-Taking Strategy: Use the process of elimination. Focus on the client's diagnosis. Recall that if the medication is used to

treat gastroparesis, it must be taken before meals to enhance digestion. Review this medication if you had difficulty with this question.
Level of Cognitive Ability: Application
Client Needs: Physiological Integrity
Integrated Concept/Process: Nursing Process/Implementation
Content Area: Pharmacology
Reference: Hodgson B, Kizior R: *Saunders nursing drug handbook 2002*, Philadelphia, 2002, WB Saunders, p. 720.

3. *Answer:* 4
Rationale: If the client experiences tardive dyskinesia (rhythmic movements of the face or limbs), the client should stop the medication and call the physician. These side effects may be irreversible. Excitability is not a side effect of this medication. Anxiety, irritability, and dry mouth are side effects that are not so harmful to the client.
Test-Taking Strategy: Use the process of elimination and focus on the issue, to call the physician. Recalling that the medication can cause tardive dyskinesia will direct you to option 4. Review the side effects of this medication if you had difficulty with this question.
Level of Cognitive Ability: Application
Client Needs: Health Promotion and Maintenance
Integrated Concept/Process: Teaching/Learning
Content Area: Pharmacology
Reference: Hodgson B, Kizior R: *Saunders nursing drug handbook 2002*, Philadelphia, 2002, WB Saunders, p. 720.

4. *Answer:* 1
Rationale: Trimethobenzamide is an antiemetic agent that is used in the treatment of nausea and vomiting. The other options are incorrect.
Test-Taking Strategy: Use the process of elimination. Recalling that trimethobenzamide is an antiemetic will easily direct you to option 1. Review the action and use of this medication if you had difficulty with this question.
Level of Cognitive Ability: Application
Client Needs: Physiological Integrity
Integrated Concept/Process: Nursing Process/Planning
Content Area: Pharmacology
Reference: Hodgson B, Kizior R: *Saunders nursing drug handbook 2002*, Philadelphia, 2002, WB Saunders, p. 720.

5. *Answer:* 3
Rationale: Ondansetron is an antiemetic that is used in the treatment of postoperative nausea and vomiting, as well as nausea and vomiting associated with chemotherapy. The other options are incorrect.
Test-Taking Strategy: Recalling that ondansetron is an antiemetic will easily direct you to option 3. Review the action and use of this medication if you had difficulty with this question.
Level of Cognitive Ability: Application
Client Needs: Physiological Integrity
Integrated Concept/Process: Nursing Process/Implementation
Content Area: Pharmacology
Reference: Hodgson B, Kizior R: *Saunders nursing drug handbook 2002*, Philadelphia, 2002, WB Saunders, p. 825.

6. *Answer:* 3
Rationale: Magnesium citrate is available as an oral solution. It is used commonly as a laxative after certain studies of the GI tract. It should be served on ice, and should not be allowed to stand for prolonged periods. This would reduce the carbonation and make the solution even less palatable. Options 1, 2, and 4 are incorrect.
Test-Taking Strategy: Use the process of elimination. Eliminate options 1 and 2 first knowing that magnesium citrate is itself a liquid. From the remaining options, it is necessary to know it should be given cold to enhance palatability. Review this medication if you had difficulty with this question.
Level of Cognitive Ability: Application
Client Needs: Physiological Integrity
Integrated Concept/Process: Nursing Process/Planning
Content Area: Pharmacology
Reference: Hodgson B, Kizior R: *Saunders nursing drug handbook 2002*, Philadelphia, 2002, WB Saunders, p. 674.

7. *Answer:* 4
Rationale: The nurse would monitor the client for blurred vision as a frequent side effect of prochlorperazine. Other frequent side effects of this phenothiazine-type antiemetic and antipsychotic are dry eyes, dry mouth, and constipation.
Test-Taking Strategy: To answer this question accurately, it is necessary to know the frequent side effects of phenothiazines. Review this medication if you had difficulty with this question.
Level of Cognitive Ability: Application
Client Needs: Physiological Integrity
Integrated Concept/Process: Nursing Process/Data Collection
Content Area: Pharmacology
Reference: Hodgson B, Kizior R: *Saunders nursing drug handbook 2002*, Philadelphia, 2002, WB Saunders, p. 923.

8. *Answer:* 1
Rationale: Pancrelipase is a pancreatic enzyme used in clients with pancreatitis as a digestive aid. The medication should reduce the amount of fatty stools (steatorrhea). Another intended effect could be improved nutritional status. It is not used to treat abdominal pain or heartburn. It could result in weight gain, but should not result in weight loss if it is aiding in digestion.
Test-Taking Strategy: Use the process of elimination. The name of the medication gives an indication of the possible uses of this medication. Use knowledge of the physiology of the pancreas to assist in directing you to the correct option. Review this medication if you had difficulty with this question.
Level of Cognitive Ability: Analysis
Client Needs: Physiological Integrity
Integrated Concept/Process: Nursing Process/Evaluation
Content Area: Pharmacology
Reference: Hodgson B, Kizior R: *Saunders nursing drug handbook 2002*, Philadelphia, 2002, WB Saunders, p. 845.

9. *Answer:* 1
Rationale: Aluminum hydroxide tablets should be chewed thoroughly before swallowing. This prevents them from entering the small intestine undissolved. They should not be swallowed whole. Antacids should be taken at least 1 hour

apart from other medications to prevent interactive effects. Constipation is a side effect of use of aluminum products, but it is not correct for the client to take a laxative with each dose of aluminum hydroxide tablets. This promotes laxative abuse; the client should first try other means to prevent constipation.
Test-Taking Strategy: Use the process of elimination. Eliminate option 4 first because this action does not promote healthy bowel function. Next eliminate option 3 using general knowledge of antacid interactive effects. Select from the remaining options using principles of digestion and medication use. Review the administration of this medication if you had difficulty with this question.
Level of Cognitive Ability: Application
Client Needs: Health Promotion and Maintenance
Integrated Concept/Process: Teaching/Learning
Content Area: Pharmacology
Reference: Lehne R: *Pharmacology for nursing care*, ed 4, Philadelphia, 2001, WB Saunders, p. 857.

10. *Answer: 2*
Rationale: Calcium carbonate is used as an antacid for the relief of heartburn and indigestion. It can also be used as a calcium supplement (option 3), or to bind phosphorus in the gastrointestinal tract with renal failure (option 4). Option 1 is incorrect, although proper calcium levels are needed for proper neurological function.
Test-Taking Strategy: Focus on the client's diagnosis. The key words in the question are "duodenal ulcer" and "optimal effects." Knowledge of the concepts related to duodenal ulcer will direct you to option 2. Review the actions and use of this medication if you had difficulty with this question.
Level of Cognitive Ability: Analysis
Client Needs: Physiological Integrity
Integrated Concept/Process: Nursing Process/Evaluation
Content Area: Pharmacology
Reference: Lehne R: *Pharmacology for nursing care*, ed 4, Philadelphia, 2001, WB Saunders, p. 806.

11. *Answer: 3*
Rationale: Sodium bicarbonate is an electrolyte modifier and antacid. It would further aggravate metabolic alkalosis. The conditions identified in the other options are not contraindications for the use of sodium bicarbonate.
Test-Taking Strategy: Use knowledge of acid-base concepts to answer this question. Focus on the name of the medication to assist in eliminating options 1, 2, and 4. Review the contraindications associated with the use of this medication if you had difficulty with this question.
Level of Cognitive Ability: Analysis
Client Needs: Physiological Integrity
Integrated Concept/Process: Nursing Process/Data Collection
Content Area: Pharmacology
Reference: Lehne R: *Pharmacology for nursing care*, ed 4, Philadelphia, 2001, WB Saunders, p. 857.

12. *Answer: 1*
Rationale: Elderly clients are especially susceptible to the central nervous system (CNS) side effects of cimetidine. The most frequent of these is confusion. Less common CNS side effects include headache, dizziness, drowsiness, and hallucinations.
Test-Taking Strategy: Use the process of elimination. Note the key words "most frequent." Use knowledge of the elderly and medication administration and knowledge of this medication to answer the question. Review this medication if you had difficulty with this question.
Level of Cognitive Ability: Application
Client Needs: Physiological Integrity
Integrated Concept/Process: Nursing Process/Implementation
Content Area: Pharmacology
Reference: Hodgson B, Kizior R: *Saunders nursing drug handbook 2002*, Philadelphia, 2002, WB Saunders, p. 238.

13. *Answer: 2*
Rationale: The medication should be scheduled for administration 1 hour before meals and at bedtime. The medication is timed to allow it to form a protective coating over the ulcer before food intake stimulates gastric acid production and mechanical irritation. The other options are incorrect.
Test-Taking Strategy: Use the process of elimination. Focusing on the client's diagnosis and recalling the action of the medication will direct you to option 2. Review this medication if you had difficulty with this question.
Level of Cognitive Ability: Application
Client Needs: Physiological Integrity
Integrated Concept/Process: Nursing Process/Implementation
Content Area: Pharmacology
Reference: Hodgson B, Kizior R: *Saunders nursing drug handbook 2002*, Philadelphia, 2002, WB Saunders, p. 1031.

14. *Answer: 4*
Rationale: A single daily dose of ranitidine is scheduled to be given at bedtime. This allows for prolonged effect and the greatest protection of the gastric mucosa. The other options are incorrect.
Test-Taking Strategy: Specific knowledge of the timing of this medication is needed to answer this question. If you had difficulty with this question, review this medication.
Level of Cognitive Ability: Application
Client Needs: Physiological Integrity
Integrated Concept/Process: Nursing Process/Implementation
Content Area: Pharmacology
Reference: Hodgson B, Kizior R: *Saunders nursing drug handbook 2002*, Philadelphia, 2002, WB Saunders, p. 961.

15. *Answer: 2*
Rationale: Omeprazole is a gastric pump inhibitor and is classified as an antiulcer agent. The intended effect of the medication is relief of pain from gastric irritation, often referred to as heartburn by clients. Options 1, 3, and 4 are incorrect.
Test-Taking Strategy: Use process of elimination. Recalling the action and use of omeprazole directs you to option 2.
Level of Cognitive Ability: Analysis
Client Needs: Physiological Integrity
Integrated Concept/Process: Nursing Process/Evaluation
Content Area: Pharmacology
Reference: Hodgson B, Kizior R: *Saunders nursing drug handbook 2002*, Philadelphia, 2002, WB Saunders, p. 824.

16. *Answer:* 1
Rationale: Cascara sagrada is a laxative that causes nausea and abdominal cramps as the most frequent side effects. Other health problems are not determined based on a single symptom.
Test-Taking Strategy: Use the process of elimination. Remember that options that are similar are not likely to be correct. This will allow you to eliminate the two gastrointestinal disorders (options 2 and 4). From the remaining options, recalling that laxatives can cause abdominal cramping will direct you to option 1. Review the effects of this medication if you had difficulty with this question.
Level of Cognitive Ability: Comprehension
Client Needs: Physiological Integrity
Integrated Concept/Process: Nursing Process/Data Collection
Content Area: Pharmacology
Reference: Hodgson B, Kizior R: *Saunders nursing drug handbook 2002*, Philadelphia, 2002, WB Saunders, p. 176.

17. *Answer:* 2
Rationale: Most rapid results from bisacodyl occur when it is taken on an empty stomach. It will not have a rapid effect if taken with a large meal. If it is taken at bedtime, the client will have a bowel movement in the morning. Taking the medication with two glasses of juice will not add to its effect.
Test-Taking Strategy: Use the process of elimination. Focus on the key words "rapid effect." Recalling that food generally slows the absorption of medication will assist in directing you to option 2. Review the administration of laxatives if you had difficulty with this question.
Level of Cognitive Ability: Application
Client Needs: Physiological Integrity
Integrated Concept/Process: Nursing Process/Implementation
Content Area: Pharmacology
Reference: Hodgson B, Kizior R: *Saunders nursing drug handbook 2002*, Philadelphia, 2002, WB Saunders, p. 125.

18. *Answer:* 3
Rationale: Senna works by changing the transport of water and electrolytes in the large intestine, which causes the accumulation of water in the mass of stool and increased peristalsis. The other options are incorrect.
Test-Taking Strategy: Knowledge regarding the action of this medication is required to answer this question. Review this medication if you had difficulty with this question.
Level of Cognitive Ability: Application
Client Needs: Physiological Integrity
Integrated Concept/Process: Nursing Process/Implementation
Content Area: Pharmacology
Reference: Hodgson B, Kizior R: *Saunders nursing drug handbook 2002*, Philadelphia, 2002, WB Saunders, p. 1000.

19. *Answer:* 4
Rationale: Loperamide is an antidiarrheal agent. It is commonly administered after loose stools. It is used in the management of acute diarrhea, and also in chronic diarrhea such as with inflammatory bowel disease. It can also be used to reduce the volume of drainage from an ileostomy. The other options are incorrect.
Test-Taking Strategy: Use the process of elimination. Knowledge that this medication is an antidiarrheal will easily direct you to the correct option. Review the action of this medication if you had difficulty with this question.
Level of Cognitive Ability: Application
Client Needs: Physiological Integrity
Integrated Concept/Process: Nursing Process/Planning
Content Area: Pharmacology
Reference: Hodgson B, Kizior R: *Saunders nursing drug handbook 2002*, Philadelphia, 2002, WB Saunders, p. 660.

20. *Answer:* 1
Rationale: The client should not exceed the recommended dose because it may be habit-forming. The medication is an antidiarrheal and therefore should not be taken with a laxative. Side effects of the medication include dry mouth and drowsiness.
Test-Taking Strategy: To answer this question accurately, it is necessary to be familiar with this medication and its habit-forming properties. Noting that atropine is an ingredient will help to eliminate options 3 and 4. From the remaining options, recalling that the medication is an antidiarrheal will assist in eliminating option 2. Review this medication if you had difficulty with this question.
Level of Cognitive Ability: Comprehension
Client Needs: Physiological Integrity
Integrated Concept/Process: Teaching/Learning
Content Area: Pharmacology
Reference: Hodgson B, Kizior R: *Saunders nursing drug handbook 2002*, Philadelphia, 2002, WB Saunders, p. 354.

21. *Answer:* 3
Rationale: Dimenhydrinate is used to treat and prevent the symptoms of dizziness, vertigo, nausea, and vomiting that accompany motion sickness. The other options are incorrect.
Test-Taking Strategy: Use the process of elimination. Recalling that dimenhydrinate is used to treat motion sickness will easily direct you to option 3. Review this medication if you had difficulty with this question.
Level of Cognitive Ability: Analysis
Client Needs: Physiological Integrity
Integrated Concept/Process: Nursing Process/Evaluation
Content Area: Pharmacology
Reference: Hodgson B, Kizior R: *Saunders nursing drug handbook 2002*, Philadelphia, 2002, WB Saunders, p. 350.

22. *Answer:* 1
Rationale: Hydroxyzine hydrochloride is an antiemetic and sedative/hypnotic. It is often used in conjunction with narcotic analgesics for added effect. It can cause pain at the injection site when administered intramuscularly. Medications administered by the IM route generally take 20 to 30 minutes to become effective. Hydroxyzine hydrochloride causes dry mouth and drowsiness as side effects.
Test-Taking Strategy: Use the process of elimination. Begin to answer this question by eliminating option 2, because intramuscular medications do not work that rapidly. From the remaining options, use knowledge regarding the medication

to assist in directing you to option 1. Review this medication if you had difficulty with this question.
Level of Cognitive Ability: Application
Client Needs: Physiological Integrity
Integrated Concept/Process: Nursing Process/Implementation
Content Area: Pharmacology
Reference: Hodgson B, Kizior R: *Saunders nursing drug handbook 2002*, Philadelphia, 2002, WB Saunders, p. 548.

23. *Answer:* 2
Rationale: Droperidol may be administered by the intramuscular or intravenous routes. It is not administered subcutaneously, untranasally or orally. Additionally, oral medications are not well tolerated by the client who is experiencing nausea.
Test-Taking Strategy: Use the process of elimination. Focus on the client's problem and use knowledge regarding the routes of administration of this medication to answer the question. Review this medication if you had difficulty with this question.
Level of Cognitive Ability: Comprehension
Client Needs: Physiological Integrity
Integrated Concept/Process: Nursing Process/Planning
Content Area: Pharmacology
Reference: Hodgson B, Kizior R: *Saunders nursing drug handbook 2002*, Philadelphia, 2002, WB Saunders, p. 383.

24. *Answer:* 3
Rationale: Propantheline is an antimuscarinic anticholinergic medication that decreases gastrointestinal secretions. It should be administered 30 minutes before meals. The other options are incorrect.
Test-Taking Strategy: Use the process of elimination. Option 4 can be eliminated immediately, as most medications cannot be administered with antacids because of interactive effects. Next, eliminate options 1 and 2 because they are similar. Review this medication if you had difficulty with this question.
Level of Cognitive Ability: Application
Client Needs: Physiological Integrity
Integrated Concept/Process: Nursing Process/Implementation
Content Area: Pharmacology
Reference: Lehne R: *Pharmacology for nursing care*, ed 4, Philadelphia, 2001, WB Saunders, p. 120.

25. *Answer:* 4
Rationale: Docusate sodium is a stool softener that promotes absorption of water into the stool, producing a softer consistency of stool. The intended effect is relief or prevention of constipation. The medication does not relieve abdominal pain, stop gastrointestinal bleeding, or decrease the amount of fat in the stools.
Test-Taking Strategy: Use the process of elimination. Recalling that docusate is a stool softener will easily direct you to option 4. Review the action of this medication if you had difficulty with this question.
Level of Cognitive Ability: Application
Client Needs: Physiological Integrity
Integrated Concept/Process: Nursing Process/Implementation
Content Area: Pharmacology
Reference: Lehne R: *Pharmacology for nursing care*, ed 4, Philadelphia, 2001, WB Saunders, p. 863.

REFERENCES

Clark J, Queener S, Karb V: *Pharmacologic basis of nursing practice*, ed 6, St Louis, 2000, Mosby.
Hodgson B, Kizior R: *Saunders nursing drug handbook 2002*, Philadelphia, 2002, WB Saunders.
Ignatavicius D, Workman M: *Medical-surgical: critical thinking for collaborative care*, ed 4, Philadelphia, 2002, WB Saunders.
Karch A: *Focus on nursing pharmacology*, Philadelphia, 2000, Lippincott.
Lehne R: *Pharmacology for nursing care*, ed 4, Philadelphia, 2001, WB Saunders.

UNIT XII

The Adult Client with a Respiratory Disorder

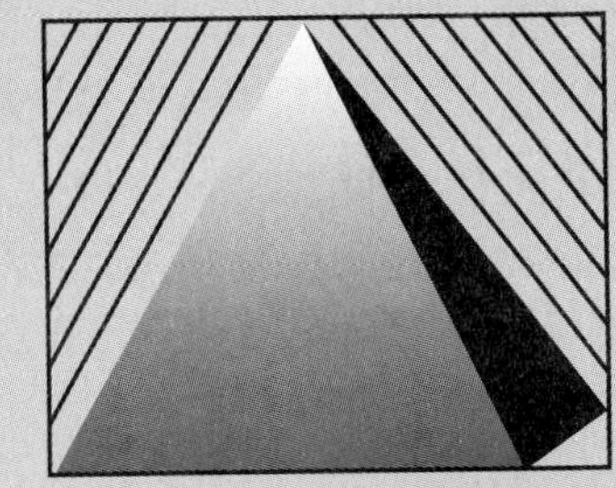

PYRAMID TERMS

Bacille Calmette-Guérin (BCG) Vaccine A vaccine containing attenuated tubercle bacilli that may be given to people in foreign countries, or to those traveling to foreign countries, to produce increased resistance to TB.

Chest Tubes Placed in the pleural space to remove air or fluid from the chest and thus restore negative pressure to reexpand the lung.

Chronic Airflow Limitation (CAL), Chronic Obstructive Lung Disease (COLD), Chronic Obstructive Pulmonary Disease (COPD) A group of diseases that includes emphysema, asthma, bronchiectasis, and bronchitis. Characterized by progressive airflow limitations into and out of the lungs, elevated airway resistance, irreversible lung distention, and arterial blood gas imbalance.

Emphysema A chronic pulmonary disease marked by a narrowing of the small airways and the trapping of air, with destructive changes in their walls. Also known as chronic obstructive pulmonary disease (COPD). In emphysema, the stimulus to breathe is a low PO_2, instead of increased PCO_2.

Endotracheal Tube A large-bore catheter inserted into the trachea through either the nose or the mouth. Used to maintain a patent airway and indicated when the client needs mechanical ventilation. The tube isolates the airway, provides access for suctioning secretions from the large airways of the pulmonary tree, and allows delivery of specific concentrations of oxygen up to 100%.

Mantoux Test The most reliable determinant of infection with tuberculosis (TB). A small amount (0.1 mL) of intermediate-strength purified protein derivative (PPD) containing 5 tuberculin units is given intradermally in the forearm. An area of induration measuring 10 mm or more in diameter 48 to 72 hours after injection indicates individual exposure to TB.

Mechanical Ventilation The use of a ventilator if the client is unable to ventilate enough to maintain proper levels of oxygen and carbon dioxide in the blood.

Multidrug-Resistant Strain (MDR-TB) A multidrug-resistant strain of TB can occur as a result of improper or noncompliant use of treatment programs and the development of mutations in the tubercle bacilli.

Mycobacterium tuberculosis The causative organism (bacillus) of tuberculosis.

Suctioning A sterile procedure that involves removal of respiratory secretions that accumulate in the tracheal bronchial airway when the client is unable to expectorate secretions. Performed to maintain a patent airway.

Tracheostomy An artificial opening into the trachea created to establish an airway. It may be temporary or permanent. Provides a patent airway by bypassing complete upper airway obstruction, as from pharyngeal tumors or laryngeal edema, by facilitating the removal of secretions, or by preventing aspiration of gastric contents.

Tuberculosis A highly communicable disease caused by *Mycobacterium tuberculosis*. It is transmitted by the airborne route via droplet infection.

PYRAMID TO SUCCESS

The Pyramid to Success focuses on maintaining a patent airway. Pyramid points also focus on infectious diseases, particularly tuberculosis, respiratory care in relation to oxygen delivery systems, the client with pneumonia, and the client with chronic obstructive pulmonary disease. The Pyramid to Success includes the care to the client with tuberculosis, especially with regard to the importance of the medication regimen, providing adequate nutrition and adequate rest to promote the healing process, and the prevention of the progression of the disease. Focus on assisting the client to cope with the social isolation issues that exist during the period of illness and on teaching the client and family the critical measures of screening and of preventing respiratory disease and the transmission of disease. The Integrated Concepts and Processes addressed in this unit include the Clinical Problem-Solving Process (Nursing Process), Caring, Communication and Documentation, Cultural Awareness, Self-Care, and Teaching/Learning.

CLIENT NEEDS

Safe, Effective Care Environment

Asepsis when caring for wounds and when performing suctioning
Client rights
Confidentiality related to the respiratory disorder
Consultations and referrals related to respiratory disorder
Establishing priorities
Handling infectious materials such as sputum or body fluids
Informed consent related to diagnostic and surgical procedures
Respiratory precautions
Standard (universal) precautions

Health Promotion and Maintenance

Health promotion programs
Health screening related to risks for respiratory disorders
Instructions related to adequate fluid and nutritional intake
Instructions related to breathing exercises, respiratory therapy, and care
Instructions related to medication administration
Instructions related to need for follow-up care
Instructions related to the prevention of transmission of infection
Prevention of respiratory disorders and infectious diseased

Psychosocial Integrity

Body image changes
Coping mechanisms
Community resources
Grief and loss
Religious and spiritual influences
Situational role changes
Support systems

Physiological Integrity

Alterations in body systems
Chronic obstructive pulmonary disease
Comfort interventions
Infectious diseases
Medication administration
Nutrition and oral hygiene
Oxygen delivery systems
Personal hygiene and rest and sleep
Pneumonia
Respiratory care
Tuberculosis

REFERENCES

Black J, Hawks J, Keene A: *Medical-surgical nursing: clinical management for positive outcomes*, ed 6, Philadelphia, 2001, WB Saunders.
Chernecky C, Berger B: *Laboratory tests and diagnostic procedures*, ed 3, Philadelphia, 2001, WB Saunders.
Clark J, Queener S, Karb V: *Pharmacologic basis of nursing practice*, ed 6, St Louis, 2000, Mosby.
DeWit S: *Fundamental concepts and skills for nursing*, Philadelphia, 2001, WB Saunders.
Hill S, Howlett H: *Success in practical nursing: personal and vocational issues*, ed 4, Philadelphia, 2001, WB Saunders.
National Council of State Boards of Nursing: *Test plan for the National Council Licensure Examination for Practical/Vocational Nurses*, Chicago, 2001, Author.
Potter P, Perry A: *Fundamentals of nursing*, ed 5, St Louis, 2001, Mosby.
Perry A, Potter P: *Clinical nursing skills and techniques*, ed 5, St Louis, 2002, Mosby.
Wilson J: *Infection control in clinical practice*, ed 2, St Louis, 2002, Balliere Tindall.

Respiratory System

I. ANATOMY AND PHYSIOLOGY

A. Primary functions
  1. Provides oxygen for metabolism in the tissues
  2. Removes carbon dioxide, the waste product of metabolism

B. Secondary functions
  1. Facilitates sense of smell
  2. Produces speech
  3. Maintains acid-base balance
  4. Maintains body water levels
  5. Maintains heat balance

C. Upper respiratory tract
  1. Nose: humidifies, warms, and filters inspired air
  2. Sinuses
    a. Air-filled cavities within the hollow bones that surround the nasal passages
    b. Provide resonance during speech
  3. Pharynx
    a. Located behind the oral and nasal cavities
    b. Divided into the nasopharynx, oropharynx, and laryngopharynx
    c. Passageway for both the respiratory and digestive tracts
  4. Larynx
    a. Located above the trachea and just below the pharynx at the root of the tongue
    b. Commonly called the voice box
    c. Contains two pairs of vocal cords, the false and true cords
    d. The opening between the true vocal cords is the glottis
    e. The glottis plays an important role in coughing, which is the most fundamental defense mechanism of the lungs
  5. Epiglottis
    a. Leaf-shaped elastic structure that is attached along one end to the top of the larynx
    b. It prevents food from entering the tracheobronchial tree by closing over the glottis during swallowing

D. Lower respiratory tract
  1. Trachea
    a. Located in front of the esophagus
    b. Branches into the right and left mainstem bronchi at the carina
  2. Mainstem bronchi
    a. Begins at the carina
    b. The right bronchus is slightly wider, shorter, and more vertical than the left bronchus
    c. The mainstem bronchi divides into five secondary or lobar bronchi that enter each of the five lobes of the lung
    d. The bronchi are lined with cilia, which propel mucus up and away from the lower airway to the trachea where it can be expectorated or swallowed
  3. Bronchioles
    a. Branch from the secondary bronchi and subdivide into the small terminal and respiratory bronchioles
    b. They contain no cartilage and depend on the elastic recoil of the lung for patency
    c. The terminal bronchioles contain no cilia and do not participate in gas exchange
  4. Alveolar ducts and alveoli
    a. Acinus is a term used to indicate all structures distal to the terminal bronchiole
    b. Alveolar ducts branch from the respiratory bronchioles
    c. Alveolar sacs, which arise from the ducts, contain clusters of alveoli, which are the basic units of gas exchange
    d. Cells in the walls of the alveoli secrete surfactant, a phospholipid protein that reduces the surface tension in the alveoli

e. Without surfactant, alveoli collapse
5. Lungs
a. Located in the pleural cavity in the thorax
b. Extend from just above the clavicles to the diaphragm, the major muscle of inspiration
c. The right lung, which is larger than the left, is divided into three lobes: the upper, middle, and lower lobe
d. The left lung, which is somewhat narrower than the right lung to accommodate the heart, is divided into two lobes
e. Innervation of the respiratory structures is accomplished by the phrenic nerve, vagus nerve, and thoracic nerves
f. The parietal pleura lines the inside of the thoracic cavity including the upper surface of the diaphragm
g. The visceral pleura covers the pulmonary surfaces
h. A thin fluid layer, which is produced by the cells lining the pleura, lubricates the visceral and parietal pleura, allowing them to glide smoothly and painlessly during respiration
i. Blood flow through the lungs occurs via the pulmonary system and the bronchial system
6. Accessory muscles of respiration includes the scalene muscles, which elevate the first two ribs; the sternocleidomastoid muscles, which raise the sternum; and the trapezius and pectoralis muscles, which fix the shoulders
7. The respiratory process
a. The diaphragm descends into the abdominal cavity during inspiration causing negative pressure in the lungs
b. The negative pressure draws air from the area of greater pressure, the atmosphere, into the area of lesser pressure, the lungs
c. In the lungs, air passes through the terminal bronchioles into the alveoli to oxygenate the body tissues
d. At the end of inspiration, the diaphragm and intercostal muscles relax and the lungs recoil
e. As the lungs recoil, pressure within the lungs becomes greater than atmospheric pressure causing the air that now contains the cellular waste products of carbon dioxide and water to move from the alveoli in the lungs to the atmosphere
f. Expiration is a passive process

II. RISK FACTORS FOR RESPIRATORY DISEASE

A. Smoking
B. Use of chewing tobacco
C. Allergies
D. Frequent respiratory illnesses
E. Chest injury
F. Surgery
G. Exposure to chemicals and environmental pollutants
H. Crowded living conditions
I. Family history of infectious disease
J. Geographic residence and travel to foreign countries

III. DIAGNOSTIC TESTS

A. Chest x-ray study
1. Description: used to provide information regarding the anatomical location and appearance of the lungs
2. Preprocedure
a. Remove all jewelry and other metal objects from the chest area
b. Assess ability to inhale and hold breath
c. Question females regarding pregnancy or the possibility of pregnancy
3. Postprocedure: assist the client to dress

B. Sputum specimen
1. Description: a specimen obtained by expectoration or tracheal **suctioning** to assist in the identification of organisms or abnormal cells
2. Preprocedure
a. Determine specific purpose of collection and check with institutional policy for appropriate collection of specimen
b. Obtain an early morning sterile specimen from **suctioning** or expectoration after a respiratory treatment, if a treatment is prescribed
c. Obtain 15 mL of sputum
d. Instruct client to rinse mouth with water before collection; instruct client to take several deep breaths and then cough deeply to obtain sputum
e. Always collect specimen before starting antibiotics
3. Postprocedure
a. If culture of sputum is prescribed, transport to laboratory immediately
b. Assist the client with mouth care

C. Bronchoscopy
1. Description: direct visual examination of the larynx, trachea, and bronchi with a fiberoptic bronchoscope
2. Preprocedure
a. Obtain informed consent
b. NPO from midnight before the procedure
c. Obtain vital signs

d. Monitor coagulation studies
e. Remove dentures or eyeglasses
f. Prepare suction equipment
g. Administer medication for sedation as prescribed
h. Have emergency resuscitation equipment readily available

3. Postprocedure
a. Monitor vital signs
b. Maintain semi-Fowler's position
c. Assess gag reflex
d. Maintain NPO status until gag reflex returns
e. Have an emesis basin readily available for client to expectorate saliva
f. Monitor for bloody sputum
g. Monitor respiratory status particularly if sedation was administered
h. Monitor for complications as bronchospasm, bacteremia, bronchial perforation indicated by facial or neck crepitus, dysrhythmias, fever, hemorrhage, hypoxemia, and pneumothorax
i. Notify physician if fever or difficulty in breathing occurs after the procedure

D. Pulmonary angiography
1. Description: an invasive fluoroscopic procedure after injection of iodine, radiopaque, or contrast material through a catheter inserted through the antecubital or femoral vein into the pulmonary artery or one of its branches
2. Preprocedure
a. Obtain informed consent
b. Assess for allergies to iodine, seafood, and other radiopaque dyes
c. Maintain NPO status for 8 hours before the procedure
d. Monitor vital signs
e. Monitor coagulation studies
f. Establish an IV access
g. Administer sedation as prescribed
h. Instruct client to lie still during the procedure
i. Instruct client that he or she may feel an urge to cough, or flushing, nausea, or salty taste after injection of the dye
j. Have emergency resuscitation equipment available
3. Postprocedure
a. Monitor vital signs
b. Avoid taking blood pressures in the extremity used for injection for 24 hours
c. Monitor peripheral neurovascular status
d. Assess insertion site for bleeding
e. Monitor for delayed reaction to the dye

E. Thoracentesis
1. Description: removal of fluid or air from the pleural space via a transthoracic aspiration
2. Preprocedure
a. Obtain informed consent
b. Obtain baseline vital signs
c. Prepare client for ultrasound or chest-x-ray study if prescribed before procedure
d. Assess coagulation studies
e. Note that client is positioned sitting upright with arms and head supported by a table at the bedside during the procedure
f. If the client cannot sit up, the client is placed lying in bed on the unaffected side with the head of the bed elevated 45 degrees
g. Inform client not to cough, breathe deeply, or move during the procedure
3. Postprocedure
a. Monitor vital signs
b. Monitor respiratory status
c. Apply a pressure dressing and assess puncture site for bleeding and crepitus
d. Monitor for signs of pneumothorax, air embolism, and pulmonary edema

F. Pulmonary function test (PFT)
1. Description: includes a number of different tests used to evaluate lung mechanics, gas exchange and acid-base disturbance through spirometric measurements, lung volumes, and arterial blood gases
2. Preprocedure
a. Determine if an analgesic that may depress the respiratory function is being administered
b. Consult with physician regarding holding bronchodilators before testing
c. Instruct client to void before procedure and to wear loose clothing
d. Remove dentures
e. Instruct client to refrain from smoking or eating a heavy meal for 4 to 6 hours before the test
3. Postprocedure: resume normal diet and any bronchodilators and respiratory treatments that were held before the procedure

G. Lung biopsy
1. Description
a. A percutaneous lung biopsy is performed to obtain tissue for analysis by culture or cytological examination
b. A needle biopsy is done to identify pulmonary lesions, changes in lung tissue, and the cause of pleural effusion
2. Preprocedure
a. Obtain informed consent
b. Maintain NPO status before the procedure

c. Inform the client that a local anesthetic will be used but that a sensation of pressure during needle insertion and aspiration may be felt
d. Administer analgesics and sedatives as prescribed
3. Postprocedure
a. Monitor vital signs
b. Apply a dressing to the biopsy site and monitor for drainage or bleeding
c. Monitor for signs of respiratory distress and notify the physician if they occur
d. Monitor for signs of pneumothorax and air emboli and notify physician if they occur
e. Prepare client for chest x-ray study if prescribed

H. Ventilation-perfusion lung scan
1. Description
a. In the perfusion scan, blood flow to the lungs is evaluated
b. The ventilation scan determines the patency of the pulmonary airways and detects abnormalities in ventilation
c. A radionuclide may be injected for the procedure
2. Preprocedure
a. Obtain informed consent
b. Assess for allergies to dye, iodine, or seafood
c. Remove jewelry around the chest area
d. Review breathing methods that may be required during testing
e. Establish an IV access
f. Administer sedation if prescribed
g. Have emergency resuscitation equipment available
3. Postprocedure
a. Monitor client for reaction to the radionuclide
b. For 24 hours after the procedure, rubber gloves are worn when urine is being discarded; they should be washed with soap and water before removing, and then the hands should be washed after the gloves are removed
c. Instruct the client to wash hands carefully with soap and water for 24 hours after the procedure

I. Arterial blood gases (ABGs) (Refer to Chapter 9 for information on ABGs.)

J. Pulse oximetry
1. Description
a. A noninvasive test that registers how saturated the client's hemoglobin is with oxygen
b. This arterial oxygen saturation (Sao_2) is recorded as a percentage
c. The normal value is 95% to 100%
d. After a hypoxic client uses up the readily available oxygen (measured as the arterial oxygen pressure, Pao_2, on arterial blood gas testing), the reserve oxygen, that oxygen attached to the hemoglobin (Sao_2), is drawn on to provide oxygen to the tissues
e. A pulse oximeter reading can alert the nurse to hypoxemia before clinical signs occur
2. Procedure
a. A sensor is placed on the client's finger, toe, nose, earlobe, or forehead to measure oxygen saturation, which is then displayed on a monitor
b. Maintain transducer at heart level
c. Do not select an extremity with an impediment to blood flow
d. Results lower than 91% necessitate immediate treatment
e. If the Sao_2 is below 85%, the body's tissues have a difficult time becoming oxygenated; an Sao_2 of less than 70% is life-threatening

IV. PROCEDURES

A. Incentive spirometry (Box 46-1)

B. Suctioning
1. Aseptic technique
2. Hyperoxygenate by Ambu bag, increasing the oxygen flow rate or by deep breaths
3. Lubricate catheter with sterile water
4. Tracheal suctioning: insert catheter 4 inches
5. Nasotracheal suctioning: insert catheter to induce cough reflex
6. Do not apply suction while inserting the catheter
7. Apply suction intermittently for 10 to 15 seconds; rotate catheter and withdraw
8. Hyperoxygenate and encourage deep breaths

C. Chest physiotherapy (CPT)
1. Description: percussion and vibration over the thorax to loosen secretions in the affected area of the lungs
2. Implementation

BOX 46-1

Client Instructions for Incentive Spirometry

Use lips to form seal around mouthpiece
Inspire deeply
Hold inspiration for a few seconds
Forcefully exhale
Avoid use of spirometry at meal times, as it may produce nausea

a. A layer of material (gown or pajamas) is placed between the hands and the client's skin
b. Best time is in the morning on rising, 1 hour before meals, or 2 to 3 hours after meals
c. Stop if pain occurs
d. Dispose of sputum properly
e. Provide mouth care after procedure
3. Contraindications
a. When bronchospasm is increased by its use
b. History of pathological fractures
c. Rib fractures
d. Chest incisions

D. Postural drainage
1. Description
a. Use of gravity to drain secretions from segments of the lungs
b. May be combined with CPT
2. Implementation
a. Position client properly (lung segment to be drained is uppermost)
b. Best time is in the morning on arising, 1 hour before meals, or 2 to 3 hours after meals
c. Stop if cyanosis or exhaustion occurs
d. Maintain position 5 to 20 minutes after procedure
e. Dispose of sputum properly
f. Provide mouth care after the procedure
3. Contraindications
a. Unstable vital signs
b. Increased intracranial pressure

V. OXYGEN

A. Implementation
1. Assess color and vital signs before and during treatment
2. Place an "Oxygen in Use" sign at client's bedside
3. Assess for presence of chronic lung problems
4. Humidify the oxygen

B. Nasal cannula (nasal prongs) (Box 46-2)
1. Description
a. Used at flow rates of l to 6 liters per minute providing approximate oxygen concentrations of 24% (at l liter per minute) to 44% (at 6 liters per minute)
b. Flow rates higher than 6 liters per minute do not significantly increase oxygenation because the anatomical reserve or dead space (oral and nasal cavities) is full
c. Used for the client with **chronic airflow limitation (CAL, COPD)** and for long-term oxygen use; however, the **CAL** client who retains carbon dioxide should never receive oxygen at a rate higher than 2 to 3 liters per minute unless on a mechanical ventilator because of the potential for apnea or respiratory arrest
d. Effective oxygen concentration can be delivered to both nose breathers and mouth breathers with the use of a nasal cannula
2. Implementation
a. Place the nasal prongs in the nostrils with the openings facing the client
b. Add humidification as prescribed when a flow rate higher than 2 liters per minute is prescribed
c. Check the water level and change the humidifier as needed
d. Monitor the client for changes in respiratory rate or depth
e. Assess mucosa as high flow rates have a drying effect and increase mucosal irritation
f. Monitor skin integrity as the oxygen tubing can irritate the skin
g. Provide water-soluble jelly to the nares PRN

C. Simple face mask (Box 46-3)
1. Description
a. A face mask used to deliver oxygen concentrations of 40% to 60% for short-term oxygen therapy or in an emergency
b. A minimal flow rate of 5 liters per minute is needed to prevent the rebreathing of exhaled air

BOX 46-2

FIO_2 Delivered via Nasal Cannula

24% at 1 liter per minute
28% at 2 liters per minute
32% at 3 liters per minute
36% at 4 liters per minute
40% at 5 liters per minute
44% at 6 liters per minute

BOX 46-3

FIO_2 Delivered via Simple Face Mask

Flow rate must be set to at least 5 liters per minute to flush the mask of carbon dioxide
40% at 5 liters per minute
45%-50% at 6 liters per minute
55%-60% at 8 liters per minute

2. Implementation
   a. Be sure mask fits securely over nose and mouth, as a poorly fitting mask reduces the FIO_2 delivered
   b. Monitor the skin and provide skin care to the area covered by the mask because pressure and moisture under the bag may cause skin breakdown
   c. Monitor the client closely for risk of aspiration because the mask limits the client's ability to clear the mouth, especially if vomiting occurs
   d. Provide emotional support to decrease anxiety to the client who feels claustrophobic
   e. Consult with physician regarding switching the client from a mask to a nasal cannula during eating

D. Partial rebreather mask (Box 46-4)
1. Description
   a. A partial rebreather mask consists of a mask with a reservoir bag that provides an oxygen concentration of 70% to 90%, with flow rates of 6 to 15 liters per minute
   b. The client rebreathes one third of the exhaled tidal volume, which is high in oxygen, thus providing a high FIO_2
2. Implementation
   a. Make sure that the reservoir does not twist or kink, which results in a deflated bag
   b. Adjust the flow rate to keep the reservoir bag inflated two-thirds full during inspiration, as deflation results in decreased oxygen delivered and rebreathing of exhaled air

E. Non-rebreather mask
1. Description
   a. A non-rebreather mask provides the highest concentration of the low-flow systems and can deliver an FIO_2 greater than 90%, depending on the client's ventilatory pattern
   b. It is most frequently used in the client with deteriorating respiratory status who might require intubation
   c. The non-rebreather mask has a one-way valve between the mask and the reservoir and two flaps over the exhalation ports
   d. The valve allows the client to draw his or her entire oxygen from the reservoir bag
   e. The flaps prevent room air from entering through the exhalation ports
   f. During exhalation air leaves through these exhalation ports while the one-way valve prevents exhaled air from reentering the reservoir bag
2. FIO_2 delivered: 60% to 100% FIO_2 at a liter flow that maintains the bag two-thirds full
3. Implementation
   a. Remove mucus or saliva from the mask
   b. Monitor the client closely
   c. Ensure that the valve and flaps are intact and functional during each breath.
   d. Valves should open during expiration and close during inhalation
   e. Suffocation can occur if the reservoir bag kinks or if the oxygen source disconnects

F. High-flow oxygen delivery systems
1. A high-flow system provides oxygen concentrations of 24% to 100% at 8 to 15 liters per minute
2. Hi-flow systems include the Venturi mask, aerosol mask, face tent, **tracheostomy** collar, and T piece
3. These devices, when properly fitted, deliver a consistent and accurate oxygen concentration that meets the client's inspiratory effort

G. Venturi mask
1. Description
   a. The Venturi mask delivers the most accurate oxygen concentration
   b. Its operation is based on a mechanism that pulls in a specific proportional amount of room air for each liter flow of oxygen
   c. An adapter is located between the bottom of the mask and the oxygen source and contains holes of different sizes, which allows only specific amounts of air to mix with the oxygen
   d. The adapter allows selection of the amount of oxygen desired
2. FIO_2 delivered: 24% to 55% FIO_2 with flow rates of 4 to 10 liters per minute
3. Implementation
   a. Monitor closely to ensure an accurate flow rate for specific FIO_2
   b. Keep the orifice for the Venturi adapter open and uncovered to ensure adequate oxygen delivery
   c. Ensure that mask fits snugly and that tubing is free of kinks, as the FIO_2 is altered if kinking occurs or if the mask fits poorly
   d. Monitor the client for dry mucous membranes because humidity or aerosol can be added to the system

BOX 46-4

FIO_2 Delivered via Partial Rebreather Mask

A flow rate high enough to maintain the bag two-thirds full during inspiration is needed

70%-90% FiO_2 is delivered at 6 to 15 liters per minute

H. Face tent, aerosol mask, **tracheostomy** collar and T piece
1. Face tent
a. Fits over the client's chin, with the top extending halfway across the face
b. The oxygen concentration varies, but the face tent is useful instead of a tight-fitting mask for the client who has facial trauma and burns
2. Aerosol mask: an aerosol mask is used for the client who requires high humidity after extubation or upper airway surgery or for the client who has thick secretions
3. **Tracheostomy** collar and T piece
a. The **tracheostomy** collar can be used to deliver high humidity and the desired oxygen to the client with a **tracheostomy**
b. A special adapter called the T piece can be used to deliver any desired FIO_2 to the client with a **tracheostomy**, laryngectomy, or **endotracheal tube**
4. FIO_2 delivered: 24% to 100% FIO_2 with flow rates at least 10 liters per minute
5. Implementation
a. Change delivery system to a nasal cannula during mealtimes
b. Ensure that aerosol mist escapes from the vents of the delivery system during inspiration and expiration
c. Empty condensation from the tubing to prevent the client from being lavaged with water and to promote an adequate flow rate
d. Ensure that there is sufficient water in the canister and change the aerosol water container as needed
e. Keep the exhalation port on T-piece open and uncovered (If the port is occluded, the client can suffocate)
f. Position the T piece so that it does not pull on the **tracheostomy** or **endotracheal tube** and cause erosion of skin at the **tracheostomy** insertion site
g. Make sure the humidifier creates enough mist; a mist should be seen during inspiration and expiration

VI. ENDOTRACHEAL TUBES

A. Description
1. Used to maintain a patent airway
2. Indicated when the client needs **mechanical ventilation**
3. If the client requires an artificial airway for longer than 10 to 14 days, a **tracheostomy** may be created to avoid mucosal and vocal cord damage that can be caused by the **endotracheal tube**
4. The cuff (located at the distal end of the tube), when inflated, produces a seal between the trachea and the cuff to prevent aspiration and ensure delivery of a set tidal volume when **mechanical ventilation** is used; an inflated cuff also prevents air from passing to the vocal cords, nose, or mouth
5. The pilot balloon permits air to be inserted into the cuff, prevents air from escaping, and is used as a guideline for determining the presence or absence of air in the cuff
6. The universal adapter enables attachment of the tube to **mechanical ventilation** tubing or other types of oxygen delivery systems

B. Orotracheal
1. Allows use of a larger-diameter tube and reduces the work of breathing
2. Indicated when the client has a nasal obstruction or a predisposition to epistaxis
3. Uncomfortable and can be manipulated by the tongue causing airway obstruction; an oral airway may be needed to keep the client from biting on the tube

C. Nasotracheal
1. Smaller-sized tube increases resistance and increases client's work of breathing
2. Discouraged in clients with bleeding disorders
3. More comfortable for the client, and client is unable to manipulate with tongue

D. Implementation
1. Placement is confirmed by chest x-ray study (correct placement is 1 to 2 cm above carina)
2. Placement is assessed by auscultating both sides of chest while manually ventilating with resuscitation bag
3. If breath sounds and chest wall movement are absent on the left side, the tube may be in the right mainstem bronchus
4. Auscultation over the stomach is performed to rule out esophageal intubation
5. If the tube is in the stomach, louder breath sounds will be heard over the stomach than over the chest, and abdominal distention will be present
6. Secure the tube immediately after intubation with adhesive tape
7. Monitor position of tube at lip or nose
8. Monitor skin and mucous membranes
9. Suction only when needed
10. The oral tube needs to be moved to the opposite side of the mouth daily to prevent pressure and necrosis of the lip and mouth area, prevent nerve damage, and facilitate

inspection and cleaning of the mouth; moving the tube to the opposite side of the mouth should be done by two health care providers

11. Prevent pulling or tugging on the tube to prevent dislodgement; suction, coughing, and speaking attempts by the client place extra stress on the tube and can cause dislodgement
12. Keep a resuscitation (Ambu) bag at bedside at all times
13. Assess pilot balloon to ensure cuff is inflated

E. Extubation
1. Hyperoxygenate the client and suction the **endotracheal tube** and the oral cavity
2. Place client in semi-Fowler's position
3. The cuff is deflated and the tube is removed at peak inspiration
4. Instruct client to cough and deep breathe to assist in removing accumulated secretions in the throat
5. Apply oxygen therapy as prescribed
6. Monitor respiratory status for signs of obstruction and notify the physician if they occur
7. Inform client that hoarseness or a sore throat is normal and to limit talking if it occurs

VII. TRACHEOSTOMY

A. Description
1. A tracheotomy is a surgical incision made into the trachea to establish an airway
2. A **tracheostomy** is the stoma or opening that results from the tracheotomy
3. The **tracheostomy** can be temporary or permanent

B. Implementation
1. Monitor respirations
2. Monitor ABGs and pulse oximetry
3. Encourage coughing and deep breathing
4. Maintain a semi- to high-Fowler's position
5. Monitor for bleeding, difficulty breathing, absence of breath sounds, and crepitus, which are indications of hemorrhage, pneumothorax, and subcutaneous **emphysema**, respectively
6. Provide respiratory treatments as prescribed
7. Suction as needed; hyperoxygenate the client before **suctioning**
8. If client is allowed to eat, sit the client up for meals and ensure that the cuff is inflated (if tube is not capped) for meals, and for 1 hour after meals
9. Assess the stoma and secretions for blood or purulent drainage
10. Follow physician's orders and agency policy for cleaning the **tracheostomy** site and inner cannula; usually half-strength hydrogen peroxide is used
11. Administer humidified oxygen as prescribed as the normal humidification process is bypassed in a client with a **tracheostomy**
12. Obtain assistance in changing **tracheostomy** ties; cut and remove old ties holding the **tracheostomy** in place
13. Keep a resuscitation (Ambu) bag, obturator, clamps and a tracheotomy set at the bedside

C. Complications (Box 46-5)

VIII. CHEST TUBE DRAINAGE SYSTEM

(Refer to Chapter 18 for information regarding chest tubes.)

IX. MECHANICAL VENTILATION

A. Description
1. Used to overcome the client's inability to ventilate or oxygenate adequately
2. It may be intermittent or continuous, short term or long term

B. Implementation
1. Assess the client first and the ventilator second
2. Assess vital signs, respiratory status, and breathing patterns
3. Monitor color, particularly in the lips and nail beds
4. Monitor the chest for bilateral expansion
5. Obtain a pulse oximetry reading
6. Assess the need for **suctioning** and observe type, color, and amount of secretions
7. Ensure that the alarms are set
8. If a cause of an alarm cannot be determined, ventilate the client manually with a resuscitation bag until the problem is corrected
9. Empty ventilator tubings when moisture collects

BOX 46-5

Complications of a Tracheostomy

Tube obstruction
Tube dislodgement
Pneumothorax
Subcutaneous emphysema
Bleeding
Infection
Tracheomalacia
Tracheal stenosis
Tracheoesophageal fistula
Trachea-innominate artery fistula

10. Turn client at least every 2 hours or get client out of bed as prescribed to prevent complications of immobility
11. Have resuscitation equipment available at the bedside

C. Causes of alarms
1. High-pressure alarm
   a. Increased secretions in the airway
   b. Wheezing or bronchospasm causing decreased airway size
   c. Displacement of the **Endotracheal tube**
   d. Obstructed **Endotracheal tube** because of water or a kink in the tubing
   e. Client coughs, gags, or bites on the tube
   f. Client is anxious or fights the ventilator
2. Low-pressure alarm
   a. Disconnection or leak in the ventilator or in the client's airway cuff
   b. The client stops spontaneous breathing

D. Complications
1. Hypotension caused by the application of positive pressure, which increases intrathoracic pressure and inhibits blood return to the heart
2. Respiratory complications such as pneumothorax or subcutaneous **emphysema** as a result of positive pressure
3. Gastrointestinal alterations as stress ulcers
4. Malnutrition
5. Infections
6. Muscular deconditioning
7. Ventilator dependence or inability to wean

E. Weaning: The process of going from ventilator dependence to spontaneous breathing

X. CHEST INJURIES

A. Rib fracture
1. Description
   a. Results from direct blunt chest trauma and causes a potential for intrathoracic injury such as pneumothorax or pulmonary contusion
   b. Pain with movement and chest splinting result in impaired ventilation and inadequate clearance of secretions
2. Data collection
   a. Pain at injury site that increases with inspiration
   b. Tenderness at site
   c. Shallow respirations
   d. Client splints chest
   e. Fractures noted on chest x-ray study
3. Implementation
   a. Note that ribs usually unite spontaneously
   b. Place client in high Fowler's position
   c. Administer pain medication as prescribed to maintain adequate ventilatory status
   d. Monitor for increased respiratory distress
   e. Instruct client to self-splint with hands and arms

B. Flail chest
1. Description
   a. A blunt chest trauma associated with accidents that may result in hemothorax and rib fractures
   b. The loose segment of the chest wall becomes paradoxical to the expansion and contraction of the rest of the chest wall
2. Data collection
   a. Paradoxical respirations (the inward movement of the thorax during inspiration with outward movement during expiration)
   b. Severe pain in chest
   c. Dyspnea
   d. Cyanosis
   e. Tachycardia
   f. Hypotension
   g. Shallow respirations
   h. Tachypnea
3. Implementation
   a. Place client in high Fowler's position
   b. Administer humidified oxygen as prescribed
   c. Monitor for increased respiratory distress
   d. Encourage coughing and deep breathing
   e. Administer pain medication as prescribed
   f. Maintain bed rest and limit activity to reduce oxygen demands
   g. Prepare for intubation with **mechanical ventilation** as prescribed

C. Pulmonary contusion
1. Description
   a. Characterized by interstitial hemorrhage associated with intraalveolar hemorrhage resulting in decreased pulmonary compliance
   b. The major complication is acute respiratory distress syndrome (ARDS)
2. Data collection
   a. Dyspnea
   b. Hypoxemia
   c. Increased bronchial secretions
   d. Hemoptysis
   e. Restlessness
   f. Decreased breath sounds
   g. Rales and wheezes
3. Implementation
   a. Maintain airway and ventilation
   b. Place client in high Fowler's position
   c. Administer oxygen as prescribed

d. Monitor for increased respiratory distress
e. Maintain bed rest and limit activity to reduce oxygen demands
f. Prepare for **mechanical ventilation** as prescribed

D. Pneumothorax
1. Description
a. The accumulation of atmospheric air in the pleural space, which results in a rise in intrathoracic pressure and reduced vital capacity
b. The loss of negative intrapleural pressure results in collapse of the lung
c. Diagnosis of pneumothorax is made by chest x-ray film
2. Data collection
a. Dyspnea
b. Tachycardia
c. Tachypnea
d. Sharp chest pain
e. Absent breath sounds on affected side
f. Decreased chest expansion unilaterally
g. Cyanosis
h. Hypotension
i. Subcutaneous **emphysema**
j. Sucking sound with open chest wound
k. Tracheal deviation to the unaffected side with tension pneumothorax
3. Implementation
a. Apply pressure dressing over open chest wound
b. Administer oxygen as prescribed
c. Place client in high Fowler's position
d. Prepare for **chest tube** placement with underwater seal drainage until the lung has fully expanded
e. Monitor the **chest tube** drainage system
f. Monitor for subcutaneous **emphysema**

XI. RESPIRATORY FAILURE

A. Description
1. Occurs when the client cannot eliminate carbon dioxide from the alveoli
2. The carbon dioxide retention results in hypoxemia
3. Oxygen reaches the alveoli but cannot be absorbed or used properly
4. The lungs can move air sufficiently but cannot oxygenate the pulmonary blood properly
5. Respiratory failure occurs as a result of a mechanical abnormality of the lungs or chest wall, a defect in the respiratory control center in the brain, or an impairment in the function of the respiratory muscles

B. Data collection
1. Dyspnea
2. Headache
3. Confusion
4. Restlessness
5. Tachycardia
6. Cyanosis
7. Dysrhythmias
8. Decreased level of consciousness
9. Alterations in respirations and breath sounds

C. Implementation
1. Identify and treat the cause of respiratory failure
2. Administer oxygen as prescribed to maintain the Pao_2 level above 60 mm Hg
3. Place the client in high Fowler's position
4. Encourage deep breathing
5. Administer bronchodilators as prescribed
6. Prepare the client for **mechanical ventilation** if supplemental oxygen cannot maintain acceptable Pao_2 levels

XII. ACUTE RESPIRATORY DISTRESS SYNDROME (ARDS)

A. Description
1. A form of acute respiratory failure caused by a diffuse lung injury leading to extravascular lung fluid
2. The interstitial edema causes compression and obliteration of the terminal airways and leads to reduced lung volume and compliance
3. The ABGs identify respiratory acidosis and hypoxemia that does not respond to an increased percentage of oxygen, and the chest x-ray study shows interstitial edema
4. Some of the causes include sepsis, fluid overload, shock, trauma, neurological injuries, burns, disseminated intravascular coagulation, drug ingestion, and the inhalation of toxic substances

B. Data collection
1. Tachypnea
2. Dyspnea
3. Decreased breath sounds
4. Deteriorating blood gas levels
5. Hypoxemia despite high concentrations of delivered oxygen
6. Decreased pulmonary compliance
7. Pulmonary infiltrates

C. Implementation
1. Identify and treat cause of the ARDS
2. Administer oxygen as prescribed
3. Place client in high Fowler's position
4. Restrict fluid intake as prescribed
5. Provide respiratory treatments as prescribed

6. Administer diuretics, anticoagulants, or steroids as prescribed
7. Prepare the client for intubation and **mechanical ventilation**

XIII. CHRONIC OBSTRUCTIVE PULMONARY DISEASE (COPD)

A. Description
   1. Also known as **chronic obstructive lung disease (COLD)** and **chronic airflow limitation (CAL)**
   2. A group of diseases that includes **emphysema**, asthma, bronchiectasis, and bronchitis
   3. Characterized by progressive airflow limitations into and out of the lungs, elevated airway resistance, irreversible lung distention, and arterial blood gas imbalance
   4. **COPD** leads to pulmonary insufficiency, pulmonary hypertension, and cor pulmonale
   5. In **emphysema**, the stimulus to breathe is a low Po_2 instead of increased Pco_2

B. Data collection
   1. Cough
   2. Exertional dyspnea
   3. Wheezing and crackles
   4. Sputum production
   5. Weight loss
   6. Barrel chest (**emphysema**)
   7. Use of accessory muscles
   8. Cyanosis
   9. Clubbing of fingers
   10. Orthopnea
   11. Cardiac dysrhythmias
   12. Congestion and hyperinflation on chest x-ray film
   13. ABGs indicate respiratory acidosis and hypoxemia
   14. PFTs demonstrate decreased vital capacity

C. Implementation
   1. Monitor vital signs
   2. Administer oxygen as prescribed at 2 to 3 liters per minute
   3. Monitor pulse oximetry
   4. Provide respiratory treatments and chest physical therapy
   5. Reposition client for breathing comfort and to mobilize secretions
   6. Instruct client in diaphragmatic or abdominal and pursed-lip breathing techniques
   7. Record the color, amount, and consistency of sputum
   8. Suction client if necessary to clear airway and prevent infection
   9. Monitor weight
   10. Encourage small, frequent meals to prevent dyspnea
   11. Encourage fluids up to 3000 mL per day to keep secretions thin unless contraindicated
   12. Place in high Fowler's position and leaning forward to aid in breathing
   13. Provide a high-calorie, high-protein, and high-carbohydrate diet with vitamin C and nitrogen
   14. Allow activity as tolerated
   15. Administer bronchodilators as prescribed and instruct client in the use of both oral and inhalant medications
   16. Administer steroids as prescribed to reduce inflammation
   17. Administer mucolytics as prescribed to thin secretions
   18. Administer antibiotics for infection if prescribed

D. Client education
   1. Stop smoking
   2. Recognize the signs and symptoms of respiratory infection and hypoxia
   3. Adhere to activity limitations, alternating rest periods with activity
   4. Avoid exposure to individuals with infections and avoid crowds
   5. Demonstrate pursed-lip and diaphragmatic or abdominal breathing
   6. Instruct in the use of medications and inhalers
   7. Instruct in the use in oxygen therapy
   8. Instruct client in nutritional requirements
   9. Avoid eating gas-producing foods, spicy foods, and extremely hot or cold foods
   10. Instruct in the importance of receiving the influenza vaccine as recommended
   11. When dusting, use a wet cloth
   12. Avoid powerful odors
   13. Avoid extremes in temperature
   14. Avoid fireplaces, pets, and feather pillows

XIV. PNEUMONIA

A. Description
   1. An infection of the pulmonary tissue including the interstitial spaces, alveoli, and bronchioles
   2. The edema associated with inflammation stiffens the lung, decreases compliance in vital capacity, and causes hypoxemia
   3. Can be community acquired or hospital acquired
   4. The chest x-ray study presents as diffuse patches throughout the lungs or consolidates in a lobe

5. A sputum culture identifies the organism
6. The white blood cells (WBCs) and erythrocyte sedimentation rate (ESR) are elevated

B. Data collection
1. Chills
2. Elevated temperature
3. Pleuritic pain
4. Rales, rhonchi, and wheezes
5. Use of accessory muscles
6. Cyanosis
7. Mental status changes
8. Sputum production
   a. Rusty, green, or bloody (pneumococcal pneumonia)
   b. Yellow-green (bronchopneumonia)

C. Implementation
1. Administer oxygen as prescribed
2. Monitor respiratory status
3. Monitor for labored respirations, cyanosis, cold and clammy skin
4. Encourage coughing and deep breathing and use of incentive spirometer
5. Place in semi-Fowler's position to facilitate breathing and lung expansion
6. Change position frequently and ambulate as tolerated to mobilize secretions
7. Provide chest physical therapy
8. Perform nasotracheal **suctioning** if client is unable to clear secretions
9. Monitor pulse oximetry
10. Monitor and record color, consistency, and amount of sputum
11. Provide a high-calorie, high-protein diet with small frequent meals
12. Encourage fluids to 3 liters a day to liquefy secretions unless contraindicated
13. Provide a balance of rest and activity increasing activity gradually
14. Administer antibiotics as prescribed
15. Administer antipyretics, bronchodilators, cough suppressants, mucolytic agents, and expectorants as prescribed
16. Prevent the spread of infection by handwashing and the proper disposal of secretions

D. Client education
1. The importance of rest, proper nutrition, and adequate fluid intake
2. Avoid chilling and exposure to individuals with respiratory infections or viruses
3. Instruct regarding medications and the use of inhalants as prescribed
4. Instruct to notify physician if chills, fever, dsypnea, hemoptysis, or increased fatigue occur
5. Instruct in the importance of receiving the influenza vaccine as recommended

XV. PLEURAL EFFUSION

A. Description
1. The collection of fluid in the pleural space
2. Any condition that interferes with either secretion or drainage of this fluid will lead to pleural effusion

B. Data collection
1. Pleuritic pain that is sharp and increases with inspiration
2. Dyspnea on exertion
3. Dry nonproductive cough caused by bronchial irritation or mediastinal shift
4. Malaise
5. Tachycardia
6. Elevated temperature
7. Decreased breath sounds
8. Chest x-ray film shows pleural effusion and a mediastinal shift away from the fluid

C. Implementation
1. Identify and treat underlying cause
2. Monitor vital signs
3. Monitor breath sounds
4. Place client in high Fowler's position
5. Encourage coughing and deep breathing
6. Prepare client for thoracentesis
7. If pleural effusion is recurrent, prepare client for pleurectomy or pleurodesis

D. Pleurectomy
1. Consists of surgically stripping the parietal pleura away from the visceral pleura
2. This produces an intense inflammatory reaction that promotes adhesion formation between the two layers during healing

E. Pleurodesis
1. Involves the instillation of a sclerosing substance into the pleural space via a thorocotomy tube
2. This creates an inflammatory response that scleroses tissues together

XVI. EMPYEMA

A. Description
1. Collection of pus within the pleural cavity
2. Fluid is thick, opaque, and foul smelling
3. The most common cause is pulmonary infection and lung abscess caused by thoracic surgery or chest trauma, where bacteria are introduced directly into the pleural space
4. Treatment focuses on emptying the empyema cavity, reexpanding the lung, and controlling the infection

B. Data collection
1. Recent febrile illnesses or trauma
2. Chest pain
3. Cough
4. Dyspnea
5. Anorexia and weight loss
6. Malaise
7. Elevated temperature and chills
8. Night sweats
9. Diminished chest wall movement on the effected side
10. Pleural exudate on chest x-ray study

C. Implementation
1. Monitor vital signs
2. Monitor breath sounds
3. Place client in semi- or high-Fowler's position
4. Encourage coughing and deep breathing
5. Administer antibiotics as prescribed
6. Instruct client to splint chest as necessary
7. Assist with **chest tube** insertion to promote drainage and lung expansion
8. If marked pleural thickening occurs, prepare client for decortication, a surgical procedure that involves removal of the restrictive mass of fibrin and inflammatory cells if prescribed

XVII. PLEURISY

A. Description
1. Inflammation of the visceral and parietal membranes
2. These membranes rub together during respiration and cause pain
3. May be caused by pulmonary infarction or pneumonia
4. Usually occurs on one side of the chest and in the lower lateral portions in the chest wall

B. Data collection
1. Knifelike pain that is aggravated on deep breathing and coughing
2. Dyspnea
3. Pleural friction rub heard on auscultation
4. Apprehension

C. Implementation
1. Monitor vital signs
2. Administer analgesics as prescribed
3. Apply hot or cold applications as prescribed
4. Encourage coughing and deep breathing
5. Instruct client to lie on affected side to splint chest

XVIII. PULMONARY EMBOLISM

A. Description
1. Occurs when a thrombus that forms in a deep vein detaches and travels to the right side of the heart and then lodges in a branch of the pulmonary artery
2. Clients prone to pulmonary embolism are those at risk for deep vein thrombosis including prolonged immobilization, surgery, obesity, pregnancy, heart failure, advanced age, and prior history of thromboembolism
3. Fat emboli can occur as a complication after a fracture of a flat long bone
4. Treatment is aimed at preventing venous status and includes range of motion (ROM) exercises and early ambulation after surgery, the use of antiembolism or pneumatic compression stockings, and preventing pressure under the popliteal space

B. Data collection
1. Dyspnea accompanied by anginal and pleuritic pain exacerbated by inspiration
2. Chest pain
3. Blood-tinged sputum
4. Tachycardia
5. Cough
6. Tachypnea
7. Hypotension
8. Shallow respirations
9. Rales on auscultation
10. Low-grade fever
11. Distended neck veins
12. Cyanosis
13. Positive Homan's sign

C. Implementation
1. Monitor vital signs
2. Administer oxygen as prescribed
3. Place client in high Fowler's position
4. Maintain bed rest and active and passive ROM exercises as prescribed
5. Encourage use of incentive spirometry as prescribed
6. Monitor pulse oximetry
7. Prepare for intubation and **mechanical ventilation** for severe hypoxemia
8. Prepare for the administration of anticoagulants such as heparin sodium (Liquaemin) or warfarin sodium (Coumadin)
9. Prepare client for embolectomy, vein ligation, or insertion of an umbrella filter as prescribed

XIX. LUNG CANCER
(REFER TO CHAPTER 40 FOR INFORMATION ON LUNG CANCER.)

A. Surgical implementation

1. Laser therapy: to relieve endobronchial obstruction
2. Thoracotomy with pneumonectomy: surgical removal of a lung for bronchiogenic carcinoma
3. Thoracotomy with lobectomy: surgical removal of one lobe of the lung for tumors confined to a single lobe
4. Thoracotomy with segmental resection: surgical removal of lobe segment for clients unable to tolerate lobectomy or pneumonectomy

B. Preoperative implementation
1. Explain the potential postoperative need for **chest tubes**
2. Note that a **chest tube** is not inserted for a pneumonectomy, and the serum fluid that accumulates in the empty thoracic cavity eventually consolidates, preventing shifts of the mediastinum, heart, and remaining lung

C. Postoperative implementation
1. Monitor vital signs
2. Monitor cardiac and respiratory status
3. Maintain **chest tube** drainage system, which will drain air and or blood that accumulates in the pleural space
4. Monitor **chest tube** insertion site for subcutaneous air and drainage
5. Administer oxygen as prescribed
6. Monitor pulse oximetry
7. Provide activity as tolerated
8. Encourage active ROM exercises to operative shoulder as prescribed
9. Maintain client position based on procedure performed
10. Check physician's orders regarding positioning; complete lateral turning is avoided

XX. LARYNGEAL CANCER (REFER TO CHAPTER 40 FOR INFORMATION ON LARYNGEAL CANCER.)

A. Surgical implementation
1. Small tumor excision or total laryngectomy: performed for infiltrate tumors that involve vocal cord paralysis and for tumors that do not respond to radiation therapy
2. Radical neck dissection
   a. Involves a laryngectomy and **tracheostomy**
   b. Performed when lymph node involvement is present

B. Preoperative implementation
1. Establish methods of communication for the client
2. Encourage the client to express feelings about changes in body image and loss of voice
3. Describe the rehabilitation program and information about the tracheotomy and **suctioning**

C. Postoperative implementation
1. Monitor vital signs
2. Assess respiratory status
3. Place client in high-Fowler's position
4. Monitor airway patency and provide frequent **suctioning** to remove bloody secretions
5. Maintain mechanical ventilator support or a **tracheostomy** collar with humidification as prescribed
6. Maintain surgical drains in the neck area if present
7. Observe for hemorrhage and edema in the neck
8. Administer oxygen via high humidity **tracheostomy** mask as prescribed
9. Monitor pulse oximetry
10. Monitor the color, amount, and consistency of sputum
11. Monitor IV fluids or total parenteral nutrition until nutrition is administered via a nasogastric, gastrostomy, or jejunostomy tube
12. Assess gag and cough reflex and ability to swallow
13. Provide oral hygiene
14. Provide stoma and laryngectomy care
15. Increase intake of fluids
16. Increase activity as tolerated
17. Provide consultation with speech and language pathologist as prescribed
18. Prepare the client for rehabilitation and speech therapy through the use of an artificial larynx followed by esophageal speech
19. Reinforce method of communication established preoperatively

D. Client education
1. Teach clean **suctioning** technique
2. Instruct client how to clean incision and provide stoma care
3. Protect neck from injury
4. Avoid swimming, showering, and using aerosol sprays
5. Demonstrate ways to prevent debris from entering the stoma
6. Instruct the client to wear a stoma guard to shield the stoma
7. Advise the client to wear loose-fitting, high-collar clothing to hide the stoma
8. Advise the client to increase humidity in the home
9. Instruct in ROM exercises for arms, shoulders, and neck daily

10. Avoid exposure to people with infections
11. Alternate rest periods with activity
12. Increase fluid intake to 3000 mL per day
13. Advise the client to obtain a Medic-Alert bracelet

XXI. CARBON MONOXIDE POISONING (REFER TO CHAPTER 38 FOR INFORMATION ON CARBON MONOXIDE POISONING.)

XXII. HISTOPLASMOSIS

A. Description
   1. A pulmonary fungal infection caused by spores of *Histoplasma capsulatum*
   2. Transmission occurs by the inhalation of spores, which are commonly located in contaminated soil
   3. Spores are also usually found in bird droppings

B. Data collection
   1. Dyspnea
   2. Chills
   3. Chest pain
   4. Elevated temperature
   5. Pulmonary infiltrates on chest x-ray
   6. Elevated WBC count
   7. Positive skin test
   8. Positive agglutination test
   9. Splenomegaly
   10. Hepatomegaly

C. Implementation
   1. Administer oxygen as prescribed
   2. Administer antiemetics, antihistamines, antipyretics, and steroids as prescribed
   3. Administer fungicidal medications as prescribed
   4. Encourage coughing and deep breathing
   5. Place client in semi-Fowler's position
   6. Monitor vital signs
   7. Monitor respiratory status
   8. Monitor for nephrotoxicity from fungicidal medications
   9. Instruct client to spray area with water before sweeping barn and chicken coups

XXIII. SARCOIDOSIS

A. Description
   1. Epithelioid cell tubercles in lung
   2. Cause is unknown
   3. High titer of Epstein-Barr may be identified
   4. Virus incidence is highest in blacks and young adults

B. Data collection
   1. Night sweats
   2. Fever
   3. Weight loss
   4. Cough
   5. Nodules on face
   6. Polyarthritis
   7. Kveim test: carcoid node antigen is injected intradermally and causes local nodular lesion in approximately 1 month

C. Implementation
   1. Administer corticosteroids as prescribed to control symptoms
   2. Monitor temperature
   3. Increase fluid intake
   4. Provide frequent periods of rest
   5. Provide small nutritious meals

XXIV. OCCUPATIONAL LUNG DISEASE (SILICOSIS)

A. Description
   1. Known as asbestosis and coal workers' pneumoconiosis
   2. Fibrotic disease of lungs caused by inhalation of inorganic dusts over long periods
   3. Common in miners and sandblasters
   4. Tuberculosis (TB) is frequent complication

B. Data collection
   1. Frequent respiratory infections
   2. Blood-streaked sputum
   3. Cough
   4. Nodular lesions in lungs seen on chest x-ray film

C. Implementation
   1. Administer antitussive as prescribed for cough
   2. Administer medications for TB as prescribed
   3. Eliminate toxic substances
   4. Administer oxygen as prescribed
   5. Encourage coughing and deep breathing

XXV. TUBERCULOSIS (TB)

A. Description
   1. A highly communicable disease caused by ***Mycobacterium tuberculosis***
   2. ***M. tuberculosis*** is a nonmotile, nonsporulating, acid-fast rod that secrets niacin; and when the bacillus reaches a susceptible site, it multiplies freely
   3. Because ***M. tuberculosis*** is an aerobic bacterium, it primarily affects the pulmonary system, especially the upper lobes where the oxygen content is greatest, but can also affect other areas of the body such as the brain, intestines, peritoneum, kidney, joints, and liver
   4. An exudative-type response causes a nonspecific pneumonitis and the development of granulomas in the lung tissue

5. **TB** has an insidious onset, and many clients are not aware of symptoms until the disease is well advanced
6. **A multidrug-resistant strain (MDR-TB)** of **TB** can exist as a result of improper or noncompliant use of treatment programs and the development of mutations in the tubercle bacilli
7. The goal of treatment is to prevent transmission, control symptoms, and prevent progression of the disease

B. Risk factors
1. Alcoholism
2. Intravenous drug use
3. Malnutrition
4. Infection
5. The elderly
6. The homeless
7. Refugees
8. Minority groups
9. Individuals from a lower socioeconomic group
10. Children younger than 5 years
11. Individuals living in crowded areas, such as long-term care facilities, prisons, and mental health facilities
12. Individuals in constant, frequent contact with an untreated or undiagnosed individual
13. Individuals with immune dysfunction, human immunodeficiency virus (HIV), or who are immunosuppressed from medication therapy
14. Drinking unpasteurized milk if the cows are infected with bovine **TB**

C. Transmission
1. Via aerosolization or airborne route by droplet infection
2. When an infected individual coughs, laughs, sneezes, or sings, droplet nuclei containing **TB** bacteria enter the air and may be inhaled by others
3. Identification of those individuals in close contact with the infected individual is important so that they can be tested and treated as necessary
4. When contacts have been identified, these people are assessed with a tuberculin test and chest x-ray study to determine infection with **TB**
5. After the infected individual has received **TB** medication for 2 to 3 weeks, the risk of transmission is greatly reduced

D. Disease progression
1. Droplets enter the lungs and the bacteria form a tubercle lesion
2. The body's defense systems encapsulate the tubercle, leaving a scar
3. If encapsulation does not occur, bacteria may enter the lymph system, travel to the lymph nodes, and cause an inflammatory response called granulomatous inflammation
4. Primary lesions form; the primary lesions may become dormant, but can be reactivated and become a secondary infection when reexposed to the bacterium
5. In an active phase, **TB** can cause necrosis and cavitation in the lesions, leading to rupture and the spread of necrotic tissue, and damage to various parts of the body

E. Client history
1. Past exposure to **TB**
2. Client's country of origin and travel to foreign countries in which there is a high incidence of **TB**
3. Recent history of influenza, pneumonia, febrile illness, cough, and foul-smelling sputum production
4. Previous tests for **TB** and what the results were
5. Recent **bacille Calmette-Guérin (BCG) vaccine** (a vaccine containing attenuated tubercle bacilli that may be given to people in foreign countries or to persons traveling to foreign countries to produce increased resistance to **TB**)
6. An individual who has received **BCG** will have a positive skin test and should be evaluated for **TB** with a chest x-ray study

F. Clinical manifestations
1. May be asymptomatic in primary infection
2. Fatigue
3. Lethargy
4. Anorexia
5. Weight loss
6. Low-grade fever
7. Chills
8. Night sweats
9. Persistent cough and the production of mucoid and mucopurulent sputum, which is occasionally streaked with blood
10. Chest tightness and a dull, aching chest pain may accompany the cough

G. Chest assessment
1. A physical examination of the chest does not provide conclusive evidence of **TB**
2. Chest x-ray study is not definitive, but the presence of multinodular infiltrates with calcification in the upper lobes suggests **TB**
3. If the disease is active, caseation and inflammation may be seen on the chest x-ray film

4. Advanced disease
   a. Dullness with percussion over involved parenchymal areas, bronchial breath sounds, rhonchi, and/or crackles
   b. Partial obstruction of a bronchus, caused by endobronchial disease or compression by lymph nodes, may produce localized wheezing and dyspnea

H. Sputum cultures
1. Sputum specimens are obtained for an acid-fast smear
2. A sputum culture identifying *M. tuberculosis* confirms the diagnosis
3. After medications are started, sputum samples are obtained again to determine the effectiveness of therapy
4. Most clients have negative cultures after 3 months of compliance to medication therapy

I. **Mantoux Test**
1. The most reliable determinant of infection with **TB**
2. A positive reaction does not mean that active disease is present but indicates exposure to **TB** or the presence of inactive (dormant) disease
3. Once the test result is positive, it will be positive in any future tests
4. A small amount (0.1 mL) of intermediate-strength purified protein derivative (PPD) containing 5 tuberculin units is administered intradermally in the forearm
5. An area of induration measuring 10 mm or more in diameter, 48 to 72 hours after injection, indicates the individual has been exposed to **TB**
6. For individuals with HIV or who are immunosuppressed, a reaction of 5 mm or greater is considered positive
7. Once an individual's skin test is positive, a chest x-ray study is necessary to rule out active **TB** or to detect old, healed lesions

J. The hospitalized client
1. The client with active **TB** is placed in respiratory isolation precautions in a well-ventilated room
2. The room should have at least six exchanges of fresh air per hour and should be ventilated to the outside environment if possible
3. The nurse wears a particulate respirator (a special individually fitted mask) when caring for the client and a gown when there is a possibility of contamination of clothing
4. Hands are always thoroughly washed before and after caring for the client
5. If the client needs to leave the room for a test or procedure, the client is required to wear a mask
6. Isolation is discontinued when the client is no longer considered infectious
7. After the infected individual has received **TB** medication for 2 to 3 weeks, the risk of transmission is greatly reduced
8. When the results of three sputum cultures are negative, the client is no longer considered infectious

K. The client at home
1. Provide the client and family with information about **TB** and allay concerns about the contagious aspect of the infection
2. Instruct the client to follow the medication regimen exactly as prescribed and always to have a supply of the medication on hand
3. Advise the client of the side effects of the medication and ways of minimizing them to ensure compliance
4. Reassure the client that after 2 to 3 weeks of medication therapy, it is unlikely that the client will infect anyone
5. Inform the client that activities should be resumed gradually
6. Instruct the client about the need for adequate nutrition and a well-balanced diet to promote healing and to prevent recurrence of infection
7. Instruct the client to increase foods rich in iron, protein, and vitamin C
8. Inform the client and family that respiratory isolation is not necessary because family members have already been exposed
9. Instruct the client to cover the mouth and nose when coughing or sneezing and to confine used tissues to plastic bags
10. Instruct the client and family about thorough handwashing
11. Inform the client that a sputum culture is needed every 2 to 4 weeks once medication therapy is initiated
12. Inform the client that when the results of three sputum cultures are negative, the client is no longer considered infectious and can usually return to their former employment
13. Advise the client to avoid excessive exposure to silicone or dust because these substances can cause further lung damage
14. Instruct the client regarding the importance of compliance to treatment, follow-up care, and sputum cultures as prescribed

L. Medications to treat TB (refer to Chapter 47)

PRACTICE QUESTIONS

1. A nurse is assisting in planning care for a client scheduled for insertion of a tracheostomy. What

equipment would the nurse plan to have at the bedside when the client returns from surgery?
1 Oral airway
2. Epinephrine
3. Obturator
4. Tracheostomy tube with the next larger size

2. A nursing instructor is observing a nursing student suctioning a client through a tracheostomy tube. Which of the following observations, if made by the instructor, would indicate an inappropriate action?
1. Hyperventilating the client with 100% oxygen before suctioning
2. Instilling 3 to 5 mL normal saline in the tracheotomy tube to loosen secretions
3. Applying suction during insertion of the catheter
4. Applying suction during withdrawal of the catheter

3. A nurse is caring for a client with an endotracheal tube attached to a ventilator. The high-pressure alarm sounds on the ventilator. The nurse prepares to perform which of the following most appropriate nursing intervention?
1. Check for a disconnection
2. Evaluate the tube cuff for a leak
3. Notify the respiratory therapist
4. Suction the client

4. A nurse is preparing to obtain a sputum specimen from the client. Which of the following nursing actions will facilitate obtaining the specimen?
1. Limiting fluids
2. Having the client take three deep breaths
3. Ask the client to spit into the collection container
4. Ask the client to obtain the specimen after eating

5. A nurse is caring for a client after a bronchoscopy and biopsy. Which of the following signs, if noted in the client, should be reported immediately?
1. Blood-streaked sputum
2. Dry cough
3. Hematuria
4. Laryngeal stridor

6. A nurse is suctioning a client via a tracheostomy tube. When suctioning, the nurse must limit the suctioning to a maximum of:
1. 5 seconds
2. 15 seconds
3. 30 seconds
4. 1 minute

7. A nurse is suctioning a client through an endotracheal tube. During the suctioning procedure the nurse notes cardiac irregularities on the monitor. Which of the following is the most appropriate nursing intervention?
1. Continue to suction
2. Ensure that the suction is limited to 15 seconds
3. Stop the procedure and reoxygenate the client
4. Notify the physician immediately

8. A nurse is preparing for removal of an endotracheal tube (ET) from a client. In preparing to assist the physician in this procedure, which initial nursing action is most appropriate?
1. Suction the ET tube
2. Deflate the cuff
3. Turn the ventilator to the off position
4. Obtain a code cart and place it at the bedside

9. A nurse is preparing to care for a client who will be weaned from a cuffed tracheostomy tube. The nurse is planning to use a tracheostomy plug and plans to insert it into the opening in the outer cannula. Which nursing intervention is required before plugging the tube?
1. Suctioning the client
2. Deflating the cuff
3. Ensuring that the client is able to swallow
4. Ensuring that the client is able to speak

10. A nurse is caring for a client with a chest tube drainage system. The nurse notes a fluctuating water level on inspiration and expiration in the submerged tube in the water seal chamber of the chest tube system. Which nursing action is most appropriate?
1. No action is necessary
2. Encourage coughing and deep breathing
3. Suction the client
4. Increase the suction

11. An emergency room nurse is caring for a client who sustained a blunt injury to the chest wall. Which of the following signs, if noted in the client, would indicate the presence of a pneumothorax?
1. Bradypnea
2. Shortness of breath
3. A low respiratory rate
4. The presence of a barrel chest

12. An oxygen delivery system is prescribed for a client with chronic airflow limitation (CAL) in order to deliver a precise oxygen concentration. Which of the following types of oxygen delivery systems would the nurse anticipate to be prescribed?
1. Venturi mask
2. Aerosol mask
3. Face tent
4. Tracheostomy collar

13. Theophylline (Theo-Dur) tablets are prescribed for a client with chronic airflow limitation (CAL), and the nurse reinforces instructions with the client about the medication. Which statement by the client indicates a need for further instructions?
1. "I need to take the medication on an empty stomach."
2. "I need to take the medication with food."
3. "I need to continue to take the medication even if I am feeling better."
4. "Periodic blood levels will need to be obtained."

14. A nurse is reinforcing instructions with a hospitalized client with a diagnosis of emphysema about positions that will enhance the effectiveness of breathing during dyspneic periods. Which of the following positions will the nurse instruct the client to assume?
   1. Side lying in bed
   2. Sitting in a recliner chair
   3. Sitting up in bed
   4. Sitting on the side of the bed leaning on an overbed table
15. A nurse is gathering data on a client with a diagnosis of tuberculosis (TB). The nurse reviews the results of which of the following diagnostic tests that will confirm this diagnosis?
   1. Bronchoscopy
   2. Chest x-ray study
   3. Sputum culture
   4. Tuberculin skin test
16. A nursing instructor asks a nursing student to describe the route of transmission of tuberculosis (TB). The nursing instructor determines that the student understands this route of transmission if the student states that TB is transmitted by:
   1. The airborne route
   2. Blood and body fluids
   3. The enteric route
   4. Hand to mouth
17. A nurse is caring for a client with emphysema who is receiving oxygen. The nurse checks the oxygen flow rate to ensure that it does not exceed:
   1. 1 liter per minute
   2. 3 liters per minute
   3. 6 liters per minute
   4. 10 liters per minute
18. A nurse is instructing a client about pursed-lip breathing, and the client asks the nurse about its purpose. The nurse tells the client that the primary purpose of pursed-lip breathing is to:
   1. Promote oxygen intake
   2. Strengthen the diaphragm
   3. Strengthen the intercostal muscles
   4. Promote carbon dioxide elimination
19. The low pressure alarm sounds on the ventilator. The nurse checks the client and then attempts to determine the cause of the alarm but is unsuccessful. Which initial action will the nurse take?
   1. Check the client's vital signs
   2. Ventilate the client manually
   3. Administer oxygen
   4. Start cardiopulmonary resuscitation (CPR)
20. A client is receiving isoetharine hydrochloride (Bronkosol) using a nebulizer. The nurse monitors for which side effect of this medication?
   1. Constipation
   2. Diarrhea
   3. Bradycardia
   4. Tachycardia
21. A nurse is caring for a client who is on strict bed rest. The nurse assists in developing a plan of care and suggests goals related to the prevention of deep vein thrombosis (DVT) and pulmonary emboli. Which of the following nursing actions would be most helpful to prevent these disorders from developing?
   1. Applying a heating pad to the lower extremities
   2. Active range of motion (ROM) exercises
   3. Placing a pillow under the knees
   4. Restricting fluids
22. A client is suspected of having a pulmonary emboli (PE). The nurse understands that which of the following is not a common clinical manifestation of PE?
   1. Decreased respirations
   2. Tachypnea
   3. Dyspnea
   4. Chest pain
23. A nurse has taught a client about the use of a respiratory inhaler. Which statement by the client indicates a need for further teaching?
   1. "I need to remove the cap and shake the inhaler well before use."
   2. "I need to press the canister down with my finger as I breath in."
   3. "I need to inhale the mist and quickly exhale."
   4. "I need to wait 1 minute between puffs if more than one puff has been prescribed."
24. A nurse is assigned to care for a client after a left pneumonectomy. The nurse would avoid positioning the client:
   1. On the side
   2. In semi-Fowler's
   3. In low-Fowler's
   4. With the head of the bed elevated 40 degrees
25. A nurse is performing nasotracheal suctioning of a client. The nurse interprets that the client is adequately tolerating the procedure if which of the following observations is made?
   1. Secretions are becoming bloody
   2. Heart rate decreases from 78 to 54 beats per minute
   3. Coughing occurs with suctioning
   4. Skin color becomes cyanotic
26. A nurse is monitoring the function of a client's chest tube that is attached to a Pleurevac drainage system. The nurse notes that the fluid in the water seal chamber rises with inspiration and falls with expiration. The nurse interprets that:
   1. The client has residual pneumothorax
   2. The system is patent
   3. Suction should be added to the system
   4. There is a leak in the system

27. A client has a chest tube attached to a Pleurevac drainage system. As part of routine nursing care, the nurse would ensure that:
    1. The connection between the chest tube and the drainage system is taped, and that an occlusive dressing is maintained at the insertion site
    2. The amount of chest tube drainage is noted and recorded every 24 hours in the client's record
    3. The suction control chamber has sterile water added every shift and that the system is kept below waist level
    4. The water seal chamber has continuous bubbling and that monitoring for crepitus is done once a shift
28. A female client is scheduled to have a chest x-ray study. Which of the following questions is of most importance to the nurse during data collection with this client?
    1. "Is there any possibility that you could be pregnant?"
    2. "Are you wearing any metal chains or jewelry?"
    3. "Can you hold your breath easily?"
    4. "Are you able to hold your arms above your head?"
29. A nurse is caring for a client after pulmonary angiography via catheter insertion into the left groin. The nurse monitors for an allergic reaction to the contrast medium by noting the presence of:
    1. Hematoma in the left groin
    2. Discomfort in the left groin
    3. Stridor
    4. Hypothermia
30. A nurse is teaching the client with chronic respiratory failure how to use a metered dose inhaler correctly. The nurse instructs the client to:
    1. Inhale through the nose
    2. Inhale quickly
    3. Take two inhalations during one breath
    4. Hold the breath after inhalation
31. A nurse is caring for a client who is suspected of having lung cancer. The nurse monitors the client for which most frequent early sign of lung cancer?
    1. Blood-streaked sputum
    2. Cough
    3. Wheezing
    4. Pleuritic pain
32. A nurse is caring for a client who has had a pulmonary resection. The nurse avoids which least effective method of splinting the client's incision for coughing and deep breathing?
    1. Applies firm, even pressure to the incision after a deep breath and before a cough
    2. Applies firm pressure with the hands to the incision before the client takes a deep breath to cough
    3. Has the client hold a pillow firmly against the incision during a cough
    4. Puts support under the incision during a cough
33. A client who has had a radical neck dissection begins to hemorrhage at the incision site. Which of the following actions by the nurse would be contraindicated?
    1. Lowering the head of the bed to a flat position
    2. Applying manual pressure over the site
    3. Monitoring the client's airway
    4. Calling the physician immediately
34. A nurse is reinforcing discharge instructions to the client with pulmonary sarcoidosis. The nurse determines that the client understands the information if the client verbalizes to report which early sign of exacerbation?
    1. Fever
    2. Weight loss
    3. Fatigue
    4. Shortness of breath
35. A nurse working on a respiratory nursing unit is caring for several clients with respiratory disorders. The nurse would identify which of the following clients as being at the least risk for infection with tuberculosis?
    1. A woman newly immigrated from Korea
    2. An uninsured man who is homeless
    3. An elderly woman admitted from a long-term care facility
    4. A man who is an inspector for the United States Postal Service
36. A nurse is reading the results of a Mantoux skin test on a client with no documented health problems. The site has no induration and a 1 mm area of ecchymosis. The nurse interprets that the result is:
    1. Positive
    2. Negative
    3. Uncertain
    4. Borderline
37. A nurse reads a client's Mantoux skin test as positive. The nurse notes that previous tests were negative. The client becomes upset and asks the nurse what this means. The nurse's response is based on the understanding that the client has:
    1. No evidence of tuberculosis
    2. Systemic tuberculosis
    3. Pulmonary tuberculosis
    4. Exposure to tuberculosis
38. A nurse is caring for a client who had a Mantoux skin test implanted 48 hours ago on admission to the nursing unit. The nurse reads the result as positive. Which of the following actions by the nurse has the highest priority?
    1. Report the findings
    2. Call the radiology department for a chest x-ray study
    3. Document the finding in the client's record
    4. Call the employee health service department

39. A nurse is caring for a client with tuberculosis who is fearful of the disease and anxious about the prognosis. In planning nursing care, the nurse would incorporate which of the following as the best strategy to assist the client in coping with the disease?
    1. Encourage the client to visit with the pastoral care department chaplain
    2. Ask family members if they wish a psychiatric consult
    3. Provide reassurance that continued compliance with medication therapy is the most proactive way to cope with the disease
    4. Allow the client to deal with the disease in an individual fashion
40. A nurse has instructed a client diagnosed with tuberculosis (TB) about how to prevent the spread of infection after discharge. The nurse determines that the client needs further reinforcement of information if the client makes which of the following statements?
    1. "It's very important to wash my hands after I touch my mask, tissues, or body fluids."
    2. "I should cough into tissues and throw them away carefully."
    3. "It's important to cover my mouth if I laugh, sneeze, or cough."
    4. "I should use disposable plates, forks, and knives."
41. A nurse is caring for the client diagnosed with tuberculosis (TB). Which of the following findings, if made by the nurse, would not be consistent with the usual clinical presentation of tuberculosis?
    1. Nonproductive or productive cough
    2. Anorexia and weight loss
    3. Chills and night sweats
    4. High-grade fever
42. A client being discharged from the hospital to home with a diagnosis of tuberculosis (TB) is worried about the possibility of infecting the family and others. The nurse interprets that the client would get the most reassurance from the knowledge that:
    1. The family does not need therapy, and the client will not be contagious after 1 month of medication therapy
    2. The family does not need therapy, and the client will not be contagious after 6 consecutive weeks of medication therapy
    3. The family will receive prophylactic therapy, and the client will not be contagious after 1 continuous week of medication therapy
    4. The family will be treated prophylactically, and the client will not be contagious after 2 to 3 consecutive weeks of medication therapy
43. A client diagnosed with tuberculosis (TB) is distressed over the loss of physical stamina and fatigue. The nurse plans to teach the client that this is:
    1. A short-lived problem, which should be gone within 1 week of medication therapy
    2. An unexpected finding with TB, but it should resolve within a month or so
    3. Expected, and the client should very gradually increase activity as tolerated
    4. Expected, and will last for at least a year
44. A nurse is teaching a client with tuberculosis (TB) about dietary elements that should be increased in the diet. The nurse suggests that the client increase the intake of:
    1. Meats and citrus fruits
    2. Grains and broccoli
    3. Eggs and spinach
    4. Potatoes and fish
45. A nurse has reinforced discharge teaching with a client who was diagnosed with tuberculosis (TB). The client has been on medication for a week and a half. The nurse evaluates that the client has understood the information if the client makes which of the following statements?
    1. "I need to continue medication therapy for 2 months."
    2. "I should not be contagious after 2 to 3 weeks of medication therapy."
    3. "I can't shop at the mall for the next 6 months."
    4. "I can return to work if a sputum culture comes back negative."
46. A client with tuberculosis asks a nurse about precautions to take after discharge from the hospital to prevent infection of others. The nurse develops a response to the client's question based on the understanding that:
    1. The client should maintain enteric precautions only
    2. The disease is transmitted by droplet nuclei
    3. Clothing and sheets should be bleached after each use
    4. Deep pile carpet should be removed from the home
47. A nurse is preparing to give a bed bath to the immobilized client with tuberculosis (TB). The nurse should plan to wear which of the following items when performing this care?
    1. Particulate respirator mask, gown, and gloves
    2. Particulate respirator and protective eyewear
    3. Surgical mask and gloves
    4. Surgical mask, gown, and protective eyewear
48. A client with tuberculosis (TB), whose status is being monitored in an ambulatory care clinic, asks the nurse when it is permissible to return to work.

The nurse replies that the client may resume employment when:
1. Three sputum cultures are negative
2. Five sputum cultures are negative
3. A sputum culture and a chest x-ray study are negative
4. A sputum culture and a Mantoux test are negative

49. A client is to begin a 6-month course of therapy with isoniazid (INH). The nurse teaches the client to:
1. Use alcohol in small amounts only
2. Report yellow eyes or skin immediately
3. Increase intake of Swiss or aged cheeses
4. Avoid vitamin supplements during therapy

50. A client has been started on long-term therapy with rifampin (Rifadin). The nurse teaches the client that the medication:
1. Should be double dosed if one dose is forgotten
2. May be discontinued independently if symptoms are gone in 3 months
3. Causes orange discoloration of sweat, tears, urine, and feces
4. Should always be taken with food or antacids

ANSWERS

1. *Answer:* 3
Rationale: A replacement tracheostomy tube of the same size and an obturator are kept at the bedside at all times in case the tracheostomy tube is dislodged. Additionally, a curved hemostat that could be used to hold the trachea open if dislodgement occurs should also be kept at the bedside. An oral airway and epinephrine would not be needed.
Test-Taking Strategy: Use the process of elimination. Eliminate option 4 first because a tracheostomy tube of the next larger size would not be appropriate for the client. Next eliminate option 2 because it is unrelated to the issue of the question. From the remaining options, recall that the airway has been altered because of the tracheostomy, so an oral airway would not be necessary. Remember that a replacement tracheostomy tube, an obturator, and a curved hemostat should be kept at the bedside of a client with a tracheostomy. Review care to the client with a tracheostomy if you had difficulty with this question.
Level of Cognitive Ability: Application
Client Needs: Physiological Integrity
Integrated Concept/Process: Nursing Process/Planning
Content Area: Adult Health/Respiratory
Reference: DeWit S: *Fundamental concepts and skills for nursing*, Philadelphia, 2001, WB Saunders, p. 537.

2. *Answer:* 3
Rationale: The client should be hyperoxygenated with 100% oxygen before suctioning and if tracheal secretions are thick and not easily removed. A total of 3 to 5 mL of sterile normal saline may be instilled into the trachea (per agency policy) to try to reduce the viscosity of the secretions and stimulate coughing. Suction is not applied during insertion of the catheter, and intermittent suction and a twirling motion of the catheter are used during withdrawal.
Test-Taking Strategy: Use the process of elimination and note the key words "inappropriate action." Visualize the procedure and think about the mechanical trauma that suctioning can cause to the tissues. This will direct you to option 3. Review this procedure if you had difficulty with this question.
Level of Cognitive Ability: Comprehension
Client Needs: Physiological Integrity
Integrated Concept/Process: Teaching/Learning
Content Area: Adult Health/Respiratory
Reference: DeWit S: *Fundamental concepts and skills for nursing*, Philadelphia, 2001, WB Saunders, p. 537.

3. *Answer:* 4
Rationale: When the high-pressure alarm sounds on a ventilator, it is most likely due to an obstruction. The obstruction can be caused by the client biting on the tube, kinking of the tubing, or mucus plugging requiring suctioning. It is also important to check the tubing for the presence of any water and determine if the client is out of rhythm with breathing with the ventilator. A disconnection or a cuff leak can cause sounding of the low pressure alarm. The respiratory therapist would be notified if the nurse could not determine the cause of the alarm.
Test-Taking Strategy: Use the process of elimination. Note the key words "high pressure alarm" in the question. Recalling that that the high-pressure alarm indicates a possible obstruction will assist in directing you to the correct option. Review nursing interventions related to care of a client on a ventilator if you had difficulty with this question.
Level of Cognitive Ability: Application
Client Needs: Physiological Integrity
Integrated Concept/Process: Nursing Process/Implementation
Content Area: Adult Health/Respiratory
Reference: Ignatavicius D, Workman M: *Medical-surgical: critical thinking for collaborative care*, ed 4, Philadelphia, 2002, WB Saunders, p. 609.

4. *Answer:* 2
Rationale: To obtain a sputum specimen, the client should brush his or her teeth to reduce mouth contamination. The client should then take three breaths and cough into a sputum specimen container. The client should be encouraged to cough and not spit so as to obtain sputum. Sputum can be thinned by fluids or by a respiratory treatment, such as inhalation of nebulized saline or water. The optimal time to obtain a specimen is on arising in the morning.
Test-Taking Strategy: Use the process of elimination. Option 1 can be eliminated first recalling that fluids assist in loosening or thinning secretions. Eliminate option 3 because of the word "spit." Spit is very different from saliva. Next eliminate option 4 because of the words "after eating." Review this procedure if you had difficulty with this question.

Level of Cognitive Ability: Application
Client Needs: Physiological Integrity
Integrated Concept/Process: Nursing Process/Implementation
Content Area: Adult Health/Respiratory
Reference: Ignatavicius D, Workman M: *Medical-surgical: critical thinking for collaborative care*, ed 4, Philadelphia, 2002, WB Saunders, p. 482.

5. *Answer:* 4
Rationale: If a biopsy was performed during a bronchoscopy, blood-streaked sputum is expected for several hours. Frank blood is indicative of hemorrhage. A dry cough may be expected. The client should be assessed for signs of complications, which can include cyanosis, dyspnea, stridor, hemoptysis, hypotension, tachycardia, and dysrhythmias. Hematuria is unrelated to this procedure.
Test-Taking Strategy: Use the process of elimination. Eliminate option 3 first because it is unrelated to the procedure. Next eliminate option 2 because a dry cough may be expected. Noting that a biopsy has been performed will assist in eliminating option 1 because blood-streaked sputum would be expected. Note that option 4, the correct option, relates to airway. If you had difficulty with this question, review postprocedure care after bronchoscopy with biopsy.
Level of Cognitive Ability: Analysis
Client Needs: Physiological Integrity
Integrated Concept/Process: Nursing Process/Data Collection
Content Area: Adult Health/Respiratory
Reference: Ignatavicius D, Workman M: *Medical-surgical: critical thinking for collaborative care*, ed 4, Philadelphia, 2002, WB Saunders, p. 486.

6. *Answer:* 2
Rationale: Hypoxemia can be caused by prolonged suctioning from stimulation of the pacemaker cells within the heart. A vasovagal response may occur causing bradycardia. The suctioning pass is limited to 15 seconds and the client is preoxygenated before suctioning.
Test-Taking Strategy: Use the process of elimination. Recall that during suctioning, the client's airway is blocked; therefore you should be able to eliminate options 3 and 4 easily. From the remaining options, eliminate option 1 because of the very short time frame. It does not seem reasonable that removal of secretions could be achieved in 5 seconds. Review the procedure for suctioning if you had difficulty with this question.
Level of Cognitive Ability: Application
Client Needs: Physiological Integrity
Integrated Concept/Process: Nursing Process/Implementation
Content Area: Adult Health/Respiratory
Reference: DeWit S: *Fundamental concepts and skills for nursing*, Philadelphia, 2001, WB Saunders, p. 537.

7. *Answer:* 3
Rationale: During suctioning, the nurse should monitor the client closely for side effects including hypoxemia, cardiac irregularities resulting from vagal stimulation, mucosal trauma, hypotension, and paroxysmal coughing. If side effects develop, especially cardiac irregularities, the procedure is stopped and the client is oxygenated.
Test-Taking Strategy: Use the process of elimination recalling that suction can cause cardiac irregularities. This principle should easily direct you to option 3. If you had difficulty with this question, review the complications and interventions associated with suctioning procedure.
Level of Cognitive Ability: Application
Client Needs: Physiological Integrity
Integrated Concept/Process: Nursing Process/Implementation
Content Area: Adult Health/Respiratory
Reference: DeWit S: *Fundamental concepts and skills for nursing*, Philadelphia, 2001, WB Saunders, p. 538.

8. *Answer:* 1
Rationale: Once the client has been weaned successfully and has achieved an acceptable level of consciousness to sustain spontaneous respiration, an ET tube may be removed. The ET tube is suctioned first and then the cuff is deflated and the tube is removed. There is no reason to have a code cart placed at the bedside. This may cause alarm and concern in the client. Additionally, the necessary resuscitative equipment should have already been at the client's bedside.
Test-Taking Strategy: Use the process of elimination and note the key word "initial" in the stem of the question. Remember airway is the first priority. Review the procedure for removal of an ET tube if you had difficulty with this question.
Level of Cognitive Ability: Application
Client Needs: Physiological Integrity
Integrated Concept/Process: Nursing Process/Implementation
Content Area: Adult Health/Respiratory
Reference: DeWit S: *Fundamental concepts and skills for nursing*, Philadelphia, 2001, WB Saunders, p. 528.

9. *Answer:* 2
Rationale: A tracheostomy tube is usually plugged by inserting the tracheostomy plug (decannulation stopper) into the opening of the outer cannula. This closes off the tracheostomy, allowing air flow and respiration to occur normally through the nose and mouth. Before plugging a cuffed tracheostomy tube, the cuff must be deflated. If it remains inflated, ventilation cannot occur and respiratory arrest could result.
Test-Taking Strategy: Focus on the issue, plugging the tracheostomy tube. Also note that the client has a cuffed tube. This will direct you to option 2. Review this procedure if you had difficulty with this question.
Level of Cognitive Ability: Application
Client Needs: Physiological Integrity
Integrated Concept/Process: Nursing Process/Implementation
Content Area: Adult Health/Respiratory
Reference: DeWit S: *Fundamental concepts and skills for nursing*, Philadelphia, 2001, WB Saunders, p. 536.

10. *Answer:* 1
Rationale: With normal breathing, the water level rises with inspiration and falls with expiration. The opposite, falls with inspiration and rises with expiration, occurs when the client is on positive pressure mechanical ventilation. This is an expected normal occurrence in a chest tube drainage system; therefore no action is necessary.
Test-Taking Strategy: Use the process of elimination and focus on the issue, water seal chamber. Recalling that the fluctuating

water level is expected will assist in easily directing you to option 1. Review chest tube drainage systems if you had difficulty with this question!
Level of Cognitive Ability: Application
Client Needs: Physiological Integrity
Integrated Concept/Process: Nursing Process/Implementation
Content Area: Adult Health/Respiratory
Reference: DeWit S: *Fundamental concepts and skills for nursing,* Philadelphia, 2001, WB Saunders, p. 531.

11. ***Answer:*** 2
Rationale: This client has sustained a blunt or a closed-chest injury. Basic symptoms of a closed pneumothorax are shortness of breath and chest pain. A larger pneumothorax may present with tachypnea, cyanosis, diminished breath sounds, and subcutaneous emphysema. There may also be hyperresonance on the affected side.
Test-Taking Strategy: Use the process of elimination. Option 4 can be eliminated because a barrel chest is a characteristic finding in a client with chronic obstructive pulmonary disease. Next, eliminate options 1 and 3 because they are similar. Review the signs of pneumothorax if you had difficulty with this question.
Level of Cognitive Ability: Comprehension
Client Needs: Physiological Integrity
Integrated Concept/Process: Nursing Process/Data Collection
Content Area: Adult Health/Respiratory
Reference: Ignatavicius D, Workman M: *Medical-surgical: critical thinking for collaborative care,* ed 4, Philadelphia, 2002, WB Saunders, p. 207.

12. ***Answer:*** 1
Rationale: The Venturi mask delivers the most accurate oxygen concentration. It is the best oxygen delivery system for the client with CAL because it delivers a precise oxygen concentration. The face tent, aerosol mask, and tracheostomy collar are also high flow oxygen delivery systems but are most often used to administer high humidity.
Test-Taking Strategy: Use the process of elimination and note the key words "precise oxygen concentration." Eliminate options 2, 3, and 4 because they are similar in that they are used to provide high humidity. Review these types of oxygen delivery systems if you had difficulty with this question.
Level of Cognitive Ability: Comprehension
Client Needs: Physiological Integrity
Integrated Concept/Process: Nursing Process/Planning
Content Area: Adult Health/Respiratory
Reference: Ignatavicius D, Workman M: *Medical-surgical: critical thinking for collaborative care,* ed 4, Philadelphia, 2002, WB Saunders, p. 167.

13. ***Answer:*** 1
Rationale: The medication should be administered with food such as milk and crackers to prevent gastrointestinal irritation. Options 2, 3, and 4 are appropriate instructions regarding the use of this medication.
Test-Taking Strategy: Use the process of elimination. Noting the options 1 and 2 are opposite in terms of administering the medication should alert you that one of these options is correct. From this point, knowledge regarding the administration of this medication is required to answer correctly. Review this medication if you had difficulty with this question.
Level of Cognitive Ability: Comprehension
Client Needs: Health Promotion and Maintenance
Integrated Concept/Process: Teaching/Learning
Content Area: Pharmacology
Reference: Hodgson B, Kizior R: *Saunders nursing drug handbook 2002,* Philadelphia, 2002, WB Saunders, p. 47.

14. ***Answer:*** 4
Rationale: Positions that will assist the client with breathing include sitting up and leaning on an overbed table, sitting up and resting with the elbows on the knees, or standing and leaning against the wall. The positions in options 1, 2, and 3 will not enhance the effectiveness of breathing.
Test-Taking Strategy: Use the process of elimination. Eliminate option 1 because side-lying will not promote appropriate lung expansion. Next, eliminate options 2 and 3 because they are similar. If you had difficulty with this question, review the positions that will decrease the work of breathing in a client with emphysema.
Level of Cognitive Ability: Application
Client Needs: Physiological Integrity
Integrated Concept/Process: Teaching/Learning
Content Area: Adult Health/Respiratory
Reference: Ignatavicius D, Workman M: *Medical-surgical: critical thinking for collaborative care,* ed 4, Philadelphia, 2002, WB Saunders, p. 547.

15. ***Answer:*** 3
Rationale: A definitive diagnosis of TB is confirmed through culture and isolation of *M. tuberculosis*. A presumptive diagnosis is made on the basis of a tuberculin skin test, a sputum smear that is positive for acid-fast bacteria, a chest x-ray study, and histological evidence of granulomatous disease on biopsy.
Test-Taking Strategy: Use the process of elimination and note the key word "confirm" in the stem of the question. Confirmation is made by identifying *M. tuberculosis*. If you had difficulty with this question, review the diagnostic procedures related to TB.
Level of Cognitive Ability: Application
Client Needs: Physiological Integrity
Integrated Concept/Process: Nursing Process/Data Collection
Content Area: Adult Health/Respiratory
Reference: Ignatavicius D, Workman M: *Medical-surgical: critical thinking for collaborative care,* ed 4, Philadelphia, 2002, WB Saunders, p. 585.

16. ***Answer:*** 1
Rationale: Tuberculosis is an infectious disease caused by the bacillus *M. tuberculosis* and spread primarily by the airborne route. Options 2, 3, and 4 are incorrect.
Test-Taking Strategy: Use the process of elimination. Recalling that TB is a respiratory disease should easily direct you to option 1. If you had difficulty with this question, review the transmission of this disease.
Level of Cognitive Ability: Comprehension
Client Needs: Physiological Integrity
Integrated Concept/Process: Teaching/Learning
Content Area: Adult Health/Respiratory

Reference: Ignatavicius D, Workman M: *Medical-surgical: critical thinking for collaborative care,* ed 4, Philadelphia, 2002, WB Saunders, p. 585.

17. *Answer:* 2
Rationale: Oxygen is used cautiously in the client with emphysema and should not exceed 3 liters per minute. Because of the long-standing hypercapnia that occurs in this disorder, the respiratory drive is triggered by low oxygen levels rather than increased carbon dioxide levels, which is the case in a normal respiratory system.
Test-Taking Strategy: Recalling the physiology associated with emphysema is required to answer this question. If you are unfamiliar with this disorder, review this content.
Level of Cognitive Ability: Application
Client Needs: Physiological Integrity
Integrated Concept/Process: Nursing Process/Data Collection
Content Area: Adult Health/Respiratory
Reference: Ignatavicius D, Workman M: *Medical-surgical: critical thinking for collaborative care,* ed 4, Philadelphia, 2002, WB Saunders, p. 541.

18. *Answer:* 4
Rationale: Pursed-lip breathing facilitates maximal expiration for clients with obstructive lung disease and promotes carbon dioxide elimination. This type of breathing allows better expiration by increasing airway pressure that keeps air passages open during exhalation. Options 1, 2, and 3 are not the purposes of this type of breathing.
Test-Taking Strategy: Use the process of elimination. Attempt to visualize the use of this breathing technique to assist in answering correctly. Recalling the respiratory conditions in which this type of breathing is helpful will also assist in directing you to option 4. Review the purpose of this breathing technique if you had difficulty with this question.
Level of Cognitive Ability: Application
Client Needs: Health Promotion and Maintenance
Integrated Concept/Process: Teaching/Learning
Content Area: Adult Health/Respiratory
Reference: Ignatavicius D, Workman M: *Medical-surgical: critical thinking for collaborative care,* ed 4, Philadelphia, 2002, WB Saunders, p. 547.

19. *Answer:* 2
Rationale: If at anytime an alarm is sounding and the nurse cannot quickly ascertain the problem, the client is disconnected from the ventilator and a manual resuscitation device is used to support respirations until the problem can be corrected. There is no reason to begin CPR. Checking vital signs is not the initial action. Although oxygen is helpful, it will not provide ventilation to the client.
Test-Taking Strategy: Use the process of elimination. Read the question carefully and note that the issue relates to adequate ventilation of the client. Focusing on this issue will direct you to option 2. If you are unfamiliar with the management of a client on a ventilator, review this content.
Level of Cognitive Ability: Application
Client Needs: Physiological Integrity
Integrated Concept/Process: Nursing Process/Implementation
Content Area: Adult Health/Respiratory
Reference: Ignatavicius D, Workman M: *Medical-surgical: critical thinking for collaborative care,* ed 4, Philadelphia, 2002, WB Saunders, p. 609.

20. *Answer:* 4
Rationale: Side effects that can occur from the use of this medication include tremors, nausea, nervousness, palpitations, tachycardia, peripheral vasodilation, and dryness of the mouth or throat.
Test-Taking Strategy: Use the process of elimination. Recalling that this medication causes sympathomimetic stimulation will direct you to option 4. If you are unfamiliar with the side effects related to this medication, review this content.
Level of Cognitive Ability: Application
Client Needs: Physiological Integrity
Integrated Concept/Process: Nursing Process/Data Collection
Content Area: Pharmacology
Reference: Hodgson B, Kizior R: *Saunders nursing drug handbook 2002,* Philadelphia, 2002, WB Saunders, p. 598.

21. *Answer:* 2
Rationale: Persons at greatest risk for pulmonary emboli are immobilized clients. Basic preventive measures include early ambulation, leg elevation, active leg exercises, elastic stockings, and intermittent pneumatic calf compression. Keeping the client well hydrated is essential because dehydration predisposes to clotting. A pillow under the knees may cause venous stasis. Heat should not be applied without a physician's prescription.
Test-Taking Strategy: Use the process of elimination and knowledge regarding preventive measures related to preventing DVT and pulmonary emboli to answer this question. Use basic principles related to care of the immobile client to assist in directing you to option 2. If you are unfamiliar with these basic measures, review this content.
Level of Cognitive Ability: Application
Client Needs: Physiological Integrity
Integrated Concept/Process: Nursing Process/Implementation
Content Area: Adult Health/Respiratory
Reference: Ignatavicius D, Workman M: *Medical-surgical: critical thinking for collaborative care,* ed 4, Philadelphia, 2002, WB Saunders, p. 591.

22. *Answer:* 1
Rationale: The most common clinical manifestations of PE are tachypnea, dyspnea, and chest pain.
Test-Taking Strategy: Use the process of elimination and note the key word "not" in the stem of the question. Note that options 1 and 2 address a similar manifestation but opposite effects. This may provide you with the clue that one of these options is the correct one. Remember, you would expect an increased respiratory rate in PE. Review the manifestations of PE if you had difficulty with this question.
Level of Cognitive Ability: Comprehension
Client Needs: Physiological Integrity
Integrated Concept/Process: Nursing Process/Data Collection
Content Area: Adult Health/Respiratory
Reference: Ignatavicius D, Workman M: *Medical-surgical: critical thinking for collaborative care,* ed 4, Philadelphia, 2002, WB Saunders, p. 592.

23. *Answer:* 3
Rationale: The client should be instructed to hold the breath at least 5 to 10 seconds before exhaling the mist. Options 1, 2, and 4 are accurate instructions regarding the use of the inhaler.
Test-Taking Strategy: Use the process of elimination and note the key words "need for further teaching." Visualizing this procedure will direct you to option 3. If you are unfamiliar with the client teaching points related to the use of an inhaler, review this content.
Level of Cognitive Ability: Comprehension
Client Needs: Health Promotion and Maintenance
Integrated Concept/Process: Teaching/Learning
Content Area: Adult Health/Respiratory
Reference: Ignatavicius D, Workman M: *Medical-surgical: critical thinking for collaborative care,* ed 4, Philadelphia, 2002, WB Saunders, p. 535.

24. *Answer:* 1
Rationale: Complete lateral positioning should be avoided after pneumonectomy. Because the mediastinum is no longer held in place on both sides by lung tissue, extreme turning may cause mediastinal shift and compression of the remaining lung.
Test-Taking Strategy: Use the process of elimination and note the key word "avoid." Eliminate options 2, 3, and 4 because they are similar. If you had difficulty with this question, review care to the client after pneumonectomy.
Level of Cognitive Ability: Application
Client Needs: Physiological Integrity
Integrated Concept/Process: Nursing Process/Implementation
Content Area: Adult Health/Respiratory
Reference: Ignatavicius D, Workman M: *Medical-surgical: critical thinking for collaborative care,* ed 4, Philadelphia, 2002, WB Saunders, p. 568.

25. *Answer:* 3
Rationale: The nurse monitors for the adverse effects of suctioning, which include cyanosis, excessively rapid or slow heart rate, or the sudden development of bloody secretions. If they occur, the nurse stops suctioning, and reports these signs to the physician immediately. Coughing is a normal response to suctioning for the client with an intact cough reflex, and does not indicate that the client is unable to tolerate the procedure.
Test-Taking Strategy: Use the process of elimination and note the key words "adequately tolerating." Cyanosis (option 4) and bradycardia (option 2) are abnormal findings and are eliminated first. From the remaining options, the use of the word "becoming" in association with bloody secretions tells you that this has not been an ongoing problem, making this an incorrect option also. Because the cough reflex is normally present, and suction triggers coughing, this is the preferable option. Review this procedure if you had difficulty with this question.
Level of Cognitive Ability: Analysis
Client Needs: Physiological Integrity
Integrated Concept/Process: Nursing Process/Evaluation
Content Area: Adult Health/Respiratory
Reference: DeWit S: *Fundamental concepts and skills for nursing,* Philadelphia, 2001, WB Saunders, p. 537.

26. *Answer:* 2
Rationale: When the chest tube is patent, the water in the water seal chamber rises with inspiration and falls with expiration. This is referred to as tidaling and indicates proper function of the system. Options 1, 3, and 4 are incorrect interpretations.
Test-Taking Strategy: Recalling the expected findings in a chest tube drainage system is required to answer this question. Review these expected findings if you had difficulty with this question.
Level of Cognitive Ability: Analysis
Client Needs: Physiological Integrity
Integrated Concept/Process: Nursing Process/Data Collection
Content Area: Adult Health/Respiratory
Reference: DeWit S: *Fundamental concepts and skills for nursing,* Philadelphia, 2001, WB Saunders, p. 532.

27. *Answer:* 1
Rationale: The nurse ensures that all system connections are securely taped to prevent accidental disconnection, and that an occlusive dressing is maintained at the chest tube insertion site. Drainage is noted and recorded every hour in the first 24 hours after insertion and every 8 hours thereafter. The system is kept below the level of the waist. Monitoring for crepitus is done once every 8 hours. Sterile water is added to the suction control chamber only as needed to replace evaporation losses. Continuous bubbling in the water seal chamber indicates an air leak in the system and requires immediate investigation and correction.
Test-Taking Strategy: Note that each option has two parts. For the option to be correct, both parts of the answer must be correct. Knowing this, eliminate options 3 and 4 first. Water needs to be added only as needed, and there should not be continuous bubbling in the water seal chamber. From the remaining options, recalling that chest tube assessment is done at least every 8 hours helps you to choose option 1 over option 2. Review the measures required in the care of a client with a chest tube if you had difficulty with this question.
Level of Cognitive Ability: Application
Client Needs: Physiological Integrity
Integrated Concept/Process: Nursing Process/Implementation
Content Area: Adult Health/Respiratory
Reference: DeWit S: *Fundamental concepts and skills for nursing,* Philadelphia, 2001, WB Saunders, p. 536.

28. *Answer:* 1
Rationale: The most important question to ask about is the client's pregnancy status, because pregnant women should not be exposed to radiation. Clients are also asked to remove any chains or metal objects that could interfere with obtaining an adequate film. A chest x-ray study is most often done at full inspiration, which gives optimal lung expansion. If a lateral view of the chest is ordered, the client is asked to raise the arms above the head. Most films are done in posteroanterior (PA) view.
Test-Taking Strategy: Note the key words "most important." Recalling the teratogenic effects of radiation on the fetus will

direct you to option 1. Review this procedure if you had difficulty with this question.
Level of Cognitive Ability: Application
Client Needs: Physiological Integrity
Integrated Concept/Process: Nursing Process/Data Collection
Content Area: Adult Health/Respiratory
Reference: DeWit S: *Fundamental concepts and skills for nursing*, Philadelphia, 2001, WB Saunders, p. 423.

29. *Answer:* 3
Rationale: Signs of allergic reaction to the contrast medium include localized itching and edema, respiratory distress, stridor, and decreased blood pressure. Hypothermia is an unrelated event. Discomfort is expected. Hematoma formation is a complication of the procedure, but does not indicate an allergic reaction.
Test-Taking Strategy: Use the ABCs—airway, breathing, and circulation—and focus on the issue, an allergic reaction. This will direct you to option 3. Review the signs of an allergic reaction to the contrast medium if you had difficulty with this question.
Level of Cognitive Ability: Application
Client Needs: Physiological Integrity
Integrated Concept/Process: Nursing Process/Data Collection
Content Area: Adult Health/Respiratory
Reference: Ignatavicius D, Workman M: *Medical-surgical: critical thinking for collaborative care*, ed 4, Philadelphia, 2002, WB Saunders, p. 642.

30. *Answer:* 4
Rationale: Instructions for using a metered-dose inhaler include to shake the canister, hold it right side up, inhale slowly and evenly through the mouth, deliver one spray per breath, and hold the breath after inhalation.
Test-Taking Strategy: Specific knowledge regarding the use of an inhaler is required to answer this question. Review this procedure if you had difficulty with this question.
Level of Cognitive Ability: Application
Client Needs: Health Promotion and Maintenance
Integrated Concept/Process: Teaching/Learning
Content Area: Adult Health/Respiratory
Reference: Potter P, Perry A: *Fundamentals of nursing*, ed 5, St Louis, 2001, Mosby, p. 896.

31. *Answer:* 2
Rationale: Cough is the most frequent early symptom of lung cancer, which begins as nonproductive and hacking and progresses to productive. In the smoker who already has a cough, a change in the character and frequency of the cough usually occurs. Wheezing and blood-streaked sputum are later signs. Pain is a very late sign and is usually pleuritic in nature.
Test-Taking Strategy: Use the process of elimination and note the key word "early." Focusing on the client's diagnosis, lung cancer, will direct you to option 2. Review the early signs of lung cancer if you had difficulty with this question.
Level of Cognitive Ability: Application
Client Needs: Physiological Integrity
Integrated Concept/Process: Nursing Process/Data Collection
Content Area: Adult Health/Respiratory
Reference: Ignatavicius D, Workman M: *Medical-surgical: critical thinking for collaborative care*, ed 4, Philadelphia, 2002, WB Saunders, p. 561.

32. *Answer:* 2
Rationale: The nurse avoids putting pressure on the chest during inspiration because it interferes with lung expansion. Acceptable methods of splinting include the use of the hands, a pillow, or a towel or drawsheet during a forced expiratory cough.
Test-Taking Strategy: Use the process of elimination and note the key words "least effective." Eliminate options 3 and 4 because they are similar. From the remaining options, visualize each method. This will direct you to option 2. Review splinting techniques if you had difficulty with this question.
Level of Cognitive Ability: Application
Client Needs: Physiological Integrity
Integrated Concept/Process: Nursing Process/Implementation
Content Area: Adult Health/Respiratory
Reference: Ignatavicius D, Workman M: *Medical-surgical: critical thinking for collaborative care*, ed 4, Philadelphia, 2002, WB Saunders, p. 1145.

33. *Answer:* 1
Rationale: If the client begins to hemorrhage from the surgical site after radical neck dissection, the nurse elevates the head of the bed to maintain airway patency and prevent aspiration. The nurse applies pressure over the bleeding site and calls the physician immediately.
Test-Taking Strategy: Use the process of elimination and note the key word "contraindicated." Option 1 would not maintain airway patency. Review care to the client after radical neck dissection if you had difficulty with this question.
Level of Cognitive Ability: Application
Client Needs: Physiological Integrity
Integrated Concept/Process: Nursing Process/Implementation
Content Area: Adult Health/Respiratory
Reference: Black J, Hawks J, Keene A: *Medical-surgical nursing: clinical management for positive outcomes*, ed 6, Philadelphia, 2001, WB Saunders, p. 1672.

34. *Answer:* 4
Rationale: Dry cough and dyspnea are typical signs and symptoms of pulmonary sarcoidosis. Others include chest pain, hemoptysis, and pneumothorax. Systemic signs and symptoms include weakness and fatigue, malaise, fever, and weight loss.
Test-Taking Strategy: Note the key word "early" in the stem of the question. Because sarcoidosis is a pulmonary problem, eliminate options 1 and 2 first. Choose option 4 over option 3, as the shortness of breath (and impaired ventilation) appears first and would cause the fatigue as a secondary symptom. Review this disorder if you had difficulty with this question.
Level of Cognitive Ability: Comprehension
Client Needs: Health Promotion and Maintenance
Integrated Concept/Process: Teaching/Learning
Content Area: Adult Health/Respiratory
Reference: Ignatavicius D, Workman M: *Medical-surgical: critical thinking for collaborative care*, ed 4, Philadelphia, 2002, WB Saunders, p. 556.

35. *Answer:* 4
Rationale: People at high risk for acquiring tuberculosis include immigrants from Asia, Africa, Latin America, and Oceania; medically underserved populations (ethnic minorities, homeless); those with HIV or other immunosuppressive disorders; residents in group settings (long-term care, correctional facilities); and health care workers.
Test-Taking Strategy: Use the process of elimination and note the key words "least risk." Begin to answer this question by eliminating options 1 and 2, as immigrants and the medically underserved are more frequently affected by the infection. From the remaining options, note that the postal inspector may or may not come in contact with many people, depending on job description. The client from the long-term care facility, however, lives in a group setting, where a large number of people share a common environment 24 hours a day. Review the risks associated with TB if you had difficulty with this question.
Level of Cognitive Ability: Comprehension
Client Needs: Physiological Integrity
Integrated Concept/Process: Nursing Process/Data Collection
Content Area: Adult Health/Respiratory
Reference: Ignatavicius D, Workman M: *Medical-surgical: critical thinking for collaborative care,* ed 4, Philadelphia, 2002, WB Saunders, p. 584.

36. *Answer:* 2
Rationale: A positive Mantoux reading has an induration measuring 10 mm or more. A small area of ecchymosis is insignificant and is probably related to injection technique.
Test-Taking Strategy: To answer this question accurately, it is necessary to know that induration is necessary for a positive response. Because the client in this question has no induration, the result is negative. Review Mantoux skin testing results if you had difficulty with this question.
Level of Cognitive Ability: Comprehension
Client Needs: Physiological Integrity
Integrated Concept/Process: Nursing Process/Data Collection
Content Area: Adult Health/Respiratory
Reference: DeWit S: *Fundamental concepts and skills for nursing,* Philadelphia, 2001, WB Saunders, p. 696.

37. *Answer:* 4
Rationale: A client who tests positive on a Mantoux skin test has either been exposed to tuberculosis or has inactive (dormant) tuberculosis. The client must then undergo a chest x-ray study and sputum culture to confirm the diagnosis.
Test-Taking Strategy: Use the process of elimination, eliminating options 2 and 3 first, because they are similar, both indicating the presence of TB. In selecting between options 1 and 4, review the case of the question noting that the Mantoux skin test is positive. From this information, it is best to eliminate option 1. Review this test if you had difficulty with this question.
Level of Cognitive Ability: Comprehension
Client Needs: Psychosocial Integrity
Integrated Concept/Process: Nursing Process/Implementation
Content Area: Adult Health/Respiratory
Reference: DeWit S: *Fundamental concepts and skills for nursing,* Philadelphia, 2001, WB Saunders, p. 696.

38. *Answer:* 1
Rationale: The nurse who interprets a Mantoux test as positive notifies the physician immediately. The physician would order a chest x-ray study to determine whether the client has clinically active tuberculosis (TB) or old, healed lesions. A sputum culture would be done to confirm the diagnosis of active TB. The client is placed on TB precautions prophylactically until a final diagnosis is made. The findings are documented in the client's record, but this action is not the highest priority. Calling employee health service would be of no benefit to the client.
Test-Taking Strategy: Use the process of elimination and note the key words "highest priority." Because the nurse may not order diagnostic tests, eliminate option 2 first. Likewise, option 4 can be eliminated, as calling employee health service is of no benefit to the client. From the remaining options, notifying the physician should have a higher priority than the documentation, even though they may both be done in the same narrow time period. Review nursing interventions related to Mantoux testing if you had difficulty with this question.
Level of Cognitive Ability: Application
Client Needs: Safe, Effective Care Environment
Integrated Concept/Process: Nursing Process/Implementation
Content Area: Adult Health/Respiratory
Reference: DeWit S: *Fundamental concepts and skills for nursing,* Philadelphia, 2001, WB Saunders, p. 696.

39. *Answer:* 3
Rationale: A primary role of the nurse in working with the client with tuberculosis is to teach the client about medication therapy. The anxious client may not absorb information optimally. The nurse continues to reinforce teaching using a variety of methods (repetition, teaching aids) and teaches the family about the medications as well. The most effective way of coping with the disease is to learn about the therapy, which will eradicate it. This gives the client a measure of power over the situation and outcome.
Test-Taking Strategy: Use the process of elimination. The question asks for the best strategy for coping with anxiety about the disease and its prognosis. Options 2 and 4 are the least useful options and may be eliminated first. Option 2 does not involve the client, and option 4 gives no active assistance to the client. To choose from the remaining options, recall that TB is a controllable disease and not necessarily a fatal one. Review the psychosocial issues related to TB if you had difficulty with this question.
Level of Cognitive Ability: Application
Client Needs: Psychosocial Integrity
Integrated Concept/Process: Nursing Process/Implementation
Content Area: Adult Health/Respiratory
Reference: Ignatavicius D, Workman M: *Medical-surgical: critical thinking for collaborative care,* ed 4, Philadelphia, 2002, WB Saunders, p. 588.

40. *Answer:* 4
Rationale: Because tuberculosis is transmitted by droplet, it cannot be carried on clothing, eating utensils, or other possessions. It is not necessary to discard any of these. It is important to perform proper handwashing after contact with body

substances, tissues, or face masks. The client should cover the mouth with a tissue when laughing, coughing, or sneezing and dispose of tissues carefully.
Test-Taking Strategy: Use the process of elimination. Recall that TB is an airborne disease and that organisms cannot be carried on inanimate objects. This will direct you to option 4. Review client teaching points related to the prevention of the spread of TB if you had difficulty with this question.
Level of Cognitive Ability: Comprehension
Client Needs: Safe, Effective Care Environment
Integrated Concept/Process: Nursing Process/Evaluation
Content Area: Adult Health/Respiratory
Reference: Ignatavicius D, Workman M: *Medical-surgical: critical thinking for collaborative care*, ed 4, Philadelphia, 2002, WB Saunders, p. 585.

41. ***Answer:*** 4
Rationale: The client with tuberculosis usually experiences cough (either productive or nonproductive), fatigue, anorexia, weight loss, dyspnea, hemoptysis, chest discomfort or pain, chills and sweats (which may occur at night), and a low-grade fever.
Test-Taking Strategy: Use the process of elimination. Options 1 and 2 can be eliminated first because they are symptoms that are common in the client with TB. From the remaining options, you need to know either that the client may get night sweats or that the fever is low grade. Review the clinical manifestations associated with TB if you had difficulty with this question.
Level of Cognitive Ability: Comprehension
Client Needs: Physiological Integrity
Integrated Concept/Process: Nursing Process/Data Collection
Content Area: Adult Health/Respiratory
Reference: Ignatavicius D, Workman M: *Medical-surgical: critical thinking for collaborative care*, ed 4, Philadelphia, 2002, WB Saunders, p. 585.

42. ***Answer:*** 4
Rationale: Family members or others who have been in close contact with a client diagnosed with TB are placed on prophylactic therapy with isoniazid (INH) for 6 to 12 months. The client is usually not communicable after taking medication for 2 to 3 consecutive weeks. However, the client must take the full course of therapy (for 6 months or longer) to prevent reinfection or drug-resistant TB.
Test-Taking Strategy: Use the process of elimination. Recalling that the family requires prophylactic therapy allows you to eliminate options 1 and 2. From the remaining options, it is necessary to know that the client is not contagious after 2 to 3 weeks of therapy. Review the concepts related to the prevention of the spread of TB if you had difficulty with this question.
Level of Cognitive Ability: Comprehension
Client Needs: Psychosocial Integrity
Integrated Concept/Process: Nursing Process/Planning
Content Area: Adult Health/Respiratory
Reference: Ignatavicius D, Workman M: *Medical-surgical: critical thinking for collaborative care*, ed 4, Philadelphia, 2002, WB Saunders, p. 588.

43. ***Answer:*** 3
Rationale: The client with TB has significant fatigue and loss of physical stamina. This can be very frightening for the client. The nurse teaches the client that this will resolve as the therapy progresses, and that the client should gradually increase activity as energy levels permit.
Test-Taking Strategy: Use the process of elimination. A helpful concept to remember in answering this question is that fatigue resulting from respiratory problems may not resolve easily and is an expected occurrence as a result of tissue hypoxia. Knowing this, you can eliminate options 1 and 2 first. Discriminate between options 3 and 4 in this way: since the client is on medication therapy for 6 to 9 months, or even up to 12 months, it is not reasonable that the fatigue would last for "at least a year." This will direct you to option 3. Review the manifestations associated with TB if you had difficulty with this question.
Level of Cognitive Ability: Application
Client Needs: Health Promotion and Maintenance
Integrated Concept/Process: Teaching/Learning
Content Area: Adult Health/Respiratory
Reference: Ignatavicius D, Workman M: *Medical-surgical: critical thinking for collaborative care*, ed 4, Philadelphia, 2002, WB Saunders, p. 588.

44. ***Answer:*** 1
Rationale: The nurse teaches the client with TB to increase intake of protein, iron, and vitamin C. Foods rich in vitamin C include citrus fruits, berries, melons, pineapple, broccoli, cabbage, green peppers, tomatoes, potatoes, chard, kale, asparagus, and turnip greens. Food sources that are rich in iron include liver and other meats, from which 10% to 30% of available iron is absorbed. Less than 10% of iron is absorbed from eggs, and less than 5 % is absorbed from grains and vegetables.
Test-Taking Strategy: To answer it correctly, you must recall that the diet in TB should be high in protein, vitamin C, and calories. Recalling which types of foods contain these various nutrients will direct you to option 1. If you had difficulty with this question, review these nutritional concepts.
Level of Cognitive Ability: Application
Client Needs: Health Promotion and Maintenance
Integrated Concept/Process: Nursing Process/Implementation
Content Area: Adult Health/Respiratory
Reference: Ignatavicius D, Workman M: *Medical-surgical: critical thinking for collaborative care*, ed 4, Philadelphia, 2002, WB Saunders, p. 588.

45. ***Answer:*** 2
Rationale: The client is continued on medication therapy for 6 to 12 months, depending on the situation. The client is generally considered not contagious after 2 to 3 weeks of medication therapy. The client is instructed to wear a mask if there will be exposure to crowds until the medication is effective in preventing transmission. The client is allowed to return to employment when the results of three sputum cultures are negative.
Test-Taking Strategy: Use the process of elimination. Knowing that the medication therapy lasts for at least 6 months helps you to eliminate option 1 first. Knowing that three sputum

cultures must be negative helps you to eliminate option 4 next. From the remaining options, recalling that the client is not contagious after 2 to 3 weeks of therapy helps you to choose option 2. If you had difficulty with this question, review the infectious period of TB.
Level of Cognitive Ability: Comprehension
Client Needs: Physiological Integrity
Integrated Concept/Process: Nursing Process/Evaluation
Content Area: Adult Health/Respiratory
Reference: Ignatavicius D, Workman M: *Medical-surgical: critical thinking for collaborative care*, ed 4, Philadelphia, 2002, WB Saunders, p. 587.

46. *Answer:* 2
Rationale: Tuberculosis is spread by droplet nuclei, or the airborne route. The disease is not carried on objects such as clothing, eating utensils, linens, or furniture. Bleaching of clothing and linens is unnecessary, although the client and family members should use good handwashing technique. It is unnecessary to remove carpeting from the home.
Test-Taking Strategy: Use the process of elimination. Knowing that TB is not carried on inanimate objects helps you to eliminate options 3 and 4 first. From the remaining options, recalling that the disease is transmitted by the airborne route will direct you to option 2. If you had difficulty with this question, review the transmission mode of TB.
Level of Cognitive Ability: Comprehension
Client Needs: Safe, Effective Care Environment
Integrated Concept/Process: Nursing Process/Planning
Content Area: Adult Health/Respiratory
Reference: Ignatavicius D, Workman M: *Medical-surgical: critical thinking for collaborative care*, ed 4, Philadelphia, 2002, WB Saunders, p. 584.

47. *Answer:* 1
Rationale: The nurse who is in contact with a client with TB should wear an individually fitted particulate respirator. The nurse would also wear gloves as per standard precautions. The nurse wears a gown when there is a possibility that the clothing could become contaminated, such as when giving a bed bath.
Test-Taking Strategy: Use the process of elimination. Knowing that the nurse should wear a particulate respirator mask helps you to eliminate options 3 and 4 first. Recalling standard precautions helps you to choose option 1 over option 2. Review care to the client with TB if you had difficulty with this question.
Level of Cognitive Ability: Application
Client Needs: Safe, Effective Care Environment
Integrated Concept/Process: Nursing Process/Planning
Content Area: Adult Health/Respiratory
Reference: Ignatavicius D, Workman M: *Medical-surgical: critical thinking for collaborative care*, ed 4, Philadelphia, 2002, WB Saunders, p. 588.

48. *Answer:* 1
Rationale: The client must have sputum cultures performed every 2 to 4 weeks after initiation of antituberculosis medication therapy. The client may return to work when the results of three sputum cultures are negative, because the client is considered noninfectious at that point.
Test-Taking Strategy: Use the process of elimination. Knowing that a positive Mantoux test never reverts to negative helps you to eliminate option 4. To discriminate among the remaining options, it is necessary to know that three negative sputum cultures are required. If this question was difficult, review these concepts.
Level of Cognitive Ability: Application
Client Needs: Safe, Effective Care Environment
Integrated Concept/Process: Nursing Process/Implementation
Content Area: Adult Health/Respiratory
Reference: Ignatavicius D, Workman M: *Medical-surgical: critical thinking for collaborative care*, ed 4, Philadelphia, 2002, WB Saunders, p. 587.

49. *Answer:* 2
Rationale: Isoniazid is hepatotoxic; therefore the client is taught to immediately report signs and symptoms of hepatitis (which includes yellow skin and sclera). For the same reason, alcohol should be avoided during therapy. The client should avoid intake of Swiss cheese, fish such as tuna, and foods containing tyramine because they may cause a reaction characterized by redness and itching of the skin, flushing, sweating, fast heartbeat, headache, or light-headedness. The client can prevent the development of peripheral neuritis by increasing the intake of pyridoxine (vitamin B_6) during the course of isoniazid therapy.
Test-Taking Strategy: Use the process of elimination. Because alcohol intake is prohibited with many medications, option 1 is eliminated first. Because the client receiving this medication typically is supplemented with vitamin B_6, option 4 is incorrect and is eliminated next. From the remaining options, knowing that the medication is hepatotoxic will direct you to option 2. If you had difficulty with this question review this medication.
Level of Cognitive Ability: Application
Client Needs: Health Promotion and Maintenance
Integrated Concept/Process: Teaching/Learning
Content Area: Adult Health/Respiratory
Reference: Hodgson B, Kizior R: *Saunders nursing drug handbook 2002*, Philadelphia, 2002, WB Saunders, p. 599.

50. *Answer:* 3
Rationale: Rifampin should be taken exactly as directed. Doses should not be doubled or skipped. The client should not stop therapy until directed to do so by a physician. The medication should be administered on an empty stomach unless it causes gastrointestinal upset, and then it may be taken with food. Antacids, if prescribed, should be taken at least 1 hour before the medication. Rifampin causes orange-red discoloration to body secretions and will permanently stain soft contact lenses.
Test-Taking Strategy: Use the process of elimination. General principles related to medication administration helps to eliminate options 1, 2, and 4. Also note the absolute word "always" in option 4. If you had difficulty with this question, review the side effects associated with this medication.
Level of Cognitive Ability: Application
Client Needs: Physiological Integrity
Integrated Concept/Process: Teaching/Learning
Content Area: Adult Health/Respiratory
Reference: Hodgson B, Kizior R: *Saunders nursing drug handbook 2002*, Philadelphia, 2002, WB Saunders, p. 971.

REFERENCES

Black J, Hawks J, Keene A: *Medical-surgical nursing: clinical management for positive outcomes*, ed 6, Philadelphia, 2001, WB Saunders.

Chernecky C, Berger B: *Laboratory tests and diagnostic procedures*, ed 3, Philadelphia, 2001, WB Saunders.

Clark J, Queener S, Karb V: *Pharmacologic basis of nursing practice*, ed 6, St Louis, 2000, Mosby.

DeWit S: *Fundamental concepts and skills for nursing*, Philadelphia, 2001, WB Saunders.

Hodgson B, Kizior R: *Saunders nursing drug handbook 2002*, Philadelphia, 2002, WB Saunders.

Ignatavicius D, Workman M: *Medical-surgical: critical thinking for collaborative care*, ed 4, Philadelphia, 2002, WB Saunders.

Potter P, Perry A: *Fundamentals of nursing*, ed 5, St Louis, 2001, Mosby.

Perry A, Potter P: *Clinical nursing skills and techniques*, ed 5, St Louis, 2002, Mosby.

Respiratory Medications

I. BROCHODILATORS

A. Description

1. Sympathomimetic bronchodilators dilate the airways of the respiratory tree, making air exchange and respiration easier for the client, and relax the smooth muscle of the bronchi (Box 47-1)
2. Xanthine bronchodilators stimulate the central nervous system and respiration, dilate coronary and pulmonary vessels, cause diuresis, and relax smooth muscle (Box 47-2)

BOX 47-1

Bronchodilators: Sympathomimetics

BETA-RECEPTOR AGONISTS
Albuterol (Proventil, Ventolin)
Bitolterol mesylate (Tornalate)
Ephedrine sulfate
Epinephrine (base) suspension (Sus-Phrine)
Epinephrine (AsthmaHaler Mist)
Epinephrine bitartrate (Bronkaid Suspension Mist)
Epinephrine (racemic) (Vaponefrin)
Epinephrine hydrochloride (Adrenalin Chloride)
Ethylnorepinephrine (Bronkephrine)
Isoetharine hydrochloride (Bronkosol)
Isoetharine mesylate (Bronkometer)
Isoproterenol hydrochloride (Isuprel Glossets, Isuprel Mistometer)
Isoproterenol sulfate (Medihaler-Iso)
Metaproterenol sulfate (Alupent, Metaprel)
Pirbuterol acetate (Maxair, Autoinhaler)
Salmeterol (Serevent)
Terbutaline sulfate (Brethine, Bricanyl, Brethaire)

ANTICHOLINERGIC
Ipratropium bromide (Atrovent)

BOX 47-2

Bronchodilators: Xanthines

Aminophylline (Generic, Truphylline, Phyllocontin)
Theophylline
Theophylline (Aerolate, Slo-phyllin, Theolair)
Theophylline (Theo-Dur, Slo-bid, Theo-24, Uni-Dur, Uniphyl)
Oxtriphylline (Choledyl, Choledyl SA)

3. Used to treat allergic rhinitis and sinusitis, acute bronchospasm, acute and chronic asthma, bronchitis, **chronic obstructive pulmonary disease,** and **emphysema**
4. Contraindicated in individuals with hypersensitivity, peptic ulcer disease, severe cardiac disease and cardiac dysrhythmias, hyperthyroidism, and uncontrolled seizure disorders
5. Used with caution in clients with hypertension, diabetes mellitus, and narrow-angle glaucoma
6. Theophylline increases the risk of digitalis toxicity and decreases the effects of lithium and phenytoin (Dilantin)
7. If theophylline and a beta-adrenergic agonist are administered together, cardiac dysrhythmias may result
8. Beta blockers, cimetidine (Tagamet), and erythromycin increase the effects of theophylline
9. Barbiturate and carbamazepine (Tegretol) decrease the effects of theophylline

B. Side effects

1. Palpitations and tachycardia
2. Dysrhythmias
3. Restlessness, nervousness, tremors
4. Anorexia, nausea, and vomiting

5. Headaches and dizziness
6. Hyperglycemia
7. Decreased clotting time
8. Mouth dryness and throat irritation with inhalers
9. Tolerance and paradoxical bronchoconstriction with inhalers

C. Implementation
1. Assess vital signs
2. Monitor for cardiac dysrhythmias
3. Assess for cough, wheezing, decreased breath sounds, and sputum production
4. Monitor for restlessness and confusion
5. Provide adequate hydration
6. Administer the medication at regular intervals around the clock to maintain a sustained therapeutic level
7. Administer oral medications with or after meals to decrease gastrointestinal (GI) irritation
8. Instruct the client not to crush enteric-coated or sustained-release tablets or capsules
9. Instruct the client to avoid caffeine products such as coffee, tea, cola, and chocolate
10. Instruct the client in the side effects of bronchodilators
11. Instruct the client how to monitor the pulse and to report any abnormalities to the physician
12. Instruct the client how to use an inhaler or nebulizer and how to monitor the amount of medication remaining in an inhaler canister
13. Instruct the client to avoid over-the-counter medications
14. Instruct the client to stop smoking and provide information regarding support resources
15. Instruct the client with diabetes mellitus to monitor blood glucose levels
16. Instruct the client with asthma to wear a Medical-Alert bracelet
17. Monitor for a therapeutic serum theophylline level of 10 to 20 μg/mL
18. Note that toxicity is likely to occur when the serum level is greater than 20 μg/mL
19. IV aminophylline or theophylline preparations should be administered slowly and always via an infusion pump

II. GLUCOCORTICOIDS (CORTICOSTEROIDS) (Box 47-3)

A. Act as an antiinflammatory and reduce edema of the airways

B. Refer to Chapter 43 for information on glucocorticoids

BOX 47-3

Glucocorticoids (Corticosteroids)

Beclomethasone dipropionate (Vanceril, Beclovent)
Triamcinolone (Azmacort)
Fluticasone (Flonase, Flovent)
Flunisolide (AeroBid)

III. INHALED NONSTEROIDAL ANTIALLERGY AGENTS (Box 47-4)

A. Description
1. An antiasthmatic, antiallergic, and mast cell stabilizer that inhibits mast cell release after exposure to antigens
2. Used for the treatment of allergic rhinitis, bronchial asthma, and exercised-induced bronchospasm
3. Contraindicated in clients with known hypersensitivity
4. Oral cromolyn sodium is used with caution in clients with impaired hepatic or renal function

B. Side effects
1. Cough or bronchospasm after inhalation
2. Nasal sting or sneezing after inhalation
3. Unpleasant taste in the mouth

C. Implementation
1. Monitor vital signs
2. Monitor respirations and assess lung sounds for rhonchi, wheezing, and rales
3. Instruct the client to drink a few sips of water before and after inhalation to prevent cough and unpleasant taste in the mouth
4. Administer oral capsules (cromolyn sodium) at least 30 minutes before meals
5. Instruct the client not to discontinue the medication abruptly because a rebound asthmatic attack can occur

IV. LEUKOTRIENE MODIFIERS (Box 47-5)

A. Description
1. Used in the prophylaxis and treatment of chronic bronchial asthma
2. Not used for acute asthma episodes

BOX 47-4

Inhaled Nonsteroidal Antiallergy Agents: Mast-Cell Stabilizers

Cromolyn sodium (Intal)
Nedocromil (Tilade)

BOX 47-5

Leukotriene Modifiers

Montelukast (Singulair)
Zafirlukast (Accolate)
Zileuton (Zyflo)

3. Inhibits bronchoconstriction caused by specific antigens
4. Reduces airway edema and smooth muscle constriction
5. Contraindicated with hypersensitivity and in breastfeeding mothers
6. Used with caution in clients with impaired hepatic function
7. Coadministration of inhaled glucocorticoids increases the risk of upper respiratory infection

B. Side effects
1. Headache
2. Nausea and vomiting
3. Dyspepsia
4. Diarrhea
5. Generalized pain, myalgia
6. Fever
7. Dizziness

C. Implementation
1. Monitor vital signs
2. Assess lung sounds for rhonchi, wheezing, and rales
3. Assess liver function laboratory values
4. Monitor for cyanosis
5. Instruct the client to take medication 1 hour before or 2 hours after meals
6. Instruct the client to increase fluid intake
7. Instruct the client not to discontinue medication and to take as prescribed even during symptom-free periods

V. ANTIHISTAMINES (Box 47-6)

A. Description
1. Called histamine antagonists or H_1-blockers; these medications compete with histamine for receptor sites, thus preventing a histamine response
2. When the H_1-receptor is stimulated, the extravascular smooth muscles, including those lining the nasal cavity are constricted
3. Decrease nasopharyngeal secretions by blocking the H_1-receptor and decrease nasal itching that causes sneezing
4. Used for the common cold, rhinitis, nausea and vomiting, motion sickness, urticaria and as a sleep aid

BOX 47-6

Antihistamines

Astemizole (Hismanal)
Azatadine maleate (Optimine)
Azelastine hydrochloride (Astelin)
Brompheniramine maleate (Dimetane)
Cetirizine hydrochloride (Zyrtec)
Chlorpheniramine maleate (Aller-Chlor, Chlor-Trimeton)
Clemastine fumarate (Tavist)
Cyproheptadine hydrochloride (Periactin)
Dexchlorpheniramine maleate (Polaramine)
Diphenhydramine (Benadryl)
Doxylamine succinate (Unisom)
Fexofenadine (Allegra)
Loratadine (Claritin)
Methdilazine hydrochloride (Tacaryl)
Phenindamine tartrate (Nolahist)
Pyrilamine maleate (Nisaval)
Tripelennamine citrate or hydrochloride (PBZ-SR)
Triprolidine hydrochloride (Myidil)

5. Can cause central nervous system (CNS) depression if taken with alcohol, narcotics, hypnotics, or barbiturates
6. Used with caution in clients with **chronic obstructive pulmonary disease (COPD)** because of their drying effect
7. Diphenhydramine (Benadryl) has an anticholinergic effect and should be avoided in clients with narrow-angle glaucoma

B. Side effects
1. Drowsiness and fatigue
2. Dizziness
3. Urinary retention
4. Blurred vision
5. Wheezing
6. Constipation
7. Dry mouth
8. GI Irritation
9. Hypotension
10. Hearing disturbances
11. Photosensitivity
12. Nervousness and irritability
13. Confusion
14. Nightmares

C. Implementation
1. Monitor vital signs
2. Monitor for signs of urinary dysfunction
3. Administer with food or milk
4. Avoid subcutaneous (SC) injection and administer intramuscular (IM) injection in a large muscle if the IM route is prescribed
5. Instruct the client to avoid hazardous activities, alcohol, and other CNS depressants 

6. Instruct the client taking medication for motion sickness to take the medication 30 minutes before the event, and then before meals and at bedtime during the event
7. Instruct the client to suck on hard candy or ice chips for dry mouth

VI. NASAL DECONGESTANTS (Box 47-7)

A. Description
  1. Stimulate the alpha-adrenergic receptors, thus producing vasoconstriction of the capillaries within the nasal mucosa
  2. Shrink nasal mucosal membranes and reduce fluid secretion
  3. Used for allergic rhinitis, hay fever, and acute coryza (profuse nasal discharge)
  4. Contraindicated or used with extreme caution in clients with hypertension, cardiac disease, hyperthyroidism, and diabetes mellitus
  5. Nasal decongestants can cause tolerance and rebound nasal congestion (vasodilation) caused by irritation of the nasal mucosa and should not be used for more than 48 hours

B. Side effects
  1. Frequent use of decongestants, especially nasal sprays or drops, can result in tolerance and rebound nasal congestion (vasodilation) caused by irritation of the nasal mucosa
  2. Nervousness
  3. Restlessness
  4. Hypertension
  5. Hyperglycemia

C. Implementation
  1. Assess the client for existing medical disorders
  2. Monitor for cardiac dysrhythmias
  3. Monitor blood glucose levels
  4. Instruct the client to avoid caffeine in large amounts because it can increase restlessness and palpitations
  5. Instruct the client in the importance of limiting the use of nasal sprays and drops

VII. EXPECTORANTS AND MUCOLYTIC AGENTS (Box 47-8)

A. Description

BOX 47-7

Nasal Decongestants

Oxymetazoline hydrochloride (Afrin)
Phenylephrine HCL (Neo-Synephrine)
Phenylpropanolamine hydrochloride (Dimetapp)
Pseudoephedrine hydrochloride (Sudafed)
Xylometazoline hydrochloride (Otrivin)

BOX 47-8

Expectorants and Mucolytic Agents

EXPECTORANTS
Guaifenesin (glycerylguaiacolate) (Anti-Tuss, Glycotuss, Humibid, Robitussin)

MUCOLYTIC
Acetylcysteine (Mucomyst)

  1. Loosen bronchial secretions so that they can be eliminated with coughing
  2. Used for dry, unproductive cough and to stimulate bronchial secretions
  3. Mucolytic agents with dextromethorphan should not be used with clients with **COPD** because they suppress the cough
  4. Acetylcysteine (Mucomyst) can increase airway resistance and should not be used in clients with asthma

B. Side effects
  1. GI irritation
  2. Skin rash
  3. Oropharyngeal irritation

C. Implementation
  1. Instruct the client to take medication with a full glass of water to loosen mucus
  2. Instruct the client to maintain an adequate fluid intake
  3. Encourage the client to cough and deep breathe
  4. Acetylcysteine (Mucomyst), administered by nebulization, should not be mixed together with another medication
  5. If acetylcysteine (Mucomyst) is administered with a bronchodilator, the bronchodilator should be administered 5 minutes before the acetylcysteine
  6. Monitor for side effects of acetylcysteine (Mucomyst) such as nausea and vomiting, stomatitis, and runny nose

VIII. ANTITUSSIVES (Box 47-9)

A. Description
  1. Act on the cough control center in the medulla to suppress the cough reflex
  2. Used for a cough that is nonproductive and irritating

B. Side effects
  1. Dizziness, drowsiness, sedation
  2. GI irritation, nausea
  3. Dry mouth
  4. Constipation
  5. Respiratory depression

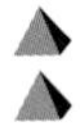

BOX 47-9

Antitussives

NARCOTICS
Codeine, codeine phosphate, codeine sulfate
Hydrocodone bitartrate (Hycodan)

NONNARCOTICS
Dextromethorphan hydrochloride (Benylin, Robitussin DM)
Diphenhydramine hydrochloride (Benylin Cough syrup, Benadryl)

C. Implementation
   1. Instruct the client that if the cough lasts longer than 1 week and a fever or rash occurs, the physician should be notified
   2. Encourage the client to take adequate fluids with the medication
   3. Encourage the client to sleep with the head of the bed elevated
   4. Instruct the client to avoid hazardous activities
   5. Note that drug dependency can occur
   6. Avoid administration to the client with a head injury or postoperative cranial surgery
   7. Avoid administration to the client using narcotics, sedative hypnotics, barbiturates, or antidepressants, because CNS depression can occur
   8. Instruct the client to avoid the use of alcohol

IX. NARCOTIC ANTAGONIST (Box 47-10)

A. Description
   1. Reverses respiratory depression in narcotic overdose
   2. Avoid use in nonnarcotic respiratory depression
B. Side effects
   1. CNS depression
   2. Nausea, vomiting
   3. Tremors
   4. Sweating
   5. Increased blood pressure
   6. Tachycardia
C. Implementation
   1. Assess vital signs, especially respirations
   2. Have oxygen and resuscitative equipment available during administration

BOX 47-10

Narcotic Antagonist

Naloxone hydrochloride (Narcan)

X. USE OF AN INHALER

A. Client instructions
B. If two different inhaled medications are prescribed, and one of the medication contains a glucocorticoid (corticosteroid), administer the bronchodilator first and the corticosteroid second
C. Wait 5 minutes after the bronchodilator before inhaling the corticosteroid

XI. TUBERCULOSIS (TB) MEDICATIONS

A. Description
   1. The most effective method for treating the disease and preventing transmission
   2. Treatment of identified lesions depends on whether the individual has active disease or has been exposed to the disease
   3. Treatment is difficult because the bacterium has a waxy substance on the capsule, which makes penetration and destruction difficult
   4. The use of a multiple medication regimen destroys organisms as quickly as possible and minimizes the emergence of medication-resistant organisms
   5. Active **TB** is treated with a combination of medications to which the organism is susceptible
   6. Individuals with active **TB** are treated for 6 to 9 months; however, clients with human immunodeficiency virus (HIV) infection will be treated for a longer period
   7. After the infected individual has received medication for 2 to 3 weeks, the risk of transmission is greatly reduced
   8. Most clients have negative sputum cultures after 3 months with compliance to medication therapy
   9. Individuals who have been exposed to active **TB** are treated with preventive isoniazid (INH) for 6 to 9 months upto 1 year
B. First-line or second-line medications
   1. First-line medications provide the most effective antituberculosis activity
   2. Second-line medications are used in combination with first-line medications, but are more toxic
   3. Current infecting organisms are proving resistant to standard first-line medications, and the resistant organisms develop because individuals with the disease fail to complete the course of treatment; surviving bacteria adapt to the medication and become resistant
   4. Multidrug therapies are instituted because of the resistant organisms

C. **Multidrug-Resistant Tuberculosis (MDR-TB)**
   1. Occurs when a client receiving two medications (first-line and second-line medications) discontinues one of the medications without the physician's knowledge
   2. The client briefly experiences some response from the single medication, but then large numbers of resistant organisms begin to grow
   3. The client, infectious again, transmits the drug-resistant organism to other individuals
   4. As this event is repeated, an organism develops that is resistant to many of the first-line **tuberculosis** medications

XII. FIRST-LINE MEDICATIONS FOR TB (Table 47-1)

A. Isoniazid (INH) (Laniazid, Nydrazid)
   1. Description
      a. Bactericidal
      b. Inhibits synthesis of mycolic acids and acts to kill actively growing organisms in the extracellular environment
      c. Inhibits growth of dormant organisms in the macrophages and caseating granulomas
      d. Active only during cell division
      e. Used in combination with other antitubercular medications
   2. Contraindications and cautions
      a. Contraindicated in clients with hypersensitivity or with acute liver disease
      b. Use with caution in clients with chronic liver disease, alcoholism, or renal impairment
      c. Use with caution in clients taking niacin, nicotinic acid (Nicobid)
      d. Use with caution in clients taking hepatotoxic medications because the risk for hepatotoxicity increases
      e. Alcohol increases the risk of hepatotoxicity
      f. Isoniazid (INH) may increase the risk of toxicity of carbamazepine (Tegretol) and phenytoin (Dilantin)
      g. Isoniazid (INH) may decrease ketoconazole (Nizoral) concentrations
   3. Side effects
      a. Hypersensitivity reactions
      b. Peripheral neuritis
      c. Neurotoxicity
      d. Hepatotoxicity
      e. Pyridoxine (vitamin B_6) deficiency
      f. Irritation at injection site with IM administration
      g. Nausea and vomiting
      h. Dry mouth
      i. Dizziness
      j. Hyperglycemia
      k. Increased liver function tests
      l. Hepatitis
   4. Implementation
      a. Assess for hypersensitivity
      b. Assess for hepatic dysfunction
      c. Assess for sensitivity to niacin, nicotinic acid (Nicobid)
      d. Monitor liver function tests
      e. Monitor for signs of hepatitis, such as anorexia, nausea, vomiting, weakness, fatigue, dark urine, or jaundice; if these symptoms occur, withhold the medication and notify the physician
      f. Monitor for tingling, numbness, or burning of the extremities
      g. Assess mental status
      h. Monitor for visual changes, and notify the physician if they occur
      i. Assess for dizziness and initiate safety precautions
      j. Monitor complete blood cell (CBC) count and blood glucose levels
      k. Administer 1 hour before or 2 hours after a meal because food may delay absorption
      l. Administer at least 1 hour before antacids, especially those antacids that contain aluminum
   5. Client education
      a. Instruct the client not to skip doses and to take medication for the full length of the prescribed therapy
      b. Instruct the client not to take any other medication without consulting the physician

TABLE 47-1

First-Line and Second-Line Medications

First-Line	Second-Line
Isoniazid (INH) (Laniazid, Nydrazid)	Capreomycin (Capastat)
Rifampin (Rifadin)	Ethionamide (Trecator-SC)
Ethambutol (Myambutol)	Aminosalicylate sodium (Tubasal)
Streptomycin	Cycloserine (Seromycin)
Pyrazinamide	Kanamycin (Kantrex)

Other Medications

Rifampin and isoniazid (Rifamate): treatment of tuberculosis after dosage of separate medications has been established

Rifampin, isoniazid, and pyrazinamide: short-course treatment of tuberculosis

c. Advise the client of the importance of follow-up physician visits, vision testing, and laboratory tests
d. Instruct the client to avoid alcohol
e. Advise the client to take medication on an empty stomach with 8 ounces of water 1 hour before or 2 hours after meals and to avoid taking antacids with the medication
f. Instruct the client to avoid tyramine-containing foods because they may cause a reaction such as red and itching skin, a pounding heartbeat, light-headedness, a hot or clammy feeling, or a headache; if these reactions occur notify the physician
g. Instruct the client in the signs of neurotoxicity, hepatitis, and hepatotoxicity
h. Instruct the client to notify the physician if signs of neurotoxicity, hepatitis and hepatotoxicity, or visual changes occur

B. Rifampin (Rifadin)
1. Description
a. Inhibits bacterial RNA synthesis
b. Binds to DNA-dependent RNA polymerase and blocks RNA transcription
c. Used in conjunction with at least one other antitubercular medication
2. Contraindications and cautions
a. Contraindicated in clients with hypersensitivity
b. Use with caution in clients with hepatic dysfunction or alcoholism
c. Use of alcohol or hepatotoxic medications may increase the risk of hepatotoxicity
d. Decreases the effects of several medications including oral anticoagulants, oral hypoglycemics, chloramphenicol (Chloromycetin), digoxin (Lanoxin), disopyramide phosphate (Norpace), mexiletine (Mexitil), quinidine polygalacturonate (Cardioquin), tocainide hydrochloride (Tonocard), fluconazole (Difulcan), methadone hydrochloride (Dolophine), phenytoin (Dilantin), and verapamil hydrochloride (Calan)
3. Side effects
a. Hypersensitivity reaction including fever, chills, shivering, headache, muscle and bone pain, and dyspnea
b. Heartburn
c. Nausea, vomiting, diarrhea
d. Increased liver function tests
e. Hepatotoxicity and hepatitis
f. Increased uric acid levels
g. Blood dyscrasias
h. Colitis
4. Implementation
a. Assess for hypersensitivity
b. Evaluate CBC, uric acid, and liver function tests
c. Assess for signs of hepatitis, and if they occur, withhold the medication and notify the physician
d. Monitor stools for signs of colitis
e. Monitor mental status
f. Assess for visual changes
5. Client education
a. Instruct the client not to skip doses and to take medication for the full length of the prescribed therapy
b. Instruct the client not to take any other medication without consulting the physician
c. Advise the client of the importance of follow-up physician visits and laboratory tests
d. Instruct the client to avoid alcohol
e. Advise the client to take medication on an empty stomach with 8 oz of water 1 hour before or 2 hours after meals and to avoid taking antacids with the medication
f. Instruct the client that urine, feces, sweat, and tears will be red-orange in color and that soft contact lenses can become permanently discolored
g. Instruct the client to notify the physician if jaundice (yellow eyes or skin) develops or if weakness, fatigue, nausea, vomiting, sore throat, fever, or unusual bleeding occurs

C. Ethambutol (Myambutol)
1. Description
a. Bacteriostatic
b. Interferes with cell metabolism and multiplication by inhibiting one or more metabolites in the susceptible organism
c. Inhibits bacterial RNA synthesis
d. Active only during cell division
e. Is slow acting and must be used in combination with other bactericidal agents
2. Contraindications and cautions
a. Contraindicated in clients with hypersensitivity, optic neuritis, and in children under 13 years old
b. Use with caution in clients with renal dysfunction, gout, ocular defects, diabetic retinopathy, cataracts, and ocular inflammatory conditions
c. Use with caution in clients taking neurotoxic medications as the risk for neurotoxicity increases
3. Side effects
a. Hypersensitivity reactions
b. Anorexia, nausea, vomiting
c. Dizziness
d. Malaise

e. Mental confusion
f. Joint pain
g. Dermatitis
h. Optic neuritis
i. Peripheral neuritis
j. Thrombocytopenia
k. Increased uric acid levels
l. Anaphylactoid reaction

4. Implementation
a. Assess for hypersensitivity
b. Evaluate results of CBC, uric acid, renal and liver function tests
c. Obtain baseline visual acuity and color discrimination, especially to the color green
d. Monitor for visual changes such as altered color perception and decreased visual acuity, and if changes occur, withhold the medication and notify the physician
e. Administer once every 24 hours and administer with food to decrease gastrointestinal (GI) upset
f. Monitor uric acid concentrations and assess for painful or swollen joints or signs of gout
g. Monitor input and output (I&O) and for adequate renal function
h. Assess mental status
i. Monitor for dizziness and initiate safety precautions
j. Assess for peripheral neuritis (numbness, tingling, or burning of the extremities) and if it occurs, notify the physician

5. Client education
a. Inform the client that he or she can prevent nausea related to the medication by taking the daily dose at bedtime, or to take prescribed antinausea medications
b. Instruct the client not to skip doses and to take the medication for the full length of the prescribed therapy
c. Instruct the client not to take any other medication without consulting the physician
d. Advise the client of the importance of follow-up physician visits, vision testing, and laboratory tests
e. Instruct the client to notify the physician immediately if any visual problems occur; if a rash, swelling and pain in the joints, or numbness or tingling occurs; or if burning in the hands or feet occurs

D. Streptomycin

1. Description
a. An aminoglycoside antibiotic that is used in conjunction with at least one other antitubercular medication
b. Bactericidal, because of receptor binding action, interfering with protein synthesis in susceptible organisms

2. Contraindications and cautions
a. Contraindicated in clients with hypersensitivity, myasthenia gravis, parkinsonism, or eighth cranial nerve damage
b. Use with caution in the elderly, in neonates because of renal insufficiency and immaturity, and in young infants because the medication may cause CNS depression
c. The risk of toxicity increases when taken with other aminoglycosides, or nephrotoxic- or ototoxic-producing medications

3. Side effects (Box 47-11)
a. Hypersensitivity
b. Visual changes
c. Increased liver and renal function tests
d. Peripheral neuritis such as burning of the face or mouth

4. Implementation
a. Assess for hypersensitivity
b. Monitor liver and renal function tests
c. Monitor for ototoxic, neurotoxic, and nephrotoxic reactions
d. Obtain baseline audiometric test and repeat every 1 to 2 months because the medication impairs the eighth cranial nerve
e. Assess hearing acuity
f. Monitor for visual changes
g. Assess hydration status and maintain adequate hydration during therapy
h. Monitor I&O
i. Assess urinalysis
j. Monitor for signs of peripheral neuritis

5. Client education
a. Instruct the client not to skip doses and to take medication for the full length of the prescribed therapy

BOX 47-11

Side Effects of Streptomycin

NEPHROTOXICITY	NEUROTOXICITY
Changes in urine output	Muscle numbness
Increased thirst	Tingling
Decreased appetite	Twitching
Nausea, vomiting	Seizures
VESTIBULAR OTOTOXICITY	**AUDITORY OTOTOXICITY**
Dizziness	Ringing in the ears
Clumsiness	Loss of hearing
Unsteadiness	A full feeling in the ears

b. Instruct the client not to take any other medication without consulting the physician
c. Advise the client of the importance of follow-up physician visits and laboratory tests
d. Instruct the client to notify physician if hearing loss, changes in vision, or urinary problems occur

E. Pyrazinamide
1. Description
a. Exact mechanism of action is unknown
b. May be bacteriostatic or bactericidal depending on its concentration at the infection site and susceptibility of infecting organism
c. Used in conjunction with at least one other antitubercular medication after failure or ineffectiveness of the primary medications occurs
2. Contraindications and cautions
a. Contraindicated in clients with hypersensitivity
b. Use with caution in clients with diabetes mellitus, renal impairment, gout, and in children
c. May decrease the effects of allopurinol (Zyloprim), colchicine, sulfinpyrazone (Anturane)
d. Cross-sensitivity is possible with isoniazid (INH), ethionamide (Trecator-SC) or niacin, nicotinic acid (Nicobid)
3. Side effects
a. Increases liver function and uric acid levels
b. Arthralgia, myalgia
c. Photosensitivity
d. Hepatotoxicity
e. Thrombocytopenia
4. Implementation
a. Assess for hypersensitivity
b. Evaluate CBC, liver function tests, and uric acid levels
c. Observe for hepatotoxic effects and if they occur, withhold the medication and notify the physician
d. Assess for painful or swollen joints
e. Evaluate blood glucose levels because diabetes mellitus may be difficult to control while on medication
5. Client education
a. Instruct the client to take the medication with food to reduce GI distress
b. Instruct the client to avoid sunlight or ultraviolet light until photosensitivity is determined
c. Instruct the client to notify physician if any side effects occur
d. Instruct the client not to skip doses and to take medication for the full length of the prescribed therapy
e. Instruct the client not to take any other medication without consulting the physician
f. Advise the client of the importance of follow-up physician visits and laboratory tests

XIII. SECOND-LINE MEDICATIONS FOR TB

A. Capreomycin sulfate (Capastat Sulfate)
1. Description
a. Mechanism of action is unknown
b. Used to treat **MDR-TB** when significant resistance to other medications is expected
c. Must be given by the IM route
2. Contraindications and cautions
a. The risk of nephrotoxicity, ototoxicity, and neuromuscular blockade is increased with the use of aminoglycosides or loop diuretics
b. Use with caution in clients with renal insufficiency, acoustic nerve impairment, hepatic disorder, myasthenia gravis, and parkinsonism
c. Do not administer to client receiving streptomycin
3. Side effects
a. Nephrotoxicity
b. Ototoxicity
c. Neuromuscular blockade
4. Implementation
a. Perform baseline audiometric testing
b. Assess renal, hepatic, and electrolyte levels before administration
c. Monitor I&O
d. Reconstituted medication may be stored for 48 hours at room temperature
e. Administer deep IM in a large muscle mass
f. Rotate injection sites
g. Observe injection site for redness, excessive bleeding, and inflammation
5. Client education
a. Instruct the client not to perform tasks that require mental alertness
b. Instruct the client to report any hearing loss, balance disturbances, respiratory difficulty, weakness or signs of hypersensitivity reactions

B. Kanamycin (Kantrex)
1. Description
a. An aminoglycoside antibiotic that is used in conjunction with at least one other antitubercular medication
b. Bactericidal, because of receptor binding action, interfering with protein synthesis in susceptible microorganisms

2. Contraindications and cautions
   a. Contraindicated in clients with hypersensitivity, neuromuscular disorders, or eighth cranial nerve damage
   b. Use with caution in the elderly, in neonates because of renal insufficiency and immaturity, and in young infants because it may cause CNS depression
   c. The risk of toxicity increases when taken with other aminoglycosides, or nephrotoxic- or ototoxic-producing medications
3. Side effects
   a. Hypersensitivity
   b. Pain and irritation at the injection site
   c. Nephrotoxicity as evidenced by increased blood urea nitrogen (BUN) and serum creatinine
   d. Ototoxicity as evidenced by tinnitus, dizziness, ringing/roaring in the ears, and reduced hearing
   e. Neurotoxicity as evidenced by headache, dizziness, lethargy, tremors, and visual disturbances
   f. Superinfections
4. Implementation
   a. Assess for hypersensitivity
   b. Monitor for ototoxic, neurotoxic, and nephrotoxic reactions
   c. Monitor liver and renal function tests
   d. Obtain baseline audiometric test and repeat every 1 to 2 months because the medication impairs the eighth cranial nerve
   e. Assess hearing acuity
   f. Monitor for visual changes
   g. Assess hydration status and maintain adequate hydration during therapy
   h. Monitor I&O
   i. Assess urinalysis
   j. Monitor for superinfection
5. Client education
   a. Instruct the client not to skip doses and to take medication for the full length of the prescribed therapy
   b. Instruct the client not to take any other medication without consulting the physician
   c. Advise the client of the importance of follow-up physician visits and laboratory tests
   d. Instruct the client to notify the physician if hearing loss, changes in vision, or urinary problems occur

C. Ethionamide (Trecator-SC)
1. Description
   a. Mechanism of action is unknown
   b. Used to treat **MDR-TB** when significant resistance to other medications is expected
2. Contraindications and cautions
   a. Contraindicated in clients with hypersensitivity
   b. Use with caution in clients with diabetes mellitus or renal dysfunction
3. Side effects
   a. Anorexia, nausea, vomiting
   b. Metallic taste in the mouth
   c. Orthostatic hypotension
   d. Jaundice
   e. Mental changes
   f. Peripheral neuritis
   g. Rash
4. Implementation
   a. Assess liver and renal function tests
   b. Monitor glucose levels in the client with diabetes mellitus
   c. Administer pyridoxine as prescribed to reduce the risk of neurotoxicity
5. Client education
   a. Instruct the client to take medication with food or meals to minimize GI irritation
   b. Instruct the client to change positions slowly
   c. Instruct the client to report signs of a rash, which can progress to exfoliative dermatitis if the medication is not discontinued
   d. Instruct the client to avoid alcohol
   e. Instruct the client to report signs of jaundice and other side effects of the medication if they occur

D. Aminosalicylate sodium (Tubasal)
1. Description
   a. Inhibits folic acid metabolism in mycobacteria
   b. Used to treat **MDR-TB** when significant resistance to other medications is expected
2. Contraindications and cautions
   a. Contraindicated with hypersensitivity to aminosalicylates, salicylates, or compounds containing para-aminophenyl group
   b. Aminobenzoates block the absorption of aminosalicylate sodium
3. Side effects 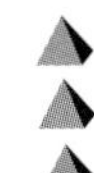
   a. Hypersensitivity
   b. Bitter taste in the mouth
   c. GI tract irritation
   d. Exfoliative dermatitis
   e. Blood dyscrasias 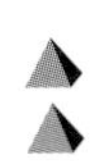
   f. Crystalluria
   g. Changes in thyroid function
4. Implementation 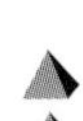
   a. Assess for hypersensitivity 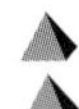

b. Offer clear water to rinse the mouth, chewing gum, or hard candy to alleviate the bitter taste
c. Encourage fluid intake to prevent crystalluria
d. Monitor I&O

5. Client education
   a. Instruct the client to discard the medication if a purplish brown discoloration occurs
   b. Instruct the client to take the medication with food
   c. Inform the client that urine may turn red on contact with hypochlorite bleach if bleach was used to clean a toilet
   d. Instruct the client not to take aspirin or over-the-counter medications without the physician's approval
   e. Inform the client with diabetes mellitus that a false-positive result can occur in glucose monitoring
   f. Instruct the client to report signs of a blood dyscrasia such as sore throat or mouth, malaise, fatigue, bruising, or bleeding

E. Cycloserine (Seromycin)
1. Description
   a. Interferes with cell wall biosynthesis
   b. Used to treat **MDR-TB** when significant resistance to other medications is expected
2. Contraindications and cautions
   a. Use of alcohol or ethionamide (Trecator-SC) increases the risk of seizures
   b. Use with caution in clients with epilepsy, depression, severe anxiety, psychosis, renal insufficiency, or the client who uses alcohol
3. Side effects
   a. Hypersensitivity
   b. CNS reactions
   c. Neurotoxicity
   d. Seizures
   e. Heart failure
   f. Headache
   g. Vertigo
   h. Altered level of consciousness (LOC)
   i. Irritability, nervousness, anxiety
   j. Confusion
   k. Mood changes, depression, thoughts of suicide
4. Implementation
   a. Monitor LOC
   b. Monitor for changes in mental status and thought processes
   c. Monitor renal and hepatic function tests
   d. Monitor serum drug level to avoid the risk of neurotoxicity; peak concentrations, measured 2 hours after dosing, should be 25 to 35 μg/mL
5. Client education
   a. Instruct the client to take the medication after meals to prevent GI upset
   b. Instruct the client to avoid alcohol
   c. Instruct the client to report signs of a rash or signs of CNS toxicity
   d. Instruct the client to avoid driving or performing tasks that require alertness until the reaction to the medication has been determined
   e. Advise the client of the need for serum drug levels weekly, as prescribed

PRACTICE QUESTIONS

1. A nurse is preparing to administer albuterol (Proventil) to a client. The nurse checks for which of the following before and during therapy?
   1. Increased urine output
   2. Nausea and vomiting
   3. Respiratory distress
   4. Complaints of headache
2. A nurse is administering a dose of isoproterenol (Isuprel) to a client. The nurse plans to monitor for which side effect of this medication?
   1. Increased pulse and blood pressure
   2. Drowsiness
   3. Hyperglycemia
   4. Hypokalemia
3. A nurse has an order to give a client metaproterenol sulfate (Alupent) two puffs and beclamethasone (Vanceril) two puffs by metered dose inhaler. The nurse administers the medication by giving the:
   1. Beclomethasone first and then the metaproterenol
   2. Metaproterenol first and then the beclomethasone
   3. Alternating a single puff of each, beginning with the beclomethasone
   4. Alternating a single puff of each, beginning with the metaproterenol
4. A client has begun therapy with oxtriphylline (Choledyl). The nurse tells the client to limit the intake of which of the following while taking this medication?
   1. Oysters, lobster, and shrimp
   2. Coffee, cola, and chocolate
   3. Cottage cheese, cream cheese, and dairy creamers
   4. Oranges and pineapple
5. A client with an order to take theophylline (Slo-bid) daily has been given medication instructions by the nurse. The nurse determines that the client needs further information about the medication if the client states to:

1. Avoid changing brands of the medication without physician approval
2. Avoid over-the-counter (OTC) cough and cold medications unless approved by physician
3. Drink at least 2 liters fluid per day
4. Take the daily dose at bedtime

6. A client is taking brompheniramine maleate (Dimetane). The nurse checks for which of the following side effects of this medication?
   1. Excitability
   2. Drowsiness
   3. Excess salivation
   4. Diarrhea
7. A client taking brompheniramine maleate (Dimetane) is scheduled for allergy skin testing and tells the nurse in the physician's office that a dose was taken this morning. The nurse determines that:
   1. A lower dose of allergen will need to be injected
   2. A higher dose of allergen will need to be injected
   3. The client should have the skin test read a day later than usual
   4. The client should reschedule the appointment
8. A client is receiving acetylcystine (Mucomyst) 20% solution diluted in 0.9% normal saline by nebulizer. The nurse should have which of the following items available for possible use after giving this medication?
   1. Suction equipment
   2. Nasogastric tube
   3. Intubation tray
   4. Ambu bag
9. A nurse is assisting to administer acetylcystine (Mucomyst) to a client admitted with acetaminophen (Tylenol) overdose. Before giving this medication, the nurse would ensure that the:
   1. Client knows how to use a nebulizer
   2. Antidote to acetaminophen is readily available
   3. Stomach is empty through emesis or lavage
   4. Solution is given full strength
10. A client has an order to take guaifenesin (Humibid) every 4 hours as needed. The nurse evaluates that the client understands the most effective use of this medication if the client states to:
    1. Take the tablet with a full glass of water
    2. Take an extra dose if the cough is accompanied by fever
    3. Watch for irritability as a side effect
    4. Crush the sustained-release tablet if immediate relief is needed
11. A postoperative client has received a dose of naloxone (Narcan) for respiratory depression shortly after transfer to the nursing unit from the postanesthesia care unit. After administration of the medication, the nurse checks the client for:
    1. Pupillary changes
    2. Sudden episodes of vomiting
    3. Sudden increase in pain
    4. Scattered lung wheezes
12. A client with suspected narcotic overdose has received a dose of naloxone (Narcan). The client subsequently becomes restless, starts to vomit, and complains of abdominal cramping. The blood pressure increases from 110/72 to 160/86 mm Hg. The nurse provides emotional support and reassurance while administering care to the client, knowing that:
    1. These effects will last only a few moments
    2. These are signs of opioid withdrawal
    3. The client may otherwise sign out against medical advice
    4. The client may next become suicidal
13. A nurse is assisting in caring for a client who is receiving a dose of naloxone (Narcan) intravenously to treat narcotic overdose. The nurse plans to have which of the following available as supportive equipment in case it is needed?
    1. Nasogastric tube
    2. Paracentesis tray
    3. Central line insertion tray
    4. Resuscitation equipment
14. A nurse is reinforcing instructions to a client about the effects of diphenhydramine (Benadryl), which has been ordered as a cough suppressant. Which statement by the client indicates the need for further instructions?
    1. "I need to avoid driving or other activities requiring mental alertness while taking this medication."
    2. "I need to use sugarless gum, candy, or oral rinses to decrease dry mouth."
    3. "I need to avoid alcohol while taking this medication."
    4. "I need to take the medication on an empty stomach."
15. A client has been prescribed a cough formula containing codeine sulfate. The nurse has given the client instructions for its use. The nurse evaluates that the client understands the instructions if the client verbalizes to self-check for:
    1. Excitability
    2. Constipation
    3. Rapid pulse
    4. Excessive urination
16. A nurse is caring for the client who has been taking hydrocodone bitartrate (Hycodan) for the last 3 months. The nurse checks the client for which of the following side effects of this medication?
    1. Psychological and physical dependence
    2. Tachycardia and hypertension
    3. Diarrhea and abdominal cramping
    4. Increased respiratory rate and bronchospasm

17. Cromolyn sodium (Intal) is prescribed for a client with allergic asthma. The nurse tells the client about this medication knowing that it acts to:
    1. Inhibit the release of mediators from mast cells after exposure to an antigen
    2. Promote the migration of eosinophils into the inflammatory site
    3. Increase the number of eosinophils
    4. Dilate the bronchi
18. Cromolyn sodium (Intal) inhaler is prescribed for the client with allergic asthma. The nurse reinforces instructions regarding the side effects knowing that which undesirable side effect is associated with this medication?
    1. Constipation
    2. Hypotension
    3. Insomnia
    4. Cough
19. Terbutaline sulfate (Brethine) is prescribed for a client with bronchitis. The nurse reviews the client's record knowing that this medication should be used with caution if which of the following existing medical conditions were present in the client?
    1. Hypothyroidism
    2. Polycystic disease
    3. Osteoarthritis
    4. Diabetes mellitus
20. Zafirlukast (Accolate) is prescribed for a client with bronchial asthma. Which of the following laboratory tests would the nurse expect to be prescribed before administration of this medication?
    1. Platelet count
    2. Complete blood cell count
    3. Liver function tests
    4. Neutrophil count

ANSWERS

1. *Answer:* 3

Rationale: Albuterol is a bronchodilator of the adrenergic type. The nurse checks the respiratory pattern, pulse, and blood pressure before and during therapy. The color, character, and amount of sputum are also noted. Options 1, 2, and 4 are not directly related to this medication.

Test-Taking Strategy: Use the ABCs—airway, breathing, and circulation—to answer the question. Option 3 is the only option that addresses airway. Review this medication if you had difficulty with this question.

Level of Cognitive Ability: Application

Client Needs: Physiological Integrity

Integrated Concept/Process: Nursing Process/Data Collection

Content Area: Pharmacology

Reference: Hodgson B, Kizior R: *Saunders nursing drug handbook 2002*, Philadelphia, 2002, WB Saunders, p. 21.

2. *Answer:* 1

Rationale: Isoproterenol is an adrenergic bronchodilator. Side effects can include tachycardia, hypertension, chest pain, dysrhythmias, nervousness, restlessness, and headache, among others. The nurse monitors for these effects during therapy.

Test-Taking Strategy: Use the process of elimination recalling that this medication is a bronchodilator. Remembering that tachycardia is a side effect should assist in selecting the option that identifies an increased pulse, option 1. Review the side effects of this medication if you had difficulty with this question.

Level of Cognitive Ability: Application

Client Needs: Physiological Integrity

Integrated Concept/Process: Nursing Process/Data Collection

Content Area: Pharmacology

Reference: Hodgson B, Kizior R: *Saunders nursing drug handbook 2002*, Philadelphia, 2002, WB Saunders, p. 601.

3. *Answer:* 2

Rationale: Metaproterenol is a bronchodilator. Beclomethasone is a glucocorticoid. Bronchodilators are always administered before glucocorticoids, when both are to be given on the same time schedule. This allows for widening of the air passages by the bronchodilator, which then makes the glucocorticoid more effective.

Test-Taking Strategy: To answer this question correctly, it is necessary to know two different things. First you must know that a bronchodilator is always given before a glucocorticoid. This would allow you to eliminate options 3 and 4, because you would not alternate the medications. To discriminate between options 1 and 2, it is necessary to know that metaproterenol is a bronchodilator, while beclomethasone is a glucocorticoid. Review these medications if you had difficulty with this question.

Level of Cognitive Ability: Application

Client Needs: Physiological Integrity

Integrated Concept/Process: Nursing Process/Implementation

Content Area: Pharmacology

Reference: Hodgson B, Kizior R: *Saunders nursing drug handbook 2002*, Philadelphia, 2002, WB Saunders, p. 701.

4. *Answer:* 2

Rationale: Oxtriphylline is a xanthine bronchodilator. The nurse teaches the client to limit the intake of xanthine containing foods while taking this medication. These include coffee, cola, and chocolate.

Test-Taking Strategy: To answer this question correctly, it is necessary to understand that oxtriphylline is a xanthine bronchodilator and to know which food items are naturally high in xanthines. Review the foods naturally high in xanthines if you had difficulty with this question.

Level of Cognitive Ability: Application

Client Needs: Health Promotion and Maintenance

Integrated Concept/Process: Nursing Process/Implementation
Content Area: Pharmacology
Reference: Lehne R: *Pharmacology for nursing care,* ed 4, Philadelphia, 2001, WB Saunders, p. 361.

5. *Answer:* 4
Rationale: The client taking a single daily dose of theophylline, a xanthine bronchodilator, should take the medication early in the morning. This enables the client to have maximal benefit from the medication during daytime activities. Additionally, this medication causes insomnia. The client should take in at least 2 liters of fluid per day to decrease viscosity of secretions. The client should check with the physician before changing brands of the medication. The client also checks with the physician before taking OTC cough, cold, or other respiratory preparations because they could cause interactive effects, increasing the side effects of theophylline and causing dysrhythmias.
Test-Taking Strategy: Use the process of elimination. Note the key words "needs further information." General principles related to medication therapy will assist in eliminating options 1 and 2. Additionally, recalling that option 3 is an important measure to thin secretions will direct you to option 4. Review this medication if you had difficulty with this question.
Level of Cognitive Ability: Comprehension
Client Needs: Health Promotion and Maintenance
Integrated Concept/Process: Teaching/Learning
Content Area: Pharmacology
Reference: Lehne R: *Pharmacology for nursing care,* ed 4, Philadelphia, 2001, WB Saunders, p. 838.

6. *Answer:* 2
Rationale: A frequent side effect of brompheniramine, an antihistamine, is drowsiness or sedation. Others include blurred vision, hypertension (and sometimes hypotension), dry mouth, constipation, urinary retention, and sweating.
Test-Taking Strategy: To answer this question correctly, it is necessary to know that this medication is an antihistamine. Recalling that antihistamines typically causes drowsiness will direct you to option 2. Review the side effects of antihistamines if you had difficulty with this question.
Level of Cognitive Ability: Application
Client Needs: Physiological Integrity
Integrated Concept/Process: Nursing Process/Data Collection
Content Area: Pharmacology
Reference: Hodgson B, Kizior R: *Saunders nursing drug handbook 2002,* Philadelphia, 2002, WB Saunders, p. 136.

7. *Answer:* 4
Rationale: Brompheniramine is an antihistamine that provides relief of symptoms caused by allergy. Antihistamines should be discontinued for at least 3 days (72 hours) before allergy skin testing to avoid false-negative readings. This client should have the appointment rescheduled for 3 days after discontinuing the medication.
Test-Taking Strategy: To answer this question correctly, it is necessary to know that this medication is an antihistamine. It is also necessary to know that antihistamines reduce the allergic response. With this in mind, option 1 is eliminated first, as it makes no sense. Options 2 and 3 are also eliminated, because the medication would still interfere with the test results. Review this medication if you had difficulty with this question.
Level of Cognitive Ability: Comprehension
Client Needs: Physiological Integrity
Integrated Concept/Process: Nursing Process/Planning
Content Area: Pharmacology
Reference: Hodgson B, Kizior R: *Saunders nursing drug handbook 2002,* Philadelphia, 2002, WB Saunders, p. 136.

8. *Answer:* 1
Rationale: Acetylcystine can be given orally or by nasogastric tube to treat acetaminophen overdose, or it may be given by inhalation for use as a mucolytic. The nurse administering this medication as a mucolytic should have suction equipment available, in case the client cannot manage to clear the increased volume of liquefied secretions.
Test-Taking Strategy: To answer this question, it is necessary to know that acetylcystine may be given for either acetaminophen overdose or as a mucolytic agent. It is also necessary to know that the inhalation route is only used for mucolytic effects. With this in mind, options 3 and 4 are eliminated, as the client does not need resuscitation. Option 2 is eliminated also, as a nasogastric tube may be used in the client with acetaminophen overdose. If you had difficulty with this question, review the purpose of this medication and the related nursing interventions.
Level of Cognitive Ability: Application
Client Needs: Physiological Integrity
Integrated Concept/Process: Nursing Process/Implementation
Content Area: Pharmacology
Reference: Hodgson B, Kizior R: *Saunders nursing drug handbook 2002,* Philadelphia, 2002, WB Saunders, p. 11

9. *Answer:* 3
Rationale: Acetylcystine can be given orally or by nasogastric tube to treat acetaminophen overdose, or it may be given by inhalation for use as a mucolytic. Before giving the medication as an antidote to acetaminophen, the nurse ensures that the client's stomach is empty through emesis or gastric lavage. The solution is diluted in cola, water, or juice to make the solution more palatable. It is then administered orally or by nasogastric tube.
Test-Taking Strategy: Use the process of elimination. Begin to answer this question by eliminating options 1 and 2. This medication is not given by the inhalation route to treat acetaminophen overdose, and acetylcysteine is the antidote (to acetaminophen). To discriminate between the remaining options, remember that the solution must be diluted and that the stomach must be emptied for maximal effect of the antidote. Review this medication if you had difficulty with this question.
Level of Cognitive Ability: Application
Client Needs: Physiological Integrity
Integrated Concept/Process: Nursing Process/Implementation
Content Area: Pharmacology
Reference: Hodgson B, Kizior R: *Saunders nursing drug handbook 2002,* Philadelphia, 2002, WB Saunders, p. 11.

10. *Answer:* 1
Rationale: Guaifenesin is an expectorant. It should be taken with a full glass of water to decrease viscosity of secretions. Sustained-release preparations should not be broken open, crushed, or chewed. The medication may occasionally cause dizziness, headache, or drowsiness as side effects. The client should contact the physician if the cough lasts longer than 1 week, or is accompanied by fever, rash, sore throat, or persistent headache.
Test-Taking Strategy: Use the process of elimination. Begin to answer this question by eliminating option 4 first. Sustained-released preparations are not crushed or broken. Option 2 is eliminated next because fever indicates infection, and an "extra dose" of an expectorant is not helpful in treating infection. From the remaining options, recalling that increased fluids helps to liquefy secretions for more effective coughing will direct you to option 1. Review this medication if you had difficulty with this question.
Level of Cognitive Ability: Comprehension
Client Needs: Health Promotion and Maintenance
Integrated Concept/Process: Nursing Process/Evaluation
Content Area: Pharmacology
Reference: Hodgson B, Kizior R: *Saunders nursing drug handbook 2002*, Philadelphia, 2002, WB Saunders, p. 521.

11. *Answer:* 3
Rationale: Naloxone is an antidote to opioids, and may also be given to the postoperative client to treat respiratory depression. When given to the postoperative client for respiratory depression, it may also reverse the effects of analgesics. Therefore the nurse must check the client for a sudden increase in the level of pain experienced.
Test-Taking Strategy: Use the process of elimination. Recalling that this medication is an antidote to narcotic analgesics will assist in directing you to option 3. Remember that this medication will cause sudden pain in the postoperative client or return of pain in the client who received narcotic analgesics. If you had difficulty with this question, review this medication.
Level of Cognitive Ability: Application
Client Needs: Physiological Integrity
Integrated Concept/Process: Nursing Process/Data Collection
Content Area: Pharmacology
Reference: Hodgson B, Kizior R: *Saunders nursing drug handbook 2002*, Philadelphia, 2002, WB Saunders, p. 771.

12. *Answer:* 2
Rationale: Signs of opioid withdrawal include increased temperature and blood pressure, abdominal cramping, vomiting, and restlessness. They can occur anywhere from a few minutes to a few hours after administration of naloxone, depending on the opioid involved, the degree of dependence, and the dose of naloxone.
Test-Taking Strategy: Use the process of elimination. Eliminate option 1 first because the symptoms identified in the question are not likely to disappear in a few moments. Option 4 is eliminated next, because there is no supporting information in the question. From the remaining options, knowing that the client with narcotic overdose may well have a history of prior chronic use, will direct you to option 2. Review the signs of opioid withdrawal if you had difficulty with this question.
Level of Cognitive Ability: Analysis
Client Needs: Psychosocial Integrity
Integrated Concept/Process: Nursing Process/Implementation
Content Area: Pharmacology
Reference: Hodgson B, Kizior R: *Saunders nursing drug handbook 2002*, Philadelphia, 2002, WB Saunders, p. 771.

13. *Answer:* 4
Rationale: The nurse should have resuscitation equipment readily available to support naloxone therapy if it is needed. Other adjuncts that may be needed include oxygen, a mechanical ventilator, and emergency medications.
Test-Taking Strategy: Use the process of elimination and note the key words "narcotic overdose." Recalling the effects of narcotics will direct you to option 4. Also, option 4 is the most global response. Review care to the client receiving naloxone if you had difficulty with this question.
Level of Cognitive Ability: Application
Client Needs: Physiological Integrity
Integrated Concept/Process: Nursing Process/Planning
Content Area: Pharmacology
Reference: Hodgson B, Kizior R: *Saunders nursing drug handbook 2002*, Philadelphia, 2002, WB Saunders, p. 772.

14. *Answer:* 4
Rationale: Diphenhydramine has several uses, including antihistamine, antitussive, antidyskinetic, and sedative/hypnotic. Instructions for use include to take the medication with food or milk to decrease gastrointestinal upset, and to use oral rinses, sugarless gum, or hard candy to minimize dry mouth. Because the medication causes drowsiness, the client should avoid the use of alcohol or central nervous system depressants, operating a car, or engaging in other activities requiring mental acuity during use.
Test-Taking Strategy: Use the process of elimination and note the key words "need for further instructions." Knowing that the medication has a sedative effect helps you to eliminate options 1 and 3 first. Next, recalling that the medication causes dry mouth helps you to eliminate option 2. If you had difficulty with this question, review the client teaching points related to this medication.
Level of Cognitive Ability: Comprehension
Client Needs: Health Promotion and Maintenance
Integrated Concept/Process: Teaching/Learning
Content Area: Pharmacology
Reference: Hodgson B, Kizior R: *Saunders nursing drug handbook 2002*, Philadelphia, 2002, WB Saunders, p. 352.

15. *Answer:* 2
Rationale: The client is taught about side effects that could occur with use of codeine sulfate. The most common side effects include drowsiness, confusion, hypotension, nausea and vomiting, and constipation. Others include bradycardia, respiratory depression, and urinary retention.
Test-Taking Strategy: Use the process of elimination. Recalling the effects of narcotics will direct you to option 2. Review these side effects if you had difficulty with this question.
Level of Cognitive Ability: Comprehension
Client Needs: Health Promotion and Maintenance
Integrated Concept/Process: Teaching/Learning

Content Area: Pharmacology
Reference: Hodgson B, Kizior R: *Saunders nursing drug handbook 2002*, Philadelphia, 2002, WB Saunders, p. 269.

16. *Answer:* 1
Rationale: Hydrocodone bitartrate is an opioid analgesic that also has antitussive properties. Side effects of this medication include physical and psychological dependence, bradycardia and hypotension, respiratory depression, nausea, vomiting, constipation, sedation, and confusion.
Test-Taking Strategy: Use the process of elimination recalling that hydrocodone bitartrate is an opioid analgesic that causes physical and psychological dependence. If this question was difficult, review information on the implications of opioid use and the side effects of this medication.
Level of Cognitive Ability: Application
Client Needs: Psychosocial Integrity
Integrated Concept/Process: Nursing Process/Data Collection
Content Area: Pharmacology
Reference: Hodgson B, Kizior R: *Saunders nursing drug handbook 2002*, Philadelphia, 2002, WB Saunders, p. 537.

17. *Answer:* 1
Rationale: Cromolyn sodium is an antiasthmatic, antiallergic, and a mast-cell stabilizer that inhibits the release of mediators from mast cells after exposure to an antigen. It can also interrupt the migration of eosinophils into the inflammatory site and decrease the number of eosinophils. These actions decrease airway hyperresponsiveness in some clients with asthma. It has no bronchodilating action.
Test-Taking Strategy: Use the process of elimination. Eliminate options 2 and 3 first because they are similar. To select between the remaining options, it is helpful to know that cromolyn sodium (Intal) has no bronchodilating action. Also, note the relationship between the words "Antigen" in the correct option and "allergic" in the question. Review the action of this medication if you had difficulty with this question.
Level of Cognitive Ability: Comprehension
Client Needs: Physiological Integrity
Integrated Concept/Process: Teaching/Learning
Content Area: Pharmacology
Reference: Hodgson B, Kizior R: *Saunders nursing drug handbook 2002*, Philadelphia, 2002, WB Saunders, p. 283.

18. *Answer:* 4
Rationale: The most common undesirable side effect associated with inhalation therapy of cromolyn sodium are bronchospasm, cough, nasal congestion, throat irritation, and wheezing. Clients receiving this medication orally may experience pruritis, nausea, diarrhea, and myalgia.
Test-Taking Strategy: Use the process of elimination and note the key word "undesirable." Use the ABCs—airway, breathing, and circulation—to select the correct option. Option 4 addresses airway. Review the side effects of this medication if you had difficulty with this question.
Level of Cognitive Ability: Application
Client Needs: Physiological Integrity
Integrated Concept/Process: Teaching/Learning
Content Area: Pharmacology
Reference: Hodgson B, Kizior R: *Saunders nursing drug handbook 2002*, Philadelphia, 2002, WB Saunders, p. 283.

19. *Answer:* 4
Rationale: Terbutaline sulfate is contraindicated in clients with hypersensitivity to sympathomimetics. It should be used with caution in clients with impaired cardiac function, diabetes mellitus, hypertension, hyperthyroidism, and clients with a history of seizures. The medication may increase blood glucose levels.
Test-Taking Strategy: Use the process of elimination and note the key words "with caution." Recalling that the medication increases blood glucose levels will direct you to option 4.. Review the contraindications and cautions associated with this medication if you had difficulty with this question.
Level of Cognitive Ability: Analysis
Client Needs: Physiological Integrity
Integrated Concept/Process: Nursing Process/Data Collection
Content Area: Pharmacology
Reference: Hodgson B, Kizior R: *Saunders nursing drug handbook 2002*, Philadelphia, 2002, WB Saunders, p. 1056.

20. *Answer:* 3
Rationale: Zafirlukast is a leukotriene receptor antagonist that is used in the prophylaxis and chronic treatment of bronchial asthma. It is used with caution in clients with impaired hepatic function. Liver function laboratory values should be obtained as a baseline and should be monitored during administration of the medication.
Test-Taking Strategy: Use the process of elimination. Eliminate options 2 and 4 first, because a complete blood count would include a neutrophil count. From this point, you would need to know that this medication would affect hepatic function. If you had difficulty with this question, review this medication.
Level of Cognitive Ability: Analysis
Client Needs: Physiological Integrity
Integrated Concept/Process: Nursing Process/Data Collection
Content Area: Pharmacology
Reference: Hodgson B, Kizior R: *Saunders nursing drug handbook 2002*, Philadelphia, 2002, WB Saunders, p. 1162.

REFERENCES

Clark J, Queener S, Karb V: *Pharmacologic basis of nursing practice*, ed 6, St Louis, 2000, Mosby.
Hodgson B, Kizior R: *Saunders nursing drug handbook 2002*, Philadelphia, 2002, WB Saunders.
Ignatavicius D, Workman M: *Medical-surgical: Critical thinking for collaborative care*, ed 4, Philadelphia, 2002, WB Saunders.
Karch A: *Focus on nursing pharmacology*, Philadelphia, 2000, Lippincott.
Lehne R: *Pharmacology for nursing care*, ed 4, Philadelphia, 2001, WB Saunders.

UNIT XIII

The Adult Client with a Cardiovascular Disorder

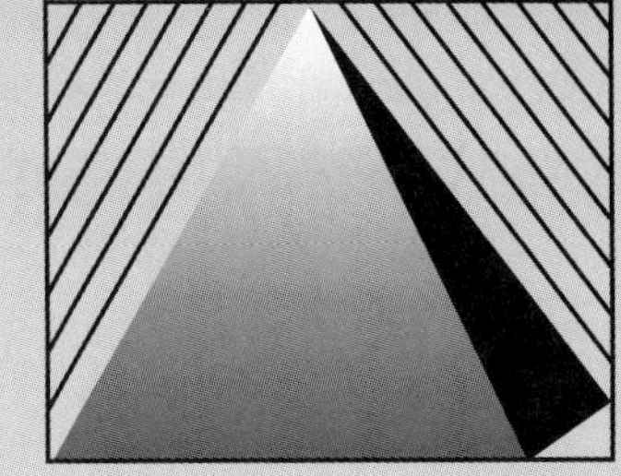

PYRAMID TERMS

Arterial Anastomoses Ensures that when one of the blood-supplying arteries is damaged, flow is maintained from the other arteries. Blood flow to the hands, feet, brain, and other organs is protected by arterial anastomoses.

Blood Pressure (BP) Measures the force exerted by the blood against the walls of the blood vessels. If the BP falls too low, blood flow to the tissues, heart, brain, and other organs become inadequate. If the BP becomes too high, the risk of vessel rupture and damage increases.

Cardiac Output The total volume of blood pumped through the heart in 1 minute.

Diastole The phase of the cardiac cycle in which the heart relaxes between contractions. It represents the period of time when the two ventricles are dilated by the blood flowing into them.

Diastolic Pressure The force of the blood exerted against the artery walls when the heart relaxes or fills. Normal diastolic pressure is 60 to 90 mm Hg.

Postural (Orthostatic) Hypotension A blood pressure fall of more than 20 mm Hg in the systolic pressure or a fall of more than 10 mm Hg in the diastolic pressure and a 10% to 20% increase in heart rate. Occurs when the client's blood pressure is not adequately maintained when moving from a lying to a sitting or standing position.

Pulse Pressure The difference between the systolic pressure and diastolic pressure. Normal pulse pressure is 30 to 40 mm Hg.

Systole The phase of contraction of the heart, especially of the ventricles, during which blood is forced into the aorta and pulmonary artery.

Systolic Pressure The maximum pressure of blood exerted against the artery walls when the heart contracts. Normal systolic pressure is 100 to 140 mm Hg.

PYRAMID TO SUCCESS

Pyramid points focus on data collection related to cardiovascular risks, health screening and promotion, complications of the various cardiovascular disorders, emergency implementation measures, and client education. Focus on the findings in angina, myocardial infarction (MI), heart failure and pulmonary edema, hypertension, and arterial and venous disorders. Focus on the care of the client after diagnostic treatments and surgical procedures. Note appropriate and therapeutic client positions, particularly with arterial and venous disorders of the extremities. Focus on treatments and medications prescribed for the various cardiovascular disorders and client teaching related to prescribed treatment plans. Be familiar with the components related to cardiac rehabilitation. The Integrated Concepts and Processes addressed in this unit include the Clinical Problem-Solving Process (Nursing Process), Caring, Communication and Documentation, Cultural Awareness, Self-Care, and Teaching/Learning.

CLIENT NEEDS

Safe, Effective Care Environment

Cardiovascular consultations and referrals
Establishing priorities
Informed consent related to treatments and procedures
Standard (universal) precautions

Health Promotion and Maintenance

Alterations in lifestyle
Assisting with the mobilization of appropriate community resources
Cardiac rehabilitation
Health screening and health promotion programs
Prevention of cardiovascular disease
Teaching related to diet therapy, exercise, and the administration of medications

Psychosocial Integrity

Accepting lifestyle changes
Body image changes
Coping mechanisms
Fear, anxiety, and denial
Support systems

Physiological Integrity

Activity limitations and rest and sleep
Assisting with basic care measures
Interventions required in emergencies
Monitoring cardiac enzymes and laboratory values related to the cardiovascular system
Monitoring for complications related to cardiovascular disorders
Nonpharmacological and pharmacological comfort interventions

REFERENCES

Black J, Hawks J, Keene A: *Medical-surgical nursing: clinical management for positive outcomes*, ed 6, Philadelphia, 2001, WB Saunders.

Chernecky C, Berger B: *Laboratory tests and diagnostic procedures*, ed 3, Philadelphia, 2001, WB Saunders.

Clark J, Queener S, Karb V: *Pharmacologic basis of nursing practice*, ed 6, St Louis, 2000, Mosby.

DeWit S: *Fundamental concepts and skills for nursing*, Philadelphia, 2001, WB Saunders.

Hill S, Howlett H: *Success in practical nursing: personal and vocational issues*, ed 4, Philadelphia, 2001, WB Saunders.

National Council of State Boards of Nursing: *Test plan for the National Council Licensure Examination for Practical/Vocational Nurses*, Chicago, 2001, Author.

Potter P, Perry A: *Fundamentals of nursing*, ed 5, St Louis, 2001, Mosby.

Perry A, Potter P: *Clinical nursing skills and techniques*, ed 5, St Louis, 2002, Mosby.

Wilson J: *Infection control in clinical practice*, ed 2, St Louis, 2002, Balliere Tindall.

48 Cardiovascular System

I. ANATOMY AND PHYSIOLOGY

A. Heart and heart layers
   1. The heart is located in the left side of the mediastinum
   2. The epicardium covers the outer surface of the heart
   3. The myocardium is the middle layer and is the actual contracting muscle of the heart
   4. The endocardium is the innermost layer and lines the inner chambers and the heart valves

B. Pericardium
   1. The pericardium encases and protects the heart from trauma and infection
   2. The parietal pericardium is the tough, fibrous outer membrane that is attached anteriorly to the lower half of the sternum, posteriorly to the thoracic vertebrae and inferiorly to the diaphragm
   3. The visceral pericardium is the thin, inner layer that closely adheres to the heart
   4. The pericardial space is between the parietal and visceral layers; it holds 5 to 20 mL of pericardial fluid that lubricates the pericardial surfaces and cushions the heart

C. Heart chambers
   1. The right atrium receives deoxygenated blood from the body via the superior and inferior vena cava
   2. The right ventricle receives blood from right atrium and pumps it to the lungs via the pulmonary artery
   3. The left atrium receives oxygenated blood from the lungs via four pulmonary veins
   4. The left ventricle is the largest and most muscular chamber; it receives oxygenated blood from the lungs via the left atrium and pumps blood into the systemic circulation via the aorta

D. Heart valves
   1. The atrioventricular valves lie between the atria and ventricles
   2. The atrioventricular valves close at the beginning of ventricular contraction and prevent blood from flowing back into the atria from the ventricles; these valves open when the ventricle relaxes
   3. The bicuspid or mitral valve is located on the left side of the heart
   4. The tricuspid valve is located on the right side of the heart
   5. The pulmonic semilunar valve lies between the right ventricle and the pulmonary artery
   6. The aortic semilunar valve lies between the left ventricle and the aorta
   7. The semilunar valves prevent blood from flowing back into the ventricles during relaxation; they open during ventricular contraction and close when the ventricles begin to relax.

E. Atrioventricular (AV) node
   1. The AV node is located in the lower aspect of the atrial septum
   2. The AV node receives electrical impulses from the sinoatrial (SA) node

F. The bundle of His (AV bundle)
   1. The bundle of His fuses with the AV node to form another pacemaker site
   2. It branches into the right bundle branch (RBB), which branches down the right side of the interventricular septum, and the left bundle branch (LBB), which extends into the left ventricle
   3. The right and left bundle branches terminate into Purkinje's fibers
   4. If the SA node fails, the bundle of His can initiate and sustain a heart rate at 40 to 60 beats per minute

G. Purkinje's fibers
   1. Purkinje's fibers are a diffuse network of conducting strands located beneath the ventricular endocardium
   2. These fibers spread the wave of depolarization through the ventricles

H. Coronary arteries
   1. The coronary arteries supply the capillaries of the myocardium with blood
   2. The right coronary artery (RCA) supplies the right atrium and ventricle, the inferior portion of the left ventricle, the posterior septal wall, the sinoatrial and the atrioventricular nodes
   3. The left coronary artery (LCA) consists of two major branches, the left anterior descending (LAD) and the circumflex arteries
   4. The LAD supplies blood to the anterior wall of the left ventricle, the anterior ventricular septum, and the apex of the left ventricle
   5. The circumflex artery supplies blood to the left atrium and the lateral and posterior surfaces of the left ventricle

I. Sinoatrial (SA) node
   1. The SA node or pacemaker initiates each heart beat
   2. Its location is at the junction of the superior vena cava and the right atrium
   3. It generates electrical impulses at approximately 60 to 100 times or beats per minute (bpm) and is controlled by the sympathetic and parasympathetic systems

J. Heart sounds
   1. The first heart sound (S_1) is heard as the AV valves close
   2. The second heart sound (S_2) is heard when the semilunar valves close

K. Heart rate
   1. The faster the heart rate, the less time the heart has for filling, and the **cardiac output** decreases
   2. An increase in heart rate increases oxygen consumption
   3. The normal heart rate is 60 to 100 bpm
   4. Sinus tachycardia is a rate of more than 100 bpm
   5. Sinus bradycardia is a rate of less than 60 bpm

L. Autonomic nervous system
   1. Stimulation of sympathetic nerve fibers releases the neurotransmitter norepinephrine producing an increased heart rate, increased conduction speed through the AV node, increased atrial and ventricular contractility, and peripheral vasoconstriction; stimulation occurs when a decrease in pressure is detected
   2. Stimulation of the parasympathetic nerve fibers releases the neurotransmitter acetylcholine, which decreases the heart rate and lessens atrial and ventricular contractility and conductivity; stimulation occurs when an increase in pressure is detected

M. **Blood pressure control**
   1. Baroreceptors, also called pressoreceptors, are located in the walls of the aortic arch and carotid sinuses
   2. Baroreceptors are specialized nerve endings that are affected by changes in the arterial **blood pressure**
   3. Increases in arterial pressure stimulate baroreceptors, and the heart rate and arterial pressure decrease
   4. Decreases in arterial pressure lead to a lessened stimulation of the baroreceptors, and vasoconstriction occurs as does an increase in heart rate
   5. Stretch receptors, located in the vena cava and the right atrium, respond to pressure changes that affect circulatory blood volume
   6. When the **blood pressure** decreases as a result of hypovolemia, a sympathetic response occurs causing increased heart rate and blood vessel constriction; when the **blood pressure** increases as a result of hypervolemia, an opposite effect occurs
   7. The antidiuretic hormone (ADH) influences **blood pressure** indirectly by regulating vascular volume
   8. Increases in blood volume result in decreased ADH release, increasing diuresis, decreasing blood volume, and thus **blood pressure**
   9. Decreases in blood volume result in increased ADH release; this promotes an increase in blood volume and thus **blood pressure**
   10. Renin, a potent vasoconstrictor, causes the **blood pressure** to increase
   11. Renin converts angiotensinogen to angiotensin I; angiotensin I is then converted to angiotensin II in the lungs
   12. Angiotensin II stimulates the release of aldosterone, which promotes water and sodium retention by the kidneys; this action increases blood volume and **blood pressure**

N. The vascular system
   1. The arteries are vessels through which the blood passes away from the heart to various parts of the body; they convey blood with high concentrations of oxygen from the left side of the heart to the tissues
   2. The arterioles control the blood flow into the capillaries

3. The capillaries allow the exchange of fluid and nutrients between the blood and the interstitial spaces
4. Venules receive blood from the capillary bed and move blood into the veins
5. Veins transport deoxygenated blood from the tissues back toward the heart and lungs for oxygenation
6. Valves help return blood to the heart against the force of gravity
7. The lymphatics drain the tissues and return the tissue fluid to the blood

II. DIAGNOSTIC TESTS AND PROCEDURES (REFER TO CHAPTER 10 FOR NORMAL LABORATORY VALUES.)

A. Cardiac enzymes
1. CK-MB (creatine kinase, myocardial muscle)
   a. An elevation in value indicates myocardial damage
   b. An elevation occurs within 4 to 6 hours and peaks 18 to 24 hours after the acute ischemic attack
   c. Normal value in conventional units is 0 to 7 units per liter (U/L)
2. Lactic acid dehydrogenase (LDH)
   a. Elevations in LDH occur within 48 hours after myocardial infarction
   b. When the serum concentration of LDH_1 is higher than LDH_2, the pattern is indicated as "flipped" signifying myocardial necrosis
   c. Normal value in conventional units is 70 to 200 IU per liter (IU/L)

B. Troponin
1. Composed of three proteins: cardiac troponin, troponin I, and troponin T
2. Troponin I, especially, has a high affinity for myocardial injury; it rises within 3 hours and persists for up to 7 days
3. Normal values are quite low, with tropinin T normally ranging from 0.0 to 0.2 ng/mL, and troponin I being less than 0.6 ng/mL; thus any rise can indicate myocardial cell damage

C. Myoglobin
1. An oxygen-binding protein found in cardiac and skeletal muscle
2. Level rises within 1 hour after cell death, peaks in 4 to 6 hours, and returns to normal within 24 to 36 hours (and in some clients even faster)

D. Complete blood cell count (CBC)
1. The red blood cell count decreases in rheumatic heart disease and infective endocarditis and increases in conditions characterized by inadequate tissue oxygenation
2. The white blood cell count increases in infectious and inflammatory diseases of the heart and after myocardial infarction because large numbers of white blood cells (WBCs) are required to dispose of the necrotic tissue resulting from the infarction
3. An elevated hematocrit can result from vascular volume depletion
4. Decrease in hematocrit and hemoglobin can indicate anemia

E. Blood coagulation factors: an increase in coagulation factors can occur during and after a myocardial infarction, which places the client at greater risk of thrombophlebitis and extension of clots in the coronary artery

F. Serum lipids
1. The lipid profile measures serum cholesterol, triglycerides, and lipoprotein levels
2. The lipid profile is used to assess the risk of developing coronary artery disease

G. Electrolytes
1. Potassium level
   a. Hypokalemia causes increased cardiac electrical instability, ventricular dysrhythmias, and increased risk of digitalis toxicity
   b. In hypokalemia, the ECG would show flattening and inversion of the T wave, the appearance of a U wave, and depression of the ST segment
   c. Hyperkalemia causes asystole and ventricular dysrhythmias
2. Sodium level
   a. The serum sodium level decreases with the use of diuretics
   b. The serum sodium level decreases in congestive heart failure, indicating water excess

H. Calcium level
1. Hypocalcemia can cause ventricular dysrhythmias, prolonged QT interval, and cardiac arrest
2. Hypercalcemia can cause a shortened QT interval, AV block, tachycardia or bradycardia, digitalis hypersensitivity, and cardiac arrest

I. Phosphorus level: Phosphorus levels should be interpreted with calcium levels because the kidneys retain or excrete one electrolyte in an inverse relationship to the other

J. Magnesium level
1. A low magnesium level can cause ventricular tachycardia and fibrillation
2. A high magnesium level can cause muscle weakness, hypotension, bradycardia, and a prolonged PR interval and wide QRS complex

K. Blood urea nitrogen (BUN): the BUN is elevated in heart disorders such as congestive heart failure and cardiogenic shock, which adversely affects renal circulation

L. Blood glucose: an acute cardiac episode can elevate the blood glucose

M. Chest x-ray study
   1. Description
      a. Done to determine the size, silhouette, and position of the heart
      b. Specific pathological changes are difficult to determine via x-ray study, but anatomical changes can be seen
   2. Implementation
      a. Prepare client for x-ray study explaining purpose and procedure
      b. Remove jewelry

N. Electrocardiogram (ECG)
   1. Description: a noninvasive common diagnostic test that evaluates the heart's function by recording electrical activity
   2. Implementation
      a. Advise the client to lie still, breathe normally, and refrain from talking during the test
      b. Reassure the client that an electrical shock will not occur
      c. Document any cardiac medications the client is taking

O. Holter monitoring
   1. Description
      a. A noninvasive test in which the client wears a Holter monitor and an ECG tracing is recorded continuously over 24 or more hours
      b. It identifies dysrhythmias if they occur and evaluates the effectiveness of antidysrhythmics or pacemaker therapy
   2. Implementation: instruct the client to resume normal daily activities and to maintain a diary documenting activities and any symptoms that may develop

P. Echocardiogram
   1. Description
      a. A noninvasive procedure, based on the principles of ultrasound
      b. It evaluates structural and functional changes in the heart
   2. Implementation: advise the client to lie still, breathe normally, and refrain from talking during the test

Q. Exercise testing (stress test)
   1. Description
      a. A noninvasive test that studies the heart during activity and detects and evaluates coronary artery disease
      b. Treadmill testing is the most commonly used mode of stress testing
      c. Stress testing may be used in conjunction with myocardial radionuclide testing at which point the procedure becomes invasive, as a radionuclide must be injected
      d. An informed consent is required if a radionuclide is injected
   2. Preprocedure implementation
      a. Obtain an informed consent if required
      b. Provide adequate rest the night before the procedure
      c. Instruct the client to eat a light meal 1 to 2 hours before the procedure
      d. Instruct the client to avoid smoking, alcohol, and caffeine before the procedure
      e. Ask the physician about taking prescribed medication on the day of the procedure
      f. Instruct the client to wear nonconstrictive, comfortable clothing and supportive shoes
   3. Postprocedure implementation
      a. Instruct the client to notify the physician if any chest pain, dizziness, or shortness of breath occurs
      b. Instruct the client to avoid taking a hot bath or shower for at least 1 to 2 hours

R. Digital subtraction angiography
   1. Description
      a. Combines x-ray techniques and a computerized subtraction technique with fluoroscopy for visualization of the cardiovascular system
      b. A contrast medium (dye) is injected
   2. Preprocedure implementation
      a. Assess client for allergy to contrast medium (dye), iodine, or seafood
      b. Obtain an informed consent
   3. Postprocedure implementation
      a. Monitor vital signs
      b. Assess injection site for bleeding or discomfort

S. Nuclear cardiology
   1. Description
      a. The use of radionuclide techniques and scanning in cardiovascular assessment
      b. The most common tests include technetium pyrophosphate scanning, thallium imaging, and multigated cardiac blood pool imaging (MUGA)
   2. Preprocedure implementation
      a. Obtain an informed consent
      b. Inform the client that a small amount of radioisotope will be injected and that the radiation exposure and risks are minimal
   3. Postprocedure implementation
      a. Assess vital signs
      b. Assess injection site for bleeding or discomfort

c. Inform the client that he or she may feel fatigued

T. Cardiac catheterization

1. Description
   a. Involves insertion of a catheter into the heart and surrounding vessels
   b. Obtains information about the structure and performance of the heart valves and circulatory system
2. Preprocedure implementation
   a. Obtain an informed consent
   b. Assess for allergies to seafood, iodine, or radiopaque dyes
   c. Withhold solid food for 6 to 8 hours and liquids for 4 hours to prevent vomiting and aspiration during the procedure
   d. Document client's height and weight because this information will be needed to determine the amount of dye to be administered
   e. Document baseline vital signs and note the quality and presence of peripheral pulses for postprocedure comparison
   f. Inform the client that a local anesthetic will be administered before catheter insertion
   g. Inform the client that he or she may feel fatigued because it is necessary to lie still and quiet on a relatively hard table for up to 2 hours
   h. Inform the client that he or she may feel a fluttery feeling as the catheter passes through the heart, a flushed, warm feeling when the dye is injected, a desire to cough, and palpitations caused by heart irritability
   i. Prepare insertion site by shaving and cleaning with an antiseptic solution if prescribed
   j. Administer preprocedure medications if prescribed
   k. Insert an IV if prescribed
3. Postprocedure implementation
   a. Monitor vital signs and cardiac rhythm for dysrhythmias every 30 minutes for 2 hours initially
   b. Monitor for chest pain and if dysrhythmias or chest pain occurs, notify the physician
   c. Monitor peripheral pulses and the color, warmth, and sensation of the extremity distal to insertion site every 30 minutes for 2 hours initially
   d. Notify the physician if the client complains of numbness and tingling; if the extremity becomes cool, pale, or cyanotic; or if sudden loss of peripheral pulses occurs
   e. Monitor the insertion site for bleeding or hematoma formation
   f. Apply a sandbag to the insertion site to provide additional pressure if required
   g. Monitor for bleeding and if bleeding occurs, apply pressure immediately and notify the physician
   h. Monitor for hematoma and if a hematoma develops, notify the physician
   i. Keep extremity extended for 4 to 6 hours, with the leg straight to prevent arterial occlusion
   j. Maintain strict bed rest for 6 to 12 hours; however the client may turn from side to side; do not elevate the head of the bed more than 15 degrees
   k. If the antecubital vessel was used, immobilize the arm on an armboard
   l. Encourage fluids if not contraindicated to promote renal excretion of the dye
   m. Monitor for nausea, vomiting, and rash or other signs of hypersensitivity to the dye

III. THERAPEUTIC MANAGEMENT

A. Percutaneous transluminal coronary angioplasty (PTCA) 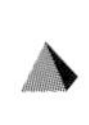

1. Description
   a. One or more arteries are dilated with a balloon catheter to open the vessel lumen and improve arterial blood flow
   b. The client can experience reocclusion after the procedure and the procedure may need to be repeated
   c. Complications can include arterial dissection or rupture, immobilization of plaque fragments, spasm, and acute myocardial infarction (MI)
   d. Firm commitment is needed on the part of client to stop smoking, lose weight, alter exercise pattern, and stop any behaviors that lead to progression of artery occlusion
2. Preprocedure implementation
   a. Maintain NPO status after midnight
   b. Prepare the groin area with antiseptic soap and shave per institutional procedure and as prescribed
   c. Assess baseline vital signs and peripheral pulses
3. Postprocedure implementation
   a. Monitor vital signs closely
   b. Monitor distal pulses in both extremities
   c. Maintain bed rest as prescribed, keeping the limb straight for 6 to 8 hours
   d. Administer anticoagulants and antiplatelets as prescribed to prevent thrombus formation

e. Monitor IV nitroglycerin if prescribed to prevent coronary spasm
f. Instruct the client in the administration of nitrates, calcium channel blockers, antiplatelets, and anticoagulants as prescribed
g. Instruct the client to take daily aspirin permanently if prescribed
h. Assist the client with planning lifestyle modifications

B. Laser-assisted angioplasty
1. Description
a. A laser probe is advanced through a cannula similar to that used for PTCA
b. Used for clients with small occlusions in the distal superficial femoral, proximal popliteal, and common iliac arteries
c. Heat from the laser vaporizes the plaque to open the occluded artery
2. Preprocedure and postprocedure care
a. Similar to the PTCA
b. Monitor for complications of coronary dissection, acute occlusion, perforation, embolism, and MI

C. Coronary artery stents
1. Description
a. Used instead of PTCA to eliminate the risk of acute coronary vessel closure and to improve long-term patency of the vessel
b. A balloon catheter bearing the stent is inserted into the coronary artery and positioned at the site of occlusion
c. When placed in the coronary artery, the stent reopens the blocked artery
2. Postprocedure implementation
a. Acute thrombosis is a major concern after the procedure, and the client is placed on antiplatelet and anticoagulation therapy for several months after the procedure
b. Monitor for complications of the procedure such as stent migration or occlusion, coronary artery dissection, and bleeding caused by anticoagulation

D. Atherectomy
1. Description
a. Removes plaque from an artery by the use of a cutting chamber on the inserted catheter or a rotating blade that pulverizes the plaque
b. Used to improve blood flow to ischemic limbs in individuals with peripheral arterial disease
2. Postprocedure implementation: monitor for complications of perforation, embolus, and restenosis

E. Transmyocardial revascularization
1. Used for clients with wide spread atherosclerosis involving vessels that are too small and numerous for replacement or balloon catheterization
2. Uses a high powered laser that creates 15 to 30 holes (channels) in the heart
3. Blood enters these small channels providing the affected region of the heart with oxygenated blood
4. Performed through a small chest incision
5. The opening on the heart's surface heals over; however, the main channels remain and perfuse the myocardium

F. Arterial revascularization
1. Description
a. Performed to increase arterial blood flow to the affected limb
b. Inflow procedures involve bypassing arterial occlusion above the superficial femoral arteries
c. Outflow procedures involve surgical bypassing of arterial occlusions at or below the superficial femoral arteries
d. Graft material is sutured above and below the occlusion to facilitate blood flow around the occlusion
2. Preoperative implementation
a. Assess baseline vital signs and peripheral pulses
b. Insert IV and urinary catheter as prescribed
c. Maintain central venous catheter and/or arterial line if inserted
3. Postoperative implementation
a. Assess vital signs
b. Monitor **blood pressure** and notify the physician if changes occur
c. Monitor for hypotension, which may indicate hypovolemia
d. Monitor for hypertension, which may place stress on the graft and facilitate clot formation
e. Maintain bed rest for 24 hours as prescribed
f. Instruct the client to keep affected extremity straight, limit movement, and avoid bending the knee and hip
g. Monitor for warmth, redness and edema, which are often expected outcomes as a result of increased blood flow
h. Monitor for graft occlusion, which often occurs within the first 24 hours
i. Assess peripheral pulses and for changes in color and temperature of the extremity
j. Monitor for a sharp increase in pain, as pain is frequently the first indicator of postoperative graft occlusion

k. If signs of graft occlusion occur, notify physician immediately
l. Encourage coughing and deep breathing and the use of incentive spirometry
m. Maintain NPO status and progress to clear liquids as prescribed
n. Use strict aseptic technique when in contact with the incision
o. Assess incision for drainage, warmth, or swelling
p. Monitor for excessive bleeding (a small amount of bloody drainage is expected)
q. Monitor the area over the graft for hardness, tenderness, and warmth, which may indicate infection; if this occurs, notify the physician immediately
r. Instruct the client about proper foot care and measures to prevent ulcer formation
s. Instruct the client to take medications as prescribed
t. Instruct the client how to care for incision
u. Assist the client in modifying lifestyle to prevent further plaque formation

G. Coronary artery bypass graft (CABG)
1. Description
a. The occluded coronary arteries are bypassed with the client's own venous or arterial blood vessels
b. The saphenous vein or internal mammary artery is used to bypass lesions in the coronary arteries
c. Performed when the client does not respond to medical management of coronary artery disease (CAD) or when disease progression is evident
2. Preoperative implementation
a. Familiarize the client and family with the cardiac surgical critical care unit
b. Instruct the client how to splint chest incision, cough and deep breathe, and perform arm and leg exercises
c. Instruct the client to inform the nurse of any postoperative pain, as pain medication will be available
d. Inform the client to expect a sternal incision, possibly a leg incision, one or two chest tubes, a Foley catheter, and several IV fluid catheters
e. Inform the client that an endotracheal tube will be in place and connected to a ventilator for 6 to 24 hours
f. Advise the client to breathe with the ventilator and not fight it
g. Inform the family that the client will not be able to talk while the endotracheal tube is in place
h. Encourage the client and family to discuss anxieties and fears related to surgery
i. Note that prescribed medications are to be discontinued before surgery (diuretics 2 to 3 days before surgery, digoxin [Lanoxin] 12 hours before surgery, and aspirin and anticoagulants 1 week before surgery)
j. Administer medications as prescribed, which may include potassium chloride, antihypertensives, antidysrhythmics, and antibiotics
3. Transfer from the cardiac surgical unit
a. Monitor vital signs, level of consciousness, and peripheral perfusion
b. Monitor for dysrhythmias
c. Auscultate lungs and assess respiratory status
d. Encourage the client to splint, cough, and deep breathe and use incentive spirometer to raise secretions and prevent atelectasis
e. Monitor temperature and WBC count, which, if elevated after 3 to 4 days, indicates infection
f. Provide adequate fluids and hydration as prescribed to liquefy secretions
g. Assess suture line and chest tube insertion sites for redness, purulent discharge, and signs of infection
h. Assess sternal suture line for instability, which may indicate an infection
i. Guide the client in a gradual resumption of activity
j. Assess the client for tachycardia, **orthostatic hypotension**, and fatigue before during and after activity
k. Discontinue activities if BP drops more that 10 to 20 mm Hg or pulse increases more than 10 beats per minute
l. Monitor episodes of pain closely
m. See Box 48-1 for home care instructions

H. Heart transplant
1. A donor heart from an individual with a comparable body weight and ABO compatibility is transplanted into a recipient in less than 6 hours of procurement
2. The surgeon removes the diseased heart, leaving the posterior portion of the atria, which serve as an anchor for the new heart
3. Because a remnant of the client's atria remains, two unrelated P waves are noted on the ECG
4. The transplanted heart is denervated and unresponsive to vagal stimulation; because the heart is denervated, clients do not experience angina

BOX 48-1

Home Care Instructions After Cardiac Surgery

Instruct the client on how to progress with activities at home

Inform the client to limit pushing or pulling activities for 6 weeks after discharge

Instruct the client about incisional care and to record signs of redness, swelling, or drainage

Inform the client that sternotomy heals in about 6 to 8 weeks

Instruct the client to avoid crossing legs, to wear elastic hose as prescribed until edema subsides, and to elevate surgical limb when sitting in a chair

Instruct the client in the use of prescribed medications

Instruct the client in dietary measures including the avoidance of saturated fats and cholesterol and the use of salt

Instruct the client that sexual intercourse can be resumed on the advice of the physician after exercise tolerance is assessed; if the client can walk one block or climb two flights of stairs without symptoms, the client can safely resume sexual activity

5. Symptoms of heart rejection include hypotension, dysrhythmias, weakness, fatigue, and dizziness
6. Endomyocardial biopsies are performed at regular scheduled intervals and whenever rejection is suspected.
7. Clients require immunosuppressive therapy for the rest of their lives
8. The heart rate approximates 100 beats per minute and responds slowly with increases in heart rate, contractility, and **cardiac output**, and to exercise and stress

IV. MANAGEMENT OF DYSRHYTHMIAS

A. Vagal maneuvers
   1. Description: induces vagal stimulation of the cardiac conduction system and are used to terminate supraventricular tachydysrhythmias
   2. Carotid sinus massage
      a. The physician instructs the client to turn the head away from the side to be massaged
      b. The physician massages over the carotid artery for 6 to 8 seconds until there is a change in cardiac rhythm
      c. Observe the cardiac monitor for a change in rhythm
      d. Record an ECG rhythm strip before, during, and after the procedure
      e. Have a defibrillator and resuscitative equipment available
      f. Monitor vital signs, cardiac rhythm, and LOC after the procedure
   3. Valsalva maneuvers
      a. The physician instructs the client to bear down or induces a gag reflex in the client both of which stimulate a vagal reflex
      b. Monitor the heart rate, rhythm, and **BP**
      c. Observe the cardiac monitor for a change in rhythm
      d. Record an ECG rhythm strip before, during, and after the procedure
      e. Provide an emesis basin if the gag reflex is stimulated and initiate precautions to prevent aspiration
      f. Have a defibrillator and resuscitative equipment available

B. Cardioversion
   1. Description
      a. Synchronized countershock to convert an undesirable rhythm to a stable rhythm
      b. An elective procedure done by the physician
      c. A lower wattage of energy is used than with defibrillation
      d. Defibrillator is synchronized to the client's R wave to avoid discharging the shock during the vulnerable period (T wave)
      e. If defibrillator were not synchronized, it would discharge on the T wave and cause ventricular fibrillation (VF)
   2. Preprocedure implementation
      a. Obtain an informed consent
      b. Administer sedation as prescribed
      c. Hold digoxin (Lanoxin) 48 hours preprocedure as prescribed to prevent postcardioversion ventricular irritability
   3. During the procedure
      a. Ensure that the skin is clean and dry in the area where the electrode paddles will be placed
      b. Oxygen is stopped during the procedure to avoid hazard of fire
      c. Be sure no one is touching the bed or the client when delivering the countershock
   4. Postprocedure implementation
      a. Maintain airway patency
      b. Administer oxygen as prescribed
      c. Assess vital signs
      d. Assess level of consciousness
      e. Monitor cardiac rhythm
      f. Monitor for indications of successful response such as conversion to sinus rhythm, strong peripheral pulses, and an adequate **BP**

C. Defibrillation
   1. Description

a. An asynchronous countershock used to terminate pulseless ventricular tachycardia (VT) or VF
b. Three rapid consecutive shocks are delivered with the first at an energy of 200 joules
c. If unsuccessful, the shock is repeated at 200 to 300 joules
d. The third and subsequent shock will be at 360 joules

2. During the procedure
    a. Oxygen is stopped during the procedure to avoid hazard of fire
    b. Be sure no one is touching the bed or the client when delivering the countershock

D. Use of paddle electrodes
1. Apply conductive pads
2. One paddle is placed at the third intercostal space to the right of the sternum; the other is placed at the fifth intercostal space on the left mid-axillary line
3. Apply firm pressure with the paddles
4. Be sure that no one is touching the bed or the client when delivering the countershock

E. Automatic external defibrillator (AED)
1. Used by laypersons and emergency medical technicians for prehospital cardiac arrest
2. Place the client on a firm, dry surface
3. Stop cardiopulmonary resuscitation (CPR)
4. Ensure that no one is touching the client to avoid motion artifact during rhythm analysis
5. Place the electrode paddles in the correct position on the client's chest
6. Press the analyzer button to identify the rhythm, which may take 30 seconds; the machine will advise whether a shock is necessary
7. Shocks are recommended for pulseless VF only
8. If shock is recommended, the shock is delivered at an energy of 200 joules for the first one
9. If unsuccessful, the shock is repeated at 200 to 300 joules
10. The third and subsequent shock will be at 360 joules
11. If unsuccessful, CPR is continued for 1 minute, and then another series of 3 shocks are delivered each at 360 joules of energy

F. Implantable cardioverter defibrillator (ICD)
1. Description
    a. Monitors cardiac rhythm and detects and terminates episodes of VT and VF
    b. It senses VT or VF and delivers 25 to 30 joules up to four times if necessary
    c. Used in clients with a history of VF or in unstable VT that is unresponsive to medications
    d. Electrodes are placed in the right atrium and ventricle and apical pericardium
    e. The generator is implanted in the abdomen
2. Client education
    a. Basic functioning of the ICD
    b. How to perform cough CPR
    c. How to take pulse and to take pulse daily and maintain a diary of pulse rates
    d. Wear loose-fitting clothing
    e. Avoid contact sports and strenuous activities
    f. Report any fever, redness, swelling, or drainage from the insertion site
    g. Report symptoms of fainting, nausea, weakness, blackouts, and rapid pulse rates to the physician
    h. During shock discharge, the client may feel faint or short of breath
    i. Instruct the client to sit or lie down if he or she feels a shock and to notify the physician
    j. Instruct the client and family how to access emergency medical system
    k. Encourage the family to learn CPR
    l. Advise the client to maintain a diary of any shocks that are delivered including the date, preceding activity, number of shocks, and whether the shocks were successful
    m. Instruct the client to avoid electromagnetic fields directly over the ICD because they can inactivate the device
    n. Instruct the client that if beeping tones are heard, to move away from the magnetic field immediately and notify the physician
    o. Keep a pacemaker identification card in the wallet and obtain and wear a Medic-Alert bracelet
    p. Inform all health care providers that an ICD is inserted

V. PACEMAKERS

A. Description: a temporary or permanent device that provides electrical stimulation and maintains the heart rate when the client's intrinsic pacemaker fails to provide a perfusing rhythm

B. Settings
1. Synchronous or demand pacemaker: senses the client's rhythm and paces only if the client's intrinsic rate falls below the set pacemaker rate
2. Asynchronous or fixed rate: paces at a preset rate regardless of the client's intrinsic rhythm

3. Overdrive pacing: to suppress the underlying rhythm in tachydysrhythmias so that the sinus node will regain control of the heart

C. Spikes
1. When a pacing stimulus is delivered to the heart, a spike (straight vertical line) is seen on the monitor or ECG strip
2. The spike should be followed by a P wave indicating atrial depolarization, or a QRS complex indicating ventricular depolarization; this pattern is referred to as "capture," indicating that the pacemaker successfully depolarized, or captured the chamber
3. If the electrode is in the ventricle, the spike is in front of the QRS complex; if the electrode is in the atria, the spike is before the P wave
4. If the electrode is in both the atria and ventricle, the spike is before both the P wave and QRS complex

D. Temporary pacemakers
1. Noninvasive temporary pacing (NTP)
   a. Used as an emergency measure or when a client is being transported and the risk of bradydysrhythmia exists
   b. A large electrode patch is placed on the chest and back
   c. Wash the skin with soap and water before applying electrodes
   d. Do not shave the hair or apply alcohol or tinctures to the skin
   e. Place the posterior electrode between the spine and left scapula behind the heart, avoiding placement over bone
   f. Place the anterior electrode between V2 and V5 position over the heart
   g. Do not place the anterior electrode over female breast tissue; rather, displace breast tissue and place under the breast
   h. Do not take the pulse or **BP** on the left side because the results will not be accurate due to the muscle twitching and electrical current
   i. Ensure that electrodes are in good contact with the skin
   j. If loss of "capture" occurs, assess the skin contact of the electrodes and increase the current until "capture" is regained
2. Transvenous invasive temporary pacing
   a. Pacing lead wire is placed through antecubital, femoral, jugular, or subclavian into the right atrium for atrial pacing, or through the right ventricle, and positioned in contact with the endocardium
   b. Monitor cardiac rhythm continuously
   c. Monitor vital signs
   d. Monitor pacemaker insertion site
   e. Restrict client movement to prevent lead wire displacement
3. Epicardial invasive temporary pacing: applied using a transthoracic approach; the lead wires are loosely threaded on the epicardial surface of the heart after cardiac surgery
4. Reducing the risk of microshock
   a. Use only inspected and approved equipment
   b. Insulate the exposed portion of wires with plastic or rubber material (fingers of rubber gloves) when wires are not attached to the pulse generator, and cover with nonconductive tape
   c. Ground all electrical equipment using a three-pronged plug
   d. Wear gloves when handling exposed wires
   e. Keep dressings dry

E. Permanent pacemakers
1. Pulse generator is internal and surgically implanted in a subcutaneous pocket under the clavicle or abdominal wall
2. The leads are passed transvenously via the cephalic or subclavian vein to the endocardium on the right side of the heart
3. May be single chambered, in which the lead wire is placed in the chamber to be paced, or may be dual chambered, with lead wires placed in the atrium and right ventricle
4. It is programmed when inserted and can be reprogrammed if necessary by noninvasive transmission from an external programmer to the implanted generator
5. Pacemakers are powered by either a lithium battery that has an average life span of 10 years, are nuclear powered with a life span of 20 years or longer, or are designed to be recharged externally
6. Provide client teaching as per Box 48-2

VI. CORONARY ARTERY DISEASE

A. Description
1. A narrowing or obstruction of the coronary arteries resulting from atherosclerosis, an accumulation of fatty plaques made of lipids in the arteries
2. Causes a decreased perfusion of myocardial tissue and inadequate myocardial oxygen supply
3. Leads to hypertension, angina, dysrhythmias, myocardial infarction, congestive heart failure, and death
4. Collateral circulation, more than one artery supplying a muscle with blood, is normally present in the coronary arteries, especially in older persons

BOX 48-2

Pacemakers: Client Education

Instruct the client about the pacemaker including the programmed rate
Instruct the client in the signs of battery failure and when to notify the physician
Instruct the client to report any fever, redness, swelling, or drainage from the insertion site
Report signs of dizziness, weakness or fatigue, swelling of the ankles or legs, chest pain, or shortness of breath
Keep pacemaker ID in wallet and obtain and wear a Medic-Alert bracelet
Instruct the client how to take pulse, to take the pulse daily, and to maintain a diary of pulse rates
Wear loose-fitting clothing
Avoid contact sports
Inform all health care providers that a pacemaker is inserted
Instruct the client to inform airport security that they have a pacemaker as the pacemaker may set off the security detector
Instruct the client that most electrical appliances can be used without any interference with the functioning of the pacemaker; however, advise the client not to operate electrical appliances directly over pacemaker site
Avoid transmitter towers and antitheft devices in stores
Instruct the client that if any unusual feelings occur when near any electrical devices, to move 5 to 10 feet away and to check the pulse
Emphasize the importance of follow-up visits with the physician

5. The development of collateral circulation takes time and occurs when chronic ischemia develops to meet metabolic demands; therefore an occlusion of a coronary artery in a younger individual is more likely to be lethal than in an older individual
6. Symptoms occur when the coronary artery is occluded to the point that inadequate blood supply to the muscle occurs causing ischemia
7. Coronary artery narrowing is significant if the lumen diameter of the left main artery is reduced at least 50%, or if any major branch is reduced at least 75%
8. The goal of treatment is to alter the atherosclerotic progression

B. Data collection
1. Findings may be normal during asymptomatic periods
2. Chest pain
3. Palpitations
4. Dyspnea
5. Syncope
6. Cough or hemoptysis
7. Excessive fatigue

C. Diagnostic studies
1. ECG
   a. When blood flow is reduced and ischemia occurs, ST segment depression or T-wave inversion is noted; the ST segment returns to normal when the blood flow returns.
   b. With infarction, cell injury results in ST segment elevation, followed by T-wave inversion
2. Cardiac catheterization
   a. Provides the most definitive source for diagnosis
   b. Would show the presence of atherosclerotic lesions
3. Blood lipid levels
   a. Blood lipid levels may be elevated
   b. Cholesterol-lowering medications may be prescribed to reduce the development of atherosclerotic plaques

D. Implementation
1. Instruct the client regarding purpose of diagnostic medical and surgical procedures and the expected preprocedure and postprocedure expectations
2. Assist the client to identify risk factors that can be modified
3. Assist the client to set goals that will promote changes in lifestyle to reduce the impact of risk factors
4. Assist the client to identify barriers to compliance with the therapeutic plan and to identify methods to overcome barriers
5. Instruct the client regarding a low-calorie, low-sodium, low-cholesterol, and low-fat diet with an increase in dietary fiber
6. Stress to the client that dietary changes are not temporary and must be maintained for life; instruct the client regarding prescribed medications
7. Provide community resources to client regarding exercise, smoking cessation, and stress reduction

E. Surgical procedures
1. Percutaneous transluminal coronary angioplasty (PTCA) to compress the plaque against the walls of the artery and dilate the vessel
2. Laser angioplasty to vaporize the plaque
3. Atherectomy to remove the plaque from the artery
4. Vascular stent to prevent the artery from closing and prevent restenosis
5. Coronary artery bypass graft to improve blood flow to the myocardial tissues that are at risk for ischemia or infarction as a result of the occluded artery

F. Medications
   1. Nitrates to dilate the coronary arteries and to decrease preload and afterload
   2. Calcium channel blockers to dilate coronary arteries and reduce vasospasm
   3. Cholesterol-lowering medications may be prescribed to reduce the development of atherosclerotic plaques
   4. Beta blockers to reduce **blood pressure** in those individuals who are hypertensive

VII. ANGINA

A. Description
   1. Chest pain resulting from myocardial ischemia caused by inadequate myocardial blood and oxygen supply
   2. Caused by an imbalance between oxygen supply and demand
   3. Causes include obstruction of coronary blood flow resulting from atherosclerosis, coronary artery spasm, and conditions increasing myocardial oxygen consumption
   4. The goal of treatment is to provide relief of an acute attack, correct the imbalance between myocardial oxygen supply and demand, to prevent the progression of the disease and further attacks to reduce the risk of MI

B. Patterns of angina
   1. Stable angina
      a. Also called exertional angina
      b. Occurs with activities as exertion or emotional stress and the pain is relieved with rest or nitroglycerin
      c. It usually has a stable pattern of onset, duration, severity, and relieving factors
   2. Unstable angina
      a. Also called preinfarction angina
      b. Occurs with an unpredictable degree of exertion or emotion and increases in occurrence, duration, and severity over time
      c. Pain may not be relieved with nitroglycerin
   3. Variant angina
      a. Also called Prinzmetal's or vasoplastic angina
      b. Results from coronary artery spasm, is similar to classic angina, but lasts longer
      c. It may occur at rest
      d. Attacks may be associated with elevation of the ST segment on the ECG
   4. Intractable angina: a chronic incapacitating angina, which is unresponsive to interventions
   5. Preinfarction angina
      a. Associated with acute coronary insufficiency
      b. Angina that lasts longer than 15 minutes
      c. A symptom of worsening cardiac ischemia
   6. Post infarction angina: occurs after an MI when residual ischemia may cause episodes of angina

C. Data collection
   1. Pain
      a. Can develop slowly or quickly
      b. Usually described as mild or moderate pain
      c. Substernal, crushing, squeezing pain
      d. May radiate to the shoulders, arms, jaw, neck, back
      e. Usually lasts less than 5 minutes; however, can last up to 15 to 20 minutes
      f. Relieved by nitroglycerin or rest
   2. Dyspnea
   3. Pallor
   4. Sweating
   5. Palpitations and tachycardia
   6. Dizziness and faintness
   7. Hypertension
   8. Digestive disturbances

D. Diagnostic studies
   1. ECG: normal during rest, with ST depression or elevation and/or T-wave inversion during an episode of pain
   2. Stress test: chest pain or changes in the ECG or vital signs during testing may indicate ischemia
   3. Cardiac enzymes: normal findings in angina
   4. Cardiac catheterization: provides a definitive diagnosis by providing information about the patency of the coronary arteries

E. Implementation
   1. Immediate management
      a. Assess pain
      b. Provide bed rest
      c. Administer oxygen at 3 liters nasal cannula as prescribed
      d. Administer nitroglycerin as prescribed to dilate the coronary arteries, reduce the oxygen requirements of the myocardium, and relieve the chest pain
      e. Obtain a 12-lead ECG
      f. Provide continuous cardiac monitoring
   2. After acute episode
      a. Instruct the client regarding purpose of diagnostic medical and surgical procedures and the expected preprocedure and postprocedure expectations
      b. Assist the client to identify angina-precipitating events
      c. Instruct the client that if chest pain occurs, to stop activity and rest, and take nitroglycerin as prescribed

d. Instruct the client that, if the pain persists, to seek medical attention
e. Instruct the client regarding prescribed medications
f. Provide diet instruction to the client, stressing that dietary changes are not temporary and must be maintained for life
g. Assist the client to identify risk factors that can be modified
h. Assist the client to set goals that will promote changes in lifestyle to reduce the impact of risk factors
i. Assist the client to identify barriers to compliance with therapeutic plan and to identify methods to overcome barriers
j. Provide community resources to client regarding exercise, smoking cessation, and stress reduction

F. Surgical procedures
1. Percutaneous transluminal coronary angioplasty (PTCA) to assess the condition of the coronary arteries and to compress the plaque, if present, against the walls of the artery and dilate the vessel
2. Laser angioplasty to vaporize the plaque if present
3. Atherectomy to remove the plaque, if present, from the artery
4. Vascular stent to prevent the artery from closing and prevent restenosis
5. Coronary artery bypass graft to improve blood flow to the myocardial tissues that are at risk for ischemia or infarction resulting from the occluded artery

G. Medications
1. Vasodilators to maintain coronary artery vasodilation and promote a greater flow of blood and oxygen to the heart
2. Calcium channel blockers to dilate coronary arteries and reduce vasospasm
3. Beta blockers to reduce the oxygen requirements of the heart and reduce **blood pressure** in those individuals who are hypertensive
4. Antiplatelet therapy to inhibit platelet aggregation and reduce the risk of developing an acute MI

VIII. MYOCARDIAL INFARCTION (MI)

A. Description
1. Occurs when myocardial tissue is abruptly and severely deprived of oxygen
2. Ischemia can lead to necrosis of myocardial tissue if blood flow is not restored
3. Infarction does not occur instantly, but evolves over several hours
4. Obvious physical changes do not occur in the heart until 6 hours after the infarction, when the infarcted area appears blue and swollen
5. After 48 hours, the infarct turns gray with yellow streaks as neutrophils invade the tissue
6. By 8 to 10 days after infarction, granulation tissue forms
7. Over 2 to 3 months, the necrotic area develops into a scar; scar tissue permanently changes the size and shape of the entire left ventricle

B. Location of MI
1. Obstruction of the LAD artery results in anterior and/or septal MIs
2. Obstruction of the circumflex artery results in posterior wall MI or lateral wall MI
3. Obstruction of the right coronary artery results in inferior wall MI

C. Risk factors
1. Atherosclerosis
2. CAD
3. Elevated cholesterol levels
4. Smoking
5. Hypertension
6. Obesity
7. Physical inactivity
8. Impaired glucose tolerance
9. Stress

D. Diagnostic studies
1. Total CK levels
   a. Rise within 3 hours after the onset of chest pain
   b. Peak within 24 hours after damage and death of cardiac tissue
2. CK-MB isoenzyme
   a. Peak elevation occurs 12 to 24 hours after the onset of chest pain
   b. Levels return to normal 48 to 72 hours later
3. Troponin levels
   a. Rise within 3 hours
   b. Remain elevated for up to 7 days
4. Myoglobin: rises within 1 hour after cell death, peaks in 4 to 6 hours, and returns to normal within 24 to 36 hours or less
5. LDH levels
   a. Rise within 12 to 24 hours after MI
   b. Peak between 40 and 72 hours and fall to normal in 7 days
   c. Serum levels of LDH_1 isoenzyme rise higher than serum levels of LDH_2
6. WBC count: an elevated white blood cell count of 10,000 to 20,000 cells/mm^3 appears on the second day post-MI and lasts up to a week

7. ECG
   a. ST segment elevation, T wave inversion, abnormal Q wave
   b. Hours to days after the MI, ST and T wave changes will return to normal, but the Q wave usually remains permanently
8. Diagnostic tests after the acute stage
   a. Exercise tolerance test or stress test may be prescribed to assess for ECG changes and ischemia and to evaluate for medical therapy or identify clients who may need invasive therapy
   b. Thallium scans may be prescribed to assess for ischemia or necrotic muscle tissue
   c. MUGA scans: may be used to evaluate left ventricular function
   d. Cardiac catheterization: performed to determine the extent and location of obstructions of the coronary arteries

E. Data collection
1. Pain
   a. Crushing substernal pain
   b. Radiates to the jaw, back, and left arm
   c. Occurs without cause, primarily early in the morning
   d. Is unrelieved by rest or nitroglycerin, and relieved only by opioids
   e. Pain lasts 30 minutes or more
2. Nausea and vomiting
3. Diaphoresis
4. Dyspnea
5. Dysrhythmias
6. Feelings of fear and anxiety
7. Pallor, cyanosis, coolness of extremities

F. Complications of MI
1. Dysrhythmias
2. Heart failure
3. Pulmonary edema
4. Cardiogenic shock
5. Thrombophlebitis
6. Pericarditis
7. Mitral valve insufficiency
8. Postinfarction angina
9. Ventricular rupture
10. Dressler's syndrome (a combination of pericarditis, pericardial effusion, and pleural effusion that can occur several weeks to months after an MI)

G. Implementation, acute stage
1. Obtain a description of the chest discomfort
2. Assess vital signs
3. Assess cardiovascular status and maintain cardiac monitoring
4. Obtain a 12-lead ECG
5. Administer nitroglycerin as prescribed
6. Administer morphine sulfate as prescribed to relieve chest discomfort that is unresponsive to nitroglycerin
7. Administer oxygen at 2 to 4 liters by nasal cannula as prescribed
8. Place the client in semi-Fowler's position to enhance comfort and tissue oxygenation
9. Establish an IV access route
10. Administer IV nitroglycerin and antidysrhythmics as prescribed
11. Monitor thrombolitic therapy, which may be prescribed within the first 6 hours of the coronary event
12. Monitor for signs of bleeding if the client is receiving thrombolitics
13. Monitor laboratory values as prescribed
14. Administer beta blockers to slow the heart rate, and increase myocardial perfusion while reducing the force of myocardial contraction as prescribed
15. Monitor for complications related to MI
16. Monitor for cardiac dysrhythmias, as tachycardia and PVCs frequently occur in the first few hours after MI
17. Assess distal peripheral pulses and skin temperature, as poor **cardiac output** may be identified by cool diaphoretic skin and diminished or absent pulses
18. Monitor I&O
19. Assess respiratory rate and breath sounds for signs of heart failure as indicated by the presence of crackles or wheezes or dependent edema
20. Monitor **blood pressure** closely after the administration of medications and if the **BP** is less than 100 mm Hg systolic or 25 mm Hg lower than the previous reading, lower the head of the bed and notify the physician
21. Provide reassurance to client and family

H. Implementation after acute episode
1. Maintain bed rest for the first 24 to 36 hours
2. Allow the client to stand to void or use a bedside commode if prescribed
3. Provide range of motion exercises to prevent thrombus formation and maintain muscle strength
4. Progress to dangling at the side of the bed or out of bed to the chair for 30 minutes three times a day as prescribed
5. Progress to ambulation in the client's room and to the bathroom and then in the hallway three times a day
6. Monitor for complications
7. Encourage the client to verbalize feelings regarding the MI

I. Cardiac rehabilitation: process of actively assisting the client with cardiac disease to achieve and maintain a vital and productive life within the limitations of the heart disease

IX. HEART FAILURE

A. Description
   1. Inability of the heart to maintain adequate circulation to meet the metabolic needs of the body because of an impaired pumping capability
   2. **Cardiac output** is diminished and peripheral tissue is not adequately perfused
   3. Congestion of the lungs and periphery may occur

B. Classification
   1. Acute: occurs suddenly
   2. Chronic: develops over time; however, a client with chronic heart failure can develop an acute episode

C. Types of heart failure
   1. Right-sided heart failure/left-sided heart failure
      a. Because the two ventricles of the heart represent two separate pumping systems, it is possible for one to fail alone for a short period
      b. Most heart failure begins with left ventricular failure and progresses to failure of both ventricles
      c. Acute pulmonary edema, a medical emergency, results from left ventricular failure
      d. If pulmonary edema is not treated, death will occur from suffocation as the client literally drowns in his or her own fluids
   2. Forward failure/backward failure
      a. In forward failure, an inadequate output of the affected ventricle causes decreased perfusion to vital organs
      b. In backward failure, blood backs up behind the affected ventricle causing increased pressure in the atrium behind the affected ventricle
   3. Low-output/high-output
      a. In low-output failure, not enough **cardiac output** is available to meet the demands of the body
      b. High-output failure occurs when a condition causes the heart to work harder to meet the demands of the body
   4. Systolic failure/diastolic failure
      a. Systolic failure leads to problems with contraction and the ejection of blood
      b. Diastolic failure leads to problems with the heart relaxing and filling with blood

D. Compensatory mechanisms
   1. Act to restore **cardiac output** to near normal levels
   2. Initially these mechanisms increase **cardiac output**; however, they eventually have a damaging effect on pump action
   3. Contribute to an increase in myocardial oxygen consumption and when this occurs, myocardial reserve is exhausted and clinical manifestations of heart failure develop
   4. Include increased heart rate, improved stroke volume, arterial vasoconstriction, sodium and water retention, and myocardial hypertrophy

E. Data collection
   1. Right-sided heart failure
      a. Signs of right-sided failure will be evident in the systemic circulation
      b. Pitting, dependent edema in feet, legs, sacrum, back, buttocks
      c. Ascites from portal hypertension
      d. Tenderness of right upper quadrant, organomegaly
      e. Distended neck veins
      f. Pulsus alternans (regular alteration of weak and strong beats noted in the pulse)
      g. Abdominal pain, bloating
      h. Anorexia, nausea
      i. Fatigue
      j. Weight gain
      k. Nocturnal diuresis
   2. Left-sided heart failure
      a. Signs of the left-sided failure will be evident in the pulmonary system
      b. Cough, which may become productive with frothy sputum
      c. Dyspnea on exertion
      d. Orthopnea
      e. Paroxysmal nocturnal dyspnea
      f. Presence of rales or crackles on auscultation
      g. Tachycardia
      h. Pulsus alternans
      i. Fatigue
      j. Pallor
      k. Cyanosis
      l. Confusion and disorientation
      m. Signs of cerebral anoxia
   3. Acute pulmonary edema
      a. Severe dyspnea and orthopnea
      b. Pallor
      c. Tachycardia
      d. Expectoration of large amounts of blood-tinged, frothy sputum
      e. Wheezing and rales
      f. Bubbling respirations

g. Acute anxiety, apprehension, restlessness
h. Profuse sweating
i. Cold, clammy skin
j. Cyanosis
k. Nasal flaring
l. Use of accessory breathing muscles
m. Tachypnea
n. Hypocapnia evidenced by muscle cramps, weakness, dizziness, and paresthesia

F. Immediate management
1. Place the client in high-Fowler's position with legs in a dependent position to reduce pulmonary congestion and relieve edema
2. Administer oxygen in high concentrations by mask or cannula as prescribed by the physician to improve gas exchange and pulmonary function
3. Prepare for intubation and ventilator support if required; monitor lung sounds for rales and decreased breath sounds
4. Suction as needed to maintain a patent airway
5. Assess level of consciousness
6. Provide reassurance to the client
7. Monitor vital signs closely noting tachycardia or pulsus alternans
8. Monitor for hypotension resulting from decreased tissue perfusion, or hypertension resulting from anxiety or history of hypertension
9. Monitor heart rate on a cardiac monitor for dysrhythmias
10. Assess for edema in dependent areas and in the sacral, lumbar, and posterior thigh region in the client in bed
11. Insert a Foley catheter as prescribed and monitor urine output closely after administration of a diuretic
12. Monitor I&O
13. Avoid administration of unnecessary IV fluids
14. Administer morphine as prescribed to provide sedation and vasodilation, and monitor for respiratory depression or hypotension after administration
15. Administer diuretics as prescribed to reduce preload, enhance renal excretion of sodium and water, reduce circulating blood volume, and reduce pulmonary congestion
16. Administer digoxin (Lanoxin) as prescribed to increase ventricular contractility and improve **cardiac output**
17. Administer bronchodilators as prescribed for severe bronchospasm or bronchoconstriction
18. Administer additional inotropic medications such as dopamine, dobutamine, or amrinone as prescribed to facilitate myocardial contractility and enhance stroke volume
19. Administer vasodilators as prescribed to reduce afterload, increase the capacity of the systemic venous bed, and decrease venous return to the heart
20. Monitor weight to determine a response to treatment
21. Assess for hepatomegaly and ascites and measure and record abdominal girth
22. Monitor peripheral pulses
23. Analyze blood gas results and evaluate electrolyte values for imbalances
24. Monitor potassium level closely, which may decrease because of the diuretic, and administer potassium supplements as prescribed to prevent digoxin toxicity

G. After the acute episode
1. Encourage the client to verbalize feelings about the necessary lifestyle changes that are required as a result of the heart failure
2. Assist the client to identify precipitating risk factors of heart failure and methods of eliminating these risk factors
3. Instruct the client in the prescribed medication regimen, which may include digoxin (Lanoxin), a diuretic, and vasodilators
4. Advise the client to notify the physician if side effects occur from the medications
5. Advise the client to avoid over-the-counter medications
6. Instruct the client to contact the physician if unable to take medications because of illness
7. Instruct the client to avoid large amounts of caffeine found in coffee, tea, cocoa, chocolate, and some carbonated beverages
8. Instruct the client on the prescribed low-sodium, low-fat, low-cholesterol diet as prescribed
9. Provide the client with a list of potassium-rich foods, as diuretics will cause hypokalemia (except for potassium-sparing diuretics)
10. Instruct the client regarding fluid restriction if prescribed, advising the client to spread out fluid intake throughout the day and to suck on hard candy to reduce thirst
11. Instruct the client to space periods of activity and rest
12. Advise the client to avoid isometric activities, which increase pressure in the heart
13. Instruct the client to monitor weight
14. Instruct the client to report signs of fluid retention such as edema or weight gain

X. CARDIOGENIC SHOCK

A. Failure of the heart to pump adequately, thereby reducing **cardiac output** and compromising tissue perfusion
B. Necrosis of more than 40% of the left ventricle occurs, usually as a result of occlusions of major coronary vessels
C. The goal of treatment is to relieve pain and decrease myocardial oxygen requirements through preload and possibly afterload reduction

XI. INFLAMMATORY DISEASES OF THE HEART

A. Pericarditis
1. Description
a. An acute or chronic inflammation of the pericardium
b. Chronic pericarditis, a chronic inflammatory thickening of the pericardium, constricts the heart causing compression
c. The pericardial sac becomes inflamed
d. Can result in loss of pericardial elasticity or an accumulation of fluid within the sac
e. Heart failure or cardiac tamponade may result
2. Data collection
a. Precordial pain in the anterior chest that radiates to the left side of the neck, shoulder, or back
b. Pain that is aggravated by breathing (particularly inspiration), coughing, and swallowing
c. Pain is worse when in the supine position and may be relieved by leaning forward
d. Pericardial friction rub (scratchy, high-pitched sound) heard on auscultation produced by the rubbing of the inflamed pericardial layers
e. Fever and chills
f. Fatigue and malaise
g. Elevated WBC count
h. ECG changes
i. Signs of right-sided heart failure in clients with chronic constrictive pericarditis
3. Implementation
a. Assess the nature of the pain
b. Position the client side-lying, high Fowler's or upright and leaning forward
c. Administer analgesics, nonsteroidal antiinflammatory drugs (NSAIDs), or corticosteriods as prescribed for pain
d. Avoid the administration of aspirin and anticoagulants because they increase the risk of tamponade
e. Auscultate for a pericardial friction rub
f. Evaluate blood culture report
g. Administer antibiotics for bacterial infection as prescribed
h. Administer diuretics and digoxin (Lanoxin) as prescribed to the client with chronic constrictive pericarditis
i. Monitor for signs of cardiac tamponade including pulsus paradoxus, jugular vein distention with clear lung sounds, muffled heart sounds, and decreased **cardiac output**
j. Notify the physician if signs of cardiac tamponade occur

B. Myocarditis
1. Description: an acute or chronic inflammation of the myocardium resulting from pericarditis, systemic infection, or allergic response
2. Data collection
a. Fever
b. Pericardial friction rub
c. A gallop rhythm
d. A murmur that sounds like fluid passing an obstruction
e. Pulsus alternans
f. Signs of heart failure
g. Fatigue
h. Dyspnea
i. Tachycardia
j. Chest pain
3. Implementation
a. Assist the client to a position of comfort such as sitting up and leaning forward
b. Administer analgesics, salicylates, NSAIDs as prescribed to reduce fever and pain
c. Administer oxygen as prescribed
d. Provide adequate rest periods
e. Limit activities to avoid overexertion and to decrease the workload of the heart
f. Administer digoxin (Lanoxin) as prescribed and monitor for signs of digoxin toxicity
g. Administer antidysrhythmics as prescribed
h. Administer antibiotics as prescribed to treat causative organism
i. Monitor for complications, which can include thrombus, congestive heart failure (CHF) or cardiomyopathy

C. Endocarditis
1. Description
a. An inflammation of the inner lining of the heart and valves
b. Occurs primarily in clients who are IV drug abusers, have had valve replacements, or have mitral valve prolapse or other structural defects

c. Ports of entry for the infecting organism includes the oral cavity (especially if the client had a dental procedure in the previous 3 to 6 months), cutaneous invasion, infections, or by invasive procedures or surgery

2. Data collection
   a. Fever
   b. Anorexia
   c. Weight loss
   d. Fatigue
   e. Cardiac murmurs
   f. Heart failure
   g. Embolic complications from vegetation fragments traveling through the circulation
   h. Petechiae
   i. Splinter hemorrhages in the nail beds
   j. Osler's nodes (reddish tender lesions) on the pads of the fingers, hands, and toes
   k. Janeway's lesions (nontender hemorrhagic lesions) on the fingers, toes, nose, or earlobes
   l. Splenomegaly
   m. Clubbing of the fingers
3. Implementation
   a. Provide adequate rest balanced with activity to prevent thrombus formation
   b. Maintain antiembolism stockings
   c. Monitor cardiovascular status
   d. Monitor for signs of heart failure
   e. Monitor for signs of emboli
   f. Monitor for splenic emboli as evidenced by sudden abdominal pain radiating to the left shoulder and the presence of rebound abdominal tenderness on palpation
   g. Monitor for renal emboli as evidenced by flank pain radiating to the groin, hematuria, and pyuria
   h. Monitor for confusion, aphasia, or dysphagia, which may be indicative of central nervous system emboli
   i. Monitor for pulmonary emboli as evidenced by pleuritic chest pain, dyspnea, and cough
   j. Assess skin, mucous membranes, and conjunctiva for petechiae
   k. Assess nail beds for splinter hemorrhages
   l. Assess for Osler's nodes on the pads of the fingers, hands, and toes
   m. Assess for Janeway's lesions on the fingers, toes, nose, or earlobes
   n. Assess for clubbing of the fingers
   o. Evaluate blood culture results
   p. Administer IV antibiotic as prescribed
   q. Plan and arrange for discharge providing resources required for the continued administration of IV antibiotics
4. Client education
   a. Instruct the client regarding the signs and symptoms of complications and to notify the physician if they occur
   b. Inform the client about the importance of good oral hygiene
   c. Instruct the client to brush teeth twice daily with a soft toothbrush followed by oral rinses
   d. Instruct the client to avoid irrigation devices, electric toothbrushes, and flossing because these activities can cause the gums to bleed, allowing the entrance of bacteria into the mucous membranes and bloodstream
   e. Advise the client of the importance of prophylactic antibiotics before any invasive procedure and the importance of informing all health care professionals of disease history

XII. CARDIAC TAMPONADE

A. Pericardial effusion occurs when the space between the parietal and visceral layers of the pericardium fill with fluid

B. Pericardial effusion places the client at risk for cardiac tamponade, an accumulation of fluid in the pericardial cavity

C. Tamponade restricts ventricular filling and **cardiac output** drops

D. Acute tamponade occurs when small volumes (20 to 50 mL) of fluid accumulate in the pericardium

XIII. VALVULAR HEART DISEASE

A. Description
1. Occurs when the heart valves cannot fully open (stenosis) or close completely (insufficiency or regurgitation)
2. Prevents efficient blood flow through the heart

B. Types
1. Mitral stenosis: valvular tissue thickens and narrows valve opening
2. Mitral insufficiency/regurgitation: valve is incompetent and prevents complete valve closure
3. Mitral valve prolapse: valve leaflets protrude into left atrium during **systole**
4. Aortic stenosis: valvular tissue thickens and narrows valve opening
5. Aortic insufficiency: valve is incompetent and prevents complete valve closure

C. Repair procedures

1. Balloon valvuloplasty
   a. Invasive nonsurgical procedure
   b. The passage of a balloon catheter from the femoral vein through the atrial septum to the mitral valve, or through the femoral artery to the aortic valve
   c. The balloon is inflated to enlarge the orifice
   d. Institute precautions for arterial puncture if appropriate
   e. Monitor for bleeding from the catheter insertion site
   f. Monitor for signs of systemic emboli
   g. Monitor for signs of a regurgitant valve by monitoring cardiac rhythm, heart sounds, and **cardiac output**
2. Mitral annuloplasty: tightening and suturing the malfunctioning valve annulus to eliminate or markedly reduce regurgitation
3. Commissurotomy/valvotomy
   a. Accomplished with cardiopulmonary bypass during open heart surgery
   b. The valve is visualized, thrombi are removed from the atria, fused leaflets are incised, and calcium is debrided from the leaflets, thus widening the orifice

D. Valve replacement procedures (Box 48-3)
1. Mechanical prosthetic valves
   a. Prosthetic valves are very durable but can fail
   b. Thromboembolism is a problem after valve replacement, and anticoagulant therapy is required for life
2. Bioprosthetic valves
   a. Biological grafts are xenografts (valves from other species), porcine valves (pig), bovine valves (cow), or homografts (human cadavers)
   b. Little risk of clot formation; therefore long-term anticoagulation is not indicated
3. Preoperative implementation: consult with physician regarding discontinuing anticoagulants 72 hours before surgery
4. Postoperative implementation
   a. Monitor closely for signs of bleeding
   b. Monitor **cardiac output** and for signs of heart pump failure
   c. Administer digoxin (Lanoxin) as prescribed to maintain **cardiac output** and prevent atrial fibrillation

XIV. CARDIOMYOPATHY

A. Description
1. A subacute or chronic disorder of the heart muscle
2. Treatment is palliative, not curative, and clients need to deal with numerous lifestyle changes and a shortened life span

B. Dilated cardiomyopathy (DCM)
1. Description
   a. Most common type
   b. Heart ejects less than 40% of the blood in the left ventricle (normal is 70%) and reduced **cardiac output** leading to heart failure occurs
2. Data collection
   a. Symptoms of left ventricular heart failure
   b. Weakness and fatigue
   c. Activity intolerance
   d. Chest pain
   e. Dysrhythmias
   f. Eventually signs of right-sided heart failure

BOX 48-3

Client Instruction After Valve Replacement

- Instruct the client that adequate rest is important and that the client will become easily fatigued
- Instruct the client in the need for anticoagulant therapy if a mechanical prosthetic valve was inserted
- Instruct the client in the hazards related to anticoagulant therapy and to notify the physician if bleeding or excessive bruising occurs
- Inform the client about the importance of good oral hygiene to reduce the risk of infective endocarditis
- Instruct the client to brush teeth twice daily with a soft toothbrush followed by oral rinses
- Instruct the client to avoid irrigation devices, electric toothbrushes, and flossing because these activities can cause the gums to bleed allowing the entrance of bacteria into the mucous membranes and bloodstream
- Instruct the client to monitor incision and to report any drainage or redness
- Inform the client to avoid any dental procedures for 6 months
- Inform the client that heavy lifting (more than 10 pounds) is to be avoided and to exercise caution when in an automobile to prevent injury to the sternal incision
- Inform the client with a prosthetic valve that a soft audible clicking sound may be heard
- Advise the client of the importance of using prophylactic antibiotics before any invasive procedure and the importance of informing all health care professionals of the valvular disease history
- Advise the client to obtain and wear a Medic-Alert bracelet

3. Implementation
   a. Symptomatic treatment of heart failure
   b. Diuretics, cardiac glycosides, and vasodilators to increase **cardiac output**
   c. Antidysrhythmics to control dysrhythmias
   d. Instruct the client to report any signs of dizziness or fainting, which may indicate a dysrhythmia
   e. Instruct the client to avoid ingestion of alcohol because of its cardiac depressant effect
   f. Heart transplant

C. Hypertropic cardiomyopathy (HCM)
1. Description
   a. Characterized by massive ventricular hypertrophy leading to hypercontraction of the left ventricle and rigid ventricle walls
   b. Causes obstruction in the left ventricular outflow
2. Data collection
   a. Exertional dyspnea
   b. Syncope
   c. Chest pain that occurs at rest, is prolonged, has no relation to exertion, and is not relieved by nitrates
   d. Dysrhythmias
3. Implementation
   a. Symptomatic treatment of symptoms similar to the care of a client with MI
   b. Conversion of atrial fibrillation if it occurs
   c. Instruct the client to report any signs of dizziness or fainting, which may indicate a dysrhythmia
   d. Instruct the client to avoid ingestion of alcohol because of its cardiac depressant effect
   e. Beta blockers and calcium antagonists to decrease the outflow obstruction and decrease heart rate
   f. Vasodilators and cardiac glycosides are contraindicated because vasodilating and positive inotropic effects augment the obstruction
   g. Ventriculomyotomy or muscle resection with mitral valve replacement

D. Restrictive cardiomyopathy
1. Description: characterized by restriction of filling of the ventricles
2. Data collection
   a. Exertional dyspnea
   b. Weakness
3. Implementation
   a. Symptomatic treatment of heart failure
   b. Exercise restriction
   c. Diuretics, cardiac glycosides, and vasodilators to increase **cardiac output**
   d. Antidysrhythmics to control dysrhythmias
   e. Instruct the client to report any signs of dizziness or fainting, which may indicate a dysrhythmia
   f. Instruct the client to avoid ingestion of alcohol because of its cardiac depressant effect

XV. VENOUS DISORDERS

A. Venous thrombosis
1. Description
   a. Thrombus can be associated with an inflammatory process
   b. When a thrombus develops, inflammation occurs, thickening the vein wall leading to embolization
2. Types
   a. Thrombophlebitis: a thrombus associated with inflammation
   b. Phlebothrombus: a thrombus without inflammation
   c. Phlebitis: vein inflammation associated with invasive procedures such as IV lines
   d. Deep vein thrombophlebitis (DVT): more serious than a superficial thrombophlebitis because of the risk for pulmonary embolism
3. Risks factors for thrombus formation
   a. Venous stasis from varicose veins, CHF, immobility
   b. Hypercoagulability disorders
   c. Injury to the venous wall from IV injections, fractures, trauma
   d. After surgery, particularly hip surgery and open prostate surgery
   e. Pregnancy
   f. Ulcerative colitis
   g. Use of oral contraceptives

B. Phlebitis
1. Data collection
   a. Red warm area radiating up an extremity
   b. Pain and soreness
   c. Swelling
2. Implementation
   a. Apply warm moist soaks as prescribed to dilate the vein and promote circulation
   b. Assess temperature of soak before applying
   c. Assess for signs of complications as tissue necrosis, infection, or pulmonary embolus

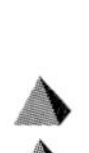

C. DVT (Box 48-4)
1. Data collection
   a. Calf or groin tenderness or pain with or without swelling
   b. Positive Homan's sign
   c. Warm skin that is tender to touch

BOX 48-4

Instructions for the Client with DVT

Educate the client regarding the hazards of anticoagulation therapy
Instruct the client to recognize the signs and symptoms of bleeding
Instruct the client to avoid prolonged sitting or standing, constrictive clothing, or crossing legs when seated
Instruct the client to elevate legs for 10 to 20 minutes every few hours each day
Plan a progressive walking program with the client as prescribed
Instruct the client how to inspect legs for edema and how to measure circumference of legs
Instruct the client about the use of antiembolism stockings as prescribed
Advise the client to avoid smoking
Advise the client to avoid any medications unless they are prescribed by the physician
Emphasize the importance of follow-up physician visits and laboratory studies
Advise the client to obtain and wear a Medic-Alert bracelet

2. Implementation
   a. Provide bed rest
   b. Elevate the affected extremity above the level of the heart as prescribed
   c. Avoid using the knee gatch or a pillow under knees
   d. Do not massage the extremity
   e. Provide thigh high compression or antiembolism stockings as prescribed to reduce venous stasis and to assist in the venous return of blood to the heart
   f. Administer intermittent or continuous warm, moist compresses as prescribed
   g. Palpate the site gently, monitoring for warmth and edema
   h. Measure and record the circumference of the thighs and calves
   i. Monitor for shortness of breath and chest pain, as it may be indicative of pulmonary emboli
   j. Administer thrombolytic therapy (t-PA, tissue plasminogen activator) may be prescribed, and needs to be initiated within 5 days after the onset of symptoms
   k. Heparin therapy may be prescribed to prevent enlargement of the existing clot and prevent the formation of new clots
   l. Monitor activated partial thromboplastin time (APTT) during heparin therapy
   m. Administer warfarin (Coumadin) as prescribed when symptoms of DVT have resolved
   n. Monitor prothrombin time (PT) and international normalized ratio (INR) during warfarin (Coumadin) therapy
   o. Monitor for the hazards and side effects associated with anticoagulant therapy
   p. Administer analgesics as prescribed to reduce pain
   q. Administer diuretics as prescribed to reduce lower extremity edema

D. Venous insufficiency
1. Description
   a. Occurs as a result of prolonged venous hypertension, which stretches the veins and damages the valves
   b. The resultant edema and venous stasis cause venous stasis ulcers, swelling, and cellulitis
   c. Treatment focuses on decreasing edema and promoting venous return from the affected extremity
   d. Treatment for venous stasis ulcers focuses on healing the ulcer and preventing stasis and ulcer recurrence
2. Data collection
   a. Stasis dermatitis or discoloration along the ankles extending up to the calf
   b. Edema
   c. The presence of ulcer formation
3. Implementation
   a. Instruct the client to wear elastic or compression stockings during the day and evening as prescribed
   b. Instruct the client to put on elastic stockings on awakening, before getting out of bed
   c. Advise the client to put on a clean pair of elastic stockings each day and that the stockings will probably need to worn for the rest of the client's lifetime
   d. Instruct the client to avoid prolonged sitting or standing, constrictive clothing, or crossing legs when seated
   e. Instruct the client to elevate legs for 10 to 20 minutes every few hours each day
   f. Instruct the client when in bed, to elevate legs above the level of the heart
   g. Instruct the client in the use of an intermittent sequential pneumatic compression system if prescribed; instruct the client to apply the compression system twice daily for 1 hour in the morning and evening
   h. Advise the client with an open ulcer that the compression system is applied over a dressing
4. Wound care

a. Provide care to the wound as prescribed by the physician
b. Assess the client's ability to care for the wound and initiate home care resources as necessary
c. If an Unna boot (a dressing constructed of gauze moistened with zinc oxide) is prescribed, it will be changed weekly by the physician
d. The wound is cleansed with normal saline before application of the Unna boot; povidone-iodine (Betadine) and hydrogen peroxide are not used because they destroy granulation tissue
e. The Unna boot is covered with an elastic wrap, which hardens to promote venous return and prevent stasis
f. Monitor for signs of arterial occlusion from an Unna boot that may be too tight
g. Keep tape off the client's skin

5. Medications
a. Apply topical agents to wound as prescribed to debride the ulcer, eliminate necrotic tissue, and promote healing
b. When applying topical agents, apply an oil-based agent such as petroleum jelly (Vaseline) on surrounding skin because debriding agents can injure healthy tissue
c. Administer antibiotics as prescribed if infection or cellulitis occurs

E. Varicose veins
1. Description
a. Distended, protruding veins that appear darkened and tortuous
b. Vein walls weaken and dilate, and valves become incompetent
2. Data collection
a. Pain in legs with dull aching after standing
b. A feeling of fullness in the legs
c. Ankle edema
3. Trendelenburg test
a. Place the client in supine position with legs elevated
b. When the client sits up, if varicosities are present, veins fill from the proximal end; veins normally fill from the distal end
4. Implementation
a. Assist with Trendelenburg test by placing the client in supine position with legs elevated
b. Emphasize the importance of antiembolism stockings as prescribed
c. Instruct the client to elevate legs as much as possible
d. Instruct the client to avoid constrictive clothing and pressure on the legs
e. Prepare the client for sclerotherapy or vein stripping as prescribed
5. Sclerotherapy
a. A solution is injected into the vein followed by the application of a pressure dressing
b. An incision and drainage of the trapped blood in the sclerosed vein is performed 14 to 21 days after the injection, followed by the application of a pressure dressing for 12 to 18 hours
6. Vein stripping
a. Varicose veins are removed if they are larger than 4 mm in diameter or if they are in clusters
b. Preoperatively assist the physician with vein marking
c. Evaluate pulses as a baseline for comparison postoperatively
d. Maintain elastic (Ace) bandages on client's legs postoperatively
e. Monitor the groin and leg for bleeding through the elastic bandages
f. Monitor extremity for edema, warmth, color, and pulses
g. Elevate legs above level of heart postoperatively
h. Encourage range of motion exercises of the legs
i. Instruct the client to avoid leg dangling or chair sitting
j. Instruct the client to elevate legs when sitting
k. Emphasize the importance of wearing elastic stockings after bandage removal

XVI. ARTERIAL DISORDERS

A. Peripheral arterial disease (PAD)
1. Description
a. A chronic disorder in which partial or total arterial occlusion deprives the lower extremities of oxygen and nutrients
b. Tissue damage occurs below the arterial occlusion
c. Atherosclerosis is the most common cause of PAD
2. Data collection
a. Intermittent claudication
b. Rest pain characterized by numbness, burning, or aching in the distal portion of the lower extremities that awakens the client at night and is relieved by placing the extremity in a dependent position
c. Lower back or buttock discomfort
d. Loss of hair and dry, scaly skin on lower extremities

e. Thickened toenails
f. Cold and gray-blue or darkened color of skin in lower extremities
g. Elevational pallor and dependent rubor in lower extremities
h. Decreased or absent peripheral pulses
i. Signs of arterial ulcer formation characterized as painful, and occurring on or between the toes, or on the upper aspect of the foot
j. **Blood pressure** measurements at the thigh, calf, and ankle are lower than the brachial pressure (normally **BP** readings in the thigh and calf are higher than those in the upper extremities)

3. Implementation
a. Assess pain
b. Monitor the extremities for color, motion, sensation, and pulses
c. Obtain **blood pressure** measurements
d. Assess for signs of ulcer formation or signs of gangrene
e. Assist in developing an individualized exercise program that is initiated gradually and slowly increased
f. Encourage prescribed exercise, which will improve arterial flow through the development of collateral circulation
g. Instruct the client to walk to the point of claudication, stop and rest, and then walk a little farther
h. As swelling in the extremities prevents arterial blood flow, instruct client to elevate their feet at rest, but to refrain from elevating them above the level of the heart, as extreme elevation slows arterial blood flow to the feet
i. In severe cases of PAD, clients with edema may sleep with the affected limb hanging from the bed or they may sit upright in a chair for comfort
j. Instruct the client with PAD to avoid crossing his or her legs, which interferes with blood flow
k. Instruct the client to avoid exposure to cold (causes vasoconstriction) to the extremities and to wear socks or insulated shoes for warmth at all times
l. Instruct the client never to apply direct heat to the limb as with a heating pad or hot water, because the decreased sensitivity in the limb will cause burning
m. Instruct the client to inspect skin on extremities daily and to report any signs of skin breakdown
n. Instruct the client to avoid tobacco and caffeine because of their vasoconstrictive effects
o. Instruct the client in the use of hemorrheologic and antiplatelet medications as prescribed
p. Inform the client of the importance of taking all medications prescribed by the physician

4. Procedures to improve arterial blood flow
a. Percutaneous transluminal angioplasty
b. Laser assisted angioplasty
c. Atherectomy
d. Bypass surgery

B. Raynaud's disease
1. Description
a. Vasospasms of the arterioles and arteries of the upper and lower extremities
b. Vasospasm causes constriction of the cutaneous vessels
c. Attacks are intermittent and occur with exposure to cold or stress
d. Affects primarily fingers, toes, ears, and cheeks

2. Data collection
a. Blanching of the extremity followed by cyanosis during vasoconstriction
b. Reddened tissue when the vasospasm is relieved
c. Numbness, tingling, swelling, and a cold temperature at the affected body part

3. Implementation
a. Monitor pulses
b. Administer vasodilators as prescribed
c. Instruct the client regarding medication therapy
d. Assist the client to identify and avoid precipitating factors as cold and stress
e. Instruct the client to avoid smoking
f. Instruct the client to wear warm clothing, socks, and gloves in cold weather
g. Advise the client to avoid injuries to fingers and hands

C. Buerger's disease
1. Description
a. Also known as thromboangiitis obliterans
b. An occlusive disease of the median and small arteries and veins
c. The distal upper and lower limbs are most commonly affected

2. Data collection
a. Intermittent claudication (pain in the muscles resulting from an inadequate blood supply)
b. Ischemic pain occurring in the digits while at rest

c. Aching pain that is more severe at night
d. Cool, numb, or tingling sensation
e. Diminished pulses in the distal extremities
f. Extremities are cool and red in the dependent position
g. Development of ulcerations in extremities

3. Implementation
   a. Instruct the client to stop smoking
   b. Monitor pulses
   c. Instruct the client to avoid injury to upper and lower extremities
   d. Administer vasodilators as prescribed
   e. Instruct the client regarding medication therapy

XVII. AORTIC ANEURYSMS

A. Description
1. Abnormal dilation of the arterial wall caused by localized weakness and stretching in the medial layer or wall of an artery
2. The aneurysm can be located anywhere along the abdominal aorta
3. The goal of treatment is to limit the progression of the disease by modifying risk factors, controlling the **BP** to prevent strain on the aneurysm, recognizing symptoms early and preventing rupture

B. Types
1. Fusiform: diffuse dilation that involves the entire circumference of the arterial segment
2. Saccular: distinct localized outpouching of the artery wall
3. Dissecting: created when blood separates the layers of the artery wall forming a cavity between them
4. False (Pseudoaneurysm)
   a. Occurs when the clot and connective tissue are outside the arterial wall
   b. Formed after complete rupture and subsequent formation of a scar sac

C. Data collection
1. Thoracic
   a. Pain extending to neck, shoulders, lower back, or abdomen
   b. Syncope
   c. Dyspnea
   d. Increased pulse
   e. Cyanosis
   f. Weakness
2. Abdominal
   a. Prominent pulsating mass in abdomen at or above umbilicus
   b. Systolic bruit over aorta
   c. Tenderness on deep palpation
   d. Abdominal or lower back pain
3. Rupturing aneurysm
   a. Severe abdominal or back pain
   b. Lumbar pain radiating to flank and groin
   c. Hypotension
   d. Increased pulse rate
   e. Signs of shock
4. Diagnostic tests
   a. Done to confirm the presence of an aneurysm
   b. Done to confirm the size and location of the aneurysm
   c. Includes abdominal ultrasound, CT scan, and arteriography
5. Implementation
   a. Monitor vital signs
   b. Assess risk factors for arterial disease process
   c. Obtain information regarding back or abdominal pain
   d. Question the client regarding sensation of palpation in the abdomen
   e. Inspect skin for presence of vascular disease or breakdown
   f. Check peripheral circulation including pulses, temperature, and color
   g. Observe for signs of rupture
   h. Note any tenderness over the abdomen
   i. Monitor for abdominal distention
6. Nonsurgical implementation
   a. Modify risk factors
   b. Instruct the client regarding the procedure for monitoring **BP**
   c. Instruct the client on the importance of regular physician visits to follow the size of the aneurysm
   d. Instruct the client that if severe back or abdominal pain or fullness, soreness over the umbilicus, sudden development of discoloration in the extremities, or a persistent elevation of **blood pressure** occurs, to notify physician immediately
   e. Instruct the client with a thoracic aneurysm to immediately report the occurrence of chest or back pain, shortness of breath, difficulty swallowing, or hoarseness

D. Pharmacological implementation
1. Administer antihypertensives to maintain **BP** within normal limits and prevent strain on the aneurysm
2. Instruct the client in the purpose of the medications
3. Instruct the client about the side effects and schedule of the medication

E. Abdominal aneurysm resection
1. Description: surgical resection or excision of the aneurysm and the excised section is replaced with a graft that is sewn end to end

2. Preoperative implementation
   a. Assess all peripheral pulses as a baseline for postoperative comparison
   b. Instruct the client on coughing and deep breathing exercises
   c. Administer bowel preparation as prescribed
3. Postoperative implementation
   a. Monitor vital signs
   b. Monitor peripheral pulses distal to the graft site
   c. Monitor for signs of graft occlusion including changes in pulses, cool to cold extremities below the graft, white or blue extremities or flanks, severe pain, or abdominal distention
   d. Limit elevation of the head of the bed to 45 degrees to prevent flexion of the graft
   e. Monitor for hypovolemia and renal failure resulting from the large amount of blood loss during surgery
   f. Monitor urine output hourly and, if it is less than 50 mL per hour, notify physician
   g. Monitor serum creatinine and BUN daily
   h. Monitor respiratory status and auscultate breath sounds to identify respiratory complications
   i. Encourage turning, coughing and deep breathing, and splinting the incision
   j. Ambulate as prescribed
   k. Maintain nasogastric tube to low suction until bowel sounds return
   l. Assess for bowel sounds and report their return to the physician
   m. Monitor for pain and administer medication as prescribed
   n. Assess incision site for bleeding or signs of infection
   o. Prepare the client for discharge by providing instructions regarding pain management, wound care, and activity restrictions
   p. Instruct the client not to lift objects weighing more than 15 to 20 pounds for 6 to 12 weeks
   q. Advise the client to avoid activities requiring pushing, pulling, or straining
   r. Instruct the client not to drive a vehicle until approved by the physician

F. Thoracic aneurysm repair
1. Description
   a. A thoracotomy or median sternotomy approach is used to enter the thoracic cavity
   b. The aneurysm is exposed and excised, and a graft or prosthesis is sewn onto the aorta
   c. Total cardiopulmonary bypass is necessary for excision of aneurysms in the ascending aorta
   d. Partial cardiopulmonary bypass is used for clients with an aneurysm in the descending aorta
2. Postoperative implementation
   a. Monitor vital signs
   b. Monitor for signs of hemorrhage such as a drop in **blood pressure** and increased pulse rate and respirations, and report to physician immediately
   c. Monitor chest tubes for an increase in chest drainage, which may indicate bleeding or separation at the graft site
   d. Assess sensation and motion of all extremities; if deficits occur, notify physician, as deficits can be due to a lack of blood supply during surgery
   e. Monitor respiratory status and auscultate breath sounds to identify respiratory complications
   f. Encourage turning, coughing and deep breathing, splinting the incision
   g. Monitor cardiac status for dysrhythmias
   h. Monitor for pain and administer medication as prescribed
   i. Assess incision site for bleeding or signs of infection
   j. Prepare the client for discharge by providing instructions regarding pain management, wound care, and activity restrictions
   k. Instruct the client not to lift objects weighing more than 15 to 20 pounds for 6 to 12 weeks
   l. Advise the client to avoid activities requiring pushing, pulling, or straining
   m. Instruct the client not to drive a vehicle until approved by the physician

XVIII. HYPERTENSION

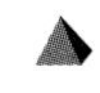

A. Description (Table 48-1)
1. Persistent elevation of the systolic **blood pressure** above 140 mm Hg and the diastolic **blood pressure** above 90 mm Hg
2. Most significant predictor of developing coronary artery disease
3. Major risk factor for coronary, cerebral, renal, and peripheral vascular disease
4. The disease is initially asymptomatic
5. The goals of treatment include to reduce the BP and to prevent or lessen the extent of organ damage
6. Nonpharmacological approaches, as lifestyle changes, may be initially prescribed and if the

TABLE 48-1

Hypertension

Organ Involvement	Complications
Eyes	Visual changes
Brain	Cerebrovascular accident
Cardiovascular system	Heart failure, hypertensive crisis
Kidneys	Renal failure

BP cannot be decreased after a reasonable period (1 to 3 months), then the client may require pharmacological treatment

B. Primary or essential hypertension
   1. No known etiology
   2. Risk factors
      a. Aging
      b. Family history
      c. Black race, with higher prevalence in males
      d. Obesity
      e. Smoking
      f. Stress

C. Secondary hypertension
   1. Treatment depends on the cause and the organs involved
   2. Occurs as a result of other disorders or conditions
   3. Precipitating disorders or conditions
      a. Cardiovascular disorders
      b. Renal disorders
      c. Endocrine system disorders
      d. Pregnancy
      e. Medications

D. Data collection
   1. May be asymptomatic
   2. Headache
   3. Visual disturbances
   4. Dizziness
   5. Chest pain
   6. Tinnitus
   7. Flushed face
   8. Epistaxis

E. Implementation
   1. Goals
      a. To reduce the **blood pressure**
      b. To prevent or lessen the extent of organ damage
   2. Question client regarding signs and symptoms indicative of hypertension
   3. Obtain **blood pressure (BP)** two or more times on both arms with the client supine and standing
   4. Compare **BP** with prior documentation
   5. Determine family history
   6. Identify current medication therapy
   7. Obtain weight
   8. Evaluate dietary patterns and sodium intake of client
   9. Monitor for visual changes or retinal damage
   10. Monitor for cardiovascular changes as distended neck veins, increased heart rate, dysrhythmias
   11. Evaluate chest x-ray film for heart enlargement
   12. Monitor neurological system
   13. Evaluate renal function
   14. Evaluate results of diagnostic and laboratory studies

F. Nonpharmacological implementation
   1. Weight reduction if necessary or maintenance of ideal weight
   2. Dietary sodium restriction to 2 grams daily as prescribed
   3. Moderate intake of alcohol and caffeine containing products
   4. Initiation of a regular exercise program
   5. Avoidance of smoking
   6. Relaxation techniques and biofeedback therapy
   7. Elimination of unnecessary medications that may contribute to the hypertension

G. Stepped-Care Approach
   1. Description
      a. If a pharmacological approach to treating hypertension is required, a single medication is prescribed and monitored for its effectiveness
      b. Medications are added to the treatment regimen until the **BP** is controlled
   2. Step 1: a single medication is prescribed, which may be a diuretic, beta-blocker, calcium channel blocker, or angiotensin-converting enzyme (ACE) inhibitor
   3. Step 2
      a. Step 1 therapy is evaluated after 1 to 3 months
      b. If the response is not adequate, compliance is evaluated
      c. The medication may be increased or a new medication prescribed, or a second medication is added to the treatment plan
   4. Step 3
      a. Compliance is evaluated
      b. Further evaluation of Step 2
      c. If a therapeutic response is not adequate, a second medication is substituted or a third medication is added to the treatment plan
   5. Step 4
      a. Compliance is evaluated
      b. Careful data collection of factors limiting the antihypertensive response is done

BOX 48-5

Client Education for Hypertension

Educate the client to prevent noncompliance with the treatment plan
Describe the disease process explaining that symptoms usually do not develop until organs have suffered damage
Initiate and assist the client in planning a regular exercise program avoiding heavy weight lifting and isometric exercises
Emphasize the importance of beginning the exercise program gradually
Encourage the client to express feelings about daily stress
Assist the client to identify ways to reduce stress
Teach relaxation techniques
Instruct the client how to incorporate relaxation techniques into their daily living pattern
Instruct the client and family in the technique for monitoring blood pressure
Instruct the client to maintain a diary of blood pressure readings
Emphasize the importance of lifelong medication and the need for follow-up treatment
Emphasize the importance of medications and instruct the client not to stop the medication without consulting with the physician
Instruct the client and family on dietary restrictions, which may include sodium, fat, calories, and cholesterol
Instruct the client how to shop and prepare low-sodium meals
Provide a list of products that contain sodium
Instruct the client to read labels of products to determine sodium content focusing on substance listed as sodium, NaCl, and MSG
Instruct the client to bake, roast, or boil foods; to avoid salt when preparing foods; and to avoid salt at the table
Instruct the client that fresh foods are best to consume and to avoid canned foods
Instruct the client about the action, side effects, and scheduling of medications
Advise the client that, if uncomfortable side effects occur, to contact the physician and not to stop the medication
Instruct the client to avoid over-the-counter medications
Stress the importance of follow-up care

c. A third or fourth medication may be added to the treatment plan

H. See Box 48-5 for client education

XIX. HYPERTENSIVE CRISIS

A. Description
1. Any clinical condition requiring immediate reduction in **blood pressure**
2. An acute and life-threatening condition
3. The accelerated hypertension requires emergency treatment as target organ damage (brain, heart, retina of the eye) can occur quickly
4. Death can be caused by stroke, renal failure, or cardiac disease

B. Data collection
1. A **diastolic pressure** above 120 mm Hg
2. Headache
3. Drowsiness
4. Confusion
5. Changes in neurological status
6. Tachycardia and tachypnea
7. Dyspnea
8. Cyanosis
9. Seizures

C. Implementation
1. Maintain a patent airway
2. Administer IV antihypertensive medications as prescribed, which may include nitroprusside (Nipride), diazoxide (Hyperstat), or trimethaphan camsylate (Arfonad)
3. Monitor vital signs assessing **BP** every 5 minutes
4. Monitor for hypotension during the administration of antihypertensives
5. Place the client in supine position if hypotension occurs
6. Have emergency medications and resuscitation equipment readily available
7. Maintain bed rest with the head of the bed at 45 degrees
8. Monitor IV therapy assessing for fluid overload
9. Monitor I&O
10. Insert Foley catheter as prescribed
11. Monitor urinary output and if oliguria or anuria occurs, notify the physician

PRACTICE QUESTIONS

1. A client is scheduled for a cardiac catheterization using a radiopaque dye. The nurse checks which most critical item before the procedure?
   1. Intake and output
   2. Peripheral pulse rates
   3. Height and weight
   4. Allergy to iodine or shellfish

2. A client is scheduled for a dipyridamole (Persantine) thallium scan. The nurse would check to make sure that the client has not had which of the following before the procedure?
   1. Milk products
   2. Caffeine
   3. Excess sugar
   4. Fatty meal
3. A client with no history of cardiovascular disease presents to the ambulatory clinic with flulike symptoms. While at the clinic, the client suddenly develops chest pain. Which of the following questions would best help the nurse to discriminate pain because of a noncardiac problem?
   1. "Have you ever had this pain before?"
   2. "Can you describe the pain to me?"
   3. "Does the pain get worse when you breathe in?'
   4. "Can you rate the pain on a scale of 1 to 10, with 10 being the worst?"
4. A client with myocardial infarction (MI) has been transferred from the coronary care unit (CCU) to the general medical unit with cardiac monitoring via telemetry. The nurse assisting in caring for the client expects to note which type of activity prescribed?
   1. Strict bed rest for 24 hours
   2. Bathroom privileges and self-care activities
   3. Unsupervised hallway ambulation with distances under 200 feet
   4. Ad lib activities because the client is monitored
5. A nurse notes bilateral 2+ edema in the lower extremities of a client with myocardial infarction admitted 2 days ago. The nurse would plan to do which of the following next?
   1. Review the intake and output records for the last 2 days
   2. Change the time of diuretic administration from morning to evening
   3. Request a sodium restriction of 1 gram per day from the physician
   4. Order daily weights beginning the next morning
6. A nurse is collecting data from a client with a primary diagnosis of heart failure. Which of the following disorders reported by the client does not play a role in exacerbating the heart failure?
   1. Recent upper respiratory infection
   2. Nutritional anemia
   3. Peptic ulcer disease
   4. Atrial fibrillation
7. A nurse is collecting data from a client with heart failure who was being sent directly to the hospital from the physician's office. The nurse reviews the physician's orders and expects to note an order for which medication?
   1. Diltiazem (Cardizem)
   2. Digoxin (Lanoxin)
   3. Propranolol (Inderal)
   4. Metoprolol (Lopressor)
8. A nurse checks the sternotomy incision of a client on the third postoperative day after cardiac surgery. The incision shows some slight "puffiness" along the edges, is nonreddened, with no apparent drainage. The client's temperature is 99° F orally. The white blood cell (WBC) count is 7500/mm^3. The nurse interprets that the incision line:
   1. Is slightly edematous but shows no active signs of infection
   2. Shows no sign of infection, although the WBC count is elevated
   3. Shows early signs of infection, although the temperature is near normal
   4. Shows early signs of infection supported by an elevated WBC count
9. A postcardiac surgery client has a urine output averaging 20 mL per hour for 2 hours. The client received a single bolus of 500 mL of IV fluid. Urine output for the subsequent hour was 25 mL. Daily laboratory results indicate the blood urea nitrogen (BUN) is 45 mg/dL and the serum creatinine is 2.2 mg/dL. The nurse interprets that the client is at risk for:
   1. Hypovolemia
   2. Urinary tract infection
   3. Glomerulonephritis
   4. Acute renal failure
10. A nurse is preparing to ambulate the client on the third postoperative day after cardiac surgery. The nurse plans to do which of the following to enable the client to best tolerate the ambulation?
    1. Encourage the client to cough and deep breathe
    2. Premedicate the client with an analgesic
    3. Provide the client with a walker
    4. Remove the telemetry equipment
11. A client is wearing a continuous cardiac monitor, which begins to alarm. The nurse sees no ECG complexes on the screen. The first action of the nurse is to:
    1. Check the client status and lead placement
    2. Press the recorder button on the ECG console
    3. Call the physician
    4. Call a code blue
12. A client with a diagnosis of rapid rate atrial fibrillation asks the nurse why the physician is going to perform carotid massage. The nurse responds that this procedure may stimulate the:
    1. Vagus nerve to slow the heart rate
    2. Vagus nerve to increase the heart rate
    3. Diaphragmatic nerve to slow the heart rate
    4. Diaphragmatic nerve to increase the heart rate
13. A nurse is caring for a client on a cardiac monitor who is alone in a room at the end of the hall. The client has a short burst of ventricular tachycardia

followed by ventricular fibrillation (VF). The client immediately loses consciousness. The nurse would immediately:
1. Call for help and initiate cardiopulmonary resuscitation (CPR)
2. Start oxygen by cannula at 10 liters per minute and lower the head of the bed
3. Go to the nurse's station quickly and call a code
4. Run to get a defibrillator from an adjacent nursing unit

14. A nurse is monitoring a client after cardioversion. Which of the following observations would be of highest priority to the nurse?
1. Oxygen flow rate
2. Status of airway
3. Blood pressure
4. Level of consciousness

15. An automatic external defibrillator is available to treat the client who goes into cardiac arrest. With this device, the nurse checks the cardiac rhythm by:
1. Applying standard ECG monitoring leads to the client and observing the rhythm
2. Holding the defibrillator paddles firmly against the chest
3. Applying the adhesive patch electrodes to the skin and moving away from the client
4. Connecting standard ECG electrodes to a transtelephonic monitoring device

16. The nurse is caring for the client immediately after insertion of a permanent demand pacemaker via the right subclavian vein. The nurse takes care not to dislodge the pacing catheter by:
1. Limiting movement and abduction of the right arm
2. Limiting movement and abduction of the left arm
3. Assisting the client to get out of bed and ambulate with a walker
4. Having the physical therapist do active range of motion to the right arm

17. A client diagnosed with thrombophlebitis 1 day ago suddenly complains of chest pain and shortness of breath and is visibly anxious. The nurse immediately checks the client for other signs and symptoms of:
1. Myocardial infarction
2. Pneumonia
3. Pulmonary embolism
4. Pulmonary edema

18. A client seeks treatment in the physician's office for unsightly varicose veins, and sclerotherapy is recommended. Before leaving the examining room, the client says to the nurse "Can you tell me again how this sclerotherapy is done?" In formulating a response, the nurse incorporates the knowledge that sclerotherapy consists of:
1. Injecting an agent into the vein to damage the vein wall and close the vein off
2. Tying off the vein at the upper end to prevent stasis from occurring
3. Tying off the vein at the lower end to prevent stasis from occurring
4. Surgical removal of the varicosity

19. A client is having a follow-up physician office visit after vein ligation and stripping. The client describes a sensation of "pins and needles" in the affected leg. Based on evaluation of this comment, the nurse:
1. Reassures the client that this is only temporary
2. Advises the client to take acetaminophen (Tylenol) until it is gone
3. States that warm packs should help
4. Reports the complaint to the physician

20. A 24-year-old man seeks medical attention for complaints of claudication in the arch of the foot. The nurse also notes superficial thrombophlebitis of the lower leg. The nurse would next check the client for:
1. Familial tendency toward peripheral vascular disease
2. Smoking history
3. Recent exposure to allergens
4. History of recent insect bites

21. A nurse has given instructions to the client with Raynaud's disease about self- management of the disease process. The nurse determines that the client needs further reinforcement if the client states that:
1. Smoking cessation is very important
2. Sources of caffeine should be eliminated from the diet
3. Taking nifedipine (Procardia) as prescribed will decrease vessel spasm
4. Moving to a warmer climate should help

22. A nurse is checking the blood pressure of a client diagnosed with primary hypertension. The nurse ensures accurate measurement by avoiding which of the following?
1. Seating the client with arm bared, supported, and at heart level
2. Measuring the blood pressure after the client is seated quietly for 5 minutes
3. Using a cuff with a rubber bladder that encircles at least 80% of the limb
4. Taking the blood pressure within 15 minutes after nicotine or caffeine ingestion

23. A client is at risk for pulmonary embolism and is on anticoagulant therapy with warfarin sodium (Coumadin). The client's prothrombin time (PT) is 20 seconds with a control of 11 seconds. The nurse determines that this result is:
1. The same as the client's own baseline level
2. Lower than the therapeutic level

3. Within the therapeutic range
4. Higher than the therapeutic range

24. A client who has been receiving heparin therapy is also started on warfarin sodium (Coumadin). The client asks the nurse why both medications are being administered. In formulating a response, the nurse incorporates the understanding that warfarin:
   1. Stimulates breakdown of specific clotting factors by the liver, and it takes 2 to 3 days for this to exert an anticoagulant effect
   2. Inhibits synthesis of specific clotting factors in the liver, and it takes 3 to 4 days for this medication to exert an anticoagulant effect
   3. Stimulates production of the body's own thrombolytic substances, and it takes 2 to 4 days for this to begin
   4. Has the same mechanism of action as heparin, and the crossover time is needed for the serum level of warfarin to be therapeutic

25. A nurse has an order to begin administering warfarin sodium (Coumadin) to a client. While implementing this order, the nurse ensures that which of the following medications is available on the nursing unit as the antidote?
   1. Vitamin K (AquaMEPHYTON)
   2. Aminocaproic acid (Amicar)
   3. Potassium chloride
   4. Protamine sulfate

26. A client is admitted to the hospital with an arterial ischemic leg ulcer. The nurse assesses the ulcer expecting to note that it:
   1. Has a pink colored base
   2. Is superficial, with uneven edges
   3. Has little granulation tissue
   4. Has brown pigmentation surrounding it

27. A nurse is assessing the neurovascular status of a client who returned to the surgical nursing unit 4 hours ago after undergoing aortoiliac bypass graft. The affected leg is warm, and the nurse notes redness and edema. The pedal pulse is palpable and unchanged from admission. The nurse interprets that the neurovascular status is:
   1. Normal, resulting from increased blood flow through the leg
   2. Slightly deteriorating and should be monitored for another hour
   3. Moderately impaired, and the surgeon should be called
   4. Adequate from an arterial approach, but venous complications are arising

28. A client with an abdominal aortic aneurysm (AAA) is not a candidate for surgery because the aneurysm is not yet large enough. The client is fearful that the aneurysm will rupture, causing death. The nurse plans to assist the client in coping with this fear by emphasizing what the client can do for self-monitoring. Which of the following items would be unnecessary for the nurse to include in discussions with the client?
   1. Antibiotic prophylaxis before invasive procedures
   2. Importance of follow-up computed tomography (CT) scans
   3. Management of hypertension
   4. Reporting abdominal or back pain

29. A client has an Unna boot applied for treatment of a venous stasis leg ulcer. The nurse notes that the client's toes are mottled and cool, and the client verbalizes some numbness and tingling of the foot. The nurse interprets that the boot:
   1. Is controlling leg edema
   2. Has been applied too tightly
   3. Is impairing venous return
   4. Has not yet dried

30. A nurse is planning care for an ambulatory client with a venous stasis leg ulcer. The nurse anticipates that which type of dressing will be used in the care of this client?
   1. Damp to dry isotonic saline dressings
   2. One-half strength Betadine dressings
   3. Dry sterile dressings
   4. Zinc oxide dressings (Unna boot)

31. A nurse is caring for a client receiving digoxin (Lanoxin) in the treatment of heart failure. The nurse would monitor the client for:
   1. Thrombocytopenia and weight gain
   2. Anorexia, nausea, and visual disturbances
   3. Diarrhea and hypotension
   4. Fatigue and muscle twitching

32. A nurse has reinforced instructions to the client who is beginning therapy with digoxin (Lanoxin). The nurse would evaluate that the client needs reinforcement if the client made which of the following statements?
   1. "I should call the doctor if my daily pulse rate is under 60 or over 100 beats per minute."
   2. "If I miss a dose, I should just take two the next day."
   3. "I shouldn't change brands without asking the doctor first."
   4. "The pills should be kept in their original container, so they don't get mixed up with my other medicines."

33. A client with angina complains that the anginal pain is prolonged and severe, and occurs at the same time each day, most often in the morning. On further data collection, the nurse notes that that the pain occurs in the absence of precipitating factors. This type of anginal pain is best described as:
   1. Stable angina
   2. Unstable angina

3. Variant angina
4. Nonanginal pain

34. A nurse is assisting in monitoring the condition of a client after pericardiocentesis for cardiac tamponade. Which of the following observations would indicate that the procedure was unsuccessful?
    1. Rising central venous pressure (CVP)
    2. Rising blood pressure (BP)
    3. Client expressions of relief
    4. Clearly audible heart sounds
35. A nurse is monitoring a client with an abdominal aortic aneurysm (AAA). Which of the following findings by the nurse is probably unrelated to the AAA?
    1. Pulsatile abdominal mass
    2. Hyperactive bowel sounds in the area
    3. Systolic bruit over the area of the mass
    4. Subjective sensation of "heart beating" in the abdomen
36. A client is taking hydrochlorothiazide (HydroDIURIL, HCTZ) without taking any form of electrolyte supplement. The nurse would encourage intake of which of the following foods?
    1. Canned pears
    2. Oranges
    3. Cranberry juice
    4. Applesauce
37. A hypertensive client who has been taking metoprolol (Lopressor) has been ordered to decrease the dose of the medication. The client asks the nurse why this must be done over 1 to 2 weeks. In formulating a response, the nurse incorporates the understanding that abrupt withdrawal could:
    1. Give the client insomnia
    2. Cause enhanced side effects of other prescribed medications
    3. Result in hypoglycemia
    4. Precipitate rebound hypertension
38. A nurse is administering medications to a client newly admitted to the nursing unit with a history of cardiac disease. The client has an order for propranolol (Inderal) 20 mg po, and albuterol (Proventil, Ventolin) 2 puffs by inhalation. The nurse should:
    1. Administer the propranolol first, followed by the albuterol
    2. Administer the albuterol first, followed by the propranolol
    3. Let the client decide which to take first, according to preference
    4. Call the physician to verify the order
39. A nurse is caring for the client with history of mild heart failure who is receiving diltiazem (Cardizem) for hypertension. The nurse would check the client for:
    1. Tachycardia and rebound hypertension
    2. Wheezing and shortness of breath
    3. Bradycardia, weight gain, and peripheral edema
    4. Chest pain and tachycardia
40. A client receiving nifedipine (Procardia) for angina complains of feeling listless, with generalized weakness and no energy. To support the client most effectively, the nurse must understand that these symptoms:
    1. Are unrelated to taking the medication
    2. Are an expected effect of the medication
    3. Indicate toxic reaction to the medication
    4. Indicate underdosing of the medication
41. A client taking nitroglycerin sublingual for the control of episodes of chest pain says to the nurse that perhaps the medication shouldn't be used unless absolutely necessary for pain. On further data collection, the nurse determines that the client knows the reasons for taking the medication, and that the client can afford to pay for the medication. The nurse should next explore with the client any concerns about:
    1. Status of the heart disease
    2. Potential myocardial infarction
    3. Developing tolerance to the medication
    4. Inconvenience of the medication schedule
42. A client has been prescribed a transdermal nitroglycerin system (Nitrodisc, Nitro-Dur) for the management of angina pectoris. The client asks the nurse why the patch must be removed at bedtime each night. In formulating a reply, the nurse incorporates the understanding that:
    1. Lack of pain relief (tolerance) occurs when worn continuously for 24 hours
    2. Hypotension occurs frequently at night unless the patch is removed
    3. The system is too irritating to the skin to be worn for 24 hours
    4. The patch always falls off from friction with the bedclothes
43. A nurse has an order to administer a dose of nitroglycerin ointment (Nitro-Bid, Nitrostat) to a client. The nurse would avoid doing which of the following in preparing the medication for administration?
    1. Using the manufacturer's papers
    2. Using the fingers to spread the ointment
    3. Applying the dose in an even layer
    4. Washing off the previous application
44. A nurse is giving a client instructions about the use of a transdermal nitroglycerin system (Nitro-Dur, Transderm-Nitro). Which statement by the client indicates a need for further instructions?
    1. "I should apply the patch with very light pressure to avoid rapid absorption."
    2. "Units are waterproof, so bathing and showering are allowed."

3. "I should not change brands, as the dosages may not be equivalent."
4. "I should not cut or trim patch to adjust dosage."

45. A hypertensive client with target organ renal damage has been prescribed minoxidil (Loniten). The client asks the nurse why the physician has also prescribed propranolol for concurrent use. The nurse's response is based on the understanding that propranolol:
1. Is used to get better control of hypertension than is possible with minoxidil alone
2. Prevents reflex tachycardia that is caused by the minoxidil
3. Exerts a protective effect on the kidney
4. Prevents fluid retention and weight gain

46. A client has begun antidysrhythmic therapy with sotalol (Brevibloc). Knowing the side effects that could affect the client's psychosocial well-being, the nurse does anticipatory counseling about the possibility of:
1. Anxiety and confusion
2. Anxiety and pain
3. Paranoia
4. Decreased libido and impotence

47. A nurse has given medication instructions to the client receiving disopyramide (Norpace). The nurse determines that the client needs clarification of the information if the client stated to:
1. Change position slowly
2. Avoid extreme heat
3. Keep tissues nearby for excessive salivation
4. Use caution with driving

48. A client has begun taking quinidine gluconate (Duraquin, Quinaglute). The nurse would check for which of the following most frequent side effects of this medication?
1. Constipation and dehydration
2. Diarrhea, nausea, and cramping
3. Tachycardia and hypertension
4. Bleeding tendencies

49. A client is beginning amiodarone (Cordarone) therapy while in the hospital. To minimize gastrointestinal side effects, the nurse would provide the client with:
1. Antidiarrheal agents
2. Antacids
3. Increased fiber and fluids
4. Soft diet

50. A nurse is reinforcing instructions to a client receiving colestipol hydrochloride (Colestid). The nurse would advise the client to increase intake of:
1. Carbohydrates
2. Fats
3. Fiber and fluids
4. Protein

ANSWERS

1. *Answer:* 4
Rationale: This procedure requires a signed consent, because it involves injection of a radiopaque dye into the blood vessel. The risk of allergic reaction and possible anaphylaxis is serious and must be assessed before the procedure. Although options 1, 2, and 3 may be a component of data collection, they are not the most critical items.
Test-Taking Strategy: Use the process of elimination and note the key words "most critical." Recalling the risk of anaphylaxis if an allergy exists will direct you to option 4. Review preprocedure interventions for a cardiac catheterization if you had difficulty with this question.
Level of Cognitive Ability: Application
Client Needs: Physiological Integrity
Integrated Concept/Process: Nursing Process/Data Collection
Content Area: Adult Health/Cardiovascular
Reference: DeWit S: *Fundamental concepts and skills for nursing,* Philadelphia, 2001, WB Saunders, p. 425.

2. *Answer:* 2
Rationale: This test is an alternative to the exercise stress test. Dipyridamole (Persantine) dilates the coronary arteries as would exercise. Before the procedure, any form of caffeine should be withheld, as well as aminophylline or theophylline. Aminophylline is the antagonist to dipyridamole.
Test-Taking Strategy: Use the process of elimination and note the key words "has not had." Remember, factors that put a strain on the heart, such as nicotine and caffeine, can interfere with cardiac diagnostic test results. Look for items such as these in similarly worded questions. Review preprocedure interventions for this test if you had difficulty with this question.
Level of Cognitive Ability: Application
Client Needs: Physiological Integrity
Integrated Concept/Process: Nursing Process/Data Collection
Content Area: Adult Health/Cardiovascular
Reference: Ignatavicius D, Workman M: *Medical-surgical: critical thinking for collaborative care,* ed 4, Philadelphia, 2002, WB Saunders, p. 648.

3. *Answer:* 3
Rationale: Chest pain is assessed using the standard pain assessment parameters, (characteristics, location, intensity, duration, precipitating and alleviating factors, and associated symptoms). Options 1, 2, and 4 may or may not help discriminate the origin of pain. Pain of pleuropulmonary origin usually worsens on inspiration.
Test-Taking Strategy: Use the process of elimination. This question is looking for a method of discriminating among the causes of pain. The three incorrect options, although appropriate to use in clinical practice, are general assessment ques-

tions only. Option 3 will discriminate between a cardiac and noncardiac cause of pain. Review pain assessment techniques if you had difficulty with this question.
Level of Cognitive Ability: Analysis
Client Needs: Physiological Integrity
Integrated Concept/Process: Nursing Process/Data Collection
Content Area: Adult Health/Cardiovascular
Reference: Ignatavicius D, Workman M: *Medical-surgical: critical thinking for collaborative care,* ed 4, Philadelphia, 2002, WB Saunders, p. 474.

4. ***Answer:*** 2
Rationale: Upon transfer from the CCU, the client is allowed self-care activities and bathroom privileges. Supervised ambulation in the hall for brief distances is encouraged, with distances gradually increased (50, 100, 200 feet).
Test-Taking Strategy: Use the process of elimination. Eliminate options 3 and 4 first, because they are excessive given that the client has just transferred from the CCU. Option 1 is not viable because the client would be doing less activity than in the CCU before transfer. Review activity prescriptions for the client with an MI if you had difficulty with this question.
Level of Cognitive Ability: Comprehension
Client Needs: Physiological Integrity
Integrated Concept/Process: Nursing Process/Planning
Content Area: Adult Health/Cardiovascular
Reference: Ignatavicius D, Workman M: *Medical-surgical: critical thinking for collaborative care,* ed 4, Philadelphia, 2002, WB Saunders, p. 811.

5. ***Answer:*** 1
Rationale: Edema, the accumulation of excess fluid in the interstitial spaces, can be measured by intake greater than output, and by a sudden increase in weight. Diuretics should be given in the morning whenever possible to avoid nocturia. Strict sodium restrictions are reserved for clients with severe symptoms.
Test-Taking Strategy: Use the process of elimination. The question asks what the nurse would do next. Focusing on the issue will direct you to option 1. Option 1 can give the nurse immediate information about fluid balance. Review data collection methods for the client with edema if you had difficulty with this question.
Level of Cognitive Ability: Application
Client Needs: Physiological Integrity
Integrated Concept/Process: Nursing Process/Implementation
Content Area: Adult Health/Cardiovascular
Reference: Ignatavicius D, Workman M: *Medical-surgical: critical thinking for collaborative care,* ed 4, Philadelphia, 2002, WB Saunders, p. 633.

6. ***Answer:*** 3
Rationale: Heart failure is precipitated or exacerbated by physical or emotional stress, dysrhythmias, infections, anemia, thyroid disorders, pregnancy, Paget's disease, nutritional deficiencies (thiamine, alcoholism), pulmonary disease, and hypervolemia.
Test-Taking Strategy: Use the process of elimination. The question asks for an item that is not related to the heart failure. Because heart failure is exacerbated by factors that increase the workload of the heart, options 1, 2 and 4 can be eliminated. Review the precipitating factors associated with heart failure if you had difficulty with this question.
Level of Cognitive Ability: Analysis
Client Needs: Health Promotion and Maintenance
Integrated Concept/Process: Nursing Process/Data Collection
Content Area: Adult Health/Cardiovascular
Reference: Ignatavicius D, Workman M: *Medical-surgical: critical thinking for collaborative care,* ed 4, Philadelphia, 2002, WB Saunders, p. 699.

7. ***Answer:*** 2
Rationale: Digoxin exerts a positive inotropic effect on the heart while slowing the overall rate through a variety of mechanisms. It is the medication of choice used to treat heart failure. Diltiazem (calcium channel blocker), propranolol, and metoprolol (beta-adrenergic blockers) have a negative inotropic effect and would worsen the failing heart.
Test-Taking Strategy: Use the process of elimination. Eliminate options 3 and 4 first because they are similar. From the remaining options, it is necessary to know that digoxin is used to treat heart failure. Review the treatment for this disorder if you had difficulty with this question.
Level of Cognitive Ability: Analysis
Client Needs: Physiological Integrity
Integrated Concept/Process: Nursing Process/Planning
Content Area: Adult Health/Cardiovascular
Reference: Hodgson B, Kizior R: *Saunders nursing drug handbook 2002,* Philadelphia, 2002, WB Saunders, p. 344.

8. ***Answer:*** 1
Rationale: Sternotomy incision sites are assessed for signs and symptoms of infection, such as redness, swelling, and induration. An elevated temperature and WBC count after 3 to 4 days usually indicate infection. A WBC count of 7500/mm^3 is within the normal range.
Test-Taking Strategy: Use the process of elimination. Eliminate options 2 and 4 because the WBC count is normal. The lack of drainage and redness helps you choose option 1 over 3. Review the signs of an incisional infection if you had difficulty with this question.
Level of Cognitive Ability: Analysis
Client Needs: Physiological Integrity
Integrated Concept/Process: Nursing Process/Data Collection
Content Area: Adult Health/Cardiovascular
Reference: Ignatavicius D, Workman M: *Medical-surgical: critical thinking for collaborative care,* ed 4, Philadelphia, 2002, WB Saunders, p. 296.

9. ***Answer:*** 4
Rationale: The client who undergoes cardiac surgery is at risk for renal injury from poor perfusion, hemolysis, low cardiac output, or vasopressor medication therapy. Renal insult is signaled by a decreased urine output, and an increased BUN and creatinine. The client may need medications to increase renal perfusion and could possibly need peritoneal dialysis or hemodialysis.
Test-Taking Strategy: Use the process of elimination. The question provides no evidence of any infection, so eliminate options 2 and 3 first. Hypovolemia is eliminated next because

of the high BUN and creatinine values, and the poor response to the bolus of fluid. Review laboratory values and postcardiac surgery complications if you had difficulty with this question.
Level of Cognitive Ability: Analysis
Client Needs: Physiological Integrity
Integrated Concept/Process: Nursing Process/Data Collection
Content Area: Adult Health/Cardiovascular
Reference: Ignatavicius D, Workman M: *Medical-surgical: critical thinking for collaborative care*, ed 4, Philadelphia, 2002, WB Saunders, p. 714.

10. *Answer:* 2
Rationale: The nurse should encourage regular use of pain medication for the first 48 to 72 hours after cardiac surgery, because analgesia will promote rest, decrease myocardial oxygen consumption resulting from pain, and allow better participation in activities such as coughing, deep breathing, and ambulation.
Test-Taking Strategy: Use the process of elimination. The question asks for the best action of the nurse to help a client tolerate ambulation. Coughing and deep breathing will not actively help endurance, so eliminate option 1. Eliminate option 4 because removal of telemetry equipment is contraindicated unless ordered. From the remaining options, noting that the client is postoperative will direct you to option 2. Review postoperative care if you had difficulty with this question.
Level of Cognitive Ability: Application
Client Needs: Physiological Integrity
Integrated Concept/Process: Nursing Process/Planning
Content Area: Adult Health/Cardiovascular
Reference: Ignatavicius D, Workman M: *Medical-surgical: critical thinking for collaborative care*, ed 4, Philadelphia, 2002, WB Saunders, p. 288.

11. *Answer:* 1
Rationale: Sudden loss of ECG complexes indicates either ventricular asystole, or possibly electrode displacement. Assessment of the client and equipment is the first action by the nurse.
Test-Taking Strategy: Use the steps of the nursing process and remember that data collection is the first step. Options 3 and 4 are incorrect because they indicate calling for assistance before collecting data. Option 2 may sound reasonable, but the ECG monitor automatically starts recording when an alarm sounds. Option 1 is the best option because you should always check the client directly before taking any action. Review care of a client on a cardiac monitor if you had difficulty with this question.
Level of Cognitive Ability: Application
Client Needs: Physiological Integrity
Integrated Concept/Process: Nursing Process/Implementation
Content Area: Adult Health/Cardiovascular
Reference: Ignatavicius D, Workman M: *Medical-surgical: critical thinking for collaborative care*, ed 4, Philadelphia, 2002, WB Saunders, p. 645.

12. *Answer:* 1
Rationale: Carotid sinus massage is one of the maneuvers used for vagal stimulation to decrease a rapid heart rate and possibly terminate a tachydysrhythmia. The other maneuvers are the Valsalva maneuver of inducing the gag reflex and asking the client to strain or bear down. Medication therapy is often needed as an adjunct to keep the rate down or maintain the normal rhythm.
Test-Taking Strategy: Use the process of elimination. Eliminate options 2 and 4 first because these options indicate increasing an already rapid rate. From the remaining options, use knowledge of anatomy and physiology. A rapid rate dysrhythmia would need to be slowed, which is the function of the vagus nerve. The diaphragmatic nerve affects respiration. If you are unfamiliar with the functions of these nerves, review this content.
Level of Cognitive Ability: Application
Client Needs: Physiological Integrity
Integrated Concept/Process: Nursing Process/Implementation
Content Area: Adult Health/Cardiovascular
Reference: Ignatavicius D, Workman M: *Medical-surgical: critical thinking for collaborative care*, ed 4, Philadelphia, 2002, WB Saunders, p. 822.

13. *Answer:* 1
Rationale: When VF occurs, the nurse remains with the client and initiates CPR until a defibrillator is available and attached to the client. Options 2, 3, and 4 are incorrect.
Test-Taking Strategy: Use the process of elimination. Eliminate options 3 and 4 first because you would never leave the client alone. From the remaining options, lowering the head of bed is appropriate (for resuscitation), but the oxygen by cannula at 10 liters is incorrect. Option 1 is the correct option. Review care to the client with VF if you had difficulty with this question.
Level of Cognitive Ability: Application
Client Needs: Physiological Integrity
Integrated Concept/Process: Nursing Process/Implementation
Content Area: Adult Health/Cardiovascular
Reference: Ignatavicius D, Workman M: *Medical-surgical: critical thinking for collaborative care*, ed 4, Philadelphia, 2002, WB Saunders, p. 644.

14. *Answer:* 2
Rationale: Nursing responsibilities after cardioversion include maintenance of a patent airway, oxygen administration, assessment of vital signs and level of consciousness, and dysrhythmia detection.
Test-Taking Strategy: Use the ABCs—airway, breathing, and circulation—to answer the question. This will direct you to option 2. Remember, airway comes first. Review care to the client after cardioversion if you had difficulty with this question.
Level of Cognitive Ability: Comprehension
Client Needs: Physiological Integrity
Integrated Concept/Process: Nursing Process/Data Collection
Content Area: Adult Health/Cardiovascular
Reference: Ignatavicius D, Workman M: *Medical-surgical: critical thinking for collaborative care*, ed 4, Philadelphia, 2002, WB Saunders, p. 690.

15. *Answer:* 3
Rationale: The nurse or rescuer puts two large adhesive patch electrodes on the client's chest in the usual defibrillator posi-

tion. The nurse stops cardiopulmonary resuscitation and orders anyone near the client to move away and not touch the client. The defibrillator then analyzes the rhythm, which may take up to 30 seconds. The machine then indicates if it is necessary to defibrillate.
Test-Taking Strategy: If you are not familiar with this piece of equipment, look first at the word "automatic" in the name. This implies that a person is not as involved in the process as with a conventional defibrillator, and may help you eliminate option 2. Because standard ECG monitoring leads do not play an active role once a resuscitation is underway (options 1 and 4), you can eliminate these similar, but incorrect, options. Although automatic external defibrillation can be done transtelephonically, it is done through the use of patch electrodes that interact via telephone lines to a base station, which controls any actual defibrillation. Review the use of this device if you had difficulty with this question.
Level of Cognitive Ability: Application
Client Needs: Physiological Integrity
Integrated Concept/Process: Nursing Process/Implementation
Content Area:Adult Health/Cardiovascular
Reference: Ignatavicius D, Workman M: *Medical-surgical: critical thinking for collaborative care,* ed 4, Philadelphia, 2002, WB Saunders, p. 691.

16. ***Answer:*** 1
Rationale: In the first several hours after insertion of either a permanent or temporary pacemaker, the most common complication is pacing electrode dislodgement. The nurse helps prevent this complication by limiting the client's activities.
Test-Taking Strategy: Use the process of elimination. The question tells you that the pacemaker was inserted on the right side. Therefore, to prevent pacing electrode dislodgement, motion must be limited on that side. Options 3 and 4 involve movement of the right arm. Limiting the movement of the left arm (option 2) is of no benefit to the client. Thus option 1 is correct. Review care to the client after pacemaker insertion if you had difficulty with this question.
Level of Cognitive Ability: Application
Client Needs: Physiological Integrity
Integrated Concept/Process: Nursing Process/Implementation
Content Area: Adult Health/Cardiovascular
Reference: Ignatavicius D, Workman M: *Medical-surgical: critical thinking for collaborative care,* ed 4, Philadelphia, 2002, WB Saunders, p. 692.

17. ***Answer:*** 3
Rationale: Pulmonary embolism is a life-threatening complication of deep vein thrombosis and thrombophlebitis. Chest pain is the most common symptom, which is sudden in onset, and may be aggravated by breathing. Other signs and symptoms include dyspnea, cough, diaphoresis, and apprehension.
Test-Taking Strategy: Use the process of elimination. This question tests your ability to analyze signs and symptoms of pulmonary embolism in a client at risk. Each of the incorrect options should be eliminated because myocardial infarction and pulmonary edema are cardiac-related problems and are therefore similar, and pneumonia is an infectious process. Review the complications of thrombophlebitis if you had difficulty with this question.
Level of Cognitive Ability: Analysis
Client Needs: Physiological Integrity
Integrated Concept/Process: Nursing Process/Data Collection
Content Area: Adult Health/Cardiovascular
Reference: DeWit S: *Fundamental concepts and skills for nursing,* Philadelphia, 2001, WB Saunders, p. 773.

18. ***Answer:*** 1
Rationale: Sclerotherapy is the injection of a sclerosing agent into a varicosity. The agent damages the vessel and causes aseptic thrombosis, which results in vein closure. With no blood flow through the vessel, there is no distention. The surgical procedure for varicose veins is vein ligation and stripping. This procedure involves tying off the varicose vein and large tributaries, and then removal of the vein with the use of hook and wires via multiple small incisions in the leg.
Test-Taking Strategy: If you are uncertain of the response to this question, look at the word "sclerotherapy." A vessel that is sclerosed is blocked. This may help you to select the correct option. At the very least, you should be able to eliminate options 2 and 3 readily, because neither of these makes sense using principles of blood flow and gravity. Also, they are very similar, and so are likely to be incorrect. Review this procedure if you had difficulty with this question.
Level of Cognitive Ability: Comprehension
Client Needs: Physiological Integrity
Integrated Concept/Process: Nursing Process/Implementation
Content Area: Adult Health/Cardiovascular
Reference: Ignatavicius D, Workman M: *Medical-surgical: critical thinking for collaborative care,* ed 4, Philadelphia, 2002, WB Saunders, p. 768.

19. ***Answer:*** 4
Rationale: Hypersensitivity or a sensation of "pins and needles" in the surgical limb may indicate temporary or permanent nerve injury after surgery. The saphenous vein and the saphenous nerve run close together in the distal third of the leg. Because complications from this surgery are relatively rare, this symptom should be reported. Options 1, 2, and 3 are incorrect actions.
Test-Taking Strategy: Use the process of elimination. Pins and needles sensations usually indicate nerve irritation or damage. Knowing this, options 2 and 3 can be eliminated as the least likely correct options. Reassuring the client about something being "only temporary" is not often a good choice, unless this is known to be absolutely true. By the process of elimination, then, the physician should be notified. Review the complications after vein ligation and stripping if you had difficulty with this question.
Level of Cognitive Ability: Application
Client Needs: Physiological Integrity
Integrated Concept/Process: Nursing Process/Implementation
Content Area: Adult Health/Cardiovascular
Reference: Ignatavicius D, Workman M: *Medical-surgical: critical thinking for collaborative care,* ed 4, Philadelphia, 2002, WB Saunders, p. 768.

20. ***Answer:*** 2
Rationale: The mixture of arterial and venous manifestations (claudication and phlebitis, respectively) in the young male

client suggests thromboangiitis obliterans (Buerger's disease). This is a relatively uncommon disorder, which is characterized by inflammation and thrombosis of smaller arteries and veins. This disorder is typically found in young adult males who smoke. The cause is unknown, but is suspected to have an autoimmune component.
Test-Taking Strategy: Use the process of elimination. You can first eliminate options 3 and 4 because they would most likely cause local skin reactions. The question asks which item you should check "next." It is often better to assess a modifiable factor before a nonmodifiable one. This will direct you to option 2. Review the causes of Buerger's disease if you had difficulty with this question.
Level of Cognitive Ability: Analysis
Client Needs: Health Promotion and Maintenance
Integrated Concept/Process: Nursing Process/Data Collection
Content Area: Adult Health/Cardiovascular
Reference: Ignatavicius D, Workman M: *Medical-surgical: critical thinking for collaborative care,* ed 4, Philadelphia, 2002, WB Saunders, p. 761.

21. ***Answer:*** 4
Rationale: Raynaud's disease responds favorably to the elimination of nicotine and caffeine. Medications such as calcium channel blockers may inhibit vessel spasm and prevent symptoms. Avoiding exposure to cold through a variety of means is very important, but moving to a warmer climate may not necessarily be beneficial because the symptoms could still occur with the use of air conditioning and during periods of cooler weather.
Test-Taking Strategy: Use the process of elimination. Note the key words "needs further reinforcement." All of the options seem reasonable. However, when you analyze each of them, note that relocation is the least favorable of all the options, from the viewpoints of practicality and encountering new environmental concerns. Review treatment measures for this disorder if you had difficulty with this question.
Level of Cognitive Ability: Comprehension
Client Needs: Health Promotion and Maintenance
Integrated Concept/Process: Nursing Process/Evaluation
Content Area: Adult Health/Cardiovascular
Reference: Ignatavicius D, Workman M: *Medical-surgical: critical thinking for collaborative care,* ed 4, Philadelphia, 2002, WB Saunders, p. 762.

22. ***Answer:*** 4
Rationale: The blood pressure should be taken with the client seated with the arm bared, positioned with support and at heart level. The client should sit with the legs on floor, feet uncrossed, and should not speak during the recording. The client should not have smoked tobacco or taken in caffeine in the 30 minutes preceding the measurement. The client should rest quietly for 5 minutes before the reading is taken. The cuff bladder should encircle at least 80% of the limb being measured. Gauges other than a mercury sphygmomanometer should be calibrated every 6 months to ensure accuracy. Finally, two or more readings should be averaged.
Test-Taking Strategy: Use the process of elimination and note the key word "avoiding." Because blood pressure measurement is a basic skill, this should be fairly easy to answer. However, remember in questions worded in this way, variables that interfere with accuracy (such as caffeine and nicotine in this instance) are likely to be the correct option. Review this procedure if you had difficulty with this question.
Level of Cognitive Ability: Application
Client Needs: Physiological Integrity
Integrated Concept/Process: Nursing Process/Data Collection
Content Area: Adult Health/Cardiovascular
Reference: DeWit S: *Fundamental concepts and skills for nursing,* Philadelphia, 2001, WB Saunders, p. 360.

23. ***Answer:*** 3
Rationale: The therapeutic range for PT is 1.5 to 2 times the control for clients at high risk for thrombus. Based on the client's control value, the therapeutic range for this individual would be 16.5 to 22 seconds.
Test-Taking Strategy: Use the process of elimination. A key to answering this question as stated is in the control value. Recalling that the purpose of anticoagulant therapy is to prolong clotting times, you can immediately eliminate options 1 and 2. Because the PT value in the question is not even double the control, option 3 is the best option. Review anticoagulant therapy and the PT level if you had difficulty with this question.
Level of Cognitive Ability: Analysis
Client Needs: Physiological Integrity
Integrated Concept/Process: Nursing Process/Evaluation
Content Area: Adult Health/Cardiovascular
Reference: Hodgson B, Kizior R: *Saunders nursing drug handbook 2002,* Philadelphia, 2002, WB Saunders, p. 1160.

24. ***Answer:*** 2
Rationale: Warfarin works in the liver. It inhibits the synthesis of four vitamin K-dependent clotting factors (X, IX, VII, and II), but it takes 3 to 4 days before the therapeutic effect of warfarin sodium is exhibited. Options 1, 3, and 4 are incorrect.
Test-Taking Strategy: Use the process of elimination. Heparin and warfarin sodium do not act in the same way, so eliminate option 4 first. Warfarin is an anticoagulant, not a thrombolytic, so option 3 is incorrect. Recalling that the liver synthesizes clotting factors helps you to choose option 2 over option 1. Review the action of warfarin sodium if you had difficulty with this question.
Level of Cognitive Ability: Comprehension
Client Needs: Physiological Integrity
Integrated Concept/Process: Nursing Process/Implementation
Content Area: Adult Health/Cardiovascular
Reference: Hodgson B, Kizior R: *Saunders nursing drug handbook 2002,* Philadelphia, 2002, WB Saunders, p. 1160.

25. ***Answer:*** 1
Rationale: The antidote to warfarin sodium is vitamin K and should be readily available for use if excessive bleeding or hemorrhage should occur.
Test-Taking Strategy: Knowledge regarding the antidote for warfarin sodium is required to answer this question. Review this medication if you had difficulty with this question.
Level of Cognitive Ability: Application
Client Needs: Physiological Integrity
Integrated Concept/Process: Nursing Process/Implementation

Content Area: Adult Health/Cardiovascular
Reference: Hodgson B, Kizior R: *Saunders nursing drug handbook 2002*, Philadelphia, 2002, WB Saunders, p. 1160.

26. *Answer:* 3
Rationale: Arterial leg ulcers tend to be deep and pale, with uneven edges and little granulation tissue. The client usually has rest pain, and the ulcer site is painful. Options 1, 2, and 4 are incorrect.
Test-Taking Strategy: Use the process of elimination. This question is asking you to discriminate between signs and symptoms of arterial and venous leg ulcers. Since arterial ulcers are caused by marked reduction in blood flow and tissue malnutrition, you can eliminate options 1 and 2. Brown discoloration (option 4) indicates clogging of peripheral tissue with waste products of metabolism and indicates a venous problem. The answer is option 3, which is also consistent with tissue malnutrition. Review the characteristics of an arterial ischemic ulcer if you had difficulty with this question.
Level of Cognitive Ability: Comprehension
Client Needs: Physiological Integrity
Integrated Concept/Process: Nursing Process/Data Collection
Content Area: Adult Health/Cardiovascular
Reference: DeWit S: *Fundamental concepts and skills for nursing*, Philadelphia, 2001, WB Saunders, p. 787.

27. *Answer:* 1
Rationale: An expected outcome of surgery is warmth, redness, and edema in the surgical extremity as a result of increased blood flow. Options 2, 3, and 4 are incorrect.
Test-Taking Strategy: Use the process of elimination. Option 3 can be easily eliminated because the pedal pulse is unchanged. Venous complications from immobilization during surgery would not be apparent within 4 hours, so eliminate option 4 next. To help you choose between options 1 and 2, think about the effects of sudden reperfusion in an ischemic limb. There would be redness from new blood flow and edema from the sudden change in pressure in the blood vessels. Thus option 1 is better than option 2. Review the expected findings after aortoiliac bypass graft if you had difficulty with this question.
Level of Cognitive Ability: Comprehension
Client Needs: Physiological Integrity
Integrated Concept/Process: Nursing Process/Data Collection
Content Area: Adult Health/Cardiovascular
Reference: DeWit S: *Fundamental concepts and skills for nursing*, Philadelphia, 2001, WB Saunders, p. 769.

28. *Answer:* 1
Rationale: Psychosocial care of the client with medical management of an AAA includes listening to the client's concerns, and reinforcing the rationales for ongoing medical surveillance. This includes periodic CT scans to monitor the size of the aneurysm, and careful adherence to medication and diet therapy for hypertension. The client is instructed to report any sensation of abdominal fullness, or complaints of abdominal or back pain to the physician without delay.
Test-Taking Strategy: Use the process of elimination and note the key word "unnecessary." Options 2 and 4 can be eliminated because they are obviously good actions. From the remaining options, remember that increased blood pressure (option 3) could cause strain and rupture. This will direct you to option 1. Review care to the client with an AAA if you had difficulty with this question.
Level of Cognitive Ability: Application
Client Needs: Physiological Integrity
Integrated Concept/Process: Nursing Process/Implementation
Content Area: Adult Health/Cardiovascular
Reference: Ignatavicius D, Workman M: *Medical-surgical: critical thinking for collaborative care*, ed 4, Philadelphia, 2002, WB Saunders, p. 757.

29. *Answer:* 2
Rationale: An Unna boot that is applied too tightly can cause signs of arterial occlusion. The nurse assesses the circulation to the foot and teaches the client to do the same. Options 1, 3, and 4 are incorrect interpretations.
Test-Taking Strategy: Note that the symptoms described in the question are signs of arterial compromise. Option 2 is the only option that is consistent with this circumstance. Review the signs of arterial compromise if you had difficulty with this question.
Level of Cognitive Ability: Analysis
Client Needs: Physiological Integrity
Integrated Concept/Process: Nursing Process/Data Collection
Content Area: Adult Health/Cardiovascular
Reference: Ignatavicius D, Workman M: *Medical-surgical: critical thinking for collaborative care*, ed 4, Philadelphia, 2002, WB Saunders, p. 767.

30. *Answer:* 4
Rationale: For the ambulatory client, the physician may apply a gauze dressing moistened with zinc oxide to the leg, which hardens like a cast (Unna boot). This dressing then prevents venous stasis and provides a sterile environment for the wound. The dressing is changed on a weekly basis. Betadine is not used; it is a strong agent that could cause further damage to friable tissues. Dry sterile dressings do not keep the wound moist. Damp-to-dry dressings are not as effective.
Test-Taking Strategy: Focus on the issue, a venous stasis ulcer. Recalling the treatment associated with this type of ulcer will direct you to option 4. Review this form of treatment if you had difficulty with this question.
Level of Cognitive Ability: Analysis
Client Needs: Physiological Integrity
Integrated Concept/Process: Nursing Process/Planning
Content Area: Adult Health/Cardiovascular
Reference: Ignatavicius D, Workman M: *Medical-surgical: critical thinking for collaborative care*, ed 4, Philadelphia, 2002, WB Saunders, p. 745.

31. *Answer:* 2
Rationale: The first signs and symptoms of digitalis toxicity in adults include abdominal pain, nausea, vomiting, visual disturbances (blurred, yellow or green vision, halos around lights), bradycardia, and other dysrhythmias.
Test-Taking Strategy: Medication side effects and toxicities are a difficult area to learn, simply because there are so many medications and so many side effects. Digoxin is a commonly

used medication, so review the signs of toxicity if you had difficulty with this question.
Level of Cognitive Ability: Application
Client Needs: Physiological Integrity
Integrated Concept/Process: Nursing Process/Data Collection
Content Area: Adult Health/Cardiovascular
Reference: Hodgson B, Kizior R: *Saunders nursing drug handbook 2002*, Philadelphia, 2002, WB Saunders, p. 344.

32. *Answer:* 2
Rationale: Client teaching includes taking the dose exactly as prescribed each day. If a client misses a dose and more than 12 hours go by, the client should omit that dose until the next scheduled one and should not double dose. A daily pulse check is imperative, and the client should know parameters for which the physician should be called. Clients are advised not to mix digoxin in pillboxes with other medications, because they may be similar in appearance. The physician should be consulted before changing brands, because the bioavailability of the medication may be different.
Test-Taking Strategy: Use the process of elimination and note the key words "needs reinforcement." Use general guidelines for medication administration to direct you to option 2. Review client teaching points related to this medication if you had difficulty with this question.
Level of Cognitive Ability: Comprehension
Client Needs: Health Promotion and Maintenance
Integrated Concept/Process: Nursing Process/Evaluation
Content Area: Adult Health/Cardiovascular
Reference: Hodgson B, Kizior R: *Saunders nursing drug handbook 2002*, Philadelphia, 2002, WB Saunders, p. 344.

33. *Answer:* 3
Rationale: Stable angina is induced by exercise and relieved by rest or nitroglycerin tablets. Unstable angina occurs at lower and lower levels of activity, or at rest , is less predictable, and is often a precursor of myocardial infarction. Variant angina, or Prinzmetal's angina, is prolonged and severe, and occurs at the same time each day, most often in the morning.
Test-Taking Strategy: Focus on the data in the question and use knowledge regarding the various types of angina to answer the question. Review the characteristics of the various types of angina if you had difficulty with this question.
Level of Cognitive Ability: Comprehension
Client Needs: Physiological Integrity
Integrated Concept/Process: Nursing Process/Data Collection
Content Area: Adult Health/Cardiovascular
Reference: Ignatavicius D, Workman M: *Medical-surgical: critical thinking for collaborative care*, ed 4, Philadelphia, 2002, WB Saunders, p. 794.

34. *Answer:* 1
Rationale: After pericardiocentesis, a rise in blood pressure and a fall in CVP is expected. The client usually expresses immediate relief. Heart sounds are no longer muffled or distant.
Test-Taking Strategy: Use the process of elimination. Note the key word "unsuccessful." Successful therapy is measured by the disappearance of the original signs and symptoms of cardiac tamponade. Therefore look for the option that identifies a sign consistent with continued tamponade. Review signs of cardiac tamponade and the expected effects of pericardiocentesis if you had difficulty with this question.
Level of Cognitive Ability: Analysis
Client Needs: Physiological Integrity
Integrated Concept/Process: Nursing Process/Evaluation
Content Area: Adult Health/Cardiovascular
Reference: Ignatavicius D, Workman M: *Medical-surgical: critical thinking for collaborative care*, ed 4, Philadelphia, 2002, WB Saunders, p. 722.

35. *Answer:* 2
Rationale: Not all clients with AAA exhibit symptoms. Those who do may describe a feeling of the "heart beating" in the abdomen when supine, or being able to feel the mass throbbing. A pulsatile mass may be palpated in the middle and upper abdomen. A systolic bruit may be auscultated over the mass. Hyperactive bowel sounds is not specifically related to an AAA.
Test-Taking Strategy: Use the process of elimination. Note the key word "unrelated." Note that options 1, 3, and 4 are similar in that they identify a circulatory component. Review the signs of AAA if you had difficulty with this question.
Level of Cognitive Ability: Analysis
Client Needs: Physiological Integrity
Integrated Concept/Process: Nursing Process/Data Collection
Content Area: Adult Health/Cardiovascular
Reference: Ignatavicius D, Workman M: *Medical-surgical: critical thinking for collaborative care*, ed 4, Philadelphia, 2002, WB Saunders, p. 757.

36. *Answer:* 2
Rationale: Hydrochlorothiazide is a potassium-losing diuretic, and clients are at risk for hypokalemia. Potassium is found in many foods, especially unprocessed foods, many vegetables, fruits, and fresh meats. Because potassium is very water-soluble, foods that are prepared in water are often lower in potassium than the same foods cooked another way (e.g., boiled vs. baked potato). Clients who need potassium added to the diet are encouraged to take in these foods. Many salt substitutes are also high in potassium.
Test-Taking Strategy: Use the process of elimination. Evaluating food choices in terms of their water content and according to how highly processed they are may be a helpful approach for some questions related to potassium. In this question, you will see that each of the incorrect options is processed to some degree and has a high water content. Review foods high in potassium if you had difficulty with this question.
Level of Cognitive Ability: Application
Client Needs: Physiological Integrity
Integrated Concept/Process: Nursing Process/Implementation
Content Area: Adult Health/Cardiovascular
Reference: Lehne R: *Pharmacology for nursing care*, ed 4, Philadelphia, 2001, WB Saunders, p. 418.

37. *Answer:* 4
Rationale: Beta-adrenergic blocking agents should be tapered slowly. This will avoid abrupt withdrawal syndrome, characterized by headache, malaise, palpitations, tremors, sweating,

rebound hypertension, dysrhythmias, and possibly myocardial infarction (in clients with cardiac disorders including angina pectoris).
Test-Taking Strategy: To answer this question correctly, you need to know that all beta-adrenergic blocking agents should be tapered slowly to prevent the effects noted above, as well as a return of the symptoms for which the medication was prescribed. The question guides you in the right direction by telling you the client was taking this medication for hypertension. Review this medication if you had difficulty with this question.
Level of Cognitive Ability: Comprehension
Client Needs: Physiological Integrity
Integrated Concept/Process: Nursing Process/Implementation
Content Area: Adult Health/Cardiovascular
Reference: Hodgson B, Kizior R: *Saunders nursing drug handbook 2002*, Philadelphia, 2002, WB Saunders, p. 724.

38. *Answer:* 4
Rationale: Propranolol is a noncardioselective beta-adrenergic blocking agent. It blocks stimulation of $beta_1$ (myocardial) and $beta_2$ (pulmonary, vascular and uterine) receptor sites. Albuterol is a sympathomimetic bronchodilator with relatively high $beta_2$ selectivity. The effects of the albuterol could be blocked by the action of propranolol. The nurse should verify the order with the physician.
Test-Taking Strategy: To answer this question successfully, you must know the basic actions of each of these medications, as well as that propranolol is a noncardioselective beta blocker. Because they oppose each other, albuterol and propranolol should be used cautiously together. The only option that indicates use of caution by the nurse is the option that verifies the order for the concurrent use of these two medications. Review this medication if you had difficulty with this question.
Level of Cognitive Ability: Application
Client Needs: Physiological Integrity
Integrated Concept/Process: Nursing Process/Implementation
Content Area: Adult Health/Cardiovascular
Reference: Hodgson B, Kizior R: *Saunders nursing drug handbook 2002*, Philadelphia, 2002, WB Saunders, p. 21.

39. *Answer:* 3
Rationale: Calcium channel blocking agents, such as diltiazem, are used cautiously in clients with conditions that could be worsened by the medication, such as aortic stenosis, bradycardia, heart failure, acute myocardial infarction, and hypotension. The nurse would assess for signs and symptoms that indicate worsening of these underlying disorders. In this question, the nurse assesses for signs and symptoms indicating heart failure.
Test-Taking Strategy: To answer this question, you must know that diltiazem is a calcium channel blocker, and that these medications decrease the rate and force of cardiac contraction. This helps you to eliminate options 1 and 4 because bradycardia is expected. Option 2 is eliminated next because these signs could indicate bronchoconstriction, which does not occur with calcium channel blockers, but rather with some beta-adrenergic blockers. Review this medication if you had difficulty with this question.
Level of Cognitive Ability: Application
Client Needs: Physiological Integrity
Integrated Concept/Process: Nursing Process/Data Collection
Content Area: Adult Health/Cardiovascular
Reference: Hodgson B, Kizior R: *Saunders nursing drug handbook 2002*, Philadelphia, 2002, WB Saunders, p. 348.

40. *Answer:* 2
Rationale: The client receiving a calcium channel blocking agent such as nifedipine may develop weakness and lethargy as an expected effect of the medication. Options 1, 3, and 4 are incorrect.
Test-Taking Strategy: To answer this question, you need to know that nifedipine is a calcium channel blocking agent, and that this medication decreases the rate and force of cardiac contraction, lowering the oxygen demand and also the cardiac output. By thinking through this process, you can reach the conclusion that decreased energy would then be an expected effect of the medication. Review this medication if you had difficulty with this question.
Level of Cognitive Ability: Comprehension
Client Needs: Physiological Integrity
Integrated Concept/Process: Nursing Process/Implementation
Content Area: Adult Health/Cardiovascular
Reference: Hodgson B, Kizior R: *Saunders nursing drug handbook 2002*, Philadelphia, 2002, WB Saunders, p. 795.

41. *Answer:* 3
Rationale: Tolerance to nitrates can develop over time. Some clients confuse tolerance with addiction. The nurse needs to explore the client's concerns and offer accurate information and support to help the client adapt to the illness and prescribed therapy.
Test-Taking Strategy: This question tells you that the client is hesitant about taking the medication and that the nurse has ruled out a lack of knowledge or financial barriers. Options 1 and 2 can be eliminated first because they are not reasons to stop taking the medication. Because the schedule is prn for chest pain, there can be no inconvenience (option 4). Thus, you are left with the psychosocial concerns of the client to explore. Review the effects of nitroglycerin if you had difficulty with this question.
Level of Cognitive Ability: Analysis
Client Needs: Health Promotion and Maintenance
Integrated Concept/Process: Nursing Process/Data Collection
Content Area: Adult Health/Cardiovascular
Reference: Hodgson B, Kizior R: *Saunders nursing drug handbook 2002*, Philadelphia, 2002, WB Saunders, p. 98.

42. *Answer:* 1
Rationale: Clients have developed tolerance when wearing a transdermal system or using nitropaste continuously for 24 hours. This is manifested by lack of pain relief by the medication. This can be avoided by having the client wear the nitrate for 12 hours, leaving 12 hours "nitrate free." Options 2, 3, and 4 are incorrect.
Test-Taking Strategy: Use the process of elimination. Option 4 should be eliminated first because of the absolute word "always." Hypotension (option 2) is not likely to occur at night when the client is supine. From the remaining options, note that option 1 is more plausible than option 3; the prod-

uct would not be very marketable if it were too irritating. Review this medication if you had difficulty with this question.
Level of Cognitive Ability: Application
Client Needs: Physiological Integrity
Integrated Concept/Process: Nursing Process/Implementation
Content Area: Adult Health/Cardiovascular
Reference: Hodgson B, Kizior R: *Saunders nursing drug handbook 2002*, Philadelphia, 2002, WB Saunders, p. 98.

43. *Answer:* 2
Rationale: The ointment is readily absorbed through the skin, so using the fingers will result in the nurse becoming hypotensive. Proper administration of nitroglycerin ointment involves the use of the dose-measuring applicator paper supplied by the manufacturer, applying in a thin, uniform even layer, and applying to a nonhairy area of the chest, abdomen, anterior thigh, or forearm. The previous dose is removed before applying, and sites are rotated to avoid inflammation.
Test-Taking Strategy: Use the process of elimination and note the key word "avoid." This question tests fundamental principles of medication administration for nitroglycerin ointment. Review this medication if you had difficulty with this question.
Level of Cognitive Ability: Application
Client Needs: Physiological Integrity
Integrated Concept/Process: Nursing Process/Implementation
Content Area: Adult Health/Cardiovascular
Reference: Hodgson B, Kizior R: *Saunders nursing drug handbook 2002*, Philadelphia, 2002, WB Saunders, p. 802.

44. *Answer:* 1
Rationale: Transdermal patches can be applied to a hairless site using firm pressure to ensure good contact with the skin, especially at the edges. The units are waterproof, but should not be trimmed to adjust the dose, because that will interfere with the absorption rate. Brands should not be switched back and forth because they may not be equivalent in dose. If the unit becomes loose or falls off, it should be replaced.
Test-Taking Strategy: Use the process of elimination. Note the key words "need for further instructions." Noting the words "light pressure" in option 1 will direct you to this option. Review this medication if you had difficulty with this question.
Level of Cognitive Ability: Analysis
Client Needs: Health Promotion and Maintenance
Integrated Concept/Process: Nursing Process/Evaluation
Content Area: Adult Health/Cardiovascular
Reference: Hodgson B, Kizior R: *Saunders nursing drug handbook 2002*, Philadelphia, 2002, WB Saunders, p. 98.

45. *Answer:* 2
Rationale: Minoxidil is a direct-acting peripheral vasodilator and acts on arterioles, with little effect on veins. It is used in severe hypertension with target organ damage, such as the kidneys. It causes reflex tachycardia, so a beta-adrenergic blocking agent must be prescribed for use at the same time. A diuretic is also needed to correct sodium and water retention that will occur.
Test-Taking Strategy: To answer this question, you must know that minoxidil is a vasodilator and that propranolol is a beta-adrenergic blocker. Option 1 is incorrect because minoxidil is not a first-line agent to use against hypertension. Propranolol does not exert a protective effect on the kidney, so option 3 is eliminated next. Knowing that beta blockers can cause fluid retention assists in eliminating option 4. Review these medications if you had difficulty with this question.
Level of Cognitive Ability: Analysis
Client Needs: Physiological Integrity
Integrated Concept/Process: Nursing Process/Implementation
Content Area: Adult Health/Cardiovascular
Reference: Hodgson B, Kizior R: *Saunders nursing drug handbook 2002*, Philadelphia, 2002, WB Saunders, p. 738.

46. *Answer:* 4
Rationale: Sotalol is classified an antidysrhythmic, but it has some of the same side effects experienced when taking other beta-adrenergic blocking agents. Fatigue, decreased libido, and impotence may result. For the total well-being of the client, medication instructions should address this aspect of therapy.
Test-Taking Strategy: Knowledge regarding the effects of this medication is needed to answer this question. Review this medication if you had difficulty with this question.
Level of Cognitive Ability: Comprehension
Client Needs: Psychosocial Integrity
Integrated Concept/Process: Nursing Process/Implementation
Content Area: Adult Health/Cardiovascular
Reference: Hodgson B, Kizior R: *Saunders nursing drug handbook 2002*, Philadelphia, 2002, WB Saunders, p. 147.

47. *Answer:* 3
Rationale: Disopyramide is an antidysrhythmic used in the treatment of atrial and ventricular tachydysrhythmias. It has fewer side effects than others in that group, but does exert an anticholinergic effect. For that reason, clients should be cautioned about dry mouth, and to keep sugarless hard candy or gum nearby, or do frequent oral rinses. Because of reduced perspiration, clients may develop heat intolerance, and they should avoid extremely warm weather. The possibility of dizziness and blurred vision mandates the use of caution when driving. Another possible side effect includes hypotension, and clients should change position slowly if this occurs.
Test-Taking Strategy: Note the key words "needs clarification." If you know that this medication is an antidysrhythmic, you can anticipate that this medication will have cardiovascular effects. This might help you eliminate options 1 and 2, as these options are cardiovascular in nature. You would need to know that this medication has an anticholinergic effect to discriminate between options 3 and 4. Review the side effects of this medication if you had difficulty with this question.
Level of Cognitive Ability: Analysis
Client Needs: Health Promotion and Maintenance
Integrated Concept/Process: Nursing Process/Evaluation
Content Area: Adult Health/Cardiovascular
Reference: Hodgson B, Kizior R: *Saunders nursing drug handbook 2002*, Philadelphia, 2002, WB Saunders, p. 348.

48. ***Answer:*** 2
Rationale: Quinidine is an antidysrhythmic, which decreases myocardial excitability and slows the velocity of conduction through the heart. The most common side effects relate to the gastrointestinal (GI) system and include diarrhea, cramping, nausea, and anorexia. Hypotension, tachycardia, and dysrhythmias are less frequent side effects that relate to the cardiovascular system.
Test-Taking Strategy: Use the process of elimination. Note the key words "most frequent side effects." If you know that quinidine is an antidysrhythmic, you may be able to eliminate option 3 as an unlikely combination. Options 1 and 2 seem to oppose each other, so it is likely that one of these is correct. In fact, quinidine causes the distressing side effects of diarrhea, nausea, and abdominal cramping. Review the side effects of this medication if you had difficulty with this question.
Level of Cognitive Ability: Application
Client Needs: Physiological Integrity
Integrated Concept/Process: Nursing Process/Data Collection
Content Area: Adult Health/Cardiovascular
Reference: Hodgson B, Kizior R: *Saunders nursing drug handbook 2002*, Philadelphia, 2002, WB Saunders, p. 951.

49. ***Answer:*** 3
Rationale: Gastrointestinal side effects occur in some clients taking amiodarone. The nurse can minimize these effects by providing a diet high in fiber and by increasing fluids, unless contraindicated. This will minimize the risk of constipation.
Test-Taking Strategy: Use the process of elimination. You can begin by eliminating a soft diet, because there is no data that indicate that the client has difficulty chewing or swallowing. Because gastrointestinal side effects are generally of two types, diarrhea or constipation, examine the remaining options. Antacids and antidiarrheals are similar in that they treat an irritated gastrointestinal tract. Therefore, eliminate these options. Review the gastrointestinal side effects of this medication if you had difficulty with this question.
Level of Cognitive Ability: Application
Client Needs: Physiological Integrity
Integrated Concept/Process: Nursing Process/Implementation
Content Area: Adult Health/Cardiovascular
Reference: Hodgson B, Kizior R: *Saunders nursing drug handbook 2002*, Philadelphia, 2002, WB Saunders, p. 49.

50. ***Answer:*** 3
Rationale: Colestipol hydrochloride is a bile acid sequestrant useful in lowering serum cholesterol levels. The medication causes constipation with possible fecal impaction. Because of this, clients are advised to carefully monitor their elimination patterns, increase intake of fiber and fluids, and to take stool softeners or possibly laxatives if needed.
Test-Taking Strategy: Use the process of elimination. Eliminate options 1, 2, and 4 because they are similar and represent a major type of food (carbohydrate, fat, protein). The correct option is the one that is different from the others, that is, fiber and fluids. Review this medication if you had difficulty with this question.
Level of Cognitive Ability: Application
Client Needs: Health Promotion and Maintenance
Integrated Concept/Process: Nursing Process/Implementation
Content Area: Adult Health/Cardiovascular
Reference: Hodgson B, Kizior R: *Saunders nursing drug handbook 2002*, Philadelphia, 2002, WB Saunders, p. 273.

REFERENCES

Black J, Hawks J, Keene A: *Medical-surgical nursing: clinical management for positive outcomes*, ed 6, Philadelphia, 2001, WB Saunders.

Chernecky C, Berger B: *Laboratory tests and diagnostic procedures*, ed 3, Philadelphia, 2001, WB Saunders.

Clark J, Queener S, Karb V: *Pharmacologic basis of nursing practice*, ed 6, St Louis, 2000, Mosby.

DeWit S: *Fundamental concepts and skills for nursing*, Philadelphia, 2001, WB Saunders.

Hodgson B, Kizior R: *Saunders nursing drug handbook 2002*, Philadelphia, 2002, WB Saunders.

Ignatavicius D, Workman M: *Medical-surgical: critical thinking for collaborative care*, ed 4, Philadelphia, 2002, WB Saunders.

Lehne R: *Pharmacology for nursing care*, ed 4, Philadelphia, 2001, WB Saunders.

Potter P, Perry A: *Fundamentals of nursing*, ed 5, St Louis, 2001, Mosby.

Perry A, Potter P: *Clinical nursing skills and techniques*, ed 5, St Louis, 2002, Mosby.

Cardiovascular Medications

I. ANTICOAGULANTS (Box 49-1)

A. Description
   1. Prevent the extension and formation of clots by inhibiting factors in the clotting cascade and decreasing blood coagulability
   2. Used for thrombosis, pulmonary embolism, and myocardial infarction (MI)
   3. Contraindicated with active bleeding, except for disseminated intravascular coagulation (DIC), bleeding disorders or blood dyscrasias, ulcers, liver and kidney disease, and spinal cord or brain injuries

BOX 49-1

Anticoagulants

ORAL
Anisindione (Miradon)
Warfarin sodium (Coumadin)

PARENTERAL
Ardeparin (Normiflo)
Dalteparin (Fragmin)
Danaproid (Orgaran)
Enoxaparin (Lovenox)
Heparin sodium (Liquaemin Sodium)

BOX 49-2

Substances to Avoid with Anticoagulants

Green leafy vegetables and foods high in vitamin K
Allopurinol (Zyloprim)
Cimetadine (Tagamet)
Corticosteroids
Nonsteroidal antiinflammatory drugs (NSAIDs)
Oral hypoglycemic agents
Phenytoin (Dilantin)
Salicylates
Sulfonamides

B. Side effects (Box 49-2)
   1. Hemorrhage
   2. Hematuria
   3. Epistaxis
   4. Ecchymosis
   5. Bleeding gums
   6. Thrombocytopenia
   7. Hypotension

C. Heparin sodium (Liquaemin Sodium)
   1. Description
      a. Prevents thrombin from converting fibrinogen to fibrin
      b. Prevents thromboembolism
      c. The therapeutic dose does not dissolve clots, but prevents new thrombus formation
   2. Blood levels
      a. Normal activated partial thromboplastin time (APTT) is 20 to 36 seconds
      b. Maintain APTT at 1.5 to 2.5 times normal
      c. At therapeutic levels, heparin will increase the APTT by a factor of 1.5 to 2
      d. APTT therapy should be measured every 4 to 6 hours during initial therapy, then on a daily basis
      e. If the APTT is too long—more than 80 seconds—the dosage should be lowered
      f. If APTT is too short—less than 60 seconds—the dosage should be increased
      g. Normal clotting time is 8 to 15 minutes; maintain the clotting time at 15 to 20 minutes
   3. Implementation
      a. Monitor clotting time and APTT
      b. Monitor platelet count

c. Observe for bleeding gums, bruises, nosebleeds, hematuria, hematemesis, occult blood in the stool, and petechiae
d. When administering heparin subcutaneously, inject into the abdomen using a small needle (25 to 28 gauge) at a 90-degree angle and do not aspirate or rub the injection site
e. Instruct the client regarding measures to prevent bleeding
f. Antidote: protamine sulfate

D. Warfarin sodium (Coumadin)
1. Description
a. Decreases prothrombin activity and prevents the use of vitamin K by the liver
b. Used for long-term anticoagulation
c. Prolongs clotting time and is monitored by the prothrombin time (PT)
d. Used mainly to prevent thromboembolitic conditions such as thrombophlebitis, pulmonary embolism, and embolism formation caused by atrial fibrillation, thrombosis, myocardial infarction (MI), or heart valve damage
e. Usually given for 2 to 3 months after an MI to decrease the incidence of deep vein thrombosis and thromboembolism
2. Blood levels
a. Average PT is 9.6 to 11.8 seconds
b. Warfarin sodium prolongs the PT
3. International normalized ratio (INR)
a. The normal INR is 1.3 to 2.0
b. The INR is determined by multiplying the observed PT ratio (the ratio of the client's PT to a control PT) by a correction factor specific to a particular thromboplastin preparation used in the testing
c. The treatment goal is to raise the INR to an appropriate value
d. An INR of 2 to 3 is appropriate for most clients, although for some clients, the target INR is 3.0 to 4.5
e. If the INR is below the recommended range, warfarin sodium dose should be increased
f. If the INR is above the recommended range, warfarin sodium dose should be reduced
4. Implementation
a. Monitor PT and INR
b. Observe for bleeding gums, bruises, nosebleeds, hematuria, hematemesis, occult blood in the stool, and petechiae
c. Instruct the client regarding measures to prevent bleeding
d. Antidote: vitamin K, phytonadione (AquaMEPHYTON)

II. THROMBOLYTIC MEDICATIONS (Box 49-3)

A. Description
1. Activate plasminogen; plasminogen generates plasmin (the enzyme that dissolves clots)
2. Used early in the course of myocardial infarct (within 4 to 6 hours of the onset of the infarct) to restore blood flow, limit myocardial damage, preserve left ventricular function, and prevent death

B. Contraindications
1. Active internal bleeding
2. History of cerebrovascular accident (CVA)
3. Intracranial problems
4. Intracranial surgery or trauma within the previous 2 months
5. History of thoracic, pelvic, or abdominal surgery in the previous 10 days
6. History of hepatic or renal disease
7. Uncontrolled hypertension
8. Recently required, prolonged cardiopulmonary resuscitation (CPR)

C. Side effects
1. Bleeding
2. Dysrhythmias
3. Fever
4. Allergic reactions

D. Implementation
1. Obtain APTT, PT, fibrinogen level, hematocrit, and platelet count
2. Monitor vital signs
3. Assess pulses
4. Monitor for bleeding
5. Monitor all excretions for occult blood
6. Monitor for neurological changes such as slurred speech, lethargy, confusion, and hemiparesis
7. Monitor for hypotension and tachycardia
8. Avoid injections if possible
9. Apply direct pressure over a puncture site for 20 to 30 minutes
10. Handle the client as little as possible when moving
11. Instruct the client to use an electric razor for shaving and to brush teeth gently

BOX 49-3

Thrombolytic Medications

Alteplase (Activase, tPA, tissue plasminogen activator)
Anistreplase (APSAC) (Eminase)
Reteplase (Retavase)
Streptokinase (Kabikinase, Streptase)
Urokinase (Abbokinase)

12. Discontinue the medication if bleeding develops and notify the physician
13. Antidote
    a. Aminocaproic acid (Amicar)
    b. Used only in acute, life-threatening conditions

III. ANTIPLATELET MEDICATIONS (Box 49-4)

A. Description
1. Inhibit the aggregation of platelets in the clotting process, thereby prolonging the bleeding time
2. May be used in conjunction with anticoagulants
3. Used in the prophylaxis of long-term complications after MI, coronary revascularization, and CVAs
4. Contraindicated in bleeding disorders and known sensitivity

B. Side effects
1. Gastrointestinal (GI) bleeding
2. Bruising
3. Hematuria
4. Tarry stools

C. Implementation
1. Determine sensitivity before administration
2. Monitor vital signs
3. Instruct the client to take medication with food if GI upset occurs
4. Monitor bleeding time
5. Monitor for side effects related to bleeding
6. Instruct the client in the use of the medication
7. Instruct the client to monitor for side effects related to bleeding and in the measures to prevent bleeding

IV. POSITIVE INOTROPIC/CARDIOTONIC MEDICATIONS (Box 49-5)

A. Description
1. Stimulates myocardial contractility and produces a positive inotropic effect
2. The increase in myocardial contractility increases cardiac, peripheral, and kidney function by increasing **cardiac output**, decreasing preload, improving blood flow to the periphery and kidneys, decreasing edema, and increasing fluid excretion; as a result, fluid retention in the lungs and extremities is decreased

B. Side effects
1. Dysrhythmias
2. Hypotension
3. Thrombocytopenia

C. Toxic/adverse reactions
1. Hepatotoxicity manifested by elevated liver enzyme levels
2. Hypersensitivity manifested by wheezing, shortness of breath, pruritis, urticaria, clammy skin, and flushing

D. Implementation
1. Monitor apical pulse and **blood pressure (BP)**
2. Monitor for hypersensitivity
3. Check lung sounds for wheezing and rales
4. Monitor for edema
5. Monitor for relief of congestive heart failure (CHF) as noted by reduction in edema, lessening of dyspnea, orthopnea, and fatigue
6. Monitor electrolytes, liver enzymes, platelet count, and renal function studies; may decrease potassium and increase liver enzymes

E. Milrinone (Primacor)
1. Side effects
    a. Headache
    b. Hypotension
    c. Angina
2. Toxic/adverse reactions: dysrhythmias
3. Implementation
    a. Monitor apical pulse and **BP**
    b. Check lung sounds for wheezing and rales
    c. Monitor for edema
    d. Monitor for relief of CHF as noted by reduction in edema, lessening of dyspnea, orthopnea, and fatigue

BOX 49-4

Antiplatelet Medications

Abciximab (ReoPro)
Aspirin (acetylsalicylic acid, ASA)
Clopidogrel bisulfate (Plavix)
Dipyridamole (Persantine)
Eptifibatide (Integril)
Ticlopidine hydrochloride (Ticlid)

BOX 49-5

Positive Inotropic/Cardiotonic Medications

AMRINONE (INOCOR)
Used for short-term management of congestive heart failure in those who have not responded adequately to cardiac glycosides, diuretics, and vasodilators

MILRINONE (PRIMACOR)
Used for short-term management of congestive heart failure or may be given before heart transplantation

V. CARDIAC GLYCOSIDES (Box 49-6)

A. Description
  1. Inhibit sodium potassium pump, thereby increasing intracellular calcium, which causes the heart muscle fibers to contract more efficiently
  2. Produces a positive inotropic action, which increases the force of myocardial contractions
  3. Produces a negative chronotropic action, which depresses the sinoatrial (SA) node, reduces conduction of the impulse through the atrioventricular (AV) node, and slows the heart rate
  4. Produces a negative dromotropic action that decreases the conduction of the heart cells
  5. The increase in myocardial contractility increases cardiac, peripheral, and kidney function by increasing **cardiac output,** decreasing preload, improving blood flow to the periphery and kidneys, decreasing edema, and increasing fluid excretion; as a result, fluid retention in the lungs and extremities is decreased
  6. Used for CHF, atrial tachycardia, atrial fibrillation, and atrial flutter
  7. Contraindicated in ventricular dysrhythmias and second- or third-degree heart block
  8. Used with caution in clients with renal disease, hypothyroidism, and hypokalemia

B. Side effects
  1. Anorexia, nausea, vomiting
  2. Headache
  3. Visual disturbances: diplopia, blurred vision, yellow-green halos
  4. Photophobia
  5. Drowsiness
  6. Bradycardia
  7. Fatigue, weakness

C. Implementation
  1. Monitor for toxicity as evidenced by anorexia, nausea, vomiting, visual disturbances, confusion, bradycardia, heart block, premature ventricular contractions (PVCs), and tachydysrhythmias
  2. Monitor serum digoxin level, electrolyte levels, and renal function tests
  3. Therapeutic digoxin range is 0.5 to 2.0 ng/mL and levels above 2.0 ng/mL are toxic
  4. An increased risk of toxicity exists in clients with hypercalcemia, hypokalemia, hypomagnesemia, or hypothyroidism
  5. Monitor potassium level, and if hypokalemia occurs (potassium below 3.5 mEq/L), notify the physician
  6. Instruct the client to avoid over-the-counter medications
  7. Monitor the client taking a potassium-wasting diuretic or corticosteroids closely for hypokalemia, because the hypokalemia can cause digoxin toxicity
  8. Note that elderly clients are more sensitive to toxicity
  9. Advise the client to eat foods high in potassium, such as fresh and dried fruits, fruit juices, vegetables, and potatoes
  10. Monitor the apical pulse
  11. If the apical pulse rate is below 60 beats per minute (bpm), medication should be held and the physician notified
  12. Teach the client how to measure pulse
  13. Teach the client to notify physician if the pulse rate is below 60 or above 100 bpm
  14. Teach the client the signs and symptoms of toxicity
  15. Antidote: digoxin immune FAB (Digibind) is used in extreme toxicity

BOX 49-6

Cardiac Glycosides

Digoxin (Lanoxicaps, Lanoxin)
Digitoxin (Crystodigin)

VI. ANTIHYPERTENSIVE MEDICATIONS (Box 49-7)

A. Thiazide diuretics (Box 49-8)
  1. Description
    a. Increase sodium and water excretion by inhibiting sodium reabsorption in the distal tubule of the kidney
    b. Used for hypertension and peripheral edema
    c. Used in clients with normal renal function
    d. Not effective for immediate diuresis
    e. Contraindicated in renal failure
    f. Used with caution in the client taking lithium because lithium toxicity can occur
    g. Used with caution in the client taking digoxin, corticosteroids, and hypoglycemic medications

BOX 49-7

Classifications of Diuretics

Thiazide diuretics
Loop diuretics
Osmotic diuretics
Potassium-sparing diuretics
Carbonic anhydrase inhibitors

BOX 49-8

Thiazide and Thiazide-Like Diuretics

THIAZIDE DIURETICS
Bendroflumethiazide (Naturetin)
Benzthiazide (Exna)
Chlorothiazide (Diuril)
Hydrochlorothiazide (Esidrix, Oretic, HydroDIURIL)
Hydroflumethiazide (Saluron, Diucardin)
Methyclothiazide (Aquatensen, Enduron)
Polythiazide (Renese)
Thichlormethiazide (Metahydrin, Naqua, Trichlorex)

THIAZIDE-LIKE DIURETICS
Chlorthalidone (Hygroton, Thalitone)
Indapamide (Lozol)
Metolazone (Zaroxolyn)
Quinethazone (Hydromox, Mykrox)

2. Side effects
   a. Hypercalcemia, hyperglycemia, hyperuricemia
   b. Hypokalemia, hyponatremia
   c. Hypovolemia
   d. Hypotension
   e. Headaches
   f. Nausea, vomiting
   g. Constipation
   h. Rashes
   i. Photosensitivity
   j. Blood dyscrasias
3. Implementation
   a. Monitor vital signs
   b. Monitor weight
   c. Monitor urine output
   d. Monitor electrolytes, glucose, calcium, and uric acid levels
   e. Check peripheral extremities for edema
   f. Instruct the client to take the medication in the morning to avoid nocturia and sleep interruption
   g. Instruct the client how to record the **BP**
   h. Instruct the client to eat foods rich in potassium
   i. Instruct the client how to take potassium supplements if prescribed
   j. Instruct the client to take medication with food to avoid GI upset
   k. Instruct the client to change positions slowly to prevent **orthostatic hypotension**
   l. Instruct the client to use sunscreen when in direct sunlight
   m. Instruct the client with diabetes mellitus to have the blood glucose checked periodically

B. Loop diuretics (Box 49-9)

BOX 49-9

Loop Diuretics

Furosemide (Lasix)
Bumetanide (Bumex)
Ethacrynic acid (Edecrin)
Torsemide (Demadex)

1. Description
   a. Inhibit sodium and chloride reabsorption from the loop of Henle and the distal tubule
   b. They have little effect on the blood glucose; however, they cause marked depletion of water and electrolytes, increased uric acid levels, and cause the excretion of calcium
   c. Are more potent than the thiazide diuretics, causing rapid diuresis, thus decreasing vascular fluid volume, decreasing **cardiac output,** and **blood pressure**
   d. Used for hypertension, edema associated with CHF, hypercalcemia, and renal disease
   e. Used with caution in the client taking digoxin or lithium
   f. Used with caution in the client on aminoglycosides, anticoagulants, corticosteroids, and amphotericin B
2. Side effects
   a. Hypokalemia, hyponatremia, hypocalcemia, hypomagnesemia
   b. Hypochloremia
   c. Thrombocytopenia
   d. Hyperuricemia
   e. **Orthostatic hypotension**
   f. Skin disturbances
   g. Ototoxicity and deafness
   h. Thiamine deficiency
   i. Dehydration
3. Implementation
   a. Monitor vital signs
   b. Monitor weight
   c. Monitor urine output
   d. Monitor electrolytes, calcium, magnesium, and uric acid levels
   e. Check the peripheral extremities for edema
   f. Monitor for signs of digoxin or lithium toxicity if the client is on these medications
   g. Instruct the client to take the medication in the morning to avoid nocturia and sleep interruption
   h. Instruct the client how to record the **BP**
   i. Instruct the client to eat foods rich in potassium
   j. Instruct the client how to take potassium supplements if prescribed

k. Instruct the client to take medication with food to avoid GI upset
l. Instruct the client to change positions slowly to prevent **orthostatic hypotension**

C. Osmotic diuretics
1. Refer to Chapter 55 for information regarding osmotic diuretics
2. Refer to Box 49-10 for a list of these medications

D. Carbonic anhydrase inhibitors (Box 49-11)
1. Description
a. Block the action of the enzyme carbonic anhydrase needed to maintain acid-base balance
b. Inhibition of this enzyme, carbonic anhydrase, causes increased sodium, potassium, and bicarbonate excretion
c. Metabolic acidosis can occur with prolonged use
d. Used to decrease intraocular pressure in open-angle (chronic) glaucoma, to produce diuresis, manage epilepsy, treat high-altitude sickness
e. Used to treat metabolic alkalosis
f. Contraindicated in narrow-angle or acute glaucoma
2. Side effects
a. Hyperglycemia, hyperuricemia, hypercalcemia
b. Hypokalemia
c. Anorexia, nausea, vomiting
d. **Orthostatic hypotension**
e. Renal calculi
f. Hemolytic anemia
3. Implementation
a. Monitor vital signs
b. Monitor weight
c. Monitor urine output
d. Monitor electrolytes, glucose, calcium, and uric acid levels
e. Monitor mental status
f. Instruct the client to monitor for signs of renal calculi

E. Potassium-sparing diuretics (Box 49-12)
1. Description
a. Act on the distal tubule to promote sodium and water excretion and potassium retention
b. Used for edema and hypertension; to increase urine output; to treat fluid retention and overload associated with CHF, hepatic cirrhosis, or nephrotic syndrome; and for diuretic-induced hypokalemia
c. Contraindicated in severe kidney or hepatic disease or in severe hyperkalemia
d. Used with caution in the client with diabetes mellitus
e. Used with caution in the client taking antihypertensives and lithium
f. Used with caution in the client taking angiotensin-converting enzyme (ACE) inhibitors, because hyperkalemia can result
g. Used with caution in the client taking potassium supplements
2. Side effects
a. Hyperkalemia
b. Nausea, vomiting, diarrhea
c. Rash
d. Dizziness, weakness
e. Headache
f. Dry mouth
g. Photosensitivity
h. Anemia
i. Thrombocytopenia
3. Implementation
a. Monitor vital signs
b. Monitor urine output
c. Monitor for signs and symptoms of hyperkalemia such as nausea, diarrhea, abdominal cramps, tachycardia followed by bradycardia, peaked narrow T wave on the electrocardiogram (ECG), or oliguria
d. Monitor for a potassium level greater than 5.1 mEq/L, which indicates hyperkalemia
e. Instruct the client to avoid foods high in potassium

BOX 49-10

Osmotic Diuretics

Mannitol (Osmitrol)
Urea (Ureaphil)

BOX 49-11

Carbonic Anhydrase Inhibitors

Acetazolamide (Diamox)
Dichlorphenamide (Daranide)
Methazolamide (Neptazane)

BOX 49-12

Potassium-Sparing Diuretics

Spironolactone (Aldactone)
Amiloride (Midamor)
Triamterene (Dyrenium)
Amiloride hydrochloride and hydrochlorothiazide (Moduretic)
Spironolactone and Hydrochlorothiazide (Aldactazide)

f. Instruct the client to avoid exposure to direct sunlight
g. Instruct the client to monitor for signs of hyperkalemia
h. Instruct the client to avoid salt substitutes because they contain potassium
i. Instruct the client to take with or after meals to decrease GI irritation

VII. PERIPHERALLY ACTING ALPHA-ADRENERGIC BLOCKERS (Box 49-13)

A. Description
   1. Decrease sympathetic vasoconstriction by reducing the effects of norepinephrine at peripheral nerve endings, resulting in vasodilation and decreased **BP**
   2. Used to maintain renal blood flow
   3. Used to treat hypertension

B. Side effects
   1. **Orthostatic hypotension**
   2. Reflex tachycardia
   3. Sodium and water retention
   4. GI disturbances
   5. Nausea
   6. Drowsiness
   7. Nasal congestion
   8. Edema
   9. Weight gain
   10. Reserpine (Serpasil) can cause depression, GI irritation, and impotence

C. Implementation
   1. Monitor vital signs
   2. Monitor for fluid retention and edema
   3. Instruct the client to change positions slowly to prevent **orthostatic hypotension**
   4. Instruct the client how to monitor the **BP**
   5. Instruct the client to monitor for edema
   6. Instruct the client to decrease salt intake
   7. Instruct the client to avoid over-the-counter medications

VIII. CENTRALLY ACTING SYMPATHOLYTICS (ADRENERGIC BLOCKERS) (Box 49-14)

A. Description
   1. Stimulate alpha receptors in the central nervous system (CNS) to inhibit vasoconstriction, thus reducing peripheral resistance
   2. Used to treat hypertension
   3. Contraindicated in impaired liver function

B. Side effects
   1. Sodium and water retention
   2. Drowsiness, dizziness
   3. Dry mouth
   4. Bradycardia
   5. Edema
   6. Impotence
   7. Hypotension
   8. Depression

C. Implementation
   1. Monitor vital signs
   2. Instruct the client not to discontinue medication, because abrupt withdrawal can cause severe rebound hypertension
   3. Monitor liver function tests

IX. ANGIOTENSIN-CONVERTING ENZYMES (ACE INHIBITORS) (Box 49-15)

A. Description
   1. Prevent peripheral vasoconstriction by blocking conversion of angiotensin I to angiotensin II
   2. Used to treat hypertension
   3. Avoid use with potassium supplements and potassium-sparing diuretics

BOX 49-13

Peripherally Acting Alpha-Adrenergic Blockers

Doxazosin mesylate (Cardura)
Prazosin (Minipress)
Terazosin (Hytrin)
Guanadrel (Hylorel)
Guanethidine (Ismelin)
Reserpine (Serpasil)
Phenoxybenzamine (Dibenzyline)
Phentolamine mesylate (Regitine)
Tolazoline (Priscoline)

BOX 49-14

Centrally Acting Sympatholytics

Clonidine (Catapres)
Methyldopa (Aldomet)
Guanabenz (Wytensin)

BOX 49-15

ACE Inhibitors

Benazepril (Lotensin)
Captopril (Capoten)
Enalapril (Vasotec)
Fosinopril (Monopril)
Lisinopril (Prinivil, Zestril)
Moexipril (Univasc)
Quinapril (Accupril)
Ramipril (Altrace)
Trandolapril (Mavik)

B. Side effects
1. Nausea, vomiting, diarrhea
2. Persistent cough
3. Hypotension
4. Hyperkalemia
5. Tachycardia
6. Headache
7. Dizziness, fatigue
8. Insomnia
9. Hypoglycemic reaction in the client with diabetes mellitus
10. Bruising, petechiae, bleeding
11. Diminished taste

C. Implementation
1. Monitor vital signs
2. Monitor protein, albumin, blood urea nitrogen (BUN), creatinine, white blood cells (WBC), potassium levels
3. Monitor for hypoglycemic reactions in the client with diabetes mellitus
4. Instruct the client to take captopril (Capoten) 20 minutes to 1 hour before a meal
5. Monitor for bruising, petechiae, or bleeding with captopril
6. Instruct the client not to discontinue medications because rebound hypertension can occur
7. Instruct the client not to take over-the-counter medications
8. Instruct the client how to take the BP
9. Instruct the client that if dizziness occurs and persists, to notify the physician
10. Inform the client that the taste of food may be diminished during the first month of therapy

X. ANTIANGINAL MEDICATIONS (Box 49-16)

A. Nitrates
1. Description
a. Produce vasodilation
b. Decrease preload and afterload and reduce myocardial oxygen consumption
c. Contraindicated in the client with marked hypotension, increased intracranial pressure (ICP), or severe anemia
d. Used with caution with severe renal or hepatic disease
e. Avoid abrupt withdrawal of long-acting preparations to prevent the rebound effect of severe pain from myocardial ischemia
2. Side effects
a. Headache
b. **Orthostatic hypotension**
c. Dizziness, weakness
d. Faintness
e. Nausea, vomiting
f. Flushing or pallor
g. Confusion
h. Rash
i. Dry mouth
j. Reflex tachycardia
k. Paradoxical bradycardia
3. Sublingual medications
a. Monitor vital signs
b. Offer sips of water before giving, because dryness may inhibit medication absorption
c. Instruct the client to place under the tongue and leave until fully dissolved
d. Instruct the client not to swallow the medication
e. Instruct the client to take 1 tablet for pain, and repeat every 5 minutes for a total of three doses
f. Instruct the client to seek medical help immediately if pain is not relieved in 15 minutes, after the three doses
g. Inform the client that a stinging or biting sensation may indicate that the tablet is fresh
h. Instruct the client to store medication in a dark, tightly closed bottle
i. Instruct the client to check the expiration date on the medication bottle, because expiration may occur within 6 months of obtaining the medication
j. Instruct the client to take acetaminophen (Tylenol) for a headache
4. Translingual medications
a. Instruct the client to direct spray against the oral mucosa
b. Instruct the client to avoid inhaling the spray
5. Sustained-released medications: instruct the client to swallow and not to chew or crush the medication
6. Transmucosal-buccal medications
a. Instruct the client to place between the upper lip and gum or in the buccal area between the cheek and gum

BOX 49-16

Antianginal Medications

Isosorbide mononitrate (Imdur, Monoket)
Isosorbide dinitrate (Iso-Bid, Isordil, Isotrate, Sorbitrate)
Nitroglycerin (Nitrostat, Nitrolingual Spray, Nitrogard, Nitrong)
Nitroglycerin ointment 2% (Nitro-Bid, Nitrol, Nitrong, Nitrodisc, Nitro-Dur, Transderm-Nitro)
Pentaerythritol tetranitrate (Pentylan Duotrate, Peritrate)

b. Inform the client that the medication will adhere to the oral mucosa and slowly dissolve
7. Transdermal patch
a. Instruct the client to apply the patch to a hairless area, using a new patch and a different site each day
b. As prescribed, instruct the client to remove the patch after 12 to 14 hours, allowing 10 to 12 "patch-free" hours each day to prevent tolerance
c. Do not apply the patch on the chest in the area of defibrillator-cardioverter paddle placement, because skin burns can result
8. Topical ointments
a. Instruct the client to remove the ointment on the skin from the previous dose
b. Instruct the client to squeeze a ribbon of ointment of the prescribed length onto the applicator paper
c. Instruct the client to spread the ointment over a 6 × 6 inch area, using the chest, back, abdomen, upper arm, or anterior thigh (avoiding hairy areas), and cover with a plastic wrap
d. Instruct the client to rotate sites and to avoid touching the ointment when applying
e. Do not apply the ointment on the chest in the area of defibrillator-cardioverter paddle placement, because skin burns can result

XI. BETA-ADRENERGIC BLOCKERS (Box 49-17)

BOX 49-17

Beta-Adrenergic Blockers

Acebutolol (Sectral)
Atenolol (Tenormin)
Betaxolol (Betoptic)
Bisoprolol fumarate (Zebeta)
Carteolol (Cartrol)
Carvedilol (Coreg)
Esmolol (Brevibloc)
Labetalol (Normodyne, Trandate, Vescal)
Levobunolol (Betagan)
Metipranolol (OptiPranolol)
Metoprolol (Lopressor, Toprol XL)
Nadolol (Corgard)
Penbutolol (Levotol)
Pindolol (Visken)
Propranolol (Inderal)
Sotalol (Betapace)
Timolol (Blocadren, Timoptic)

A. Description
1. Inhibit response to beta-adrenergic stimulation, thus decreasing **cardiac output**
2. Block the release of the catecholamines, epinephrine, and norepinephrine, thus decreasing the heart rate and **blood pressure**
3. Decrease the workload of the heart and decrease oxygen demands
4. Used for angina, dysrhythmias, hypertension, migraine headaches, prevention of MI, and glaucoma
5. Contraindicated in the client with asthma, bradycardia, CHF, severe renal or hepatic disease, hyperthyroidism, and CVA
6. Used with caution in the client with diabetes mellitus, because it may mask symptoms of hypoglycemia
7. Used with caution in the client on antihypertensives

B. Side effects
1. Bradycardia
2. Bronchospasm
3. Hypotension
4. Weakness, fatigue
5. Nausea, vomiting
6. Dizziness
7. Hyperglycemia
8. Agranulocytosis
9. Behavioral or psychotic response
10. Depression
11. Nightmares

C. Implementation
1. Monitor vital signs
2. Hold the medication if the pulse or **BP** is not within the prescribed parameters
3. Monitor for signs of CHF
4. Assess for respiratory distress and for signs of wheezing and dyspnea
5. Instruct the client to report dizziness, lightheadedness, or nasal congestion
6. Instruct the client not to stop the medication because rebound hypertension, rebound tachycardia, or an anginal attack can occur
7. Advise the client on insulin that early signs of hypoglycemia, such as tachycardia and nervousness, can be masked by the beta blocker
8. Instruct the client on insulin to monitor the blood glucose level
9. Instruct the client how to take a pulse and **BP**
10. Instruct the client to change positions slowly to prevent **orthostatic hypotension**
11. Instruct the client to avoid over-the-counter cold medications and nasal decongestants

XII. CALCIUM CHANNEL BLOCKERS (Box 49-18)

A. Description
1. Decrease cardiac contractility (negative inotropic effect by relaxing smooth muscle) and the workload of the heart, thus decreasing the need for oxygen
2. Promote vasodilation of the coronary and peripheral vessels
3. Used for angina, dysrhythmias, or hypertension
4. Used with caution in the client with CHF, bradycardia, or AV block

B. Side effects
1. Bradycardia
2. Hypotension
3. Reflex tachycardia as a result of hypotension
4. Headache
5. Dizziness, light-headedness
6. Fatigue
7. Peripheral edema
8. Constipation
9. Flushing of the skin
10. Changes in liver and kidney function

C. Implementation
1. Monitor vital signs
2. Monitor for signs of CHF
3. Monitor liver enzyme levels
4. Monitor kidney function tests
5. Instruct the client not to discontinue the medication
6. Instruct the client how to take a pulse
7. Instruct the client to notify the physician if dizziness or fainting occurs
8. Instruct the client not to crush or chew sustained-released tablets

XIII. PERIPHERAL VASODILATORS (Box 49-19)

A. Description
1. Decrease peripheral resistance by exerting a direct action on the arteries or on both the arteries and veins

BOX 49-18

Calcium Channel Blockers

Amlodipine (Norvasc)
Bepridil (Bepadin, Vascor)
Diltiazem (Cardizem, Cardizem SR)
Felodipine (Plendil)
Isradipine (DynaCirc)
Nicardipine (Cardene)
Nifedipine (Procardia, Procardia XL, Adalat CC)
Nisoldipine (Sular)
Verapamil (Calan, Isoptin)

BOX 49-19

Peripheral Vasodilators

ALPHA-ADRENERGIC BLOCKER
Tolazoline (Priscoline)

BETA-ADRENERGIC AGONIST
Isoxsuprine (Vasodilan)

DIRECT-ACTING PERIPHERAL VASODILATOR
Ergoloid mesylates (Hydergine)

ALPHA BLOCKER
Doxazosin mesylate (Cardura)
Prazosin hydrochloride (Minipress)
Terazosin hydrochloride (Hytrin)

CALCIUM CHANNEL BLOCKER
Nifedipine (Procardia)
Nimodipine (Nimotop)

HEMORRHEOLOGIC
Pentoxifylline (Trental)
Increases microcirculation and tissue perfusion

2. Increase blood flow to the extremities
3. Used in peripheral vascular disorders of venous and arterial vessels
4. Most effective for disorders resulting from vasospasm (Raynaud's disease)
5. These medications may decrease some of the symptoms of cerebral vascular insufficiency

B. Side effects
1. Light-headedness, dizziness
2. **Postural hypotension**
3. Tachycardia
4. Palpitations
5. Flushing
6. GI distress

C. Implementation
1. Monitor vital signs, especially the **BP** and heart rate
2. Monitor for **orthostatic hypotension** and tachycardia
3. Monitor for signs of inadequate blood flow to the extremities such as pallor, coldness of the extremities, and pain
4. Instruct the client that it may take up to 3 months for a desired therapeutic response
5. Advise the client not to smoke because smoking increases vasospasm
6. Instruct the client to avoid aspirin or aspirin-like compounds unless approved by the physician
7. Instruct the client to take the medication with meals if GI disturbances occur

8. Instruct the client to avoid alcohol because it may cause a hypotensive reaction
9. Encourage the client to change positions slowly to avoid **orthostatic hypotension**

XIV. ANTILIPEMIC MEDICATIONS

A. Description
1. Reduce serum levels of cholesterol, triglycerides, or low-density lipoprotein (LDL)
2. When cholesterol, triglycerides, and LDL are elevated, the client is at increased risk for coronary artery disease
3. In many cases diet alone will not lower blood lipid levels; therefore antilipemic medications will be prescribed

B. Bile sequestrants (Box 49-20)
1. Description
   a. Binds with acids in the intestines
   b. Bile acid sequestrants should not be used as the only therapy in clients with elevated triglycerides, because they typically raise triglyceride levels
2. Side effects
   a. Constipation
   b. Peptic ulcer
3. Implementation
   a. Cholestyramine (Questran) comes in a gritty powder that must be mixed thoroughly in juice or water before administration
   b. Monitor the client for early signs of peptic ulcer such as nausea and abdominal discomfort followed by abdominal pain and distention
   c. Instruct the client that the medication must be taken with and followed by sufficient fluids

C. HMG-CoA reductase inhibitors (Box 49-21)
1. Description
   a. Lovastatin (Mevacor) is highly protein bound and should not be administered with anticoagulants
   b. Lovastatin should not be administered with gemfibrozil (Lopid)
   c. Administer lovastatin with caution to the client on immunosuppressive medications
2. Side effects
   a. Nausea
   b. Diarrhea or constipation
   c. Abdominal pain or cramps
   d. Flatulence
   e. Dizziness
   f. Headache
   g. Blurred vision
   h. Rash
   i. Pruritis
   j. Elevated liver enzymes
   k. Causes GI disturbances, headaches, muscle cramps, and fatigue
3. Implementation
   a. Monitor serum liver enzymes
   b. Instruct the client to receive an annual eye examination because the medication causes cataract formation
   c. If lovastatin is not effective in lowering the lipid level after 3 months, it should be discontinued

D. Other antilipemic medications (Box 49-22)
1. Description
   a. Gemfibrozil should not be taken with anticoagulants because they compete for protein sites, and if the client is on an anticoagulant, the anticoagulant dose should be reduced during antilipemic therapy and the INR monitored closely
   b. Do not administer gemfibrozil with lovastatin
   c. Clofibrate (Atromid-S) should not be used long term because of its side effects such as dysrhythmias, angina, thromboembolism, and gallbladder stones
2. Implementation
   a. Monitor vital signs
   b. Monitor liver enzyme levels

BOX 49-20

Bile Acid Sequestrants

Cholestyramine (Questran)
Colestipol (Colestid)

BOX 49-21

HMG-CoA Reductase Inhibitors

Atorvastatin (Lipitor)
Cerivastatin (Baycol)
Fluvastatin (Lescol)
Lovastatin (Mevacor)
Pravastatin (Pravachol)
Simvastatin (Zocor)

BOX 49-22

Other Antilipemic Medications

Clofibrate (Atromid-S)
Fenofibrate (Tricor)
Gemfibrozil (Lopid)
Nicotinic acid (Niacor, Niacin)

c. Monitor serum cholesterol and triglyceride levels
d. Instruct the client to restrict intake of fats, cholesterol, carbohydrates, and alcohol
e. Instruct the client to follow an exercise program
f. Instruct the client that it will take several weeks before the lipid level declines
g. Instruct the client to have an annual eye examination and to report any changes in vision
h. Instruct the client with diabetes mellitus taking gemfibrozil to monitor blood glucose levels regularly
i. Instruct the client to increase fluid intake
j. Note that nicotinic acid has numerous side effects that include GI disturbances, flushing of the skin, elevated liver enzymes, hyperglycemia, and hyperuricemia
k. Instruct the client that aspirin may assist in reducing the side effects of nicotinic acid
l. Instruct the client to take nicotinic acid with meals to reduce GI discomfort

PRACTICE QUESTIONS

1. A nurse reinforces discharge instructions to a postoperative client taking warfarin sodium (Coumadin). Which statement, if made by the client, indicates the need for further teaching?
   1. "I will take Ecotrin for my headaches because it is coated."
   2. "I will be certain to limit my alcohol consumption."
   3. "I will take my pills every day at the same time."
   4. "I have already called my family to pick up a Medic-Alert bracelet."
2. A client taking digoxin (Lanoxin) has a serum potassium level of 3.0 mEq/L and is complaining of anorexia. The physician orders a digoxin level to rule out digoxin toxicity. The nurse checks the results of the test knowing that the therapeutic serum level for digoxin is which of the following?
   1. 0.1 to 0.5 ng/mL
   2. 0.3 to 0.8 ng/mL
   3. 0.5 to 2.0 ng/mL
   4. 1.0 to 3.0 ng/mL
3. Heparin sodium (Liquaemin) by subcutaneous (SC) injection is prescribed for a client. When administering the medication, the nurse would:
   1. Use a 23- to 25-gauge, 1-inch needle
   2. Aspirate before injection
   3. Apply heat after the injection
   4. Administer with a 25- to 27-gauge, $\frac{5}{8}$-inch needle
4. A client with a cardiac irregularity is being treated with procainamide (Pronestyl). The client complains of dizziness and tells the nurse that this has been occurring for the past few days. The initial nursing action is to:
   1. Administer a PRN nitroglycerin tablet
   2. Check the client's apical pulse and obtain a blood pressure
   3. Contact the physician
   4. Tell the client that this is an expected side effect
5. A 51-year-old client is admitted with a diagnosis of myocardial infarction. The client is started on streptokinase (Streptase) therapy. The nurse knows that teaching has been effective when the client's wife states that the purpose of the medication is to:
   1. Thin the blood
   2. Slow the clotting of the blood
   3. Dissolve any clots in the coronary arteries
   4. Prevent further clots from forming in the coronary arteries
6. A client is being treated for moderate hypertension and has been taking diltiazem (Cardizem) for several months. The client is seen by the physician and Prinzmetal's angina is diagnosed. The nurse planning care for the client understands that which action of the medication will provide a therapeutic effect for this new diagnosis?
   1. Increases oxygen demands within the myocardium
   2. Prevents influx of calcium ions in vascular smooth muscle
   3. Leads to an increase in calcium absorption in the vascular smooth muscle
   4. Increases the force of contraction of ventricular tissues
7. A nurse is caring for a client who is taking propranolol (Inderal). Which of the following data would indicate an adverse reaction associated with this medication?
   1. A baseline blood pressure of 150/80 mm Hg followed by a blood pressure of 138/72 mm Hg after two doses of the medication
   2. A baseline resting heart rate of 88 beats per minute followed by a resting heart rate of 72 beats per minute after two doses of the medication
   3. The development of audible expiratory wheezes
   4. The development of complaints of insomnia
8. A client is admitted to the emergency department with an acute anterior wall myocardial infarction. Streptokinase (Streptase) therapy is prescribed for the client. The spouse is concerned about the dangers of this treatment. Which of the following statements by the nurse is most appropriate?
   1. "Your loved one is very ill. The physician has made the best decision for you."
   2. "There is no reason to worry. We use this medication all of the time."

3. "I'm certain you made the correct decision to use this medication."
4. "You have concerns about whether this treatment is the best option."

9. A physician prescribed digoxin (Lanoxin) 0.25 mg for a client with atrial fibrillation. The medication is available as 0.125 mg tablets. The nurse calculates that the client will receive two tablets of digoxin. When the nurse administers the medication, the client looks at the medication and states, "Every time I get chest pain, I will take one of these heart pills." After double-checking the dosage calculation the nurse decides to:
   1. Not administer the medication as prescribed and calculated
   2. Administer one-half tablet of the medication instead of the dosage calculated
   3. Administer the medication as prescribed and calculated, and monitor for untoward effects such as seizures
   4. Administer the medication as prescribed and calculated and proceed with further client teaching

10. A nurse is caring for an elderly client who will be discharged home. Furosemide (Lasix) is prescribed for the client. The nurse reinforces instructions to the client about the medication. Which of the following statements, if made by the client, indicates the need for further instructions?
    1. "I will take my medication every morning with breakfast."
    2. "I will call my doctor if my ankles swell or my rings get tight."
    3. "I need to drink lots of coffee and tea to keep myself healthy."
    4. "I will sit up slowly before standing each morning."

11. Isosorbide mononitrate (Imdur) is prescribed for a client with angina pectoris. The client tells the nurse that the medication is causing a chronic headache. The nurse most appropriately suggests that the client:
    1. Contact the physician
    2. Discontinue the medication
    3. Cut the dose in half
    4. Take the medication with food

12. A client is being discharged with a prescription for propanolol (Inderal).When reinforcing instructions to the client about the medication, the nurse would include which of the following?
    1. Gentle exercising will prevent orthostatic hypotension
    2. Hot baths and showers are advised to increase vasodilation
    3. Medication should be taken on an empty stomach to enhance absorption
    4. Medication should be withheld if the pulse rate drops below 60 beats per minute

13. Heparin sodium (Liquaemin) is prescribed for the client. The nurse expects that the physician will order which of the following to monitor for a therapeutic effect of the medication?
    1. Prothrombin time (PT)
    2. Activated partial thromboplastin time (APTT)
    3. Hematocrit
    4. Hemoglobin

14. A client has suffered an acute myocardial infarction and is receiving tissue plasminogen activator (TPA). Which of the following is a priority nursing intervention while caring for the client?
    1. Have heparin sodium (Liquaemin) available
    2. Monitor for renal failure
    3. Monitor for signs of bleeding
    4. Monitor psychosocial status

15. A nurse is reinforcing instructions to the client about the use of a nitrate patch for the treatment of angina pectoris. Which of the following will the nurse include in the instructions to prevent client tolerance to nitrates?
    1. Do not remove the patches
    2. Have a 12-hour "no nitrate" time
    3. Have a 24-hour "no nitrate" time
    4. Keep nitrates on 24 hours, then off 24 hours

16. A client was admitted to the medical unit with nausea and bradycardia. The family handed the nurse a small white envelope labeled "heart pill." The envelope is sent to pharmacy and reveals digoxin (Lanoxin). The family stated, "That doctor doesn't know how to take care of my family." The most therapeutic response by the nurse would be:
    1. "You are concerned that your loved one receives the best care."
    2. "You're right! I've never seen a doctor put pills in an envelope."
    3. "I think you're wrong. That physician has been in practice over 30 years."
    4. "Don't worry about this. I'll take care of everything."

17. A client with a diagnosis of congestive heart failure is seen in the clinic. The client is being treated with a variety of medications including digoxin (Lanoxin) and furosemide (Lasix). Which of the following findings on data collection would lead the nurse to suspect that the client is hypokalemic?
    1. Diarrhea
    2. Intermittent intestinal colic
    3. Muscle weakness and leg cramps
    4. Tingling of fingers and toes

18. A nurse is reinforcing dietary instructions to a client who is taking triamterene (Dyrenium). The nurse instructs the client that it is appropriate to consume which of the following food items daily?
    1. Avocado
    2. Banana

3. Baked potato
4. Apple

19. Hydrochlorothiazide (HydroDIURIL) is prescribed for the client. The nurse checks the client's record for documentation of which of the following before administering the medication?
    1. Penicillin allergy
    2. Hyperkalemia
    3. Sulfa allergy
    4. History of osteoporosis
20. Cholestyramine resin (Questran) is prescribed for a client with an elevated triglycerides and a serum cholesterol of 398 mg/dL. The nurse reinforces instructions to the client about the medication. Which of the following statements, if made by the client, indicates the need for further instructions?
    1. "Constipation and bloating might be a problem."
    2. "I'll continue to watch my diet and reduce my fats."
    3. "I'll continue my nicotinic acid from the health food store."
    4. "Walking a mile each day will help the whole process."
21. A client is experiencing impotence after taking guanfacine (Tenex). The client states, "I would sooner have a stroke than keep living with the side effects of this medication." The most appropriate response by the nurse is:
    1. "I can understand completely."
    2. "That doctor should change your prescription."
    3. "You wouldn't really want to have a stroke."
    4. "You are concerned about the side effects of your medication."
22. A physician tells the nurse that a potassium-sparing diuretic is being prescribed for the client with congestive heart failure. The nurse reviews the physician's orders expecting that which of the following medications will be prescribed?
    1. Spironolactone (Aldactone)
    2. Furosemide (Lasix)
    3. Ethacrynic acid (Edecrin)
    4. Hydrochlorothiazide (HydroDIURIL)
23. A client with coronary artery disease complains of substernal chest pain. After checking the client's heart rate and blood pressure, the nurse administers nitroglycerin 0.4 mg sublingually. After 5 minutes, the client states, "My chest still hurts." If the vital signs have remained stable, the nurse should:
    1. Wait another 10 minutes and then administer a second nitroglycerin tablet
    2. Apply 10 liters of oxygen via nasal cannula
    3. Administer another nitroglycerin tablet
    4. Call the resuscitation team immediately
24. A client is admitted to the hospital with a diagnosis of paroxysmal nocturnal dyspnea (PND). The nurse reviews the physician's orders expecting that which of the following medications will be prescribed for this condition?
    1. Lidocaine (Xylocaine)
    2. Propranolol (Inderal)
    3. Bumetanide (Bumex)
    4. Urokinase (Abbokinase)
25. A client arrives in the emergency department after complaining of unrelieved chest pain for 2 days. The pain has subsided slightly but never disappeared. When the nurse approaches the client with a nitroglycerin sublingual tablet, the client states, "I don't need that. My dad takes that for his heart. There's nothing wrong with my heart." Which of the following best describes the client's response?
    1. Obsessive-compulsive
    2. Denial
    3. Phobic
    4. Angry
26. A nurse is collecting data from a client being admitted to the nursing unit with a diagnosis of syncope. The client tells the nurse that he/she has been taking enalapril (Vasotec), atenolol (Tenormin), and aspirin (ASA) daily. The client admits that the medications were prescribed by different physicians. The admitting physician wrote in the client's order sheet "administer medications as taken at home." Which of the following is the most appropriate action for the nurse to take?
    1. Give the medications as ordered by the physician
    2. Send the client's medication bottles to the pharmacy for identification and then administer the medications as ordered
    3. Contact the physician, describe the medications, and request order clarification
    4. Refuse to give any medications and wait until the physician makes rounds to clarify the orders
27. A 66-year-old client is seen in the clinic complaining of not feeling well. The client is taking several medications for the control of heart disease and hypertension. These medications include atenolol (Tenormin), digoxin (Lanoxin), and chlorothiazide (Diuril). A tentative diagnosis of digoxin toxicity is made. The nurse collects data from the client knowing that which of the following would support this diagnosis?
    1. Chest pain, hypotension, and paresthesia
    2. Constipation, dry mouth, and sleep disorder
    3. Double vision, loss of appetite, and nausea
    4. Dyspnea, edema, and palpitations
28. A 79-year-old client is being treated with bumetanide (Bumex) for congestive heart failure. The vital signs are blood pressure 100/60 mm Hg, pulse 96 beats per minute, and respirations 24 breaths per minute. The nurse checks which of the following priority items before administering the medication?

1. Blood pressure
2. Weight
3. Urine output
4. Temperature

29. Atorvastatin (Lipitor) has been prescribed for a client with an elevated cholesterol level. The nurse collects a health history from the client knowing that the medication is contraindicated in which of the following conditions?
1. Cirrhosis
2. Coronary artery disease
3. Diabetes mellitus
4. Hypothyroidism

30. Warfarin sodium (Coumadin) is prescribed for the client. The nurse expects that the physician will order which of the following to monitor for a therapeutic effect of the medication?
1. Prothrombin time (PT)
2. Activated partial thromboplastin time (APTT)
3. Red blood cell (RBC) count
4. Platelet count

ANSWERS

1. *Answer:* 1
Rationale: Ecotrin is an aspirin-containing product and should be avoided. Excessive alcohol consumption should be avoided when taking warfarin sodium. Taking prescribed medication at the same time increases client compliance. The Medic-Alert bracelet provides health care personnel with emergency information.
Test-Taking Strategy: Use the process of elimination. Note the key words "need for further teaching." Recalling that warfarin sodium is an anticoagulant and that Ecotrin is an aspirin-containing product will direct you to option 1. Review client teaching points related to warfarin sodium if you had difficulty with this question.
Level of Cognitive Ability: Comprehension
Client Needs: Health Promotion and Maintenance
Integrated Concept/Process: Nursing Process/Evaluation
Content Area: Pharmacology
Reference: Hodgson B, Kizior R: *Saunders nursing drug handbook 2002*, Philadelphia, 2002, WB Saunders, p.82.

2. *Answer:* 3
Rationale: The therapeutic serum digoxin level ranges from 0.5 to 2.0 ng/mL.
Test-Taking Strategy: Knowledge of the therapeutic serum digoxin level is necessary to answer the question. Review this level if you had difficulty with this question.
Level of Cognitive Ability: Comprehension
Client Needs: Physiological Integrity
Integrated Concept/Process: Nursing Process/Data Collection
Content Area: Pharmacology
Reference: Hodgson B, Kizior R: *Saunders nursing drug handbook 2002*, Philadelphia, 2002, WB Saunders, p. 344.

3. *Answer:* 4
Rationale: For SC heparin sodium injection, a 25- to 27-gauge, 3/8- to 5/8-inch needle is used to prevent tissue trauma and inadvertent intramuscular injection. A 1-inch needle would inject the heparin sodium into the muscle. The application of heat may vary the absorption of the heparin. Aspiration before injection is avoided with heparin sodium.
Test-Taking Strategy: Use the process of elimination. Recalling the anatomy of muscle and subcutaneous layers of tissue will assist in directing you to option 4. If you had difficulty with this question, review the principles related to heparin administration.
Level of Cognitive Ability: Application
Client Needs: Physiological Integrity
Integrated Concept/Process: Nursing Process/Implementation
Content Area: Pharmacology
Reference: Hodgson B, Kizior R: *Saunders nursing drug handbook 2002*, Philadelphia, 2002, WB Saunders, p. 528.

4. *Answer:* 2
Rationale: Dizziness is a sign of toxicity. Additional signs of toxicity from procainamide include confusion, drowsiness, decreased urination, nausea, vomiting, and tachydysrhythmias. The initial nursing action is to check the client's apical pulse and obtain a blood pressure. The physician may need to be notified, but data collection is necessary first. Options 1 and 4 are incorrect actions.
Test-Taking Strategy: Use the process of elimination. Note the key word "initial." Use the steps of the nursing process and note that option 2 is the only option that addresses data collection. Review the toxic effects of this medication if you had difficulty with this question.
Level of Cognitive Ability: Application
Client Needs: Physiological Integrity
Integrated Concept/Process: Nursing Process/Implementation
Content Area: Pharmacology
Reference: Hodgson B, Kizior R: *Saunders nursing drug handbook 2002*, Philadelphia, 2002, WB Saunders, p. 344.

5. *Answer:* 3
Rationale: Streptokinase converts plasminogen in the blood to plasmin. Plasmin is an enzyme that digests or dissolves fibrin clots wherever they exist. Options 1, 2, and 4 describe mechanisms of action of heparin sodium (Liquaemin) and warfarin sodium (Coumadin).
Test-Taking Strategy: Use the process of elimination. Remember that streptokinase dissolves clots. This will direct you to option 3. Review this medication if you had difficulty with this question.
Level of Cognitive Ability: Comprehension
Client Needs: Physiological Integrity
Integrated Concept/Process: Teaching/Learning

Content Area: Pharmacology
Reference: Hodgson B, Kizior R: *Saunders nursing drug handbook 2002*, Philadelphia, 2002, WB Saunders, p. 1026.

6. *Answer:* 2
Rationale: Diltiazem is a calcium channel blocker that inhibits calcium influx through the slow channels of the membrane of smooth muscle cells. Calcium channel blockers decrease myocardial oxygen demands and blocks calcium channels, thereby decreasing the force of contraction of the ventricular tissue.
Test-Taking Strategy: Knowledge of the mechanisms involved in Prinzmetal's angina (coronary artery spasm) is required to understand why calcium channel blockers would be prescribed. Review the action of calcium channel blockers if you had difficulty with this question.
Level of Cognitive Ability: Comprehension
Client Needs: Physiological Integrity
Integrated Concept/Process: Nursing Process/Planning
Content Area: Pharmacology
Reference: Hodgson B, Kizior R: *Saunders nursing drug handbook 2002*, Philadelphia, 2002, WB Saunders, p. 348.

7. *Answer:* 3
Rationale: Audible expiratory wheezes may indicate a serious adverse reaction, bronchospasm. Beta blockers may induce this reaction, particularly in clients with chronic obstructive pulmonary disease (COPD) or asthma. A normal decrease in blood pressure and heart rate is expected. Insomnia is a frequent mild side effect and should be monitored.
Test-Taking Strategy: Use the process of elimination. Eliminate options 1 and 2 first because these are expected responses from the medication. From the remaining options, noting the key words "adverse reaction" will assist in directing you to option 3. Review the adverse effects of this medication if you had difficulty with this question.
Level of Cognitive Ability: Analysis
Client Needs: Physiological Integrity
Integrated Concept/Process: Nursing Process/Data Collection
Content Area: Pharmacology
Reference: Hodgson B, Kizior R: *Saunders nursing drug handbook 2002*, Philadelphia, 2002, WB Saunders, p. 57.

8. *Answer:* 4
Rationale: Paraphrasing is restating the client's or family member's own words. Option 1 represents a communication block that denies the person's right to an opinion. Option 2 is offering a false reassurance. In option 3, the nurse is expressing approval, which can be harmful to the client-nurse or family-nurse relationship.
Test-Taking Strategy: Use therapeutic communication techniques. Remembering to address client feelings first will easily direct you to option 4. Review these therapeutic techniques if you had difficulty with this question.
Level of Cognitive Ability: Application
Client Needs: Psychosocial Integrity
Integrated Concept/Process: Communication and Documentation
Content Area: Pharmacology
Reference: Potter P, Perry A: *Fundamentals of nursing*, ed 5, St Louis, 2001, Mosby, p. 459.

9. *Answer:* 4
Rationale: It is appropriate to treat atrial fibrillation with the prescribed and calculated dose of digoxin as indicated in the question. The issue of the question is that the client verbalizes inaccurate and unsafe knowledge regarding this medication and the treatment for chest pain. This client needs further teaching regarding the safe administration of medications for episodes of chest pain. Options 1, 2, and 3 are incorrect actions.
Test-Taking Strategy: Perform the calculation first and determine that the dose that the nurse is to give is correct. From this point, eliminate options 1 and 2. From the remaining options, note the issue of the question, the need for client teaching. This should direct you to option 4. Review the client teaching points related to digoxin if you had difficulty with this question.
Level of Cognitive Ability: Application
Client Needs: Health Promotion and Maintenance
Integrated Concept/Process: Nursing Process/Planning
Content Area: Pharmacology
Reference: Hodgson B, Kizior R: *Saunders nursing drug handbook 2002*, Philadelphia, 2002, WB Saunders, p. 344.

10. *Answer:* 3
Rationale: Tea and coffee are stimulants as well as mild diuretics. These are a poor choice for hydration. Taking the medication at the same time each day improves compliance. Since furosemide is a diuretic, the morning is the best time to take the medication so as not to interrupt sleep. Notification of the health care provider is appropriate if edema is noted in the hands, feet, or face, or if the client is short of breath. Sitting up slowly prevents postural hypotension.
Test-Taking Strategy: Use the process of elimination. Note the key words "need for further instructions." Tea and coffee are stimulants and diuretics can potentially worsen dehydration. Additionally, coffee and tea are not healthy foods. This should alert you that this is the correct option for this question, as stated. Review client teaching points related to this medication if you had difficulty with this question.
Level of Cognitive Ability: Comprehension
Client Needs: Health Promotion and Maintenance
Integrated Concept/Process: Teaching/Learning
Content Area: Pharmacology
Reference: Hodgson B, Kizior R: *Saunders nursing drug handbook 2002*, Philadelphia, 2002, WB Saunders, p. 487.

11. *Answer:* 4
Rationale: Headache is a frequent side effect of isosorbide mononitrate and usually disappears during continued therapy. If a headache occurs during therapy, the client should be instructed to take the medication with food or meals. It is not necessary to contact the physician unless the headaches persist with therapy. It is not appropriate to instruct the client to discontinue therapy or adjust the dosages.
Test-Taking Strategy: Use the process of elimination. Eliminate options 2 and 3 first because it is not within the scope of nursing practice to instruct a client to discontinue or adjust

dosages. From the remaining options, recalling that the headache can be relieved with the administration of food with the medication will assist in directing you to option 4. Review this medication if you had difficulty with this question.
Level of Cognitive Ability: Application
Client Needs: Health Promotion and Maintenance
Integrated Concept/Process: Teaching/Learning
Content Area: Pharmacology
Reference: Hodgson B, Kizior R: *Saunders nursing drug handbook 2002*, Philadelphia, 2002, WB Saunders, p. 602.

12. *Answer:* 4
Rationale: Most beta blockers may be administered with food or on an empty stomach, but propranolol is best absorbed if taken with meals or directly after eating. Exercise will not prevent orthostatic hypotension. Hot showers and baths are not advised because of their vasodilating effect. The client needs to be instructed how to take pulse rate and to notify the physician if the heart rate falls below 60 beats per minute.
Test-Taking Strategy: Use the process of elimination. Recalling that bradycardia can occur with propranolol will easily direct you to option 4. If you had difficulty with this question, review this medication.
Level of Cognitive Ability: Application
Client Needs: Health Promotion and Maintenance
Integrated Concept/Process: Teaching/Learning
Content Area: Pharmacology
Reference: Hodgson B, Kizior R: *Saunders nursing drug handbook 2002*, Philadelphia, 2002, WB Saunders, p. 57.

13. *Answer:* 2
Rationale: The PT will assess for the therapeutic effect of warfarin sodium (Coumadin) and the APTT will assess the therapeutic effect of heparin sodium. Heparin sodium doses are determined based on these laboratory results. The hemoglobin and hematocrit assess red blood cell concentrations.
Test-Taking Strategy: Use the process of elimination. Eliminate options 3 and 4 because these laboratory values are unrelated to heparin sodium therapy. From the remaining options, knowledge of the appropriate test for monitoring therapeutic values of both heparin sodium and warfarin sodium is required to answer this question. Review this content if you had difficulty with this question.
Level of Cognitive Ability: Comprehension
Client Needs: Physiological Integrity
Integrated Concept/Process: Nursing Process/Data Collection
Content Area: Pharmacology
Reference: Hodgson B, Kizior R: *Saunders nursing drug handbook 2002*, Philadelphia, 2002, WB Saunders, p. 1160.

14. *Answer:* 3
Rationale: TPA is a thrombolytic. Hemorrhage is a complication of any type of thrombolytic medication. The client should be monitored for bleeding. Monitoring for renal failure and the client's psychosocial status are important; however, they are not the priority. Heparin sodium is given after thrombolytic therapy, but the question is not asking for the associated medications after TPA therapy.
Test-Taking Strategy: Use the process of elimination and note the key word "priority." Use the principles of prioritizing and knowledge regarding this medication to direct you to option 3. Additionally, remember that bleeding is a priority. Review this medication if you had difficulty with this question.
Level of Cognitive Ability: Application
Client Needs: Physiological Integrity
Integrated Concept/Process: Nursing Process/Implementation
Content Area: Pharmacology
Reference: Lehne R: *Pharmacology for nursing care*, ed 4, Philadelphia, 2001, WB Saunders, p. 575.

15. *Answer:* 2
Rationale: To help prevent tolerance, clients need a 12-hour "no nitrate" time. In addition to having a 12-hour "no nitrate" time, the client must rotate the nitrate patch and wash the hands to prevent topical absorption through the fingers. Options 1, 3, and 4 are incorrect.
Test-Taking Strategy: Use the process of elimination. Option 1 can be easily eliminated based on the issue of the question. Eliminate options 3 and 4 next because they are similar. Review the administration of nitrate patches if you had difficulty with this question.
Level of Cognitive Ability: Application
Client Needs: Health Promotion and Maintenance
Integrated Concept/Process: Teaching/Learning
Content Area: Pharmacology
Reference: Hodgson B, Kizior R: *Saunders nursing drug handbook 2002*, Philadelphia, 2002, WB Saunders, p. 98.

16. *Answer:* 1
Rationale: Option 1 is a therapeutic nonjudgmental response. Option 2 creates doubt about the physician's practice without actually knowing the circumstances. Option 3 is argumentative and nontherapeutic. Option 4 dismisses the family's concerns and disempowers the family.
Test-Taking Strategy: Use therapeutic communication techniques to answer the question. Remember that reflection of the client's or family's concerns is most therapeutic. Review therapeutic communication techniques if you had difficulty with this question.
Level of Cognitive Ability: Application
Client Needs: Psychosocial Integrity
Integrated Concept/Process: Communication and Documentation
Content Area: Pharmacology
Reference: Potter P, Perry A: *Fundamentals of nursing*, ed 5, St Louis, 2001, Mosby, p. 460.

17. *Answer:* 3
Rationale: Clients on potassium-wasting diuretics are at high risk of hypokalemia. Clinical manifestations of hypokalemia include fatigue, anorexia, nausea, vomiting, muscle weakness, leg cramps, decreased bowel motility, paresthesias, and dysrhythmias. Diarrhea and intestinal colic are signs of hyperkalemia. Tingling of the fingers and toes is a sign of hypocalcemia.
Test-Taking Strategy: Knowledge regarding the signs of hypokalemia is required to answer the question. If you had difficulty with this question, review the signs of this electrolyte imbalance.
Level of Cognitive Ability: Comprehension

Client Needs: Physiological Integrity
Integrated Concept/Process: Nursing Process/Data Collection
Content Area: Pharmacology
Reference: DeWit S: *Fundamental concepts and skills for nursing*, Philadelphia, 2001, WB Saunders, p. 446.

18. *Answer:* 4
Rationale: Triamterene is a potassium-sparing diuretic, which means that the client must avoid the intake of foods high in potassium. Options 1, 2, and 3 are high-potassium food items.
Test-Taking Strategy: Knowledge that triamterene is a potaassium-sparing diuretic and knowledge of those food items high in potassium is required to answer this question. If you are unfamiliar with this medication and those foods high in potassium, review this content.
Level of Cognitive Ability: Application
Client Needs: Physiological Integrity
Integrated Concept/Process: Teaching/Learning
Content Area: Pharmacology
Reference: Hodgson B, Kizior R: *Saunders nursing drug handbook 2002*, Philadelphia, 2002, WB Saunders, p. 1118.

19. *Answer:* 3
Rationale: Thiazide diuretics such as hydrochlorothiazide are sulfa-based medications, and a client with a sulfa allergy is at risk for an allergic reaction. Options 1, 2, and 4 are not associated with the use of this medication.
Test-Taking Strategy: Knowledge of the chemical make-up of thiazide diuretics is necessary to answer this question. Recalling that these medications contain a sulfa-ring in their makeup will easily direct you to option 3. Review the contraindications associated with the thiazide diuretics if you had difficulty with this question.
Level of Cognitive Ability: Application
Client Needs: Safe, Effective Care Environment
Integrated Concept/Process: Nursing Process/Data Collection
Content Area: Pharmacology
Reference: Hodgson B, Kizior R: *Saunders nursing drug handbook 2002*, Philadelphia, 2002, WB Saunders, p. 535.

20. *Answer:* 3
Rationale: Nicotinic acid should be avoided because it may lead to liver abnormalities. All lipid-lowering medications can also cause liver abnormalities, so a combination of nicotinic acid and cholestyramine is to be avoided. Constipation and bloating are the two most common side effects. Both walking and the reduction of fats in the diet are therapeutic measures to reduce cholesterol and triglyceride levels.
Test-Taking Strategy: Use the process of elimination. Recalling that over-the-counter medications should be avoided when a client is taking a prescription medication will easily direct you to option 3. Review client teaching points related to this medication if you had difficulty with this question.
Level of Cognitive Ability: Comprehension
Client Needs: Health Promotion and Maintenance
Integrated Concept/Process: Nursing Process/Evaluation
Content Area: Pharmacology
Reference: Hodgson B, Kizior R: *Saunders nursing drug handbook 2002*, Philadelphia, 2002, WB Saunders, p. 790.

21. *Answer:* 4
Rationale: Reflection of the client's own comment lets the client know that you are hearing the concerns without judging. The nurse cannot understand what the client is experiencing (option 1). Option 2 devalues the physician's judgment. Option 3 is confrontational and unsupportive.
Test-Taking Strategy: Use therapeutic communication techniques. Select nonjudgmental responses that reflect the fact you are listening to the client's concerns. Review these techniques if you had difficulty with this question.
Level of Cognitive Ability: Application
Client Needs: Psychosocial Integrity
Integrated Concept/Process: Communication and Documentation
Content Area: Pharmacology
Reference: Potter P, Perry A: *Fundamentals of nursing*, ed 5, St Louis, 2001, Mosby, p. 460.

22. *Answer:* 1
Rationale: Spironolactone is a potassium-sparing diuretic that promotes sodium excretion while conserving potassium. Options 2, 3, and 4 identify diuretics that do not conserve potassium.
Test-Taking Strategy: Knowledge that spironolactone is a potassium-sparing diuretic is required to answer this question. Review the potassium-sparing diuretics if you are unfamiliar with them and had difficulty with this question.
Level of Cognitive Ability: Analysis
Client Needs: Physiological Integrity
Integrated Concept/Process: Nursing Process/Planning
Content Area: Pharmacology
Reference: Hodgson B, Kizior R: *Saunders nursing drug handbook 2002*, Philadelphia, 2002, WB Saunders, p. 1022.

23. *Answer:* 3
Rationale: Nitroglycerin tablets are usually ordered one every 5 minutes PRN for chest pain for a total dose of 3 tablets. Waiting 10 minutes is inappropriate if the client is having chest pain. Oxygen at 10 liters is an unsafe dose. There is no need to call the resuscitation team at this time.
Test-Taking Strategy: Focus on the information provided in the question and use knowledge regarding the administration of nitroglycerin for chest pain. Recalling that a nitroglycerin tablet can be administered for three doses 5 minutes apart if the vital signs remain stable will easily direct you to option 3. Review the administration of nitroglycerin if you had difficulty with this question.
Level of Cognitive Ability: Application
Client Needs: Physiological Integrity
Integrated Concept/Process: Nursing Process/Implementation
Content Area: Pharmacology
Reference: Hodgson B, Kizior R: *Saunders nursing drug handbook 2002*, Philadelphia, 2002, WB Saunders, p. 800.

24. *Answer:* 3
Rationale: The PND may be due to increased venous return when lying in bed. When this occurs, a diuretic is prescribed. Bumetanide is a diuretic. Propranolol is a beta blocker. Lidocaine is an antidysrhythmic, and urokinase is a thrombolytic.

Test-Taking Strategy: Knowledge of the pathophysiology associated with PND and the classifications of the medications in each of the options will easily direct you to option 3. Review PND and the actions of the medications identified in the options if you had difficulty with this question.
Level of Cognitive Ability: Analysis
Client Needs: Physiological Integrity
Integrated Concept/Process: Nursing Process/Planning
Content Area: Pharmacology
Reference: Hodgson B, Kizior R: *Saunders nursing drug handbook 2002*, Philadelphia, 2002, WB Saunders, p. 138.

25. *Answer:* 2
Rationale: Denial is the most common reaction when a client has a myocardial infarction or anginal pain. No angry behavior was identified in the question. Phobias and obsessive-compulsive disorders are mental health diagnoses.
Test-Taking Strategy: Use the process of elimination. Eliminate options 1 and 3 first because these are medical diagnoses. Recalling that denial is the most common reaction when a person has chest pain will easily direct you to option 2. Review psychosocial responses in the client experiencing chest pain if you had difficulty with this question.
Level of Cognitive Ability: Analysis
Client Needs: Psychosocial Integrity
Integrated Concept/Process: Nursing Process/Data Collection
Content Area: Pharmacology
Reference: Ignatavicius D, Workman M: *Medical-surgical: critical thinking for collaborative care*, ed 4, Philadelphia, 2002, WB Saunders, p. 794.

26. *Answer:* 3
Rationale: The nurse is ultimately responsible for giving the correct medication. When medication orders are vague, the nurse must contact the physician. Often, the physician is unaware of other medications prescribed by other physicians. The nurse would not administer the medication without verification. Waiting until the physician makes rounds delays necessary treatment.
Test-Taking Strategy: Use the process of elimination. Options 1 and 2 are easily eliminated because they are similar. Eliminate option 4 because it is not appropriate to wait to clarify an unclear physician's order. Review the safeguards related to physician's orders if you had difficulty with this question.
Level of Cognitive Ability: Application
Client Needs: Safe, Effective Care Environment
Integrated Concept/Process: Nursing Process/Implementation
Content Area: Pharmacology
Reference: DeWit S: *Fundamental concepts and skills for nursing*, Philadelphia, 2001, WB Saunders, p. 107.

27. *Answer:* 3
Rationale: Double vision, loss of appetite, and nausea are signs of digoxin toxicity. Additional signs of digoxin toxicity include bradycardia, difficulty reading, visual alterations such as green and yellow vision, seeing spots or halos, confusion, vomiting, diarrhea, decreased libido, and impotence.
Test-Taking Strategy: Knowledge regarding the signs of digoxin toxicity is required to answer the question. Remembering that gastrointestinal and visual disturbances are signs of toxicity will direct you to option 3. If you had difficulty with this question, review the signs of digoxin toxicity.
Level of Cognitive Ability: Comprehension
Client Needs: Physiological Integrity
Integrated Concept/Process: Nursing Process/Data Collection
Content Area: Pharmacology
Reference: Hodgson B, Kizior R: *Saunders nursing drug handbook 2002*, Philadelphia, 2002, WB Saunders, p. 344.

28. *Answer:* 1
Rationale: Hypotension is a common side effect with this medication and an increased risk exists in an elderly client. Options 2 and 3 will also require monitoring but are not the priority. The temperature is unrelated to administering this medication.
Test-Taking Strategy: Use the process of elimination and focus on the key word "priority." Use the ABCs—airway, breathing, and circulation. Blood pressure reflects circulation. Review the side effects of this medication if you had difficulty with this question.
Level of Cognitive Ability: Application
Client Needs: Physiological Integrity
Integrated Concept/Process: Nursing Process/Data Collection
Content Area: Pharmacology
Reference: Hodgson B, Kizior R: *Saunders nursing drug handbook 2002*, Philadelphia, 2002, WB Saunders, p. 138.

29. *Answer:* 1
Rationale: Atorvastin is an antihyperlipidemic medication. It is contraindicated in pregnancy, lactation, liver disease, biliary cirrhosis or obstruction, severe renal dysfunction, and in clients who are hypersensitive to the medication. Options 2, 3, and 4 are not contraindications to the use of this medication.
Test-Taking Strategy: Knowledge regarding the contraindications associated with use of this medication is required to answer this question. Review these contraindications if you had difficulty with this question.
Level of Cognitive Ability: Comprehension
Client Needs: Physiological Integrity
Integrated Concept/Process: Nursing Process/Data Collection
Content Area: Pharmacology
Reference: Hodgson B, Kizior R: *Saunders nursing drug handbook 2002*, Philadelphia, 2002, WB Saunders, p. 87.

30. *Answer:* 1
Rationale: The PT will assess for the therapeutic effect of warfarin sodium (Coumadin) and the APTT will assess the therapeutic effect of heparin sodium. The RBC count and platelet count will assess red blood cell concentrations and the client's potential for bleeding, respectively. Warfarin sodium doses are determined based on the results of the PT.
Test-Taking Strategy: Use the process of elimination. Eliminate options 3 and 4 first because these laboratory values are unrelated to warfarin sodium therapy. From the remaining options, knowledge of the appropriate test for monitoring the therapeutic values of both heparin sodium and warfarin sodium is required to answer this question. Review this medication if you had difficulty with this question.

Level of Cognitive Ability: Comprehension
Client Needs: Physiological Integrity
Integrated Concept/Process: Nursing Process/Data Collection
Content Area: Pharmacology
Reference: Hodgson B, Kizior R: *Saunders nursing drug handbook 2002*, Philadelphia, 2002, WB Saunders, p. 1160.

REFERENCES

Clark J, Queener S, Karb V: *Pharmacologic basis of nursing practice*, ed 6, St Louis, 2000, Mosby.

Hodgson B, Kizior R: *Saunders nursing drug handbook 2002*, Philadelphia, 2002, WB Saunders.

Ignatavicius D, Workman M: *Medical-surgical: critical thinking for collaborative care*, ed 4, Philadelphia, 2002, WB Saunders.

Karch A: *Focus on nursing pharmacology*, Philadelphia, 2000, Lippincott.

Lehne R: *Pharmacology for nursing care*, ed 4, Philadelphia, 2001, WB Saunders.

UNIT XIV

The Adult Client with a Renal System Disorder

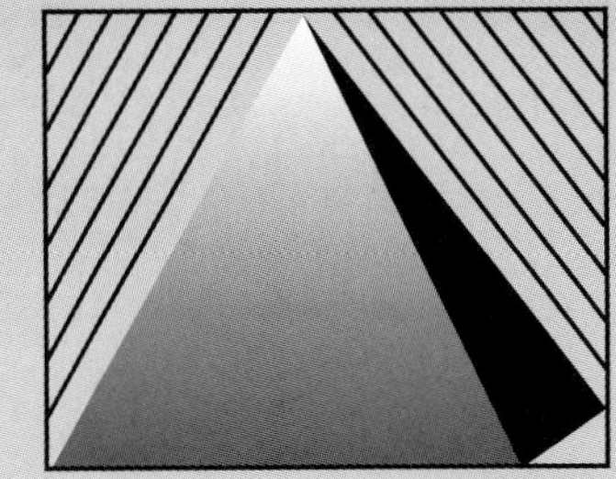

PYRAMID TERMS

Anuria Urine output of less than 100 mL a day.

Hemodialysis The process of cleansing the client's blood. The diffusion of dissolved particles from one fluid compartment into another across a semipermeable membrane. The client's blood flows through one fluid compartment and the dialysate is in another fluid compartment.

Internal Arteriovenous Fistula (AV Fistula) Access of choice for chronic dialysis clients. Created surgically during which an artery in the arm is anastomosed to a vein. This creates an opening, or fistula, between a large artery and a large vein. The flow of arterial blood into the venous system causes the veins to become engorged (maturity). The fistula requires 1 to 2 weeks to mature before it can be used. Maturity is necessary so that the engorged vein can be punctured with a large bore needle for the dialysis procedure.

Nephrolithiasis Refers to the formation of kidney stones. Kidney stones are formed in the renal parenchyma.

Oliguria Urine output of less than 400 mL a day.

Peritoneal Dialysis The peritoneum is the dialyzing membrane (semipermeable membrane) and substitutes for kidney function during renal failure. Works on the principles of diffusion and osmosis, and the dialysis occurs via the transfer of fluid and solute from the bloodstream through the peritoneum.

Renal Failure The loss of kidney function. The types of renal failure are acute renal failure and chronic renal failure. The signs and symptoms of renal failure occur because of the retention of wastes, the retention of fluids, and the inability of the kidneys to regulate electrolytes.

Urolithiasis The formation of urinary stones or calculi. Urinary calculi are formed in the ureter.

PYRAMID TO SUCCESS

Pyramid points focus on the preprocedure and postprocedure care of the client undergoing diagnostic tests and procedures related to the renal system. Be familiar with renal failure, dialysis procedures such as hemodialysis and continuous ambulatory peritoneal dialysis (CAPD), dialysis access devices, urinary diversions, and postoperative care to the client after urinary or renal surgery. Focus on the care to the client after prostatectomy and the treatment measures for the client with urinary or renal calculi. Additionally, pyramid points address measures that promote urinary elimination, prevent infection, and maintain skin integrity. The Integrated Concepts and Processes addressed in this unit include the Clinical Problem-Solving Process (Nursing Process), Caring, Communication and Documentation, Cultural Awareness, Self-Care, and Teaching/Learning.

CLIENT NEEDS

Safe, Effective Care Environment

Accident prevention related to complications associated with disorder
Asepsis related to wound care
Client rights
Confidentiality related to renal disorder
Consultations and referrals related to renal disorder
Establishing priorities
Informed consent related to diagnostic and surgical procedures
Renal organ donation
Standard (universal) precautions related to care of the client

Health Promotion and Maintenance

Instructions regarding home care measures
Instructions regarding the prevention of the recurrence of a urinary and renal disorder
Instructions regarding prescribed treatments related to urinary or renal disorder
Instructions regarding postoperative management

Psychosocial Integrity

Body image disturbances
Coping mechanisms
Community resources
Loss of function of a body part that occurs in clients with a renal disorder
Religious and spiritual influences
Support systems

Physiological Integrity

Adequate rest and sleep
Care related to dialysis access devices
Care to the client after prostatectomy
Comfort interventions
Diagnostic tests and laboratory results
Elimination measures
Fluid and electrolyte disorders
Medication administration
Personal hygiene
Prescribed nutrition and fluid measures
Skin integrity
Treatment measures for the client with urinary or renal calculi
Urinary diversions

REFERENCES

Black J, Hawks J, Keene A: *Medical-surgical nursing: clinical management for positive outcomes*, ed 6, Philadelphia, 2001, WB Saunders.

Chernecky C, Berger B: *Laboratory tests and diagnostic procedures*, ed 3, Philadelphia, 2001, WB Saunders.

Clark J, Queener S, Karb V: *Pharmacologic basis of nursing practice*, ed 6, St Louis, 2000, Mosby.

DeWit S: *Fundamental concepts and skills for nursing*, Philadelphia, 2001, WB Saunders.

Hill S, Howlett H: *Success in practical nursing: personal and vocational issues*, ed 4, Philadelphia, 2001, WB Saunders.

National Council of State Boards of Nursing: *Test plan for the National Council Licensure Examination for Practical/Vocational Nurses*, Chicago, 2001, Author.

Potter P, Perry A: *Fundamentals of nursing*, ed 5, St Louis, 2001, Mosby.

Perry A, Potter P: *Clinical nursing skills and techniques*, ed 5, St Louis, 2002, Mosby.

Wilson J: *Infection control in clinical practice*, ed 2, St Louis, 2002, Balliere Tindall.

Renal System

I. ANATOMY AND PHYSIOLOGY

A. Kidneys
  1. Attached to the abdominal wall at the level of the last thoracic and first three lumbar vertebra
  2. Enclosed in the renal capsule
  3. The cortex is the outer layer of the renal capsule
  4. The medulla is surrounded by the cortex
  5. The nephron makes up the functional unit of the kidney
  6. Functions of kidneys
     a. Maintains homeostasis of the blood
     b. Excretes end products of body metabolism
     c. Controls fluid and electrolyte balance
     d. Excretes bacterial toxins, water-soluble drugs, and drug metabolites
     e. Secrete renin and erythropoietin, which play a role in the function of the parathyroid hormones and vitamin D
  7. Nephron
     a. Functional renal unit
     b. Composed of glomerulus and tubules
  8. Glomerulus
     a. Is encased in Bowman's capsule
     b. Filters the fluid out of blood
  9. Tubules
     a. Includes proximal, distal, and Henle's loop
     b. Fluid is converted to urine in the tubules and then moves to the pelvis of the kidney
     c. Fluid moves to the pelvis of the kidney, flows through the ureter and empties into the bladder

B. Bladder
  1. The ureterovesical sphincter prevents the reflux of urine from the bladder to the ureter
  2. The total capacity of the bladder is 1 liter

C. Prostate gland
  1. Surrounds the male urethra
  2. Contains a duct that opens into the prostatic portion of the urethra and secretes the alkaline portion of seminal fluid

D. Urine production
  1. As fluid flows through the proximal tubules, water and solutes are reabsorbed
  2. Water and solutes that are not reabsorbed become urine
  3. The process of selective reabsorption determines the amount of water and solutes to be secreted

E. Homeostasis of water
  1. The antidiuretic hormone (ADH) is primarily responsible for the reabsorption of water by kidneys
  2. ADH is produced by the hypothalamus and secreted from the posterior lobe of the pituitary gland
  3. Secretion of ADH is stimulated by dehydration or high sodium intake and by a decrease in blood volume
  4. ADH increases the permeability to water of the distal convoluted tubules and collecting duct
  5. Water is drawn out of the tubules by osmosis into a high salt concentration of fluid in the medulla and its capillaries; water returns to the blood, and concentrated urine remains in the tubule to be excreted
  6. When the client lacks ADH, diabetes insipidus develops
  7. Clients with diabetes insipidus produce very large amounts of dilute urine and without treatment have difficulty drinking sufficient water to survive

F. Homeostasis of sodium
   1. When the amount of sodium increases, extra water is retained to preserve osmotic pressure
   2. An increase in sodium and water produces an increase in the blood volume and blood pressure (BP)
   3. When the BP increases, glomerular filtration increases and extra water and salt are lost; blood volume is reduced and returns the BP to normal
   4. Reabsorption of sodium in the distal convoluted tubules is controlled by the hormones of the renin-angiotensin system
   5. Renin is secreted when the BP or concentration of fluid in the distal convoluted tubule is low
   6. Renin is an enzyme and splits angiotensin I from angiotensinogen and converts to angiotensin II as blood flows through the lung
   7. Angiotensin II, a potent vasoconstrictor, stimulates the secretion of aldosterone
   8. Aldosterone stimulates the distal convoluted tubules to reabsorb more sodium and excrete more potassium
   9. The additional sodium increases water reabsorption and increases blood volume and the BP, returning it to normal; the stimulus for the secretion of renin is then removed

G. Homeostasis of potassium
   1. Increases in potassium stimulate the secretion of aldosterone
   2. Aldosterone stimulates the distal convoluted tubules to secrete potassium; this acts to return the potassium concentration to normal

H. Homeostasis of acidity (pH)
   1. Blood pH is controlled by maintaining the concentration of buffer systems
   2. Carbonic acid and sodium bicarbonate form the most important buffer for neutralizing acids in the plasma
   3. The concentration of carbonic acid is controlled by the respiratory system
   4. The concentration of sodium bicarbonate is controlled by the kidneys
   5. Normal pH is 7.35 to 7.45, maintained by keeping the ratio of concentrations of sodium bicarbonate to carbon dioxide constant at 20:1
   6. Strong acids are neutralized by sodium bicarbonate to produce carbonic acid and the sodium salts of the strong acid; this process quickly restores the ratio and thus blood pH
   7. The carbonic acid produced dissociates into carbon dioxide and water and because the concentration of carbon dioxide is maintained at a constant level by the respiratory system, the excess carbonic acid is rapidly excreted
   8. Sodium combined with the strong acid is actively reabsorbed in the distal convoluted tubules in exchange for hydrogen or potassium ions; the strong acid is neutralized by the secretion of ammonia and is excreted as ammonia or potassium salts

II. DIAGNOSTIC TESTS (Box 50-1 and Box 50-2)

A. Urinalysis
   1. Description: a urine test for evaluation of the renal system and for determining renal disease
   2. Implementation
      a. Wash perineal area
      b. Use a clean container
      c. Obtain 10 to 15 mL of the first morning sample
      d. Note that refrigerated samples may alter the specific gravity
      e. If the client is menstruating, indicate on the laboratory requisition form

B. Specific gravity determination
   1. Description: a urine test that measures the kidney's ability to concentrate urine
   2. Implementation
      a. Obtain a freshly voided specimen
      b. Fill the specific gravity container one-half to two-thirds full
      c. Place the hydrometer (urinometer) in the urine and spin gently
      d. Read the scale at the level of the meniscus

BOX 50-1

Risk Factors Associated with Renal Disorders

Frequent urinary tract infections
High-sodium diet
Contact sports
Trauma and injury
History of hypertension
Family history of renal disease
Medication use
Associated medical conditions

BOX 50-2

Normal Renal Function Tests

BUN (Blood urea nitrogen), 8 to 25 mg/dL
Serum creatinine, 0.6 to 1.3 mg/dL
Creatinine clearance, 100 to 120 mL/minute
Uric acid, serum, 2.5 to 8.0 mg/dL
Uric acid, urine, 250 to 750 mg/24 hours

C. Urine culture and sensitivity
1. Description: a urine test that identifies the presence of microorganisms and determines the specific antibiotics that will appropriately treat the existing microorganism
2. Implementation
a. Clean perineal area and urinary meatus with bacteriostatic solution
b. Collect midstream sample in a sterile container
c. Send the collected specimen to laboratory immediately
d. Note that urine from clients who forced fluids may be too dilute to provide a positive culture
e. Identify any sources of potential contaminants during the collection of the specimen such as the hands, skin, clothing, hair, and vaginal or rectal secretions

D. Creatinine clearance test
1. Description
a. A blood and timed urine specimen that evaluates kidney function
b. Blood is drawn at the start of the test and the morning of the day that the 24-hour urine specimen collection is complete
2. Implementation
a. Encourage adequate fluids before and during the test
b. Instruct the client as prescribed to avoid tea, coffee, and medications during testing
c. If the client is taking adrenocorticotropic hormone (ACTH), cortisone, or thyroxine, check with the physician regarding administration of these medications during testing
d. Maintain the urine specimen on ice or refrigerate and check with the laboratory regarding the addition of a preservative to the specimen during collection

E. Vanillylmandelic acid (VMA) test
1. Description
a. A 24-hour urine collection to diagnose pheochromocytoma, a tumor of the adrenal gland
b. The test identifies an assay of urinary catecholamines in the urine
2. Implementation
a. Instruct the client to avoid foods such as caffeine, cocoa, vanilla, cheese, gelatin, licorice, and fruits for at least 2 days before beginning the urine collection and during the collection, and to avoid taking medications for 2 to 3 days before beginning the test as prescribed
b. Instruct the client to avoid stress and to maintain adequate food and fluids during the test
c. Save all urine, label the container, add preservative, and place specimen on ice or refrigerate
d. Check with the laboratory regarding medication restrictions

F. 17-Ketosteroids test
1. Description: a 24-hour urine collection to diagnose endocrine imbalances of adrenal glands, ovaries, and testes
2. Implementation
a. Encourage fluids and a normal diet during testing
b. Add preservative and place specimen collection on ice or refrigerate
c. Note that obesity and severe mental and physical stress may affect the test results
d. Note that levels may increase during the third trimester of pregnancy

G. Uric acid test
1. Description: a 24-hour urine collection to diagnose gout and kidney disease
2. Implementation
a. Encourage fluids and a regular diet during testing
b. Place specimen on ice or refrigerate and check with the laboratory regarding the addition of a preservative

H. Kidneys, ureters, and bladder (KUB) radiograph
1. Description: an x-ray film, which views the urinary system and adjacent structures; used to detect urinary calculi
2. Implementation: there is no specific preparation

I. Intravenous pyelogram (IVP) ▲
1. Description
a. The injection of a radiopaque dye, which outlines the renal system
b. Performed to identify abnormalities in the system
2. Implementation preprocedure
a. Obtain an informed consent
b. Assess the client for allergies to iodine, seafood, and radiopaque dyes ▲
c. Withhold food and fluids after midnight on the night before the test
d. Administer laxatives as prescribed
e. Inform the client about possible throat irritation, flushing of the face, warmth, or a salty taste, which may be experienced during the test
3. Implementation postprocedure
a. Monitor vital signs
b. Instruct the client to drink at least 1 liter of fluids unless contraindicated ▲
c. Monitor the venipuncture site for bleeding
d. Monitor urinary output

J. Renal angiography
 1. Description: the injection of a radiopaque dye through a catheter for examination of the renal arterial supply
 2. Implementation preprocedure
  a. Obtain an informed consent
  b. Assess the client for allergies to iodine, seafood, and radiopaque dyes
  c. Inform the client about the possible burning feeling or the feeling of heat along the vessel after the dye is injected
  d. Withhold food and fluids after midnight on the night before the test
  e. Instruct the client to void immediately before the procedure
  f. Administer enemas as prescribed
  g. Shave injection sites as prescribed
  h. Assess and mark the peripheral pulses
 3. Implementation postprocedure
  a. Assess vital signs and peripheral pulses
  b. Provide bed rest and use of a sandbag at insertion site for 4 to 8 hours
  c. Assess the color and temperature of the involved extremity
  d. Inspect the catheter insertion site for bleeding or swelling
  e. Encourage fluids unless contraindicated
  f. Monitor urinary output

K. Renal scan
 1. Description: an intravenous (IV) injection of a radioisotope for visual imaging of renal blood flow
 2. Implementation preprocedure
  a. Obtain an informed consent
  b. Assess for allergies
  c. Assist with administering radioisotope as necessary
  d. Instruct the client that he or she will be required to remain motionless
  e. Instruct the client that imaging may be repeated at various intervals before the test is complete
 3. Implementation postprocedure
  a. Encourage fluids unless contraindicated
  b. Assess the client for signs of delayed allergic reaction, such as itching and hives
  c. Note that the radioactivity is eliminated in 24 hours
  d. Follow standard precautions when caring for incontinent clients and double-bag client linens per agency policy

L. Cystometrogram (CMG)
 1. Description: a graphic recording of the pressures exerted at varying phases of filling of the bladder
 2. Implementation preprocedure: inform the client about the voiding requirements during the procedure
 3. Implementation postprocedure: monitor client voiding after the procedure

M. Cystoscopy
 1. Description: the bladder mucosa is examined for inflammation, calculi, or tumors by means of a cystoscope
 2. Implementation preprocedure: obtain an informed consent
 3. Implementation postprocedure
  a. Encourage the intake of fluids
  b. Assess urine for color and consistency
  c. Note that pink-tinged or tea-colored urine is common
  d. Monitor for bright red urine or clots and notify physician if this occurs

N. Renal biopsy
 1. Description: insertion of a needle into the kidney to obtain a sample of tissue for examination
 2. Implementation preprocedure
  a. Assess vital signs
  b. Assess baseline clotting studies
  c. Obtain informed consent
  d. Withhold food and fluids after midnight on the night before the test
 3. Implementation during procedure: position client prone with a pillow under the abdomen and shoulders
 4. Implementation postprocedure
  a. Monitor vital signs
  b. Monitor hemoglobin and hematocrit
  c. Place the client in the supine position and on bed rest for 8 hours as prescribed
  d. Provide pressure to the biopsy site for 30 minutes
  e. Check the biopsy site for bleeding
  f. Encourage fluid intake of 1500 to 2000 mL as prescribed
  g. Instruct the client to avoid heavy lifting and strenuous activity for 2 weeks

III. RENAL FAILURE

A. Description
 1. The loss of kidney function
 2. The types of **renal failure** include **acute renal failure** or **chronic renal failure**
 3. The signs and symptoms of **renal failure** are caused by the retention of wastes, the retention of fluids, and the inability of the kidneys to regulate electrolytes

B. **Acute renal failure (ARF)**
 1. Description

a. The sudden loss of kidney function caused by renal cell damage from ischemia or toxic substances
b. **Acute renal failure** occurs abruptly and can be reversible
c. It leads to hypoperfusion, cell death, and decompensation in renal function
d. The prognosis is dependent on the cause and condition of the client
e. Near normal or normal kidney function may resume gradually

2. Causes
a. Infection
b. Renal artery occlusion
c. Obstruction
d. Acute kidney disease
e. Dehydration
f. Diuretic therapy
g. Ischemia from hypovolemia, heart failure, septic shock, and blood loss
h. Toxic substances as medications, particularly antibiotics

3. Oliguric phase
a. Duration is 8 to 15 days and the longer the duration, the less chance for recovery
b Sudden drop in urine output; urine output less than 400 mL per day
c. Urine specific gravity of 1.010 to 1.016
d. Anorexia, nausea, and vomiting
e. Hypertension
f. Decreased skin turgor
g. Pruritus
h. Tingling of the extremities
i. Drowsiness progressing to disorientation to coma
j. Edema
k. Dysrhythmias
l. Signs of congestive heart failure (CHF) and pulmonary edema
m. Signs of pericarditis
n. Signs of acidosis

4. Diuretic phase
a. Urine output rises slowly and then diuresis occurs (4 to 5 liters per day)
b. High volume of urine output indicates recovery of damages nephrons
c. Hypotension
d. Tachycardia
e. Improvement in level of consciousness (LOC)

5. Recovery phase (convalescent)
a. A slow process; complete recovery may take 1 to 2 years
b. Urine volume is normal
c. Increase in strength
d. Increase in LOC
e. BUN is stable and normal
f. Client can develop **chronic renal failure (CRF)**

C. **Chronic renal failure**

1. Description
a. The progressive loss and ongoing deterioration in kidney function that occurs slowly over time
b. It occurs in four stages, is irreversible, and results in uremia or end-stage renal disease
c. **Chronic renal failure** requires dialysis or kidney transplantation to maintain life
d. Hypervolemia can occur because of the inability of the kidneys to excrete sodium and water, or hypovolemia can occur because of the inability of the kidneys to conserve sodium and water

2. Causes
a. May follow **acute renal failure**
b. Renal artery occlusion
c. Chronic urinary obstruction
d. Recurrent infections
e. Hypertension
f. Metabolic disorders
g. Diabetes mellitus
h. Autoimmune disorders

3. Data collection
a. Anorexia and nausea
b. Headache
c. Weakness and fatigue
d. Hypertension
e. Confusion, lethargy followed by convulsions and coma
f. Kussmaul respirations
g. Diarrhea or constipation
h. Muscle twitching and numbness of extremities
i. Decreased urine output
j. Decreased urine specific gravity
k. Proteinuria
l. Anemia
m. Azotemia
n. Fluid overload and signs of heart failure
o. Uremic frost

D. Implementation

1. Monitor vital signs
2. Monitor intake and urine output (hourly in ARF)
3. Monitor weight noting that an increase of ½ to 1 lb daily indicates fluid retention
4. Monitor BUN, creatinine, and electrolyte values
5. Monitor for acidosis and treat with sodium bicarbonate as prescribed
6. Assess urinalysis for protein, hematuria, casts, and specific gravity
7. Monitor LOC

8. Assess for signs of infection, as client may not demonstrate a temperature or an increased white blood cell count
9. Assess for dysrhythmias, as a potassium level above 6 mEq/L will cause peaked T waves and widened QRS complex
10. Monitor for fluid overload; assess lungs for rales and rhonchi
11. Monitor for edema
12. Administer prescribed diet; usually a moderate protein intake (to decrease the workload on the kidney) and a high carbohydrate, low-potassium, and low-phosphorus diet is prescribed
13. Restrict sodium intake as prescribed based on the electrolyte level
14. Daily fluid allowances may be 400 mL to 1000 mL plus measured urinary output
15. Administer sodium polystyrene sulfonate (Kayexalate) to lower potassium level as prescribed
16. Be alert to nephrotoxic medications such as antibiotics, which may be prescribed
17. Prepare the client for dialysis if prescribed

E. Special problems in renal failure
1. Hypertension
   a. Failure of the kidneys to maintain homeostasis of the blood pressure
   b. Monitor vital signs
   c. Maintain fluid and sodium restrictions as prescribed
   d. Administer diuretics and antihypertensives as prescribed
   e. Administer propranolol (Inderal), a beta-adrenergic antagonist, as prescribed, which decreases renin release (renin causes vasoconstriction)
2. Hypervolemia
   a. Monitor vital signs
   b. Monitor input and output (I&O) and weight
   c. Monitor for edema
   d. Monitor electrolytes
   e. Monitor for hypertension
   f. Monitor for CHF and pulmonary edema
   g. Administer diuretics as prescribed
   h. Instruct the client to avoid foods with salts
   i. Instruct the client to avoid antacids or cold remedies containing sodium bicarbonate
3. Hypovolemia
   a. Monitor vital signs
   b. Monitor I&O
   c. Monitor electrolytes
   d. Monitor for hypotension
   e. Monitor for dehydration
   f. Provide replacement therapy based on electrolyte results
   g. Provide sodium supplements as prescribed depending on electrolyte value
4. Potassium retention
   a. Monitor vital signs and apical rate
   b. Monitor potassium level
   c. Monitor for dysrhythmias (peaked T waves and widened QRS complex) indicating hyperkalemia
   d. Provide a low-potassium diet
   e. Administer medications as prescribed to lower the potassium
   f. Prepare the client for dialysis
5. Phosphorus retention
   a. Phosphorus rises and calcium levels decline, which leads to stimulation of parathyroid hormone causing bone demineralization
   b. Treatment is aimed at lowering serum phosphorus levels
   c. Administer aluminum hydroxide preparations or other phosphate binders, as prescribed that bind phosphorus in the intestine and allow the phosphorus to be eliminated
   d. Administer aluminum hydroxide preparations at meals and not with other medications because they bind medications in the intestinal tract
   e. Administer stool softeners and laxatives as prescribed to prevent constipation because aluminum hydroxide preparations are constipating
6. Low calcium
   a. Occurs because of the high phosphorus level and because of the inability of the diseased kidney to activate vitamin D
   b. The absence of vitamin D causes poor absorption of calcium from the intestinal tract
   c. Monitor calcium level
   d. Administer calcium supplements as prescribed
   e. Administer activated vitamin D as prescribed
7. Metabolic acidosis
   a. The kidneys are unable to excrete hydrogen ions and manufacture bicarbonate and acidosis occurs
   b. Administer alkalyzers such as sodium bicarbonate as prescribed
   c. Note that clients with **CRF** adjust to low bicarbonate levels and do not become acutely ill

8. Anemia
   a. A decreased rate of production of red blood cells (RBCs) occurs as a result of the diseased kidney and the decreased secretion of erythropoeitin
   b. Monitor hemoglobin and hematocrit
   c. Administer epoetin alfa (Epogen) as prescribed to stimulate production of RBCs
   d. Administer folic acid (vitamin B_9) as prescribed instead of oral iron, as oral iron is not well absorbed by the GI tract in **CRF** and causes nausea and vomiting
   e. Administer blood transfusions if prescribed, but blood transfusions are prescribed only when necessary because they decrease the stimulus to produce RBCs
   f. Monitor bleeding
   g. Instruct the client to use a soft toothbrush
   h. Administer stool softeners as prescribed
   i. Avoid administration of acetylsalicylic acid (aspirin) as the medication is excreted by the kidneys and, if administered, high toxic levels will occur and prolong bleeding time
9. GI bleeding
   a. Urea is broken down to ammonia by the intestinal bacteria, and ammonia is a mucosal irritant that causes ulceration and bleeding
   b. Monitor hemoglobin and hematocrit
   c. Monitor stools for occult blood
10. Infection and injury
   a. Infection and injury needs to be monitored and avoided because tissue breakdown causes increased potassium levels
   b. Monitor for signs of infection
   c. Avoid urinary catheters and provide strict asepsis during insertion and catheter care
   d. Instruct the client to avoid fatigue, which decreases body resistance
   e. Instruct the client to avoid persons with infections
   f. Administer antibiotics as prescribed, monitoring for nephrotoxic effects
11. Pruritis
   a. Urate crystals are excreted through the skin to eliminate excess wastes from the body
   b. Uremic frost (the deposit of crystals) is seen in advanced stages of **renal failure**
   c. Monitor for skin breakdown, rash, and uremic frost
   d. Provide good skin care and oral hygiene
   e. Avoid the use of soaps
   f. Administer antipruritics as prescribed
12. Muscle cramps
   a. Occurs in the extremities and hands and can be due to the low sodium level
   b. Monitor electrolytes
   c. Administer electrolyte replacements as prescribed
   d. Administer heat and massage as prescribed
13. Ocular irritation
   a. Calcium deposits in the conjunctiva cause burning and watering
   b. Administer medications to control phosphate level as prescribed
   c. Administer lubricating eye drops
14. Insomnia and fatigue
   a. The diseased kidneys cause a build up of wastes causing fatigue in the client
   b. Provide adequate rest periods
   c. Administer mild CNS depressants as prescribed
15. Neurological changes
   a. The buildup of active particles and fluids causes changes in the brain cells and leads to confusion and impairment in the decision making ability
   b. Monitor for confusion and monitor LOC
   c. Protect the client from injury
   d. Provide a safe and hazard-free environment
   e. Use side rails as needed
   f. Provide a calm and restful environment
   g. Provide comfort measures and backrubs
16. Psychosocial problems: monitor client for psychological problems such as depression, anxiety, suicidal behavior, denial, dependency/independence conflict, changes in body image

IV. HEMODIALYSIS

A. Description
   1. The diffusion of dissolved particles from one fluid compartment into another across a semipermeable membrane
   2. The client's blood flows through one fluid compartment and the dialysate is in another fluid compartment

B. Functions of **hemodialysis**
   1. Cleanses the blood of accumulated waste products
   2. Removes the byproducts of protein metabolism such as urea, creatinine, and uric acid
   3. Removes excessive fluids
   4. Maintains or restores the body's buffer system
   5. Maintains or restores electrolyte levels

C. Principles of **hemodialysis**

1. The semipermeable membrane is made of a thin porous cellophane
2. The pore size of the membrane allows small particles to pass through such as urea, creatinine, uric acid, and water molecules
3. Proteins, bacteria, and blood cells are too large to pass through the membrane
4. The client's blood flows into the dialyzer; the movement of substances occurs from the blood to the dialysate
5. Diffusion: the movements of particles from an area of greater concentration to lesser concentration
6. Osmosis: the movement of fluids across a semipermeable membrane from an area of lesser to an area of greater concentration
7. Ultrafiltration: the movement of fluid across a semipermeable membrane as a result of an artificially created pressure gradient

D. Dialysate bath
1. Composed of water and major electrolytes
2. The dialysate bath need not be sterile because bacteria are too large to pass through; however, the dialysate must meet specific standards

E. Implementation
1. Monitor vital signs
2. Monitor laboratory values before, during, and after dialysis
3. Assess the client for fluid overload before the procedure
4. Assess patency of blood access device
5. Weigh the client before and after procedure to determine fluid loss
6. Hold antihypertensives and other medications that can affect the BP prior to the procedure as prescribed
7. Monitor for shock and hypovolemia during the procedure
8. Provide adequate nutrition (client may eat before the procedure)

V. COMPLICATIONS OF HEMODIALYSIS (Box 50-3)

A. Disequilibrium syndrome
1. Description

BOX 50-3

Complications of Hemodialysis

Hypotension and shock
Muscle cramping
Electrolyte changes
Sepsis
Loss of blood
Hepatitis
Disequilibrium syndrome
Dialysis encephalopathy

a. A rapid change in the composition of the extracellular fluid (ECF) occurs during hemodialysis
b. Solutes are removed from the blood faster than from the cerebrospinal fluid (CSF) and brain; fluid is pulled into the brain causing cerebral edema

2. Data collection
a. Nausea
b. Vomiting
c. Headache
d. Hypertension
e. Restlessness and agitation
f. Confusion
g. Seizures

3. Implementation
a. Monitor for signs of disequilibrium syndrome
b. Notify the physician if signs of disequilibrium syndrome occur
c. Prepare to dialyze the client for a shorter period at reduced blood flow rates to prevent occurrence

B. Dialysis encephalopathy
1. Description: an aluminum toxicity that occurs as a result of aluminum in the H_2O sources used in the dialysate bath and the ingestion of aluminum containing antacids (phosphate binders)
2. Data collection
a. Progressive neurological impairment
b. Mental cloudiness
c. Speech disturbances
d. Dementia
e. Muscle incoordination
f. Bone pain
g. Seizures
3. Implementation
a. Monitor for signs of dialysis encephalopathy
b. Notify the physician if signs of dialysis encephalopathy occurs
c. Administer aluminum chelating agents as prescribed so that the aluminum is freed up and dialyzed from the body

VI. ACCESS FOR HEMODIALYSIS

A. Subclavian and femoral catheter
1. Description
a. A subclavian (subclavian vein) or femoral (femoral vein) catheter may be inserted for short-term or temporary use in **ARF**
b. May be used until a fistula or graft matures, or when the client has fistula or graft access failure caused by infection or clotting
2. Implementation

a. Monitor insertion site for hematoma, bleeding, dislodging, and infection
b. Do not use these catheters for any reason other than dialysis
3. Subclavian vein catheter
a. The catheter is capped between dialysis treatments
b. The catheter may be left in place for up to 6 weeks if complications do not occur
4. Femoral vein catheter
a. The client should not sit up more than 45 degrees or lean forward because the catheter may kink and occlude
b. Monitor extremity for circulation, temperature, and pulses
c. Prevent pulling or disconnecting of the catheter when giving care
d. Maintain patency of the catheter

B. External arteriovenous shunt (AV shunt) (Figure 50-1)
1. Description
a. Access is formed by the surgical insertion of two Silastic cannulas into an artery and a vein in the forearm or leg, to form an external blood path
b. The cannulas are connected to form a U shape; blood flows from the client's artery through the shunt into the vein.
c. A tube leading to the membrane compartment is connected to the arterial cannula
d. Blood fills the membrane compartment and flows back to the client by way of a tube connected to the venous cannula
e. When dialysis is complete, the cannulas are clamped and reattached to form their U shape
2. Advantages
a. Can be used immediately after creation
b. No venipuncture is necessary for dialysis
3. Disadvantages
a. External danger of disconnecting or dislodging
b. Risk of hemorrhage, infection, or clotting
c. Skin erosion around the catheter site can occur
4. Implementation
a. Avoid wetting the shunt
b. A dressing is completely wrapped around the shunt and kept dry and intact
c. Cannula clamps need to be available at the client's bedside
d. Do not take a blood pressure, draw blood, place an IV, or administer injections in the shunt extremity
e. Monitor for hemorrhage, infection, and clotting
f. Monitor skin integrity around insertion site
g. Note that the shunt is patent if warm
h. Auscultate and palpate for a bruit, although a bruit may not be heard and is not always felt with the shunt
i. Notify the physician immediately if signs of clotting, hemorrhage, or infection occur
5. Signs of clotting
a. Fold back Ace wrap to expose Silastic tubing and assess for signs of clotting
b. Fibrin-white flecks noted in the tubing
c. The separation of serum and cells
d. The absence of a previously heard bruit
e. Coolness of the tubing or extremity
f. Client complaints of a tingling sensation

C. Internal arteriovenous fistula (AV fistula) (Figure 50-2)
1. Description
a. Access of choice for chronic dialysis clients
b. Created surgically in which an artery in the arm is anastamosed to a vein; this creates an opening or fistula between a large artery and a large vein
c. The flow of arterial blood into the venous system causes the veins to become engorged (maturity)
d. Maturity takes about 1 to 2 weeks and is required before the fistula can be used, so

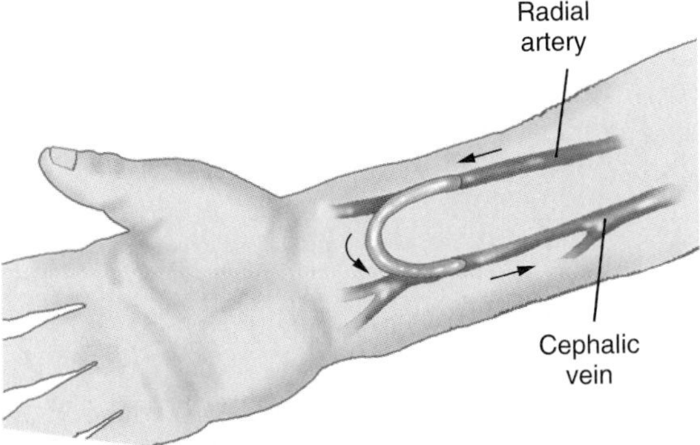

FIG. 50-1 Arteriovenous shunt. (From Sanders MJ et al: *Mosby's paramedic textbook*, ed 2, St Louis, 2000, Mosby.)

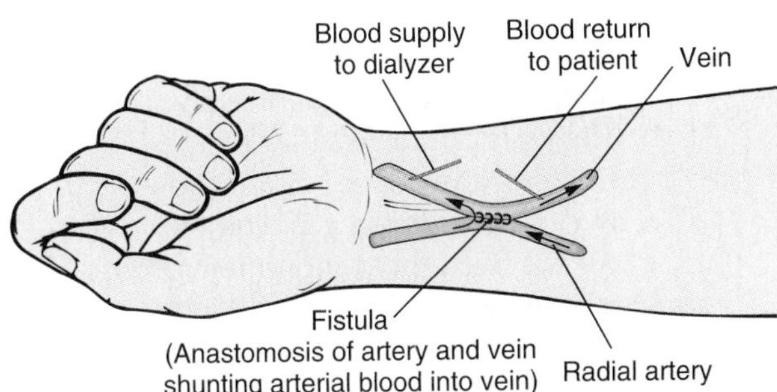

FIG. 50-2 Arteriovenous fistula. (From Lewis SM, Heitkemper MM, Dirksen SR: *Medical-surgical nursing*, ed 5, St Louis, 2000, Mosby.)

that the engorged vein can be punctured for the dialysis procedure using a large-bore needle
e. Subclavian or femoral catheters, **peritoneal dialysis**, or an external AV shunt can be used for dialysis while the fistula is maturing
2. Advantages
a. Because the fistula is internal, there is less danger of clotting and bleeding
b. The fistula can be used indefinitely
c. Decreased incidence of infection
d. No external dressing is required
e. Allows freedom of movement
3. Disadvantages
a. Cannot be used immediately after insertion
b. Needle insertions are required for dialysis
c. Infiltration of the needles during dialysis can occur and cause hematomas
d. An aneurysm can form in the fistula
e. Arterial steal syndrome can develop (too much blood is diverted to the vein and arterial perfusion to the hand is compromised)
f. CHF can occur from the increased blood flow in the venous system

D. Internal arteriovenous graft (AV graft)
1. Description
a. The internal graft is used primarily for chronic dialysis clients who do not have adequate blood vessels for the creation of a fistula
b. An artificial graft made of Gore-Tex or a bovine (cow) carotid artery is used create an artificial vein for blood flow
c. The procedure involves the anastomosis of the graft to the artery, a tunneling under the skin, and anastomosis to a vein
d. The graft can be used 2 weeks after insertion
e. Complications of the graft include clotting, aneurysms, and infection
2. Advantages
a. Because the graft is internal, there is less danger of clotting and bleeding
b. The graft can be used indefinitely
c. Decreased incidence of infection
d. No external dressing is required
e. Allows freedom of movement
3. Disadvantages
a. Cannot be used immediately after insertion
b. Needle insertions are required for dialysis
c. Infiltration of the needles during dialysis can occur and cause hematomas
d. An aneurysm can form in the fistula
e. Arterial steal syndrome can develop (too much blood is diverted to the vein and arterial perfusion to the hand is compromised)
f. CHF can occur from the increased blood flow in the venous system

E. Implementation: AV fistula and AV graft
1. Do not take a blood pressure, draw blood, place an IV, or administer injections in the fistula extremity
2. Monitor for clotting
a. Complaints of tingling or discomfort in the extremity
b. Inability to palpate or auscultate a bruit or thrill over the fistula or graft
c. Monitor for arterial steal syndrome
d. Palpate or auscultate for bruit or thrill over the fistula or graft
e. Palpate pulses below the fistula/graft and monitor for hand swelling as an indication of ischemia
f. Monitor for infection
g. Monitor lung and heart sounds for signs of CHF
h. Notify the physician immediately if signs of clotting, or infection or arterial steal syndrome occur

VII. PERITONEAL DIALYSIS (Figure 50-3)

A. Description
1. The peritoneum is the dialyzing membrane (semipermeable membrane) and substitutes for kidney function during kidney failure
2. Works on the principles of diffusion and osmosis, and the dialysis occurs via the transfer of fluid and solute from the bloodstream through the peritoneum
3. The peritoneal membrane is large and porous, allowing solutes and fluid to move via an osmotic gradient from an area of higher concentration in the body to lower concentration in the dialyzing fluid
4. The peritoneal cavity is rich in capillaries; therefore it provides a ready access to the blood supply

B. Contraindications for peritoneal dialysis
1. Peritonitis
2. Recent abdominal surgery
3. Abdominal adhesions
4. Impending renal transplantation

C. Dialysate solution
1. Solution is sterile and contains electrolytes, minerals, and glucose

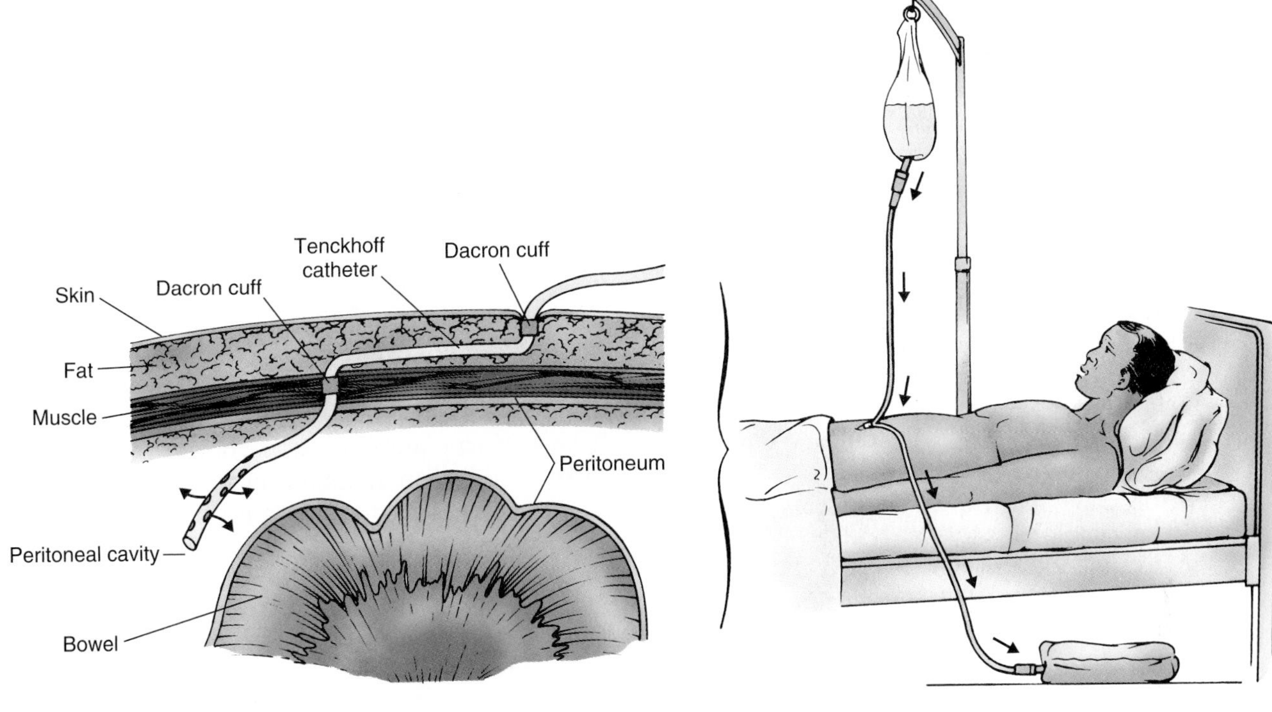

FIG. 50-3 Manual peritoneal dialysis via an implanted abdominal catheter (Tenckhoff catheter). (From Ignatavicius D, Workman M: *Medical-surgical: critical thinking for collaborative care*, ed 4, Philadelphia, 2002, WB Saunders.)

2. The higher the glucose concentration, the greater the amount of fluid removed during an exchange
3. Increasing the glucose concentration increases the concentration of active particles that cause osmosis, and increases the rate of ultrafiltration and the amount of fluid removed
4. Potassium: if hyperkalemia is not a problem, 4 mEq of potassium may be added to each bag of solution
5. Heparin: added to the dialysate solution to prevent clotting of the catheter
6. Antibiotics: prophylactic antibiotics may be added to dialysate to prevent peritonitis
7. Insulin: may be added to the dialysate for the client with diabetes mellitus

VIII. ACCESS FOR PERITONEAL DIALYSIS

A. Description
1. A surgical insertion of a siliconized rubber catheter into the abdominal cavity is required to allow infusion of dialysis fluid
2. The preferred insertion site is 3 to 5 cm below the umbilicus, as this area is relatively avascular and has less fascial resistance
3. The catheter is tunneled under the skin for stabilization and to reduce the risk of infection
4. Over a period of 1 to 2 weeks after insertion, there is an ingrowth of fibroblasts and blood vessels into the cuffs of the catheter, which fix the catheter in place and provide an extra barrier against dialysate leakage and bacterial invasion

B. Types of **peritoneal dialysis**
1. Continuous ambulatory **peritoneal dialysis** (CAPD)
   a. Closely resembles renal function because it is a continuous process
   b. Does not require a machine for the procedure
   c. Promotes client independence
   d. The client performs self-dialysis 24 hours a day, 7 days a week
   e. Four dialysis cycles are administered in 24 hours, including an 8-hour dwell overnight
   f. 1.5 to 2.0 liters of dialysate is instilled into the abdomen four times daily and allowed to dwell as prescribed
   g. The dialysis bag, attached to the catheter, is folded and carried in the client's clothing until time for outflow

h. After dwell, the bag is placed lower than the insertion site so fluid drains by gravity flow
i. When full, the bag is changed, and new dialysate is instilled into the abdomen, and the process continues
2. Automated **peritoneal dialysis** (APD)
a. Similar to CAPD in that it is a continuous dialysis process
b. Requires a peritoneal cycling machine
c. Can be done as intermittent peritoneal dialysis (IPD), continuous cycling peritoneal dialysis (CCPD), or nightly peritoneal dialysis (NPD)

C. **Peritoneal dialysis** infusion
1. Description
a. One infusion (inflow), dwell, and outflow, is considered one exchange
b. Uses an open system that presents a risk of infection
c. Inflow: the infusion of 1 to 2 liters of dialysate is infused by gravity into the peritoneal space, which usually takes approximately 10 to 20 minutes
d. Dwell time: the amount of time that the dialysate solution remains in the peritoneal space; prescribed by the physician
e. Outflow: fluid drains out of body by gravity into the drainage bag
2. Implementation before treatment
a. Monitor vital signs
b. Obtain weight
c. Have the client void if possible
d. Assess electrolyte and glucose levels
3. Implementation during treatment
a. Monitor vital signs
b. Monitor for signs of infection
c. Monitor for respiratory distress, pain, or discomfort
d. Monitor for signs of pulmonary edema
e. Monitor for hypotension and hypertension
f. Monitor for malaise, nausea, vomiting
g. Assess the catheter site dressing for wetness or bleeding
h. Monitor dwell time as prescribed by the physician and initiate outflow
i. Do not allow dwell time to extend beyond the physician's order, as this increases the risk for hyperglycemia
j. Turn the client from side to side or have client sit upright if flow is slow to start
k. Monitor outflow, which should be a continuous stream after the clamp is opened
l. Monitor outflow for color and clarity
m. Monitor I&O accurately
n. If outflow is less than inflow, the difference is equal to the amount absorbed or retained by the client during dialysis and should be counted as intake

IX. COMPLICATIONS OF PERITONEAL DIALYSIS

A. Peritonitis 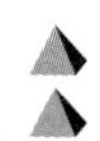
1. Maintain meticulous sterile technique with hooking up or clamping off bags and when caring for catheter insertion site
2. Follow institutional procedure for hooking up or clamping off bags, which may include scrubbing the connection sites with an antiseptic
3. Monitor temperature closely
4. Monitor for fever, cloudy outflow, and rebound abdominal tenderness
5. If peritonitis is suspected, obtain a culture of the outflow to determine the infective organism
6. Administer antibiotics as prescribed

B. Abdominal pain
1. Pain during inflow is common during the first few exchanges and is caused by peritoneal irritation and usually disappears after a week or two
2. The cold temperature of dialysate aggravates the discomfort, and the dialysate should be warmed before use only with a special dialysate warmer pad
3. Place a heating pad on the abdomen during the inflow to relieve discomfort

C. Insufficient outflow
1. May be caused by catheter migration out of the peritoneal area; if this occurs, catheter must be repositioned by the physician
2. Insufficient outflow can also be caused by a full colon
3. Maintain drainage bag below the client's abdomen
4. Change the client during outflow position by turning or ambulating
5. Check for kinks in the tubing
6. Encourage a high-fiber diet
7. Administer stool softeners as prescribed

D. Leakage around the catheter site
1. Over a period of 1 to 2 weeks after insertion of the catheter, an ingrowth of fibroblasts and blood vessels into the cuffs of the catheter occurs, which fixes the catheter in place and provides an extra barrier against dialysate leakage and bacterial invasion
2. It may take up to 2 weeks for the client to tolerate a full 2-liter exchange without leakage around the catheter site

E. Characteristics of outflow
1. During the first or initial exchanges, the outflow may be bloody; outflow should be clear and colorless thereafter

2. A brown outflow indicates bowel perforation
3. If the outflow is the same color as urine, bladder perforation has occurred
4. Cloudy outflow indicates peritonitis

X. UREMIC SYNDROME

A. Description
1. The accumulation of nitrogenous waste products in the blood due to the inability of the kidneys to filter out these waste products
2. It may occur as a result of **acute or chronic renal failure**

B. Data collection
1. **Oliguria**
2. The presence of protein, red blood cells, casts in the urine
3. A urine specific gravity of 1.010
4. Elevated levels of urea, uric acid, potassium, and magnesium in the urine
5. Hypotension or hypertension
6. Alterations in LOC
7. Electrolyte imbalances
8. Stomatitis
9. Nausea or vomiting
10. Diarrhea or constipation

C. Implementation
1. Monitor vital signs
2. Monitor electrolyte values
3. Monitor I&O
4. Provide diet low in protein unless the client is on **peritoneal dialysis**
5. Limit sodium, nitrogen, potassium, and phosphate intake as prescribed

XI. CYSTITIS/URINARY TRACT INFECTIONS (UTI) (Box 50-4)

A. Description
1. Inflammation of the bladder from infection or obstruction of the urethra
2. The most common causative organisms are *Escherichia coli, Enterobacter, Pseudomonas,* and *Serratia*
3. More common in females because they have a shorter urethra than males, and the location of the urethra in the female is close to the rectum
4. Sexually active and pregnant women are most vulnerable to cystitis

B. Data collection
1. Frequency and urgency
2. Burning on urination
3. Voiding in small amounts
4. Inability to void
5. Incomplete emptying of the bladder
6. Lower abdominal discomfort or back discomfort
7. Cloudy, dark, foul-smelling urine
8. Hematuria
9. Bladder spasms
10. Malaise, chills, fever
11. Nausea and vomiting

C. Implementation
1. Obtain a urine specimen for culture and sensitivity to identify bacterial growth before administering prescribed antibiotics
2. Instruct the client to drink fluids up to 3000 mL a day, especially if the client is taking a sulfonamide, because these medications can form crystals in concentrated urine
3. Maintain acid urine pH (5.5) by an acid-ash diet; instruct the client in foods to consume on an acid-ash diet
4. Use strict aseptic technique when inserting a urinary catheter
5. Maintain closed urinary drainage systems for clients with indwelling catheters
6. Provide meticulous perineal care for clients with indwelling catheters
7. Administer medications as prescribed, which may include analgesics, antiseptics, antispasmodics, antibiotics, and antimicrobials
8. Note that if the client is prescribed an aminoglycoside, a sulfonamide or nitrofurantoin (Macrodantin), that the actions of these medications are diminished by acidic urine
9. Discourage caffeine products as coffee, tea, and cola
10. Instruct the client to avoid alcohol
11. Provide heat to the abdomen or sitz baths for complaints of discomfort

BOX 50-4

Causes of Cystitis

Hormonal changes influencing alterations in vaginal flora
Loss of bactericidal properties of prostatic secretions in the male
Sexual intercourse
Poor-fitting diaphragms
Use of spermicides
Synthetic underwear and pantyhose
Wet bathing suits
Allergens or irritants such as soaps, sprays, bubble bath, perfumed sanitary napkins
Invasive urinary tract procedures
Indwelling urethral catheters
Bladder distention
Urinary stasis
Calculus

12. Instruct the client to take medications as prescribed
13. Instruct the client to take antibiotics on schedule and to take entire course of medications as prescribed, which may be a course of 10 to 14 days
14. Instruct the client in the importance of follow-up urine culture after treatment
15. Preventive measures are listed in Box 50-5

XII. UROSEPSIS

A. Description
   1. A gram-negative bacteremia originating in the urinary tract
   2. The most common organism responsible is *E. coli*
   3. The most common cause is the presence of an indwelling catheter or an untreated UTI in a client that is medically compromised
   4. The major problem is the ability of this bacterium to develop resistant strains
   5. Urosepsis can lead to septic shock if not treated aggressively

B. Data collection: fever is the most common and earliest manifestation

C. Implementation
   1. Obtain a urine specimen for urine culture and sensitivity
   2. Administer IV antibiotics as prescribed usually until the client has been afebrile for 3 to 5 days
   3. Administer oral antibiotics as prescribed after the 3- to 5-day afebrile period

BOX 50-5

Prevention of Cystitis

Teach the client good perineal care and to wipe from front to back
Instruct the client to avoid bubble baths and tub baths and avoid vaginal deodorants
Instruct the client to void every 2 to 3 hours
Instruct the client to void and drink a glass of water after intercourse
Instruct the female client to wear cotton pants and to avoid wearing tight clothes and panty hose with slacks, and to avoid sitting in a wet bathing suit for prolonged periods of time
Encourage menopausal women to use estrogen vaginal creams to restore pH
Instruct women to use water-soluble lubricants for coitus, especially after menopause

XIII. URETHRITIS

A. Description
   1. An inflammation of the urethra that is commonly associated with sexually transmitted diseases (STD) and may be seen with cystitis
   2. In men, it is most often caused by gonorrhea and chlamydial infection
   3. In women, it is most often caused by feminine hygiene sprays, perfumed toilet paper and sanitary napkins, spermicidal jellies, UTIs, and changes in the vaginal mucosal lining

B. Data collection
   1. Males
      a. Burning on urination
      b. Frequency
      c. Urgency
      d. Nocturia
      e. Difficulty voiding
      f. Discharge from the penis
   2. Females
      a. Frequency
      b. Urgency
      c. Nocturia
      d. Painful urination
      e. Difficulty voiding
      f. Lower abdominal discomfort

C. Implementation
   1. Encourage fluids
   2. Prepare the client for testing to determine if STD is present
   3. Administer antibiotics as prescribed
   4. Instruct the client in the administration of sitz baths
   5. If stricture occurs, prepare client for dilation of the urethra and instillation of an antiseptic solution
   6. Instruct the client to avoid intercourse until the symptoms subside or treatment of the STD is complete
   7. Instruct the female client to avoid the use of perfumed toilet paper, sanitary napkins, and feminine hygiene sprays

XIV. URETERITIS AND PYELONEPHRITIS

A. Ureteritis
   1. An inflammation of the ureter that is commonly associated with pyelonephritis
   2. Chronic pyelonephritis causes the ureter to become fibrotic and narrowed by strictures

B. Pyelonephritis
   1. An inflammation of the renal pelvis and the parenchyma commonly caused by bacterial invasion

2. Acute pyelonephritis often occurs after bacterial contamination of the urethra or after an invasive procedure of the urinary tract
3. Chronic pyelonephritis most commonly occurs after chronic obstruction with reflux or chronic disorders
4. *E. coli* is the most common bacterial-causing organism

C. Acute pyelonephritis
1. Usually a short course that recurs as a relapse of a previous infection or as a new infection
2. Can progress to bacteremia or chronic pyelonephritis
3. Data collection
   a. Fever and chills
   b. Nausea
   c. Flank pain on the affected side
   d. Costovertebral (CVA) tenderness
   e. Headache
   f. Muscular pain
   g. Dysuria
   h. Frequency and urgency
   i. Cloudy or bloody or foul-smelling urine
   j. Increased white blood cells (WBCs) in the urine

D. Chronic pyelonephritis
1. A slow, progressive disease that is usually associated with recurrent acute attacks
2. Causes contraction of the kidney and dysfunctioning of the nephrons, which are replaced by scar tissue
3. Can lead to **renal failure**
4. Data collection
   a. It is frequently diagnosed incidentally when a client is being evaluated for hypertension
   b. Poor urine concentrating ability
   c. Pyuria
   d. Azotemia
   e. Proteinuria
   f. Anemia
   g. Acidosis

E. Implementation
1. Monitor vital signs
2. Monitor I&O
3. Monitor weight
4. Encourage fluids up to 3000 mL a day
5. Encourage adequate rest
6. Instruct the client in high-calorie, low-protein diet
7. Provide warm, moist compresses to flank area
8. Encourage the client to take warm baths
9. Administer analgesics, antipyretics, and antiemetics as prescribed
10. Administer antibiotics as prescribed
11. Administer urinary antiseptics as prescribed
12. Monitor for signs of **renal failure**

XV. GLOMERULONEPHRITIS 

A. Description
1. A term that includes a variety of disorders, most of which are caused by an immunological reaction
2. It results in proliferative and inflammatory changes within the glomerular structure
3. Destruction, inflammation, and sclerosis of the glomeruli of both kidneys occur
4. Inflammation of the glomeruli results from an antigen-antibody reaction produced from an infection elsewhere in the body
5. Loss of kidney function develops

B. Causes
1. Immunological diseases
2. Streptococcal infection group A beta hemolytic
3. History of pharyngitis or tonsillitis 2 to 3 weeks before symptoms
4. Autoimmune diseases

C. Types
1. Acute: occurs 2 to 3 weeks after a streptococcal infection
2. Chronic: can occur after the acute phase or slowly over time

D. Complications
1. Heart failure
2. Hypertensive encephalopathy
3. Pulmonary edema
4. Renal failure

E. Data collection
1. Gross hematuria
2. Dark, smoky, cola-colored or red-brown urine
3. Proteinuria, which produces a persistent and excessive foam in the urine
4. Urinary debris
5. Mid to high specific gravity
6. Low urinary pH
7. **Oliguria** or **anuria**
8. Headache
9. Chills and fever
10. Fatigue and weakness
11. Anorexia, nausea, and vomiting
12. Pallor
13. Edema in the face and periorbital area, feet, or generalized
14. Shortness of breath, ascites, pleural effusion, and CHF
15. Abdominal or flank pain
16. Hypertension
17. Reduced visual acuity
18. Increased BUN and creatinine
19. Increased antistreptolysin O titer (used to diagnosis disorders caused by streptococcal infections)

F. Implementation
1. Monitor vital signs
2. Monitor I&O and urine closely
3. Monitor daily weight
4. Monitor for edema
5. Monitor for fluid overload, ascites, pulmonary edema, and CHF
6. Restrict fluid intake as prescribed
7. Provide a high-calorie and low-protein diet
8. Restrict sodium intake as prescribed if edema is present
9. Provide bed rest and limit activity
10. Instruct the client to obtain treatment for infections, specifically sore throats and upper respiratory infections
11. Administer diuretics, antihypertensives, and antibiotics as prescribed
12. Monitor for signs of **renal failure**, cardiac failure, hypertensive encephalopathy
13. Initiate seizure precautions as indicated and provide safety measures
14. Instruct the client to report signs of bloody urine, headache, or edema

XVI. NEPHROTIC SYNDROME

A. Description: a set of clinical manifestations arising from protein wasting secondary to diffuse glomerular damage

B. Data collection
1. Proteinuria
2. Hypoalbuminemia
3. Edema
4. Hyperlipidemia
5. Waxy pallor to the skin
6. Anemia
7. Anorexia
8. Malaise
9. Irritability
10. Amenorrhea or abnormal menses
11. Hematuria may be present
12. Hypertension

C. Implementation
1. Monitor vital signs
2. Monitor I&O
3. Bed rest if severe edema is present
4. Normal to low-protein diet as prescribed with adequate carbohydrate and calorie intake
5. Monitor daily weights
6. Provide mild sodium restriction as prescribed
7. Monitor potassium level, as potassium may be restricted from the diet if the potassium level increases
8. Administer diuretics as prescribed
9. Administer corticosteroids and cytotoxic medications as prescribed
10. Administer plasma volume expanders such as albumin, plasma, and dextran to raise the osmotic pressure
11. Administer anticoagulants as prescribed for those clients who develop renal vein thrombosis

XVII. HYDRONEPHROSIS

A. Description
1. Distention of the renal pelvis and calices caused by an obstruction of normal urine flow
2. The urine becomes trapped proximal to the obstruction
3. The causes include calculus, tumors, scar tissue, or kinks in the ureter

B. Data collection
1. Hypertension
2. Headache
3. Flank pain
4. Electrolyte imbalances

C. Implementation
1. Monitor vital signs frequently
2. Monitor for fluid and electrolyte imbalances including dehydration after the obstruction is relieved
3. Monitor for diuresis, which can lead to fluid depletion
4. Monitor daily weights
5. Monitor urine for specific gravity, albumin, and glucose
6. Administer fluid replacement as prescribed

XVIII. GENITOURINARY TUBERCULOSIS

A. Description
1. Usually a late manifestation of tuberculosis and is caused by the spread of *Mycobacterium tuberculosis* from the lungs through the bloodstream
2. *M. tuberculosis* is the cause of tuberculosis and is most often seen in the poor, the malnourished, those living in close housing, and in the immunosuppressed client

B. Data collection
1. Frequency and pain on urination
2. Bladder spasms
3. Fatigue
4. Weight loss
5. Tubercle bacilli in urine culture
6. Lesions noted on x-ray study
7. Tuberculosis nodules noted on the prostate

C. Implementation

1. Administer antitubercular medications as prescribed
2. Use precautions when handling urine specimens because the bacillus in the urine is infectious
3. Instruct the client to use precautions to prevent the spread of the disease
4. Instruct the client to use condoms during intercourse to prevent the spread of the disease

XIX. POLYCYSTIC KIDNEY DISEASE

A. Description
1. A cystic formation and hypertrophy of both kidneys that leads to cystic rupture, infection, formation of scar tissue, and damaged nephrons
2. There is no known way to arrest the progress of the destructive cysts
3. The ultimate result of this disease is **renal failure**

B. Types
1. Infantile polycystic disease: an inherited autosomal-recessive trait that results in the death of the infant within a few months after birth
2. Adult polycystic disease: autosomal-dominant trait that results in end-stage **renal failure**

C. Data collection
1. Flank, lumbar, or abdominal pain
2. Fever and chills
3. UTIs
4. Hematuria, proteinuria, and pyuria
5. Calculi
6. Hypertension
7. Palpable abdominal masses and enlarged kidneys

D. Implementation
1. Monitor for gross hematuria, which indicates cyst rupture
2. Increase sodium and water because waste, rather than retention of sodium, occurs
3. Provide bed rest if ruptured cysts and bleeding occur
4. Prepare the client for percutaneous cyst puncture for relief of obstruction or for draining an abscess
5. Prepare the client for dialysis or renal transplantation
6. Encourage the client to seek genetic counseling

XX. UROLITHIASIS AND NEPHROLITHIASIS

A. Description
1. Calculi or stones can form anywhere in the urinary tract; however, the most frequent site is the kidney
2. Problems that can occur as a result of calculi are pain, obstruction, and tissue trauma with secondary hemorrhage and infection
3. A KUB, IVP, computed tomography (CT) scan, and renal ultrasonography will determine the stone location
4. A stone analysis will be done after passage to determine the type of stone and assist in determining treatment
5. **Urolithiasis** refers to the formation of urinary stones; urinary calculi are formed in the ureter
6. **Nephrolithiasis** refers to the formation of kidney stones; kidney stones are formed in the renal parenchyma
7. When a calculus occludes the ureter and blocks the flow of urine, the ureter dilates, which is known as hydroureter
8. If the obstruction is not removed, urinary stasis results in infection, impairment of renal function on the side of the blockage, and hydronephrosis and irreversible kidney damage

B. Causes
1. Family history of stone formation
2. Diet high in calcium, vitamin D, milk, protein, oxalate, purines, or alkali
3. A high intake of purine-rich food
4. Obstruction and urinary stasis
5. Dehydration
6. Use of diuretics, which can cause volume depletion
7. UTIs and prolonged urinary catheterization
8. Immobilization
9. Hypercalcemia and hyperparathyroidism
10. Elevated uric acid

C. Data collection
1. Renal colic originates in the lumbar region and radiates around the side and down toward the testicle in the male, and to the bladder in the female
2. Ureteral colic radiates toward the genitalia and thigh
3. Sharp, severe pain of sudden onset
4. Dull, aching kidney
5. Nausea and vomiting, pallor, and diaphoresis during acute pain
6. Urinary frequency with alternating retention
7. Signs of UTI
8. Low-grade fever
9. RBCs, WBCs, and bacteria in urinalysis
10. Hematuria

D. Implementation
1. Monitor vital signs
2. Monitor I&O

3. Assess for fever, chills, and infection
4. Monitor for nausea, vomiting, and diarrhea
5. 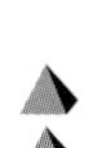 Encourage fluids up to 3000 mL per day unless contraindicated to facilitate the passage of the stone and prevent infection
6. Strain all urine for the presence of stones
7. Send stones to the laboratory for analysis
8. Provide warm baths and heat to flank area
9. Administer analgesics at regularly scheduled intervals as prescribed to relieve pain
10. Assess the client's response to pain medication
11. Administer IV fluids as prescribed to increase the flow of urine and facilitate the passage of the stone
12. Assist the client in performing relaxation techniques to assist in relieving pain
13. Instruct the client in the diet specific to the stone composition
14. Maintain urinary pH depending on type of stone
15. Turn and reposition immobilized clients
16. Prepare the client for surgical procedures if prescribed

E. Stone composition (Box 50-6 and Box 50-7)
   1. Calcium phosphate stones
      a. Caused by supersaturation of urine with calcium and phosphate
      b. Diet includes acid ash foods because calcium stones have an alkaline chemistry
      c. Dietary prescription may include to decrease intake of foods high in calcium and phosphate to reduce urinary calcium content, and to avoid excess vitamin D intake to prevent stones from forming
   2. Calcium oxalate stones
      a. Caused by supersaturation of urine with calcium and oxalate
      b. Diet includes acid ash foods because calcium stones have an alkaline chemistry
      c. Dietary prescription may include decreasing intake of foods high in calcium
      d. Dietary prescription may include to avoid oxalate food sources to reduce urinary oxalate content and the formation of stones
      e. Oxalate-rich foods include tea, almonds, cashews, chocolate, cocoa, beans, spinach, and rhubarb
   3. Struvite stones
      a. Also called triple phosphate stones and are made of magnesium and ammonium phosphate
      b. Caused by urea splitting by bacteria
      c. Struvite stones tend to form in alkaline urine
      d. Diet includes acid ash foods
      e. Dietary prescription includes limiting high phosphate foods such as dairy products, red and organ meats, and whole grains to reduce urinary phosphate content
   4. Uric acid stones
      a. Cause by excess dietary purine or gout
      b. Uric acid stones tend to form in acidic urine
      c. Dietary prescription may include alkaline ash foods and decreased intake of purine sources as organ meats, gravies, red wines, and sardines to reduce urinary purine content
      d. Allopurinol (Zyloprim) may be prescribed to lower uric acid levels
   5. Cystine stones
      a. Caused by cystine crystal formation
      b. Cystine stones tend to form in acidic urine
      c. Diet includes alkaline ash foods

BOX 50-6

Alkaline Ash Diet

OUTCOME
Increases the pH
Reduces the acidity of the urine

FOODS TO INCLUDE
Milk
Fruits except cranberries, plums, and prunes
Rhubarb
Most vegetables
Small amounts of beef, halibut, veal, trout, and salmon

BOX 50-7

Acid-Ash Diet

OUTCOME
Decreases pH
Makes the urine more acid

FOODS TO INCLUDE
Cheese
Eggs
Meat, fish, oysters, poultry
Bread, cereal, whole grains
Pastries
Cranberries, prunes, plums, tomatoes
Peas
Corn and legumes

d. Dietary prescription may also include a low intake of methionine, an essential amino acid that forms cystine, and the client would be instructed to avoid meat, milk, cheese, and eggs
e. Dietary measures also focus on encouraging fluid intake, up to 3 liters a day unless contraindicated, to help dilute the urine and prevent cystine crystals from forming

XXI. SURGICAL MANAGEMENT OF KIDNEY STONES

A. Cystoscopy
1. May be done for stones located in the bladder or lower ureter
2. There is no incision
3. One or two ureteral catheters are inserted past the stone
4. The stone may be manipulated and dislodged by the procedure
5. The catheters may mechanically guide the stones downward as they are removed
6. Catheters are left in place for 24 hours to drain the urine trapped proximal to the stone and to dilate the ureter
7. A continuous chemical irrigation may be prescribed to dissolve the stone

B. Extracorporeal shock wave lithotripsy (ESWL)
1. Noninvasive mechanical procedure for breaking up stones that are located in the kidney or upper ureter so that they can pass spontaneously or be removed by other methods
2. Fluoroscopy is used to visualize the stone
3. There is no incision or drains
4. Ultrasonic waves are delivered through a bath of warm water to the areas of the stone to disintegrate it
5. Stones are passed in the urine within a few days
6. Preprocedure: NPO for 8 hours before procedure
7. Postprocedure
   a. Monitor vital signs
   b. Monitor I&O
   c. Monitor for bleeding
   d. Monitor for pain and signs of urinary obstruction
   e. Instruct the client to increase fluid intake to wash out the stone fragments
   f. Inform the client that ambulation is important

C. Percutaneous lithotripsy
1. Performed for stones in the bladder, ureters, or kidney
2. An invasive procedure in which a guide is inserted under fluoroscopy near the area of the stone
3. An ultrasonic wave is aimed at the stone to break it into fragments
4. May be performed via cystoscopy or nephroscopy
5. No incision is required for cystoscopy; however, a small flank incision is needed for nephrostomy
6. The client may possibly have an indwelling catheter
7. A nephrostomy tube may be placed to administer chemical irrigation to break up the stone; nephrostomy tube may remain in place for 1 to 5 days
8. Encourage the client to drink 3000 to 4000 mL of fluid per day after the procedure
9. Monitor for and instruct client to monitor for complications of infection, hemorrhage, and extravasation of fluid into the retroperitoneal cavity

D. Ureterolithotomy
1. An open surgical procedure, performed if lithotripsy is not effective
2. Performed if the location of the stone is in the ureter
3. Incision into the ureter is made through a lower abdominal or flank incision to remove the stone
4. The client may have a Penrose drain, ureteral stent catheter, and an indwelling bladder catheter

E. Pyelolithotomy
1. A flank incision into the kidney is made to remove stones from the renal pelvis
2. A large flank incision is required
3. The client will have a Penrose drain and indwelling catheter

F. Nephrolithotomy
1. Incision into the kidney is made to remove the stone
2. A large flank incision is required
3. The client may have a nephrostomy tube and an indwelling catheter

G. Partial or total nephrectomy
1. Performed if there is extensive kidney damage, renal infection, or severe obstruction, and to prevent stone recurrence
2. Postoperative implementation
   a. The plan of care will be based on incision location and type of drainage tubes
   b. Monitor incision, particularly if a Penrose drain is in place, as it will drain large amounts of urine
   c. Protect the skin from urine

d. Place an ostomy pouch over the Penrose drain to protect the skin if urinary drainage is excessive
e. Monitor nephrostomy tube, which may be attached to a drainage bag for a free flow of urine
f. If urethral catheters are in place, do not irrigate
g. Monitor indwelling Foley catheter for drainage
h. Encourage fluid intake to ensure 2500 to 3000 mL or more of urine output per day
i. Monitor I&O closely
j. Determine composition of stone from laboratory analysis
k. Instruct the client in dietary restrictions if required
l. Instruct the client about medications that may be needed long term to reduce the development of calculi
m. Medications prescribed for calcium stones may include phosphates, thiazide diuretics, and allopurinol (Zyloprim)
n. Vitamin B_6 or magnesium oxide may be prescribed for clients with oxalate stones
o. Allopurinol (Zyloprim) may be prescribed for oxalate and uric acid stones
p. Long-term antibiotic use may be prescribed for struvite or cystine stones

XXII. KIDNEY TUMORS

A. Description
1. May be benign or malignant, bilateral or unilateral
2. Common sites of metastasis include bone, lungs, liver, spleen, or other kidney
3. The exact cause of renal carcinoma is unknown

B. Data collection
1. Dull flank pain
2. Palpable renal mass
3. Painless gross hematuria

C. Radical nephrectomy
1. Description
a. Removal of the entire kidney, adjacent adrenal gland, and renal artery and vein
b. Radiation therapy and possibly chemotherapy may follow radical nephrectomy
2. Postoperative implementation
a. Monitor vital signs
b. Monitor abdomen for distention caused by bleeding
c. Observe bed linens under the client for bleeding
d. Monitor for hypotension, decreases in urinary output, and alterations in LOC as indicating signs of hemorrhage
e. Monitor for signs of adrenal insufficiency
f. In clients with adrenal insufficiency, a large urinary output followed by hypotension and subsequent **oliguria** occurs
g. Administer IV fluids and packed RBCs as prescribed
h. Monitor I&O and daily weight
i. Monitor for a urinary output of 30 to 50 mL an hour to ensure adequate renal perfusion
j. Monitor urine for specific gravity
k. Maintain semi-Fowler's position
l. Monitor for signs of respiratory complications related to surgery
m. Encourage coughing and deep breathing exercises
n. Monitor bowel sounds for paralytic ileus
o. Apply antiembolism stockings as prescribed
p. Do not irrigate or manipulate the nephrostomy tube if in place
q. Administer pain medications as prescribed

XXIII. BLADDER TRAUMA

A. Description
1. Occurs after a blunt or penetrating injury to the lower abdomen
2. Penetrating wounds occur as a result of a stabbing, gunshot wound, or from other objects piercing the abdominal wall
3. A fractured pelvis that causes bone fragments to puncture the bladder is the most common cause of bladder trauma
4. When a blunt trauma occurs, it causes compression of the abdominal wall and the bladder

B. Data collection
1. **Anuria**
2. Hematuria
3. Pain over costovertebral area (CVA)
4. Nausea and vomiting

C. Implementation
1. Monitor vital signs
2. Monitor for hematuria, hemorrhage, and signs of shock
3. Promote bed rest
4. Monitor pain level
5. Prepare client for insertion of a suprapubic catheter to aid in urinary drainage if prescribed
6. Prepare client for surgical repair of the laceration if prescribed

XXIV. EPIDIDYMITIS

A. Description
1. An acute or chronic inflammation of the epididymis that occurs as a result of a urinary tract infection, sexually transmitted diseases, prostatitis, or long-term use of a Foley catheter
2. The infective organism passes upward through urethra and ejaculatory duct, along vas deferens to the epididymis

B. Data collection
1. Scrotal pain
2. Groin pain
3. Swelling in scrotum and groin
4. Pus and bacteria in the urine
5. Fever and chills
6. Abscess development

C. Implementation
1. Encourage fluid intake
2. Encourage bed rest with the scrotum elevated to prevent traction on the spermatic cord to facilitate drainage and to relieve pain
3. Instruct the client in the intermittent application of cold compresses to scrotum
4. Instruct the client in the use of sitz baths
5. Instruct the client in the administration of antibiotics for self and sexual partner if chlamydia or gonorrhea is the cause
6. Instruct the client to avoid lifting, straining, and sexual contact until the infection subsides

XXV. PROSTATITIS

A. Description
1. An inflammation of the prostate gland that can be caused by an infectious agent (bacterial) or by tissue hyperplasia (abacterial)
2. Bacterial prostatitis occurs as a result of the organism reaching the prostate via the urethra or bloodstream
3. Abacterial prostatitis usually occurs after a viral illness or a decrease in sexual activity

B. Data collection
1. Bacterial
   a. Fever and chills
   b. Dysuria
   c. Urethral discharge
   d. Boggy tender prostate
   e. Urethral discharge on palpation of prostrate
   f. WBCs found in prostatic secretions
2. Abacterial
   a. Backache
   b. Dysuria
   c. Perineal pain
   d. Frequency
   e. Hematuria
   f. Irregularly enlarged, firm, and tender prostate

C. Implementation
1. Encourage adequate fluid intake
2. Instruct the client in the use of sitz baths to promote comfort
3. Administer antibiotics, analgesics, antispasmodics, and stool softeners as prescribed
4. Inform the client of activities to drain the prostate such as intercourse, masturbation, and prostatic massage
5. Instruct the client to avoid spicy foods, coffee, alcohol, prolonged auto rides, and sexual intercourse during an acute inflammation

XXVI. BENIGN PROSTATIC HYPERTROPHY OR HYPERPLASIA (BPH)

A. Description
1. A slow enlargement of the prostate gland with hypertrophy and hyperplasia of normal tissue
2. The enlargement causes narrowing of the urethra and results in partial or complete obstruction
3. The cause is unknown and the disorder usually occurs in men older than 50 years

B. Data collection
1. Urgency, frequency, and hesitancy
2. Changes in size and force of urinary stream
3. Retention
4. Dribbling
5. Nocturia
6. Hematuria
7. Urinary stasis
8. Urinary tract infections

C. Implementation
1. Encourage fluids of up to 2000 to 3000 mL per day unless contraindicated
2. Prepare for bladder drainage via urinary catheterization for distention
3. Avoid administering medications such as anticholinergics, which cause urinary retention
4. Administer androgen-depriving agents such as finasteride (Proscar) as prescribed
5. Prepare the client for surgery as prescribed (Box 50-8)

BOX 50-8

Surgical Interventions for BPH

Transurethral resection (TUR)
Retropubic prostatectomy
Suprapubic prostatectomy
Perineal prostectomy

D. Transurethral resection (TUR)
   1. Insertion of a scope into urethra to excise prostatic tissue
   2. Bleeding is common after TUR and monitoring for hemorrhage is an important nursing intervention
   3. A continuous bladder irrigation (CBI) will be prescribed in the postoperative period to maintain the urine at a pink color
   4. Bladder spasms are common after surgery and antispasmodics for the bladder spasms may be prescribed
   5. Dribbling or incontinence may occur in the postoperative period, and it is important for the nurse to instruct the client to monitor for recurrence
   6. Sterility may or may not occur after the surgical procedure

E. Suprapubic prostatectomy
   1. Removal of the prostate by an abdominal incision with a bladder incision
   2. The client will have an abdominal dressing, which may drain copious amounts of urine, and the abdominal dressing will need to be changed frequently
   3. Severe hemorrhage is possible and monitoring for blood loss is an important nursing intervention
   4. Bladder spasms are common and antispasmodics may be prescribed for the bladder spasms
   5. CBI will be prescribed and administered to keep the urine pink in color
   6. A longer healing process is involved as compared with the TUR
   7. Sterility occurs with this procedure

F. Retropubic prostatectomy
   1. Removal of the prostate gland by a low abdominal incision without opening the bladder
   2. Less bleeding occurs with this procedure and the client experiences fewer bladder spasms
   3. There is minimal abdominal drainage
   4. CBI may be used
   5. Sterility occurs with this procedure

G. Perineal prostatectomy
   1. The prostate gland is removed through an incision made between the scrotum and anus
   2. Minimal bleeding occurs with this procedure
   3. The client needs to be monitored closely for infection, as the risk of infection is increased with this type of prostectomy
   4. Urinary incontinence is common
   5. The procedure causes sterility
   6. It is important to teach the client how to perform perineal exercises
   7. It is important to avoid inserting rectal tubes and taking the temperature rectally
   8. The administration of enemas also needs to be avoided

H. Postoperative implementation
   1. Monitor vital signs
   2. Monitor urinary output
   3. Increase fluids to 2000 to 3000 mL a day unless contraindicated
   4. Ambulate the client as early as possible and as soon as urine begins to clear
   5. Monitor urine for hemorrhage and clots
   6. Monitor for arterial bleeding as evidenced by bright red urine with numerous clots, and if it occurs, increase CBI and notify the physician immediately
   7. Monitor for venous bleeding as evidenced by burgundy-colored urine output, and if it occurs, inform the physician, who may apply traction on the catheter
   8. Monitor hemoglobin and hematocrit levels
   9. Expect red to light pink urine for 24 hours, which will turn to amber in 3 days
   10. Inform the client that a continuous feeling of an urge to void is normal
   11. Instruct the client to avoid attempts to void around the catheter, as it will cause bladder spasms
   12. Administer antibiotics, analgesics, stool softeners, and antispasmodics as prescribed
   13. Monitor 3-way Foley catheter, which will have a 30- to 45-mL retention balloon (Box 50-9)
   14. Maintain continuous bladder irrigation (CBI) with normal saline or prescribed solution to keep the catheter free of obstruction

I. Postoperative suprapubic prostatectomy
   1. Monitor suprapubic and Foley catheter drainage
   2. Monitor CBI if prescribed
   3. Note that the Foley catheter will be removed 2 to 4 days after surgery if the client has a suprapubic catheter
   4. Clamp the suprapubic catheter after the Foley catheter is removed and instruct client to attempt to void
   5. After the client has voided, assess residual urine in the bladder by unclamping the suprapubic tube
   6. Prepare for removal of suprapubic catheter when client consistently empties bladder and residual urine is 75 mL or less
   7. Monitor suprapubic incision dressing, which may become saturated with urine until the incision heals

BOX 50-9

Postoperative Care After TURP and Related Surgical Procedures

CONTINUOUS BLADDER IRRIGATION (CBI)

A three-way (lumen) irrigation to decrease bleeding and to keep the bladder free from clots:
One lumen for inflating the balloon (30 mL)
One lumen for instillation (inflow)
One lumen for outflow

IMPLEMENTATION

Maintain traction on the catheter if applied to prevent bleeding by pulling the catheter taut and taping it to the abdomen or thigh
Instruct the client to keep the leg straight if traction is applied to the catheter and taped to the thigh
Catheter traction is not released without a physician's order and is usually released after any bright red drainage has diminished
Use normal saline or prescribed solution only to prevent water intoxication
Run the solution at a rate as prescribed to keep the urine pink in color
Run the solution rapidly if bright red drainage or clots are present
Run the solution as about 40 gtts per minute when the bright red drainage clears
If the urinary catheter becomes obstructed, turn off the CBI and irrigate the catheter with 30 to 50 mL of normal saline if prescribed; notify physician if obstruction does not resolve
Monitor for TUR syndrome or severe hyponatremia (water intoxication) caused by the excessive absorption of bladder irrigation (altered mental status, bradycardia, increased blood pressure, and confusion)
Discontinue CBI and Foley catheter as prescribed, which is usually 24 to 48 hours after surgery
Monitor for continence and urinary retention when the catheter is removed
Inform the client that some burning, frequency, and dribbling may occur after catheter removal
Inform the client that he should be voiding 150 to 200 mL of clear yellow urine every 3 to 4 hours by 3 days after surgery
Inform the client that he may pass small clots and tissue debris for several days
Teach the client to avoid heavy lifting, stressful exercise, driving, Valsalva maneuver, and sexual intercourse for 2 to 6 weeks to prevent strain, and to call the physician if bleeding occurs or there is a decrease in urinary stream
Instruct the client to drink 2000 to 3000 mL of fluid each day, preferably before 8 PM
Instruct the client to avoid alcohol, caffeinated beverages, and spicy foods to avoid overstimulation of the bladder
Instruct the client, that if the urine becomes bloody, to rest and increase fluid intake and, that if the bleeding does not subside, to notify the physician

J. Postoperative retropubic prostatectomy
   1. Note that because the bladder is not entered, there is no urinary drainage on the abdominal dressing
   2. Monitor for infection
   3. Assess for urinary or purulent drainage on the dressing; if this occurs notify the physician
   4. Monitor for fever and increased pain, which may indicate an infection

K. Postoperative perineal prostatectomy
   1. Note that the client will have an incision, which may or may not have a drain
   2. Avoid rectal thermometers, rectal tubes, and enemas, as they may cause trauma and bleeding

XXVII. KIDNEY TRANSPLANTATION

A. Description
   1. Implantation of a human kidney from a compatible donor into a recipient
   2. Performed for irreversible kidney failure
   3. Immunosuppressive medications must be taken by the recipient for life

B. Living related donors
   1. Most desirable source of kidneys for transplant is living related donors who match client closely
   2. Screened for ABO blood group, tissue-specific antigen, human leukocyte antigen (HLA) suitability, and mixed lymphocyte culture index (histocompatibility)
   3. Donor must be in excellent health with two properly functioning kidneys
   4. The emotional well-being of the donor is determined
   5. Complete understanding of donation process and outcome is necessary

C. Cadaver donors
   1. Must meet criteria of brain death
   2. Must be under 60 years of age
   3. Must have normal renal function
   4. No malignant disease outside of the CNS can be present
   5. No generalized infection can be present
   6. No abdominal or renal trauma can be present
   7. Normal BP must be present
   8. Potential donor must have a negative hepatitis B antigen and negative human immunodeficiency virus antibody

9. Continuous ventilation and heartbeat are maintained until the kidneys are surgically removed
10. Once potential donor has demonstrated cerebral death, it is crucial to restore intravascular volume, wean from vasopressors, and establish diuresis

D. Warm ischemic time
1. The time elapsed between the cessation of, perfusion and cooling of the kidney, and the time required for anastomosis of the kidney
2. Maximal allowable warm ischemic time is 30 to 60 minutes
3. Kidney can be cooled and then the maximum time for transplantation is increased to 24 to 48 hours

E. Preoperative implementation
1. Verify histocompatability tests of identical twin or family member
2. Administer immunosuppressive medications to recipient as prescribed for 2 days before the transplantation
3. Maintain protective isolation
4. Verify that **hemodialysis** of recipient was completed 24 hours before transplantation
5. Ensure client is free of any infections
6. Assess renal function studies
7. Encourage discussion of feelings of both donor and recipient

F. Postoperative implementation
1. Kidney begins to function immediately or may be delayed a few days
2. **Hemodialysis** is performed until adequate kidney function is established
3. Monitor vital signs
4. Monitor I&O
5. Monitor urine output every hour
6. Monitor daily laboratory studies, urine for blood and specific gravity, daily weight, pulse oximetry, BUN, and creatinine levels
7. Maintain the client in semi-Fowler's position
8. Monitor for patency of Foley catheter
9. Note that urine is pink and bloody initially, but gradually returns to normal within several days to weeks
10. Monitor for gross hematuria and clots, which are not expected; notify the physician if they occur
11. Monitor 3-way Foley irrigation, if prescribed, to prevent blood clot formation
12. Note that the Foley catheter should be removed as soon as possible to prevent infection
13. Maintain protective isolation precautions and monitor for infection
14. Monitor IV fluids closely and for fluid overload
15. Begin oral fluids in 21 to 24 hours as prescribed
16. Monitor for bowel sounds and initiate diet as prescribed when bowel sounds return
17. Maintain good oral hygiene monitoring for stomatitis and bacterial and fungal infections
18. Encourage coughing and deep breathing exercises
19. Maintain strict aseptic technique with wound care
20. Administer medications as prescribed, which may include antifungal medications, antibiotics, immunosuppressive agents, and corticosteroids
21. Assess for organ rejection (Box 50-10)
22. Promote live donor and recipient relationship
23. Monitor client and recipient for depression

G. Graft rejection: except for identical twin donor and recipient, the major postoperative complication is graft rejection
1. Data collection
   a. Fever
   b. Malaise
   c. Elevated WBC
   d. Graft tenderness
   e. Signs of deteriorating renal function
   f. Acute hypertension
   g. Anemia
2. Hyperacute rejection
   a. Occurs immediately after surgery to 48 hours after surgery
   b. Implementation: removal of rejected kidney
3. Acute rejection
   a. Occurs within 6 weeks but can occur as late as 2 years

BOX 50-10

Client Instructions After Kidney Transplantation

Instruct the client to avoid prolonged periods of sitting
Instruct the client to recognize the signs and symptoms of infection and rejection
Instruct the client to avoid contact sports
Instruct the client to avoid exposure to people with infections
Instruct the client in the signs and symptoms of infection and to monitor for infection
Instruct the client in the use of medications as prescribed and in the importance of maintenance of immunosuppressive therapy for life

b. Potentially reversible with increased immunosuppression
c. Implementation: high doses of steroids; if steroids are ineffective, monoclonal antibodies may be administered
4. Chronic rejection
a. Occurs slowly months to years after transplantation
b. Can be irreversible
c. Mimics CRF
d. Implementation: immunosuppressive medications

PRACTICE QUESTIONS

1. A nurse has inserted an indwelling Foley catheter and inflates the balloon. The client immediately complains of pain. Which of the following represents the best plan by the nurse?
   1. Tell the client that the discomfort will pass
   2. Withdraw 1 mL from the balloon of the catheter
   3. Deflate the balloon and push it farther into the bladder
   4. Deflate the balloon and replace it with another catheter
2. A nurse has an order to obtain a urinalysis from a client with an indwelling urinary catheter. The nurse would plan to avoid which of the following, which could contaminate the specimen?
   1. Obtaining the specimen from the urinary drainage bag
   2. Clamping the tubing of the drainage bag
   3. Aspirating a sample from the port on the drainage bag
   4. Wiping the port with an alcohol swab before inserting the syringe
3. A nurse is caring for the client who has had a renal biopsy. Which of the following interventions would the nurse avoid in the care of the client after this procedure?
   1. Encouraging fluids to at least 3 liters in the first 24 hours
   2. Administering PRN narcotics
   3. Testing serial samples with dipsticks for occult blood
   4. Ambulating the client in the room and hall for short distances
4. An elderly client with cystitis also has an indwelling urinary catheter. The nurse would plan to ensure that the nursing assistant does not:
   1. Use soap and water to cleanse the perineal area
   2. Keep the drainage bag below the level of the bladder
   3. Use the drainage tubing port to obtain urine samples
   4. Let the drainage tubing rest under the leg
5. A nurse is assisting the client with cystitis with diet selection with an acid-ash diet. The nurse encourages the client to eat which of the following foods?
   1. Low-fat milk
   2. Baked haddock
   3. Garden peas
   4. Apples
6. A client with acute pyelonephritis who was started on antibiotic therapy 24 hours ago is still complaining of burning with urination. The nurse would check the physician's orders to see if which of the following medications is prescribed?
   1. Phenazopyridine (Pyridium)
   2. Bethanechol chloride (Urecholine)
   3. Oxybutynin chloride (Ditropan)
   4. Propantheline bromide (Pro-Banthine)
7. A client who has a history of gout is also diagnosed with urolithiasis. The stones are determined to be of uric acid type. The nurse gives the client instructions in foods to limit, which include:
   1. Liver
   2. Apples
   3. Carrots
   4. Milk
8. A nurse is caring for a client who has been diagnosed as having a kidney mass. The client asks the nurse the reason for renal biopsy, when other tests such as CT scan and ultrasound are available. In formulating a response, the nurse incorporates the knowledge that renal biopsy:
   1. Helps differentiate between a solid mass and a fluid-filled cyst
   2. Provides an outline of the renal vascular system
   3. Gives specific cytological information about the lesion
   4. Determines whether the mass is growing rapidly or slowly
9. A female client is admitted to the Emergency Department after a fall from a horse. The physician orders insertion of a Foley catheter. The nurse notes blood at the urinary meatus while preparing for the procedure. The nurse should:
   1. Use extra povidone-iodine solution in cleansing the meatus
   2. Use a smaller size catheter
   3. Administer pain medication before inserting the catheter
   4. Notify the physician
10. A male client has a tentative diagnosis of urethritis. The nurse collects data from the client knowing that which of the following are manifestations of the disorder?
    1. Hematuria and penile discharge
    2. Hematuria and pyuria
    3. Dysuria and proteinuria
    4. Dysuria and penile discharge

11. A nurse is assisting in planning a teaching session with the female client diagnosed with urethritis resulting from infection with chlamydia. The nurse would plan to include which of the following points in the teaching session?
    1. The most serious complication of this infection is sterility
    2. The infection can be prevented by using spermicide to alter the pH in the perineal area
    3. Medication therapy should be continued for 2 weeks without interruption
    4. Sexual partners during the last 12 months should be notified and treated
12. A male client who is admitted for an unrelated medical problem is diagnosed with urethritis resulting from chlamydial infection. The nursing assistant assigned to the client asks the nurse what measures are necessary to prevent contraction of the infection during care. The nurse tells the assistant that:
    1. Enteric precautions should be instituted for the client
    2. Contact isolation should be initiated, as the disease is highly contagious
    3. Universal precautions are quite sufficient, as the disease is transmitted sexually
    4. Gloves and mask should be used when in the client's room
13. A client with chlamydial infection has received instructions on self-care and prevention of further infection. The nurse evaluates that the client needs further reinforcement if the client states to:
    1. Reduce the chance of reinfection by limiting the number of sexual partners
    2. Use latex condoms to prevent disease transmission
    3. Return to the clinic as requested for follow-up culture in 1 week
    4. Use doxycycline prophylactically to prevent symptoms of chlamydia
14. A nurse is caring for a client with epididymitis. The nurse anticipates which of the following findings on data collection?
    1. Fever, diarrhea, groin pain, and ecchymosis
    2. Fever, nausea and vomiting, and painful scrotal edema
    3. Diarrhea, groin pain, and scrotal edema
    4. Nausea and vomiting, and scrotal edema with ecchymosis
15. A client is in extreme pain from scrotal swelling that is caused by epididymitis. The nurse administers an intramuscular narcotic analgesic in the left arm to relieve the pain. The nurse should plan to do which of the following actions next?
    1. Tell the client to do ROM to the left arm to absorb the medication into the bloodstream
    2. Check the name bracelet of the client
    3. Put the side rails up on the bed
    4. Dim the lights in the room
16. A nurse is caring for the client with epididymitis. The nurse would avoid using which of the following treatment modalities in the care of the client?
    1. Bed rest
    2. Scrotal elevation
    3. Sitz bath
    4. Use of heating pad
17. A client has epididymitis as a complication of urinary tract infection. The nurse is giving the client instructions to prevent a recurrence. The nurse would evaluate that the client needs further instruction if the client states to:
    1. Drink increased amounts of fluids
    2. Continue to take antibiotics until all symptoms are gone
    3. Limit the force of the stream during voiding
    4. Use condoms to eliminate risk from chlamydia and gonorrhea
18. A client with acute prostatitis has difficulty voiding, which is accompanied by pain. The client asks the nurse "Can't you just put a catheter in so I won't be in this misery when I try to go?" The nurse's response is based on the understanding that catheterization:
    1. Will prolong the course of the inflammation
    2. Could result in obstruction from rebound edema once the catheter is removed
    3. Is avoided whenever possible to avoid pushing organisms up into the bladder
    4. Could puncture the prostate gland because it is so inflamed
19. A nurse is collecting data from a client who has had benign prostatic hyperplasia (BPH) in the past. To determine if the client is currently experiencing difficulty, the nurse asks the client about the presence of which of the following early symptoms?
    1. Urge incontinence
    2. Nocturia
    3. Decreased force of the stream of urine
    4. Urinary retention
20. A client who has a cold is seen in the Emergency Department with inability to void. Because the client has a history of benign prostatic hyperplasia (BPH), the nurse determines that the client should be questioned about use of which of the following medications?
    1. Diuretics
    2. Antibiotics
    3. Antitussives
    4. Decongestants
21. A client is diagnosed with benign prostatic hyperplasia (BPH), and is scheduled for transrectal ultrasound and drawing of a prostate-specific antigen (PSA) level. The client says to the nurse "I can't remember. Can you tell me again why I need these

tests to be done?" The nurse would respond that the tests:
1. Help to rule out the presence of cancer
2. Predict the course of BPH
3. Pinpoint the likelihood of developing urinary obstruction
4. Give an indication of whether intermittent self-catheterization is needed

22. A client who has had a prostatectomy has learned perineal exercises to gain control of the urinary sphincter. The nurse evaluates that the client needs further instruction if the client states to perform which of the following as part of these exercises?
1. Tighten the muscles as if trying to prevent urination
2. Contracting the abdominal, gluteal, and perineal muscles
3. Tightening the rectal sphincter while relaxing abdominal muscles
4. Performing the Valsalva maneuver

23. A client newly diagnosed with chronic renal failure (CRF) has many learning needs about the disease. The nurse prepares a teaching plan for this client to help the client adapt to the disease. The nurse recognizes that which of the following items pertaining to the client's situation is least likely to interfere with the client's ability to learn?
1. Anxiety
2. Memory deficits
3. Short attention span
4. Presence of family

24. A client with renal failure has a medication order for epoetin alfa (Epogen). The nurse would administer this medication:
1. Subcutaneously
2. Intramuscularly
3. With a full glass of water
4. Diluted in juice to enhance taste

25. A nurse is working with the client newly diagnosed with chronic renal failure (CRF) to set up a schedule for hemodialysis. The client states, "This is impossible! How can I even think about leading a normal life again if this is what I'm going to have to do?" The nurse determines that the client is exhibiting:
1. Withdrawal
2. Depression
3. Anger
4. Projection

26. A client newly diagnosed with chronic renal failure has recently begun hemodialysis. Knowing that the client is at risk for disequilibrium syndrome, the nurse monitors the client during dialysis for:
1. Hypertension, tachycardia, and fever
2. Hypotension, bradycardia, and hypothermia
3. Restlessness, irritability, and generalized weakness
4. Headache, deteriorating level of consciousness, and seizures

27. A client with chronic renal failure has been on dialysis for 3 years. The client is receiving the usual combination of medications for the disease, including aluminum hydroxide as a phosphate-binding agent. The client now presents with mental cloudiness, dementia, and complaints of bone pain. The nurse interprets that these data are compatible with:
1. Phosphate overdose
2. Aluminum intoxication
3. Advancing uremia
4. Folic acid deficiency

28. A hemodialysis client with a left arm fistula is at risk for steal syndrome. The nurse monitors this client for which of the following manifestations?
1. Warmth, redness, and pain in the left hand
2. Pallor, diminished pulse, and pain in the left hand
3. Edema and purplish discoloration of the left arm
4. Aching pain, pallor, and edema of the left arm

29. A nurse is reviewing the medical record of a client with a diagnosis of pyelonephritis. Which of the following disorders, if noted on the client's record, would the nurse identify as a risk factor for this disorder?
1. Hypoglycemia
2. Coronary artery disease
3. Diabetes mellitus
4. Orthostatic hypotension

30. A nurse is reviewing the client's record and notes that the physician has documented that the client has a renal disorder. On review of the laboratory results, the nurse would most likely expect to note which of the following?
1. Elevated blood urea nitrogen (BUN)
2. Decreased hemoglobin
3. Decreased red blood cell (RBC) count
4. Decreased white blood cell (WBC) count

31. A nursing assistant collects a urine specimen from a client and is planning to deliver the specimen to the laboratory after completing morning care to other assigned clients. The licensed practical nurse (LPN) instructs the nursing assistant to place the collected specimen in the refrigerator. The nursing assistant asks the LPN about the reason that the urine needs refrigeration. The LPN bases the response on the fact that when urine is allowed to stand unrefrigerated:
1. The urine becomes more acidic
2. Bacteria and white blood cells (WBCs) decompose
3. The urine clumps
4. The pH decreases

32. A nurse is collecting a 24-hour urine specimen from the client. Which of the following is an inaccurate action when collecting the specimen?
1. Ask the client to void, save the specimen, and note the start time

2. Discard the urine specimen at the start time
3. Place the specimen on ice or refrigerated
4. Ask the client to void at the end of the collection and add this to the collection

33. Which of the following would the nurse include in the plan of care for a client after a renal scan?
1. Place the client on radiation precautions for 18 hours
2. Save all urine in a radiation safe container for 18 hours
3. Limit contact with the client for 20 minutes per hour
4. No special precautions except to wear gloves if coming in contact with the client's urine

34. A client is scheduled for an intravenous pyelogram (IVP). Before the test, the priority nursing action would be to:
1. Administer an oral preparation of radiopaque dye
2. Restrict fluids
3. Determine a history of allergies
4. Administer a sedative

35. A nurse instructs the client to obtain a clean-catch urine culture. Which of the following statements, if made by the client, would indicate that the client understands the procedure for collecting the specimen?
1. "I need to empty the bladder into a container so that the full amount of urine can be determined."
2. "A urine specimen will be obtained from a catheter."
3. "I need to cleanse the labia using cleansing towels, void into toilet, and then void into sterile specimen container."
4. "I need to clean the labia with toilet paper and void into sterile specimen container."

36. After a renal biopsy, the client complains of pain at the biopsy site that radiates to the front of the abdomen. The nurse interprets this complaint and further monitors the client for:
1. Bleeding
2. Infection
3. Renal colic
4. A normal expected pain

37. A client is admitted to the hospital and has a diagnosis of early stage of chronic renal failure (CRF). Which of the following would the nurse expect to note on data collection of the client?
1. Polyuria
2. Polydypsia
3. Oliguria
4. Anuria

38. A nurse is reviewing the medication record of a client diagnosed with chronic renal failure. The nurse notes that the client is receiving aluminum hydroxide (Amphojel). The nurse determines that the purpose of this medication is to:
1. Combine with phosphorus and help eliminate phosphates from the body
2. Prevent ulcers
3. Promote the elimination of potassium from the body
4. Prevent constipation

39. A nurse is assisting a client on a low-potassium diet to select food items from the menu. Which of the following food items, if selected by the client, would indicate an understanding of this dietary restriction ?
1. Cantaloupe
2. Spinach
3. Lima beans
4. Strawberries

40. A nurse is caring for an 88-year-old woman suspected of having a urinary tract infection (UTI). Which of the following, if noted in the client, would alert the nurse to the possibility of the presence of a UTI?
1. Fever
2. Frequency
3. Confusion
4. Urgency

41. A nurse is providing dietary instructions to a client with a diagnosis of acute glomerulonephritis. Which of the following dietary measures would be included in the instructions?
1. Limit fluid intake
2. Restrict protein intake
3. Increase intake of high fiber foods
4. Increase intake of potassium-rich foods

42. A client passes a urinary stone and laboratory analysis of the stone indicates that it is composed of calcium oxate. Based on this analysis, which of the following would the nurse include in the dietary instructions?
1. Increase intake of meat, fish, plums, and cranberries
2. Avoid citrus fruits and citrus juices
3. Avoid green leafy vegetables such as spinach
4. Increase intake of dairy products

43. A nurse is performing an admission assessment on a client with a diagnosis of bladder cancer. Which of the following symptoms would the nurse most likely expect to note on assessment of this client?
1. Hematuria
2. Burning
3. Urgency
4. Frequency

44. A client with benign prostatic hyperplasia (BPH) undergoes a transurethral resection (TUR). The client is receiving continuous postoperative bladder irrigations. The nurse assesses the client for signs of transurethral resection (TUR) syndrome. Which of the following data would indicate the onset of this syndrome?

1. Bradycardia and confusion
2. Tachycardia and diarrhea
3. Decreased urinary output and bladder spasms
4. Increased urinary output and anemia

45. A client with prostatitis secondary to kidney infection has received instructions on management of the condition at home and prevention of recurrence. The nurse evaluates that the client understood the instructions if the client verbalized to:

1. Keep fluid intake to a minimum to decrease the need to void
2. Exercise as much as possible to stimulate circulation
3. Stop antibiotic therapy when pain subsides
4. Use warm sitz baths and analgesics to increase comfort

ANSWERS

1. *Answer:* 4

Rationale: The appropriate procedure, if the client complains of pain after insertion, is to remove the catheter after deflating the balloon and replace it with another one. This is preferred to option 3, which could make the client more at risk for developing urinary tract infection, as the catheter would be advanced after part of it was resting against the client's external genitalia. Options 1 and 2 are incorrect.

Test-Taking Strategy: Use the process of elimination. Options 1 and 2 are the least plausible and should be eliminated first. You would be able to discriminate correctly between options 3 and 4 using principles of aseptic technique. Review this procedure if you had difficulty with this question.

Level of Cognitive Ability: Application

Client Needs: Safe, Effective Care Environment

Integrated Concept/Process: Nursing Process/Implementation

Content Area: Adult Health/Renal

Reference: Potter P, Perry A: *Fundamentals of nursing,* ed 5, St Louis, 2001, Mosby, p. 459.

2. *Answer:* 1

Rationale: A urine specimen is not taken from the urinary drainage bag. Urine undergoes chemical changes while sitting in the bag and does not necessarily reflect current client status. In addition, it may become contaminated with bacteria from opening the system.

Test-Taking Strategy: This question tests a basic principle of asepsis. If this question was difficult in any way, review this technique.

Level of Cognitive Ability: Application

Client Needs: Safe, Effective Care Environment

Integrated Concept/Process: Nursing Process/Implementation

Content Area: Adult Health/Renal

Reference: DeWit S: *Fundamental concepts and skills for nursing,* Philadelphia, 2001, WB Saunders, p. 551.

3. *Answer:* 4

Rationale: After renal biopsy, the nurse ensures that the client remains in bed for at least 24 hours. Vital signs and puncture site assessments are done frequently during this time. Fluids are encouraged to reduce possible clot formation at the biopsy site. A Hematest is done on serial urine samples with urine dipsticks to evaluate bleeding. Narcotic analgesics are often needed to manage the renal colic pain that some clients feel after this procedure.

Test-Taking Strategy: Use the process of elimination. Begin to answer this question by recalling that pain and bleeding are potential concerns after this procedure. This would allow you to eliminate options 2 and 3 as possible responses. To discriminate between the last two options, you would need to recall that encouraging fluids will reduce clotting at the site, whereas ambulation could initiate or enhance bleeding at the biopsy site. Review care to the client after a renal biopsy if you had difficulty with this question.

Level of Cognitive Ability: Application

Client Needs: Physiological Integrity

Integrated Concept/Process: Nursing Process/Implementation

Content Area: Adult Health/Renal

Reference: Ignatavicius D, Workman M: *Medical-surgical: critical thinking for collaborative care,* ed 4, Philadelphia, 2002, WB Saunders, p. 1610.

4. *Answer:* 4

Rationale: Proper care of an indwelling catheter is especially important to prevent prolonged infection or reinfection in the client with cystitis. The nurse and all caregivers must use strict aseptic technique when emptying the drainage bag or obtaining urine specimens. The perineal area is cleansed thoroughly using mild soap and water at least twice a day and after a bowel movement. The drainage bag is kept below the level of the bladder to prevent urine from being trapped in the bladder; for the same reason, the drainage tubing is not placed under the client's leg. The tubing must drain freely at all times.

Test-Taking Strategy: Use the process of elimination. The wording of the question guides you to look for an incorrect response. Eliminate option 1 first, as this is a basic standard of care for the client with an indwelling catheter. Option 3 is also consistent with principles of asepsis and is eliminated next. To discriminate between options 2 and 4, recall that option 2 promotes drainage, whereas option 4 could impede drainage. Thus the answer to the question is option 4, according to the wording of the question. Review care to the client with an indwelling catheter if you had difficulty with this question.

Level of Cognitive Ability: Application

Client Needs: Safe, Effective Care Environment
Integrated Concept/Process: Nursing Process/Implementation
Content Area: Adult Health/Renal
Reference: DeWit S: *Fundamental concepts and skills for nursing,* Philadelphia, 2001, WB Saunders, p. 559.

5. *Answer:* 2
Rationale: Foods that are allowed on an acid-ash diet include meat, fish, shellfish, cheese, eggs, poultry, grains, cranberries, prunes, plums, corn, lentils, as well as foods with high amounts of chlorine, phosphorus, and sulfur. Foods that are not included are all milk and milk products; all other vegetables except corn and lentils; all fruits except cranberries, plums, and prunes; and foods containing high amounts of sodium, potassium, calcium, and magnesium.
Test-Taking Strategy: Use the process of elimination. This question is difficult to answer without specific knowledge of the types of foods that may be included in the acid-ash diet. Knowing that most fruits and vegetables are not included on the list may help you to eliminate options 3 and 4. To discriminate between options 1 and 2, it is necessary to know that foods such as meat, fish, cheese, and eggs are included, but milk and milk products are not. Review this diet if you had difficulty with this question.
Level of Cognitive Ability: Application
Client Needs: Health Promotion and Maintenance
Integrated Concept/Process: Nursing Process/Implementation
Content Area: Adult Health/Renal
Reference: Black J, Hawks J, Keene A: *Medical-surgical nursing: clinical management for positive outcomes,* ed 6, Philadelphia, 2001, WB Saunders, p. 825.

6. *Answer:* 1
Rationale: The pain experienced with pyelonephritis usually resolves as antibiotic therapy becomes effective. However, clients may be treated for urinary tract pain with phenazopyridine, which is a urinary analgesic. Bethanechol chloride is a cholinergic agent used with neurogenic bladder or for urinary retention. Oxybutinin and propantheline bromide are antispasmodics that are used to treat bladder spasm.
Test-Taking Strategy: Specific knowledge of the classifications of these medications is necessary to answer this question correctly. Review these medications if you had difficulty with this question.
Level of Cognitive Ability: Application
Client Needs: Physiological Integrity
Integrated Concept/Process: Nursing Process/Data Collection
Content Area: Pharmacology
Reference: Ignatavicius D, Workman M: *Medical-surgical: critical thinking for collaborative care,* ed 4, Philadelphia, 2002, WB Saunders, p. 1646.

7. *Answer:* 1
Rationale: Foods containing high amounts of purines should be avoided in the client with uric acid stones. This includes limiting or avoiding organ meats, such as liver, brain, heart, kidney, and sweetbreads. Other foods to avoid include herring, sardines, anchovies, meat extracts, consommés, and gravies. Foods that are low in purines include all fruits, many vegetables, milk, cheese, eggs, refined cereals, sugars and sweets, coffee, tea, chocolate, and carbonated beverages.
Test-Taking Strategy: To answer this question, begin by examining the options and classifying the types of food sources they represent. Options 2 and 3 represent foods that are grown, whereas options 1 and 4 represent foods that derive from animal sources. Because purines are end products of protein metabolism, eliminate options 2 and 3 first. To discriminate between options 1 and 4, you would need to know that organ meats such as liver provide a greater quantity of protein than milk. With this in mind, choose option 1 over option 4. Review the foods that are high in purines if you had difficulty with this question.
Level of Cognitive Ability: Application
Client Needs: Health Promotion and Maintenance
Integrated Concept/Process: Nursing Process/Implementation
Content Area: Adult Health/Renal
Reference: DeWit S: *Fundamental concepts and skills for nursing,* Philadelphia, 2001, WB Saunders, p. 494.

8. *Answer:* 3
Rationale: Renal biopsy is a definitive test that gives specific information about whether the lesion is benign or malignant. An ultrasound discriminates between a fluid-filled cyst and a solid mass. Renal arteriography outlines the renal vascular system.
Test-Taking Strategy: Use the process of elimination. Begin to answer this question by eliminating options 1 and 2 first. Basic knowledge of the purposes of biopsy helps you discard these quickly. To discriminate between options 3 and 4, remember that with biopsy the cells are examined under a microscope. This examination then yields specific information about the type of neoplastic cell. While some types of cancer grow more quickly than others, it is not possible to determine this for any one individual by biopsy. Thus you would choose option 3 as the better answer. Review the purpose of this test if you had difficulty with this question.
Level of Cognitive Ability: Application
Client Needs: Physiological Integrity
Integrated Concept/Process: Nursing Process/Implementation
Content Area: Adult Health/Renal
Reference: Ignatavicius D, Workman M: *Medical-surgical: critical thinking for collaborative care,* ed 4, Philadelphia, 2002, WB Saunders, p. 1610.

9. *Answer:* 4
Rationale: The presence of blood at the urinary meatus may indicate urethral trauma or disruption. The nurse notifies the physician, knowing that the client should not be catheterized until the cause of the bleeding is determined by diagnostic testing.
Test-Taking Strategy: This question is straightforward in wording and intent. Basic knowledge of catheter insertion allows you to easily eliminate each of the incorrect options. Review this procedure and the indications of urethral trauma if you had difficulty with this question.
Level of Cognitive Ability: Application
Client Needs: Physiological Integrity
Integrated Concept/Process: Nursing Process/Implementation
Content Area: Adult Health/Renal

Reference: DeWit S: *Fundamental concepts and skills for nursing,* Philadelphia, 2001, WB Saunders, p. 559.

10. ***Answer:*** 4
Rationale: Urethritis in the male client often results from chlamydial infection and is characterized by dysuria, which is accompanied by a clear to mucopurulent discharge. Because this disorder often coexists with gonorrhea, diagnostic tests are done for both and include culture and rapid assays.
Test-Taking Strategy: Use the process of elimination. Begin to answer this question by eliminating options 1 and 2. Urethritis is generally accompanied by dysuria in the male client, which is present only in options 3 and 4. Knowing that the problem originates in the urethra, not the kidney, you would then eliminate the option with proteinuria, which indicates a problem with kidney function. This leaves option 4 as the correct answer. The male client with urethritis has dysuria and discharge from the penis. Review the signs of urethritis if you had difficulty with this question.
Level of Cognitive Ability: Comprehension
Client Needs: Physiological Integrity
Integrated Concept/Process: Nursing Process/Data Collection
Content Area: Adult Health/Renal
Reference: Ignatavicius D, Workman M: *Medical-surgical: critical thinking for collaborative care,* ed 4, Philadelphia, 2002, WB Saunders, p. 1621.

11. ***Answer:*** 1
Rationale: The most serious complication of chlamydial infection is sterility. The infection can be prevented by the use of latex condoms. It is treated with doxycycline for 7 days, or with azithromycin (Zithromax) as a single dose. All sexual partners during the 30 days before diagnosis should be notified, examined, and treated as necessary.
Test-Taking Strategy: Use the process of elimination. Eliminate option 2 first as a possible answer using principles of infection control. Knowing that most courses of antibiotic therapy extend from 7 to 10 days in general may help you to eliminate option 3 next. To discriminate accurately between options 1 and 4, it is necessary to know either that sterility is a serious and permanent complication, or that partners within the last month should be notified and treated as needed. Review the complications of this infection if you had difficulty with this question.
Level of Cognitive Ability: Application
Client Needs: Health Promotion and Maintenance
Integrated Concept/Process: Teaching/Learning
Content Area: Adult Health/Renal
Reference: Ignatavicius D, Workman M: *Medical-surgical: critical thinking for collaborative care,* ed 4, Philadelphia, 2002, WB Saunders, p. 447.

12. ***Answer:*** 3
Rationale: Chlamydia is a sexually transmitted disease and is frequently called nongonococcal urethritis in the male client. It requires no special precautions. Caregivers cannot acquire the disease during administration of care, and using universal precautions is the only measure that needs to be used.
Test-Taking Strategy: This question is straightforward in nature. A basic knowledge of infection control and disease transmission guides you to select option 3 as correct. If this question was difficult for you, review transmission of this disorder and standard (universal) precautions.
Level of Cognitive Ability: Application
Client Needs: Safe, Effective Care Environment
Integrated Concept/Process: Nursing Process/Implementation
Content Area: Adult Health/Renal
Reference: Ignatavicius D, Workman M: *Medical-surgical: critical thinking for collaborative care,* ed 4, Philadelphia, 2002, WB Saunders, p. 447.

13. ***Answer:*** 4
Rationale: Antibiotics are not taken prophylactically to prevent acquisition of urethritis from chlamydia. The risk of reinfection can be reduced by limiting the number of sexual partners, and by the use of condoms. In some instances, follow-up culture is requested in 4 to 7 days to confirm a cure.
Test-Taking Strategy: Use the process of elimination. The wording of the question guides you to look for an incorrect response. Options 1 and 2 are the most obviously correct and are therefore eliminated as possible answers to the question. Knowing the basic principles of antibiotic therapy allows you to discard option 4, as antibiotics are not used intermittently at will for prophylaxis of this infection. Review the client teaching points related to this infection if you had difficulty with this question.
Level of Cognitive Ability: Comprehension
Client Needs: Health Promotion and Maintenance
Integrated Concept/Process: Nursing Process/Evaluation
Content Area: Adult Health/Renal
Reference: Ignatavicius D, Workman M: *Medical-surgical: critical thinking for collaborative care,* ed 4, Philadelphia, 2002, WB Saunders, p. 1621.

14. ***Answer:*** 2
Rationale: Typical signs and symptoms of epididymitis include scrotal pain and edema, which are often accompanied by fever, nausea and vomiting, and chills. It is most often caused by infection, although sometimes it can be caused by trauma. It needs to be correctly distinguished from testicular torsion.
Test-Taking Strategy: Use the process of elimination. Any disorder that ends in "itis" results from inflammation or infection. Therefore, an expected finding would be elevated temperature. With this in mind, you may eliminate options 3 and 4, as they do not contain fever as part of the response. Knowing that ecchymosis results from bleeding, which is not part of this clinical picture, helps you to choose option 2 over option 1. Review the signs of this infection if you had difficulty with this question.
Level of Cognitive Ability: Analysis
Client Needs: Physiological Integrity
Integrated Concept/Process: Nursing Process/Data Collection
Content Area: Adult Health/Renal
Reference: Ignatavicius D, Workman M: *Medical-surgical: critical thinking for collaborative care,* ed 4, Philadelphia, 2002, WB Saunders, p. 1803.

15. ***Answer:*** 3
Rationale: The client who receives a narcotic analgesic should immediately have the side rails raised on the bed to prevent

injury after the medication has taken effect. Dimming the light in the room is the next most helpful action. The name bracelet should have been checked before administering the medication. It is unnecessary to do range of motion at the site of injection.
Test-Taking Strategy: Use the process of elimination. Begin to answer this question by eliminating option 2, as this should have been done before administering the medication. Option 1 is not necessary and may be eliminated next. To discriminate between options 3 and 4, note that the question asks you for the action to be taken "next." With this in mind, you would choose option 3. Although option 4 is a correct answer, it would be done upon leaving the room. As part of protecting the client's safety after administration of a narcotic analgesic, you would put the side rails up first. Review care to the client receiving pain medication if you had difficulty with this question.
Level of Cognitive Ability: Application
Client Needs: Physiological Integrity
Integrated Concept/Process: Nursing Process/Implementation
Content Area: Adult Health/Renal
Reference: DeWit S: *Fundamental concepts and skills for nursing,* Philadelphia, 2001, WB Saunders, p. 317.

16. *Answer:* 4
Rationale: Common interventions used in the treatment of epididymitis include bed rest, elevation of the scrotum with a Bellevue bridge, ice packs, sitz baths, analgesics, and antibiotics. A heating pad would not be used because direct application of heat could increase blood flow to the area and increase the swelling.
Test-Taking Strategy: Use the process of elimination. Begin to answer this question by eliminating options 1 and 2, as they are obviously the most helpful in the care of the client. In examining options 3 and 4, note that they both address the application of heat to the client. A sitz bath uses a milder temperature and the heat is moist and soothing. Knowing that direct heat may increase inflammation with tissue that is already at risk would guide you to choose option 4 as the item to avoid. Review care to the client with epididymitis if you had difficulty with this question.
Level of Cognitive Ability: Application
Client Needs: Physiological Integrity
Integrated Concept/Process: Nursing Process/Implementation
Content Area: Adult Health/Renal
Reference: Ignatavicius D, Workman M: *Medical-surgical: critical thinking for collaborative care,* ed 4, Philadelphia, 2002, WB Saunders, p. 1803.

17. *Answer:* 2
Rationale: The client who experiences epididymitis from urinary tract infection (UTI) should increase intake of fluids to flush the urinary system. Because organisms can be forced into the vas deferens and epididymis from strain or pressure during voiding, the client may limit the force of the stream. Condom use can help to prevent urethritis and epididymitis from sexually transmitted diseases. Antibiotics are always taken until the full course of therapy is completed.
Test-Taking Strategy: Use the process of elimination. The wording of the question guides you to look for an incorrect response. Because option 1 is consistent with good practices in the prevention of UTI, this option may be eliminated first. To eliminate options 3 and 4, it is necessary to know that the force of stream should be limited to prevent backflow into the epididymis, and that condoms are helpful in preventing this disorder from occurring as a complication of an STD. Remember that antibiotics are not stopped when symptoms subside, but must be taken until the full course of therapy is completed. Review care to the client with epididymitis if you had difficulty with this question.
Level of Cognitive Ability: Comprehension
Client Needs: Health Promotion and Maintenance
Integrated Concept/Process: Nursing Process/Evaluation
Content Area: Adult Health/Renal
Reference: Ignatavicius D, Workman M: *Medical-surgical: critical thinking for collaborative care,* ed 4, Philadelphia, 2002, WB Saunders, p. 1803.

18. *Answer:* 3
Rationale: Occasionally, the client with acute prostatitis needs urinary catheterization if the client cannot void at all. Otherwise, catheterization is avoided to prevent introducing bacteria into the bladder by pushing them up the urethra. Catheterization does not prolong the course of the inflammation, nor does it cause rebound edema when it is discontinued. There is no reported risk of prostate gland puncture from this procedure, although it may be painful.
Test-Taking Strategy: Use the process of elimination. Option 4 is the least plausible of all the choices and is eliminated first. Option 1 is also not very plausible and may be eliminated next. In comparing the remaining two responses, knowledge of transmission of infection would guide you to choose option 3 over option 2. Review this procedure if you had difficulty with this question.
Level of Cognitive Ability: Comprehension
Client Needs: Physiological Integrity
Integrated Concept/Process: Nursing Process/Implementation
Content Area: Adult Health/Renal
Reference: Ignatavicius D, Workman M: *Medical-surgical: critical thinking for collaborative care,* ed 4, Philadelphia, 2002, WB Saunders, p. 1902.

19. *Answer:* 3
Rationale: Decreased force in the stream of urine is an early sign of BPH. The stream later becomes weak and dribbling. The client may then develop hematuria, frequency, urgency, urge incontinence, and nocturia. If untreated, complete obstruction and urinary retention can occur.
Test-Taking Strategy: Use the process of elimination. Note that the question asks for an early symptom. If you know that benign prostatic hyperplasia can lead to urinary obstruction, you can then work backwards from the most severe symptom to the least, which should also be the earliest. Option 4 is obviously the most severe of symptoms and therefore is eliminated first. Options 1 and 2 are also more severe than option 3, which guides you to select option 3 as the answer to the question. Review the signs of benign prostatic hyperplasia if you had difficulty with this question.
Level of Cognitive Ability: Application
Client Needs: Physiological Integrity

Integrated Concept/Process: Nursing Process/Data Collection
Content Area: Adult Health/Renal
Reference: Ignatavicius D, Workman M: *Medical-surgical: critical thinking for collaborative care,* ed 4, Philadelphia, 2002, WB Saunders, p. 1784.

20. ***Answer:*** 4
Rationale: In the client with BPH, episodes of urinary retention can be triggered by certain medications, such as decongestants, anticholinergics, and antidepressants. The client should be questioned about use of these medications if presenting with urinary retention. Retention can also be precipitated by other factors such as alcoholic beverages, infection, bed rest and becoming chilled.
Test-Taking Strategy: Use the process of elimination. The question is asking about medications that could exacerbate or contribute to urinary retention in the client with BPH. Diuretics should help voiding; therefore option 1 is easily eliminated. Antibiotics should have no effect at all; thus option 2 is eliminated as well. To discriminate between options 3 and 4, it is necessary to know that medications that contain anticholinergics may cause urinary retention. This would guide you to choose option 4 over option 3. Antitussives have no effect on urinary retention. Review the causes of urinary retention in the client with BPH if you had difficulty with this question.
Level of Cognitive Ability: Analysis
Client Needs: Physiological Integrity
Integrated Concept/Process: Nursing Process/Data Collection
Content Area: Adult Health/Renal
Reference: Ignatavicius D, Workman M: *Medical-surgical: critical thinking for collaborative care,* ed 4, Philadelphia, 2002, WB Saunders, p. 1783.

21. ***Answer:*** 1
Rationale: A transrectal ultrasound and PSA level help to rule out the possibility of prostate cancer. They do not predict the course of BPH or the development of complications such as urinary obstruction. These tests have nothing to do with determining need for self-catheterization.
Test-Taking Strategy: Use the process of elimination. Begin to answer this question by eliminating options 2 and 3. These diagnostic tests do not predict the course of the disease or the likelihood of developing complications (such as obstruction). Diagnostic tests also will not determine whether self-catheterization is needed. This leaves option 1 as the correct answer. You would also choose this option just by knowing that biopsy is done to rule out cancer. Review the purpose of this test if you had difficulty with this question.
Level of Cognitive Ability: Application
Client Needs: Physiological Integrity
Integrated Concept/Process: Nursing Process/Implementation
Content Area: Adult Health/Renal
Reference: Ignatavicius D, Workman M: *Medical-surgical: critical thinking for collaborative care,* ed 4, Philadelphia, 2002, WB Saunders, p. 1784.

22. ***Answer:*** 4
Rationale: The Valsalva maneuver is avoided after prostatectomy because it increases the risk of bleeding in the postoperative period. An acceptable exercise is tightening the abdominal, gluteal, and perineal muscles, as if trying to prevent urination. Another acceptable exercise is tightening the rectal sphincter while relaxing the abdominal muscles; this prevents the Valsalva maneuver from occurring.
Test-Taking Strategy: Use the process of elimination. Notice that the type of movement in the exercises described in options 1, 2, and 3 are all muscle tightening. On the other hand, the Valsalva maneuver in option 4 involves bearing down or pushing. Knowing that the answer to the question is not likely to be one that is similar to other options, you would choose the Valsalva maneuver (option 4) as the item to avoid. Review the purpose of perineal exercises if you had difficulty with this question.
Level of Cognitive Ability: Comprehension
Client Needs: Health Promotion and Maintenance
Integrated Concept/Process: Nursing Process/Evaluation
Content Area: Adult Health/Renal
Reference: Ignatavicius D, Workman M: *Medical-surgical: critical thinking for collaborative care,* ed 4, Philadelphia, 2002, WB Saunders, p. 1789.

23. ***Answer:*** 4
Rationale: The client with CRF may have several barriers to learning. Anxiety about the disease and its ramifications may frequently interfere with learning. Physiological effects of the disease process also impair the client's mental functioning. Specifically, the client may exhibit a short attention span and have memory deficits. This usually improves after hemodialysis has begun. The presence of family is helpful, as the family needs to understand the disease and treatment, and may help reinforce information with the client after the formal teaching session is over.
Test-Taking Strategy: Use the process of elimination. This question asks for the least interfering variable. Knowing that anxiety commonly interferes with learning, you would eliminate option 1 first. Options 2 and 3 are similar, in that they reflect neurological impairment. In this case, they are due to physiological effects of the disease on the nervous system. Recall that similar options are not likely to be correct. This would leave option 4 as the correct answer. The presence of family does not automatically interfere with learning; in fact, they may be quite helpful. Review the psychosocial aspects of care for the client with CRF if you had difficulty with this question.
Level of Cognitive Ability: Analysis
Client Needs: Psychosocial Integrity
Integrated Concept/Process: Nursing Process/Evaluation
Content Area: Adult Health/Renal
Reference: Ignatavicius D, Workman M: *Medical-surgical: critical thinking for collaborative care,* ed 4, Philadelphia, 2002, WB Saunders, p. 1681.

24. ***Answer:*** 1
Rationale: Epoetin alfa is a erythropoietin that has been manufactured through the use of recombinant DNA technology. It is used to treat anemia in the client with chronic renal failure. The drug may be administered subcutaneously or intravenously.
Test-Taking Strategy: Specific knowledge of epoetin alfa is necessary to answer this question. Review this medication if you had difficulty with this question.
Level of Cognitive Ability: Application

Client Needs: Physiological Integrity
Integrated Concept/Process: Nursing Process/Implementation
Content Area: Pharmacology
Reference: Ignatavicius D, Workman M: *Medical-surgical: critical thinking for collaborative care,* ed 4, Philadelphia, 2002, WB Saunders, p. 1673.

25. *Answer:* 3
Rationale: Psychosocial reactions to chronic renal failure and hemodialysis are varied and may include anger. Other reactions include personality changes, emotional lability, withdrawal, and depression. The individual client's response may vary depending on the client's personality and support systems. The client in this question is exhibiting anger. The client has not projected blame on the nurse, nor does the client's statement reflect withdrawal or depression.
Test-Taking Strategy: Knowledge of basic communication theory helps you answer this question correctly. Review the psychosocial aspects of care for the client with CRF if you had difficulty with this question.
Level of Cognitive Ability: Analysis
Client Needs: Psychosocial Integrity
Integrated Concept/Process: Nursing Process/Data Collection
Content Area: Adult Health/Renal
Reference: Ignatavicius D, Workman M: *Medical-surgical: critical thinking for collaborative care,* ed 4, Philadelphia, 2002, WB Saunders, p. 1681.

26. *Answer:* 4
Rationale: Disequilibrium syndrome is characterized by headache, mental confusion, decreasing level of consciousness, nausea, vomiting, twitching, and possible seizure activity. It is caused by rapid removal of solutes from the body during hemodialysis. At the same time, the blood-brain barrier interferes with the efficient removal of wastes from brain tissue. As a result, water goes into cerebral cells because of the osmotic gradient, causing brain swelling and onset of symptoms. It most often occurs in clients who are new to dialysis and is prevented by dialyzing for shorter times or at reduced blood flow rates.
Test-Taking Strategy: Familiarity with the causes and symptoms of disequilibrium syndrome is necessary to answer this question correctly. Review this syndrome if you had difficulty with this question.
Level of Cognitive Ability: Application
Client Needs: Physiological Integrity
Integrated Concept/Process: Nursing Process/Data Collection
Content Area: Adult Health/Renal
Reference: Ignatavicius D, Workman M: *Medical-surgical: critical thinking for collaborative care,* ed 4, Philadelphia, 2002, WB Saunders, p. 140.

27. *Answer:* 2
Rationale: Aluminum intoxication may occur when there is accumulation of aluminum, an ingredient in many phosphate-binding antacids. It results in mental cloudiness, dementia, and bone pain from infiltration of the bone with aluminum. This condition was formerly known as dialysis dementia. It may be treated with aluminum chelating agents, which make aluminum available to be dialyzed from the body. It can be prevented by avoiding or limiting the use of phosphate-binding agents that contain aluminum.
Test-Taking Strategy: To answer this question correctly, it is necessary to understand the potential implications of long-term use of aluminum-containing phosphate-binding agents by the hemodialysis client. Review the signs of aluminum intoxication if you had difficulty with this question.
Level of Cognitive Ability: Analysis
Client Needs: Physiological Integrity
Integrated Concept/Process: Nursing Process/Data Collection
Content Area: Adult Health/Renal
Reference: Ignatavicius D, Workman M: *Medical-surgical: critical thinking for collaborative care,* ed 4, Philadelphia, 2002, WB Saunders, p. 1693.

28. *Answer:* 2
Rationale: Steal syndrome results from vascular insufficiency after creation of a fistula. The client exhibits pallor and diminished pulse distal to the fistula, and the client complains of pain distal to the fistula, which is due to tissue ischemia. Warmth, redness, and pain would more likely characterize a problem with infection. The patterns described in options 3 and 4 are not indicative of Steal syndrome.
Test-Taking Strategy: Knowledge of steal syndrome and its signs and symptoms is needed to answer this question correctly. Review these signs if you had difficulty with this question.
Level of Cognitive Ability: Analysis
Client Needs: Physiological Integrity
Integrated Concept/Process: Nursing Process/Data Collection
Content Area: Adult Health/Renal
Reference: Ignatavicius D, Workman M: *Medical-surgical: critical thinking for collaborative care,* ed 4, Philadelphia, 2002, WB Saunders, p. 1693.

29. *Answer:* 3
Rationale: Risk factors associated with pyelonephritis include diabetes mellitus, hypertension, chronic renal calculi, chronic cystitis, structural abnormalities of the urinary tract, presence of urinary stones, and indwelling or frequent urinary catheterization.
Test-Taking Strategy: Use the process of elimination. Eliminate options 1 and 4 first as least likely being associated as risk factors. From the remaining options, remember that diabetes mellitus can cause renal complications. This will assist in directing you to the correct option. Review these risk factors if you had difficulty with this question.
Level of Cognitive Ability: Comprehension
Client Needs: Health Promotion and Maintenance
Integrated Concept/Process: Nursing Process/Data Collection
Content Area: Adult Health/Renal
Reference: Ignatavicius D, Workman M: *Medical-surgical: critical thinking for collaborative care,* ed 4, Philadelphia, 2002, WB Saunders, p. 1647.

30. *Answer:* 1
Rationale: The BUN is the most frequently used laboratory test to determine renal function. The BUN starts to rise when the glomerular filtration rate falls below 40% to 60%. A decreased hemoglobin and RBC count may be noted if bleeding from the urinary tract occurs or if erythropoietic function by the

kidney is impaired. An increased WBC is most likely to be noted in renal disease.
Test-Taking Strategy: Use the process of elimination. Note the key words "most likely expect to note" in the stem of the question. Eliminate option 4 first. Although options 2 and 3 may be noted in some renal disorders, option 1 is the most likely laboratory finding. Review these significant laboratory tests if you had difficulty with this question.
Level of Cognitive Ability: Comprehension
Client Needs: Physiological Integrity
Integrated Concept/Process: Nursing Process/Data Collection
Content Area: Adult Health/Renal
Reference: Chernecky C, Berger B: *Laboratory tests and diagnostic procedures*, ed 3, Philadelphia, 2001, WB Saunders, p. 1039.

31. *Answer:* 2
Rationale: Refrigeration preserves the elements of urine, but the delay can cause crystals to precipitate. If the specimen stands at room temperature, the warmth causes bacteria and WBCs to decompose. When urine is allowed to stand unrefrigerated, the urea breaks down to ammonia and becomes more alkaline. The pH decreases in an acidic condition.
Test-Taking Strategy: Use the process of elimination. Careful reading will assist you to easily eliminate option 3. Eliminate options 1 and 4 next because they are similar. pH decreases in acidic conditions. This leaves option 2 as the likely option. Review this procedure if you had difficulty with this question.
Level of Cognitive Ability: Comprehension
Client Needs: Physiological Integrity
Integrated Concept/Process: Teaching/Learning
Content Area: Adult Health/Renal
Reference: DeWit S: *Fundamental concepts and skills for nursing*, Philadelphia, 2001, WB Saunders, p. 551.

32. *Answer:* 1
Rationale: Because the 24-hour urine test is a timed quantitative determination, it is essential to start the test with an empty bladder. The urine collection should be refrigerated or placed on ice to prevent changes in urine. Fifteen minutes before the end of the collection time, the client should be asked to void and this specimen is added to the collection.
Test-Taking Strategy: Use the process of elimination. Note that options 1 and 2 are addressing the same issue and are different in regards to this procedure. This would lead you to think that one of these options is the correct option. Try to think about the purpose of this timed test and eliminate option 2 because it would make sense that this test should be started when the client has an empty bladder. Review this procedure if you had difficulty with this question.
Level of Cognitive Ability: Application
Client Needs: Physiological Integrity
Integrated Concept/Process: Nursing Process/Implementation
Content Area: Adult Health/Renal
Reference: DeWit S: *Fundamental concepts and skills for nursing*, Philadelphia, 2001, WB Saunders, p. 418.

33. *Answer:* 4
Rationale: No specific precautions must be taken after a renal scan. If the client is able, urination into a commode is acceptable without risk from the small amount of radioactive material to be excreted. The nurse wears gloves to maintain body secretion precautions.
Test-Taking Strategy: Use the process of elimination. Knowing that there is generally no danger from the small amount of radioactive material used in this procedure will easily direct you to option 4. Review this procedure if you had difficulty with this question.
Level of Cognitive Ability: Application
Client Needs: Safe, Effective Care Environment
Integrated Concept/Process: Nursing Process/Implementation
Content Area: Adult Health/Renal
Reference: Chernecky C, Berger B: *Laboratory tests and diagnostic procedures*, ed 3, Philadelphia, 2001, WB Saunders, p. 906.

34. *Answer:* 3
Rationale: The iodine-based dye used during the IVP can cause allergic reactions such as itching, hives, rash, tight feeling in the throat, shortness of breath, and bronchospasm. Assessing for allergies is the priority.
Test-Taking Strategy: Note the key word "priority" in the stem of the question. Use the nursing process as a guide. Options 1, 2, and 4 address implementation. Option 3 is the only option that addresses data collection. Review this test if you had difficulty with this question.
Level of Cognitive Ability: Application
Client Needs: Physiological Integrity
Integrated Concept/Process: Nursing Process/Implementation
Content Area: Adult Health/Renal
Reference: Chernecky C, Berger B: *Laboratory tests and diagnostic procedures*, ed 3, Philadelphia, 2001, WB Saunders, p. 653.

35. *Answer:* 3
Rationale: Urine specimens for cultures should be obtained using proper cleansing and voiding techniques to avoid contamination from external sources. The use of paper towels will contaminate the specimen. The procedure described in option 1 would not provide a clean specimen. It is not necessary to obtain the specimen via catheter.
Test-Taking Strategy: Use the process of elimination. Note the key words "clean catch." These words should assist in eliminating options 1 and 4 and direct you to option 3. If you had difficulty with this question, review the procedure for this type of urine collection.
Level of Cognitive Ability: Comprehension
Client Needs: Safe, Effective Care Environment
Integrated Concept/Process: Nursing Process/Evaluation
Content Area: Adult Health/Renal
Reference: DeWit S: *Fundamental concepts and skills for nursing*, Philadelphia, 2001, WB Saunders, p. 551.

36. *Answer:* 1
Rationale: If pain originates at the biopsy site and begins to radiate to the flank area and around the front of the abdomen, bleeding should be suspected. Hypotension, a decreasing hematocrit, and gross or microscopic hematuria would also indicate bleeding. Signs of infection would not appear immediately after a biopsy. Pain of this nature is not normal. There is no data to support the presence of renal colic.
Test-Taking Strategy: Use the process of elimination. You can easily eliminate options 3 and 4. Recalling that signs of infection

may not appear immediately after biopsy will assist in directing you to option 1. Review the complications after renal biopsy if you had difficulty with this question.
Level of Cognitive Ability: Analysis
Client Needs: Physiological Integrity
Integrated Concept/Process: Nursing Process/Data Collection
Content Area: Adult Health/Renal
Reference: Ignatavicius D, Workman M: *Medical-surgical: critical thinking for collaborative care,* ed 4, Philadelphia, 2002, WB Saunders, p. 426.

37. ***Answer:*** 1
Rationale: Polyuria occurs early in CRF and if untreated can cause severe dehydration. Polyuria progresses to anuria and the client loses all normal functions of the kidney. Oliguria and anuria are not early signs and polydypsia is unrelated to CRF.
Test-Taking Strategy: Use the process of elimination. Note the key word "early" in the question. Eliminate options 3 and 4 because they are similar. From the remaining options, select option 1 because this option relates to renal function and is the correct answer to this question. Review the early and the later signs of CRF if you had difficulty with this question.
Level of Cognitive Ability: Comprehension
Client Needs: Physiological Integrity
Integrated Concept/Process: Nursing Process/Data Collection
Content Area: Adult Health/Renal
Reference: Ignatavicius D, Workman M: *Medical-surgical: critical thinking for collaborative care,* ed 4, Philadelphia, 2002, WB Saunders, p. 1681.

38. ***Answer:*** 1
Rationale: Amphojel binds with phosphate in the intestines to be excreted in the feces, thus lowering phosphorus levels. It can cause constipation and it does not promote the elimination of potassium. It may be used in the treatment of hyperacidity associated with gastric ulcers, but this is not the purpose of its use in the client with renal failure.
Test-Taking Strategy: Knowledge regarding the purpose of this medication in CRF is required to answer this question. Review this medication if you had difficulty with this question.
Level of Cognitive Ability: Comprehension
Client Needs: Physiological Integrity
Integrated Concept/Process: Nursing Process/Implementation
Content Area: Adult Health/Renal
Reference: Hodgson B, Kizior R: *Saunders nursing drug handbook 2002,* Philadelphia, 2002, WB Saunders, p.36.

39. ***Answer:*** 3
Rationale: Cantaloupe (¼ small), spinach (½ cup cooked) and strawberries (1 ¼ cups) are high potassium foods and average 7 mEq per serving. Lima beans (⅓ cup) average 3 mEq per serving.
Test-Taking Strategy: Use the process of elimination remembering that many fruits and green leafy vegetables are high in potassium. This may assist in directing you to option 3. Review the foods low in potassium if you had difficulty with this question.
Level of Cognitive Ability: Comprehension
Client Needs: Health Promotion and Maintenance
Integrated Concept/Process: Nursing Process/Evaluation
Content Area: Adult Health/Renal
Reference: Ignatavicius D, Workman M: *Medical-surgical: critical thinking for collaborative care,* ed 4, Philadelphia, 2002, WB Saunders, p. 153.

40. ***Answer:*** 3
Rationale: In an elderly client, the only symptom of a UTI may be something as vague as increasing mental confusion or frequent unexplained falls. Frequency and urgency may commonly occur in an elderly client, and fever can be associated with a variety of conditions.
Test-Taking Strategy: Use the process of elimination. Note the client's age in the question. Eliminate options 2 and 4 because they may commonly occur in an elderly client. Eliminate option 1 next because fever can be associated with a variety of conditions. Review clinical manifestations of UTI that occur in elderly people if you had difficulty with this question.
Level of Cognitive Ability: Comprehension
Client Needs: Physiological Integrity
Integrated Concept/Process: Nursing Process/Data Collection
Content Area: Adult Health/Renal
Reference: Black J, Hawks J, Keene A: *Medical-surgical nursing: clinical management for positive outcomes,* ed 6, Philadelphia, 2001, WB Saunders, p. 807.

41. ***Answer:*** 2
Rationale: In acute glomerulonephritis it is important to protect the kidneys while they are recovering function. The diet is generally high calorie and low protein. This diet avoids protein catabolism and allows the kidneys to rest.
Test-Taking Strategy: Knowledge regarding the treatment measures in acute glomerulonephritis is required to answer this question. Recalling that protein would increase the workload of the kidneys will assist in directing you to option 2. Review this disorder if you had difficulty with this question.
Level of Cognitive Ability: Application
Client Needs: Health Promotion and Maintenance
Integrated Concept/Process: Nursing Process/Implementation
Content Area: Adult Health/Renal
Reference: Ignatavicius D, Workman M: *Medical-surgical: critical thinking for collaborative care,* ed 4, Philadelphia, 2002, WB Saunders, p. 403.

42. ***Answer:*** 3
Rationale: Oxalate is found in dark-green foods such as spinach. Other foods that raise urinary oxalate are rhubarb, strawberries, chocolate, wheat bran, nuts, beets, and tea.
Test-Taking Strategy: Using knowledge regarding the foods that raise urinary oxalate will assist in answering this question. Remembering the green leafy foods are high in oxalate will assist in directing you to option 3. Review these foods if you had difficulty with this question.
Level of Cognitive Ability: Application
Client Needs: Health Promotion and Maintenance
Integrated Concept/Process: Nursing Process/Implementation
Content Area: Adult Health/Renal
Reference: Williams S: *Basic nutrition and diet therapy,* ed 11, St Louis, 2001, Mosby, p. 415.

43. *Answer:* 1
Rationale: Gross, painless hematuria is most frequently the first manifestation of bladder cancer. As the disease progresses the client may experience dysuria, frequency, and urgency.
Test-Taking Strategy: Use the process of elimination. The issue of the question relates specifically to bladder cancer. Focusing on this issue should easily direct you to option 1. Review the specific manifestations associated with bladder cancer if you had difficulty with this question.
Level of Cognitive Ability: Comprehension
Client Needs: Physiological Integrity
Integrated Concept/Process: Nursing Process/Data Collection
Content Area: Adult Health/Renal
Reference: Ignatavicius D, Workman M: *Medical-surgical: critical thinking for collaborative care*, ed 4, Philadelphia, 2002, WB Saunders, p. 1638.

44. *Answer:* 1
Rationale: TUR syndrome is caused by increased absorption of nonelectrolyte irrigating fluid used during surgery. The client may show signs of cerebral edema and increased intracranial pressure such as increased blood pressure, bradycardia, confusion, disorientation, muscle twitching, visual disturbances, and nausea and vomiting.
Test-Taking Strategy: Knowledge regarding TUR syndrome is required to answer this question. Recalling that increased intracranial pressure is the concern easily directs you to option 1. Review this disorder if you had difficulty with this question.
Level of Cognitive Ability: Analysis
Client Needs: Physiological Integrity
Integrated Concept/Process: Nursing Process/Data Collection
Content Area: Adult Health/Renal
Reference: Ignatavicius D, Workman M: *Medical-surgical: critical thinking for collaborative care*, ed 4, Philadelphia, 2002, WB Saunders, p. 1788.

45. *Answer:* 4
Rationale: Treatment of prostatitis includes medication with antibiotics, analgesics, and stool softeners. The client is also taught to rest, increase fluid intake; and use sitz baths for comfort. Antimicrobial therapy is always continued until the prescription is completely finished.
Test-Taking Strategy: Use the process of elimination. Eliminate option 3 first because stopping medication therapy before the end of the course is contraindicated. Option 1 is also eliminated, as fluid intake should be increased. To discriminate between the last two options, it is necessary to understand that sitz baths provide comfort, or that rest is helpful in the healing process. Knowledge of either of these concepts would help you to choose option 4 as the correct answer. Review the measures to prevent prostatitis if you had difficulty with this question.
Level of Cognitive Ability: Analysis
Client Needs: Health Promotion and Maintenance
Integrated Concept/Process: Nursing Process/Evaluation
Content Area: Adult Health/Renal
Reference: Ignatavicius D, Workman M: *Medical-surgical: critical thinking for collaborative care*, ed 4, Philadelphia, 2002, WB Saunders, p. 1802.

REFERENCES

Black J, Hawks J, Keene A: *Medical-surgical nursing: clinical management for positive outcomes*, ed 6, Philadelphia, 2001, WB Saunders.

Chernecky C, Berger B: *Laboratory tests and diagnostic procedures*, ed 3, Philadelphia, 2001, WB Saunders.

Clark J Queener S, Karb V: *Pharmacologic basis of nursing practice*, ed 6, St Louis, 2000, Mosby.

DeWit S: *Fundamental concepts and skills for nursing*, Philadelphia, 2001, WB Saunders.

Hodgson B, Kizior R: *Saunders nursing drug handbook 2002*, Philadelphia, 2002, WB Saunders.

Ignatavicius D, Workman M: *Medical-surgical: critical thinking for collaborative care*, ed 4, Philadelphia, 2002, WB Saunders.

Lehne R: *Pharmacology for nursing care*, ed 4, Philadelphia, 2001, WB Saunders.

Potter P, Perry A: *Fundamentals of nursing*, ed 5, St Louis, 2001, Mosby.

Perry A, Potter P: *Clinical nursing skills and techniques*, ed 5, St Louis, 2002, Mosby.

Renal Medications

I. URINARY TRACT ANTISEPTICS (Box 51-1)

A. Description
   1. Inhibit the growth of bacteria in the urine
   2. Act as disinfectants within the urinary tract
   3. Used to treat urinary tract infections
   4. These medications do not achieve effective antibacterial concentrations in blood or tissues and therefore cannot be used for infections at sites outside the urinary tract

B. Side effects and nursing considerations
   1. Nitrofurantoin
      a. Gastrointestinal effects such as anorexia, nausea, vomiting, and diarrhea; administration with milk or meals will minimize gastrointestinal (GI) distress
      b. Pulmonary reactions such as dyspnea, chest pain, chills, fever, cough, and alveolar infiltrates; these resolve in 2 to 4 days after cessation of treatment
      c. Hematological effects such as agranulocytosis, leukopenia, thrombocytopenia, and megaloblastic anemia
      d. Peripheral neuropathy such as muscle weakness, tingling sensations, and numbness
      e. Neurological effects such as headache, vertigo, drowsiness, nystagmus
      f. Imparts a harmless brown color to the urine
      g. Contraindicated in clients with renal impairment
      h. Instruct the client in the expected side effects and those warranting notifying the physician
   2. Methenamine
      a. Relatively safe and well tolerated
      b. May cause gastric distress
      c. Chronic high-dose therapy can cause bladder irritation
      d. Can cause crystalluria and should not be used in clients with renal impairment
      e. Decomposition of medication generates ammonia; thus it should not be used for clients with liver dysfunction
      f. Requires acidic urine with pH of 5.5 or less
      g. Ingestion of large amounts of fluid will reduce antibacterial effects by diluting the medication and raising the urinary pH
      h. Should not be combined with sulfonamides because of the risk of crystalluria and urinary tract injury
      i. Clients taking this medication should not be given alkalinizing agents
   3. Nalidixic acid
      a. Gastrointestinal disturbances: nausea, vomiting, and abdominal discomfort
      b. Rash
      c. Visual disturbances
      d. Photosensitivity reactions
      e. May produce intracranial hypertension in pediatric clients and should not be administered to children under age 3 months
      f. When used for more than 2 weeks, complete blood cell (CBC) counts and liver function tests should be performed

BOX 51-1

Urinary Tract Antiseptics

Nitrofurantoin (Furadantin, Furalan, Macrobid)
Nitrofurantoin macrocrystals (Macrodantin)
Methenamine (Mandelamine, Hiprex, Urex)
Nalidixic acid (NegGram)
Clinoaxcin (Cinobac)
Norfloxacin (Noroxin)

   g. Can intensify the effects of oral anticoagulants
   h. Contraindicated in clients with a history of convulsive disorders
4. Clinoaxcin
   a. Side effects are similar to nalidixic acid
   b. Dosage should be reduced in clients with renal impairment; failure to do so could result in accumulation of the medication to toxic levels
5. Norfloxacin
   a. Can cause fatigue, headache, nausea, constipation, rash, and elevated liver function tests
   b. Encourage the client to consume a high fluid intake
   c. Advise the client to take medication 1 hour before or 2 hours after meals because food may hamper absorption

II. SULFONAMIDES (Box 51-2)

A. Description
   1. Suppress bacterial growth by inhibiting the synthesis of folic acid
   2. Active against a broad spectrum of microbes

B. Side effects and nursing considerations
   1. Hypersensitivity reactions: rash, fever, and photosensitivity
   2. Stevens-Johnson syndrome, the most severe hypersensitivity response, producing symptoms that include widespread lesions of the skin and mucous membranes with fever, malaise, and toxemia
   3. Should be discontinued if a rash is observed
   4. Can cause hemolytic anemia, agranulocytosis, leukopenia, and thrombocytopenia
   5. Instruct the client to take medication on an empty stomach with a full glass of water
   6. Instruct the client to avoid prolonged exposure to sunlight, wear protective clothing, and apply a sunscreen to exposed skin
   7. Adults should maintain a daily urine output of 1200 mL by consuming 8 to 10 glasses of water each day to minimize the risk of renal damage from the medication
   8. Can intensify the effects of warfarin sodium (Coumadin), phenytoin (Dilantin), and oral hypoglycemics
   9. Administer with caution in clients with renal impairment
   10. Contraindicated if a hypersensitivity exists to sulfonamides, sulfonylureas, thiazide, or loop diuretics
   11. Contraindicated in infants under age 2 months and in pregnant women or to mothers who are breastfeeding

BOX 51-2

Sulfonamides

Sulfadiazine
Sulfadoxine; pyrimethamine (Fansidar)
Sulfamethizole (Thiosulfil Forte)
Sulfamethoxazole (Gantanol, Urobak)
Sulfamethoxazole; phenazopyridine (Azo Gantanol)
Sulfasalazine (Azulifidine)
Sulfisoxazole (Gantrisin)
Sulfisoxazole; phenazopyridine (Azo Gantrisin)

III. TRIMETHOPRIM (PROLOPRIM, TRIMPEX)

A. Description
   1. Active against a broad spectrum of microbes
   2. Suppresses bacterial synthesis of DNA, RNA, and proteins

B. Side effects and nursing considerations
   1. Itching and rash are the most frequent side effects
   2. GI reactions such as epigastric distress, nausea and vomiting, glossitis, and stomatitis occur occasionally
   3. Megaloblastic anemia, thrombocytopenia, and neutropenia may occur in individuals with preexisting folic acid deficiency
   4. If early signs of bone marrow suppression occur such as sore throat, fever, or pallor, a CBC should be performed
   5. Contraindicated in women who are pregnant or are breastfeeding
   6. Contraindicated in clients with a folate deficiency

IV. TRIMETHOPRIM-SULFAMETHOXAZOLE

A. Description
   1. A fixed-dose combination product (TMP-SMZ) that is a powerful broad-spectrum antimicrobial preparation
   2. Trade names include Bactrim, Cotrim, and Septra

B. Side effects and nursing considerations
   1. Nausea, vomiting, and rash are the most common side effects
   2. Can cause megaloblastic anemia in clients who are folate deficient
   3. Can cause central nervous system (CNS) effects such as headache, depression, and hallucinations
   4. Hyperkalemia can occur

5. Toxicity: hypersensitivity reactions, blood dyscrasias, and renal damage
6. Contraindicated during pregnancy and lactation, for infants under age 2 months, in clients with a folate deficiency, and in clients with a history of hypersensitivity to sulfonamides and chemically related medications

V. CHOLINERGIC (Box 51-3)

A. Description
   1. Used to treat nonobstructive urinary retention and neurogenic bladder
   2. Used to increase bladder tone and function

B. Side effects
   1. Headache
   2. Hypotension
   3. Flushing and sweating
   4. Increased salivation
   5. Abdominal cramps
   6. Nausea and vomiting
   7. Diarrhea
   8. Urinary urgency
   9. Bronchoconstriction

C. Nursing considerations
   1. Do not administer if the client has a urinary obstruction
   2. Never administer by the intramuscular (IM) or intravenous (IV) route
   3. Monitor intake and output (I&O)
   4. Monitor for increased bladder tone and function
   5. Monitor for cholinergic overdose
   6. Have atropine sulfate (antidote) readily available

VI. ANTISPASMOTICS

A. Description
   1. Oxybutynin chloride (Ditropan) relaxes smooth muscles of the urinary tract
   2. Propantheline bromide (Pro-Banthine) decreases bladder muscle spasms

B. Oxybutynin chloride (Ditropan)
   1. Side Effects
      a. Leukopenia
      b. Anxiety
      c. Anorexia, nausea, vomiting
      d. Palpitations
      e. Sinus bradycardia
   2. Nursing considerations
      a. Do not administer in clients with known hypersensitivity, GI or genitourinary (GU) obstruction, glaucoma, severe colitis, or myasthenia gravis
      b. Instruct the client to avoid hazardous activities

C. Propantheline bromide (Pro-Banthine)
   1. Side effects
      a. Palpitations
      b. Blurred vision
      c. Confusion in elderly clients
      d. Tachycardia
      e. Constipation
      f. Dry mouth
      g. Urinary hesitancy and urgency
      h. Decreased sweating
   2. Nursing considerations
      a. Monitor I&O
      b. Provide gum or hard candy for dry mouth
      c. Do not administer to clients with narrow-angle glaucoma, obstructive uropathy, GI disease, or ulcerative colitis

VII. URINARY ANALGESIC (Box 51-4)

A. Description
   1. Used for pain from urinary tract irritation or infection
   2. Administered with an antibiotic because it does not treat infection; it only treats pain

B. Side effects
   1. Nausea
   2. Headache
   3. Vertigo

C. Nursing considerations
   1. Instruct the client that the urine will turn red or orange
   2. Contraindicated in renal or hepatic disease

VIII. HEMATOPOIETIC GROWTH FACTOR (Box 51-5)

A. Description
   1. Used to stimulate red blood cell (RBC) production

BOX 51-3

Cholinergic

Bethanechol chloride (Duvoid, Urecholine)

BOX 51-4

Urinary Analgesic

Phenazopyridine hydrochloride (Pyridium)

BOX 51-5

Hematopoietic Growth Factor

Epoetin alfa (Epogen, Procrit)

2. Reverses anemia associated with **chronic renal failure**
3. Initial effects can be seen within 1 to 2 weeks, and the hematocrit reaches normal levels (30% to 33%) in 2 to 3 months

B. Side effect: major side effect is hypertension

C. Nursing considerations
1. Monitor the CBC
2. Monitor vital signs, especially the blood pressure for hypertension
3. The extent of hypertension is directly related to the rate of rise in the hematocrit
4. Contraindicated in clients with uncontrolled hypertension or hypersensitivity to mammalian cell-derived products or human albumin
5. Use with caution in clients with cancers of myeloid origin

IX. PREVENTING ORGAN REJECTION (Box 51-6)

A. Description
1. Cyclosporine acts on T lymphocytes to suppress production of interleukin-2, gamma interferon, and other cytokines
2. Tracrolimus inhibits calcineurin and thereby prevents T cells from producing interleukin-2, gamma interferon, and other cytokines
3. Azathioprine (Imuran) suppresses cell-mediated and humoral immune responses by inhibiting the proliferation of B and T lymphocytes
4. Mycophenolate mofetil causes selective inhibition of B and T lymphocyte proliferation
5. Muromonab-CD3 blocks all T-cell functions
6. Therapeutic effect of antithymocyte globulin results from a decrease in the number and activity of thymus-derived lymphocytes
7. Dacliximab and basiliximab bind to IL-2 receptors on lymphocytes resulting in diminished cell-mediated immune reactions

B. Cyclosporine (Sandimmune, Neoral)
1. Used to prevent rejection of allogenic kidney transplant
2. Prednisone is usually administered concurrently
3. Oral administration is preferred; IV administration is reserved for clients who cannot take the medication orally
4. Blood levels should be measured periodically
5. The most common adverse effects are nephrotoxicity, infection, hypertension, tremor, and hirsutism
6. The client should be informed about the possibility of renal and liver damage and the need for periodic blood urea nitrogen (BUN), creatinine, and liver function tests
7. The client should be instructed to monitor for early signs of infection and to report these signs immediately
8. Instruct the client to dispense the oral liquid into a glass container using a specially calibrated pipette, mix well, and drink immediately; rinse the glass container with diluent and drink it to ensure ingestion of the complete dose; dry the outside of the pipette and return to its cover for storage
9. Instruct the client to mix the concentrated medication solution with milk, chocolate milk, or orange juice just before administration
10. Assure the client that hirsutism is reversible
11. Grapefruit juice can raise cyclosporine levels, thereby increasing the risk of toxicity
12. Phenytoin (Dilantin), phenobarbital, rifampin (Rifadin), and TMP-SMZ can decrease cyclosporine levels
13. Ketoconazole (Nizoral), erythromycin, and amphotericin B (Fungizone) can elevate cyclosporine levels
14. Renal damage can be intensified by the concurrent use of other nephrotoxic medications
15. Contraindicated in the presence of hypersensitivity, pregnancy, breastfeeding, recent inoculation with live virus vaccines, and recent contact with an active infection such as chickenpox or herpes zoster
16. Is embryotoxic, and women of childbearing age should use a mechanical form of contraception and avoid oral contraceptives

BOX 51-6

Preventing Organ Rejection

IMMUNOSUPPRESSANTS
Cyclosporine (Sandimmune, Neoral)
Tracrolimus (Prograf)

CYTOTOXIC MEDICATIONS
Azathioprine (Imuran)
Mycophenolate Mofetil (CellCept)

GLUCOCORTICOID
Prednisone (Deltasone)

ANTIBODIES
Antithymocyte globulin (Atgam)
Basiliximab (Simulect)
Dacliximab (Zenapax)
Muromonab-CD3 (Orthoclone OKT3)

C. Tacrolimus (Prograf)
   1. Nephrotoxicity is the major concern
   2. Other common reactions include neurotoxicity, GI effects, hypertension, hyperkalemia, and hyperglycemia
   3. Increases the risk of infection and lymphomas
   4. Concurrent use of glucocorticoids is recommended

D. Azathioprine (Imuran)
   1. Used as an adjunct to cyclosporine and glucocorticoids to help suppress transplant rejection
   2. Can cause neutropenia and thrombocytopenia from bone marrow suppression
   3. Contraindicated in pregnancy and is associated with an increased incidence of neoplasms

E. Mycophenolate mofetil (CellCept)
   1. Used in combination with cyclosporine and glucocorticoids
   2. Major adverse effects include diarrhea, severe neutropenia, vomiting, and sepsis
   3. Associated with an increased risk of infection and malignancies
   4. Absorption is decreased by the use of magnesium and aluminum antacids and by cholestyramine (Questran, Prevalite)
   5. Contraindicated in pregnancy

F. Muromonab-CD3 (Orthoclone OKT3)
   1. Used to prevent acute allograft rejection of kidney transplants
   2. Adverse reactions include fever, chills, dyspnea, chest pain, and nausea and vomiting

G. Antithymocyte globulin (Atgam)
   1. Used to prevent rejection of renal transplants
   2. Usually administered with glucocorticoids and azathioprine
   3. Adverse reactions include chills, fever, leukopenia, and skin reactions

H. Dacliximab (Zenapax) and basiliximab (Simulect)
   1. Used to prevent acute rejection of transplanted kidneys
   2. Used in combination with other immunosuppressants such as cyclosporine and glucocorticoids
   3. Administered by the IV route
   4. Contraindicated in the client with an allergy to protein
   5. Dacliximab (Zenapax)
      a. Initial dose administered within 24 hours before transplantation
      b. Side effects include chest pain, GI distress, edema, shortness of breath, pain in the joints, and slow wound healing
   6. Basiliximab (Simulect)
      a. Initial dose administered within 2 hours before transplantation
      b. Side effects are similar to those for dacliximab; additionally, headache, insomnia, dizziness, and tremor can occur

PRACTICE QUESTIONS

1. Cinoxacin (Cinobac) is prescribed for the client with a urinary tract infection. The nurse tells the client to take the medication:
   1. 1 hour before meals
   2. With meals
   3. At bed time
   4. In the morning before breakfast
2. Laboratory analysis of a urine for culture and sensitivity reveals a gram-negative bacterial infection. Nalidixic acid (NegGram) is prescribed for the client. The nurse questions the prescription if the client has which of the following disorders?
   1. Diabetes mellitus
   2. Seizure disorder
   3. Coronary artery disease
   4. Peptic ulcer disease
3. Norfloxacin (Noroxin) is prescribed for a client with *Pseudomonas* infection of the urinary tract. The nurse tells the client to take the medication:
   1. With meals
   2. At bed time
   3. 2 hours after meals
   4. With a snack in the late afternoon
4. Nitrofurantoin (Macrodantin) is prescribed for the client with an acute urinary tract infection. Which of the following food items would the nurse instruct the client to avoid during the administration of this medication?
   1. Orange juice
   2. Cranberry juice
   3. Prune juice
   4. Rhubarb
5. Methenamine mandelate (Mandelamine) is prescribed for the client with a gram-positive urinary tract infection. The nurse questions the prescription if which of the following preexisting disorders is noted in the client's record?
   1. Cirrhosis
   2. Diabetes mellitus
   3. Peripheral vascular disease
   4. Hypothyroidism
6. A client receiving nitrofurantoin (Macrodantin) calls the physician's office complaining of side effects related to the medication. Which of the following side effects indicates the need to stop treatment with this medication?
   1. Anorexia
   2. Nausea

3. Cough and chest pain
4. Diarrhea

7. Nitrofurantoin (Macrodantin) is prescribed for an adult client for treatment of acute urinary tract infection (UTI). Which of the following is the appropriate adult dose?
   1. 50 mg three to four times a day
   2. 100 mg three times a day
   3. 300 mg administered at bedtime
   4. 1 g distributed evenly throughout the day
8. Methenamine (Mandelamine) is prescribed for the client with a chronic urinary tract infection. The nurse administers the medication knowing that the mechanism of action is which of the following?
   1. Inhibits the replication of bacterial DNA
   2. Denatures bacterial proteins
   3. Decreases bladder muscles and spasms
   4. Relaxes smooth muscles of the urinary tract
9. Nalidixic acid (NegGram) is prescribed for the client with a urinary tract infection. Reviewing the client's record, the nurse notes that the client is taking warfarin (Coumadin) on a daily basis. Which of the following prescriptions would the nurse anticipate because the client is on this oral anticoagulant?
   1. An increase in the anticoagulation dosage
   2. A reduction in the anticoagulation dosage
   3. The need to discontinue the Coumadin during therapy
   4. The need to administer an alternative medication to treat the urinary tract infection
10. Nalidixic acid (NegGram) is prescribed for the adult client with urinary tract infection. The normal adult dosage for this medication is:
    1. 1 g four times a day for 1 week
    2. 500 mg a day administered at bedtime
    3. 250 mg administered BID
    4. 100 mg administered TID
11. Cinoxacin (Cinobac), a urinary antiseptic, is prescribed for the client. The nurse reviews the client's record knowing that this medication would be administered with caution in which of the following disorders?
    1. Hepatic disease
    2. Renal disease
    3. Diabetes insipidus
    4. Congestive heart failure
12. A nurse is reinforcing discharge instructions to a client receiving sulfisoxazole (Gantrisin). Which of the following would be included in the plan of care for instructions?
    1. Restrict fluid intake
    2. Maintain a high fluid intake
    3. Decrease the dosage when symptoms are improving to prevent an allergic response
    4. If the urine turns dark brown, call the physician immediately
13. Sulfamethoxazole (Gantanol) is prescribed for a client with a urinary tract infection. The client is a diabetic and is receiving tolbutamide (Orinase). Based on the administration of these two medications in combination, which of the following would the nurse anticipate might be prescribed?
    1. A decreased dosage of the tolbutamide
    2. An increased dosage of the tolbutamide
    3. A decreased dosage of the sulfamethoxazole
    4. An increased dosage of the sulfamethoxazole
14. Trimethoprim-sulfamethoxazole (Bactrim) is prescribed for the client. The nurse tells the client to report which of the following symptoms if it develops during the course of this medication therapy?
    1. Headache
    2. Nausea
    3. Diarrhea
    4. Sore throat
15. Phenazopyridine (Pyridium) is prescribed for the client for symptomatic relief of pain resulting from a lower urinary tract infection. The nurse tells the client:
    1. To take the medication before meals
    2. That a reddish-orange discoloration of the urine may occur
    3. To discontinue the medication if a headache occurs
    4. To take the medication at bedtime
16. Bethanechol (Urecholine) is prescribed for the client with urinary retention. The nurse reviews the client's record knowing that which of the following preexisting disorders would be a contraindication to the administration of this medication?
    1. Neurogenic atony
    2. Urinary strictures
    3. Gastroesophageal reflux
    4. Gastric atony
17. Bethanechol (Urecholine) is prescribed for the client. The nurse tells the client to take the medication:
    1. With meals
    2. 2 hours after meals
    3. With a snack in the afternoon
    4. At bedtime with crackers and cheese
18. Bethanechol (Urecholine) is prescribed for the client. The normal adult oral dosage of this medication ranges from:
    1. 10 to 50 mg three to four times a day
    2. 50 to 100 mg three to four times a day
    3. 100 mg every 4 hours
    4. 100 mg at bedtime
19. A nurse is administering 5 mg of bethanechol (Urecholine) subcutaneously to a client with urinary retention. Which of the following would the nurse prepare to have readily available when administering this medication?

1. Protamine sulfate
2. Vitamin K
3. Atropine sulfate
4. Mucomyst

20. A nurse administering bethanechol (Urecholine) is monitoring for acute toxicity associated with the medication. Which of the following is not a manifestation associated with overdose?
    1. Salivation
    2. Sweating
    3. Bradycardia
    4. Severe hypertension
21. Bethanechol (Urecholine) is prescribed for the client with urinary retention. An injectable form of bethanechol is available for use. The nurse informs the client of the physician's order knowing that the medication will be administered:
    1. Intravenously
    2. Intramuscularly
    3. Intradermally
    4. Subcutaneously
22. Oxybutynin (Ditropan) is prescribed for the client with neurogenic bladder. The nurse monitors the client knowing that which of the following would indicate a possible toxic effect related to this medication?
    1. Bradycardia
    2. Pallor
    3. Restlessness
    4. Drowsiness
23. Propantheline bromide (Pro-Banthine) is prescribed for the client with bladder spasms. Which of the following disorders, if noted in the client's record, alerts the nurse to question the prescription for this medication?
    1. Glaucoma
    2. Hypothyroidism
    3. Myxedema
    4. Coronary artery disease
24. After kidney transplantation, cyclosporine (Sandimmune) is prescribed for the client. Which of the following laboratory results indicates an adverse effect from the use of this medication?
    1. Decreased white blood cell (WBC) count
    2. Decreased hemoglobin
    3. Elevated blood urea nitrogen (BUN)
    4. Decreased creatinine
25. A nurse is providing dietary instructions to a client who has been prescribed cyclosporine (Sandimmune). Which of the following food items would the nurse instruct the client to avoid?
    1. Orange juice
    2. Grapefruit juice
    3. Red meats
    4. Green leafy vegetables
26. Cyclosporine (Sandimmune) is prescribed for the client after kidney transplantation. The nurse would be most concerned if the nurse noted that the client is presently taking which of the following prescribed medications?
    1. Digoxin (Lanoxin)
    2. Propranolol (Inderal)
    3. Phenytoin (Dilantin)
    4. Prednisone (Deltasone)
27. A nurse is caring for a client who will be receiving amphotericin B (Fungizone). The nurse notes that the client is also taking cyclosporine (Sandimmune) to prevent rejection of a kidney transplant performed 2 years ago. Which of the following prescriptions would the nurse anticipate to be prescribed for this client during the concurrent administration of these medications?
    1. An increased amount of amphotericin B
    2. A decreased amount of amphotericin B
    3. An increased amount of cyclosporine
    4. A decreased amount of cyclosporine
28. A nurse reinforces instructions to the client prescribed to take cyclosporine (Sandimmune) oral solution. Which of the following instructions would the nurse reinforce?
    1. Dilute the medication in a Styrofoam cup before administration
    2. Avoid diluting the concentrate for administration
    3. Mix the concentration with chocolate milk
    4. Mix the concentration with grapefruit juice
29. A nurse reinforces instructions regarding the administration of cyclosporine (Sandimmune) to a client. Which of the following statements, if made by the client, would indicate the need for further instruction?
    1. "I need to mix the concentrate well and drink it immediately."
    2. "After taking the medication, I need to rinse the container with diluent and drink it to ensure that I have taken the complete dose."
    3. "I will purchase a dropper from the pharmacy to calibrate the amount of medication that I need."
    4. "I will mix the concentrate with orange juice to improve the taste."
30. A nurse is monitoring a client receiving cyclosporine (Sandimmune). Which of the following indicates to the nurse that the client is experiencing an adverse effect from this medication?
    1. Nausea
    2. Alopecia
    3. Tremor
    4. Hypotension
31. Tacrolimus (Prograf) is prescribed for a client for prevention of organ rejection after renal transplantation. Which of the following would the nurse

expect to be prescribed for this client during administration of this medication?

1. Prednisone (Deltasone)
2. Erythromycin (E-Mycin)
3. Fluconazole (Diflucan)
4. Phenytoin (Dilantin)

32. Tacrolimus (Prograf) is prescribed for the client. Which of the following disorders, if noted on the client's record, indicates that the medication needs to be administered with caution?
    1. Diabetes insipidus
    2. Coronary artery disease
    3. Renal insufficiency
    4. Ulcerative colitis
33. A nurse is reviewing the laboratory results documented in the record of a client receiving tacrolimus (Prograf). Which of the following indicates to the nurse that the client is experiencing an adverse effect of the medication?
    1. White blood cell (WBC) count of 6000/μL
    2. Blood glucose of 200 mg/dL
    3. Potassium level 3.8 mEq/L
    4. Platelet count 300,000 cells/μL
34. Muromonab-CD3 (Orthoclone OKT3) is prescribed for a client to manage allograft rejection after renal transplantation. The nurse administers the medication knowing that the primary mechanism of action of this medication is that it:
    1. Binds to the CD3 site and blocks all T-cell functions.
    2. Inhibits the proliferation of B lymphocytes.
    3. Crosslinks DNA, causing cell injury and death
    4. Suppresses B lymphocytes
35. Mycophenolate mofetil (CellCept) is prescribed for a client as prophylaxis for organ rejection after allogeneic renal transplantation. Which of the following instructions does the nurse reinforce regarding administration of this medication?
    1. Administer after meals
    2. Open the capsule and mix with food for administration
    3. Contact the physician if a sore throat occurs
    4. Take the medication with a magnesium-type antacid
36. Azathioprine (Imuran) is prescribed for the client to suppress rejection of a renal transplant. The nurse administers the medication knowing that the mechanism of action of this medication is that it:
    1. Inhibits the proliferation of B and T lymphocytes
    2. Crosslinks DNA
    3. Blocks all T-cell functions
    4. Decreases the activity of thymus-derived lymphocytes
37. A client with chronic renal failure (CRF) is receiving epoetin alfa (Epogen). The nurse is reviewing the laboratory results and notes that which of the following results indicates a therapeutic effect of the medication?
    1. White blood cell (WBC) count of 6000/μL
    2. Hematocrit count of 32%
    3. Platelet count of 400,000 cells/μL
    4. Blood urea nitrogen (BUN) of 15 mg/dL
38. Epoetin alfa (Epogen) has been prescribed for the client with chronic renal failure (CRF). The nurse will prepare to administer this medication by which of the following routes?
    1. PO
    2. IM
    3. Intradermally
    4. Subcutaneously
39. A nurse is monitoring the client receiving epoetin alfa (Epogen) for adverse effects of the medication. The nurse notes that which of the following indicates an adverse effect?
    1. Hypotension
    2. Hypertension
    3. Depression
    4. Bradycardia
40. A nurse is reviewing the laboratory studies of a client receiving epoetin alfa (Epogen). The nurse expects to note a therapeutic effect of this medication:
    1. After 1 week of therapy
    2. Immediately
    3. 3 days after therapy
    4. 2 weeks after therapy
41. A nurse is reinforcing instructions to a client regarding how to administer epoetin alfa (Epogen) by subcutaneous route. The nurse tells the client to:
    1. Shake the bottle before use
    2. Keep the vial of medication at room temperature
    3. Use only 1 dose per vial
    4. Use alcohol to clean the top of the vial when reused
42. Aluminum hydroxide gel (Amphojel) is prescribed for the client with chronic renal failure (CRF). The nurse instructs the client to take this medication:
    1. On an empty stomach
    2. At bedtime
    3. With meals
    4. In the morning upon arising

ANSWERS

1. *Answer:* 2

Rationale: Cinobac is a urinary antiseptic and is administered with meals to decrease gastrointestinal side effects. Options 1, 3, and 4 are incorrect.

Test-Taking Strategy: Use the process of elimination. Eliminate options 1, 3, and 4 because they are similar in that all of these options indicate taking the medication on an empty stomach. Review this medication if you had difficulty with this question.

Level of Cognitive Ability: Application

Client Needs: Health Promotion and Maintenance

Integrated Concept/Process: Nursing Process/Implementation

Content Area: Pharmacology

Reference: Black J, Hawks J, Keene A: *Medical-surgical nursing: clinical management for positive outcomes*, ed 6, Philadelphia, 2001, WB Saunders, p. 804.

2. *Answer:* 2

Rationale: NegGram is used for acute and chronic urinary tract infections, especially gram-negative bacterial infections. The medication is contraindicated in clients with a history of seizures. It is used with caution in clients with liver or renal disorders.

Test-Taking Strategy: Knowledge regarding the contraindications associated with this medication is required to answer the question. Review this medication if you had difficulty with this question.

Level of Cognitive Ability: Application

Client Needs: Safe, Effective Care Environment

Integrated Concept/Process: Nursing Process/Implementation

Content Area: Pharmacology

Reference: Lehne R: *Pharmacology for nursing care*, ed 4, Philadelphia, 2001, WB Saunders, p. 976.

3. *Answer:* 3

Rationale: Noroxin is administered 1 hour before or 2 hours after meals because food may hamper absorption. The normal dosage is 400 mg PO BID for 7 to 10 days for mild infections and for 10 to 21 days for severe infections.

Test-Taking Strategy: Use the process of elimination. Eliminate options 1 and 4 first because they are similar. To discriminate between the remaining options, knowledge that this medication is administered more than once a day will direct you to option 3. Review this medication if you had difficulty with this question.

Level of Cognitive Ability: Application

Client Needs: Health Promotion and Maintenance

Integrated Concept/Process: Nursing Process/Implementation

Content Area: Pharmacology

Reference: Hodgson B, Kizior R: *Saunders nursing drug handbook 2002*, Philadelphia, 2002, WB Saunders, p. 810.

4. *Answer:* 4

Rationale: When a client is receiving Macrodantin, the urinary pH must be maintained in an acid range. The client needs to be instructed to consume an acid-ash diet. Rhubarb will reduce the acidity of the urine and should be avoided when the client requires an acid-ash diet.

Test-Taking Strategy: Use the process of elimination. Note the key word "avoid" in the stem of the question. Knowledge that this medication requires that the urinary pH be maintained in an acid range will assist in directing you to option 4. Review this medication if you had difficulty with this question.

Level of Cognitive Ability: Application

Client Needs: Health Promotion and Maintenance

Integrated Concept/Process: Nursing Process/Implementation

Content Area: Pharmacology

Reference: Hodgson B, Kizior R: *Saunders nursing drug handbook 2002*, Philadelphia, 2002, WB Saunders, p. 800.

5. *Answer:* 1

Rationale: Mandelamine is contraindicated in clients with renal or hepatic disease or in clients with severe dehydration. The nurse would question the physician's prescription for this medication in the client with cirrhosis.

Test-Taking Strategy: Use the process of elimination. Knowledge that this medication is contraindicated in hepatic disease will easily direct you to option 1. Review this medication if you had difficulty with this question.

Level of Cognitive Ability: Application

Client Needs: Safe, Effective Care Environment

Integrated Concept/Process: Nursing Process/Implementation

Content Area: Pharmacology

Reference: Lehne R: *Pharmacology for nursing care*, ed 4, Philadelphia, 2001, WB Saunders, p. 976.

6. *Answer:* 3

Rationale: Gastrointestinal (GI) effects are the most frequent adverse reactions to this medication and can be minimized by administering the medication with milk or meals. Pulmonary reactions, manifested as dyspnea, chest pain, chills, fever, cough, and the presence of alveolar infiltrates on x-ray film, would indicate the need to stop the treatment. These symptoms would resolve in 2 to 4 days after discontinuation of this medication.

Test-Taking Strategy: Use the process of elimination. Eliminate options 1, 2, and 4 because they are GI-related side effects. Review this medication if you had difficulty with this question.

Level of Cognitive Ability: Analysis

Client Needs: Physiological Integrity

Integrated Concept/Process: Nursing Process/Data Collection

Content Area: Pharmacology

Reference: Hodgson B, Kizior R: *Saunders nursing drug handbook 2002*, Philadelphia, 2002, WB Saunders, p. 800.

7. *Answer:* 1

Rationale: For treatment of acute UTI, the adult dosage is 50 mg three to four times a day. For prophylaxis of recurrent UTI, low doses are used, such as 50 to 100 mg at bedtime for adults.

Test-Taking Strategy: Use the process of elimination. Knowledge regarding the normal adult dosage of Macrodantin is required to answer this question. Review this medication if you had difficulty with this question.

Level of Cognitive Ability: Comprehension

Client Needs: Physiological Integrity

Integrated Concept/Process: Nursing Process/Implementation

Content Area: Pharmacology

Reference: Hodgson B, Kizior R: *Saunders nursing drug handbook 2002*, Philadelphia, 2002, WB Saunders, p. 800.

8. *Answer:* 2
Rationale: Methenamine, under acidic conditions, decomposes into ammonia and formaldehyde. The formaldehyde denatures bacterial proteins, causing death. Nalidixic acid (NegGram) is a medication that inhibits the replication of bacterial DNA. Antispasmodics relax smooth muscle of the urinary tract and decrease bladder muscle spasms.
Test-Taking Strategy: Use the process of elimination. Eliminate options 3 and 4 because they are similar. From the remaining options, it is necessary to know the action of this medication. If you had difficulty with this question review this medication.
Level of Cognitive Ability: Comprehension
Client Needs: Physiological Integrity
Integrated Concept/Process: Nursing Process/Implementation
Content Area: Pharmacology
Reference: Lehne R: *Pharmacology for nursing care,* ed 4, Philadelphia, 2001, WB Saunders, p. 972.

9. *Answer:* 2
Rationale: Nalidixic acid can intensify the effects of oral anticoagulants. When an oral anticoagulant is combined with nalidixic acid, a reduction in the anticoagulant dosage may be needed.
Test-Taking Strategy: Use the process of elimination. Option 3 can be eliminated as the least likely choice. Eliminate option 1 as the next least likely prescription. From the remaining options, the most likely choice, based on the situation presented, is option 2. Review this medication if you had difficulty with this question.
Level of Cognitive Ability: Analysis
Client Needs: Physiological Integrity
Integrated Concept/Process: Nursing Process/Implementation
Content Area: Pharmacology
Reference: Lehne R: *Pharmacology for nursing care,* ed 4, Philadelphia, 2001, WB Saunders, p. 976.

10. *Answer:* 1
Rationale: Nalidixic acid is dispensed in tablets of 250 mg, 500 mg, and 1 g, and in a suspension of 50 mg/mL for oral use. Adult dosage is 1 gram four times a day for 1 week. It should not be administered to children less than 3 months old because it may produce intracranial hypertension in pediatric clients.
Test-Taking Strategy: Knowledge regarding the normal adult dosage of nalidixic acid is required to answer this question. Review this medication if you had difficulty with this question.
Level of Cognitive Ability: Comprehension
Client Needs: Physiological Integrity
Integrated Concept/Process: Nursing Process/Implementation
Content Area: Pharmacology
Reference: Lehne R: *Pharmacology for nursing care,* ed 4, Philadelphia, 2001, WB Saunders, p. 976.

11. *Answer:* 2
Rationale: Cinoxacin should be administered with caution in clients with renal impairment. The dosage should be reduced, and failure to do so could result in accumulation of cinoxacin to toxic levels. The disorders in options 1, 3, and 4 are not contraindications to this medication.
Test-Taking Strategy: Use the process of elimination. Knowledge that this medication is to be used with caution in clients with renal impairment will easily direct you to option 2. Review the contraindications associated with this medication if you had difficulty with this question.
Level of Cognitive Ability: Analysis
Client Needs: Physiological Integrity
Integrated Concept/Process: Nursing Process/Data Collection
Content Area: Pharmacology
Reference: Black J, Hawks J, Keene A: *Medical-surgical nursing: clinical management for positive outcomes,* ed 6, Philadelphia, 2001, WB Saunders, p. 804.

12. *Answer:* 2
Rationale: Each dose of Gantrisin should be administered with a full glass of water, and the client should maintain a high fluid intake. The medication is more soluble in alkaline urine. The client should not be instructed to taper or discontinue the dose. Some forms of Gantrisin such as Azo Gantrisin cause the urine to turn dark brown or red. This does not indicate the need to notify the physician.
Test-Taking Strategy: Use the process of elimination. General principles related to medication administration will assist in eliminating option 3. From the remaining options, recalling that this medication is a sulfonamide will direct you to option 2. Review this medication if you had difficulty with this question.
Level of Cognitive Ability: Application
Client Needs: Health Promotion and Maintenance
Integrated Concept/Process: Teaching/Learning
Content Area: Pharmacology
Reference: Lehne R: *Pharmacology for nursing care,* ed 4, Philadelphia, 2001, WB Saunders, p. 965.

13. *Answer:* 1
Rationale: Sulfonamides can intensify the effects of warfarin (Coumadin), phenytoin (Dilantin), and oral hypoglycemics such as tolbutamide (Orinase). When combined with sulfonamides, these medications may require a reduction in dosage.
Test-Taking Strategy: Use the process of elimination. Options 3 and 4 can be eliminated as the least likely choices. From the remaining options, the most likely choice, based on the situation presented, would be option 1. Review medication interactions associated with sulfonamides if you had difficulty with this question.
Level of Cognitive Ability: Analysis
Client Needs: Physiological Integrity
Integrated Concept/Process: Nursing Process/Planning
Content Area: Pharmacology
Reference: Lehne R: *Pharmacology for nursing care,* ed 4, Philadelphia, 2001, WB Saunders, p. 963.

14. *Answer:* 4
Rationale: Clients taking trimethoprim-sulfamethoxazole should be informed about early signs of blood disorders that can occur from this medication. These signs include sore throat, fever, or pallor; the client should be instructed to notify the physician if these symptoms occur. The other options do not require physician notification.

Test-Taking Strategy: Knowledge that this medication can cause blood dyscrasias is required to answer the question. Review this medication if you had difficulty with this question.
Level of Cognitive Ability: Application
Client Needs: Health Promotion and Maintenance
Integrated Concept/Process: Nursing Process/Implementation
Content Area: Pharmacology
Reference: Lehne R: *Pharmacology for nursing care,* ed 4, Philadelphia, 2001, WB Saunders, p. 968.

15. *Answer:* 2
Rationale: The client should be instructed that a reddish-orange discoloration of urine may occur. The client should also be instructed that this discoloration can stain fabric. The medication should be taken after meals to reduce the possibility of gastrointestinal upset. A headache is an occasional side effect of the medication and does not warrant discontinuation of the medication.
Test-Taking Strategy: Use the process of elimination. Eliminate options 1 and 4 first because they are similar. From the remaining options, eliminate option 3 because the nurse would not advise the client to discontinue this medication. Review this medication if you had difficulty with this question.
Level of Cognitive Ability: Application
Client Needs: Health Promotion and Maintenance
Integrated Concept/Process: Nursing Process/Implementation
Content Area: Pharmacology
Reference: Lehne R: *Pharmacology for nursing care,* ed 4, Philadelphia, 2001, WB Saunders, p. 901.

16. *Answer:* 2
Rationale: Urecholine can be hazardous to clients with urinary tract obstruction or weakness of the bladder wall. The medication has the ability to contract the bladder and thereby increase pressure within the urinary tract. Elevation of pressure within the urinary tract could rupture the bladder in clients with these conditions.
Test-Taking Strategy: Knowledge regarding the contraindications associated with this medication is required to answer this question. Noting that the medication is used for urinary retention may assist in directing you to option 2. Review this medication if you had difficulty with this question.
Level of Cognitive Ability: Analysis
Client Needs: Physiological Integrity
Integrated Concept/Process: Nursing Process/Data Collection
Content Area: Pharmacology
Reference: Lehne R: *Pharmacology for nursing care,* ed 4, Philadelphia, 2001, WB Saunders, p. 116.

17. *Answer:* 2
Rationale: Administration of bethanechol with meals can cause nausea and vomiting in the client. To avoid this problem, oral doses should be administered 1 hour before meals or 2 hours after meals.
Test-Taking Strategy: Use the process of elimination. Note that options 1, 3, and 4 are similar in that they all suggest administering the medication with a food item. Review this medication if you had difficulty with this question.
Level of Cognitive Ability: Application
Client Needs: Health Promotion and Maintenance
Integrated Concept/Process: Nursing Process/Implementation
Content Area: Pharmacology
Reference: Lehne R: *Pharmacology for nursing care,* ed 4, Philadelphia, 2001, WB Saunders, p. 115.

18. *Answer:* 1
Rationale: The normal adult dosage of bethanechol ranges from 10 to 50 mg three to four times daily.
Test-Taking Strategy: Knowledge regarding the normal dosage of this medication is required to answer this question. Learn this dosage if you had difficulty with this question.
Level of Cognitive Ability: Comprehension
Client Needs: Physiological Integrity
Integrated Concept/Process: Nursing Process/Implementation
Content Area: Pharmacology
Reference: Lehne R: *Pharmacology for nursing care,* ed 4, Philadelphia, 2001, WB Saunders, p. 115.

19. *Answer:* 3
Rationale: Cholinergic overdose can occur with bethanechol. The antidote is atropine sulfate administered SC or by IV, which should be readily available for use if overdose occurs. Protamine sulfate is the antidote for heparin. Vitamin K is the antidote for warfarin sodium (Coumadin). Mucomyst is the antidote for acetaminophen (Tylenol) overdose.
Test-Taking Strategy: Use the process of elimination. Knowledge regarding the antidotes for certain medication overdoses is required to answer this question. Review these antidotes if you had difficulty with this question.
Level of Cognitive Ability: Application
Client Needs: Physiological Integrity
Integrated Concept/Process: Nursing Process/Implementation
Content Area: Pharmacology
Reference: Lehne R: *Pharmacology for nursing care,* ed 4, Philadelphia, 2001, WB Saunders, p. 115.

20. *Answer:* 4
Rationale: Overdose produces manifestations of excessive muscarinic stimulation such as salivation, sweating, involuntary urination and defecation, bradycardia, and severe hypotension. Treatment includes supportive measures and the administration of atropine SC or IV.
Test-Taking Strategy: Knowledge of the signs of cholinergic overdose is required to answer this question. Review these signs if you had difficulty with this question.
Level of Cognitive Ability: Analysis
Client Needs: Physiological Integrity
Integrated Concept/Process: Nursing Process/Data Collection
Content Area: Pharmacology
Reference: Lehne R: *Pharmacology for nursing care,* ed 4, Philadelphia, 2001, WB Saunders, p. 115.

21. *Answer:* 4
Rationale: The injectable form of bethanechol is intended for SC administration only. Bethanechol must never be injected IM or IV because the resulting high drug levels can cause severe toxicity such as bloody diarrhea, bradycardia, profound hypotension, and cardiovascular collapse.

Test-Taking Strategy: Knowledge regarding the route of administration of this medication is required to answer this question. Review this medication and administration route if you had difficulty with this question.
Level of Cognitive Ability: Application
Client Needs: Physiological Integrity
Integrated Concept/Process: Nursing Process/Implementation
Content Area: Pharmacology
Reference: Lehne R: *Pharmacology for nursing care*, ed 4, Philadelphia, 2001, WB Saunders, p. 116.

22. ***Answer:*** 3
Rationale: Overdose produces central nervous system excitation such as nervousness, restlessness, hallucinations, and irritability. Other signs of overdose include either hypotension or hypertension, confusion, tachycardia, flushed or red face, and signs of respiratory depression. Drowsiness is a frequent side effect of the medication, but does not indicate overdose.
Test-Taking Strategy: Knowledge regarding the manifestations related to overdose is required to answer this question. Review this medication if you had difficulty with this question.
Level of Cognitive Ability: Application
Client Needs: Physiological Integrity
Integrated Concept/Process: Nursing Process/Data Collection
Content Area: Pharmacology
Reference: Hodgson B, Kizior R: *Saunders nursing drug handbook 2002*, Philadelphia, 2002, WB Saunders, p. 836.

23. ***Answer:*** 1
Rationale: Pro-Banthine is contraindicated in clients with narrow angle glaucoma, obstructive uropathy, gastrointestinal disease, or ulcerative colitis. Options 2, 3, and 4 are not contraindications to the use of this medication.
Test-Taking Strategy: Use the process of elimination. Eliminate options 2 and 3 because they are similar. From the remaining options, it is necessary to know the contraindications associated with the medication. Review these contraindications if you had difficulty with this question.
Level of Cognitive Ability: Analysis
Client Needs: Physiological Integrity
Integrated Concept/Process: Nursing Process/Data Collection
Content Area: Pharmacology
Reference: Lehne R: *Pharmacology for nursing care*, ed 4, Philadelphia, 2001, WB Saunders, p. 120.

24. ***Answer:*** 3
Rationale: Nephrotoxicity can occur from the use of Sandimmune. Nephrotoxicity is evaluated by monitoring for an elevated BUN and serum creatinine level. Sandimmune does not depress the bone marrow.
Test-Taking Strategy: Use the process of elimination. Eliminate options 1 and 2 first because they are unrelated to renal function. Next, eliminate option 4 because the creatinine level would be elevated, not decreased. Option 3 is the only option that indicates an increased level of a renal function test. Review these contraindications if you had difficulty with this question.
Level of Cognitive Ability: Analysis
Client Needs: Physiological Integrity
Integrated Concept/Process: Nursing Process/Data Collection
Content Area: Pharmacology
Reference: Lehne R: *Pharmacology for nursing care*, ed 4, Philadelphia, 2001, WB Saunders, p. 749.

25. ***Answer:*** 2
Rationale: A compound present in grapefruit juice inhibits metabolism of cyclosporine. As a result, consuming grapefruit juice can raise cyclosporine levels by 50% to 100%, thereby greatly increasing the risk of toxicity.
Test-Taking Strategy: Use the process of elimination. Note the key word "avoid." Knowledge regarding substances that inhibit the metabolism of cyclosporine is required to answer this question. Review this medication if you had difficulty with this question.
Level of Cognitive Ability: Application
Client Needs: Health Promotion and Maintenance
Integrated Concept/Process: Teaching/Learning
Content Area: Pharmacology
Reference: Lehne R: *Pharmacology for nursing care*, ed 4, Philadelphia, 2001, WB Saunders, p. 749.

26. ***Answer:*** 3
Rationale: Medications known to lower cyclosporine levels include phenytoin, phenobarbital, rifampin, and trimethoprim-sulfamethoxazole. Cyclosporine levels should be monitored and the dosage adjusted in clients taking these medications.
Test-Taking Strategy: Knowledge regarding the medications that lower cyclosporine levels is required to answer this question. Review this information related to cyclosporine if you had difficulty with this question.
Level of Cognitive Ability: Analysis
Client Needs: Physiological Integrity
Integrated Concept/Process: Nursing Process/Data Collection
Content Area: Pharmacology
Reference: Lehne R: *Pharmacology for nursing care*, ed 4, Philadelphia, 2001, WB Saunders, p. 754.

27. ***Answer:*** 4
Rationale: Amphotericin B as well as erythromycin and ketoconazole can elevate cyclosporine levels. When either of these medications is combined with cyclosporine, the dosage of cyclosporine must be reduced to prevent accumulation to toxic levels.
Test-Taking Strategy: Knowledge regarding the medications that elevate cyclosporine levels is required to answer this question. Review this information related to cyclosporine if you had difficulty with this question.
Level of Cognitive Ability: Analysis
Client Needs: Physiological Integrity
Integrated Concept/Process: Nursing Process/Planning
Content Area: Pharmacology
Reference: Hodgson B, Kizior R: *Saunders nursing drug handbook 2002*, Philadelphia, 2002, WB Saunders, p. 59.

28. ***Answer:*** 3
Rationale: To improve palatability, the client should be taught to mix the concentrated medication solution with chocolate milk or orange juice just before administration. Grapefruit juice can raise cyclosporine levels. Instruct client to dispense

the oral liquid into a glass container using a specially calibrated pipette; mix well and drink immediately; rinse the container with diluent and drink it to ensure ingestion of the complete dose; dry the outside of the pipette, and return it to its cover for storage.
Test-Taking Strategy: Knowledge regarding the administration of the oral concentrate is required to answer this question. Review this procedure if you had difficulty with this question.
Level of Cognitive Ability: Application
Client Needs: Health Promotion and Maintenance
Integrated Concept/Process: Teaching/Learning
Content Area: Pharmacology
Reference: Lehne R: *Pharmacology for nursing care,* ed 4, Philadelphia, 2001, WB Saunders, p. 754.

29. *Answer:* 3
Rationale: The client needs to be instructed to dispense the oral liquid into a glass container using a specially calibrated pipette. The client should not use any other type of dropper to calibrate the amount of prescribed medication. Options 1, 2, and 4 are correct client statements.
Test-Taking Strategy: Use the process of elimination. Note the key words "indicate the need for further instruction." Knowledge regarding the administration of the oral concentrate is required to answer this question. Review this procedure if you had difficulty with this question.
Level of Cognitive Ability: Comprehension
Client Needs: Health Promotion and Maintenance
Integrated Concept/Process: Nursing Process/Evaluation
Content Area: Pharmacology
Reference: Lehne R: *Pharmacology for nursing care,* ed 4, Philadelphia, 2001, WB Saunders, p. 754.

30. *Answer:* 3
Rationale: The most common adverse effects of cyclosporine are nephrotoxicity, infection, hypertension, tremor, and hirsutism. Of these, nephrotoxicity and infection are the most serious.
Test-Taking Strategy: Knowledge regarding the adverse effects associated with cyclosporine is required to answer this question. Review these effects if you had difficulty with this question.
Level of Cognitive Ability: Analysis
Client Needs: Physiological Integrity
Integrated Concept/Process: Nursing Process/Data Collection
Content Area: Pharmacology
Reference: Lehne R: *Pharmacology for nursing care,* ed 4, Philadelphia, 2001, WB Saunders, p. 754.

31. *Answer:* 1
Rationale: Prograf is an alternative medication to cyclosporine for prevention of organ rejection in clients receiving transplant. The medication is somewhat more effective than cyclosporine but is also more toxic. Concurrent use of glucocorticoids is recommended during administration of this medication.
Test-Taking Strategy: Knowledge that glucocorticoids are administered concurrently with some medications used to prevent organ rejection will easily direct you to option 1. Review this medication if you had difficulty with this question.
Level of Cognitive Ability: Analysis
Client Needs: Physiological Integrity
Integrated Concept/Process: Nursing Process/Planning
Content Area: Pharmacology
Reference: Hodgson B, Kizior R: *Saunders nursing drug handbook 2002,* Philadelphia, 2002, WB Saunders, p. 1040.

32. *Answer:* 3
Rationale: Tacrolimus is used with caution in immunosuppressed clients and in clients with renal or hepatic function impairment. It is contraindicated in clients with hypersensitivity to this medication or hypersensitivity to cyclosporine.
Test-Taking Strategy: Many medications affect renal and hepatic function. If you had to select an option and were unsure of the correct answer, select the option that addresses renal or hepatic function. Review the cautions and contraindications associated with the administration of this medication if you had difficulty with this question.
Level of Cognitive Ability: Analysis
Client Needs: Physiological Integrity
Integrated Concept/Process: Nursing Process/Data Collection
Content Area: Pharmacology
Reference: Lehne R: *Pharmacology for nursing care,* ed 4, Philadelphia, 2001, WB Saunders, p. 751.

33. *Answer:* 2
Rationale: Nephrotoxicity is a major concern with this medication. Other common reactions include neurotoxicity evidenced by headache, tremor, and insomnia; gastrointestinal effects such as diarrhea, nausea, and vomiting; hypertension; hyperkalemia; and hyperglycemia evidenced by an elevated blood glucose level.
Test-Taking Strategy: Use the process of elimination noting that options 1, 3, and 4 represent normal values. Option 2 is the only abnormal value reflecting an elevation. Review these normal laboratory values if you had difficulty with this question.
Level of Cognitive Ability: Analysis
Client Needs: Physiological Integrity
Integrated Concept/Process: Nursing Process/Data Collection
Content Area: Pharmacology
Reference: Hodgson B, Kizior R: *Saunders nursing drug handbook 2002,* Philadelphia, 2002, WB Saunders, p. 1040.

34. *Answer:* 1
Rationale: Orthoclone is a monoclonal antibody. Upon binding to the CD3 site, the antibody blocks all T-cell function. Options 2, 3, and 4 are not actions of this medication.
Test-Taking Strategy: Knowledge regarding the action of this medication is required to answer this question. Review this medication if you had difficulty with this question.
Level of Cognitive Ability: Comprehension
Client Needs: Physiological Integrity
Integrated Concept/Process: Nursing Process/Implementation
Content Area: Pharmacology
Reference: Lehne R: *Pharmacology for nursing care,* ed 4, Philadelphia, 2001, WB Saunders, p. 753.

35. *Answer:* 3
Rationale: Mycophenolate mofentil should be administered on an empty stomach. The capsules should not be opened or

crushed. The client should contact the physician if unusual bleeding or bruising, sore throat, mouth sores, abdominal pain, or fever occurs. Antacids containing magnesium and aluminum may decrease the absorption of the medication and therefore should not be taken with the medication. The medication is given in combination with corticosteroids and cyclosporine.
Test-Taking Strategy: Knowledge regarding the teaching points associated with the administration of this medication is required to answer this question. Review this medication if you had difficulty with this question.
Level of Cognitive Ability: Application
Client Needs: Health Promotion and Maintenance
Integrated Concept/Process: Teaching/Learning
Content Area: Pharmacology
Reference: Lehne R: *Pharmacology for nursing care,* ed 4, Philadelphia, 2001, WB Saunders, p. 752.

36. ***Answer:*** 1
Rationale: Imuran suppresses cell mediated and humoral immune responses by inhibiting the proliferation of B and T lymphocytes. It is generally used as an adjunct to cyclosporine and glucocorticoids to help suppress transplant rejection.
Test-Taking Strategy: Knowledge regarding the action of this medication is required to answer this question. Review this medication if you had difficulty with this question.
Level of Cognitive Ability: Comprehension
Client Needs: Physiological Integrity
Integrated Concept/Process: Nursing Process/Implementation
Content Area: Pharmacology
Reference: Lehne R: *Pharmacology for nursing care,* ed 4, Philadelphia, 2001, WB Saunders, p. 795.

37. ***Answer:*** 2
Rationale: Epoetin alfa is used to reverse anemia associated with CRF. Therapeutic effect is seen when the hematocrit is between 30% and 33%.
Test-Taking Strategy: Use the process of elimination. Relate the name of the medication "Epogen" to the potential action or effect. The only laboratory test that would reflect the effect of this medication is identified in option 2. Review the therapeutic effect of this medication if you had difficulty with this question.
Level of Cognitive Ability: Analysis
Client Needs: Physiological Integrity
Integrated Concept/Process: Nursing Process/Evaluation
Content Area: Pharmacology
Reference: Lehne R: *Pharmacology for nursing care,* ed 4, Philadelphia, 2001, WB Saunders, p. 603.

38. ***Answer:*** 4
Rationale: Epoetin alfa is administered parenterally either by IV or SC route. Administration is by IV bolus for dialysis clients and by IV bolus or SC injection for nondialysis clients. It cannot be given orally because it is a glycoprotein and would be degraded in the gastrointestinal tract.
Test-Taking Strategy: Knowledge regarding administration of this medication is required to answer this question. Review this medication if you had difficulty with this question.
Level of Cognitive Ability: Application
Client Needs: Physiological Integrity
Integrated Concept/Process: Nursing Process/Implementation
Content Area: Pharmacology
Reference: Lehne R: *Pharmacology for nursing care,* ed 4, Philadelphia, 2001, WB Saunders, p. 603.

39. ***Answer:*** 2
Rationale: Epoetin alfa is generally well tolerated. The most significant adverse effect is hypertension. Occasionally, a tachycardia may occur as a side effect. It may also cause an improved sense of well-being.
Test-Taking Strategy: Knowledge regarding the significant adverse effect associated with epoetin alfa is required to answer this question. Review this medication if you had difficulty with this question.
Level of Cognitive Ability: Analysis
Client Needs: Physiological Integrity
Integrated Concept/Process: Nursing Process/Data Collection
Content Area: Pharmacology
Reference: Lehne R: *Pharmacology for nursing care,* ed 4, Philadelphia, 2001, WB Saunders, p. 603.

40. ***Answer:*** 4
Rationale: Epoetin alfa stimulates erythropoiesis. It takes 2 to 6 weeks after initiation of therapy before a clinically significant increase in hematocrit is observed. Therefore this medication is not intended for clients who require immediate correction of severe anemia, and it is not a substitute for emergency transfusions.
Test-Taking Strategy: Knowledge that the medication stimulates erythropoiesis will assist in directing you to option 4. Review this medication and its therapeutic effects if you had difficulty with this question.
Level of Cognitive Ability: Analysis
Client Needs: Physiological Integrity
Integrated Concept/Process: Nursing Process/Evaluation
Content Area: Pharmacology
Reference: Lehne R: *Pharmacology for nursing care,* ed 4, Philadelphia, 2001, WB Saunders, p. 608.

41. ***Answer:*** 3
Rationale: The client should be instructed not to shake the bottle. The medication should be refrigerated at all times. All partially used vials should be discarded, and the client should use only 1 dose per vial and not reenter the vial. Unused portions need to be discarded.
Test-Taking Strategy: Use the process of elimination. Note that options 3 and 4 are identifying opposite actions. This should provide you with the clue that one of these options may be the correct one. Review the teaching points related to this medication if you had difficulty with this question.
Level of Cognitive Ability: Application
Client Needs: Health Promotion and Maintenance
Integrated Concept/Process: Nursing Process/Implementation
Content Area: Pharmacology
Reference: Lehne R: *Pharmacology for nursing care,* ed 4, Philadelphia, 2001, WB Saunders, p. 608.

42. ***Answer:*** 3
Rationale: The client who is receiving Amphojel should take the medication with meals. The phosphate-binding effect is

best when it is taken with food. If tablets are used, they should be chewed well before swallowing.

Test-Taking Strategy: Use the process of elimination. Note that options 1, 2, and 4 are similar in that they all suggest administering the medication without a food item. Review this medication if you had difficulty with this question.

Level of Cognitive Ability: Application
Client Needs: Health Promotion and Maintenance
Integrated Concept/Process: Nursing Process/Implementation
Content Area: Pharmacology
Reference: Lehne R: *Pharmacology for nursing care,* ed 4, Philadelphia, 2001, WB Saunders, p. 856.

REFERENCES

Black J, Hawks J, Keene A: *Medical-surgical nursing: clinical management for positive outcomes,* ed 6, Philadelphia, 2001, WB Saunders.

Chernecky C, Berger B: *Laboratory tests and diagnostic procedures,* ed 3, Philadelphia, 2001, WB Saunders.

Clark J, Queener S, Karb V: *Pharmacologic basis of nursing practice,* ed 6, St Louis, 2000, Mosby.

DeWit S: *Fundamental concepts and skills for nursing,* Philadelphia, 2001, WB Saunders.

Hodgson B, Kizior R: *Saunders nursing drug handbook 2002,* Philadelphia, 2002, WB Saunders.

Ignatavicius D, Workman M: *Medical-surgical: critical thinking for collaborative care,* ed 4, Philadelphia, 2002, WB Saunders.

Lehne R: *Pharmacology for nursing care,* ed 4, Philadelphia, 2001, WB Saunders.

Potter P, Perry A: *Fundamentals of nursing,* ed 5, St Louis, 2001, Mosby.

Smeltzer S, Bare B: *Brunner & Suddarth's Textbook of medical-surgical nursing, ed 9,* Philadelphia, 2000, Lippincott Williams & Wilkins.

UNIT XV

The Adult Client with an Eye or Ear Disorder

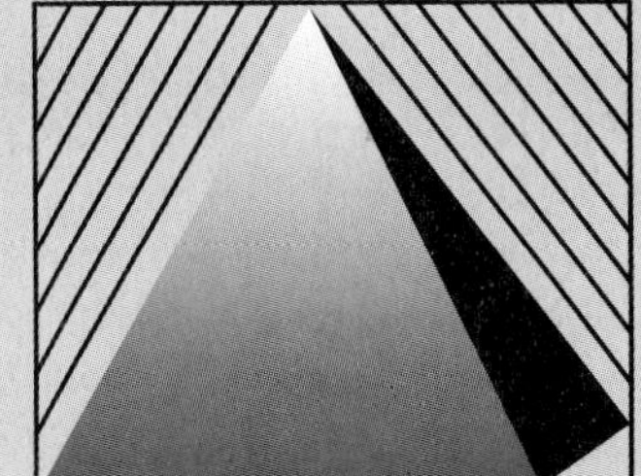

PYRAMID TERMS

Astigmatism Corneal curvature; eye may be hyperopic or myopic.

Cataracts An opacity of the lens that distorts the image projected onto the retina and that can progress to blindness.

Conductive Hearing Loss When sound waves are blocked to the inner ear fibers because of external ear or middle ear disorders. Disorders can often be corrected with no damage to hearing, or minimal permanent hearing loss.

Cycloplegia Refers to paralysis of the ciliary muscles. Cycloplegia causes blurred vision because the shape of the lens can no longer be adjusted to near vision.

Fenestration The stapes is removed with a small hole drilled in the footplate, and a prosthesis is connected between the incus and foot plate. Sounds cause the prosthesis to vibrate in the same manner as did the stapes.

Glaucoma Increased intraocular pressure as a result of inadequate drainage of aqueous humor from the canal of Schlemm or overproduction of aqueous humor. The condition damages the optic nerve and can result in blindness.

Hyperopia Farsightedness; objects converge to a point behind the retina. Vision beyond 20 feet is normal but near vision is poor. Correction is done by a convex lens.

Legally Blind If the best visual acuity with corrective lenses in the better eye is 20/200 or less, or if visual acuity is less than 20 degrees of the visual field in the better eye.

Meniere's Syndrome A syndrome also called endolymphatic hydrops, which refers to dilation of the endolymphatic system either by overproduction or decreased reabsorption of endolymphatic fluid. It is characterized by tinnitus, unilateral sensorineural hearing loss, and vertigo.

Miosis Refers to a constricted pupil.

Miotics Medications that cause contraction of the pupil.

Mydriasis Refers to a dilated pupil.

Mydriatics Medications that dilate the pupil.

Myopia Nearsightedness; rays coming from an object are focused in front of the retina. Near vision is normal but distant vision is defective. A biconcave lens is used for correction.

Otosclerosis Disease of the labyrinthine capsule of the middle ear that results in a bony overgrowth of tissue surrounding the ossicles. Causes the development of irregular areas of new bone formation and fixation of the bones. Stapes fixation leads to a conductive hearing loss.

Presbycusis Common cause of sensorineural hearing loss associated with aging.

Retinal Detachment Occurs when the layers of the retina separate as a result of accumulation of fluid between them, or when both retinal layers elevate away from choroid as a result of a tumor. Partial separation becomes complete if untreated. When detachment becomes complete, blindness occurs.

Sensorineural Hearing Loss A pathological process of the inner ear or of the sensory fibers that leads to the cerebral cortex. It is often permanent and measures must be taken to reduce further damage or to attempt to amplify sound as a means of improving hearing to some degree.

PYRAMID TO SUCCESS

Pyramid points focus on nursing interventions for clients with impairment in sight or hearing and on the nursing care related to disorders such as cataracts, glaucoma, and retinal detachment. Pyramid points also focus on emergency interventions for eye and ear disorders and injuries. Review nursing care related to organ donation for the donor and the recipient. Pyramid points also focus on client instructions related to medication administration, sensory perceptual alterations and safety issues, and available support systems. The Integrated Concepts and Processes addressed in this unit include the Clinical Problem-Solving Process (Nursing Process), Caring, Communication and Documentation, Cultural Awareness, Self-Care, and Teaching/Learning.

CLIENT NEEDS

Safe, Effective Care Environment

Accident prevention related to sensory impairments
Asepsis with procedures and treatments
Client rights
Communication techniques for impaired vision and hearing
Establishing priorities
Informed consent for invasive procedures
Organ donation
Standard (universal) precautions

Health Promotion and Maintenance

Aging process
Expected body image changes
Home care instructions after procedures related to the eye and ear
Instructions regarding the administration of eye and ear medications
Reinforcement regarding the importance of compliance to the prescribed therapy
The prevention and early detection of health problems and diseases related to the eye and ear

Psychosocial Integrity

Ability to cope with feelings of isolation and loss of independence
Available community resources
Family support systems
Sensory perceptual alterations
Threat to vision or hearing loss

Physiological Integrity

Care of assistive devices such as glasses, contact lenses, and hearing aids
Cataracts
Complications related to procedures
Expected responses to therapy
Glaucoma
Hearing or visual loss
Initial treatment for eye and ear emergencies
Organ donation
Pharmacological medications, actions, agents, side effects, and adverse effects
Retinal detachment
Self-care limitations

REFERENCES

Black J, Hawks J, Keene A: *Medical-surgical nursing: clinical management for positive outcomes*, ed 6, Philadelphia, 2001, WB Saunders.

Chernecky C, Berger B: *Laboratory tests and diagnostic procedures*, ed 3, Philadelphia, 2001, WB Saunders.

Clark J, Queener S, Karb V: *Pharmacologic basis of nursing practice*, ed 6, St Louis, 2000, Mosby.

DeWit S: *Fundamental concepts and skills for nursing*, Philadelphia, 2001, WB Saunders.

Hill S, Howlett H: *Success in practical nursing: personal and vocational issues*, ed 4, Philadelphia, 2001, WB Saunders.

National Council of State Boards of Nursing: *Test plan for the National Council Licensure Examination for Practical/Vocational Nurses*, Chicago, 2001, Author.

Potter P, Perry A: *Fundamentals of nursing*, ed 5, St Louis, 2001, Mosby.

Perry A, Potter P: *Clinical nursing skills and techniques*, ed 5, St Louis, 2002, Mosby.

Wilson J: *Infection control in clinical practice*, ed 2, St Louis, 2002, Balliere Tindall.

The Eye and the Ear

I. ANATOMY AND PHYSIOLOGY OF THE EYE

A. The eye
 1. The eye is 1 inch in diameter
 2. It is located in the anterior portion of the orbit
 3. The orbit is the bony structure of the skull that surrounds the eye and offers protection to the eye

B. Layers of the eye
 1. External layer
  a. The fibrous coat that supports the eye
  b. Contains the sclera, which is an opaque white tissue
  c. Contains the cornea, which is a dense transparent layer
 2. Middle layer
  a. The second layer of the eyeball
  b. Is vascular and heavily pigmented
  c. Consists of the choroid, ciliary body, and iris
  d. The choroid is the dark brown membrane located between the sclera and the retina
  e. The choroid lines most of the sclera and is attached to the retina, but can easily detach from the sclera
  f. The choroid contains many blood vessels and supplies nutrients to the retina
  g. The ciliary body connects the choroid with the iris and secretes aqueous humor that helps give the eye its shape
  h. The iris is the colored portion of the eye, is located in front of the lens, and has a central circular opening called the pupil
 3. Internal layer
  a. Consists of the retina
  b. The retina is a thin, delicate structure in which the fibers of the optic nerve are distributed
  c. The retina is bordered externally by the choroid and sclera and internally by the vitreous
  d. The retina contains blood vessels and photoreceptors called rods and cones

C. Vitreous body
 1. Contains a gelatinous substance that occupies the vitreous chamber, which is the space between the lens and the retina
 2. It transmits light and gives shape to the posterior eye

D. Vitreous
 1. A gel-like substance that maintains the shape of the eye
 2. Provides additional physical support to the retina

E. Rods and cones
 1. Rods are responsible for peripheral vision and function at reduced levels of illumination
 2. Cones function at bright levels of illumination and are responsible for color vision and central vision

F. Optic disk
 1. A creamy pink to white depressed area in the retina
 2. The optic nerve enters and exits the eyeball at this area
 3. This area is called the blind spot because it contains only nerve fibers, lacks photoreceptor cells, and is insensitive to light

G. Macula lutea
 1. A small, oval, yellowish pink area located lateral and temporal to the optic disk
 2. The central depressed part of the macula is the fovea centralis where most acute vision occurs

H. Aqueous humor
 1. A clear watery fluid that fills the anterior and posterior chambers of the eye

2. Produced by the ciliary processes and the fluid drains into the canal of Schlemm
3. The anterior chamber lies between the cornea and the iris
4. The posterior chamber lies between iris and lens

I. Canal of Schlemm
1. A passageway that extends completely around the eye
2. Permits fluid to drain out of the eye into the systemic circulation so a constant intraocular pressure is maintained

J. Lens
1. A transparent circular structure behind the iris and in front of vitreous body
2. Bends rays of light so that the light falls on the retina

K. Pupils
1. Control the amount of light that enters the eye and reaches the retina
2. Darkness produces dilation
3. Light produces constriction

L. Conjunctivae
1. The thin transparent mucous membrane
2. Lines the posterior surface of each eyelid and is located over the sclera

M. Lacrimal gland
1. Produces tears
2. Tears are drained throughout the punctum into the lacrimal duct and sac

N. Eye muscles
1. Muscles do not work independently but work in conjunction with the muscle that produces the opposite movement
2. Rectus muscles: exert their pull when the eye turns temporally
3. Oblique muscles: exert their pull when the eye turns nasally

O. Nerves
1. Cranial nerve III: oculomotor
2. Cranial nerve IV: trochlear
3. Cranial nerve VI: abducens
4. Cranial nerve II: optic nerve (nerve of sight)

P. Blood vessels
1. Ophthalmic artery: major artery supplying the structures in the eye
2. Ophthalmic veins: venous drainage occurs through the veins

II. ANATOMY AND PHYSIOLOGY OF THE EAR

A. Functions
1. Hearing
2. Maintenance of balance

B. External ear
1. Embedded in the temporal bone bilaterally at the level of the eyes
2. Extends from the auricle through the external canal to the tympanic membrane or eardrum
3. Includes the mastoid process, which is the body ridge located over the temporal bone

C. Middle ear
1. Consists of the medial side of the tympanic membrane
2. Contains three bony ossicles
   a. Malleus
   b. Incus
   c. Stapes
3. The tympanic membrane is a thick transparent sheet of tissue that provides a barrier between the external and the middle ear
4. The middle ear is protected from the inner ear by the round and the oval window membranes
5. The eustachian tube opens into the middle ear and allows for equalization of pressure on both sides of the tympanic membrane

D. Inner ear
1. Contains the semicircular canals, the cochlea, and the distal end of the eighth cranial nerve
2. The semicircular canals contain fluid and hair cells connected to sensory nerve fibers of the vestibular portion of eighth cranial nerve
3. Maintains sense of balance or equilibrium
4. Cochlea: spiral-shaped organ of hearing
5. Organ of Corti: receptor and organ of hearing
6. Eighth cranial nerve
   a. Cochlear branch: transmits neuroimpulses from the cochlea to the brain where they are interpreted as sound
   b. Vestibular branch: maintains balance and equilibrium

E. Hearing and equilibrium
1. The external ear conducts sound waves to the middle ear
2. The middle ear, also called the tympanic cavity, conducts sound vibrations to the inner ear
3. The middle ear is filled with air, which is kept at atmospheric pressure by the opening of the eustachian tube
4. The inner ear contains sensory receptors for sound and for equilibrium
5. The receptors in the inner ear transmit sound waves and changes in body position to the nerve impulses

III. ASSESSMENT OF VISION

A. Acuity
1. Visual acuity tests measure the client's distance and near vision
2. Snellen chart
   a. A simple tool to record visual acuity

b. The client stands 20 feet from the chart and covers one eye and uses the other eye to read the line that appears most clearly
c. If the client is able to do this accurately, the client reads the next lower line
d. This sequence is repeated until the client is unable to correctly identify more than half the characters on the line
e. The procedure is repeated for the other eye
f. The findings are recorded as a comparison between what the client can read at 20 feet
g. A result 20/50 means that the client is able to read at 20 feet from the chart what a healthy eye can read at 50 feet
h. Clients who wear corrective lenses other than for reading should have their vision tested with the lens in place

B. Confrontational test: performed to examine visual fields or peripheral vision
C. Extraocular muscle function: the client holds the head still and is asked to move eyes and to follow a small object through the six cardinal positions of gaze
D. Color vision: the standard tests for color vision involve picking numbers or letters out of a complex and colorful picture such as with the use of an Ishihara's chart
E. Pupils
1. Round and of equal size
2. Increasing light causes pupillary constriction
3. Decreasing light causes pupillary dilation
4. Constriction of both pupils is a normal response to direct light
5. The client is asked to look straight ahead while the examiner quickly brings a beam of a flashlight in from the side and directing it onto the eye
6. The constriction of the eye is a direct response to the shining of a flashlight into that eye; constriction of the opposite eye is known as a consensual response

F. Sclera and cornea
1. Normal sclera color is white
2. A yellow color to the sclera may indicate jaundice or systemic problems
3. In a dark-skinned person, the sclera may appear yellow; pigmented dots may be present
4. The cornea is transparent, smooth, shiny, and bright
5. Cloudy areas or specks on the cornea may be the result of an accident or eye injury

G. Ophthalmoscopy
1. An instrument is used to examine the external structures and the interior of the eye
2. The room is darkened so that the pupil will dilate

IV. DIAGNOSTIC TESTS FOR THE EYE

A. Fluorescein angiography
1. Description: detailed imaging and recording of ocular circulation by a series of photographs after the administration of a dye
2. Implementation preprocedure
a. Assess the client for allergies and previous reactions to dyes
b. Obtain an informed consent
c. A mydriatic medication, which causes pupil dilation, is instilled in the eye 1 hour before the test
d. The dye is injected into a vein of the client's arm
e. Inform the client that the dye may cause the skin to appear yellow for several hours after the test and is gradually eliminated through the urine
f. The client may experience nausea, vomiting, sneezing, paresthesia of the tongue, or pain at the injection site
g. If hives appear, oral or intramuscular antihistamines such as diphenhydramine (Benadryl) are administered as prescribed
3. Implementation postprocedure
a. Encourage rest
b. Encourage fluids to remove the dye from the client's system
c. Remind the client that the yellow skin appearance will disappear
d. Instruct the client that the urine will appear bright green until the dye is excreted
e. Instruct the client to avoid direct sunlight for a few hours after the test
f. Instruct the client that the photophobia will continue until pupil dilation returns to normal

B. Computed tomography (CT)
1. Description
a. A beam of x-ray scans the skull and orbits of the eye
b. Contrast material is not usually administered
2. Implementation
a. No special client preparation or follow-up care is required
b. Instruct the client that he or she will be positioned in a confined space and will need to keep the head still during procedure

C. Slit lamp
1. Description
a. Allows examination of the anterior ocular structures under microscopic magnification
b. The client leans on a chin rest to stabilize the head while a narrowed beam of light is

aimed so it illuminates only a narrow segment of the eye

2. Implementation
   a. Explain the procedure the client
   b. Advise the client about the brightness of the light and the need to look forward at a point over the examiner's ear

D. Corneal staining
1. Description
   a. Instillation of a topical dye into the conjunctival sac to outline irregularities of the corneal surface that are not easily visible
   b. The eye is viewed through a blue filter, and a bright green color indicates areas of a nonintact corneal epithelium
2. Implementation
   a. If the client wears contact lenses, they must be removed
   b. The client is instructed to blink after the dye has been applied to distribute the dye evenly across the cornea

E. Tonometry
1. Description
   a. The test is primarily used to assess for an increase in intraocular pressure and potential **glaucoma**
   b. Normal ocular pressure is 10 to 21 mm Hg
2. Implementation
   a. Each eye is anesthetized
   b. The client is asked to stare forward at a point above the examiner's ear
   c. A flattened cone is brought in contact with the cornea
   d. The amount of pressure needed to flatten the cornea is measured
   e. The client must be instructed to avoid rubbing the eye after the examination if the eye has been anesthetized because the potential for scratching the cornea exists

V. ASSESSMENT OF THE EAR

A. Otoscopic examination
1. A speculum is introduced into the external canal to visualize the tympanic membrane
2. The normal external canal is pink and intact without lesions and with various amounts of cerumen and fine little hairs
3. The tympanic membrane is transparent, opaque, pearly gray, slightly concave, and is intact and free from lesions

B. Auditory assessment
1. Sound is transmitted by air conduction and bone conduction
2. Air conduction take two to three times longer than bone conduction
3. Hearing loss is categorized as **conductive, sensorineural**, and mixed **conductive** and **sensorineural**
4. **Conductive hearing loss** is caused by any physical obstruction to the transmission of sound waves
5. **Sensorineural hearing loss** is a result of a defect in the organ of hearing, in the eighth cranial nerve, or in the brain itself
6. A mixed **conductive, sensorineural hearing loss** results in profound hearing loss
7. Tuning fork tests: the Weber and the Rinne tuning fork tests assist in distinguishing **conductive hearing loss** from **sensorineural hearing loss**

C. Vestibular assessment
1. Test for falling: a significant sway is a positive Romberg sign
2. Test for past pointing
   a. The normal test response is that the client can easily return to the point of reference
   b. Clients with vestibular function problems lack a normal sense of position and are unable to return their extended fingers to the point of reference; instead, they deviate either to the right or left of the reference point
3. Gaze nystagmus evaluation: any spontaneous nystagmus, a constant and involuntary cyclic movement of the eyeball in any direction, represents problems with the vestibular system
4. Hallpike maneuver
   a. Assesses for positional vertigo or induced dizziness
   b. The client assumes a supine position and the head is rotated to one side for 1 minute.
   c. A positive test results in nystagmus after 5 to 10 seconds

VI. DIAGNOSTIC TESTS FOR THE EAR

A. Tomography
1. Description
   a. Assesses the mastoid, middle ear, and inner ear structures; aids in the diagnosis of **conductive** and **sensorineural hearing loss**
   b. Multiple x-rays of the head are performed; especially helpful in the diagnosis of acoustic tumors
2. Implementation
   a. All jewelry is removed
   b. Lead eye shields are used to cover the cornea to diminish the radiation dose to the eyes
   c. The client must remain still in a supine position
   d. No follow-up care is required

B. Audiometry
1. Description
a. Measures hearing acuity using pure tone audiometry and speech audiometry
b. Pure tone audiometry is used to identify problems with hearing, speech, music, and other sounds in the environment
c. In speech audiometry, the client's ability to hear spoken words is measured
d. After testing, audiogram patterns are depicted on a graph to determine the type and level of the hearing loss
2. Implementation: instruct client to identify the sounds as they are heard

C. Caloric test (bithermal test)
1. Description
a. Performed to evaluate the client experiencing dizziness
b. Nystagmus, nausea, vomiting, or ataxia may indicate a pathological condition of the labyrinth system, whereas a decreased response may indicate that the vestibular system is affected
2. Implementation
a. Warm water causes a greater response than cold water
b. Warm-water caloric testing (irrigation) precedes cool-water caloric testing (irrigation)
c. The client must assume a supine position with the eyes closed and head elevated to 30 degrees
d. After the procedure, the client begins taking clear fluids slowly and cautiously because nausea and vomiting may occur
e. Assistance with ambulation may also be necessary after the procedure

VII. DISORDERS OF THE EYE

A. Risk factors related to eye disorders (Box 52-1)

B. **Legally blind**
1. Description: if the best visual acuity with corrective lenses in the better eye is 20/200 or less, or if visual acuity is less than 20 degrees of the visual field

BOX 52-1

Risk Factors of Eye Disorders

Aging process
Trauma
Hereditary
Congenital
Diabetes mellitus
Medications

2. Implementation
a. When speaking to the client who has limited sight or blindness, the nurse uses a normal tone of voice
b. Orient the client to the environment
c. Use a focal point and provide further orientation to the environment from that focal point
d. Allow the client to touch objects in the room
e. Use the clock placement of foods on the meal tray to orient the client
f. When ambulating, allow the client to grasp the nurse's arm at the elbow; the arm is kept close to the nurse's body so that the client can detect the direction of movement
g. Instruct the client to remain one step behind the nurse when ambulating
h. Instruct the client in the use of the cane used for the blind client, which is differentiated from other canes by its straight shape and white color with red tip
i. Instruct the client that the cane is held in the dominant hand several inches off the floor
j. Instruct the client that the cane sweeps the ground where the client's foot will be placed next, to determine the presence of obstacles
k. Alert the client when approaching
l. Provide radios, TVs, and clocks that give the time orally or provide Braille watches
m. Promote independence as much as is possible

C. **Cataracts**
1. Description
a. An opacity of the lens that distorts the image projected onto the retina and that can progress to blindness
b. Causes include the aging process (senile **cataracts**), inherited (congenital **cataracts**), injury (traumatic **cataracts**), and as a result of another eye disease (secondary **cataracts**)
c. Intervention is indicated when visual acuity has been reduced to a level that the client finds to be unacceptable or adversely affecting lifestyle
2. Data collection
a. Opaque or cloudy white pupil
b. Gradual loss of vision
c. Blurred vision
d. Decreased color perception
e. Vision that is better in dim light with pupil dilation
3. Implementation

a. Surgical removal of the lens, one eye at a time
b. Extracapsular extraction: the lens is lifted out without removing the lens capsule; may be performed by phacoemulsification in which the lens is broken up by ultrasonic vibrations and extracted
c. Intracapsular extraction: the lens is removed within its capsule through a small incision
d. A lens implantation may be performed at the time of the surgical procedure

4. Preoperative implementation: administer preoperative eye medications including **mydriatics** and cycloplegics as prescribed
5. Postoperative implementation
   a. Elevate head of bed 30 to 45 degrees
   b. Turn the client to back or nonoperative side
   c. Maintain eye patch; orient client to the environment
   d. Position the client's personal belongings to the nonoperative side
   e. Use side rails for safety
   f. Assist with ambulation
6. Client education (Box 52-2)

BOX 52-2

Client Education After Cataract Surgery

Avoid eye straining
Avoid rubbing or placing pressure on the eyes
Avoid rapid movements, straining, sneezing, coughing, bending, vomiting, lifting objects weighing more than 5 pounds
Instruct the client in measures to prevent constipation
Instruct the client and significant other on dressing changes and prescribed eye drops and medications
Wipe excess drainage or tearing with a sterile wet cotton ball from the inner to the outward canthus
Instruct the client and significant other in the use of an eye shield at bedtime
Instruct the client that if a lens implant was not performed, the eye cannot accommodate and glasses must be worn at all times
Instruct the client that cataract glasses act as magnifying glasses and replace central vision only
Instruct the client that cataract glasses magnify and objects will appear closer; therefore, they need to accommodate, judge distance, and climb stairs carefully
Instruct the client that contact lenses will provide sharp visual acuity but that dexterity is needed to insert them
Advise the client to contact physician for any decrease in vision, severe eye pain, or increase in eye discharge

D. **Glaucoma**
1. Description
   a. Increased intraocular pressure as a result of inadequate drainage of aqueous humor from canal of Schlemm or overproduction of aqueous humor
   b. The condition damages the optic nerve and can result in blindness
2. Types (Box 52-3)
3. Data collection
   a. Progressive loss of peripheral vision
   b. Elevated intraocular pressure (normal pressure is 10 to 21 mm Hg)
   c. Vision worsening in the evening with difficulty adjusting to dark rooms
   d. Blurred vision and progressive loss of central vision
   e. Halos around white lights
   f. Frontal headaches and eye pain
4. Implementation: acute **glaucoma**
   a. Treated as a medical emergency and medications are administered as prescribed to lower intraocular pressure
   b. Prepare the client for peripheral iridectomy, which allows aqueous humor to flow from the posterior to anterior chamber
5. Implementation: chronic **glaucoma**
   a. Instruct the client on the importance of medications (**miotics**) to constrict the pupils, and carbonic anhydrase inhibitors and beta blockers to decrease the production of aqueous humor
   b. Instruct the client on the need for lifelong medication use
   c. Instruct the client to wear a Medic-Alert bracelet
   d. Instruct the client to avoid anticholinergic medications
   e. Instruct the client to report eye pain, halos around the eyes, and changes in vision to the physician
   f. Instruct the client that when maximal medical therapy has failed to halt the progres-

BOX 52-3

Types of Glaucoma

Acute closed-angle or narrow-angle glaucoma: results from obstruction to outflow of aqueous humor
Chronic closed-angle glaucoma: follows an untreated attack of acute closed-angle glaucoma
Chronic open-angle glaucoma: results from overproduction or obstruction to the outflow of aqueous humor
Acute: a rapid onset of intraocular pressure greater than 50 to 70 mm Hg
Chronic: a slow, progressive, gradual onset of intraocular pressure greater that 30 to 50 mm Hg

sion of visual field loss and optic nerve damage, surgery will be recommended
   g. Prepare the client for trabeculoplasty as prescribed to facilitate aqueous humor drainage
   h. Prepare the client for trabeculectomy as prescribed, which allows drainage of aqueous humor into the conjunctival spaces by the creation of an opening

E. **Retinal detachment**
1. Description
   a. Occurs when the layers of the retina separate because of the accumulation of fluid between them, or when both retinal layers elevate away from choroid as a result of a tumor
   b. Partial separation becomes complete if untreated
   c. When detachment becomes complete, blindness occurs
2. Data collection
   a. Flashes of light
   b. Floaters
   c. Increase in blurred vision
   d. Sense of a curtain being drawn over the eyes
   e. Loss of a portion of the visual field
3. Immediate implementation
   a. Provide bed rest
   b. Cover both eyes with patches to prevent further detachment
   c. Position the client's head as prescribed
   d. Protect the client from injury
   e. Avoid jerky head movements and minimize eye stress
   f. Speak to the client before approaching
   g. Prepare client for surgical procedures as prescribed
4. Surgical procedures
   a. Draining fluid from the subretinal space so that the retina can return to the normal position
   b. Sealing retinal breaks by cryosurgery, a cold probe applied to the sclera, to stimulate an inflammatory response leading to adhesions
   c. Diathermy, the use of electrode needle and heat through the sclera, to stimulate an inflammatory response
   d. Laser therapy, to stimulate an inflammatory response, to seal small retinal tears before the detachment occurs
   e. Scleral buckling, to hold the choroid and retina together with a splint, until scar tissue forms, closing the tear
   f. Insertion of gas or silicone oil to encourage attachment because these agents have a specific gravity less than vitreous or air, and can float against the retina
5. Postoperative implementation
   a. Maintain eye patches bilaterally as prescribed
   b. Monitor for hemorrhage
   c. Prevent nausea and vomiting and monitor for restlessness, which can cause hemorrhage
   d. Monitor for sudden, sharp eye pain (notify the physician)
   e. Encourage deep breathing but avoid coughing
   f. Provide bed rest for 1 to 2 days as prescribed
   g. Position client as prescribed
   h. If gas has been inserted, position as prescribed on the abdomen and turn the head so the unaffected eye is down
   i. Assist the client with activities of daily living
   j. Avoid sudden head movements or anything that increases intraocular pressure
   k. Instruct the client to limit reading for 3 to 5 weeks
   l. Instruct the client to avoid squinting, straining and constipation, lifting heavy objects, and bending from the waist
   m. Instruct the client to wear dark glasses during the day and an eye patch at night
   n. Encourage follow-up care because of the danger of recurrence or occurrence in the other eye

F. Hyphema
1. Description
   a. The presence of blood in the anterior chamber that occurs as a result of an injury
   b. The condition usually resolves in 5 to 7 days
2. Implementation
   a. Encourage rest with client in semi-Fowler's position
   b. Avoid sudden eye movements for 3 to 5 days to decrease likelihood of bleeding
   c. Administer **cycloplegic** eye drops as prescribed to place the eye at rest
   d. Instruct the client in the use of eye shields or eye patches as prescribed
   e. Instruct the client to restrict reading and watching television

G. Contusions
1. Description
   a. Bleeding into the soft tissue as a result of an injury
   b. Causes a black eye, and the discoloration disappears in approximately 10 days

c. Visual acuity is usually not affected
d. Pain, photophobia, edema, and diplopia may occur
2. Implementation
a. Place ice on the eye immediately
b. Instruct the client to receive an eye examination

H. Foreign bodies
1. Description: an object such as dust that enters the eye
2. Implementation
a. Have the client look upward, expose the lower lid, wet a cotton-tipped applicator with sterile normal saline, and gently twist the swab over the particle and remove it
b. If the particle cannot be seen, have the client look downward, place a cotton-tipped applicator horizontally on the outer surface of the upper eye lid, grasp the lashes, and pull the upper lid outward and over the cotton applicator; if particle is seen, gently twist swab over it to remove

I. Penetrating objects
1. Description: an injury that occurs to the eye in which an object penetrates the eye
2. Implementation
a. Never remove the object because it may be holding ocular structures in place
b. The object must be removed by the physician
c. Cover the object with a cup
d. Do not allow the client to bend
e. Do not place pressure on eye
f. Client is to be seen by a physician immediately

J. Chemical burns
1. Description: an eye injury in which a caustic substance enters the eye
2. Implementation
a. Flush the eyes at the site of injury with water for at least 15 to 20 minutes
b. At the scene of the accident, obtain a sample of the chemical involved
c. At the emergency room, the eye is irrigated with gentle solutions such as normal saline or an ophthalmic irrigation solution
d. The solution is directed across the cornea and toward the lateral canthus
e. Prepare the client for visual acuity assessment
f. Apply antibiotic ointment as prescribed
g. Cover the eye with a patch as prescribed

K. Enucleation and exenteration
1. Description
a. Enucleation: removal of the entire eyeball
b. Exenteration: removal of the eyeball and surrounding tissues and bone
c. Performed for the removal of ocular tumors
d. After the eye is removed, a ball implant is inserted to provide a firm base for socket prosthesis and to facilitate the best cosmetic result
e. A prosthesis is fitted approximately 1 month after surgery
2. Preoperative implementation
a. Provide emotional support to the client
b. Encourage the client to verbalize feelings related to loss
3. Postoperative implementation
a. Monitor vital signs
b. Monitor pressure patch or dressing
c. Report changes in vital signs or the presence of bright red drainage on the pressure patch or dressing

L. Organ donation
1. Donor eyes
a. Obtained from cadavers
b. Must be enucleated soon after death because of rapid cell death
c. Must be stored in a preserving solution
d. Storage, handling, and coordination of donor tissue with surgeons are provided by a network of state eye bank associations across the country
2. Care to deceased client as a potential eye donor
a. Raise the head of the bed 30 degrees
b. Instill antibiotic eye drops as prescribed
c. Close the eyes and apply a small ice pack to the closed eyes
d. The family and physician are contacted to discuss the option of eye donation
3. Preoperative care to the recipient
a. Recipient may be told of the tissue availability only several hours to 1 day before the surgery
b. Assist in alleviating client anxiety
c. Monitor the eyes for signs of infection
d. Report the presence of any redness, watery, or purulent drainage or edema around the eye
e. Instill antibiotic drops into the eye as prescribed to reduce the number of microorganisms present
4. Postoperative care to the recipient
a. The eye is covered with a pressure patch and protective shield that is left in place until the next day
b. Do not remove or change the dressing without a physician's order
c. Monitor vital signs
d. Monitor level of consciousness

e. Assess dressing
f. Position the client on nonoperative side to reduce intraocular pressure
g. Orient the client frequently
h. Monitor for complications of bleeding, wound leakage, infection, and graft rejection
i. Instruct the client how to apply a patch and eye shield
j. Instruct the client to wear the eye shield at night for 1 month and whenever around small children or pets
k. Advise client not to rub the eye

5. Graft rejection
   a. Can occur at any time
   b. Inform the client of the signs of rejection
   c. Signs include redness, swelling, decreased vision, and pain (RSVP)
   d. Treated with topical corticosteroids

VIII. DISORDERS OF THE EAR

A. Risk factors related to ear disorders (Box 52-4)

B. **Conductive hearing loss**
1. Description
   a. When sound waves are blocked to the inner ear fibers because of external ear or middle ear disorders
   b. Disorders can often be corrected with no damage to hearing, or minimal permanent hearing loss
2. Causes
   a. Any inflammatory process or obstruction of the external or middle ear
   b. Tumors
   c. **Otosclerosis**
   d. A buildup of scar tissue on the ossicles from previous middle ear surgery

C. **Sensorineural hearing loss**
1. Description
   a. A pathological process of the inner ear or of the sensory fibers that lead to the cerebral cortex
   b. Is often permanent and measures must be taken to reduce further damage or to attempt to amplify sound as a means of improving hearing to some degree
2. Causes
   a. Damage to the inner ear structures
   b. Damage to cranial nerve VIII
   c. Prolonged exposure to loud noise
   d. Medications
   e. Trauma
   f. Inherited disorders
   g. Metabolic and circulatory disorders
   h. Infections
   i. Surgery
   j. **Meniere's syndrome**

D. Mixed hearing loss: client has both **sensorineural** and **conductive hearing loss**

E. Signs of hearing loss and facilitating communication (Box 52-5 and Box 52-6)

F. Cochlear implantation
1. Used for **sensorineural hearing loss**
2. A small computer converts sound waves into electrical impulses that directly stimulate nerve fibers
3. Electrodes are placed by the internal ear with a computer device attached to the external ear

G. Hearing aids
1. Used for the client with **conductive hearing loss**
2. Can help the client with **sensorineural** loss, although it is not as effective
3. A difficulty that exists is the amplification of background noise as well as voices
4. Client education (Box 52-7)

H. **Presbycusis**
1. Description
   a. Associated with aging
   b. Leads to degeneration or atrophy of the ganglion cells in the cochlea and a loss of elasticity of the basilar membranes

BOX 52-4
Risk Factors of Ear Disorders

Infection
Trauma
Ototoxicity
Medications
Tumors
Aging process

BOX 52-5
Signs of Hearing Loss

Frequently asking people to repeat statements
Straining to hear
Turning head or leaning forward to favor one ear
Shouting in conversation
Ringing in the ears
Failing to respond when not looking in the direction of the sound
Irritability
Answering questions incorrectly
Raising the volume of the television or radio
Avoiding large groups
Better understanding of speech when in small groups
Withdrawing from social interactions

BOX 52-6

Facilitating Communication

Using written words if the client is able to see, read, and write
Providing plenty of light in the room
Facing the client when speaking
Talking in a room without distracting noises
Moving close to the client and speaking slowly and clearly
Getting the attention of the client before you begin to speak
Keeping hands and other objects away from the mouth when talking to the client
Talking in lower tones, because shouting is not helpful
Rephrasing sentences and repeating information
Validating with the client the understanding of statements made, by asking the client to repeat what was said
Reading lips
Encouraging the client to wear glasses when talking to someone to improve vision for lip reading
Sign language, which combines speech with hand movements that signify letters, words, or phrases
Use of telephone amplifiers
Installing flashing lights that are activated by ringing of the telephone or doorbell
Using specially trained dogs that help the client to be aware of sound and to alert the client of potential dangers

BOX 52-7

Client Education Regarding a Hearing Aid

Encourage the client to start using the hearing aid slowly to develop an adjustment to the device
Adjust the volume to the minimal hearing level to prevent feedback squeaking
Teach the client to concentrate on the sounds that are to be heard and to filter out background noise
Instruct the client to clean the ear mold with mild soap and water
Avoid excessive wetting of hearing aid and try to keep the hearing aid dry
Clean the ear cannula of the hearing aid with a toothpick or pipe cleaner
Turn off the hearing aid and remove the battery when not in use
Keep extra batteries on hand
Keep hearing aid in a safe place
Prevent hair sprays, oils, or other hair and face products from coming in contact with the receiver of the hearing aid

c. Leads to compromise of the vascular supply to the inner ear with changes in several areas of the ear structure

2. Data collection
    a. Hearing loss is gradual and bilateral
    b. Client states they have no problem with hearing, but they cannot understand what the words are
    c. Client thinks that the speaker is mumbling

I. External otitis
1. Description
    a. Infective inflammatory or allergic responses involving the structure of the external auditory canal or the auricles
    b. An irritating or infective agent comes in contact with the epithelial layer of the external ear that leads to either an allergic response or signs and symptoms of an infection
    c. The skin becomes red, swollen, and tender to touch on movements
    d. The extensive swelling of the canal can lead to **conductive hearing loss** because of obstruction
    e. It is more common in children, occurs more often in hot, humid environments, and is termed "swimmer's ear"
    f. Prevention includes the elimination of irritating or infecting agents
2. Data collection
    a. Pain, itching, redness, and edema
    b. Plugged feeling in the ear
    c. Exudate
    d. Hearing loss
3. Implementation
    a. Apply heat locally for 20 minutes three times a day
    b. Encourage bed rest to assist in reducing pain
    c. Administer antibiotics or corticosteriods as prescribed
    d. Administer analgesics such as aspirin or acetaminophen (Tylenol) for the pain as prescribed
    e. Instruct the client that ears should be kept clean and dry
    f. Instruct the client to use ear plugs for swimming
    g. Instruct the client that cotton-tipped applicators should not be used to dry ears because their use can lead to trauma to the canal
    h. Instruct the client that irritating agents such as hair products or ear phones should be discontinued

J. Otitis media
1. Description: acute or chronic infective inflammatory or allergic responses involving the structure of the middle ear
2. Chronic otitis media

a. Surgical treatment is necessary to restore hearing
b. The type of surgery can vary and includes either a simple reconstruction of the tympanic membrane, a myringoplasty, or replacement of the ossicles within the middle ear
c. A tympanoplasty, a reconstruction of the middle ear, may be attempted to improve **conductive hearing loss**

3. Data collection
   a. Pain from pressure in the ear
   b. Hearing loss
   c. Tinnitus, dizziness, or vertigo
   d. Fever, headache, malaise
   e. Nausea and vomiting
   f. Bulging tympanic membrane
   g. Fluid behind the tympanic membrane
4. Implementation
   a. Provide bed rest to limit head movements and prevent pain
   b. Administer localized heat as prescribed
   c. Administer antibiotics as prescribed
   d. Administer analgesics such as aspirin and acetaminophen (Tylenol) as prescribed
   e. Administer oral and nasal antihistamines and decongestants to decrease mucus production and decrease levels of fluid in the middle ear
5. Myringotomy
   a. Surgically performed perforation of the tympanic membrane
   b. Allows drainage of middle ear fluids and thus alleviates pain
   c. Client education (Box 52-8)

BOX 52-8

Client Education After Myringotomy

Avoid strenuous activities
Avoid rapid head movements, bouncing, or bending
Avoid straining on bowel movement
Avoid drinking through a straw
Avoid traveling by air
Avoid forceful coughing
Avoid contact with persons with colds
Instruct the client that if they need to blow nose, blow one side at a time with mouth open
Avoid washing hair, showering, or getting head wet for 1 week
Instruct the client to keep ears dry for 6 weeks by keeping a ball of cotton coated with petroleum jelly in the ear and to change cotton ball daily
Instruct the client to change ear dressing every 24 hours as prescribed
Instruct the client to report excessive ear drainage to the physician

6. Needle aspiration: to remove fluid from middle ear
7. Insertion of a grommet: placed through the tympanic membrane to allow continuous drainage of the middle ear
8. Postoperative implementation for middle ear surgery
   a. Inform the client that initial hearing after surgery is diminished because of the packing in the ear canal, and that hearing improvement will occur after the ear canal packing is removed
   b. Keep the dressing clean and dry
   c. Keep the client flat with operative ear up for at least 12 hours as prescribed
   d. Administer antibiotics as prescribed
   e. Instruct the client that he or she may return to work in approximately 3 weeks after surgery as prescribed

K. Mastoiditis
1. Description
   a. May be acute or chronic and results from untreated or inadequately treated chronic or acute otitis media
   b. The pain is not relieved by myringotomy
2. Data collection
   a. Swelling behind the ear and pain with minimal movement of the head
   b. Cellulitus on the skin or external scalp over the mastoid process
   c. A reddened, dull, thick, immobile tympanic membrane with or without perforation
   d. Tender and enlarged postauricular lymph nodes
   e. Low-grade fever, malaise, anorexia
3. Implementation
   a. Prepare the client for surgical removal of infected material is necessary
   b. Simple or modified radical mastoidectomy with tympanoplasty is the most common treatment
   c. Once tissue that is infected is removed, tympanoplasty is performed to reconstruct the ossicles and the tympanic membranes in an attempt to restore normal hearing
4. Postoperative implementation
   a. Monitor for dizziness
   b. Monitor for signs of meningitis as evidenced by a stiff neck and vomiting
   c. Prepare for a wound dressing change 24 hours after surgery
   d. Monitor the surgical incision for edema, drainage, and redness
   e. Position the client flat with operative side up as prescribed

f. Restrict the client to bed with bedside commode privileges for 24 hours as prescribed
g. Assist client with getting out of bed to prevent falling or injuries from dizziness
h. With reconstruction of ossicles via graft, precautions are taken to prevent dislodging of graft

L. **Otosclerosis**
1. Description
a. Disease of the labyrinthine capsule of the middle ear that results in a bony overgrowth of tissue surrounding the ossicles
b. Causes the development of irregular areas of new bone formation and causes the fixation of the bones
c. Stapes fixation leads to a **conductive hearing loss**
d. If the disease involves the inner ear, **sensorineural hearing loss** is present
e. It is not uncommon to have bilateral involvement, although hearing loss may be worse in one ear
f. The cause is unknown, although it is thought to have a familial tendency
g. Nonsurgical intervention promotes improvement of hearing through amplification
h. Surgical intervention involves removal of the bony growth that is causing the hearing loss
i. A partial stapedectomy or complete stapedectomy with prosthesis (**fenestration**) may be surgically performed
2. Data collection
a. Slowly progressing **conductive hearing loss**
b. Bilateral hearing loss
c. A ringing or roaring type of constant tinnitus
d. Loud sounds heard in the ear when chewing
e. Pinkish discoloration (Schwartze's sign) of the tympanic membrane, which indicates vascular changes within the ear

M. **Fenestration**
1. Description
a. Removal of the stapes with a small hole drilled in the footplate, and a prosthesis is connected between the incus and foot plate
b. Sounds cause the prosthesis to vibrate in the same manner as did the stapes
c. Complications include complete hearing loss, prolonged vertigo, infection, or facial nerve damage
2. Preoperative implementation
a. Instruct the client in measures to prevent middle ear or external ear infections
b. Instruct the client to avoid excessive nose blowing
c. Instruct the client not to clean the ear canal with any foreign object
d. Instruct the client to remove hearing aid 2 weeks before surgery to ensure the integration of local tissue
3. Postoperative implementation
a. Inform the client that hearing is initially worse after the surgical procedure because of swelling and that no noticeable improvement in hearing may occur for as long as 6 weeks
b. Inform the client that the Gelfoam ear packing interferes with hearing but is used to decrease bleeding
c. Assist with ambulating during the first 1 to 2 days after surgery
d. Provide side rails when the client is in bed
e. Administer antibiotics, antivertiginous, and pain medications as prescribed
f. Monitor for facial nerve damage, weakness, changes in tactile sensation, changes in taste sensation, vertigo, nausea, and vomiting
g. Instruct the client to move the head slowly when changing positions to prevent vertigo
h. Instruct the client to avoid persons with upper respiratory tract infections
i. Instruct the client to avoid showering and getting head and wound wet
j. Instruct the client to refrain from using small objects to clean the external ear canal
k. Instruct the client to avoid rapid, extreme changes in pressure caused by quick head movements, sneezing, nose blowing, straining, and changes in altitude
l. Instruct the client to avoid changes in middle ear pressure because they could dislodge the graft or prosthesis

N. Labyrinthitis
1. Description: infection of the labyrinth that occurs as a complication of acute or chronic otitis media
2. Data collection
a. Hearing loss that may be permanent on the affected side
b. Tinnitus
c. Spontaneous nystagmus to the affected side
d. Vertigo
e. Nausea and vomiting
3. Implementation

a. Monitor for signs of meningitis, the most common complication, as evidenced by headache, stiff neck, lethargy
b. Administer systemic antibiotics as prescribed
c. Advise the client to stay in bed in a darkened room
d. Administer antiemetics and antivertiginous medications as prescribed
e. Instruct the client that the vertigo subsides as the inflammation resolves
f. Instruct the client that balance problems that persist may require gait training through physical therapy

O. **Meniere's syndrome**
1. Description
a. A syndrome also called endolymphatic hydrops, which refers to dilation of the endolymphatic system either by overproduction or decreased reabsorption of endolymphatic fluid
b. Symptoms occur in attacks and last for several days and the client becomes totally incapacitated during the attacks
c. Initial hearing loss is reversible, but as the frequency of attacks continues, hearing loss becomes permanent
d. Repeated damage to the cochlea caused by increased fluid pressure leads to the permanent hearing loss
2. Data collection
a. Feelings of fullness in the ear
b. Tinnitus, as a continuous low-pitched roar or humming sound, is present much of the time, but worsens just before and during severe attacks
c. Hearing loss is worse during an attack
d. Vertigo, as periods of whirling, which might cause the client to fall to the ground
e. Vertigo, which is so intense, that even while lying down, the client holds the bed or ground in an attempt to prevent the whirling
f. Nausea and vomiting
g. Nystagmus
h. Severe headaches
3. Nonsurgical implementation
a. Prevent injury during vertigo attacks
b. Provide bed rest in a quiet environment
c. Instruct the client to move head slowly to prevent worsening of the vertigo
d. Initiate salt and fluid restrictions as prescribed
e. Instruct the client to stop smoking
f. Administer nicotinic acid as prescribed for its vasodilatory effect
g. Administer antihistamines as prescribed, which will reduce the production of histamine and the inflammation
h. Administer antiemetics, tranquilizers, and sedatives as prescribed, to calm the client and allow the client to rest, and to control vertigo, nausea, and vomiting
4. Surgical implementation
a. Performed when medical therapy is ineffective and the functional level of the client has decreased significantly
b. Endolymphatic drainage and insertion of a shunt may be performed early in the course of the disease to assist with the drainage of excess fluids
c. Resection of the vestibular nerve or total removal of the labyrinth or a labyrinthectomy may be performed
5. Postoperative implementation
a. Monitor packing and dressing on the ear
b. Speak to the client on the side of the unaffected ear
c. Monitor neurological status
d. Maintain side rails
e. Assist with ambulating
f. Encourage the use of a bedside commode
g. Administer antivertiginous and antiemetic medications as prescribed

P. Acoustic neuroma
1. Description
a. A benign tumor of the vestibular or acoustic nerve
b. The tumor may cause damage to hearing and to facial movements and sensations
c. Treatment includes surgical removal of the tumor via craniotomy
d. Care is taken to preserve the function of facial nerve
e. The tumor rarely recurs after surgical removal
f. Postoperative nursing care is similar to postoperative craniotomy care
2. Data collection
a. Symptoms usually begin with tinnitus and progresses to gradual **sensorineural hearing loss**
b. As the tumor enlarges, damage to adjacent cranial nerves occurs

Q. Trauma
1. Description
a. The tympanic membrane has a limited stretching ability and gives way under high pressure
b. Foreign objects placed in the external canal may exert pressure on the tympanic membrane and cause perforation

c. If the object continues through the canal, the bony structure of the stapes, incus, and malleus may be damaged
d. A blunt injury to the basal skull and ear can damage the middle ear structures through fractures extending to the middle ear
e. Excessive nose blowing and rapid changes of pressure that occur with nonpressurized air flights can increase pressure in the middle ear
f. Depending on the damage to the ossicles, hearing loss may or may not return

2. Implementation
a. Tympanic membrane perforations usually heal within 24 hours
b. Surgical reconstruction of the ossicles and tympanic membrane through tympanoplasty or myringoplasty may be performed to improve hearing

R. Cerumen and foreign bodies
1. Description
a. Cerumen or wax is the most common cause of impacted canals
b. Foreign bodies can include vegetables, beads, pencil erasers, or insects
2. Data collection
a. Sensation of fullness in the ear with or without hearing loss
b. Pain, itching, or bleeding
3. Cerumen
a. Irrigation may be performed to remove cerumen
b. Irrigation is contraindicated in clients with a history of tympanic membrane perforation
4. Foreign bodies
a. With a foreign object of vegetable matter, irrigation is used with care because this material expands with hydration
b. Insects are killed before removal, unless they can be coaxed out by flashlight or a humming noise
c. Mineral oil or alcohol may be instilled to suffocate the insect, which is then removed using ear forceps
d. A small ear forceps is used to remove the object to avoid pushing the object further into the canal and damaging the tympanic membrane

PRACTICE QUESTIONS

1. A nurse is asked to test the visual acuity of a client using a Snellen chart. The nurse prepares to perform the test knowing that which of the following identifies the accurate procedure for this visual acuity test?
   1. Both eyes are tested together followed by the testing of the right and then the left eye
   2. The right eye is tested followed by the left eye, then both eyes are tested
   3. The client is asked to stand at a distance of 40 feet from the chart and is asked to read the largest line on the chart
   4. The client is asked to stand at a distance of 40 feet from the chart and to read the line that can be read 200 feet away by an individual with unimpaired vision
2. A client's vision is tested with a Snellen chart. The results of the tests are documented as 20/60. The nurse interprets this as:
   1. The client can read at a distance of 60 feet what a client with normal vision can read at 20 feet
   2. The client is legally blind
   3. The client's vision is normal
   4. The client can read at a distance of 20 feet what a client with normal vision can read at 60 feet
3. A nurse notes that after several eye examinations, the physician has documented a diagnosis of legal blindness in the client's chart. Which of the following would the nurse expect to note documented as the result of the Snellen chart test?
   1. 20/20 vision
   2. 20/40 vision
   3. 20/60 vision
   4. 20/200 vision
4. A nurse is preparing the client for eye testing and the examiner is planning to test the eyes using the confrontational method. The nurse tells the client that this test is performed to:
   1. Examine visual fields or peripheral vision
   2. Check for glaucoma
   3. Check for color blindness
   4. Examine pupil constriction
5. Tonometry is performed on the client with a suspected diagnosis of glaucoma. The nurse reviews the test results as documented in the client's chart and understands that normal intraocular pressure is:
   1. 2 to 7 mm Hg
   2. 10 to 21 mm Hg
   3. 22 to 30 mm Hg
   4. 31 to 35 mm Hg
6. A nurse is assisting in developing a plan of care for the client scheduled for cataract surgery. The nurse makes suggestions regarding the plan knowing that which of the following problems is most specifically associated with this type of surgery?
   1. Self-care deficit
   2. Alteration in nutrition
   3. Sensory perceptual alteration
   4. Anxiety
7. A nurse is reviewing the health record of a client diagnosed with a cataract. The chief clinical mani-

festation that the nurse would expect to note in the early stages of cataract formation is:
1. Eye pain
2. Floating spots
3. Blurred vision
4. Diplopia

8. A nurse is assigned to administer the prescribed eye drops for a client preparing for cataract surgery. Which of the following types of eye drops will the nurse expect to be prescribed?
1. An osmotic diuretic
2. A miotic agent
3. A mydriatic medication
4. A thiazide diuretic

9. A nurse is assigned to care for a client after a cataract extraction. The nurse plans to position the client:
1. On the operative side
2. On the nonoperative side
3. Prone
4. Supine

10. During the early postoperative stage, the cataract extraction client complains of nausea and severe eye pain over the operative site. What is the initial nursing action in this situation?
1. Report the client's complaints
2. Administer the ordered pain medication and antiemetic
3. Reassure the client that this is normal
4. Turn the client on their operative side

11. A client is being discharged from the ambulatory care unit after cataract removal. The nurse reinforces instructions regarding home care. Which of the following, if stated by the client, indicates effective teaching?
1. "I will take aspirin if I have any discomfort."
2. "I will sleep on the side that I was operated on."
3. "I will wear my eye shield at night and my glasses during the day."
4. "I will not lift anything if it weighs more than 10 pounds."

12. A client is diagnosed with glaucoma. Which of the following data gathered by the nurse indicate a risk factor associated with glaucoma?
1. A history of migraine headaches
2. Frequent urinary tract infections
3. Cardiovascular disease
4. Frequent upper respiratory infections

13. A client with glaucoma asks the nurse if complete vision will return. The most appropriate response is:
1. "Although some vision has been lost and cannot be restored, further loss may be prevented by adhering to the treatment plan."
2. "Your vision will return as soon as the medication begins to work."
3. "Your vision will never return to normal."
4. "Your vision loss is temporary and will return in about 3 to 4 weeks."

14. A nurse is assisting in developing a teaching plan for the client with glaucoma. Which of the following instructions would the nurse suggest to include in the plan of care?
1. Decrease fluid intake to control the intraocular pressure
2. Avoid reading the newspaper and watching the TV
3. Decrease the amount of salt in the diet
4. Eye medications will need to be administered for the rest of your life

15. A nurse is assigned to care for a client with a detached retina. Which of the following findings would the nurse expect to be documented in the client's record?
1. Pain in the affected eye
2. Blurred vision
3. A sense of a curtain falling across the field of vision
4. A yellow discoloration of the sclera

16. A nurse is assigned to care for a client with a diagnosis of detached retina. Which of the following findings would indicate that bleeding has occurred as a result of retinal detachment?
1. Complaints of a burst of black spots or floaters
2. A sudden sharp pain in the eye
3. Total loss of vision
4. A reddened conjunctiva

17. A client with retinal detachment is admitted to the nursing unit in preparation for a scleral buckling procedure. Which of the following would the nurse anticipate to be prescribed?
1. Bathroom privileges only
2. Elevating the head of the bed to 45 degrees
3. Placing an eye patch over the client's affected eye
4. Wearing dark glasses to read or watch TV

18. A client arrives in the emergency room after an automobile accident. The client's forehead hit the steering wheel and a hyphema is diagnosed. The nurse would prepare to position the client:
1. Flat on bed rest
2. On bed rest in a semi-Fowler's position
3. In the lateral position on the affected side
4. In the lateral position on the unaffected side

19. A client sustains a contusion of the eyeball after a traumatic injury with a blunt object. The nurse prepares to initiate which of the following immediately?
1. Notify the physician
2. Irrigate the eye with cool water
3. Apply ice to the affected eye
4. Accompany the client to the emergency room

20. A client arrives in the emergency room with a penetrating eye injury from wood chips while cutting wood. The nurse checks the eye and notes the piece

of wood protruding form the eye. The nurse immediately prepares the client for which of the following?
1. Removal of the piece of wood using a sterile eye clamp
2. Application of an eye patch
3. Visual acuity tests
4. Irrigation of the eye with sterile saline

21. A client sustains a chemical eye injury from a splash of battery acid. The nurse prepares the client for which of the following immediate measures?
1. Assessment of visual acuity
2. Irrigation of the eye with sterile normal saline
3. Swabbing the eye with antibiotic ointment
4. Covering the eye with a pressure patch

22. A nurse is caring for a client after enucleation. The nurse notes the presence of bright red drainage on the dressing. Which of the following actions is most appropriate?
1. Report the findings
2. Continue to monitor vital signs
3. Document the finding
4. Mark the drainage on the dressing and monitor for any increase in bleeding

23. A nurse is preparing to administer ear drops to an adult client. The nurse administers the ear drops knowing that which of the following is the appropriate procedure?
1. Pull the pinna up and back
2. Pull the earlobe down and back
3. Instruct the client to stand and lean to one side
4. Tilt the client's head forward and down

24. A nurse is preparing to perform a voice test to check the client's hearing. The nurse performs the procedure knowing that which of the following describes the accurate procedure?
1. Stand 4 feet away from the client to ensure that the client can hear at this distance
2. Quietly whisper a statement and ask the client to repeat it
3. Whisper a statement with the examiner's back facing the client
4. Whisper a statement while the client blocks both ears

25. A nurse is assisting the physician with performing a Weber tuning fork test on a client. The nurse understands that this test checks for:
1. Visual loss
2. Cataract development
3. Hearing loss
4. Nystagmus

26. A nurse is caring for a client that is hearing impaired. Which of the following approaches will facilitate communication?
1. Speak frequently
2. Speak loudly
3. Speak directly into the impaired ear
4. Speak in a normal tone

27. A client arrives at the emergency room with a foreign body in the left ear that has been determined to be an insect. Which of the following interventions would the nurse anticipate to be prescribed initially?
1. Irrigation of the ear
2. Instillation of diluted alcohol
3. Instillation of antibiotic ear drops
4. Instillation of corticosteroid ointment

28. A nurse notes that the physician has documented a diagnosis of presbycusis on the client's chart. The nurse understands that this condition is most accurately described as:
1. A sensorineural loss that occurs with aging
2. A conductive hearing loss that occurs with aging
3. Tinnitus that occurs with aging
4. Nystagmus that occurs with aging

29. A nurse is reinforcing discharge instructions for a client who had a fenestration procedure for the treatment of otosclerosis. Which of the following, if stated by the client, would indicate that teaching was effective?
1. "I should drink liquids through a straw for the next 2 to 3 weeks."
2. "It is OK to take a shower and wash my hair."
3. "I will take stool softeners as prescribed by my doctor."
4. "I can resume my tennis lessons starting next week."

30. A client with Meniere's disease is experiencing severe vertigo. The nurse instructs the client to do which of the following to assist in controlling the vertigo?
1. Increase fluid intake to 3000 mL a day
2. Avoid sudden head movements
3. Lie still and watch the TV
4. Increase sodium in the diet

31. A nurse is assigned to care for a client hospitalized with Meniere's disease. The nurse expects that which of the following would most likely be prescribed for the client?
1. Low cholesterol diet
2. Low sodium diet
3. Low carbohydrate diet
4. Low fat diet

32. A nurse is caring for a client after craniotomy for removal of an acoustic neuroma. The nurse understands that assessment of which of the following cranial nerves would identify a complication specifically associated with this surgery?
1. Cranial nerve I, olfactory
2. Cranial nerve III, oculomotor
3. Cranial nerve IV, trochlear
4. Cranial nerve VII, facial nerve

33. A nurse is monitoring a client with a blunt head injury sustained from a motor vehicle accident. Which of the following would indicate a basal skull fracture as a result of the injury?
   1. Purulent drainage from the auditory canal
   2. Bloody or clear drainage from the auditory canal
   3. Epistaxis
   4. Periorbital edema
34. A nurse is reviewing the record of a client with mastoiditis. The nurse would expect to note which of the following documented regarding the results of the otoscopic examination?
   1. A pink tympanic membrane
   2. A pearly-colored tympanic membrane
   3. A red, dull, thick and immobile tympanic membrane
   4. A transparent and clear tympanic membrane
35. A client is diagnosed with a disorder involving the inner ear. The nurse caring for the client understands that which of the following is the most common client complaint associated with a disorder involving the inner ear?
   1. Hearing loss
   2. Pruritus
   3. Tinnitus
   4. Burning in the ear
36. A nurse is assigned to care for a client with a diagnosis of Meniere's disease. The nurse plans care knowing that this condition is a disorder of the:
   1. External ear canal
   2. Tympanic membrane
   3. Middle ear
   4. Inner ear
37. A nurse is caring for a client who will be undergoing surgical treatment for Meniere's disease. The nurse plans care understanding that surgical treatment for this disorder is performed to:
   1. Provide relief from accumulation of inner ear fluid in the endolymphatic sac
   2. Repair the tympanic membrane
   3. Replace the stapes footplate
   4. Provide relief from accumulation of fluid in the middle ear
38. A nurse is assigned to care for a client with Meniere's disease. The nurse reviews the physician's orders. The nurse plans care knowing that which of the following would not be prescribed for the client?
   1. Increased fluid intake
   2. Low-sodium diet
   3. Vasodilating medications
   4. Mild sedative
39. A nurse is reviewing the health care record of a client with a diagnosis of otosclerosis. The nurse would expect to note documentation of which early symptom of this disorder?
   1. Ringing in the ears
   2. Blurred vision
   3. Headache
   4. Vertigo
40. Surgery has been recommended for the client with otosclerosis and the client tells the nurse that surgery is not desired. The client asks the nurse about alternative methods to improve hearing. The most appropriate response is which of the following?
   1. "There are no other methods to improve hearing."
   2. "You need to have surgery since it has been recommended."
   3. "A hearing aid may improve your hearing."
   4. "Your physician is the best. You need to do what the physician suggests."
41. A nurse is caring for a hospitalized client with an acute attack from Meniere's disease. The client verbalizes concern because the client has experienced a hearing loss as a result of the attack. Which of the following responses would the nurse make to the client regarding the hearing loss?
   1. "It will take several weeks before the hearing returns."
   2. "The hearing loss will fluctuate for 1 week."
   3. "The attack leaves a hearing loss in the involved ear."
   4. "The hearing will return to normal."
42. A nurse is reviewing the physician's orders on a client admitted to the hospital with a diagnosis of an acute attack of Meniere's disease. Which of the following orders, if noted on the client's chart, would the nurse question?
   1. Administration of a sedative
   2. Administration of an antihistamine
   3. Administration of a vasoconstrictor
   4. Bed rest
43. A nurse is reinforcing discharge instructions to the client who was hospitalized for an acute attack of Meniere's disease. Which of the following statements, if made by the client, indicates a need for further education?
   1. "I need to take the diuretics to decrease the fluid in the ear."
   2. "I need to take the antihistamine as prescribed."
   3. "I need to take a vasodilator."
   4. "It is not necessary to restrict salt in my diet."
44. A client with a diagnosis of otosclerosis is admitted to the ambulatory care unit for stapedectomy. The nurse reinforces instructions for the client regarding home care after the procedure. Which of the following statements, if made by the client, indicates a need for further education?
   1. "I need to keep water out of the ear canal for at least 3 weeks."
   2. "I need to avoid air travel for at least 6 months."

3. "I need to notify the physician if I experience any persistent dizziness."
4. "I need to avoid bending and lifting heavy objects for at least 3 weeks."

45. A nurse is reinforcing discharge instructions with a client who is being discharged after a fenestration procedure for the treatment of otosclerosis. Which of the following will be included in the list of instructions prepared for the client?
    1. "It is OK to begin your golf lessons."
    2. "It is alright to take a shower daily."
    3. "You need to avoid air travel."
    4. "You need to avoid bending activities for 1 week."

46. A myringotomy is performed on a client in the ambulatory care center. The ambulatory care nurse calls the client 24 hours after the procedure to evaluate the status of the client. The client reports to the nurse that a small amount of brownish drainage has been coming from the ear. Which of the following instructions would the nurse provide to the client?
    1. Contact the physician
    2. Lie on the unaffected side to prevent the drainage from occurring
    3. Continue to monitor the drainage because this is normal and may occur for 24 to 48 hours after the surgery
    4. Place a cotton plug in the ear to absorb the drainage

47. A nurse is reinforcing instructions to a client regarding the use of a hearing aid. Which of the following statements, if made by the client, indicates a need for further education?
    1. "I should keep an extra battery available at all times."
    2. "I should wash the ear mold frequently with mild soap and water."
    3. "I should turn the hearing aid off after removing it from the ear."
    4. "I should not wear the hearing aid during an ear infection."

48. A nurse assesses the client with a blunt head injury sustained from a motor vehicle accident. The nurse notes the presence of bloody drainage from the auditory canal. Which of the following nursing actions would be most appropriate?
    1. Document the findings
    2. Place a gauze pad over the ear to absorb the drainage
    3. Report the findings
    4. Continue to monitor the drainage

49. A client with Meniere's disease has been given suggestions for methods to control vertigo. The nurse evaluates that the client understood the information presented if the client stated to:
    1. Cut down smoking to 10 cigarettes per day
    2. Increase sodium in the diet
    3. Increase fluid intake to 3000 mL a day
    4. Avoid sudden head movements

ANSWERS

1. *Answer:* 2

Rationale: Visual acuity is tested in one eye at a time, then in both eyes together with the client comfortably seated. Begin with the right eye while the left eye is covered, then test the left eye with the right eye covered, followed by testing both eyes together. Visual acuity is measured with or without corrective lenses and the client stands at a distance of 20 feet from the chart.

Test-Taking Strategy: Use the process of elimination. Remember that normal visual acuity as measured by a Snellen chart is 20/20 vision. This should assist you to eliminate options 3 and 4. It is best to test each eye separately first, then test both eyes together. This most accurately assesses visual acuity. Review this basic procedure if you had difficulty with this question.

Level of Cognitive Ability: Application

Client Needs: Health Promotion and Maintenance

Integrated Concept/Process: Nursing Process/Data Collection

Content Area: Adult Health/Eye

Reference: DeWit S: *Fundamental concepts and skills for nursing*, Philadelphia, 2001, WB Saunders, p. 379.

2. *Answer:* 4

Rationale: Vision that is 20/20 is normal; that is, the client is able to read from 20 feet what a person with normal vision can read from 20 feet. A client with a visual acuity of 20/60 can only read at a distance of 20 feet what a person with normal vision can read at 60 feet.

Test-Taking Strategy: Use the process of elimination. Understanding how to interpret the results of this visual acuity test is necessary to answer this question. Review this visual acuity test if you had difficulty with this question.

Level of Cognitive Ability: Comprehension

Client Needs: Health Promotion and maintenance

Integrated Concept/Process: Nursing Process/Evaluation

Content Area: Adult Health/Eye

Reference: DeWit S: *Fundamental concepts and skills for nursing*, Philadelphia, 2001, WB Saunders, p. 379.

3. *Answer:* 4

Rationale: Legal blindness is defined as 20/200 or less with corrected vision (glasses or contact lenses) or less than 20 degrees of visual field in the better eye. Options 1, 2, and 3 are incorrect descriptions.

Test-Taking Strategy: Knowledge regarding the definition of legal blindness is required to answer this question. Review this definition if you had difficulty with this question.
Level of Cognitive Ability: Comprehension
Client Needs: Physiological Integrity
Integrated Concept/Process: Nursing Process/Data Collection
Content Area: Adult Health/Eye
Reference: DeWit S: *Fundamental concepts and skills for nursing,* Philadelphia, 2001, WB Saunders, p. 155.

4. *Answer:* 1
Rationale: The confrontational method of eye testing is used to examine visual fields or peripheral vision. Tonometry is used to check for glaucoma. An Ishihara chart is used to check color vision. A flashlight is used to assess pupillary response to light.
Test-Taking Strategy: Knowledge regarding the procedure for checking peripheral vision by the confrontational method is required to answer this question. Review the purpose of this test if you had difficulty with this question.
Level of Cognitive Ability: Application
Client Needs: Health Promotion and Maintenance
Integrated Concept/Process: Nursing Process/Implementation
Content Area: Adult Health/Eye
Reference: Ignatavicius D, Workman M: *Medical-surgical nursing: critical thinking for collaborative care,* ed 4, Philadelphia, 2002, WB Saunders, p. 1016.

5. *Answer:* 2
Rationale: Tonometry is the method of measuring intraocular fluid pressure using a calibrated instrument that indents or flattens the corneal apex. Pressures between 10 and 21 mm Hg are considered within the normal range.
Test-Taking Strategy: Knowledge regarding the normal intraocular pressure is required to answer this question. Review this normal value if you had difficulty with this question.
Level of Cognitive Ability: Comprehension
Client Needs: Physiological Integrity
Integrated Concept/Process: Nursing Process/Data Collection
Content Area: Adult Health/Eye
Reference: Black J, Hawks J, Keene A: *Medical-surgical nursing: clinical management for positive outcomes,* ed 6, Philadelphia, 2001, WB Saunders, p. 195.

6. *Answer:* 3
Rationale: The most specifically associated problem for the client scheduled for cataract surgery is sensory perceptual alteration (visual) related to lens extraction and replacement. Options 1 and 2 may also be concerns but would occur as a result of a sensory perceptual alteration. Option 4 can occur with any type of surgical procedure.
Test-Taking Strategy: Use the process of elimination focusing on the type of surgery. Remember disorders of the eye or ear relate to sensory perceptual alterations. Review the problems associated with these disorders if you had difficulty with this question.
Level of Cognitive Ability: Comprehension
Client Needs: Psychosocial Integrity
Integrated Concept/Process: Nursing Process/Planning
Content Area: Adult Health/Eye
Reference: DeWit S: *Fundamental concepts and skills for nursing,* Philadelphia, 2001, WB Saunders, p. 841.

7. *Answer:* 3
Rationale: A gradual painless blurring of central vision is the chief clinical manifestation of a cataract. Early symptoms include slightly blurred vision and a decrease in color perception. Options 1, 2, and 4 are not specifically associated with a cataract.
Test-Taking Strategy: Use the process of elimination. Note the key word "chief." Recall the pathophysiology related to cataract development. As a cataract develops, the lens of the eye becomes opaque. This description will assist in directing you to the correct option. If you had difficulty with this question review the signs associated with cataract development.
Level of Cognitive Ability: Comprehension
Client Needs: Physiological Integrity
Integrated Concept/Process: Nursing Process/Data Collection
Content Area: Adult Health/Eye
Reference: DeWit S: *Fundamental concepts and skills for nursing,* Philadelphia, 2001, WB Saunders, p. 841.

8. *Answer:* 3
Rationale: A mydriatic medication produces mydriasis or dilation of the pupil. Mydriatic medications are used preoperatively in the cataract client. These medications act by dilating the pupils. They also constrict blood vessels. A miotic agent would constrict the pupil. An osmotic agent would act to decrease intraocular pressure. A thiazide diuretic would promote the excretion of body fluid. A thiazide diuretic is not likely to be prescribed for a client with a cataract.
Test-Taking Strategy: Knowledge regarding the actions of the specific medications identified in the options is required to answer this question. Read the question carefully noting that the client is being prepared for eye surgery. Dilation of the eye is necessary before cataract extraction. Review the preparation of a client for cataract surgery if you had difficulty with this question.
Level of Cognitive Ability: Comprehension
Client Needs: Physiological Integrity
Integrated Concept/Process: Nursing Process/Planning
Content Area: Adult Health/Eye
Reference: Ignatavicius D, Workman M: *Medical-surgical nursing: critical thinking for collaborative care,* ed 4, Philadelphia, 2002, WB Saunders, p. 1027.

9. *Answer:* 2
Rationale: After cataract extraction, clients should be positioned on their backs in semi-Fowler's position or on the nonoperative side to prevent edema in the surgical site. Options 1, 3, and 4 are incorrect positions and will cause swelling at the surgical site.
Test-Taking Strategy: Use the process of elimination. Remember edema to the surgical site can occur after the trauma of surgery. Think about the principles of gravity and the prevention of the accumulation of fluid around the surgical site. This will assist in directing you to the correct option. If you had difficulty with this question, review postoperative care of a client after cataract surgery.
Level of Cognitive Ability: Application

Client Needs: Physiological Integrity
Integrated Concept/Process: Nursing Process/Planning
Content Area: Adult Health/Eye
Reference: Ignatavicius D, Workman M: *Medical-surgical nursing: critical thinking for collaborative care,* ed 4, Philadelphia, 2002, WB Saunders, p. 1034.

10. *Answer:* 1
Rationale: Severe pain or pain accompanied by nausea is an indicator of increased intraocular pressure and should be reported to the physician immediately. Options 2, 3, and 4 are incorrect.
Test-Taking Strategy: Use the process of elimination. Note the key word "severe." Eliminate option 3 as this is not a normal condition. The client should not be turned to their operative side; therefore eliminate option 4. Noting the key word in the question should direct you to eliminating option 2. If you had difficulty with this question, review the postoperative complications of cataract surgery requiring physician notification.
Level of Cognitive Ability: Application
Client Needs: Physiological Integrity
Integrated Concept/Process: Nursing Process/Implementation
Content Area: Adult Health/Eye
Reference: Ignatavicius D, Workman M: *Medical-surgical nursing: critical thinking for collaborative care,* ed 4, Philadelphia, 2002, WB Saunders, p. 1034.

11. *Answer:* 3
Rationale: The client is instructed to wear a metal or plastic shield to protect the eye from accidental injury and is instructed not to rub the eye. Glasses may be worn during the day. Aspirin or medications containing aspirin are not to be administered or taken by the client, and the client is instructed to take acetaminophen (Tylenol) as needed for pain. The client is instructed not to sleep on the side of the body that was operated on. The client is not to lift more than 5 pounds.
Test-Taking Strategy: Note the key words "indicates effective teaching." Use the process of elimination and knowledge regarding the postoperative care after this procedure. If you had difficulty with this question, review these client instructions.
Level of Cognitive Ability: Comprehension
Client Needs: Health Promotion and Maintenance
Integrated Concept/Process: Teaching/Learning
Content Area: Adult Health/Eye
Reference: Ignatavicius D, Workman M: *Medical-surgical nursing: critical thinking for collaborative care,* ed 4, Philadelphia, 2002, WB Saunders, p. 1035.

12. *Answer:* 3
Rationale: Hypertension, cardiovascular disease, diabetes, and obesity are associated with the development of glaucoma. Smoking, ingestion of caffeine or large amounts alcohol, illicit drugs, corticosteroids, altered hormone levels, posture, and eye movements may cause varying transient increases in intraocular pressure.
Test-Taking Strategy: Use knowledge regarding the risk factors associated with glaucoma to answer this question. If you had difficulty with this question review the risk factors associated with this disorder.
Level of Cognitive Ability: Comprehension
Client Needs: Health Promotion and Maintenance
Integrated Concept/Process: Nursing Process/Data Collection
Content Area: Adult Health/Eye
Reference: DeWit S: *Fundamental concepts and skills for nursing,* Philadelphia, 2001, WB Saunders, p. 841.

13. *Answer:* 1
Rationale: Vision loss to glaucoma is irreparable. Reassure the client that although some vision has been lost and cannot be restored, further loss may be prevented by adhering to the treatment plan. Options 2 and 4 are incorrect. Option 3 does not provide reassurance to the client.
Test-Taking Strategy: Use the process of elimination. Knowledge regarding the effects of glaucoma on vision is required to answer this question. Read the options carefully. Eliminate option 3 as this option does not provide a reassuring response and will produce anxiety in the client. Note that option 1 is more global; that is, it addresses the importance of compliance with the treatment plan. Review this disorder if you had difficulty with this question.
Level of Cognitive Ability: Application
Client Needs: Psychosocial Integrity
Integrated Concept/Process: Nursing Process/Implementation
Content Area: Adult Health/Eye
Reference: DeWit S: *Fundamental concepts and skills for nursing,* Philadelphia, 2001, WB Saunders, p. 841.

14. *Answer:* 4
Rationale: Administration of eye drops is a critical component of the treatment plan for the client with glaucoma. The client needs to be instructed that lifelong medication use is necessary. Limiting fluids and reducing salt will not decrease intraocular pressure. Option 2 is not necessary.
Test-Taking Strategy: Use the process of elimination. Knowing that medications are an integral component of the treatment plan will assist in directing you to the correct option. Review the treatment associated with the care of the client with glaucoma if you had difficulty with this question.
Level of Cognitive Ability: Application
Client Needs: Health Promotion and Maintenance
Integrated Concept/Process: Nursing Process/Planning
Content Area: Adult Health/Eye
Reference: DeWit S: *Fundamental concepts and skills for nursing,* Philadelphia, 2001, WB Saunders, p. 841.

15. *Answer:* 3
Rationale: A characteristic clinical manifestation of retinal detachment described by clients is the feeling that a shadow or curtain is falling across the field of vision. There is no pain associated with detachment of the retina. A retinal detachment is an ophthalmic emergency and even more so if visual acuity is still normal. Options 2 and 4 are not specifically associated with a detached retina.
Test-Taking Strategy: Knowledge regarding the clinical manifestations associated with retinal detachment is required to answer this question. Retinal detachment can occur suddenly and is an ophthalmic emergency. Review the clinical manifestations associated with this condition if you had difficulty with this question.

Level of Cognitive Ability: Comprehension
Client Needs: Physiological Integrity
Integrated Concept/Process: Nursing Process/Data Collection
Content Area: Adult Health/Eye
Reference: Ignatavicius D, Workman M: *Medical-surgical nursing: critical thinking for collaborative care,* ed 4, Philadelphia, 2002, WB Saunders, p. 1040.

16. *Answer:* 1
Rationale: Complaints of a sudden burst of black spots or floaters indicates that bleeding has occurred as a result of the detachment. Options 2, 3, and 4 are not specifically associated with bleeding as a result of detached retina.
Test-Taking Strategy: Knowledge regarding the signs of hemorrhage associated with retinal detachment is required to answer this question. Hemorrhage is a serious complication associated with retinal detachment. Review the clinical manifestations associated with the complications of a detached retina if you had difficulty with this question.
Level of Cognitive Ability: Analysis
Client Needs: Physiological Integrity
Integrated Concept/Process: Nursing Process/Data Collection
Content Area: Adult Health/Eye
Reference: Ignatavicius D, Workman M: *Medical-surgical nursing: critical thinking for collaborative care,* ed 4, Philadelphia, 2002, WB Saunders, p. 1040.

17. *Answer:* 3
Rationale: The nurse places an eye patch over the client's affected eye to reduce eye movement. Some clients may need bilateral patching. Depending on the location and size of the retinal break, activity restrictions including watching TV, may be needed immediately. These restrictions are necessary to prevent further tearing or detachment and to promote drainage of any subretinal fluid. The nurse positions the client as prescribed by the physician.
Test-Taking Strategy: Use the process of elimination. Eliminate options that suggest activity such as in options 1 and 4. Remember that the eye needs to be protected and rested. This should direct you to the correct option. If you had difficulty with this question, review care to the client with retinal detachment.
Level of Cognitive Ability: Comprehension
Client Needs: Physiological Integrity
Integrated Concept/Process: Nursing Process/Planning
Content Area: Adult Health/Eye
Reference: Ignatavicius D, Workman M: *Medical-surgical nursing: critical thinking for collaborative care,* ed 4, Philadelphia, 2002, WB Saunders, p. 1040.

18. *Answer:* 2
Rationale: A hyphema is the presence of blood in the anterior chamber. It is produced when a force is sufficient to break the integrity of the blood vessels in the eye. It can be caused by direct injury such as penetrating injury from a BB pellet, or indirectly such as from striking the forehead on a steering wheel during an accident. The client is treated by bed rest in a semi-Fowler's position to assist gravity in keeping the hyphema away from the optical center of the cornea.
Test-Taking Strategy: Use the process of elimination. Placing the client flat will produce an increase in pressure at the injured site. Note that option 2 is the only option that identifies a position different from the other options. Review care to the client with hyphema if you had difficulty with this question.
Level of Cognitive Ability: Application
Client Needs: Physiological Integrity
Integrated Concept/Process: Nursing Process/Implementation
Content Area: Adult Health/Eye
Reference: Ignatavicius D, Workman M: *Medical-surgical nursing: critical thinking for collaborative care,* ed 4, Philadelphia, 2002, WB Saunders, p. 1043.

19. *Answer:* 3
Rationale: Treatment for a contusion begins at the time of injury. Ice is applied immediately. The client should receive a thorough eye examination to rule out the presence of other eye injuries. Eye irrigation is not indicated in a contusion. Options 1 and 4 will delay immediate treatment. After the application of ice, the physician would be notified.
Test-Taking Strategy: Knowledge regarding the initial treatment after a contusion to the eye is required to answer this question. Use the process of elimination noting the key word "immediately." Review this content if you had difficulty with this question.
Level of Cognitive Ability: Application
Client Needs: Physiological Integrity
Integrated Concept/Process: Nursing Process/Implementation
Content Area: Adult Health/Eye
Reference: Ignatavicius D, Workman M: *Medical-surgical nursing: critical thinking for collaborative care,* ed 4, Philadelphia, 2002, WB Saunders, p. 1043.

20. *Answer:* 3
Rationale: If the laceration is the result of a penetrating injury, an object may be noted protruding from the eye. This object must never be removed except by the ophthalmologist, because it may be holding ocular structures in place. Application of an eye patch or irrigation of the eye may disrupt the foreign body and cause further tearing of the cornea.
Test-Taking Strategy: Use the process of elimination. Note the key word "penetrating." This should indicate that a laceration has occurred and that interventions are directed at preventing further disruption of the integrity of the eye. The only accurate option among the choices is to prepare for testing visual acuity. Review this content if you had difficulty with this question.
Level of Cognitive Ability: Application
Client Needs: Physiological Integrity
Integrated Concept/Process: Nursing Process/Implementation
Content Area: Adult Health/Eye
Reference: Ignatavicius D, Workman M: *Medical-surgical nursing: critical thinking for collaborative care,* ed 4, Philadelphia, 2002, WB Saunders, p. 1044.

21. *Answer:* 2
Rationale: Emergency care after a chemical burn to the eye includes irrigating the eye immediately with sterile normal saline or ocular irrigating solution. The irrigation should be

maintained for at least 10 minutes. After this emergency treatment, visual acuity is assessed. Options 3 and 4 are not immediate measures.
Test-Taking Strategy: Use the process of elimination. Read the question carefully noting the type of injury to the eye. The question asks about emergency care; therefore in this type of injury, it is necessary to irrigate the eye first. Review this content if you had difficulty with this question.
Level of Cognitive Ability: Application
Client Needs: Physiological Integrity
Integrated Concept/Process: Nursing Process/Implementation
Content Area: Adult Health/Eye
Reference: Ignatavicius D, Workman M: *Medical-surgical nursing: critical thinking for collaborative care*, ed 4, Philadelphia, 2002, WB Saunders, p. 1562.

22. *Answer:* 1
Rationale: If the nurse notes the presence of bright red drainage on the dressing, it must be reported to the physician, as this can indicate hemorrhage. Options 2, 3, and 4 will delay necessary treatment.
Test-Taking Strategy: Use the process of elimination. Note the key words "bright red." Bright red drainage indicates active bleeding. The physician needs to be notified if this type of drainage occurs. Review postoperative complications associated with an enucleation if you had difficulty with this question.
Level of Cognitive Ability: Application
Client Needs: Physiological Integrity
Integrated Concept/Process: Nursing Process/Implementation
Content Area: Adult Health/Eye
Reference: Black J, Hawks J, Keene A: *Medical-surgical nursing: clinical management for positive outcomes*, ed 6, Philadelphia, 2001, WB Saunders, p. 1825.

23. *Answer:* 1
Rationale: The nurse tilts the client's head slightly away and pulls the pinna up and back. Instructing the client to stand and lean to one side is inappropriate and unsafe.
Test-Taking Strategy: Use the process of elimination noting that the question addresses an adult client. Use basic knowledge regarding the administration of ear medications in selecting the correct option. In the adult, the pinna is pulled up and back. Review this procedure if you had difficulty with this question.
Level of Cognitive Ability: Application
Client Needs: Physiological Integrity
Integrated Concept/Process: Nursing Process/Implementation
Content Area: Adult Health/Ear
Reference: DeWit S: *Fundamental concepts and skills for nursing*, Philadelphia, 2001, WB Saunders, p. 666.

24. *Answer:* 2
Rationale: The examiner stands 1 to 2 feet away from the client and asks the client to block one external ear canal. The nurse quietly whispers a statement and asks the client to repeat it. Each ear is tested separately. Options 3 and 4 are not measures that would effectively check hearing. Option 1 would check distance hearing.
Test-Taking Strategy: Use the process of elimination. Eliminate options 3 and 4, as they are not measures that would effectively check hearing. Eliminate option 1, as distance hearing is not the issue of the question. Review this hearing test if you had difficulty with this question.
Level of Cognitive Ability: Application
Client Needs: Health Promotion and Maintenance
Integrated Concept/Process: Nursing Process/Implementation
Content Area: Adult Health/Ear
Reference: DeWit S: *Fundamental concepts and skills for nursing*, Philadelphia, 2001, WB Saunders, p. 163.

25. *Answer:* 3
Rationale: The Weber tuning fork test assesses for conductive or sensorineural hearing loss. Options 1, 2, and 4 are incorrect.
Test-Taking Strategy: Use the process of elimination. Recalling that this is a test to determine the type of hearing loss will easily direct you to option 3. Review the purpose of this test if you had difficulty with this question.
Level of Cognitive Ability: Comprehension
Client Needs: Physiological Integrity
Integrated Concept/Process: Nursing Process/Data Collection
Content Area: Adult Health/Ear
Reference: DeWit S: *Fundamental concepts and skills for nursing*, Philadelphia, 2001, WB Saunders, p. 374.

26. *Answer:* 4
Rationale: Speak in a normal tone to the client with impaired hearing and do not shout. Talk directly to the client while facing the client and speak clearly. If the client does not seem to understand what is said, express it differently. Moving closer to the client and toward the better ear may facilitate communication, but avoid talking directly into the impaired ear.
Test-Taking Strategy: Knowledge regarding effective communication techniques for the hearing impaired is required to answer this question. If you had difficulty with this question, review these techniques.
Level of Cognitive Ability: Application
Client Needs: Physiological Integrity
Integrated Concept/Process: Communication and Documentation
Content Area: Adult Health/Ear
Reference: DeWit S: *Fundamental concepts and skills for nursing*, Philadelphia, 2001, WB Saunders, p. 93.

27. *Answer:* 2
Rationale: Insects are killed before removal unless they can be coaxed out by a flashlight or a humming noise. Mineral oil or diluted alcohol is instilled into the ear to suffocate the insect, which is then removed by using ear forceps. When the foreign object is vegetable matter, irrigation is not used because this material expands with hydration and the impaction becomes worse. Options 1, 3, and 4 may be prescribed after the initial treatment if necessary and if inflammation or infection is a concern.
Test-Taking Strategy: Use the process of elimination and knowledge regarding care to the client with a foreign body in the ear to answer this question. If you had difficulty with this question review the treatment for this occurrence.

Level of Cognitive Ability: Comprehension
Client Needs: Physiological Integrity
Integrated Concept/Process: Nursing Process/Planning
Content Area: Adult Health/Ear
Reference: Ignatavicius D, Workman M: *Medical-surgical nursing: critical thinking for collaborative care,* ed 4, Philadelphia, 2002, WB Saunders, p. 1063.

28. *Answer:* 1
Rationale: Presbycusis is a type of hearing loss that occurs with aging. It is a gradual sensorineural loss caused by nerve degeneration in the inner ear or auditory nerve. Options 2, 3, and 4 are not accurate descriptions.
Test-Taking Strategy: Knowledge regarding the description of presbycusis is required to answer this question. If you are unfamiliar with this condition, review this age-related disorder.
Level of Cognitive Ability: Comprehension
Client Needs: Physiological Integrity
Integrated Concept/Process: Nursing Process/Data Collection
Content Area: Adult Health/Ear
Reference: Ignatavicius D, Workman M: *Medical-surgical nursing: critical thinking for collaborative care,* ed 4, Philadelphia, 2002, WB Saunders, p. 1048.

29. *Answer:* 3
Rationale: After ear surgery, clients need to avoid straining when having a bowel movement. Clients need to be instructed to avoid drinking with a straw, air travel, and excessive coughing for 2 to 3 weeks. Clients need to avoid getting their head wet, washing their hair, and showering for 1 week. Clients need to avoid rapidly moving the head, bouncing, and bending over for 3 weeks.
Test-Taking Strategy: Use the process of elimination. Note the key words "teaching was effective." Consider the anatomical area of the client condition and the surgical procedure in eliminating the incorrect options. If you had difficulty with this question review client instructions after ear surgery.
Level of Cognitive Ability: Comprehension
Client Needs: Health Promotion and Maintenance
Integrated Concept/Process: Teaching/Learning
Content Area: Adult Health/Ear
Reference: Black J, Hawks J, Keene A: *Medical-surgical nursing: clinical management for positive outcomes,* ed 6, Philadelphia, 2001, WB Saunders, p. 1846.

30. *Answer:* 2
Rationale: The nurse instructs the client to make slow head movements to prevent worsening of the vertigo. Dietary changes such as salt and fluid restrictions that reduce the amount of endolymphatic fluid is sometimes prescribed. Watching TV can increase the vertigo.
Test-Taking Strategy: Identify the issue of the question. The issue is vertigo. Note the relationship between vertigo and the correct option, avoiding sudden head movements. If you had difficulty with this question review measures that will reduce vertigo in the client with Meniere's disease.
Level of Cognitive Ability: Application
Client Needs: Physiological Integrity
Integrated Concept/Process: Nursing Process/Implementation
Content Area: Adult Health/Ear
Reference: DeWit S: *Fundamental concepts and skills for nursing,* Philadelphia, 2001, WB Saunders, p. 374.

31. *Answer:* 2
Rationale: Dietary changes such as salt and fluid restrictions that reduce the amount of endolymphatic fluid are sometimes prescribed. Options 1, 3, and 4 are not specific dietary prescriptions for this condition.
Test-Taking Strategy: Knowledge regarding the pathophysiology related to Meniere's disease is required to answer this question. From this point, use the process of elimination. Review the pathophysiology related to this condition and the treatment if you had difficulty with this question.
Level of Cognitive Ability: Comprehension
Client Needs: Physiological Integrity
Integrated Concept/Process: Nursing Process/Planning
Content Area: Adult Health/Ear
Reference: Ignatavicius D, Workman M: *Medical-surgical nursing: critical thinking for collaborative care,* ed 4, Philadelphia, 2002, WB Saunders, p. 1048.

32. *Answer:* 4
Rationale: Treatment for acoustic neuroma is surgical removal via a craniotomy. Extreme care is taken to preserve remaining hearing and preserve the function of the facial nerve. Acoustic neuromas rarely recur after surgical removal.
Test-Taking Strategy: Use knowledge regarding the anatomical location of acoustic neuromas to answer this question. If you had difficulty with this question, review the complications associated with this surgical procedure.
Level of Cognitive Ability: Analysis
Client Needs: Physiological Integrity
Integrated Concept/Process: Nursing Process/Data Collection
Content Area: Adult Health/Ear
Reference: Ignatavicius D, Workman M: *Medical-surgical nursing: critical thinking for collaborative care,* ed 4, Philadelphia, 2002, WB Saunders, p. 1001.

33. *Answer:* 2
Rationale: Bloody or clear watery drainage from the auditory canal indicates a cerebrospinal leak after trauma and suggests a basal skull fracture. This warrants immediate attention. Option 1 is indicative of an infectious process. Options 3 and 4 are not specifically associated with a basal skull fracture.
Test-Taking Strategy: Knowledge regarding the signs associated with a basal skull fracture is required to answer this question. If you had difficulty with this question, review these signs.
Level of Cognitive Ability: Analysis
Client Needs: Physiological Integrity
Integrated Concept/Process: Nursing Process/Data Collection
Content Area: Adult Health/Ear
Reference: Ignatavicius D, Workman M: *Medical-surgical nursing: critical thinking for collaborative care,* ed 4, Philadelphia, 2002, WB Saunders, p. 929.

34. *Answer:* 3
Rationale: Otoscopic examination in a client with mastoiditis reveals a red, dull, thick and immobile tympanic membrane

with or without perforation. Postauricular lymph nodes are tender and enlarged. Clients also have a low-grade fever, malaise, anorexia, swelling behind the ear, and pain with minimal movement of the head. Options 1, 2, and 4 are not findings that would be noted in this examination in the client with mastoiditis
Test-Taking Strategy: Knowledge regarding assessment findings associated with mastoiditis is required to answer this question. If you had difficulty with this question, review these findings.
Level of Cognitive Ability: Comprehension
Client Needs: Physiological Integrity
Integrated Concept/Process: Nursing Process/Data Collection
Content Area: Adult Health/Ear
Reference: DeWit S: *Fundamental concepts and skills for nursing*, Philadelphia, 2001, WB Saunders, p. 374.

35. *Answer:* 3
Rationale: Tinnitus is the most common complaint of clients with otological disorders, especially those involving the inner ear. Symptoms of tinnitus range from mild ringing in the ear, which can go unnoticed during the day, to a loud roaring in the ear, which can interfere with the client's thinking process and attention span. Hearing loss may or may not occur. Options 2 and 4 are not specifically associated with inner ear problems.
Test-Taking Strategy: Knowledge regarding symptoms associated with inner ear disorders is required to answer this question. Use the process of elimination recalling the functions of the inner ear to select the correct option. Review inner ear problems and the associated findings if you had difficulty with this question.
Level of Cognitive Ability: Comprehension
Client Needs: Physiological Integrity
Integrated Concept/Process: Nursing Process/Data Collection
Content Area: Adult Health/Ear
Reference: DeWit S: *Fundamental concepts and skills for nursing*, Philadelphia, 2001, WB Saunders, p. 374.

36. *Answer:* 4
Rationale: Meniere's disease is a disorder of the labyrinth of the inner ear. This disorder does not affect the external ear, tympanic membrane, or middle ear.
Test-Taking Strategy: Use the process of elimination. Knowledge that a symptom of Meniere's disease is tinnitus will assist in directing you to option 4. Review this disorder if you had difficulty with this question.
Level of Cognitive Ability: Comprehension
Client Needs: Physiological Integrity
Integrated Concept/Process: Nursing Process/Planning
Content Area: Adult Health/Ear
Reference: Ignatavicius D, Workman M: *Medical-surgical nursing: critical thinking for collaborative care*, ed 4, Philadelphia, 2002, WB Saunders, p. 1048.

37. *Answer:* 1
Rationale: Surgical treatment for Meniere's disease involves relief from accumulation of inner ear fluid in the endolymphatic sac. Procedures may be directed toward relief of pressure by the bony structures surrounding the sac, or toward opening the sac and diverting the flow of endolymph by means of a shunt to the mastoid bone or to the subarachnoid space. Options 2, 3, and 4 are procedures that are unrelated to Meniere's disease.
Test-Taking Strategy: Use the process of elimination. Knowledge that Meniere's disease affects the inner ear will assist in directing you to option 1. If you are unfamiliar with this disorder and the surgical procedures, review this content.
Level of Cognitive Ability: Comprehension
Client Needs: Physiological Integrity
Integrated Concept/Process: Nursing Process/Planning
Content Area: Adult Health/Ear
Reference: Ignatavicius D, Workman M: *Medical-surgical nursing: critical thinking for collaborative care*, ed 4, Philadelphia, 2002, WB Saunders, p. 1048.

38. *Answer:* 1
Rationale: A low-sodium diet, restriction of fluids, and vasodilating medications are used in the treatment of Meniere's disease to assist in reducing the accumulation of inner ear fluid in the endolymphatic sac. Mild sedation may be prescribed.
Test-Taking Strategy: Use the process of elimination. Recalling that in Meniere's disease an accumulation of inner ear fluid occurs will assist in directing you to option 1. If you are unfamiliar with this disease, review this content.
Level of Cognitive Ability: Comprehension
Client Needs: Physiological Integrity
Integrated Concept/Process: Nursing Process/Planning
Content Area: Adult Health/Ear
Reference: Ignatavicius D, Workman M: *Medical-surgical nursing: critical thinking for collaborative care*, ed 4, Philadelphia, 2002, WB Saunders, p. 1068.

39. *Answer:* 1
Rationale: Otosclerosis involves the formation of spongy bone in the capsule of the labyrinth of the ear, often causing the auditory ossicles to become fixed and less able to pass vibrations when sound enters the ear. An early symptom is ringing in the ears, but the most noticeable symptom is progressive hearing loss. Options 2, 3, and 4 are not associated with this condition.
Test-Taking Strategy: Use the process of elimination. Note the key word "early." Knowledge that this disorder involves the ear will assist in eliminating options 2 and 3. Focusing on the key word will assist in directing you to option 1. If you had difficulty with this question review this disorder.
Level of Cognitive Ability: Comprehension
Client Needs: Physiological Integrity
Integrated Concept/Process: Nursing Process/Data Collection
Content Area: Adult Health/Ear
Reference: Ignatavicius D, Workman M: *Medical-surgical nursing: critical thinking for collaborative care*, ed 4, Philadelphia, 2002, WB Saunders, p. 1048.

40. *Answer:* 3
Rationale: Clients with otosclerosis who do not desire surgery may have their hearing loss relieved by the use of a hearing aid. Options 1, 2, and 4 are inappropriate responses.
Test-Taking Strategy: Use therapeutic communication techniques. Eliminate options 2 and 4 first because they are

similar and provide advice to the client. Next eliminate option 1 because it is incorrect and nontherapeutic. Review the surgical treatment for otosclerosis if you had difficulty with this question.
Level of Cognitive Ability: Application
Client Needs: Psychosocial Integrity
Integrated Concept/Process: Nursing Process/Implementation
Content Area: Adult Health/Ear
Reference: Ignatavicius D, Workman M: *Medical-surgical nursing: critical thinking for collaborative care,* ed 4, Philadelphia, 2002, WB Saunders, p. 1048.

41. ***Answer:*** 3
Rationale: After the acute phase, remission occurs, but symptoms will recur with two or three acute attacks per year. As this pattern of attacks and remissions develops, fewer symptoms occur during the acute phase. A complete remission eventually occurs with some degree of hearing loss varying from slight to complete. It takes several weeks before all symptoms subside after an attack, leaving a loss of hearing in the involved ear. Options 1, 2, and 4 are incorrect.
Test-Taking Strategy: Use the process of elimination. Knowledge that a hearing loss occurs to some degree in an acute attack of Meniere's disease is required to answer this question. If you are unfamiliar with the effects of Meniere's disease on hearing, review this content.
Level of Cognitive Ability: Application
Client Needs: Physiological Integrity
Integrated Concept/Process: Nursing Process/Implementation
Content Area: Adult Health/Ear
Reference: Ignatavicius D, Workman M: *Medical-surgical nursing: critical thinking for collaborative care,* ed 4, Philadelphia, 2002, WB Saunders, p. 1069.

42. ***Answer:*** 3
Rationale: Medical interventions during the acute phase of Meniere's disease include using atropine or diazepam (Valium) to decrease the autonomic nervous system function. Diphenhydramine (Benadryl) may be prescribed for its antihistamine effects, and a vasodilator will also be prescribed. The client will remain on bed rest during the acute attack, and, when allowed to be out of bed, the client will need assistance with walking, sitting, or standing.
Test-Taking Strategy: Knowledge regarding the pathophysiology associated with Meniere's disease is required to answer this question. Use the process of elimination in considering the correct response. If you are unfamiliar with the treatment measures for this disorder, review this content.
Level of Cognitive Ability: Analysis
Client Needs: Physiological Integrity
Integrated Concept/Process: Nursing Process/Implementation
Content Area: Adult Health/Ear
Reference: Ignatavicius D, Workman M: *Medical-surgical nursing: critical thinking for collaborative care,* ed 4, Philadelphia, 2002, WB Saunders, p. 1069.

43. ***Answer:*** 4
Rationale: Management during remission includes diuretics to decrease the fluid and thereby decrease pressure in the endolymphs. Antihistamines, vasodilators, and diuretics may be prescribed for the client. A low-salt diet is prescribed for the client to reduce fluid. The major goal of treatment is to preserve the client's hearing, and careful medical management helps achieve this in most clients with Meniere's disease.
Test-Taking Strategy: Knowledge that Meniere's disease occurs as a result of a disturbance in the fluid of the endolymphatic system is required to answer this question. This knowledge and use of the process of elimination will easily direct you to option 4. If you are unfamiliar with the management of this disorder during remission, review this content.
Level of Cognitive Ability: Comprehension
Client Needs: Health Promotions and Maintenance
Integrated Concept/Process: Teaching/Learning
Content Area: Adult Health/Ear
Reference: Ignatavicius D, Workman M: *Medical-surgical nursing: critical thinking for collaborative care,* ed 4, Philadelphia, 2002, WB Saunders, p. 1069.

44. ***Answer:*** 2
Rationale: After stapedectomy, the client is instructed to keep water out of the ear canal for at least 3 weeks and to avoid swimming for 6 weeks. The client is also instructed to avoid coughing and sneezing and to avoid bending and lifting heavy objects or other strenuous activities for at least 3 weeks. Air travel is avoided for 4 weeks. If the client develops sudden hearing loss, fever, or severe persistent vertigo or dizziness, the physician should be notified.
Test-Taking Strategy: Use the process of elimination. Note the key words "indicates a need for further education." Read each option carefully noting the time frame and the activities described in the options. Eliminate options 1 and 4 first because of the similar time frames. Eliminate option 3 next because of the word "persistent." Review the client teaching points after this procedure if you had difficulty with this question.
Level of Cognitive Ability: Comprehension
Client Needs: Health Promotion and Maintenance
Integrated Concept/Process: Teaching/Learning
Content Area: Adult Health/Ear
Reference: Ignatavicius D, Workman M: *Medical-surgical nursing: critical thinking for collaborative care,* ed 4, Philadelphia, 2002, WB Saunders, p. 1075.

45. ***Answer:*** 3
Rationale: After ear surgery, clients need to avoid straining when having a bowel movement. Clients need to be instructed to avoid drinking with a straw, air travel, and excessive coughing for 2 to 3 weeks. Clients need to avoid getting their head wet, washing their hair, and showering for 1 week. Clients need to avoid rapidly moving the head, bouncing, and bending over for 3 weeks.
Test-Taking Strategy: Use the process of elimination. Note that the question asks for the instruction that will be included in the plan of care. Consider the anatomical area of the client condition and the surgical procedure in eliminating the incorrect options. If you had difficulty with this question, review client instructions after ear surgery.
Level of Cognitive Ability: Application
Client Needs: Health Promotion and Maintenance
Integrated Concept/Process: Teaching/Learning

Content Area: Adult Health/Ear
Reference: Black J, Hawks J, Keene A: *Medical-surgical nursing: clinical management for positive outcomes,* ed 6, Philadelphia, 2001, WB Saunders, p. 1846.

46. *Answer:* 3
Rationale: A small amount of brownish or reddish drainage is normal for 24 to 48 hours after the surgery. Excessive drainage, especially clear fluid should be reported immediately. Options 1, 2, and 4 are inaccurate instructions.
Test-Taking Strategy: Knowledge regarding the normal expectations after this procedure is required to answer this question. Read each option carefully and use the process of elimination. If you are unfamiliar with the normal findings after myringotomy, review this content.
Level of Cognitive Ability: Application
Client Needs: Physiological Integrity
Integrated Concept/Process: Nursing Process/Implementation
Content Area: Adult Health/Ear
Reference: Ignatavicius D, Workman M: *Medical-surgical nursing: critical thinking for collaborative care,* ed 4, Philadelphia, 2002, WB Saunders, p. 1065.

47. *Answer:* 3
Rationale: Nurses should have a basic knowledge of the care to a hearing aid to assist the client in its use. The client should be instructed to turn the hearing aid off before removing it from the ear to prevent squealing feedback. The hearing aid should be turned off when not in use, and the client should keep an extra battery available at all times. The client should wash the ear mold frequently with mild soap and water with the use of a pipe cleaner to cleanse the cannula. The client should not wear the hearing aid during an ear infection.
Test-Taking Strategy: Use the process of elimination to answer this question. Read each option carefully. Knowledge regarding squealing feedback will assist in directing you to the correct option. If you had difficulty with this question, review the use of the hearing aid.
Level of Cognitive Ability: Comprehension
Client Needs: Health Promotion and Maintenance
Integrated Concept/Process: Self-Care
Content Area: Adult Health/Ear
Reference: DeWit S: *Fundamental concepts and skills for nursing,* Philadelphia, 2001, WB Saunders, p. 310.

48. *Answer:* 3
Rationale: Bloody or clear watery drainage from the auditory canal indicates a cerebrospinal leak after trauma and suggests a basal skull fracture. This warrants immediate attention and the physician should be notified. Options 1, 2 and 4 are inappropriate nursing actions.
Test-Taking Strategy: Use the process of elimination to answer the question. Eliminate options 1 and 4 first because they are similar. Knowledge that the presence of bloody or clear drainage from the auditory canal suggests the presence of a basal skull fracture will easily direct you to option 3. If you had difficulty with this question, review the complications after a head injury.
Level of Cognitive Ability: Application
Client Needs: Physiological Integrity
Integrated Concept/Process: Nursing Process/Implementation
Content Area: Adult Health/Ear
Reference: Ignatavicius D, Workman M: *Medical-surgical nursing: critical thinking for collaborative care,* ed 4, Philadelphia, 2002, WB Saunders, p. 929.

49. *Answer:* 4
Rationale: The client should move the head slowly to prevent worsening of the vertigo. Salt and fluid restrictions are sometimes prescribed to reduce the amount of endolymphatic fluid. Clients are advised to stop smoking because of its vasoconstrictive effects.
Test-Taking Strategy: Use the process of elimination. Identify the issue of the question, which is vertigo. Note the relationship between vertigo and the correct option, avoiding sudden head movements. If you had difficulty with this question, review measures that will reduce vertigo in the client with Meniere's disease.
Level of Cognitive Ability: Comprehension
Client Needs: Health Promotion and Maintenance
Integrated Concept/Process: Nursing Process/Evaluation
Content Area: Adult Health/Ear
Reference: Ignatavicius D, Workman M: *Medical-surgical nursing: critical thinking for collaborative care,* ed 4, Philadelphia, 2002, WB Saunders, p. 1068.

REFERENCES

Black J, Hawks J, Keene A: *Medical-surgical nursing: clinical management for positive outcomes,* ed 6, Philadelphia, 2001, WB Saunders.
Chernecky C, Berger B: *Laboratory tests and diagnostic procedures,* ed 3, Philadelphia, 2001, WB Saunders.
Clark J, Queener S, Karb V: *Pharmacologic basis of nursing practice,* ed 6, St Louis, 2000, Mosby.
DeWit S: *Fundamental concepts and skills for nursing,* Philadelphia, 2001, WB Saunders.
Hodgson B, Kizior R: *Saunders nursing drug handbook 2002,* Philadelphia, 2002, WB Saunders.
Ignatavicius D, Workman M: *Medical-surgical nursing: critical thinking for collaborative care,* ed 4, Philadelphia, 2002, WB Saunders.
Lehne R: *Pharmacology for nursing care,* ed 4, Philadelphia, 2001, WB Saunders.
Potter P, Perry A: *Fundamentals of nursing,* ed 5, St Louis, 2001, Mosby.
Perry A, Potter P: *Clinical nursing skills and techniques,* ed 5, St Louis, 2002, Mosby.

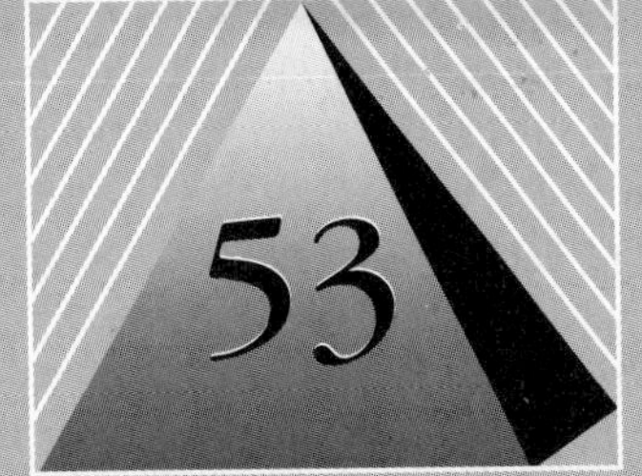

Ophthalmic and Otic Medications

I. OPHTHALMIC MEDICATION ADMINISTRATION (Box 53-1)

A. Guidelines for the use of eye medications

1. Eye medications are usually in the form of drops or ointments
2. To prevent overflow of medication into the nasal and pharyngeal passages, thus reducing systemic absorption, instruct the client to occlude the nasolacrimal duct with one finger for 1 to 2 minutes after instilling the medication
3. When two or more eye medications are to be administered, wait at least 3 minutes between medications
4. Wash hands before administering eye medications to avoid contaminating the eye or medication dropper or applicator, and after administering eye medications to rinse off any residue
5. Use a separate bottle or tube of medication for each client to avoid accidental cross contamination
6. Place prescribed dose of eye medication in the lower conjunctival sac, never directly onto the cornea
7. Avoid touching any part of the eye with the dropper or applicator
8. Administer drops or liquid preparations before ointments
9. Administer glucocorticoid preparations before other medications
10. Monitor the pulse of the client receiving an ophthalmic beta blocker and instruct the client to do the same; if the pulse is below 50 to 60 beats per minute (adult), withhold the next dose of eye medication an ' notify the physician
11. Instruct the client how to instill medication correctly and supervise instillation until the client can do it safely
12. Instruct the client to read the medication labels carefully to ensure administration of the correct medication and correct strength
13. Remind the client to keep these medications out of the reach of children
14. Instruct the client to avoid driving or operating hazardous equipment if vision is blurred
15. Inform the client that he or she may be unable to drive home after eye examinations when medications to dilate the pupil **(mydriatics)** or medications to paralyze the ciliary muscle **(cycloplegics)** are used
16. If photophobia occurs, instruct the client to wear sunglasses and avoid bright lights
17. Instruct the client to administer a missed dose of the eye medication as soon as remembered, unless the next dose is scheduled to be administered in 1 to 2 hours
18. Inform the client with **glaucoma** that the disorder cannot be cured, only controlled
19. Reinforce the importance of using medications to treat **glaucoma** as prescribed and not to discontinue these medications without consulting the physician
20. Inform the client that medications used to treat **glaucoma** may cause pain and blurred vision, especially when therapy is begun

BOX 53-1

Abbreviations

Left eye (OS)
Right eye (OD)
Both eyes (OU)

21. Instruct the client to report the development of any eye irritation
22. Inform the client using eye gel to store the gel at room temperature or in the refrigerator but not to freeze it
23. Instruct the client to discard unused eye gel kept at room temperature after 8 weeks
24. Inform the client that soft contact lenses may absorb certain eye medications and that preservatives in eye medications may discolor the contact lenses
25. Advise the client wearing contact lenses to question the physician carefully about special precautions to observe
26. In infants, inform the parents that atropine sulfate eye drops may contribute to abdominal distention
27. Instruct the parents to keep a record of the bowel movements of the infant being administered atropine sulfate eye drops
28. Auscultate bowel sounds of the infant or child receiving atropine sulfate eye drops

B. Instillation of eye medications
   1. Drops
      a. Wash hands
      b. Put gloves on
      c. Check the name, strength, and expiration date of the medication
      d. Instruct the client to tilt the head backward, open the eyes, and look up
      e. Pull the lower lid down against the cheekbone
      f. Hold the bottle like a pencil with the tip downward
      g. Holding the bottle, gently rest the wrist of the hand on the client's cheek
      h. Squeeze the bottle gently to allow the drop to fall into the conjunctival sac
      i. Instruct the client to close the eyes gently and not to squeeze the eyes shut
      j. Wait 3 to 5 minutes before instilling another drop, if more than one drop is prescribed, to promote maximal absorption of the medication
      k. Do not allow the medication bottle, dropper, or applicator to come in contact with the eyeball
   2. Ointments
      a. Hold the ointment tube near, but not touching, the eye or eyelashes
      b. Squeeze a thin ribbon of ointment along the lining of the lower conjunctival sac from the inner to the outer canthus
      c. Instruct the client to close the eyes gently
      d. Instruct the client that vision may be blurred by the ointment

II. MYDRIATIC/CYCLOPLEGIC AND ANTICHOLINERGIC MEDICATIONS (Box 53-2)

A. Description
   1. **Mydriatics** and **cycloplegics** dilate the pupils **(mydriasis)** and relax the ciliary muscles **(cycloplegia)**
   2. Anticholinergics block responses of the sphincter muscle in the ciliary body, producing **mydriasis** and **cycloplegia**
   3. Used preoperatively or for eye examinations to produce **mydriasis**
   4. Contraindicated in clients with **glaucoma** because of the risk of increased intraocular pressure
   5. **Mydriatics** are contraindicated in cardiac dysrhythmias and cerebral atherosclerosis and should be used with caution in elderly clients and in clients with prostatic hypertrophy, diabetes mellitus, or parkinsonism

B. Side effects
   1. Tachycardia
   2. Photophobia
   3. Conjunctivitis
   4. Dermatitis

C. Atropine toxicity
   1. Dry mouth
   2. Blurred vision
   3. Photophobia
   4. Tachycardia
   5. Fever
   6. Urinary retention
   7. Constipation
   8. Headache, brow pain
   9. Confusion
   10. Hallucinations, delirium
   11. Coma
   12. Worsening of narrow-angle **glaucoma**

D. Systemic reactions of anticholinergics
   1. Dry mouth and skin
   2. Fever

BOX 53-2

Mydriatic/Cycloplegic Eye Medications

Atropine sulfate (Isopto Atropine, Ocu-Tropine, Atropair, Atropisol)
Scopolamine hydrobromide (Isopto Hyoscine)
Cyclopentolate HCl (Cyclogyl, AK-Pentolate, Pentolair)
Homatropine hydrobromide (Isopto Homatrine, AK-Homatropine, Spectro-Homatrine)
Tropicamide (Mydriacyl, I-Picamide, Tropicacyl)
Phenylephrine HCl (AK-Dilate, Dilatair, Mydfrin, Ocu-Phrin)

3. Thirst
4. Confusion
5. Hyperactivity

E. Implementation
1. Monitor for allergic response
2. Assess for risk of injury
3. Assess for constipation and urinary retention
4. Instruct the client that a burning sensation may occur on instillation
5. Instruct the client not to drive or operate machinery for 24 hours after instillation of the medication unless otherwise directed by the physician
6. Instruct the client to wear sunglasses until the effects of the medication wear off
7. Instruct the client to notify the physician if blurring of vision, loss of sight, difficulty breathing, sweating, or flushing occurs
8. Instruct the client to report eye pain to the physician

F. Alpha-adrenergic blocker
1. Medication: dapiprazole HCl (Rev-Eyes)
2. Use: to counteract **mydriasis**

III. ANTIINFECTIVE EYE MEDICATIONS (Box 53-3)

A. Description: kill or inhibit the growth of bacteria, fungi, and viruses

B. Side effects
1. Superinfection
2. Global irritation

C. Implementation
1. Assess for risk of injury
2. Instruct the client how to apply the eye medication
3. Instruct the client to continue treatment as prescribed
4. Instruct the client to wash hands thoroughly and frequently
5. Advise the client that if improvement does not occur, to notify the physician

IV. ANTIINFLAMMATORY EYE MEDICATIONS (Box 53-4)

A. Description
1. Control inflammation, thereby reducing vision loss and scarring
2. Used for uveitis, allergic conditions, and inflammation of the conjunctiva, cornea, and lids

B. Side effects
1. **Cataracts**
2. Increased intraocular pressure
3. Impaired healing
4. Masking signs and symptoms of infection

C. Implementation
1. Refer to implementation, antiinfective medications
2. Note that dexamethasone (Maxidex) should not be used for eye abrasions and wounds

V. TOPICAL ANESTHETICS FOR THE EYE (Box 53-5)

A. Description
1. Produce corneal anesthesia
2. Used for anesthesia for eye examinations, surgery, or to remove foreign bodies from the eye

B. Side effects
1. Temporary stinging or burning of the eye
2. Temporary loss of corneal reflex

BOX 53-3
Antiinfective Eye Medications

ANTIBACTERIAL
Chloramphenicol (Chloromycetin, Chloroptic)
Ciprofloxacin (Cipro)
Erythromycin (Ilotycin)
Gentamicin sulfate (Garamycin, Genoptic)
Norfloxacin (Chibroxin)
Tobramycin (Nebcin, Tobrex)
Silver nitrate 1%

ANTIFUNGAL
Natamycin (Natacyn ophthalmic)

ANTIVIRAL
Idoxuridine (Herplex Liquifilm)
Trifluridine (Viroptic)
Vidarabine (Vira-A ophthalmic)

BOX 53-4
Antiinflammatory Eye Medications

Dexamethasone (Maxidex)
Diclofenac sodium (Voltaren)
Flurbiprofen sodium (Ocufen)
Suprofen (Profenal)
Ketorolac tromethamine (Acular)
Prednisolone acetate (Predforte, Econopred)
Prednisolone sodium phosphate (AK-Pred, Inflamase Mild, Inflamase Forte)
Rimexolone (Vexol)

BOX 53-5
Topical Anesthetics for the Eye

Proparacaine HCl (Ophthaine, Ophthetic)
Tetracaine HCl (Pontocaine)

C. Implementation
1. Assess for risk of injury
2. Note that the medications should not be given to the client for home use and are not to be self-administered by the client
3. Note that the blink reflex is temporarily lost and that the corneal epithelium needs to be protected
4. Provide an eye patch to protect the eye from injury until the corneal reflex returns

VI. EYE LUBRICANTS (Box 53-6)

A. Description
1. Replace tears or add moisture to the eyes
2. Moisten contact lenses or an artificial eye
3. Protect the eyes during surgery or diagnostic procedures
4. Used for keratitis, during anesthesia, or in a disorder that results in unconsciousness or decreased blinking

B. Side effects
1. Burning on instillation
2. Discomfort or pain on instillation

C. Implementation
1. Inform the client that burning may occur on instillation
2. Be alert to allergic responses to the preservatives in the lubricants

VII. MIOTICS (Box 53-7)

A. Description
1. Reduce intraocular pressure by constricting the pupil and contracting the ciliary muscle, thereby increasing the blood flow to the retina and decreasing retinal damage and loss of vision
2. Open the anterior chamber angle and increase the outflow of aqueous humor
3. **Miotic** cholinergic medications reduce intraocular pressure by mimicking the action of acetylcholine
4. **Miotic** acetylcholine inhibitors reduce intraocular pressure by inhibiting the action of cholinesterase
5. Used for chronic open-angle **glaucoma** or acute and chronic closed-angle **glaucoma**
6. Used to achieve **miosis** during eye surgery
7. Contraindicated in clients with **retinal detachment**, adhesions between the iris and lens, or in inflammatory diseases
8. Use with caution in clients with asthma, hypertension, corneal abrasion, hyperthyroidism, coronary artery disease, urinary tract obstruction, gastrointestinal (GI) obstruction, ulcer disease, parkinsonism, and bradycardia

B. Side effects
1. **Myopia**
2. Headache
3. Eye pain
4. Decreased vision in poor light
5. Local irritation
6. Systemic effects
   a. Flushing
   b. Diaphoresis
   c. GI upset and diarrhea
   d. Frequent urination
   e. Increased salivation
   f. Muscle weakness
   g. Respiratory difficulty
7. Toxicity
   a. Vertigo and syncope
   b. Bradycardia
   c. Hypotension
   d. Cardiac dysrhythmias
   e. Tremors
   f. Seizures

C. Implementation
1. Assess vital signs
2. Assess for risk of injury
3. Assess the client for the degree of diminished vision
4. Monitor for side effects and toxic effects
5. Monitor for postural hypotension and instruct the client to change positions slowly
6. Assess breath sounds for rales and rhonchi because cholinergic medications can cause bronchospasms and increased bronchial secretions

BOX 53-6

Eye Lubricants

Hydroxypropyl methylcellulose (Lacril, Isopto Plain)
Petroleum-based ointment (Artificial Tears, Liquifilm Tears)

BOX 53-7

Miotics

Acetylcholine chloride (Miochol)
Carbachol (Miostat)
Pilocarpine HCl (Isopto Carpine, Pilocar)
Pilocarpine nitrate (Pilofrin , Liquifilm, Pilagan)
Echothiophate iodide (Phospholine Iodide)
Demecarium bromide (Humorsol)
Isoflurophate (Floropryl)

7. Maintain oral hygiene because of the increase in salivation
8. Have atropine sulfate available as an antidote for pilocarpine
9. Instruct the client or family regarding the correct administration of eye medications
10. Instruct the client not to stop the medication suddenly
11. Instruct the client to avoid activities such as driving while vision is impaired
12. Instruct clients with **glaucoma** to read labels on over-the-counter medications and to avoid atropine-like medications because atropine will increase intraocular pressure

VIII. OCUSERT SYSTEM

A. Description
1. Ocusert is a thin eye wafer (disk) impregnated with time-release pilocarpine
2. It is devised to overcome the need for frequent application of pilocarpine
3. It is placed in the upper or lower cul-de-sac of the eye
4. The pilocarpine is released over 1 week
5. The disk is replaced every 7 days
6. Drawbacks of its use include sudden leakage of pilocarpine, migration of the system over the cornea, and unnoticed loss of the system

B. Implementation
1. Assess the client's ability to insert the medication disk
2. Store the medication in the refrigerator
3. Instruct the client to discard damaged or contaminated disks
4. Inform the client that temporary stinging is expected but to notify the physician if blurred vision or brow pain occurs
5. Instruct the client to check for the presence of the disk in the conjunctival sac daily at bedtime and on arising
6. Because vision may change in the first few hours after the eye system is inserted, instruct the client to replace the disk at bedtime

IX. BETA-ADRENERGIC-BLOCKING EYE MEDICATIONS (Box 53-8)

A. Description
1. Reduce intraocular pressure by decreasing sympathetic impulses and decreasing aqueous humor production without affecting **accommodation** or pupil size
2. Used to treat chronic open-angle **glaucoma**

BOX 53-8

Beta-Adrenergic Blocking Eye Medications

Betaxolol HCl (Betoptic)
Carteolol HCl (Ocupress)
Levobunolol HCl (Betagan)
Metipranolol HCl (OptiPranolol)
Timolol maleate (Timoptic)

3. Contraindicated in the client with asthma because systemic absorption can cause increased airway resistance
4. Use with caution in the client receiving oral beta blockers

B. Side effects
1. Ocular irritation
2. Visual disturbances
3. Bradycardia
4. Hypotension
5. Bronchospasm

C. Implementation
1. Monitor vital signs, especially blood pressure and pulse before administering medication
2. If the pulse is 60 or below or if the systolic blood pressure is below 90 mm Hg, withhold the medication and contact the physician
3. Monitor for shortness of breath
4. Assess for risk of injury
5. Monitor input and output (I&O)
6. Instruct the client to notify the physician if shortness of breath occurs
7. Instruct the client not to discontinue the medication abruptly
8. Instruct the client to change positions slowly to avoid orthostatic hypotension
9. Instruct the client to avoid hazardous activities
10. Instruct the client to avoid over-the-counter medications without the physician's approval

D. Adrenergic medications (Box 53-9)
1. Decrease the production of aqueous humor and lead to a decrease in intraocular pressure
2. Used to treat **glaucoma**

BOX 53-9

Adrenergic Medications

Apraclonidine Hcl (Iopidine)
Brimonidine tartrate (Alphagan)
Dipivefrin HCl (Propine)
Epinephrine borate (Epinal, Eppy)
Epinephrine HCl (Epifrin, Glaucon)

X. CARBONIC ANHYDRASE INHIBITORS (Box 53-10)

A. Description
1. Interfere with the production of carbonic acid, which leads to decreased aqueous humor formation and decreased intraocular pressure
2. Used for long-term treatment of open-angle **glaucoma**
3. Contraindicated in the client allergic to sulfonamides

B. Side effects
1. Appetite loss
2. GI upset
3. Paresthesias in the fingers, toes, and face
4. Polyuria
5. Hypokalemia
6. Renal calculi
7. Photosensitivity
8. Lethargy and drowsiness
9. Depression

C. Implementation
1. Monitor vital signs
2. Assess visual acuity
3. Assess for risk of injury
4. Monitor I&O
5. Monitor weight
6. Maintain oral hygiene
7. Monitor for side effects such as lethargy, anorexia, drowsiness, polyuria, nausea, and vomiting
8. Monitor electrolytes for hypokalemia
9. Increase fluid intake unless contraindicated
10. Advise the client to avoid prolonged exposure to sunlight
11. Encourage the use of artificial tears for dry eyes
12. Instruct the client not to discontinue the medication abruptly
13. Instruct the client to avoid hazardous activities while vision is impaired

XI. OSMOTIC MEDICATIONS (Box 53-11)

A. Description
1. Lower intraocular pressure

BOX 53-10

Carbonic Anhydrase Inhibitors: Eye Medications

Acetazolamide (Diamox, AK-Zol)
Dichlorphenamide (Daranide)
Dorzolamide HCl (Trusopt)
Methazolamide (Neptazane)
Brinzolamide (Azopt)

BOX 53-11

Osmotic Medications for the Eye

Glycerin (Glyrol, Osmoglyn)
Mannitol (Osmitrol)
Urea (Ureaphil)

2. Used in emergency treatment of acute closed-angle **glaucoma**
3. Used preoperatively and postoperatively to decrease vitreous humor volume

B. Side effects
1. Headache
2. Nausea, vomiting, diarrhea
3. Disorientation
4. Electrolyte imbalances

C. Implementation
1. Assess vital signs
2. Assess visual acuity
3. Assess for risk of injury
4. Monitor I&O
5. Monitor weight
6. Monitor electrolyte imbalances
7. Increase fluid intake unless contraindicated
8. Monitor for changes in level of orientation

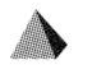

XII. OTIC MEDICATION ADMINISTRATION (Box 53-12)

A. Administering drops
1. In an adult, pull the pinna up and back to straighten the external canal to instill ear drops

BOX 53-12

Medications That Affect Hearing

ANTIBIOTICS
Amikacin sulfate (Amikin)
Chloramphenicol (Chloromycetin, Chloroptic, Ophthochlor)
Erythromycin (E-Mycin, ERYC, Ery-Tab, PCE Dispertabs, Ilotycin)
Gentamicin sulfate (Garamycin)
Streptomycin sulfate (Streptomycin)
Tobramycin sulfate (Nebcin)
Vancomycin HCl (Vancocin)

DIURETICS
Acetazolamide (Diamox)
Furosemide (Lasix)
Ethacrynic acid (Edecrin)

OTHERS
Cisplatin (Platinol, Platinol-AQ)
Nitrogen mustard
Quinine sulfate (Quinamm)
Quinidine (Cardioquin, Quinaglute, Quinidex)

2. Pull the ear down and back for infants and children younger than 3 years old; up and back for older children

B. Irrigation of the ear
   1. Irrigation of the ear needs to be prescribed by the physician
   2. Ensure that there is direct visualization of the tympanic membrane
   3. Warm irrigating solution to 100° F because solutions that are not close to the client's body temperature will cause ear injury, nausea, and vertigo
   4. Irrigation must be done gently to avoid damage to the eardrum
   5. When irrigating, do not direct irrigation solution directly toward the eardrum
   6. If a perforation of the eardrum is suspected, irrigation is not done

XIII. ANTIINFECTIVE EAR MEDICATIONS (Box 53-13)

A. Description
   1. Kill or inhibit the growth of bacteria
   2. Used for otitis media or otitis externa
   3. Contraindicated if a prior hypersensitivity exists

B. Side effects: overgrowth of nonsusceptible organisms

C. Implementation
   1. Monitor vital signs
   2. Assess for allergies
   3. Asses for pain
   4. Monitor for nephrotoxicity
   5. Instruct the client to report dizziness, fatigue, fever, or sore throat, which may be indicative of a superimposed infection
   6. Instruct the client to complete the entire course of the medication
   7. Instruct the client to keep ear canals dry

BOX 53-13

Antiinfective Ear Medications

Amoxicillin trihydrate (Amoxil)
Ampicillin trihydrate (Polycillin)
Cefaclor (Ceclor)
Clindamycin HCl (Cleocin)
Trimethoprim (TMP) and sulfamethoxazole (SMZ) (Bactrim, Cotrim, and Septra)
Erythromycin (Ilotycin, E-Mycin)
Penicillin V potassium (Pen-V)
Loracarbef (Lorabid)
Clarithromycin (Biaxin)
Chloramphenicol (Chloromycetin Otic)
Polymyxin B sulfate (Aerosporin)
Tetracycline HCl (Achromycin)
Acetic acid and aluminum acetate (Otic Domeboro)

XIV. ANTIHISTAMINES AND DECONGESTANTS (Box 53-14)

A. Description
   1. Produce vasoconstriction
   2. Stimulate the receptors of the respiratory mucosa
   3. Reduce respiratory tissue hyperemia and edema to open obstructed eustachian tubes
   4. Used for acute otitis media

B. Side effects
   1. Drowsiness
   2. Blurred vision
   3. Dry mucous membranes

C. Implementation
   1. Inform the client that drowsiness, blurred vision, and dry mouth may occur
   2. Instruct the client to increase fluid intake unless contraindicated and to suck on hard candy to alleviate dry mouth
   3. Instruct the client to avoid hazardous activities if drowsiness occurs

XV. LOCAL ANESTHETICS

A. Description
   1. Block nerve conduction at or near the application site to control pain
   2. Used for pain associated with ear infections

B. Medication: benzocaine (Americaine Otic; Tympagesic)

C. Side effects
   1. Allergic reaction
   2. Irritation

D. Implementation
   1. Monitor for effectiveness if used for pain relief
   2. Assess for irritation or allergic reaction

BOX 53-14

Antihistamines and Decongestants

Triprolidine and pseudoephedrine (Actifed)
Naphazoline HCl (Allerest, Albalon)
Chlorpheniramine (Chlor-Trimeton, Teldrin)
Brompheniramine maleate (Bromphen, Dimetane)
Terfenadine (Seldane)
Clemastine fumarate (Tavist)
Cetirizine HCl (Zyrtec)
Astemizole (Hismanal)

BOX 53-15

Ceruminolytic Medications

Carbamide peroxide (Debrox)
Boric acid (Ear-Dry)
Trolamine polypeptide oleate-condensate (Cerumenex)

XVI. CERUMINOLYTIC MEDICATIONS (Box 53-15)

A. Description
  1. Emulsify and loosen cerumen deposits
  2. Used to loosen and remove impacted wax from the ear canal

B. Side effects
  1. Irritation
  2. Redness or swelling of the ear canal

C. Implementation
  1. Instruct the client not to use drops more often than prescribed
  2. Moisten a cotton plug with medication before insertion
  3. Keep the container tightly closed and away from moisture
  4. Avoid touching the ear with the dropper
  5. Thirty minutes after instillation, gently irrigate the ear as prescribed with warm water using a soft rubber bulb ear syringe
  6. Irrigation may be done with hydrogen peroxide solution as prescribed, to flush cerumen deposits out of the ear canal
  7. For a chronic cerumen impaction, 1 to 2 drops of mineral oil will soften the wax
  8. Instruct the client to notify physician if redness, pain, or swelling persists

PRACTICE QUESTIONS

1. In preparation for cataract surgery, the nurse is to administer cyclopentolate HCl (Cyclogyl) eye drops. The nurse administers the medication knowing that the purpose of this medication is to:
   1. Provide lubrication to the operative eye
   2. Produce miosis of the operative eye
   3. Dilate the pupil of the operative eye
   4. Constrict the pupil of the operative eye

2. A nurse is reinforcing instructions to the client regarding the administration of the prescribed eye drops. Which of the following statements by the client indicates a need for further education?
   1. "I can tilt my head back, pull down on the lower lid, and place the drop in the lower lid."
   2. "I can lie down, pull down on the lower lid, and place the drop in the lower lid."
   3. "I can lie down, pull up on the upper lid, and place the drop in the lower lid."
   4. "I can lie on my side opposite to the eye I am going to place the drop, put the drop in the corner of the lid nearest my nose, and then slowly turn to my other side while blinking."

3. A nurse is preparing to administer ear drops to an infant. The nurse plans to:
   1. Pull up and back on the ear and direct the solution onto the eardrum
   2. Pull down and back on the ear and direct the solution onto the eardrum
   3. Pull down and back on the ear and direct the solution toward the wall of the canal
   4. Pull up and back on the ear lobe and direct the solution toward the wall of the canal

4. To minimize the systemic effects that eye drops can produce, the nurse plans to instruct the client to:
   1. Eat before instilling the drops
   2. Swallow several times after instilling the drops
   3. Blink vigorously to encourage tearing after instilling the drops
   4. Occlude the nasolacrimal duct with a finger for several minutes after instilling the drops

5. A client is receiving both epinephrine HCl (Epifrin, Glaucon) and timolol maleate (Timoptic) eye drops. When instructing the client on the administration of the eye drops the nurse plans to tell the client to:
   1. Administer the epinephrine HCl first, followed by the timolol maleate
   2. Administer the timolol maleate first, followed by the epinephrine HCl
   3. Administer epinephrine HCl in the morning and the timolol maleate in the evening
   4. Wait 3 minutes between the instillation of each medication

6. A licensed practical nurse (LPN) is assigned to care for a client with glaucoma. The LPN reviews the client's medication record and would notify the registered nurse (RN) if which of the following medications was noted on the client's record?
   1. Carbachol (Miostat)
   2. Pilocarpine HCl (Isopto Carpine)
   3. Pilocarpine (Ocusert Pilo-20, Ocusert Pilo-40)
   4. Atropine sulfate

7. A miotic medication has been prescribed for the client with glaucoma. The client asks the nurse about the purpose of the medication. The nurse tells the client that:
   1. "The medication will lower the pressure in your eye and increase the blood flow to the retina."
   2. "The medication will help to dilate the eye to prevent pressure from occurring."
   3. "The medication will relax the muscles of the eye and prevent blurred vision."
   4. "The medication will help to block the responses that are sent to the muscles in the eye."

8. Pilocarpine HCl (Isopto Carpine) is prescribed for the client with glaucoma. Which of the following medications does the nurse plan to have available in the event of systemic toxicity?
   1. Naloxone HCl (Narcan)
   2. Pindolol (Visken)
   3. Atropine sulfate
   4. Mesoridazine besylate (Serentil)
9. Betaxolol HCl (Betoptic) eye drops have been prescribed for the client with glaucoma. Which of the following nursing actions is most appropriate related to monitoring for the side effects of this medication?
   1. Monitor temperature
   2. Monitor blood pressure
   3. Monitor urine for sugar and acetone
   4. Monitor peripheral pulses
10. A nurse is assisting the physician with performing an ear irrigation on an assigned client. The nurse would plan to:
   1. Position the client to turn his or her head so that the ear to be irrigated is facing upward
   2. Warm the irrigating solution to 100° F
   3. Cool the irrigating solution to 85° F
   4. Position the client with the affected side up after the irrigation

ANSWERS

1. *Answer:* 3

Rationale: Cyclopentolate is a rapidly acting mydriatic and cycloplegic medication. It is effective in 25 to 75 minutes, and accommodation returns in 6 to 24 hours. Cyclopentolate is used for preoperative mydriasis. Options 1, 2, and 4 are not actions of this medication.

Test-Taking Strategy: Use the process of elimination. Options 2 and 4 are similar because miosis refers to constricted pupil. Note that the question identifies a client being prepared for eye surgery. The pupil would need to be dilated for the surgical procedure. Review the action and purpose of this medication if you had difficulty with this question.

Level of Cognitive Ability: Comprehension

Client Needs: Physiological Integrity

Integrated Concept/Process: Nursing Process/Implementation

Content Area: Adult Health/Eye

Reference: Lehne R: *Pharmacology for nursing care,* ed 4, Philadelphia, 2001, WB Saunders, p. 1147.

2. *Answer:* 3

Rationale: The client can either lie down or sit with the head tilted back. The lower lid should be pulled downward with the thumb or fingers. The client holds the bottle like a pencil, with the tip downward, and squeezes the bottle gently, allowing 1 drop to fall into the sac. The client gently closes the eye. An alternative method for clients who blink very easily is to place the client in the supine position with the head turned to one side. The eye to receive the eye drops should be uppermost. With the eye slightly closed, drop the prescribed dose on the inner canthus of the eye. Have the client turn from side to midline and to other side while blinking. The eye drops will move via gravity and surface tension into the conjunctival sac.

Test-Taking Strategy: Use the process of elimination. Note the key words "a need for further education." Knowing that the client places drops into the eye by pulling down on the lower lid will direct you to the correct option. Review the procedure for the administration of eye medications if you had difficulty with this question.

Level of Cognitive Ability: Comprehension

Client Needs: Health Promotion and Maintenance

Integrated Concept/Process: Teaching/Learning

Content Area: Adult Health/Eye

Reference: DeWit S: *Fundamental concepts and skills for nursing,* Philadelphia, 2001, WB Saunders, p. 666.

3. *Answer:* 3

Rationale: When administering ear drops to an infant, pull the ear down and straight back. In the adult or a child older than 3 years, pull up and back on the ear to straighten the auditory canal. Administer the medication by aiming it at the wall of the canal rather than directly onto the eardrum.

Test-Taking Strategy: Use the process of elimination. Eliminate options 1 and 2 because you would not direct ear solution directly onto the eardrum. Remember that in a child younger than 3 years, pulling the ear down and straight back is the correct procedure for administering ear medications. Review the procedure for administering ear medications if you had difficulty with this question.

Level of Cognitive Ability: Application

Client Needs: Physiological Integrity

Integrated Concept/Process: Nursing Process/Implementation

Content Area: Child Health

Reference: DeWit S: *Fundamental concepts and skills for nursing,* Philadelphia, 2001, WB Saunders, p. 668.

4. *Answer:* 4

Rationale: Applying pressure on the nasolacrimal duct prevents systemic absorption of the medication. Options 1, 2 and 3 will not prevent this occurrence.

Test-Taking Strategy: Use the process of elimination. Eliminate options 1 and 2 because eating and swallowing are similar and are unrelated to the systemic absorption of an eye medication. Blinking vigorously to produce tearing may result in the loss of the administered medication. Review this procedure if you had difficulty with this question.

Level of Cognitive Ability: Application

Client Needs: Health Promotion and Maintenance

Integrated Concept/Process: Teaching/Learning

Content Area: Adult Health/Eye

Reference: DeWit S: *Fundamental concepts and skills for nursing,* Philadelphia, 2001, WB Saunders, p. 667.

5. *Answer:* 4
Rationale: When two or more medications are to be administered, the client should wait 3 minutes between instillations. Options 1, 2, and 3 are incorrect.
Test-Taking Strategy: Use the process of elimination. Knowledge regarding the administration of more than one eye medication is helpful to answer this question. Note that option 4 is different from the other options and provides specific information related to the question. Review the administration of eye medications if you had difficulty with this question.
Level of Cognitive Ability: Application
Client Needs: Health Promotion and Maintenance
Integrated Concept/Process: Teaching/Learning
Content Area: Adult Health/Eye
Reference: DeWit S: *Fundamental concepts and skills for nursing*, Philadelphia, 2001, WB Saunders, p. 666.

6. *Answer:* 4
Rationale: Atropine sulfate is a mydriatic and cycloplegic medication and its use is contraindicated in clients with glaucoma. Mydriatic medications dilate the pupil and can cause an increase in intraocular pressure in the eye. Options 1, 2, and 3 are miotic agents used in the treatment of glaucoma.
Test-Taking Strategy: Use the process of elimination. Knowledge regarding the classifications of the medications identified in the options will assist you in answering the question. Remember that my"d"riatics, "d"ilate, and these medications are contraindicated in glaucoma. Review these medications if you had difficulty with this question.
Level of Cognitive Ability: Analysis
Client Needs: Safe, Effective Care Environment
Integrated Concept/Process: Nursing Process/Implementation
Content Area: Adult Health/Eye
Reference: Hodgson B, Kizior R: *Saunders nursing drug handbook 2002*, Philadelphia, 2002, WB Saunders, p. 90.

7. *Answer:* 1
Rationale: Miotics are used to lower the intraocular pressure, thereby increasing blood flow to the retina and decreasing retinal damage and loss of vision. Options 2, 3, and 4 all describe actions related to mydriatic medications, which primarily dilate the pupils and relax the ciliary muscles.
Test-Taking Strategy: Use the process of elimination. Knowledge regarding the action of miotics is required to answer this question. Note that the client has glaucoma. This should provide you with the clue to direct you to the correct option. Remember, prevention of increased intraocular pressure is the goal in clients with glaucoma. Review this type of medication if you had difficulty with this question.
Level of Cognitive Ability: Application
Client Needs: Health Promotion and Maintenance
Integrated Concept/Process: Nursing Process/Implementation
Content Area: Adult Health/Eye
Reference: Lehne R: *Pharmacology for nursing care*, ed 4, Philadelphia, 2001, WB Saunders, p. 1126.

8. *Answer:* 3
Rationale: Systemic absorption of pilocarpine HCl can produce toxicity and includes manifestations of vertigo, bradycardia, tremors, hypotension, and seizures. Atropine sulfate must be available in the event of systemic toxicity. Mesoridazine besylate is an antipsychotic medication. Pindolol is a beta-adrenergic blocker. Naloxone HCl is an opioid antagonist used to reverse narcotic-induced respiratory depression.
Test-Taking Strategy: Knowledge regarding antidotes related to various medications is required to answer this question. Atropine sulfate is the antidote for systemic reactions that occur with pilocarpine. Review antidotes if you had difficulty with this question.
Level of Cognitive Ability: Analysis
Client Needs: Physiological Integrity
Integrated Concept/Process: Nursing Process/Planning
Content Area: Adult Health/Eye
Reference: Hodgson B, Kizior R: *Saunders nursing drug handbook 2002*, Philadelphia, 2002, WB Saunders, p. 886.

9. *Answer:* 2
Rationale: This medication is an antiglaucoma medication and a beta-adrenergic blocker. Hypotension manifested as dizziness, nausea, diaphoresis, headache, fatigue, constipation, and diarrhea are systemic effects of the medication. The nurse would monitor the client's blood pressure. Options 1, 3, and 4 are not related to side effects associated with this medication.
Test-Taking Strategy: Knowledge regarding the systemic effects related to this medication is required to answer the question. Use the ABCs—airway, breathing, and circulation. Although option 4 is also related to circulation monitoring, the blood pressure is the more global option. Review the side effect of this medication if you had difficulty with this question.
Level of Cognitive Ability: Application
Client Needs: Physiological Integrity
Integrated Concept/Process: Nursing Process/Implementation
Content Area: Adult Health/Eye
Reference: Hodgson B, Kizior R: *Saunders nursing drug handbook 2002*, Philadelphia, 2002, WB Saunders, p. 120.

10. *Answer:* 2
Rationale: Irrigation solutions that are not close to the client's body temperature can be uncomfortable and may cause injury, nausea, and vertigo. Position the client so that the ear to be irrigated is facing downward, as this allows gravity to assist in the removal of the ear wax and solution. After the irrigation, the client is to lie on the affected side for a while to finish the drainage of the irrigating solution.
Test-Taking Strategy: Use the process of elimination. Knowledge regarding the procedure for ear irrigation is necessary to answer the question. Visualizing the procedure will assist in eliminating options 1 and 4. Recalling that the irrigating solution should be close to body temperature will assist in eliminating option 3. Review this procedure if you had difficulty with this question.
Level of Cognitive Ability: Application
Client Needs: Physiological Integrity
Integrated Concept/Process: Nursing Process/Planning
Content Area: Adult Health/Ear
Reference: DeWit S: *Fundamental concepts and skills for nursing*, Philadelphia, 2001, WB Saunders, p. 796.

REFERENCES

Clark J, Queener S, Karb V: *Pharmacologic basis of nursing practice*, ed 6, St Louis, 2000, Mosby.

Hodgson B, Kizior R: *Saunders nursing drug handbook 2002*, Philadelphia, 2002, WB Saunders.

Ignatavicius D, Workman M: *Medical-surgical nursing: critical thinking for collaborative care*, ed 4, Philadelphia, 2002, WB Saunders.

Karch A: *Focus on nursing pharmacology*, Philadelphia, 2000, Lippincott.

Lehne R: *Pharmacology for nursing care*, ed 4, Philadelphia, 2001, WB Saunders.

UNIT XVI

The Adult Client with a Neurological Disorder

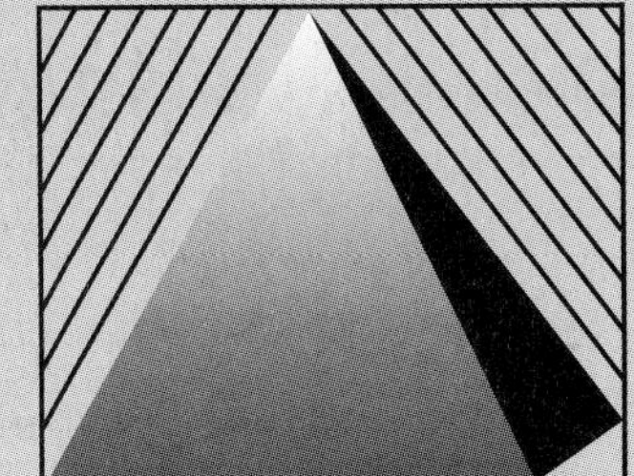

PYRAMID TERMS

Agnosia The inability to use an object correctly.

Apraxia The inability to carry out a purposeful activity.

Decerebrate Posturing (Abnormal Extension Response) Client stiffly extends one or both arms and possibly the legs. Indicates a brainstem lesion.

Decorticate Posturing (Abnormal Flexion Response) Client flexes one or both arms on the chest and may stiffly extend the legs. Indicates a nonfunctioning cortex.

Flaccid Posturing Client displays no motor response in any extremity.

Glasgow Coma Scale A method of assessing a client's neurological condition. A scoring system based on a scale of 1 to 15 points. A score below 8 indicates coma is present. Eye-opening is the most important indicator.

Hemianopia Blindness in half the visual field.

Homonymous Hemianopia Blindness in the same visual field of both eyes.

Increased Intracranial Pressure An increase in intracranial pressure caused by trauma, hemorrhage, growths or tumors, hydrocephalus, edema, or inflammation. Can impede circulation to the brain and absorption of cerebrospinal fluid, and affect the functioning of nerve cells and lead to brainstem compression and death.

Unconscious Client A state of depressed cerebral functioning with unresponsiveness to sensory and motor function. Some of the causes include head trauma, cerebral toxins, shock, hemorrhage, tumor, or infections.

PYRAMID TO SUCCESS

Pyramid points related to neurological disorders focus on safety issues, care to the unconscious client, monitoring for increased intracranial pressure, monitoring level of consciousness, positioning clients, implementation during a seizure, cerebrovascular accident (CVA) client, Parkinson's disease, and care to the client with myasthenia gravis. Altered body image and psychosocial issues that occur as a result of the neurological disorder are also a focus of the Pyramid to Success. The Integrated Concepts and Processes addressed in this unit include the Clinical Problem-Solving Process (Nursing Process), Caring, Communication and Documentation, Cultural Awareness, Self-Care, and Teaching/Learning.

CLIENT NEEDS

Safe, Effective Care Environment

Accident prevention related to neurological deficits
Advance directives
Advocacy
Asepsis with procedures and treatments
Client rights
Confidentiality
Consultation and referrals
Establishing priorities
Informed consent for invasive procedures
Standard (universal) precautions

Health Promotion and Maintenance

Expected body image changes resulting from neurological deficits
Home care instructions regarding care related to neurological disorder
Prevention and early detection of health problems associated with neurological deficits
Reinforcement regarding the importance of prescribed therapy

Psychosocial Integrity

Ability to cope with feelings of isolation and loss of independence
Body image changes
Coping mechanisms
Cultural, religious, and spiritual influences
Grief and loss
Sensory and perceptual alterations
Support systems and use of community resources

Physiological Integrity

Assessing level of consciousness
Complications related to procedures
Emergency care
Head injuries
Increased intracranial pressure
Implementation during a seizure
Measures to promote comfort
Myasthenia gravis
Parkinson's disease
Pharmacological medications, actions, agents, side effects, and adverse effects
Positioning clients
Promoting normal elimination patterns
Promoting self-care measures
Spinal cord injuries
The CVA client
Use of assistive devices for mobility

REFERENCES

Black J, Hawks J, Keene A: *Medical-surgical nursing: clinical management for positive outcomes,* ed 6, Philadelphia, 2001, WB Saunders.
Chernecky C, Berger B: *Laboratory tests and diagnostic procedures,* ed 3, Philadelphia, 2001, WB Saunders.
Clark J, Queener S, Karb V: *Pharmacologic basis of nursing practice,* ed 6, St Louis, 2000, Mosby.
DeWit S: *Fundamental concepts and skills for nursing,* Philadelphia, 2001, WB Saunders.
Hill S, Howlett H: *Success in practical nursing: personal and vocational issues,* ed 4, Philadelphia, 2001, WB Saunders.
National Council of State Boards of Nursing: *Test plan for the National Council Licensure Examination for Practical/Vocational Nurses,* Chicago, 2001, Author.
Potter P, Perry A: *Fundamentals of nursing,* ed 5, St Louis, 2001, Mosby.
Perry A, Potter P: *Clinical nursing skills and techniques,* ed 5, St Louis, 2002, Mosby.
Wilson J: *Infection control in clinical practice,* ed 2, St Louis, 2002, Balliere Tindall.

54

Neurological System

I. ANATOMY AND PHYSIOLOGY OF THE BRAIN AND SPINAL CORD

A. Cerebrum
   1. Consists of the right and left hemispheres
   2. Each hemisphere receives sensory information from the opposite side of the body and controls the skeletal muscles of the opposite side
   3. Governs sensory and motor activity
   4. Governs thought and learning

B. Cerebral cortex (Box 54-1)
   1. Outer gray layer
   2. Divided into four lobes
   3. Responsible for the conscious activities of the cerebrum

C. Basal ganglia
   1. Cell bodies in white matter
   2. Assists cerebral cortex in producing smooth voluntary movements

D. Diencephalon
   1. Thalamus
      a. Relays sensory impulses to the cortex
      b. Provides a thalamic pain gate
      c. Part of the reticular activating system
   2. Hypothalamus

BOX 54-1

Cerebral Cortex

Frontal lobe: Broca's area for speech; prefrontal lobe controls morals, emotions, and judgments
Parietal lobe: interprets pain, touch, temperature, and pressure
Temporal lobe: auditory center; Wenicke's area for sensory and speech
Occipital lobe: visual area

      a. Regulates autonomic responses of the sympathetic and parasympathetic nervous system
      b. Regulates stress response, sleep, appetite, body temperature, fluid balance, and emotions
      c. Responsible for the production of hormones secreted by the pituitary gland and hypothalamus

E. Brainstem
   1. Midbrain
      a. Responsible for motor coordination
      b. Visual reflex and auditory relay centers
   2. Pons
      a. Contains respiratory centers
      b. Regulates breathing
   3. Medulla oblongata
      a. Contains all afferent and efferent tracts
      b. Contains cardiac, respiratory, vomiting, and vasomotor centers
      c. Controls heart rate, respiration, blood vessel diameter, sneezing, swallowing, vomiting, and coughing

F. Cerebellum
   1. Coordinates smooth muscle movement
   2. Coordinates posture, equilibrium, and muscle tone

G. The spinal cord
   1. Provides neuron and synapse networks to produce involuntary responses to sensory stimulation
   2. Allows for control of the number of pain impulses that pass through the spinal cord on their way to the brain
   3. Carries sensory information to, and motor information from, the brain
   4. Extends from the first cervical to the second lumbar vertebra

5. Protected by the meninges, cerebrospinal fluid, and adipose tissue
6. Horns
   a. Inner column of gray matter contains two anterior and two posterior horns
   b. Posterior horns connect with afferent (sensory) nerve fibers
   c. Anterior horns contain efferent (motor) nerve fibers
7. Nerve tracts
   a. White matter contains the nerve tract
   b. Ascending tracts (sensory pathway)
   c. Descending tract (motor pathway)

H. Meninges
1. Dura mater is the tough and fibrous membrane
2. Arachnoid membrane is the delicate membrane and contains subarachnoid fluid
3. Pia mater is the vascular membrane
4. Subarachnoid space is formed by the arachnoid membrane and the pia mater

I. Cerebrospinal fluid
1. Secreted in the ventricles and circulates through the ventricles to the subarachnoid layer of the meninges where it is reabsorbed
2. Circulates in the subarachnoid space
3. Normal pressure is 60 to 180 mm H_2O
4. Normal volume is 125 to 150 mL
5. Acts as a protective cushion
6. Aids in the exchange of nutrients and wastes

J. Ventricles
1. Four ventricles
2. Communicate between the subarachnoid space
3. Produce and circulate cerebrospinal fluid

K. Blood supply
1. Right and left internal carotids
2. Right and left vertebral arteries
3. These arteries supply the brain via an anastamosis at the base of the brain called the circle of Willis

L. Neurotransmitters
1. Acetylcholine
2. Norepinephrine
3. Dopamine
4. Serotonin
5. Amino acids
6. Polypeptides

M. Neurons
1. The cell body
2. Contains the axons and dendrites
3. Neurons carrying impulses to the central nervous system (CNS) are called sensory neurons
4. Neurons carrying impulses away from the CNS are called motor neurons
5. Synapse is the chemical transmission of impulses from one neuron to another

N. Axons and dendrites
1. The axon conducts impulses from the cell body
2. The dendrites receive stimuli from the body and transmit them to the axon
3. Protected and insulated by Schwann cells
4. The Schwann cell sheath is called the neurolemma
5. Neurons do not reproduce after the neonatal period
6. If an axon or dendrite is damaged, it will die and be slowly replaced only if the neurolemma is intact and the cell body has not died

O. Spinal nerves
1. Thirty-one pairs of spinal nerves
2. Mixed nerve fibers are formed by the joining of the anterior motor and posterior sensory roots
3. Posterior roots contain afferent (sensory) nerve fibers
4. Anterior roots contain efferent (motor) nerve fibers

P. Autonomic nervous system
1. Sympathetic (adrenergic) fibers dilate pupils, increase heart rate and rhythm, contract blood vessels, and relax smooth muscles of the bronchi
2. Parasympathetic (cholinergic) fibers produce the opposite effect

II. DIAGNOSTIC TESTS

A. Skull and spinal x-ray studies
1. Description
   a. X-ray films of the skull reveal the size and shape of the skull bones, suture separation in infants, fractures or bony defects, erosion, or calcification
   b. Spinal x-ray studies identify fractures, dislocation, compression, curvature, erosion, narrowed spinal cord, and degenerative processes
2. Implementation preprocedure
   a. Provide nursing support for the confused, combative, or ventilator-dependent client
   b. Maintain immobilization of the neck if a spinal fracture is suspected
   c. Remove metal items from body parts
   d. If the client has thick and heavy hair, this should be documented, as it may affect interpretation of the x-ray film
3. Implementation postprocedure: maintain immobilization until results are known

B. Computed tomography (CT) scan
   1. Description
      a. A type of brain scanning that may or may not require an injection of a dye
      b. Used to detect intracranial bleeding, space-occupying lesions, cerebral edema, infarctions, hydrocephalus, cerebral atrophy, and shifts of brain structures
   2. Implementation preprocedure
      a. Obtain informed consent if a dye is used
      b. Monitor for allergies to iodine, contrast dyes, or shellfish if a dye is used
      c. Instruct client that they will need to lie still and flat during the test
      d. Instruct client that they will need to hold their breath when requested
      e. Initiate an intravenous (IV) line if prescribed
      f. Remove objects from the head such as wigs, barrettes, earrings, and hairpins
      g. Monitor for claustrophobia
      h. Inform client that they may hear mechanical noises as the scanning occurs
      i. Inform client that they may feel a hot, flushed sensation and a metallic taste in the mouth when the dye is injected
      j. Note that some clients may be given the dye even if they report an allergy, and are pretreated with an antihistamine and corticosteroids before the injection, to reduce the severity of a reaction
   3. Implementation postprocedure
      a. Provide replacement fluids, as diuresis from the dye is expected
      b. Monitor for allergic reaction to dye
      c. Monitor dye injection site for bleeding or hematoma, and monitor extremity for color, warmth, and the presence of distal pulses
C. Magnetic resonance imaging (MRI)
   1. Description
      a. A noninvasive procedure that identifies types of tissues and identifies tumors and vascular abnormalities
      b. Similar to the CT scan but provides more detailed pictures
   2. Implementation preprocedure
      a. Remove all metal objects from the client
      b. Determine if client has a pacemaker, implanted defibrillator, or metal implants such as a hip prosthesis or vascular clips, as these clients cannot have this test performed
      c. Remove IV fluid pumps during the test
      d. Provide precautions for the client with pulse oximetry, as it can cause a burn during testing if coiled around the body or a body part
      e. Provide data collection of the client with claustrophobia
      f. Administer medication as prescribed for the client with claustrophobia
      g. Determine if the use of a contrast agent is to be used and follow the prescription related to the administration of food, fluids, and medications
      h. Instruct the client that they will need to remain still during the procedure
   3. Implementation postprocedure
      a. Client may resume normal activities
      b. Expect diuresis if a contrast agent was used
D. Lumbar puncture
   1. Description
      a. Insertion of a spinal needle through L3-L4 interspace into the lumbar subarachnoid space to obtain cerebrospinal fluid (CSF), measure CSF fluid or pressure, or to instill air, dye, or medications
      b. Contraindicated in clients with **increased intracranial pressure**, as the procedure will cause a rapid decrease in pressure within the CSF around the spinal cord, leading to brain herniation
   2. Implementation preprocedure
      a. Obtain an informed consent
      b. Have client empty the bladder
   3. Implementation during the procedure
      a. Position the client in lateral recumbent position and have client draw knees up to the abdomen and chin onto the chest
      b. Assist with the collection of specimens (label the specimens in sequence)
      c. Maintain strict asepsis
   4. Implementation postprocedure
      a. Monitor vital signs and neurological signs
      b. Position the client flat as prescribed
      c. Encourage fluids
      d. Monitor input and output (I&O)
E. Myelogram
   1. Description: injection of dye or air into subarachnoid space to detect abnormalities of the spinal cord and vertebrae
   2. Implementation preprocedure
      a. Obtain informed consent
      b. Provide hydration for at least 12 hours before the test
      c. Monitor for allergies to iodine
      d. If the client is taking a phenothiazine, hold the medication, as this medication lowers the seizure threshold
      e. Premedicate for sedation as prescribed

3. Implementation postprocedure
   a. Vital signs and neurological assessment frequently as prescribed
   b. If a water-based dye is used, elevate the head 15 to 30 degrees for 8 hours as prescribed
   c. If an oil-based dye is used, keep client flat 6 to 8 hours as prescribed
   d. If air is used, keep the head lower than the trunk
   e. Administer analgesics for headache or backache as prescribed
   f. Encourage fluids
   g. Monitor I&O
   h. Monitor for bladder distention and voiding

F. Cerebral angiography
1. Description: injection of a contrast agent through the femoral artery into the carotid arteries to visualize the cerebral arteries and monitor for lesions
2. Implementation preprocedure
   a. Obtain informed consent
   b. Monitor client allergies to iodine and shellfish
   c. Encourage hydration for 2 days before the test
   d. NPO 4 to 6 hours before test as prescribed
   e. Obtain a baseline neurological assessment
   f. Mark the peripheral pulses
   g. Remove metal items from the hair
   h. Administer premedication as prescribed
3. Implementation postprocedure
   a. Monitor neurological status and vital signs frequently until stable
   b. Monitor for swelling in the neck and for difficulty swallowing and notify physician if these symptoms occur
   c. Maintain bed rest for 12 hours as prescribed
   d. Elevate the head of the bed 15 to 30 degrees only if prescribed
   e. Keep the bed flat if the femoral artery is used
   f. Monitor peripheral pulses
   g. Immobilize the puncture site for 12 hours as prescribed
   h. Apply sandbags and a pressure dressing to the injection site as prescribed
   i. Place ice to the puncture site as prescribed
   j. Encourage fluids

G. Electroencephalography (EEG)
1. Description: a graphic recording of the electrical activity of the superficial layers of the cerebral cortex
2. Implementation preprocedure
   a. Wash the client's hair
   b. Inform the client that electrodes are attached to the head and that electricity does not enter the head
   c. Withhold stimulants, antidepressants, tranquilizers, and anticonvulsants for 24 to 48 hours before the test as prescribed
   d. Allow the client to have breakfast if prescribed
   e. Premedicate for sedation as prescribed
3. Implementation postprocedure
   a. Wash client's hair
   b. Maintain side rails and safety precautions if the client was sedated

H. Caloric testing (oculovestibular testing)
1. Description: provides information about the function of the vestibular portion of the eighth cranial nerve and aids in the diagnosis of cerebellum and brainstem lesions
2. Procedure
   a. Patency of the external canal is confirmed
   b. Cold or warm water is introduced into the external auditory canal
   c. Stimulation of the auditory canal with warm water produces a horizontal nystagmus toward the side of the irrigated ear when the vestibular eighth cranial nerve is normal
   d. Stimulation of the auditory canal with cold water produces a horizontal nystagmus away from the side of the irrigated ear if the brainstem is intact

III. NEUROLOGICAL ASSESSMENT

A. Assessment of risk factors
1. Trauma
2. Hemorrhage
3. Tumors
4. Infection
5. Toxicity
6. Metabolic disorders
7. Hypoxic conditions
8. Deficiency conditions
9. Hypertension
10. Cigarette smoking
11. Stress

B. Assessment of the cranial nerves
1. Cranial nerve I (olfactory) sensory, smell
   a. Have the client close eyes and occlude one nostril with finger
   b. Ask the client to identify nonirritating odors such as coffee, tea, cloves, soap, chewing gum, and peppermint
   c. Repeat the test on the other nostril
2. Cranial nerve II (optic) sensory, vision

a. Monitor visual acuity with a Snellen chart or newspaper, or ask the client to count how many fingers the examiner is holding up
b. Check visual fields by confrontation
c. Have the client sit directly in front of examiner and stare at examiner's nose
d. Examiner slowly moves his or her finger from the periphery toward the center until the client says it can be seen
e. Check color vision by asking the client to name the color of several nearby objects

3. Cranial nerve III (oculomotor); Cranial nerve IV (trochlear); cranial nerve VI (abducens)
   a. The motor functions of these nerves overlap; therefore they need to be tested together
   b. First, inspect the eyelids for ptosis (drooping), then assess ocular movements and note any eye deviation
   c. Test accommodation and direct and consensual light reflexes
   d. Cranial nerve III (oculomotor) motor: assesses pupillary constriction, upper eyelid elevation and most eye movement
   e. Cranial nerve IV (trochlear): motor: assesses downward and inward eye movement
   f. Cranial nerve VI (abducens) assesses lateral eye movement
4. Cranial nerve V (trigeminal) sensory and motor
   a. Assesses sensation to the cornea, nasal and oral mucosa, facial skin and mastication
   b. To test motor function, ask the client to close jaws tightly then try to separate the clenched jaw
   c. Test the corneal reflex by lightly touching the client's cornea with a cotton wisp
   d. Check sensory function by asking the client to close eyes, then lightly touch forehead, cheeks, and chin noting if the touch can be felt equally on both sides
5. Cranial nerve VII (facial) sensory and motor
   a. Test taste perception on the anterior two thirds of the tongue
   b. Have the client show teeth
   c. Attempt to close client's eyes against resistance and ask client to puff out cheeks
   d. Place sugar, salt, or vinegar on the front of the tongue and have the client identify these substances by taste
6. Cranial nerve VIII (acoustic) sensory
   a. The ability to hear tests the cochlear portion
   b. The sense of equilibrium tests the vestibular portion
   c. Check the client's ability to hear a watch ticking or a whisper
   d. Observe the client's balance and observe for swaying when walking or standing
7. Cranial nerve IX (glossopharyngeal) sensory and motor
   a. Assesses swallowing ability
   b. Assesses sensation to the pharyngeal soft palate and tonsillar mucosa, and taste perception on the posterior third of the tongue and salivation
8. Cranial nerve X (vagus) sensory and motor
   a. Assesses swallowing and phonation, sensation to the exterior ear's posterior wall and sensation behind the ear
   b. Assesses sensation to the thoracic and abdominal viscera
9. Cranial nerve IX (glossopharyngeal); cranial nerve X (vagus)
   a. Have the client identify a taste at the back of tongue
   b. Inspect the soft palate and observe for symmetrical elevation when the client says "aah"
   c. Touch the posterior pharyngeal wall with a tongue depressor to elicit a gag reflex
10. Cranial nerve XI (spinal accessory) motor
   a. Assesses uvula and soft palate movement, sternocleidomastoid and trapezius muscles
   b. Assesses upper portion of trapezius muscle, which governs shoulder movement and neck rotation
   c. Palpate and inspect the sternocleidomastoid muscle as the client pushes the chin against the examiner's hand
   d. Palpate and inspect the trapezius muscle as the client shrugs shoulders against the examiner's resistance
11. Cranial nerve XII (hypoglossal) motor
   a. Assesses tongue movements involved in swallowing and speech
   b. Observe the tongue for asymmetry, atrophy, deviation to one side, and fasciculations
   c. Ask the client to push tongue against a tongue depressor, then have client move tongue rapidly in and out and from side to side

C. Assessment of level of consciousness (LOC)
   1. Assesses cerebral function
   2. Monitor client behavior to determine LOC such as confusion, delirium, unconsciousness, stupor, coma

D. Assessment of vital signs: monitor for blood pressure or pulse changes that may indicate **increased intracranial pressure (ICP)**
E. Assessment of respirations (Box 54-2)
F. Monitoring of temperature
  1. An elevated temperature increases the brain's metabolic rate
  2. An early rise in temperature indicates a dysfunction of the hypothalamus or brainstem
  3. A slow rise in temperature may indicate infection
G. Assessment of pupils
  1. Size
  2. Equality
  3. Reactions to light described as brisk, slow, or fixed
  4. Unusual eye movements
  5. Unilateral pupil dilation indicates compression of the third cranial nerve
  6. Mid position, fixed pupil indicates midbrain injury
  7. Pinpoint, fixed indicates pontine damage
H. Assessment of motor function
  1. Muscle tone including strength and equality
  2. Voluntary and involuntary movements
  3. Purposeful and nonpurposeful movements
I. Monitoring for posturing (Figure 54-1)
  1. Posturing indicates deterioration of the condition
  2. Flexor (**decorticate posturing**)
    a. Client flexes one or both arms on the chest and may stiffly extend the legs
    b. Indicates a nonfunctioning cortex
  3. Extensor (**decerebrate posturing**)
    a. Client stiffly extends one or both arms and possibly the legs
    b. Indicates a brainstem lesion
  4. **Flaccid posturing**: client displays no motor response in any extremity
J. Assessment of reflexes (Box 54-3)
K. Assessment of meningeal irritation (Box 54-4)
  1. Nuchal rigidity
  2. Irritability
  3. Fever
L. Assessment of the autonomic system
  1. Sympathetic functions/adrenergic responses

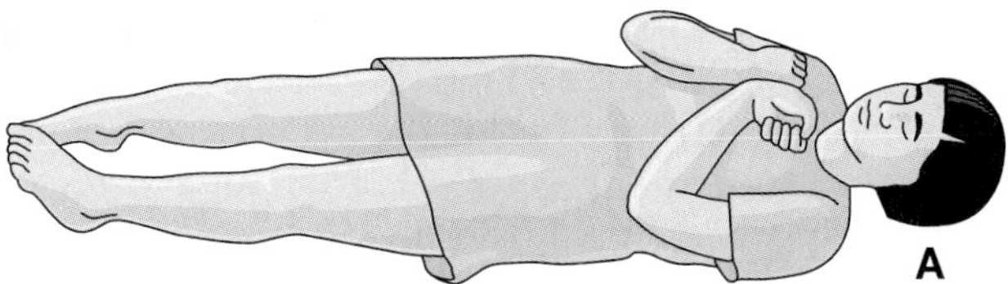

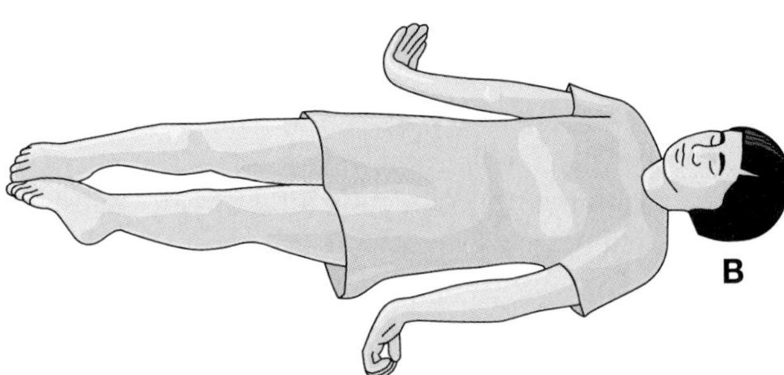

FIG. 54-1 Posturing. **A,** Decorticate. **B,** Decerebrate. (From Ignatavicius D, Workman M: *Medical-surgical nursing: critical thinking for collaborative care*, ed 4, Philadelphia, 2002, WB Saunders.)

BOX 54-2

Types of Respirations

CHEYNE-STOKES
Rhythmical with periods of apnea
Can indicate a metabolic dysfunction or dysfunction in the cerebral hemisphere or basal ganglia

NEUROGENIC HYPERVENTILATION
Regular rapid and deep sustained respirations
Indicates a dysfunction to the low midbrain and middle pons

APNEUSTIC
Irregular respirations with pauses at the end of inspiration and expiration
Indicates a dysfunction to the mid or caudal pons

ATAXIC
Totally irregular in rhythm and depth
Indicates a dysfunction in the medulla

CLUSTER
Clusters of breaths with irregularly spaced pauses
Indicates a dysfunction in the medulla and pons

BOX 54-3

Reflexes

BABINSKI REFLEX
Dorsiflexion of the ankle and great toe with fanning of the other toes
Indicates a disruption of the pyramidal tract

CORNEAL REFLEX
Loss of the blink reflex
Indicates a dysfunction of cranial nerve V

GAG REFLEX
Loss of the gag reflex
Indicates a dysfunction of cranial nerves IX and X

BOX 54-4

Signs of Meningeal Irritation

Brudzinski's sign: flexion of the head causes flexion of both thighs at the hips and knee flexion

Kernig's sign: flex thigh and knee to right angles and when extended, causes spasm of hamstring and pain

a. Increased pulse and blood pressure
b. Dilated pupils
c. Decreased peristalsis
d. Increased perspiration

2. Parasympathetic function/cholinergic responses
    a. Decreased pulse and blood pressure
    b. Constricted pupils
    c. Increased salivation
    d. Increased peristalsis
    e. Dilated blood vessels
    f. Bladder contraction

M. Assessment of sensory function
1. Touch
2. Pressure
3. Pain
4. Bladder control
5. Bowel control

N. **Glasgow Coma Scale** (Box 54-5)
1. A method of assessing a client's neurological condition
2. A scoring system based on a scale of 1 to 15 points

BOX 54-5

Glasgow Coma Scale

MOTOR RESPONSE POINTS
Obeys a simple response = 6
Localizes painful stimuli = 5
Normal flexion (withdrawal) = 4
Abnormal flexion (decorticate posturing) = 3
Extensor response (decerebrate posturing) = 2
No motor response to pain = 1

VERBAL RESPONSE POINTS
Oriented = 5
Confused conversation = 4
Inappropriate words = 3
Responds with incomprehensible sounds = 2
No verbal response = 1

EYE OPENING POINTS
Spontaneous = 4
In response to sound = 3
In response to pain = 2
No response even to painful stimuli = 1

3. A score below 8 indicates coma is present
4. Eye opening is the most important indicator

IV. THE UNCONSCIOUS CLIENT

A. Description
1. A state of depressed cerebral functioning with unresponsiveness to sensory and motor function
2. Some of the causes include head trauma, cerebral toxins, shock, hemorrhage, tumor, or infections

B. Data collection
1. Unarousable
2. Primitive or no response to painful stimuli
3. Altered respirations
4. Decreased cranial nerve and reflex activity

C. Implementation (Box 54-6)

V. INCREASED INTRACRANIAL PRESSURE

A. Description
1. An **increase in intracranial pressure** caused by trauma, hemorrhage, growths or tumors, hydrocephalus, edema, or inflammation
2. Can impede circulation to the brain, impede the absorption of CSF, affect the functioning of nerve cells and lead to brainstem compression and death

B. Data collection
1. Monitor LOC, which is the most sensitive and earliest indication of **increasing ICP**
2. Declining LOC from restlessness to confusion and coma
3. Headache
4. Abnormal respirations
5. Rise in blood pressure with widening pulse pressure
6. Slowing of pulse
7. Elevated temperature
8. Vomiting
9. Pupil changes
10. Changes in motor function from weakness to hemiplegia, a positive Babinski reflex, posturing such as decorticate, decerebrate, and seizures
11. Late signs of **increased ICP** include increased systolic blood pressure, widened pulse pressure, and slowed heart rate

C. Implementation
1. Elevate the head of the bed 30 to 40 degrees as prescribed
2. Avoid Trendelenburg position
3. Prevent flexion of the neck and hips
4. Monitor respiratory status and prevent hypoxia

BOX 54-6

Care to the Unconscious Client

Monitor patency of airway and keep an airway and emergency equipment at the bedside
Monitor blood pressure, pulse, and heart sounds
Monitor respiratory and circulatory status
Suction prn
Monitor neurological status including LOC, pupillary reactions, motor and sensory function
Place the client in semi-Fowler's position
Change position of client every 2 hours avoiding injury when turning
Avoid Trendelenburg position
Use side rails at all times
Monitor for edema
Monitor for dehydration
Monitor I&O and daily weight
Maintain NPO status until consciousness returns
Maintain nutrition, fluid, and electrolyte balance
Check gag and swallowing reflex before resuming diet and begin with ice chips and fluids
Monitor intravenous or enteral feedings as prescribed
Monitor bowel sounds
Monitor elimination patterns
Monitor for constipation, impaction, and paralytic ileus
Maintain urinary output to prevent stasis, infection, and calculi formation
Monitor status of skin integrity
Initiate measures to prevent skin breakdown
Provide frequent mouth care
Remove dentures and contact lens
Monitor eyes for corneal reflex and irritation and instill artificial tears or cover with eye patches
Monitor drainage from the ears or nose for the presence of cerebrospinal fluid
Assume that the unconscious client can hear
Avoid restraints
Do not leave the client unattended if unstable
Initiate seizure precautions if necessary
Provide range of motion exercises to prevent contractures
Use of a footboard or high top sneakers to prevent foot drop
Use splints to prevent wrist deformities
Initiate physical therapy as appropriate

5. Avoid the administration of morphine to prevent the occurrence of hypoxia
6. Maintain mechanical ventilation as prescribed maintaining the $PaCO_2$ at 30 to 35 mm Hg, which will result in vasoconstriction of the cerebral blood vessels, decreased blood flow, and thus decreased **ICP**
7. Maintain body temperature
8. Prevent shivering, which can raise **ICP**
9. Decrease environmental stimuli
10. Monitor electrolyte levels and acid base balance
11. Monitor I&O
12. Limit fluid intake to 1200 mL per day
13. Instruct the client to avoid straining activities such as coughing and sneezing
14. Instruct the client to avoid Valsalva maneuver

D. Surgical intervention (Box 54-7)

BOX 54-7

Surgical Intervention for ICP: Ventriculoperitoneal Shunt

Shunts CSF from the ventricles into the peritoneum
Postprocedure implementation:
Position client supine and turn from back to unoperated side
Monitor for signs of increasing intracranial pressure resulting from shunt failure
Monitor for signs of infection

VI. HYPERTHERMIA

A. Description
1. A temperature of 106° F, which increases the cerebral metabolism and increases the risk of hypoxia
2. The causes include infection, heat stroke, exposure to high environmental temperatures, and dysfunction of the thermoregulatory center

B. Data collection
1. Temperature of 106° F
2. Shivering
3. Nausea and vomiting

C. Implementation
1. Maintain a patent airway
2. Initiate seizure precautions
3. Monitor I&O and monitor skin and mucous membranes for signs of dehydration
4. Monitor lung sounds
5. Monitor for cardiac irregularities
6. Monitor peripheral pulses for systemic blood flow
7. Induce normothermia with fluids, cool baths, fans, or hypothermia blanket

D. Inducing normothermia
1. Prevent shivering, which will increase CSF pressure and oxygen consumption
2. Monitor neurological changes
3. Monitor for infection and respiratory complications, as hypothermia may mask signs of infection

4. Monitor for cardiac irregularities
5. Monitor I&O
6. Administer medications as prescribed to prevent shivering
7. Prevent trauma to the skin and tissues
8. Apply lotion to the skin frequently
9. Inspect for frostbite

E. Medications to prevent shivering (Box 54-8)

VII. HEAD INJURY

A. Description
1. A trauma to the skull resulting in mild to extensive damage to the brain
2. Immediate complications include cerebral bleeding, hematomas, uncontrolled **increased ICP**, infections, and seizures
3. Changes in personality or behavior, cranial nerve deficits, and any other residual deficits depend on the area and extent of the brain damage

B. Types of head injuries (Box 54-9)
1. Open
   a. Scalp lacerations
   b. Fractures in the skull
   c. Interruption of the dura mater
2. Closed
   a. Concussions
   b. Contusions
   c. Fractures

C. Hematoma
1. Description: can occur as a result of a subarachnoid or intracerebral hemorrhage
2. Data collection
   a. Assessment findings will be dependent on the injury
   b. Clinical manifestations usually result from increased ICP
   c. Changing neurological signs in the client
   d. LOC
   e. Airway and breathing pattern
   f. Vital signs for signs of **increasing ICP**
   g. Headache, nausea and vomiting
   h. Visual disturbances, pupillary changes, papilledema, extraocular eye movements
   i. Nuchal rigidity
   j. CSF drainage from the ears or nose
   k. Weakness and paralysis
   l. Posturing
   m. Decreased sensation or absence of feeling
   n. Reflex activity
   o. Seizure activity
3. Implementation
   a. Monitor respiratory status and maintain a patent airway, as increased CO_2 levels increase cerebral edema
   b. Monitor neurological status and vital signs including temperature
   c. Monitor for **ICP**
   d. Maintain head elevation to reduce venous pressure
   e. Prevent neck flexion
   f. Initiate normothermia measures for increased temperature
   g. Monitor cranial nerve function, reflexes, motor and sensory function

BOX 54-8

Medications to Prevent Shivering

Chlorpromazine HCl (Thorazine): depresses thermoregulation in the hypothalamus and reduces peripheral vasoconstriction, muscle tone, and shivering

Meperidine HCl (Demerol): relaxes the smooth muscle and reduces shivering

BOX 54-9

Types of Head Injuries

CONCUSSION

A jarring of the brain within the skull with temporary loss of consciousness

CONTUSION

A bruising type injury to brain

It may occur with subdural or extradural collections of blood

SKULL FRACTURES

Linear
Depressed
Compound
Comminuted

EPIDURAL HEMATOMA

The most serious type of hematoma

Forms rapidly and results from an arterial bleed

Forms between the dura and the skull from a tear in the meningeal artery

A surgical emergency

SUBDURAL HEMATOMA

Forms slowly and results from a venous bleed

Occurs under the dura as a result of tears in the veins crossing the subdural space

SUBARACHNOID HEMORRHAGE

Bleeding directly into the brain, ventricles, or subarachnoid space

INTRACEREBRAL HEMORRHAGE

Multiple hemorrhages around a contused area

h. Initiate seizure precautions
i. Monitor for pain and restlessness
j. Avoid morphine sulfate as it is a respiratory depressant and may **increase ICP**
k. Monitor for drainage from the nose or ears, as this fluid may be CSF
l. Do not attempt to clean nose, suction, or allow client to blow nose if drainage occurs
m. Do not clean ear if drainage is noted but apply a loose dry sterile dressing
n. Check drainage for presence of CSF
o. Notify the physician if drainage from ears or nose is noted
p. Instruct the client to avoid coughing as this **increases ICP**
q. Monitor for signs of infection
r. Prevent complications of immobility

D. Craniotomy
1. Description
a. A surgical procedure that involves an incision through the cranium to remove accumulated blood or a tumor
b. Complications of the procedure include **increased ICP** from cerebral edema, hemorrhage, or obstruction of the normal flow of CSF
c. Additional complications include hematomas, hypovolemic shock, hydrocephalus, respiratory and neurogenic complications, pulmonary edema, and wound infections
d. Complications related to fluid and electrolyte imbalances include diabetes insipidus and syndrome of inappropriate secretion of antidiuretic hormone
2. Preoperative implementation
a. Explain the procedure to client and family
b. Ensure that informed consent has been obtained
c. Prepare to shave client's head as prescribed and cover head with appropriate covering
d. Stabilize the client before surgery
3. Postoperative implementation (Box 54-10)
4. Postoperative positioning (Box 54-11)

VIII. SPINAL CORD INJURY

A. Description (Box 54-12)
1. Trauma to the spinal cord causing partial or complete disruption of the nerve tracts and neurons
2. The injury can range from a concussion to a contusion, laceration, or compression of the cord
3. Spinal cord edema develops and necrosis of the spinal cord can develop as a result of compromised capillary circulation and venous return
4. Loss of motor function, sensation, reflex activity, and bowel and bladder control may result
5. The most common causes include motor vehicle accidents, falls, sporting, and industrial accidents and gunshot or stab wounds
6. Complications related to the injury include respiratory failure, autonomic dysreflexia, spinal shock, further cord damage, and death

BOX 54-10

Nursing Care After Craniotomy

Monitor vital signs and neurological status every 30 minutes to every hour
Monitor for increased intracranial pressure
Monitor for decreased level of consciousness, motor weakness or paralysis, aphasia, visual changes, and personality changes
Check physician orders regarding client positioning
Avoid extreme hip or neck flexion and maintain head in midline neutral position
Provide a quiet environment
Monitor head dressing frequently for signs of drainage
Mark the area of drainage once each nursing shift for baseline comparison
Monitor the Hemovac or Jackson-Pratt drain, which may be in place for 24 hours
Maintain suction on the Hemovac or drain
Measure drainage from the Hemovac or drain every 8 hours and record the amount and color
Notify the physician if drainage is greater than the normal of 30 to 50 mL per shift
Notify the physician immediately of excessive amounts of drainage or a saturated head dressing
Record strict measurement of hourly I&O
Maintain fluid restriction to 1500 mL per day as prescribed
Monitor electrolyte values
Monitor for cardiac irregularities, which may occur as a result of fluid and electrolyte imbalance
Apply ice packs or cool compresses as prescribed for periorbital edema and ecchymosis of one or both eyes, which is not an unusual occurrence
Provide range of motion exercises every 8 hours
Place antiembolism stockings on the client as prescribed
Administer anticonvulsants, antacids, corticosteroids, and antibiotics as prescribed
Administer analgesics such as codeine and acetaminophen as prescribed for pain

BOX 54-11

Client Positioning After Craniotomy

Positions prescribed after craniotomy vary with the type of surgery and the specific postoperative physician's orders

Always check the physician's orders regarding client positioning

Incorrect positioning may cause serious and possibly fatal complications

REMOVAL OF A BONE FLAP FOR DECOMPRESSION

To facilitate brain expansion, the client should be turned from the back to the unoperated side, but not to the side operated on

POSTERIOR FOSSA SURGERY

To protect the operative site from pressure and minimize tension on the suture line, position client on the side, with a pillow under the head for support, and not on the back

INFRATENTORIAL SURGERY

Involves surgery below the brain's tentorium

The physician may order a flat position without head elevation or may order the head of the bed to be elevated at 30 to 45 degrees

Do not elevate the head of the bed in the acute phase of care after surgery without a physician's order

SUPRATENTORIAL SURGERY

Involves surgery above the brain's tentorium

The physician may order the head of the bed to be elevated at 30 degrees to promote venous outflow through the jugular veins

Do not lower the head of the bed in the acute phase of care after surgery without a physician's order

BOX 54-12

Effects of the Spinal Cord Injury

QUADRIPLEGIA

Injury occurring from C1 through C8

Paralysis involving all four extremities

PARAPLEGIA

Injury occurring from T1 through L4

Paralysis involving only the lower extremities

B. Most frequently involved vertebrae
   1. Cervical 5, 6, and 7
   2. Thoracic 12
   3. Lumbar 1
C. Transection of the Cord
   1. Complete transection of the cord
      a. The spinal cord is completely severed with total loss of sensation, movement, and reflex activity below the level of injury
      b. If the cord has not suffered irreparable damage, early treatment is needed to prevent partial damage from developing into total and permanent damage
   2. Partial transection of the cord
      a. The spinal cord is partially damaged or severed
      b. Symptoms depend on the extent and location of the damage
D. Types of injuries
   1. Anterior cord syndrome
      a. Damage to the anterior portion of the gray and white matter of the spinal cord
      b. Motor function, pain, and temperature sensation are lost below the level of injury; however, the sensations of touch, position, and vibration remain intact
   2. Posterior cord injury
      a. Damage to the posterior portion of the gray and white matter of the spinal cord
      b. Motor function remains intact, but the client experiences a loss of vibratory sense, crude touch, and position sensation
   3. Central cord syndrome
      a. Occurs from a lesion in the central portion of the spinal cord
      b. Loss of motor function is more pronounced in the upper extremities and varying degrees and patterns of sensation remain intact
   4. Brown-Sequard syndrome
      a. Results from penetrating injuries that cause hemisection of the spinal cord or injuries that affect half the cord
      b. Motor function, proprioception, vibration, and deep touch sensations are lost on the same side of the body (ipsilateral) as the lesion
      c. On the opposite side of the body (contralateral) from the injury, sensations of pain, temperature, and light touch are affected
E. Assessment of spinal cord injuries
   1. Depends on the level of the cord injury
   2. The level of spinal cord injury is the lowest spinal cord segment with intact motor and sensory function

3. Respiratory status
4. Motor and sensory changes below the level of injury
5. Total sensory loss and motor paralysis below the level of injury
6. Loss of reflexes below the level of injury
7. Loss of bladder and bowel control
8. Urinary retention and bladder distention
9. Presence of sweat, which does not occur on paralyzed areas

F. Cervical injuries
1. C2-3 injury is usually fatal
2. C4 is the major innervation to the diaphragm by the phrenic nerve
3. Involvement above C4 causes respiratory difficulty and paralysis of all four extremities
4. Client may have movement in the shoulder if the injury is at C5 or below

G. Thoracic level injuries
1. Loss of movement of the chest, trunk, bowel, bladder, and legs depending on the level of injury
2. Leg paralysis (paraplegia)
3. Autonomic dysreflexia with lesions above T6 and in cervical lesions
4. Visceral distention from a distended bladder or impacted rectum may cause reactions such as sweating, bradycardia, hypertension, nasal stuffiness, "goose flesh"

H. Lumbar and sacral level injuries
1. Loss of movement and sensation of the lower extremities
2. S2 and S3 center on micturition, therefore below this level, the bladder will contract but not empty (neurogenic bladder)
3. Injury above S2 in males allows them to have an erection, but they are unable to ejaculate because of sympathetic nerve damage
4. Injury between S2 and S4 damages the sympathetic and parasympathetic response preventing erection or ejaculation

I. Emergency implementation
1. Emergency management is critical, as improper handling can cause further damage and loss of neurological function
2. Maintain patent airway
3. Always suspect spinal cord injury until this injury is ruled out
4. Immobilize the client on a spinal back board with the head in a neutral position to prevent an incomplete injury from becoming complete
5. Prevent head flexion, rotation, or extension
6. During immobilization, maintain traction and alignment on head by placing hands on either side of the head by the ears
7. Maintain an extended position
8. Log roll the client
9. No part of the body should be twisted or turned, nor should the client be allowed to assume a sitting position
10. In the emergency room, a client who has sustained a severe cervical injury should be placed immediately in skeletal traction via skull tongs or halo vest to immobilize the cervical spine and reduce the fracture and dislocation

J. Implementation during hospitalization
1. Respiratory system
   a. Monitor respiratory status, as paralysis of the intercostal and abdominal muscles occur with C4 injuries
   b. Monitor arterial blood gases and maintain mechanical ventilation if prescribed to prevent respiratory arrest, especially with cervical injuries
   c. Encourage deep breathing and the use of an incentive spirometer
   d. Monitor for signs of infection particularly pneumonia
2. Cardiovascular system
   a. Monitor for cardiac irregularities
   b. Monitor for signs of hemorrhage or bleeding around the fracture site
   c. Monitor for signs of shock such as hypotension, tachycardia, and a weak and thready pulse
   d. Monitor lower extremities for deep vein thrombosis
   e. Measure circumference of calf and thigh
   f. Apply thigh-high antiembolism stockings as prescribed
   g. Remove antiembolism stockings daily to assess skin
   h. Monitor for orthostatic hypotension when repositioning the client
3. Neuromuscular system
   a. Monitor neurological status
   b. Monitor motor and sensory status to determine the level of injury
   c. Monitor motor ability by testing client's ability to squeeze hands, spread fingers, move toes, turn feet
   d. Monitor sensation by pinching skin, or pricking with a pin starting at shoulders and working down extremities
   e. Monitor for signs of autonomic dysreflexia and spinal shock
   f. Immobilize the client to promote healing and prevent further injury
   g. Monitor pain
   h. Initiate measures to reduce pain
   i. Administer analgesics as prescribed

j. Monitor for complications of immobility
k. Prepare the client for decompression laminectomy, spinal fusion, or insertion of steel rods if prescribed
l. Collaborate with physical therapist and occupational therapist to determine appropriate exercise techniques, to assess the need for hand and wrist splints, and to develop an appropriate plan to prevent foot drop

4. Gastrointestinal system
   a. Monitor abdomen for distention and hemorrhage
   b. Monitor bowel sounds and monitor for paralytic ileus
   c. Prevent bowel retention
   d. Initiate a bowel control program as appropriate
   e. Maintain adequate nutrition and a high-fiber diet
5. Renal system
   a. Prevent bladder retention
   b. Initiate a bladder control program as appropriate
   c. Maintain fluid and electrolyte balance
   d. Maintain adequate fluid intake of 2000 mL daily
   e. Monitor for urinary tract infection and calculi
6. Integumentary system
   a. Monitor skin integrity
   b. Turn the client every 2 hours
7. Psychosocial integrity
   a. Monitor psychosocial status
   b. Encourage the client to express feelings of anger and depression
   c. Discuss sexual concerns of the client
   d. Promote self-care, setting realistic goals based on the client's potential functional level
   e. Encourage contact with appropriate community resources

K. Spinal shock
1. Description
   a. Also known as neurogenic shock
   b. A sudden depression of reflex activity in the spinal cord below the level of injury (areflexia)
   c. Occurs within the first hour of injury and lasts days to months
   d. Muscles become completely paralyzed and flaccid and reflexes are absent
   e. **Spinal shock** ends when the reflexes are regained
2. Data collection
   a. Flaccid paralysis
   b. Hypotension
   c. Bradycardia
   d. Loss of reflex activity below the level of injury
   e. Paralytic ileus
3. Implementation
   a. Monitor for signs of **spinal shock** after spinal cord injury
   b. Monitor for hypotension and bradycardia
   c. Monitor for reflex activity
   d. Monitor bowel sounds
   e. Monitor for bowel and bladder retention
   f. Provide supportive measures as prescribed based on the presence of symptoms
   g. Monitor for the return of reflexes

L. Autonomic dysreflexia
1. Description
   a. Also known as hyperreflexia
   b. Commonly caused by visceral distention from a distended bladder or impacted rectum
   c. A neurological emergency that must be treated immediately to prevent a hypertensive stroke
   d. It generally occurs after the period of **spinal shock** is resolved
   e. Occurs with lesions above T6 and in cervical lesions
2. Data collection
   a. Hypertension
   b. Bradycardia
   c. Flushing of the face and neck
   d. Severe, throbbing headache
   e. Nasal stuffiness
   f. Piloerection (gooseflesh)
   g. Sweating
   h. Nausea
   i. Restlessness
   j. Dilated pupils and blurred vision
3. Implementation
   a. Notify the physician if signs of **autonomic dysreflexia** occur
   b. Monitor for potential cause and remove the stimulus
   c. Monitor vital signs, particularly blood pressure every 15 minutes
   d. Raise the head of the bed to high Fowler's position
   e. Loosen tight clothing
   f. Monitor for bladder distention and prepare for urinary catheterization
   g. If a urinary catheter is present, check for kinks in the tubing and for drainage
   h. Monitor for a fecal impaction and disimpact immediately
   i. Administer antihypertensives as prescribed

M. Cervical traction for cervical injuries (Figure 54-2)
   1. Description
      a. Skeletal traction used to stabilize fractures or dislocations of the cervical or upper thoracic spine
      b. Two types of equipment used for cervical traction are skull tongs and halo traction
   2. Skull tongs
      a. Skull tongs are inserted into the outer aspect of the client's skull and traction is applied
      b. Weights are attached to the tongs and the client is used as countertraction
      c. Monitor neurological status of the client
      d. Determine the amount of weight prescribed to be added to the traction
      e. Ensure that weights hang securely and freely at all times
      f. Ensure that ropes for the traction remain within the pulley
      g. Maintain body alignment and maintain care of the client on Roto-Rest bed, Stryker, or Foster frame as prescribed
      h. Turn the client every 2 hours
      i. Monitor insertion site of the tongs for infection
      j. Provide sterile pin site care as prescribed
   3. Halo traction
      a. Consists of a head piece with four pins, two anterior and two posterior, inserted into the client's skull, then a halo jacket or cast is applied
      b. Once the fracture is stable, the headpiece can be attached to a body jacket called a halo vest
      c. Monitor the client's neurological status for changes in movement or decreased strength
      d. Never move or turn the client by holding or pulling on the halo device
      e. Monitor for tightness of the jacket by ensuring that one finger can be placed under the jacket
      f. Monitor skin integrity to ensure that the jacket, vest, or cast is not causing pressure
      g. Provide sterile pin site care as prescribed
   4. Client education for halo vest (Box 54-13)

N. Implementation for thoracic and lumbar/sacral injuries
   1. Bed rest
   2. Immobilization with a fiberglass or plastic body cast
   3. Use of a brace or corset when the client is out of bed

O. Surgical implementation for thoracic and lumbar/sacral injuries
   1. Decompressive laminectomy
      a. Removal of one or more laminae
      b. Allows for cord expansion from edema
      c. Performed if conventional methods fail to prevent neurological deterioration
   2. Spinal fusion and Harrington rod insertion
      a. Used for thoracic spinal injuries
      b. Insertion of a metal or steel rod to stabilize thoracic spine
   3. Postoperative implementation
      a. Monitor for respiratory impairment
      b. Monitor vital signs, motor function, sensation, and circulatory status in lower extremities

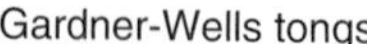

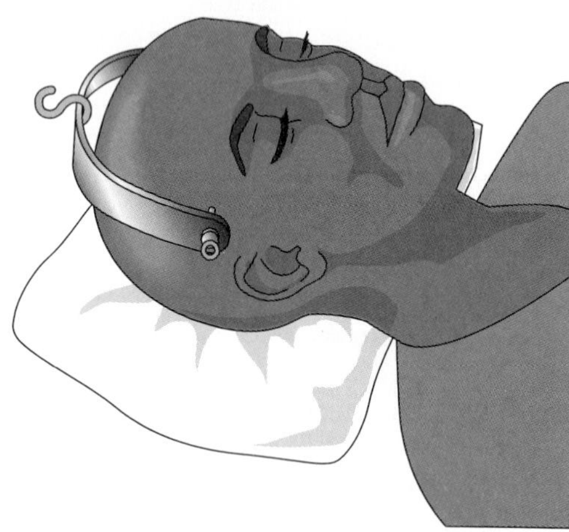

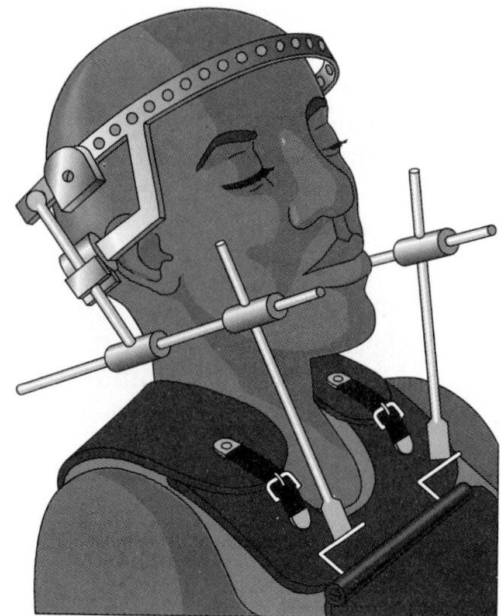

FIG. 54-2 Types of cervical traction. (From Ignatavicius D, Workman M: *Medical-surgical nursing: critical thinking for collaborative care*, ed 4, Philadelphia, 2002, WB Saunders.)

BOX 54-13

Client Education for a Halo Vest

Notify the physician if halo vest or ring bolts loosen
Use fleece or foam inserts to relieve pressure points
Keep vest lining dry
Clean the pin site daily
Notify the physician if redness, swelling, drainage, open areas, pain, tenderness, or a clicking sound occurs from the pin site
A sponge bath or tub bath is allowed; showers are prohibited
Inspect the skin under the vest daily for breakdown using a flashlight
Do not use any products other than shampoo on the hair
When shampooing the hair, cover the vest with plastic
When getting out of bed, roll onto the side and push on the mattress with arms
Never use the metal frame for turning or lifting
Use a rolled towel or pillowcase between the back of the neck and the bed, or next to the cheek when lying on the side, and raise the head of the bed to increase sleep comfort
Adapt clothing to fit over the halo
Eat foods high in protein and calcium to promote bone healing
Have the correct size wrench available at all times for an emergency
If cardiopulmonary resuscitation is required, the anterior portion of the vest will be loosened and the posterior portion will remain in place to provide stability

c. Encourage breathing exercises
d. Monitor for signs of fluid and electrolyte imbalance
e. Observe for complications of immobility
f. Keep the client flat
g. Provide cast care if client is in a full body cast
h. Turn and reposition frequently by log rolling side to back to side using turning sheets and pillows between legs to maintain alignment
i. Administer pain medication as prescribed
j. Maintain NPO status until client is actively passing flatus
k. Monitor bowel sounds
l. Provide the use of a fracture bed pan
m. Monitor I&O
n. Provide diet high in protein, iron, and thiamine and low in calcium

P. Medications
1. Dexamethasone (Decadron)
 a. Used for its antiinflammatory and edema reducing effects
 b. May interfere with healing
2. Dextran
 a. A plasma expander
 b. Used to increase capillary blood flow within the spinal cord and to prevent or treat hypotension
3. Dantrolene (Dantrium)/Baclofen (Lioresal)
 a. Used for clients with upper motor neuron injuries
 b. Controls muscle spasticity

IX. CEREBRAL ANEURYSM

A. Description
1. Dilation of the walls of a weakened cerebral artery
2. Can lead to rupture

B. Data collection
1. Pain
2. Diplopia
3. Blurred vision
4. Tinnitus
5. Nausea
6. Hemiparesis
7. Nuchal rigidity
8. Irritability
9. Seizures

C. Implementation
1. Maintain a patent airway (suction only with a physician order)
2. Administer oxygen as prescribed
3. Monitor vital signs and for hypertension or dysrhythmias
4. Avoid rectal temperatures
5. Maintain bed rest in semi-Fowler's position or side-lying position
6. Maintain a darkened room without stimulation
7. Limit visitors
8. Maintain fluid restrictions
9. Monitor I&O
10. Avoid stimulants in the diet

X. SEIZURES

A. Description
1. An abnormal, sudden, excessive discharge of electrical activity within the brain
2. Epilepsy is a disorder characterized by chronic seizure activity and indicates brain or CNS irritation
3. Causes include genetic factors, trauma, tumors, circulatory or metabolic disorders, toxicity, or infections
4. Status epilepticus involves a rapid succession of epileptic spasms without intervals of consciousness, is a potential complication that

can occur with any type of seizure, and may result in brain damage

B. Types of seizures (Table 54-1)
   1. Generalized seizures
      a. Tonic-clonic (grand mal)
      b. Absence (petit mal)
      c. Myoclonic
      d. Atonic or akinetic (drop attacks)
   2. Partial seizures
      a. Simple partial
      b. Complex partial

C. Data collection
   1. Seizure history
   2. Type of seizure
   3. Occurrences before, during, and after the seizure
   4. Prodromal signs as mood changes, irritability, and insomnia
   5. Aura, a sensation that warns the client of the impending seizure
   6. Loss of motor activity or bowel and bladder function or loss of consciousness during the seizure
   7. Occurrences during the postictal state such as headache, LOC, sleepiness, impaired speech or thinking

D. Implementation
   1. Note the time and duration of the seizure
   2. Monitor behavior at the onset of the seizure, if the client experienced an aura, if a change in facial expression occurred, or if a sound or cry occurred from the client
   3. If the client is standing, place the client on the floor and protect the head and body
   4. Maintain a patent airway (do not force the jaws open)
   5. Administer oxygen
   6. Prepare to suction
   7. Turn the client's head to the side
   8. Prevent injury during the seizure
   9. Remain with the client
   10. Do not restrain the client
   11. Loosen restrictive clothing
   12. Note the type, character, and progression of movements during the seizure
   13. Monitor for incontinence
   14. Administer medications IV diazepam (Valium), phenytoin (Dilantin), and phenobarbital sodium (Luminal) as prescribed to stop the seizure
   15. Document the characteristics of the seizure

TABLE 54-1

Types of Seizures

Generalized Seizures	Partial Seizures
TONIC-CLONIC (GRAND MAL) May begin with an aura; the tonic phase involves the stiffening or rigidity of the muscles of the arms and legs and usually lasts 10 to 20 seconds followed by loss of consciousness The clonic phase consists of hyperventilation and jerking of the extremities and usually lasts about 30 seconds Full recovery from the seizure may take several hours	**SIMPLE PARTIAL** Produces sensory symptoms accompanied by motor symptoms which are localized or confined to a specific area The client remains conscious and may report an aura
ABSENCE (PETIT - MAL) Brief seizure lasting seconds and the individual may or may not lose consciousness No loss or change in muscle tone occurs Seizures may occur several times during a day The victim appears to be day dreaming These type of seizures are more common in children	**COMPLEX PARTIAL** A psychomotor seizure; the area of the brain most involved is the temporal lobe Characterized by periods of altered behavior which the client is not aware of; the client loses consciousness for a few seconds
MYOCLONIC A seizure that presents as a brief generalized jerking or stiffening of extremities The victim may fall to ground from the seizure	
ATONIC OR AKINETIC (DROP ATTACKS) A sudden momentary loss of muscle tone The victim may fall to ground as a result of the seizure	

16. Monitor behavior after seizure such as the state of consciousness, motor ability, and speech ability
17. Instruct the client on the importance of lifelong medication and the need for follow-up medication blood levels
18. Instruct the client to avoid alcohol, excessive stress, and fatigue
19. Encourage the client to contact available community resources such as the Epilepsy Foundation

XI. CEREBROVASCULAR ACCIDENT (CVA)

A. Description
1. A sudden focal neurological deficit resulting from cerebrovascular disease
2. A syndrome in which the cerebral circulation is interrupted causing neurological deficits
3. Cerebral anoxia lasting longer than 10 minutes causes cerebral infarction with irreversible change
4. Surrounding cerebral edema and congestion causes further dysfunction
5. Diagnosis is determined by CT scan, EEG, and cerebral arteriography
6. The permanent disability cannot be determined until the cerebral edema subsides
7. The order in which function may return is facial, swallowing, lower limb, speech, and arms

B. Causes
1. Thrombosis
2. Embolism
3. Hemorrhage from rupture of a vessel
4. Transient ischemia attack

C. Risk factors
1. Atherosclerosis
2. Hypertension
3. Anticoagulation therapy
4. Diabetes mellitus
5. Stress
6. Obesity
7. Oral contraceptives

D. Data collection (Table 54-2 and Box 54-14)
1. Airway patency
2. Slow bounding pulse
3. Cheyne-Stokes respirations
4. Hypertension
5. Headache, nausea, and vomiting
6. Dizziness and vertigo

BOX 54-14

Assessment Findings in a CVA

Agnosia: inability to use an object correctly
Apraxia: inability to carry out a purposeful activity
Hemianopia: blindness in half of the visual field
Homonymous hemianopia: blindness in the same side of both eyes
Pyramid point: with visual problems, client must turn head to scan complete range of vision

TABLE 54-2

Left and Right Hemisphere Lesions

Findings depend on area of brain affected
Lesions in the cerebral hemisphere result in manifestations on the contralateral side, which is the side of the body opposite the cerebrovascular

LEFT HEMISPHERE LESION	RIGHT HEMISPHERE LESION
Aphasia both expressive and receptive	Disoriented to time, place, and person
Agraphia - difficulty writing	Cannot recognize faces
Alexia - reading problems	Spatial - perceptual deficits
No memory deficit	Neglect of left side
Deficits in the right visual field as reading problems and inability to discriminate words and letters	Client unaware of paralyzed side
No hearing deficit	Loss of depth perception
Behavior slow, cautious, and disorganized	Impulsive
Anxious when attempting a new task	Unaware of neurological deficits
Depression	Confabulates
Sense of guilt	Euphoric, impaired sense of humor
Quick anger and frustration	Constantly smiles
Feelings of worthlessness	Denies illness
Worries over the future	Poor judgment
	Overestimates ability
	Loss of ability to hear tonal variations

7. Facial drooping
8. Nuchal rigidity
9. Diplopia and nystagmus
10. Papilledema
11. Blindness
12. Ataxia
13. Dysarthria
14. Dysphagia
15. Speech changes
16. Decreased sensation to pressure, heat, and cold
17. Bowel and bladder dysfunctions
18. Emotional changes
19. Paralysis

E. Aphasia
   1. Expressive
      a. Damage in Broca's area of the frontal brain
      b. Client understands what is said, but is unable to verbally communicate
   2. Receptive
      a. Injury involving Wernicke's area in the temporoparietal area
      b. Client unable to understand the spoken and often written word
   3. Global or mixed: language dysfunction in both the areas of expression and reception
   4. Implementation for aphasia
      a. Provide repetitive directions
      b. Break tasks down to one step at a time
      c. Repeat names of objects frequently used
      d. Use a picture board or communication board

F. Implementation during the acute phase of cerebrovascular accident (CVA)
   1. Maintain a patent airway and administer oxygen as prescribed
   2. Monitor vital signs
   3. Maintain a blood pressure of 150/100 mm Hg to maintain cerebral perfusion after a CVA
   4. Suction but never suction nasally and for no longer than 10 seconds to prevent **increasing ICP**
   5. Monitor for **increasing ICP**, as the client is at most risk during first 72 hours
   6. Position client on side with head of bed elevated 15 to 30 degrees as prescribed
   7. Monitor LOC, pupillary response, motor and sensory response, cranial nerve function, and reflexes
   8. Maintain a quiet environment and provide minimal handling of the client to prevent further bleeding
   9. Administer IVs as prescribed
   10. Insert Foley catheter as prescribed
   11. Maintain fluid and electrolyte balance
   12. Prepare to administer anticoagulants, antiplatelets, diuretics, antihypertensives, and anticonvulsants as prescribed
   13. Establish a form of communication system

G. Implementation in the postacute phase of CVA
   1. Continue with implementation from the acute phase
   2. Position the client 2 hours on the unaffected side, 20 minutes on the affected side
   3. Position the client in the prone position if prescribed, for 30 minutes three times daily
   4. Provide skin, mouth, and eye care
   5. Perform passive range of motion exercises to prevent contractures
   6. Place antiembolism stockings on client
   7. Measure thighs and calves for increase in size and monitor for positive Homan's sign
   8. Monitor gag reflex and ability to swallow
   9. Provide sips of fluids and slowly advance diet to foods that are easy to chew and swallow
   10. Provide soft and semisoft foods and fluids rather than thin liquids, as clients are better able to tolerate these types of food
   11. When eating, position client sitting in a chair, or sitting up in bed with the head and neck positioned slightly forward and flexed
   12. Place food in the back of the mouth on the unaffected side to prevent trapping of food in affected cheek

H. Implementation in the chronic phase of CVA
   1. Provide eye care for visual deficits
   2. Approach the client from the nonaffected side
   3. Place the client's personal objects within the visual field
   4. Instruct the client with visual problems to turn head from side to side
   5. Place a patch over affected eye if the client has diplopia
   6. Increase mobility as tolerated
   7. Encourage fluids and high-fiber diet
   8. Administer stool softeners as prescribed
   9. Encourage the client to express feelings
   10. Encourage independence in activities of daily living
   11. Monitor need for assistive devices such as a cane, walker, splints, or braces
   12. Teach transfer technique from bed to chair, and chair to bed
   13. Provide gait training
   14. Initiate physical and occupational therapy
   15. Referral to speech and language pathologist

XII. MULTIPLE SCLEROSIS (MS)

A. Description
   1. A chronic, progressive, noncontagious, degenerative disease of the CNS characterized by demyelinization of the neurons
   2. It usually occurs between the ages of 20 and 40 years and consists of periods of remissions and exacerbations
   3. Causes are unknown but thought to be due to autoimmune response or viral infection
   4. Precipitating factors include pregnancy, fatigue, stress, infection, and trauma
   5. EEG findings are abnormal
   6. A lumbar puncture indicates increased gamma globulin but the serum globulin level is normal

B. Data collection
   1. Fatigue and weakness
   2. Ataxia and vertigo
   3. Tremors and spasticity of the lower extremities
   4. Parasthesias
   5. Blurred vision and diplopia
   6. Nystagmus
   7. Dysphasia
   8. Decreased perception to pain, touch, and temperature
   9. Bladder and bowel disturbances including urgency, frequency, retention, and incontinence
   10. Abnormal reflexes including hyperreflexia, absent reflexes and positive **Babinski reflex**
   11. Emotion changes as apathy, euphoria, irritability, and depression
   12. Memory changes and confusion

C. Implementation (Box 54-15)

BOX 54-15

Medications Used with Multiple Sclerosis

Corticosteroids: used to reduce edema and the inflammatory response; used to decrease the length of time the client's symptoms are exacerbated and improve the degree of recovery

Immunosuppressives: used for the treatment of chronic progressive MS to stabilize the disease process

Baclofen (Lioresal), dantrolene (Dantrium), or diazepam (Valium): used to lessen muscle spasticity

Carbamazepine (Tegretol): used to treat paresthesia

Propranolol (Inderal) and Clonazepam (Clonopin): used to treat cerebellar ataxia

Behanechol (Urecholine): used to prevent urinary retention

Oxybutynin chloride (Ditropan): used to increase bladder capacity

   1. Provide bed rest during exacerbation
   2. Protect the client from injury by providing safety measures
   3. Place an eye patch on eye for diplopia
   4. Monitor for potential complications as urinary tract infections, calculi, decubiti ulcers, respiratory tract infections, and contractures
   5. Promote regular elimination by bladder and bowel training
   6. Encourage independence
   7. Assist the client to establish a regular exercise and rest program
   8. Monitor the need for and provide assistive devices
   9. Initiate physical and speech therapy
   10. Instruct the client to avoid fatigue, stress, infection, overheating, and chilling
   11. Instruct the client to balance moderate activity with rest periods
   12. Instruct the client to increase fluids and eat a balanced diet including low-fat, high-fiber, and foods high in potassium
   13. Instruct the client in safety measures related to sensory loss such as regulating the temperature of bath water and avoiding heating pads
   14. Instruct the client in safety measures related to motor loss such as avoiding the use of scatter rugs and using assistive devices such as a walker or cane
   15. Instruct the client in the self-administration of prescribed medications
   16. Provide information about National Multiple Sclerosis Society

XIII. MYASTHENIA GRAVIS

A. Description
   1. A neuromuscular disease characterized by marked weakness and abnormal fatigue of the voluntary muscles
   2. A defect in the transmission of nerve impulses at the myoneural junction occurs
   3. Causes include insufficient secretion of acetylcholine, excessive secretion of cholinesterase, or unresponsiveness of the muscle fibers to acetylcholine

B. Data collection
   1. Weakness and fatigue
   2. Difficulty chewing
   3. Dysphagia
   4. Ptosis
   5. Diplopia
   6. Weak, hoarse voice
   7. Difficulty breathing
   8. Diminished breath sounds
   9. Respiratory paralysis and failure

C. Implementation
   1. Monitor respiratory status and ability to cough and deep breathe adequately
   2. Monitor for respiratory failure
   3. Maintain suctioning and emergency equipment at bedside
   4. Monitor vital signs
   5. Monitor speech and swallowing abilities to prevent aspiration
   6. Encourage the client to sit up when eating
   7. Monitor muscle status
   8. Instruct the client to conserve strength
   9. Plan short activities, which coincide with times of maximal muscle strength
   10. Monitor for myasthenic and cholinergic crisis
   11. Administer anticholinesterase medications as prescribed
   12. Instruct the client to avoid stress, infection, fatigue, and over-the counter drugs
   13. Instruct the client to wear a Medic-Alert bracelet
   14. Inform the client about services from the Myasthenia Gravis Foundation

D. Anticholinesterase medications
   1. Action: increase levels of acetycholine at myoneural junction
   2. Medications
      a. Neostigmine (Prostigmin)
      b. Pyridostigmine (Mestinon)
      c. Physostigmine (Antilirium)
      d. Edrophonium (Tensilon)
   3. Side effects
      a. Sweating
      b. Salivation
      c. Nausea
      d. Diarrhea and abdominal cramps
      e. Bradycardia
      f. Hypotension
   4. Implementation
      a. Administer medications on time
      b. Administer medication 30 minutes before meals with milk and crackers to reduce GI upset
      c. Monitor and record muscle strength
      d. Note that excessive doses lead to cholinergic crisis
      e. Have the antidote (atropine) available

E. Myasthenic crisis
   1. Description
      a. Acute exacerbation of disease
      b. Caused by a rapid, unrecognized progression of the disease, an inadequate amount of medication, infection, fatigue, or stress
   2. Data collection
      a. Weakness
      b. Dyspnea
      c. Dysphagia
      d. Restlessness
      e. Difficulty speaking
   3. Implementation
      a. Monitor for signs of myasthenic crisis
      b. Increase anticholinesterase medication

F. Cholinergic crisis
   1. Description
      a. Depolarization of the motor end plates
      b. Caused by overmedication with anticholinesterase
   2. Data collection
      a. Restlessness
      b. Weakness
      c. Dysphagia
      d. Dyspnea
      e. Nausea, vomiting, and diarrhea
      f. Fasciculations
      g. Sweating
      h. Salivation
      i. Increased bronchial secretions
   3. Implementation
      a. Hold anticholinesterase medication
      b. Prepare to administer the antidote, atropine sulfate, if prescribed

G. Tensilon test
   1. Description: test done to diagnose myasthenia gravis and to differentiate between myasthenic crisis and cholinergic crisis
   2. To diagnose myasthenia gravis
      a. Tensilon injection is given to the client
      b. Positive for myasthenia: client shows improvement in muscle strength after the administration of Tensilon
      c. Negative for myasthenia: client shows no improvement in muscle strength, and strength may even deteriorate after injection of Tensilon
   3. To differentiate crisis
      a. Myasthenic crisis: Tensilon is administered and if strength improves, the client needs more medication
      b. Cholinergic crisis: Tensilon is administered and if weakness is more severe, an overdose of medication has occurred; administer atropine sulfate, the antidote, as prescribed

XIV. PARKINSON'S DISEASE

A. Description
   1. A degenerative disease caused by the depletion of dopamine that interferes with the inhibition of excitatory impulses
   2. It results in a dysfunction of the extrapyramidal system

3. It is a slow progressive disease that results in a crippling disability
4. The debilitation can result in falls, self-care deficits, depression, and failure of body systems
5. Mental deterioration occurs late in the disease

B. Data collection
1. Bradykinesia, abnormal slowness of movement and sluggishness of physical and mental responses
2. Aching shoulders and arms
3. Monotonous speech
4. Handwriting that becomes progressively smaller
5. Tremors in hands and fingers at rest (pill rolling)
6. Tremors increasing when fatigued and decreasing with purposeful activity or sleep
7. Rigidity with jerky interrupted movements
8. Restlessness and pacing
9. Blank facial expression
10. Drooling
11. Difficulty swallowing and speaking
12. Loss of coordination and balance
13. Shuffling steps, stooped position, and propulsive gait

C. Implementation (Box 54-16)
1. Monitor neurological status
2. Monitor ability to swallow and chew
3. Provide high-calorie, high-protein, high-fiber soft diet with small, frequent feedings
4. Increase fluids to 2000 mL per day
5. Promote independence along with safety measures
6. Avoid rushing client with activities
7. Assist with ambulation
8. Provide assistive devices
9. Instruct the client to wear low-heeled shoes
10. Encourage the client to lift feet when walking and to avoid prolonged sitting
11. Provide a firm mattress and position client prone, without a pillow, to facilitate proper posture
12. Instruct proper posture by teaching client to hold hands behind back to keep spine and neck erect
13. Monitor for constipation
14. Promote physical therapy and rehabilitation
15. Administer anticholinergic medications as prescribed to treat tremors and rigidity and to inhibit the action of acetylcholine
16. Administer antiparkinsonian medications to increase the level of dopamine in the CNS
17. Instruct the client to avoid foods high in vitamin B_6, as they block the effects of antiparkinsonian medications
18. Instruct the client to avoid monoamine oxidase inhibitors, as they will precipitate hypertensive crisis

BOX 54-16

Medications to Treat Parkinson's Disease

Amantadine HCl (Symadine, Symmetrel)
Ethopropazine HCl (Parsidol)
Levodopa (Dopar, Larodopa)
Carbidopa and levodopa (Sinemet)
Trihexphenidyl HCl (Artane)
Procyclidine HCl (Kemadrin)
Benztropine mesylate (Cogentin)
Bromocriptine (Parlodel)

XV. TRIGEMINAL NEURALGIA

A. Description
1. A sensory disorder of the fifth cranial nerve
2. Results in severe, recurrent, sharp, facial pain along the trigeminal nerve

B. Data collection
1. Pain on the lips, gums, nose, or across the cheeks
2. Situations that stimulate symptoms include cold temperatures, washing the face, chewing, food, or fluids of extreme temperatures

C. Implementation (Box 54-17)
1. Identify and instruct the client to avoid situations that cause pain
2. Instruct the client to avoid hot or cold foods and fluids
3. Provide small feedings of liquid and soft foods
4. Instruct the client to chew food on unaffected side
5. Administer medications as prescribed

D. Surgical implementation
1. An alcohol injection along affected portion of the nerve to produce anesthesia of the nerve may provide relief of pain for up to 16 months
2. Retrogasserian rhizotomy or total severance of the sensory root of the trigeminal nerve
3. Jannetta procedure, which surgically relocates the artery that is compressing the trigeminal nerve

BOX 54-17

Medications to Treat Trigeminal Neuralgia

Carbamazepine (Tegretol)
Phenytoin (Dilantin)
Baclofen (Lioresal)

4. Electrocoagulation or percutaneous radiofrequency rhizotomy to create a heat lesion

XVI. BELL'S PALSY (FACIAL PARALYSIS)

A. Description
   1. A lower motor neuron lesion of the seventh cranial nerve that may occur as a result of trauma, hemorrhage, meningitis, or a tumor
   2. It results in paralysis of one side of the face
   3. Recovery usually occurs in a few weeks without residual effects

B. Data collection
   1. Inability to raise eyebrows, frown, smile, close eyelids, or puff out cheeks
   2. Upward movement of the eye when attempting to close the eyelid
   3. Loss of taste

C. Implementation
   1. Encourage active facial exercises to prevent the loss of muscle tone
   2. Provide a face sling to prevent stretching of weak muscles
   3. Protect the eyes from dryness and prevent injury
   4. Promote good oral care
   5. Instruct the client to chew on the unaffected side
   6. Administer analgesics and steroids as prescribed

XVII. GUILLAIN-BARRÉ SYNDROME

A. Description
   1. An acute infectious neuronitis of the cranial and peripheral nerves
   2. The immune system overreacts to the infection and destroys the myelin sheath
   3. It is usually preceded by a mild upper respiratory infection or gastroenteritis
   4. The recovery is a slow process and can take years
   5. The major concern is difficulty breathing

B. Data collection
   1. Paresthesias
   2. Weakness of lower extremities
   3. Gradual progressive weakness of upper extremities and facial muscles
   4. Can progress to respiratory failure
   5. Cardiac dysrhythmias
   6. CSF reveals an elevated protein level
   7. EEG is abnormal

C. Implementation
   1. Care is directed toward the treatment of symptoms
   2. Monitor respiratory status
   3. Provide respiratory treatments
   4. Prepare to initiate respiratory support
   5. Monitor cardiac status
   6. Monitor for complications of immobility
   7. Provide client and family support

XVIII. AMYOTROPHIC LATERAL SCLEROSIS

A. Description
   1. Also known as Lou Gehrig's disease
   2. A progressive degenerative disease involving the motor system
   3. The sensory and autonomic system are not involved and mental status changes do not result from the disease
   4. The cause of the disease may be related to an excess of glutamate, a chemical responsible for relaying messages between the motor neurons
   5. As the disease progresses, muscle weakness and atrophy develop until a flaccid quadriplegia develops
   6. Eventually the respiratory muscles become affected, leading to respiratory compromise, pneumonia, and death
   7. There is no known cure and the treatment is symptomatic

B. Data collection
   1. Fatigue
   2. Fatigue while talking
   3. Muscle weakness
   4. Muscle atrophy
   5. Tongue atrophy
   6. Dysphagia
   7. Weakness of the hands and arms
   8. Fasciculations of the face
   9. Nasal quality of speech
   10. Dysarthria

C. Implementation
   1. Care is directed toward the treatment of symptoms
   2. Monitor respiratory status
   3. Provide respiratory treatments
   4. Prepare to initiate respiratory support
   5. Monitor for complications of immobility
   6. Provide the client and family support

XIX. ENCEPHALITIS

A. Description
   1. An inflammation of the brain parenchyma and often the meninges
   2. Affects the cerebrum, brainstem and/or cerebellum
   3. Most often caused by a viral agent, although bacteria, fungi or parasites may also be involved

4. Viral encephalitis is almost always preceded by a viral infection

B. Transmission
1. Arboviruses can be transmitted to humans through the bite of an infected mosquito or tick
2. Echovirus, coxsackievirus, poliovirus, herpes zoster, and viruses that cause mumps and chickenpox are common enteroviruses associated with encephalitis
3. Herpes simplex type 1 virus can cause viral encephalitis
4. Amebic meningoencephalitis can enter the nasal mucosa of people swimming in warm fresh-water ponds and lakes

C. Data collection
1. Presence of cold sores, lesions, or ulcerations of the oral cavity
2. History of insect bites and swimming in fresh water
3. Exposure to infectious diseases
4. Travel to areas where disease in prevalent
5. Fever
6. Nausea, vomiting
7. Stiff neck
8. Changes in LOC and mental status
9. Symptoms of **increased ICP**
10. Motor dysfunction and focal neurological deficits

D. Implementation
1. Monitor vital and neurological signs
2. Monitor LOC using the **Glasgow Coma Scale**
3. Monitor mental status changes and personality and behavior changes
4. Monitor for signs of **increased ICP**
5. Monitor for presence of nuchal rigidity and a positive Kernig's or Brudzinski's sign indicating meningeal irritation
6. Assist the client to turn, cough, and deep breathe frequently
7. Elevate the head of the bed 30 to 45 degrees
8. Monitor for muscle and neurological deficits
9. Administer acyclovir (Zovirax) as prescribed
10. Initiate rehabilitation as needed for motor dysfunction or neurological deficits

XX. MENINGITIS

A. Description
1. Inflammation of the arachnoid and pia mater of the brain and spinal cord
2. Caused by bacterial and viral organisms, although fungal and protozoal meningitis also occurs
3. Predisposing factors include skull fractures, brain or spinal surgery, sinus or upper respiratory infections, the use of nasal sprays, as well as individuals with a compromised immune system
4. CSF fluid is analyzed to determine the diagnosis and type of meningitis

B. Transmission
1. Direct contact including droplet spread
2. Occurs in areas of high population density, crowded living areas, and prisons

C. Data collection
1. Mild lethargy
2. Memory changes
3. Short attention span
4. Personality and behavior changes
5. Severe headache
6. Generalized muscle aches and pains
7. Nausea and vomiting
8. Fever and chills
9. Tachycardia
10. Deterioration in level of consciousness
11. Red, macular rash with meningococcal meningitis
12. Abdominal and chest pain with viral meningitis
13. Photophobia
14. Signs of meningeal irritation such as nuchal rigidity and a positive Kernig's and Brudzinski's sign

D. Implementation
1. Monitor vital signs and neurological signs
2. Monitor for signs of **increasing ICP**
3. Initiate seizure precautions
4. Monitor for seizure activity
5. Monitor or signs of meningeal irritation
6. Perform cranial nerve assessment
7. Monitor vascular status
8. Maintain isolation precautions as necessary with bacterial meningitis
9. Maintain urine and stool precautions with viral meningitis
10. Maintain respiratory isolation for the client with pneumococcal meningitis
11. Elevate the head of the bed 30 degrees and avoid neck flexion and extreme hip flexion
12. Prevent stimulation and restrict visitors
13. Administer analgesics as prescribed
14. Administer antibiotics as prescribed

PRACTICE QUESTIONS

1. A client has an impairment of cranial nerve II. Specific to this impairment, the nurse would plan to do which of the following to ensure client safety?
   1. Provide a clear path for ambulation without obstacles

2. Test the temperature of the shower water
3. Speak loudly to the client
4. Check the temperature of the food on the dietary tray

2. The client has a cerebellar lesion. The nurse would evaluate that the client was adapting successfully to this problem if the client demonstrated proper use of which of the following items?
   1. Adaptive eating utensils
   2. Walker
   3. Raised toilet seat
   4. Slider board
3. A nurse is planning care for the client who displays confusion secondary to a neurological problem. Which of the following approaches by the nurse would be least helpful in assisting this client?
   1. Giving simple, clear directions
   2. Providing a stable environment
   3. Providing sensory cues
   4. Encouraging multiple visitors at one time
4. A client with a neurological impairment experiences urinary incontinence. Which of the following nursing actions would be most helpful in helping the client adapt to this alteration?
   1. Establishing a toileting schedule
   2. Inserting a Foley catheter
   3. Using adult diapers
   4. Padding the bed with an absorbent cotton pad
5. The nurse has obtained a personal and family history for the client with a neurological disorder. Which of the following factors in the client's history does not give the client added risk for neurological problems?
   1. Previous back injury
   2. Allergy to pollen
   3. History of hypertension
   4. History of headaches
6. A client with right leg hemiplegia has a nursing diagnosis of Impaired Physical Mobility. The nurse would evaluate that the family needs reinforcement of teaching if the nurse observed which of the following being done by the family?
   1. Encouraging the client to stand unassisted on the leg
   2. Active range of motion (ROM) to the affected leg
   3. Passive ROM to the affected leg
   4. Application of a premolded splint
7. A nurse is preparing the client who is scheduled to have a cerebral angiogram performed. The nurse would check the client for:
   1. Allergy to salmon
   2. Allergy to iodine or shellfish
   3. Claustrophobia
   4. Excessive weight
8. A client admitted with a neurological problem indicates to the nurse that magnetic resonance imaging (MRI) may be done. The nurse interprets that the client may be ineligible for this diagnostic procedure based on the client's history of:
   1. Hypertension
   2. Chronic obstructive pulmonary disorder
   3. Heart failure
   4. Prosthetic valve replacement
9. A client is having a lumbar puncture (LP) performed. The nurse would position the client in which of the following positions for the procedure?
   1. Side-lying, with legs pulled up and head bent down onto chest
   2. Sims position
   3. Prone, in slight Trendelenburg
   4. Prone, with a pillow under the abdomen
10. The client is somewhat nervous about having magnetic resonance imaging (MRI). Which of the following statements by the nurse would provide the most reassurance to the client about the procedure?
    1. "It is necessary to remove any metal or metal-containing objects before having the MRI done to avoid the metal being drawn into the magnetic field."
    2. "The MRI machine is a long, hollow narrow tube, and may make you feel somewhat claustrophobic."
    3. "Even though you are alone in the scanner, you will be in voice communication with the technologist during the procedure."
    4. "You will be able to eat before the procedure unless you get nauseous easily. If so, you should eat lightly."
11. A client has just undergone computed tomography (CT) scanning with a contrast medium. The nurse would evaluate that the client understands postprocedure care if the client verbalized to:
    1. Eat lightly for the remainder of the day
    2. Rest quietly for the remainder of the day
    3. Hold medications for at least 4 hours
    4. Consume extra fluids for the day
12. A nurse is admitting the client to the short-stay unit after a myelogram. A water-based contrast agent was used. The nurse would plan which of the following activity restrictions for the client?
    1. Bed rest for 6 to 8 hours, with head of bed elevated 15 to 30 degrees
    2. Bed rest for 2 to 4 hours, with head of bed elevated 15 to 30 degrees
    3. Bed rest for 6 to 8 hours, with the head of bed flat
    4. Bed rest for 2 to 4 hours, with the head of bed flat
13. A nurse is administering mouth care to an unconscious client. The nurse should avoid doing which of the following?
    1. Positioning the client on the side
    2. Using products with lemon or alcohol

3. Cleansing the mucous membranes with Toothettes
4. Brushing the teeth with a small toothbrush

14. A nurse is trying to help the family of an unconscious client cope with the situation. Which of the following interventions would the nurse plan to incorporate into the routine care for the client?
    1. Discouraging the family from touching the client
    2. Explaining equipment and procedures on an ongoing basis
    3. Ensuring adherence to visiting hours to ensure client's rest
    4. Encouraging family not to "give in" to their feelings of grief
15. The nurse is suctioning the unconscious client with a tracheostomy. The nurse should avoid which of the following actions?
    1. Keeping a supply of suction catheters at the bedside
    2. Auscultating breath sounds to determine need for suctioning
    3. Hyperoxygenating the client before, during, and after suctioning
    4. Making sure not to suction for longer than 30 seconds
16. A nurse has applied a hypothermia blanket to a client with a fever. The nurse would inspect the skin frequently to detect which complication of hypothermia blanket use?
    1. Skin breakdown
    2. Frostbite
    3. Arterial insufficiency
    4. Venous insufficiency
17. A nurse is caring for an unconscious client who is experiencing persistent hyperthermia with no signs and symptoms of infection. The nurse interprets that there may be damage to the client's thermoregulatory center in the:
    1. Cerebrum
    2. Cerebellum
    3. Hippocampus
    4. Hypothalamus
18. A client seeking treatment for an episode of hyperthermia is being discharged to home. The nurse would evaluate that the client needs clarification of discharge instructions if the client stated to:
    1. Stay in a cool environment when possible
    2. Increase fluid intake for the next 24 hours
    3. Monitor voiding for adequacy of urine output
    4. Resume full activity level immediately
19. A nurse is caring for the client with increased intracranial pressure (ICP). The nurse would monitor for which of the following trends in vital signs if the intracranial pressure is rising?
    1. Increasing temperature, increasing pulse, increasing respirations, decreasing blood pressure (BP)
    2. Increasing temperature, decreasing pulse, decreasing respirations, increasing BP
    3. Decreasing temperature, decreasing pulse, increasing respirations, decreasing BP
    4. Decreasing temperature, increasing pulse, decreasing respirations, increasing BP
20. A nurse is positioning the client with increased intracranial pressure (ICP). Which of the following positions would the nurse avoid?
    1. Head turned to the side
    2. Head midline
    3. Neck in neutral position
    4. Head of bed elevated 30 to 45 degrees
21. A client recovering from a head injury is arousable and participating in care. The nurse would evaluate that the client understands measures to prevent elevations in intracranial pressure (ICP) if the nurse observed the client doing which of the following activities?
    1. Exhaling during repositioning
    2. Isometric exercises
    3. Blowing nose
    4. Coughing vigorously
22. A family of an unconscious client with increased intracranial pressure is talking at the client's bedside. They are discussing the gravity of the client's condition and wondering if the client will ever recover. The nurse intervenes, based on the understanding that:
    1. The family needs immediate crisis intervention
    2. The family could benefit from a conference with the physician
    3. It is possible the client can hear the family
    4. The client might have wanted a visit from the hospital chaplain
23. A nurse is providing care to the client with increased intracranial pressure (ICP). Which of the following approaches may not be beneficial in controlling the client's ICP from an environmental viewpoint?
    1. Maintaining a calm atmosphere
    2. Reducing environmental noise
    3. Clustering nursing activities to be done all at one time
    4. Allowing the client uninterrupted time for sleep
24. A client has clear fluid leaking from the nose after basilar skull fracture. The nurse determines that this is cerebrospinal fluid (CSF) if the fluid:
    1. Clumps together on the dressing and has a pH of 7
    2. Separates into concentric rings and tests positive for glucose
    3. Is grossly bloody in appearance and has a pH of 6
    4. Is clear in appearance and tests negative for glucose
25. A client is admitted for observation after an auto accident with probable minor head injury. The

nurse would plan on leaving the cervical collar in place until:
1. The physician makes rounds
2. The family comes to visit
3. The result of spinal x-ray films are known
4. The nurse needs to do physical care

26. A client was seen and treated in the Emergency Department for treatment of a concussion. The nurse evaluates that the family needs reinforcement of the discharge instructions if they verbalize to call the physician for which of the following client signs and symptoms?
1. Difficulty speaking
2. Difficulty awakening
3. Vomiting
4. Minor headache

27. A nurse is caring for a client who has undergone craniotomy with a supratentorial incision. The nurse would use which of the following postoperative positions?
1. Head of bed flat, head and neck midline
2. Head of bed flat, head turned to the nonoperated side
3. Head of bed elevated 30 to 45 degrees, head and neck midline
4. Head of bed elevated 30 to 45 degrees, head turned to the operated side

28. A nurse is preparing to give the postcraniotomy client medication for incisional pain. The family asks the nurse why the client is receiving codeine sulfate and not "something stronger." In formulating a response, the nurse incorporates the understanding that codeine:
1. Is one of the strongest narcotic analgesics available
2. Cannot lead to physical or psychological dependence
3. Does not cause gastrointestinal upset or constipation as other narcotics do
4. Does not alter respirations or mask neurological signs as other narcotics do

29. A nurse is assisting in preparing home care instructions for the postcraniotomy client. Which of the following items would the nurse not include in the instructions?
1. Tub bath or shower is permitted, but keep the scalp dry until sutures are removed
2. Use a check-off system for anticonvulsant medications to avoid missing doses
3. The client after craniotomy will not hear sounds clearly unless they are loud
4. If the client is prone to seizures or gets dizzy spells, someone should be with the client while walking

30. A nurse notes documentation of a nursing diagnosis of Body Image Disturbance for the client after craniotomy. The nurse would evaluate that the client has not met the outcome criteria by discharge if the client:
1. Wears a turban to cover the incision
2. States an intention to purchase a hairpiece until hair has grown back
3. Verbalizes that periorbital bruising will disappear over time
4. Indicates that facial puffiness will be a permanent problem

31. A client with a cervical spine injury has Crutchfield tongs applied in the Emergency Department. The nurse would avoid which of the following when planning care for this client?
1. Use of a Roto-Rest bed
2. Assessment of the integrity of the weights and pulleys
3. Comparing the amount of ordered traction with the amount in use
4. Removing the weights to reposition the client

32. A client with spinal cord injury becomes angry and belligerent whenever the nurse tries to administer care. The nurse should:
1. Advise the client that rehabilitation progresses more quickly with cooperation
2. Acknowledge the client's anger and continue to encourage participation in care
3. Leave the client alone until ready to participate
4. Ask the family to deliver the care

33. A nurse has completed reinforcing discharge instructions for the client with application of a halo vest. The nurse would evaluate that the client needs further clarification of the instructions if the client stated to:
1. Use caution because the vest alters balance
2. Wash the skin daily under the lamb's wool liner of the vest
3. Use a straw for drinking
4. Drive only during the daytime

34. A client with a spinal cord injury expresses little interest in food and is very particular about the choice of meals that are actually eaten. The nurse interprets that:
1. Meal choices represent an area of client control, and should be encouraged as much as is nutritionally reasonable
2. Anorexia is a sign of clinical depression, and a referral to a psychologist is needed
3. The client has compulsive habits, which should be ignored as long as they are not harmful
4. The client probably has a naturally slow metabolism, and the decreased nutritional intake won't matter

35. A client with paraplegia has a diagnosis of Risk for Injury related to spasticity of leg muscles. Which of the following items would the nurse not include in a plan to minimize the risk of injury to the client?

1. Removing potentially harmful objects near the spastic limbs
2. Performing range of motion to the affected limbs
3. Use of padded restraints to immobilize the limb
4. Use of prn orders for muscle relaxants such as baclofen (Lioresal)

36. A nurse is teaching the paraplegic client measures to promote skin integrity. Which of the following instructions will be least helpful to the client?
   1. Shifting weight every 2 hours while in a wheelchair
   2. Using a mirror to inspect for redness and breakdown twice a week
   3. Checking the bottom sheet for wetness and wrinkles
   4. Using a pressure relief pad while in a wheelchair
37. A client who is paraplegic after spinal cord injury has been taught muscle strengthening exercises for the upper body. The nurse would evaluate that the client will derive the least muscle strengthening benefit from which of the following activities?
   1. Doing push-ups in a prone position
   2. Extending the arms while holding weights
   3. Doing active range of motion to finger joints
   4. Squeezing rubber balls
38. A nurse is caring for the client who has suffered spinal cord injury. The nurse monitors the client for signs of autonomic dysreflexia and suspects this complication if which of the following are noted?
   1. Severe, throbbing headache
   2. Pallor of the face and neck
   3. Sudden tachycardia
   4. Severe and sudden hypotension
39. A family of a client with a spinal cord injury rushes to the nursing station saying that the client needs immediate help. On entering the room, the nurse notes that the client is diaphoretic with a flushed face and neck, and complains of severe headache. The pulse is 40 and BP is 230/100 mm Hg. The nurse acts quickly, knowing the client is experiencing:
   1. Spinal shock
   2. Malignant hypertension
   3. Pulmonary embolism
   4. Autonomic dysreflexia
40. A client with spinal cord injury is prone to experiencing autonomic dysreflexia. The nurse would avoid which of the following measures to minimize the risk of recurrence?
   1. Strict adherence to a bowel retraining program
   2. Limiting bladder catheterization to once every 12 hours
   3. Keeping the linen wrinkle-free under the client
   4. Avoiding unnecessary pressure on the lower limbs
41. A client with spinal cord injury suddenly experiences an episode of autonomic dysreflexia. After checking vital signs, the nurse immediately:
   1. Lowers the head of the bed and administers an antihypertensive agent
   2. Removes the noxious stimulus and administers an antihypertensive agent
   3. Lowers the head of the bed and removes the noxious stimulus
   4. Raises the head of the bed and removes the noxious stimulus
42. A nurse is planning care for the client in spinal shock. Which of the following actions would be least helpful in minimizing the effects of vasodilation below the level of the injury?
   1. Monitoring vital signs before and during position changes
   2. Using vasopressor medications as prescribed
   3. Moving the client quickly as one unit
   4. Applying TEDs or compression stockings
43. A nurse is caring for a client with intracranial aneurysm who was previously alert. Which of the following findings would not be an early indication that the level of consciousness (LOC) is deteriorating?
   1. Slight slurring of speech
   2. Ptosis of the left eyelid
   3. Mild drowsiness
   4. Less frequent spontaneous speech
44. A nurse is planning to put aneurysm precautions in place for the client with a cerebral aneurysm. Which of the following items would not be included as part of the precautions?
   1. Avoidance of pushing or straining, such as with defecation
   2. Maintaining head of bed at 15 degrees
   3. Limiting cigarettes to three per day
   4. Provision of physical aspects of care by the nurse
45. A nurse is monitoring the client who is experiencing seizure activity. The nurse would not need to obtain information about which of the following items as part of routine monitoring of seizures?
   1. Duration of the seizure
   2. What the client ate in the 2 hours preceding seizure activity
   3. Seizure progression and type of movements
   4. Changes in pupil size or eye deviation
46. A nurse is planning to institute seizure precautions for a client who is being admitted from the Emergency Department. Which of the following measures would the nurse avoid in planning for the client's safety?
   1. Placing airway, oxygen, and suction equipment at the bedside
   2. Padding the side rails of the bed

3. Putting a padded tongue blade at the head of the bed
4. Having IV equipment ready for insertion of IV access

47. A nurse is caring for the client who begins to experience seizure activity while in bed. Which of the following actions by the nurse would be contraindicated?
   1. Loosening restrictive clothing
   2. Removing pillow and raising padded side rails
   3. Restraining the client's limbs
   4. Positioning the client to the side if possible, with head flexed forward
48. A nurse has given medication instructions to the client receiving phenytoin (Dilantin). The nurse evaluates that the client has adequate understanding if the client states:
   1. The medication dose may be self-adjusted depending on side effects
   2. Alcohol is not contraindicated while taking this medication
   3. Good oral hygiene is needed, including brushing and flossing
   4. The morning dose of the medication should be taken before a serum drug level is drawn
49. A nurse is planning care for the client with hemiparesis of the right arm and leg. The nurse incorporates in the care plan to place objects:
   1. Within the client's reach, on the right side
   2. Within the client's reach, on the left side
   3. Just out of the client's reach, on the right side
   4. Just out of the client's reach, on the left side
50. A client with a cerebrovascular accident (CVA) has residual dysphagia. When a diet order is initiated, the nurse avoids doing which of the following?
   1. Giving the client thin liquids
   2. Thickening liquids to the consistency of oatmeal
   3. Placing food on the unaffected side of the mouth
   4. Allowing plenty of time for chewing and swallowing
51. A nurse has instructed the family of a client diagnosed with cerebrovascular accident (CVA) who has homonymous hemianopsia about measures to help the client overcome the deficit. The nurse would evaluate that the family understands the measures to use if they stated to:
   1. Place objects in the client's impaired field of vision
   2. Approach the client from the impaired field of vision
   3. Remind the client to turn the head to scan the lost visual field
   4. Discourage the client from wearing own eyeglasses
52. A nurse is trying to communicate with a client with aphasia resulting from cerebrovascular accident (CVA). Which of the following actions by the nurse would be least helpful to the client?
   1. Speaking to the client at a slower rate
   2. Completing the sentences that the client cannot finish
   3. Looking directly at the client during attempts at speech
   4. Allowing plenty of time for the client to respond
53. A client with diplopia has been taught to use an eye patch to promote better vision and prevent injury. The nurse would evaluate that the client has correct understanding of the use of the patch if the client states to:
   1. Use the patch only when vision is especially troublesome
   2. Wear the patch for 1 hour at a time
   3. Wear the patch continuously, alternating eyes each day
   4. Wear the patch continuously, alternating eyes each week
54. A client receives a dose of edrophonium (Tensilon) intravenously. The client shows improvement in muscle strength for a period of time after the injection. The nurse interprets that this finding is compatible with:
   1. Multiple sclerosis
   2. Amyotrophic lateral sclerosis
   3. Myasthenia gravis
   4. Muscular dystrophy
55. A client with myasthenia gravis is having difficulty speaking. The speech is dysarthritic and has a nasal tone. The nurse would plan to avoid using which of the following communication strategies when working with this client?
   1. Repeating what the client said to verify the message
   2. Encouraging the client to speak quickly
   3. Using a communication board when necessary
   4. Asking yes-and-no questions when able
56. A client has experienced an episode of myasthenic crisis. The nurse would identify whether the client has precipitating factors such as:
   1. Too little exercise
   2. Increased intake of fatty foods
   3. Omitted doses of medication
   4. Excess medication
57. A nurse is teaching the client with myasthenia gravis about prevention of myasthenic and cholinergic crises. The nurse tells the client that this is most effectively done by:
   1. Doing all chores early in the day while less fatigued
   2. Taking medications on time to maintain therapeutic blood levels
   3. Doing muscle-strengthening exercises
   4. Eating large, well-balanced meals

58. A nurse has instructed the client with myasthenia gravis about ways to manage own health at home. The nurse would evaluate that the client needs more information if the client made which of the following statements?
   1. "I should take my medications an hour before mealtime."
   2. "I've made arrangements to get a portable resuscitation bag and home suction equipment."
   3. "Going to the beach will be a nice, relaxing form of activity."
   4. "Here's the Medic-Alert bracelet I obtained."
59. A client with Parkinson's disease is embarrassed about the symptoms of the disorder, and is bored and lonely. The nurse would plan which of the following approaches as most therapeutic in assisting the client to cope with the disease?
   1. Plan only a few activities for the client during the day
   2. Assist the client with activities of daily living (ADLs) as much as possible
   3. Encourage and praise perseverance in exercising and performing ADLs
   4. Cluster activities at the end of the day when the client is most bored
60. A client with Parkinson's disease is experiencing a parkinsonian crisis. The nurse would immediately place the client:
   1. In a quiet, dim room with respiratory and cardiac support available
   2. In a high Fowler's position, with a nasogastric tube at the bedside
   3. In a room near the nursing station which is near the code cart
   4. In a bed with padded side rails, with limb restraints nearby
61. A nurse has given instructions to the client with Parkinson's disease about maintaining mobility. The nurse would evaluate that the client understood the directions if the client stated to:
   1. Exercise in the evening to combat fatigue
   2. Rock back and forth to start movement with bradykinesia
   3. Sit in soft, deep chairs
   4. Buy clothes with many buttons to maintain finger dexterity
62. A nurse has given suggestions to the client with trigeminal neuralgia about strategies to minimize episodes of pain. The nurse would evaluate that the client needs reinforcement of information if the client made which of the following statements?
   1. "I will wash my face with cotton pads."
   2. "I'll have to start chewing on the unaffected side."
   3. "I should rinse my mouth sometimes if tooth brushing is painful."
   4. "I'll try to eat my food either very warm or very cold."

ANSWERS

1. *Answer:* 1

Rationale: Cranial nerve II is the optic nerve, which governs vision. The nurse can provide safety for the visually impaired client by clearing the path of obstacles when ambulating. Testing the shower water temperature would be useful if there was impairment of peripheral nerves. Speaking loudly may help overcome deficit of cranial nerve VIII (vestibulocochlear). Cranial nerve VII (facial) and IX (glossopharyngeal) control taste from the anterior two thirds and posterior one third of the tongue, respectively.

Test-Taking Strategy: Knowledge of the cranial nerves is needed to answer this question accurately. Review these cranial nerves if you had difficulty with this question.

Level of Cognitive Ability: Application

Client Needs: Safe, Effective Care Environment

Integrated Concept/Process: Nursing Process/Planning

Content Area: Adult Health/Neurological

Reference: Black J, Hawks J, Keene A: *Medical-surgical nursing: clinical management for positive outcomes,* ed 6, Philadelphia, 2001, WB Saunders, p. 1869.

2. *Answer:* 2

Rationale: The cerebellum is responsible for balance and coordination. A walker would provide stability for the client during ambulation. Adaptive eating utensils may be beneficial when the client has partial paralysis of the hand. A raised toilet seat is useful when the client does not have the mobility or ability to flex the hips. A slider board is used in transferring a client from a bed to stretcher or wheelchair.

Test-Taking Strategy: Use the process of elimination. To answer this question correctly, you must know that the cerebellum controls balance and coordination. This would immediately help you eliminate options 3 and 4. To help you choose between options 1 and 2, adaptive eating utensils are used when there is loss of fine motor coordination, such as with cerebrovascular accident. The walker would help the client maintain balance. Review care to the client with a cerebellar lesion if you had difficulty with this question.

Level of Cognitive Ability: Comprehension

Client Needs: Health Promotion and Maintenance

Integrated Concept/Process: Nursing Process/Evaluation

Content Area: Adult Health/Neurological

Reference: Black J, Hawks J, Keene A: *Medical-surgical nursing: clinical management for positive outcomes,* ed 6, Philadelphia, 2001, WB Saunders, p. 1856.

3. *Answer:* 4

Rationale: Clients with cognitive impairment from neurological dysfunction respond best to a stable environment, which is limited in the amounts and type of sensory input. The nurse can provide sensory cues and give clear, simple directions in a positive manner. Confusion and agitation can be minimized by reducing environmental stimuli (such as television, multiple

visitors) and keeping familiar personal articles (such as family pictures) at the bedside.
Test-Taking Strategy: Use the process of elimination. This question asks for the least helpful action, which makes you look for an incorrect response. The client who is confused can handle limited amounts of information at one time, which makes option 4 the correct answer to this question. Review care to the neurological client if you had difficulty with this question.
Level of Cognitive Ability: Application
Client Needs: Psychosocial Integrity
Integrated Concept/Process: Nursing Process/Implementation
Content Area: Adult Health/Neurological
Reference: Black J, Hawks J, Keene A: *Medical-surgical nursing: clinical management for positive outcomes,* ed 6, Philadelphia, 2001, WB Saunders, p. 1918.

4. *Answer:* 1
Rationale: A bladder retraining program, such as use of a toileting schedule, may be helpful to clients experiencing urinary incontinence. A Foley catheter should be used only when necessary because of the risk of infection. Use of diapers or pads is the least acceptable alternative, because the risk of skin breakdown is great.
Test-Taking Strategy: This question can be answered most easily by looking at it from a client safety viewpoint. Because Foley catheters carry risk of infection, and the use of diapers or pads carries the risk of skin breakdown, the only acceptable answer is the toileting schedule. Review care to the client with a neurological impairment if you had difficulty with this question.
Level of Cognitive Ability: Application
Client Needs: Physiological Integrity
Integrated Concept/Process: Nursing Process/Implementation
Content Area: Adult Health/Neurological
Reference: Black J, Hawks J, Keene A: *Medical-surgical nursing: clinical management for positive outcomes,* ed 6, Philadelphia, 2001, WB Saunders, p. 835.

5. *Answer:* 2
Rationale: Previous neurological problems such as headaches or back injuries place the client more at risk for development of a neurological disorder. Chronic diseases such as hypertension and diabetes mellitus also place the client at greater risk. Assessment of allergies is a routine part of the health history, regardless of the nature of the client's problem.
Test-Taking Strategy: Use the process of elimination. This question is fairly straightforward. Each of the incorrect options for the question has an actual or potential neurological association. Allergies indicate a disturbance of the immune system. Review the risks associated with neurological problems if you had difficulty with this question.
Level of Cognitive Ability: Comprehension
Client Needs: Physiological Integrity
Integrated Concept/Process: Nursing Process/Data Collection
Content Area: Adult Health/Neurological
Reference: Black J, Hawks J, Keene A: *Medical-surgical nursing: clinical management for positive outcomes,* ed 6, Philadelphia, 2001, WB Saunders, p. 1880.

6. *Answer:* 1
Rationale: The question is worded to elicit an unsafe action on the part of the family. Depending on the client's functional ability, either passive or active ROM is indicated to keep the joint moving freely. Application of a premolded splint would also keep the limb aligned and in good position. The client should not attempt to stand unsupported on a weak or paralyzed limb. The inability to bear weight will cause the client to fall.
Test-Taking Strategy: This question tests fundamental concepts of impaired mobility and corrective actions. If you had any difficulty with this question, review these concepts.
Level of Cognitive Ability: Analysis
Client Needs: Health Promotion and Maintenance
Integrated Concept/Process: Nursing Process/Evaluation
Content Area: Adult Health/Neurological
Reference: Black J, Hawks J, Keene A: *Medical-surgical nursing: clinical management for positive outcomes,* ed 6, Philadelphia, 2001, WB Saunders, p. 1957.

7. *Answer:* 2
Rationale: The client undergoing cerebral angiography is assessed for possible allergy to the contrast dye, which can be determined by questioning the client about allergies to iodine or shellfish. Salmon is irrelevant to the question. Claustrophobia and excessive weight are areas of concern with magnetic resonance imaging.
Test-Taking Strategy: This concept is fundamental for angiography of any group of blood vessels. Review this diagnostic test if you had difficulty with this question.
Level of Cognitive Ability: Application
Client Needs: Physiological Integrity
Integrated Concept/Process: Nursing Process/Data Collection
Content Area: Adult Health/Neurological
Reference: DeWit S: *Fundamental concepts and skills for nursing,* Philadelphia, 2001, WB Saunders, p. 409.

8. *Answer:* 4
Rationale: The client having an MRI has all metallic objects removed because of the magnetic field generated by the device. A careful history is done to determine if any metal objects are inside the client, such as orthopedic hardware, pacemakers, artificial heart valves, aneurysm clips, or intrauterine devices. These may heat up, become dislodged, or malfunction during this procedure. The client may be ineligible if there is significant risk.
Test-Taking Strategy: Use the process of elimination. You will note that each of the incorrect options is a medical disorder. The correct answer is the name of a surgical procedure where an artificial valve (sometimes metal) is implanted. An important concept with regard to MRI is the avoidance of any metal objects in the vicinity of the machine. Review the contraindications related to this procedure if you had difficulty with this question.
Level of Cognitive Ability: Comprehension
Client Needs: Physiological Integrity
Integrated Concept/Process: Nursing Process/Data Collection
Content Area: Adult Health/Neurological
Reference: DeWit S: *Fundamental concepts and skills for nursing,* Philadelphia, 2001, WB Saunders, p. 409.

9. *Answer:* 1
Rationale: The client undergoing LP is positioned lying on the side, with the legs pulled up to the abdomen, and with the head bent down onto the chest. This position helps to open the spaces between the vertebrae.
Test-Taking Strategy: Use the process of elimination. Knowing that an LP is the introduction of a needle into the subarachnoid space, it is reasonable that the position of the client must facilitate this. The correct answer is the only position that flexes the vertebrae for easier needle insertion. Review positioning procedures for an LP if you had difficulty with this question.
Level of Cognitive Ability: Application
Client Needs: Physiological Integrity
Integrated Concept/Process: Nursing Process/Implementation
Content Area: Adult Health/Neurological
Reference: DeWit S: *Fundamental concepts and skills for nursing,* Philadelphia, 2001, WB Saunders, p. 409.

10. *Answer:* 3
Rationale: The MRI scanner is a hollow tube that gives some clients a feeling of claustrophobia. Metal objects must be removed before the procedure, so they are not drawn in to the magnetic field. The client may eat and take all prescribed medications before the procedure. If a contrast medium is used, the client may wish to eat lightly if the client has a tendency to get nauseated easily. The client lies supine on a padded table, which moves into the imager. The client must lie still during the procedure. The imager makes tapping noises while scanning. The client is alone in the imager, but the nurse can reassure the client that the technician is in voice communication with the client at all times during the procedure.
Test-Taking Strategy: Use the process of elimination. The statements in each of the options are correct. However, the question asks which of them will give the most reassurance to the client. While all statements are factually true, the correct option is the only one that provides a measure of reassurance to the client. Review MRI if you had difficulty with this question.
Level of Cognitive Ability: Application
Client Needs: Psychosocial Integrity
Integrated Concept/Process: Nursing Process/Implementation
Content Area: Adult Health/Neurological
Reference: DeWit S: *Fundamental concepts and skills for nursing,* Philadelphia, 2001, WB Saunders, p. 409.

11. *Answer:* 4
Rationale: After CT scanning, the client may resume all usual activities. The client should be encouraged to take in extra fluids to replace those lost with diuresis from the contrast dye.
Test-Taking Strategy: Use the process of elimination. Looking at the available choices, option 3 makes the least sense and should be eliminated first. Knowing that there is no special aftercare lets you eliminate options 1 and 2 next. Review the procedure related to CT scanning if you had difficulty with this question.
Level of Cognitive Ability: Comprehension
Client Needs: Health Promotion and Maintenance
Integrated Concept/Process: Nursing Process/Evaluation
Content Area: Adult Health/Neurological
Reference: DeWit S: *Fundamental concepts and skills for nursing,* Philadelphia, 2001, WB Saunders, p. 409.

12. *Answer:* 1
Rationale: After a myelogram, the client is placed on bed rest for 6 to 8 hours after the procedure. When a water-based contrast medium is used, the client is positioned with the head of bed elevated 15 to 30 degrees. With use of an oil-based medium, the head of bed is positioned flat (even though the contrast is aspirated out after the procedure).
Test-Taking Strategy: Use the process of elimination. This question is asking for knowledge of two separate items (e.g., length of bed rest and head position). With a myelogram procedure, if you reason that the longer the bed rest, the less likelihood of complications, then you can narrow your choices to options 1 and 3. If you can remember that "oil rises, so keep the head low," you will be able to choose correctly. Review postprocedure care after a myelogram if you had difficulty with this question.
Level of Cognitive Ability: Application
Client Needs: Physiological Integrity
Content Area: Adult Health/Neurological
Integrated Concept/Process: Nursing Process/Planning
Reference: Black J, Hawks J, Keene A: *Medical-surgical nursing: clinical management for positive outcomes,* ed 6, Philadelphia, 2001, WB Saunders, p. 1899.

13. *Answer:* 2
Rationale: The unconscious client is positioned on the side during mouth care to prevent aspiration. The teeth are brushed at least twice daily using a small toothbrush. The gums, tongue, roof of mouth, and oral mucous membranes are cleansed with Toothettes to avoid encrustation and infection. The lips are coated with water-soluble lubricant to prevent drying, cracking, and encrustation. The use of products with lemon or alcohol should be avoided, as they have a drying effect.
Test-Taking Strategy: Use the process of elimination. The question asks what the nurse should avoid. Standard mouth care procedures include use of toothbrush and Toothettes, so these may be eliminated first. Knowing that the unconscious client is at risk of aspiration tells you that option 1 is also correct. This leaves option 2 as incorrect, because repeated use of these products could dry and crack the oral mucous membranes. Review care to the unconscious client if you had difficulty with this question.
Level of Cognitive Ability: Application
Client Needs: Physiological Integrity
Integrated Concept/Process: Nursing Process/Implementation
Content Area: Adult Health/Neurological
Reference: DeWit S: *Fundamental concepts and skills for nursing,* Philadelphia, 2001, WB Saunders, p. 302.

14. *Answer:* 2
Rationale: Families often need assistance to cope with the sudden severe illness of a loved one. The nurse can help the family of an unconscious client by assisting them to work through their feelings of grief. The nurse should explain all equipment, treatments, and procedures, and supplement or reinforce information given by the physician. Family should be encour-

aged to touch and speak to the client, and to become involved in the client's care to the extent they are comfortable. The nurse should allow the family to stay with the client to the extent possible, and should encourage them to eat and sleep adequately to maintain their strength.
Test-Taking Strategy: Use the process of elimination. The options seem to revolve around two themes: the adjustment of the family to the situation, and the involvement or interaction with the client and care. Each of the incorrect options either inhibits the family's coping, or distances the family from the client or the client's care. Avoid selecting these types of options. Review the psychosocial needs of the family of an unconscious client if you had difficulty with this question.
Level of Cognitive Ability: Application
Client Needs: Psychosocial Integrity
Integrated Concept/Process: Nursing Process/Implementation
Content Area: Adult Health/Neurological
Reference: DeWit S: *Fundamental concepts and skills for nursing,* Philadelphia, 2001, WB Saunders, p. 752.

15. *Answer:* 4
Rationale: Suction equipment should be kept at the bedside of an unconscious client, regardless of whether an artificial airway is used. The nurse auscultates breath sounds every 2 to 4 hours, or more frequently if there is need. The client should be hyperoxygenated before, during, and after suctioning to minimize cerebral hypoxia. The client should not be suctioned for longer than 10 seconds at one time to prevent cerebral hypoxia and a rise in intracranial pressure.
Test-Taking Strategy: Use the process of elimination. The question is worded to make you seek an incorrect nursing action. Each of the first three options is standard suctioning procedure. The only option that is different and dangerous is option 4. If you had difficulty with this question, review suctioning procedure.
Level of Cognitive Ability: Application
Client Needs: Physiological Integrity
Integrated Concept/Process: Nursing Process/Implementation
Content Area: Adult Health/Neurological
Reference: DeWit S: *Fundamental concepts and skills for nursing,* Philadelphia, 2001, WB Saunders, p. 573.

16. *Answer:* 1
Rationale: When a hypothermia blanket is used, the skin is inspected frequently for pressure points, which over time could lead to skin breakdown.
Test-Taking Strategy: Use the process of elimination. Options 3 and 4 may be eliminated first, as they are other health problems. The temperature of the blanket is not cold enough to produce frostbite. This leaves skin breakdown as the correct answer. Review the complications associated with the use of a hypothermia blanket if you had difficulty with this question.
Level of Cognitive Ability: Application
Client Needs: Physiological Integrity
Integrated Concept/Process: Nursing Process/Implementation
Content Area: Adult Health/Neurological
Reference: DeWit S: *Fundamental concepts and skills for nursing,* Philadelphia, 2001, WB Saunders, p. 801.

17. *Answer:* 4
Rationale: Hypothalamic damage causes hyperthermia, which may also be called "central fever." It is characterized by a persistent high fever with no diurnal variation. There is also an absence of sweating.
Test-Taking Strategy: Use the process of elimination. Knowledge of the location of the brain's thermoregulatory center is needed to answer this question. Eliminate options 1 and 2 first, as they are responsible for higher mental functions and balance, respectively. A quick trick may be to remember that hyperthermia is due to the hypothalamus. Review the anatomy and physiology of the brain if you had difficulty with this question.
Level of Cognitive Ability: Comprehension
Client Needs: Physiological Integrity
Integrated Concept/Process: Nursing Process/Data Collection
Content Area: Adult Health/Neurological
Reference: DeWit S: *Fundamental concepts and skills for nursing,* Philadelphia, 2001, WB Saunders, p. 336.

18. *Answer:* 4
Rationale: Discharge instructions for the client hospitalized for hyperthermia include prevention of heat-related disorders, increased fluid intake for 24 hours, self-monitoring of voiding, and the importance of staying in a cool environment and resting.
Test-Taking Strategy: Use the process of elimination. This question is worded to elicit the least appropriate activity on discharge. Options 2 and 3 relate to maintaining and monitoring fluid balance and are therefore eliminated. A cool environment is appropriate, so this option is also eliminated. Resumption of full activity is not helpful; rather rest periods are indicated, so this is the correct option. Review home care instructions for the client with hyperthermia if you had difficulty with this question.
Level of Cognitive Ability: Comprehension
Client Needs: Health Promotion and Maintenance
Integrated Concept/Process: Nursing Process/Evaluation
Content Area: Adult Health/Neurological
Reference: DeWit S: *Fundamental concepts and skills for nursing,* Philadelphia, 2001, WB Saunders, p. 336.

19. *Answer:* 2
Rationale: A change in vital signs may be a late sign of increased ICP. Trends include increasing temperature and blood pressure, and decreasing pulse and respirations. Respiratory irregularities may also arise.
Test-Taking Strategy: Use the process of elimination. This question looks complex, but can be logically answered. If you remember that temperature rises, then you are able to eliminate options 3 and 4. If you know that the client becomes bradycardic, or know that the blood pressure rises, you are able to make the correct choice. Review the signs of increased intracranial pressure if you had difficulty with this question.
Level of Cognitive Ability: Application
Client Needs: Physiological Integrity
Integrated Concept/Process: Nursing Process/Data Collection
Content Area: Adult Health/Neurological
Reference: Black J, Hawks J, Keene A: *Medical-surgical nursing: clinical management for positive outcomes,* ed 6, Philadelphia, 2001, WB Saunders, p. 1970.

20. *Answer:* 1
Rationale: The head of the client with increased ICP should be positioned in a neutral, midline position. The nurse should avoid flexing or extending the neck, or turning the neck side to side. The head of bed should be raised to 30 to 45 degrees. Use of proper positions promotes venous drainage from the cranium to keep intracranial pressure lowered.
Test-Taking Strategy: This question is asking which position will be detrimental to the client with increased ICP. Such a position would interfere either with arterial circulation to the brain or with venous drainage from the brain. The only position that meets one of those criteria is option 1. Review client positioning with ICP if you had difficulty with this question.
Level of Cognitive Ability: Application
Client Needs: Physiological Integrity
Integrated Concept/Process: Nursing Process/Implementation
Content Area: Adult Health/Neurological
Reference: Black J, Hawks J, Keene A: *Medical-surgical nursing: clinical management for positive outcomes,* ed 6, Philadelphia, 2001, WB Saunders, p. 1969.

21. *Answer:* 1
Rationale: Activities that increase intrathoracic and intraabdominal pressures cause indirect elevation of the ICP. Some of these activities include isometric exercises, Valsalva maneuver, coughing, sneezing, and blowing the nose. Exhaling during activities such as repositioning or pulling up in bed opens the glottis, which prevents intrathoracic pressure from rising.
Test-Taking Strategy: Use the process of elimination. Evaluate each of the options in terms of the tension it puts on the body. Doing so will help you eliminate each of the incorrect options systematically. Review the measures that will reduce or prevent increased intracranial pressure if you had difficulty with this question.
Level of Cognitive Ability: Comprehension
Client Needs: Health Promotion and Maintenance
Integrated Concept/Process: Nursing Process/Evaluation
Content Area: Adult Health/Neurological
Reference: Black J, Hawks J, Keene A: *Medical-surgical nursing: clinical management for positive outcomes,* ed 6, Philadelphia, 2001, WB Saunders, p. 1969.

22. *Answer:* 3
Rationale: Some clients who have awakened from an unconscious state have reported they remember hearing specific voices and conversations. Family and staff should assume the client's sense of hearing is still intact, and act accordingly. Research has also shown that positive outcomes are associated with coma stimulation, that is, speaking to and touching the client.
Test-Taking Strategy: Use the process of elimination. The nurse would not infer that the client wants a visit from the chaplain based on the family speaking over the client at the bedside, so eliminate that option first. The family demonstrates no evidence of crisis, and they seem to be well informed. This eliminates options 1 and 2. Option 3 is the only correct choice. Review care to the unconscious client if you had difficulty with this question.
Level of Cognitive Ability: Application
Client Needs: Psychosocial Integrity
Integrated Concept/Process: Nursing Process/Implementation
Content Area: Adult Health/Neurological
Reference: Black J, Hawks J, Keene A: *Medical-surgical nursing: clinical management for positive outcomes,* ed 6, Philadelphia, 2001, WB Saunders, p. 752.

23. *Answer:* 3
Rationale: Nursing interventions should be spaced out over the shift to minimize the risk of a sustained rise in ICP. If possible, activities known to raise the ICP should be avoided where possible. Other interventions to control the ICP include maintaining a calm, quiet environment, and avoiding emotional stress and interruption of sleep.
Test-Taking Strategy: Use the process of elimination. This question tests the concept that stimulation raises the ICP. If you know this, you will be able to eliminate each of the incorrect options. Review nursing care to the client with increased intracranial pressure if you had difficulty with this question.
Level of Cognitive Ability: Application
Client Needs: Physiological Integrity
Integrated Concept/Process: Nursing Process/Implementation
Content Area: Adult Health/Neurological
Reference: Black J, Hawks J, Keene A: *Medical-surgical nursing: clinical management for positive outcomes,* ed 6, Philadelphia, 2001, WB Saunders, p. 1969.

24. *Answer:* 2
Rationale: Leakage of CSF from the ears or nose may accompany basilar skull fracture. It can be distinguished from other body fluids because the drainage will separate into bloody and yellow concentric rings on dressing material, called Halo's sign. The fluid also tests positive for glucose.
Test-Taking Strategy: The key to answering this question lies in knowing that CSF contains glucose, whereas other secretions, such as mucus, do not. Knowing that CSF separates into rings will also help you with this particular question. Review testing for CSF fluid if you had difficulty with this question.
Level of Cognitive Ability: Analysis
Client Needs: Physiological Integrity
Integrated Concept/Process: Nursing Process/Evaluation
Content Area: Adult Health/Neurological
Reference: Black J, Hawks J, Keene A: *Medical-surgical nursing: clinical management for positive outcomes,* ed 6, Philadelphia, 2001, WB Saunders, p. 1989.

25. *Answer:* 3
Rationale: There is a significant association between cervical spine injury and head injury. For this reason, the nurse leaves any form of spinal immobilization in place until lateral cervical spine x-ray studies rule out fracture or other damage.
Test-Taking Strategy: This question is straightforward. The reason for spinal immobilization is to protect the spine from movement, which could cause further damage if the cervical spine was injured. If x-ray study results are negative, there is no reason to leave the collar in place. Review emergency care of the client with a suspected cervical injury if this question was difficult.
Level of Cognitive Ability: Application
Client Needs: Physiological Integrity
Integrated Concept/Process: Nursing Process/Implementation

Content Area: Adult Health/Neurological
Reference: Black J, Hawks J, Keene A: *Medical-surgical nursing: clinical management for positive outcomes*, ed 6, Philadelphia, 2001, WB Saunders, p. 2269.

26. *Answer:* 4
Rationale: A concussion after head injury is a temporary loss of consciousness (from a few seconds to a few minutes) without evidence of structural damage. After concussion, the family is taught to monitor the client and to call the physician or return the client to the Emergency Department if several signs and symptoms are noted. These include confusion, difficulty awakening or speaking, one-sided weakness, vomiting, or severe headache. Minor headache is expected.
Test-Taking Strategy: To answer this question, you need to be familiar with neurological signs and symptoms of increased intracranial pressure (ICP). Vomiting and neurological deficits (in this case, speaking), indicate increased ICP. Decreasing LOC (difficulty arousing) is an early sign of increasing ICP. For these reasons, eliminate each of these options, and choose the minor headache, which is expected. Review care to the client with a concussion if you had difficulty with this question.
Level of Cognitive Ability: Analysis
Client Needs: Health Promotion and Maintenance
Integrated Concept/Process: Nursing Process/Evaluation
Content Area: Adult Health/Neurological
Reference: Black J, Hawks J, Keene A: *Medical-surgical nursing: clinical management for positive outcomes*, ed 6, Philadelphia, 2001, WB Saunders, p. 1950.

27. *Answer:* 3
Rationale: After supratentorial surgery, the head is kept at a 30- to 45-degree angle. The head and neck should not be angled either anteriorly or laterally, but rather should be kept in a neutral (midline) position. This will promote venous return through the jugular veins, which will help prevent a rise in intracranial pressure.
Test-Taking Strategy: This question tests knowledge of differences in positioning the craniotomy client with an infratentorial versus supratentorial incision. If you know that with supra- "keep the head up", and with infra- "keep the head down", you can eliminate options 1 and 2. Knowing how to position the head for optimal venous drainage helps you to select option 3 over option 4. Review client positioning after craniotomy if you had difficulty with this question.
Level of Cognitive Ability: Application
Client Needs: Physiological Integrity
Integrated Concept/Process: Nursing Process/Implementation
Content Area: Adult Health/Neurological
Reference: Black J, Hawks J, Keene A: *Medical-surgical nursing: clinical management for positive outcomes*, ed 6, Philadelphia, 2001, WB Saunders, p. 1937.

28. *Answer:* 4
Rationale: Codeine sulfate is the narcotic analgesic of choice for clients after craniotomy. It is often combined with a non-narcotic analgesic such as acetaminophen for added effect. It does not alter the respiratory rate or mask neurological signs as do other narcotics. Side effects of codeine include gastrointestinal upset and constipation. The medication can lead to physical and psychological dependence with chronic use.
Test-Taking Strategy: Use the process of elimination. This question tests your knowledge of codeine as a narcotic analgesic. General knowledge about narcotic analgesics as a class helps you to eliminate options 2 and 3. Because codeine is not the strongest narcotic available, eliminate option 1 next. This leaves the correct option, which is codeine's advantage of not masking neurological signs. Review this medication if you had difficulty with this question.
Level of Cognitive Ability: Application
Client Needs: Physiological Integrity
Integrated Concept/Process: Nursing Process/Implementation
Content Area: Pharmacology
Reference: Black J, Hawks J, Keene A: *Medical-surgical nursing: clinical management for positive outcomes*, ed 6, Philadelphia, 2001, WB Saunders, p. 1937.

29. *Answer:* 3
Rationale: Seizures are a potential complication that can occur for up to 1 year after surgery. For this reason, the client must diligently take anticonvulsant medications and avoid missing doses. The family should learn seizure precautions and accompany the client while ambulating if dizziness or seizures tend to occur. The suture line is kept dry until sutures are removed to prevent infection. After a craniotomy, the client is typically sensitive to loud noises and can find them irritating (e.g., loud television). Awareness control of environmental noise by others is helpful to this client.
Test-Taking Strategy: Use the process of elimination. Begin to answer this question by eliminating option 1 first, as it is a general teaching point appropriate after many types of surgery. Recalling that seizures are a potential postoperative risk for up to a year after surgery, assists in eliminating options 2 and 4. This leaves option 3 as the correct answer. Many clients after craniotomy have sensitivity to or are irritated by loud noises. Review home care instructions after craniotomy if you had difficulty with this question.
Level of Cognitive Ability: Application
Client Needs: Health Promotion and Maintenance
Integrated Concept/Process: Nursing Process/Implementation
Content Area: Adult Health/Neurological
Reference: Black J, Hawks J, Keene A: *Medical-surgical nursing: clinical management for positive outcomes*, ed 6, Philadelphia, 2001, WB Saunders, p. 1937.

30. *Answer:* 4
Rationale: After craniotomy, clients may experience difficulty with altered personal appearance. The nurse can help by listening to client concerns, and by clarifying any misconceptions about facial edema, periorbital bruising, and hair loss (which are temporary). The nurse can encourage the client to participate in self-grooming and use personal articles of clothing. Finally, the nurse can suggest the use of a turban, followed by a hairpiece, to help the client adapt to the temporary change in appearance.
Test-Taking Strategy: Use the process of elimination. The wording of this question suggests an incorrect statement or a maladaptive response. Options 1 and 2 both indicate adaptive

responses and are therefore eliminated. Knowing that facial edema and bruising are temporary helps you to choose option 4 over option 3. Review care to the client after craniotomy if you had difficulty with this question.
Level of Cognitive Ability: Analysis
Client Needs: Psychosocial Integrity
Integrated Concept/Process: Nursing Process/Evaluation
Content Area: Adult Health/Neurological
Reference: Black J, Hawks J, Keene A: *Medical-surgical nursing: clinical management for positive outcomes,* ed 6, Philadelphia, 2001, WB Saunders, p. 1937.

31. *Answer:* 4
Rationale: Crutchfield tongs are applied after drilling holes in the client's skull with the patient under local anesthesia. Weights are attached to the tongs, which exert pulling pressure on the longitudinal axis of the cervical spine. Serial x-ray films of the cervical spine are taken, with weights being gradually added until the film reveals that the vertebral column is realigned. After that, weights may be gradually reduced to a point that maintains alignment. The client with Crutchfield tongs is placed on a Stryker frame or Roto-Rest bed. The nurse ensures that weights hang freely, and the amount of weight matches the current order. The nurse also inspects the integrity and position of the ropes and pulleys. The nurse does not remove the weights to administer care.
Test-Taking Strategy: Use the process of elimination. The question asks for an action that is to be avoided, so the correct answer is an item that would be contraindicated. Knowing the basics of traction is sufficient to answer this question. Remember traction weights are not removed. Review nursing care related to the client with cervical tongs if you had difficulty with this question.
Level of Cognitive Ability: Application
Client Needs: Physiological Integrity
Integrated Concept/Process: Nursing Process/Planning
Content Area: Adult Health/Neurological
Reference: Black J, Hawks J, Keene A: *Medical-surgical nursing: clinical management for positive outcomes,* ed 6, Philadelphia, 2001, WB Saunders, p. 2053.

32. *Answer:* 2
Rationale: Adjusting to paralysis is difficult both physically and psychosocially for the client and family. The nurse recognizes that the client goes through the grieving process in adjusting to the loss, and may move back and forth among the stages of grief. The nurse acknowledges the client's feelings while continuing to meet the client's physical needs and encouraging independence.
Test-Taking Strategy: Use the process of elimination. This question can be answered easily by examining the impact or outcome of each of the options. The nurse cannot neglect the client until the client is ready (option 3), so this can be eliminated first. The family is also in crisis and needs the nurse's support (option 4), and should not be relied on for care. Option 1 represents a factual, but noncaring approach to the client, which is also not therapeutic. This leaves option 2 as the best choice of the available responses. Also, option 2 acknowledges the client's feelings. Review the psychosocial needs of a client with a spinal cord injury if you had difficulty with this question.
Level of Cognitive Ability: Application
Client Needs: Psychosocial Integrity
Integrated Concept/Process: Nursing Process/Implementation
Content Area: Adult Health/Neurological
Reference: Black J, Hawks J, Keene A: *Medical-surgical nursing: clinical management for positive outcomes,* ed 6, Philadelphia, 2001, WB Saunders, p. 2065.

33. *Answer:* 4
Rationale: The Halo vest alters balance and can cause fatigue because of its weight. The client should cleanse the skin daily under the vest to protect the skin from ulceration, and should use powder or lotions sparingly or not at all. The wool liner should be changed if odor becomes a problem. The client should have food cut into small pieces to facilitate chewing and use straws for drinking. Pin care is done as instructed. The client should not drive because the device impairs the range of vision.
Test-Taking Strategy: Use the process of elimination. To answer this question successfully, it is necessary to know that a Halo vest is used to allow mobility for the client who needs continuous cervical traction. It maintains the head and spine in a neutral position. With this in mind, it may be fairly easy to choose option 4 as the correct answer to the question as stated. The inability to turn the head without turning the torso would make driving contraindicated. Review client education points related to a Halo vest if you had difficulty with this question.
Level of Cognitive Ability: Analysis
Client Needs: Health Promotion and Maintenance
Integrated Concept/Process: Nursing Process/Evaluation
Content Area: Adult Health/Neurological
Reference: Black J, Hawks J, Keene A: *Medical-surgical nursing: clinical management for positive outcomes,* ed 6, Philadelphia, 2001, WB Saunders, p. 2054.

34. *Answer:* 1
Rationale: Depression is frequently seen in the client with spinal cord injury and may be exhibited as a loss of appetite. The client should be allowed to choose the types of food eaten, and when they are eaten as much as is feasible, as it is one of the few areas of control that the client has left.
Test Testing Strategy: Use the process of elimination. The nurse does not make the diagnosis of clinical depression, which makes this an unreasonable choice. For the same reason, the option related to compulsive habits should be eliminated. There is no evidence in the question to demonstrate that the client has a slow metabolic rate, so this is eliminated next. The option that is left is the correct choice, that is, leaving the client as much control as possible. Review the psychosocial needs of the client with a spinal cord injury if you had difficulty with this question.
Level of Cognitive Ability: Analysis
Client Needs: Psychosocial Integrity
Integrated Concept/Process: Nursing Process/Data Collection
Content Area: Adult Health/Neurological
Reference: Black J, Hawks J, Keene A: *Medical-surgical nursing: clinical management for positive outcomes,* ed 6, Philadelphia, 2001, WB Saunders, p. 2065.

35. *Answer:* 3
Rationale: Range of motion exercises are beneficial in stretching muscles, which may diminish spasticity. Removing potentially harmful objects is a good safety measure. Use of muscle relaxants is also indicated if the spasms cause discomfort to the client or pose a risk to client safety. Use of limb restraints will not alleviate spasticity and could harm the client.
Test-Taking Strategy: Use the process of elimination. The wording of the question guides you to look for a response that is potentially harmful to the client. Each of the incorrect options can be eliminated systematically if you evaluate the options by looking for those interventions that would pose a risk to the client. Restraints should be avoided. Review the safety needs for the client with paraplegia if you had difficulty with this question.
Level of Cognitive Ability: Application
Client Needs: Safe, Effective Care Environment
Integrated Concept/Process: Nursing Process/Planning
Content Area: Adult Health/Neurological
Reference: Black J, Hawks J, Keene A: *Medical-surgical nursing: clinical management for positive outcomes,* ed 6, Philadelphia, 2001, WB Saunders, p. 2058.

36. *Answer:* 2
Rationale: To prevent pressure ulcers from developing, the paraplegic client should shift weight in the wheelchair every 2 hours, and use a pressure relief pad. While the client is in bed, the bottom sheet should be free of wrinkles and wetness. The client should use a mirror to inspect the skin twice a day (morning and evening) to assess for redness, edema, and breakdown. General additional measures include a nutritious diet and meticulous skin care.
Test-Taking Strategy: Use the process of elimination. This question asks for a "least helpful" measure. Each option appears reasonable on first inspection. With a closer look, however, you will notice that the time frame for inspecting the skin is much too infrequent, making this the correct response to the question as stated. Review care of the paraplegic client if you had difficulty with this question.
Level of Cognitive Ability: Application
Client Needs: Health Promotion and Maintenance
Integrated Concept/Process: Nursing Process/Implementation
Content Area: Adult Health/Neurological
Reference: Black J, Hawks J, Keene A: *Medical-surgical nursing: clinical management for positive outcomes,* ed 6, Philadelphia, 2001, WB Saunders, p. 2061.

37. *Answer:* 3
Rationale: Range of motion to the finger joints prevents contractures, but does not actively strengthen muscle groups needed for self-mobilization with paraplegia. Other activities that are more effective include push-ups from a prone position, sit-ups from a sitting position, extending the arms while holding weights, and squeezing rubber balls or crumpling newspaper.
Test-Taking Strategy: Use the process of elimination. This question can be answered by thinking about the energy expenditure of the muscle groups involved in the activities listed in each option. The one that will involve the least energy expenditure (and therefore the least amount of muscle development) is the range of motion exercises, which makes it the correct answer to this question as stated. Review care to the paraplegic client if you had difficulty with this question.
Level of Cognitive Ability: Analysis
Client Needs: Health Promotion and Maintenance
Integrated Concept/Process: Nursing Process/Evaluation
Content Area: Adult Health/Neurological
Reference: Black J, Hawks J, Keene A: *Medical-surgical nursing: clinical management for positive outcomes,* ed 6, Philadelphia, 2001, WB Saunders, p. 2060.

38. *Answer:* 1
Rationale: The client with spinal cord injury is at risk for autonomic dysreflexia with an injury above the level of T7. It is characterized by severe, throbbing headache, flushing of the face and neck, bradycardia, and sudden severe hypertension. Other signs include nasal stuffiness, blurred vision, nausea, and sweating. It is a life-threatening syndrome triggered by a noxious stimulus below the level of the injury.
Test-Taking Strategy: Use the process of elimination. To answer this question correctly, it is necessary to know what causes autonomic dysreflexia. It results from the sudden exaggerated response of the sympathetic nervous system to a noxious stimulus. A massive sympathetic nervous system response causes severe hypertension. This would account for the throbbing headache (the correct answer) and cause flushing of the face and neck. Baroreceptors sense the sudden hypertension, causing a reflex bradycardia. The pulse and blood pressure changes with autonomic dysreflexia are actually the opposite of what would occur with hypovolemic shock. Review the signs of autonomic dysreflexia if you had difficulty with this question.
Level of Cognitive Ability: Analysis
Client Needs: Physiological Integrity
Integrated Concept/Process: Nursing Process/Data Collection
Content Area: Adult Health/Neurological
Reference: Black J, Hawks J, Keene A: *Medical-surgical nursing: clinical management for positive outcomes,* ed 6, Philadelphia, 2001, WB Saunders, p. 2064.

39. *Answer:* 4
Rationale: The client with spinal cord injury is at risk for autonomic dysreflexia with an injury above the level of T7. It is characterized by severe, throbbing headache, flushing of the face and neck, bradycardia, and sudden severe hypertension. Other signs include nasal stuffiness, blurred vision, nausea and sweating. It is a life-threatening syndrome triggered by a noxious stimulus below the level of the injury.
Test-Taking Strategy: Use the process of elimination. Begin to answer this question by eliminating options 1 and 3. The client in spinal shock would be hypotensive (not hypertensive), and the client's clinical picture does not match pulmonary embolism. (It also may be useful to know that autonomic dysreflexia does not occur until spinal shock resolves.) Recalling that malignant hypertension occurs with anesthesia would direct you to eliminate this option as well. Review the signs of autonomic dysreflexia if you had difficulty with this question.

Level of Cognitive Ability: Analysis
Client Needs: Physiological Integrity
Integrated Concept/Process: Nursing Process/Data Collection
Content Area: Adult Health/Neurological
Reference: Black J, Hawks J, Keene A: *Medical-surgical nursing: clinical management for positive outcomes,* ed 6, Philadelphia, 2001, WB Saunders, p. 2050.

40. *Answer:* 2
Rationale: The most frequent cause of autonomic dysreflexia is a distended bladder. Straight catheterization should be done every 4 to 6 hours, and Foley catheters should be checked frequently to prevent kinks in the tubing. Constipation and fecal impaction are other causes, so maintaining bowel regularity is important. Other causes include stimulation of the skin from tactile, thermal, or painful stimuli. The nurse administers care to minimize risk in these areas.
Test-Taking Strategy: The easiest way to answer questions of this nature is to remember that autonomic dysreflexia is caused by noxious stimuli to the bowel, bladder, or skin. With this in mind, you can easily eliminate each of the incorrect options for this question. Review the measures to minimize the risk of autonomic dysreflexia if you had difficulty with this question.
Level of Cognitive Ability: Application
Client Needs: Physiological Integrity
Integrated Concept/Process: Nursing Process/Implementation
Content Area: Adult Health/Neurological
Reference: Black J, Hawks J, Keene A: *Medical-surgical nursing: clinical management for positive outcomes,* ed 6, Philadelphia, 2001, WB Saunders, p. 2065.

41. *Answer:* 4
Rationale: Key nursing actions are to sit the client up in bed, remove the noxious stimulus, and bring the blood pressure under control with antihypertensive medication per protocol. The nurse can also clearly label the client's chart identifying the risk for autonomic dysreflexia. Client and family should be taught to recognize and later manage the signs and symptoms of this syndrome.
Test-Taking Strategy: Use the process of elimination. Note the word "immediately" in the stem. This is a clue that the first item in each option must be the first action. If you know to raise the head of the client's bed first (to try to minimize cerebral hypertension), this eliminates each of the incorrect options. Review immediate nursing interventions for the client experiencing autonomic dysreflexia if you had difficulty with this question.
Level of Cognitive Ability: Application
Client Needs: Physiological Integrity
Integrated Concept/Process: Nursing Process/Implementation
Content Area: Adult Health/Neurological
Reference: Black J, Hawks J, Keene A: *Medical-surgical nursing: clinical management for positive outcomes,* ed 6, Philadelphia, 2001, WB Saunders, p. 2065.

42. *Answer:* 3
Rationale: Reflex vasodilation below the level of spinal cord injury places the client at risk of orthostatic hypotension, which may be profound. Measures to minimize this include measuring vital signs before and during position changes, use of tilt table in early mobilization, and changing the client's position slowly. Venous pooling can be reduced by using TEDs or pneumatic boots. Vasopressor medications are used as per protocol.
Test-Taking Strategy: Use the process of elimination. Reflex vasodilation below the level of the injury causes hypotension. The question asks which is the least helpful in minimizing the hypotensive effect. Options 1, 2, and 4 are helpful and are thus eliminated. Knowing that quick position changes and movement would aggravate hypotension helps you be sure that you have selected the correct option. Review care to the client with spinal shock if you had difficulty with this question.
Level of Cognitive Ability: Application
Client Needs: Physiological Integrity
Integrated Concept/Process: Nursing Process/Implementation
Content Area: Adult Health/Neurological
Reference: Black J, Hawks J, Keene A: *Medical-surgical nursing: clinical management for positive outcomes,* ed 6, Philadelphia, 2001, WB Saunders, p. 2055.

43. *Answer:* 2
Rationale: Ptosis of the eyelid is due to pressure on and dysfunction of cranial nerve III. Once this occurs, it is ongoing and does not relate to LOC. Early changes in LOC relate to alertness and verbal responsiveness. Less frequent speech, slight slurring of speech, and mild drowsiness are early signs of decreasing LOC.
Test-Taking Strategy: Use the process of elimination. The question asks for which assessment is not an early sign of LOC deterioration. Thus the answer is either a later sign or one that is unrelated. If you know that LOC includes orientation, awareness, and verbal responsiveness, you would eliminate each of the incorrect options systematically. Review the early signs of decreasing LOC if you had difficulty with this question.
Level of Cognitive Ability: Analysis
Client Needs: Physiological Integrity
Integrated Concept/Process: Nursing Process/Data Collection
Content Area: Adult Health/Neurological
Reference: Black J, Hawks J, Keene A: *Medical-surgical nursing: clinical management for positive outcomes,* ed 6, Philadelphia, 2001, WB Saunders, p. 1875.

44. *Answer:* 3
Rationale: Aneurysm precautions include placing the client on bed rest in a quiet setting. Lights are kept dim to minimize environmental stimulation. Any activity that increases blood pressure or impedes venous return from the brain is prohibited, such as pushing, pulling, sneezing, coughing, or straining. The nurse provides all physical care to minimize increases in blood pressure. For the same reason, visitors, radio, television, and reading materials are prohibited or limited. Stimulants such as caffeine and nicotine are prohibited; decaffeinated coffee or tea may be used.
Test-Taking Strategy: Use the process of elimination. To answer this question you must understand that a global principle in aneurysm precautions is to limit the amount of

stimulation (in any form) that the client receives, and to prevent increased intracranial pressure (ICP). Options 1 and 2 are effective in promoting venous drainage from the brain (to keep ICP down) and are part of the precautions. Option 4 limits the amount of stimulation and exertion by the client and is also part of the precautions. Nicotine must be completely eliminated, which makes this the answer to the question. Review aneurysm precautions if you had difficulty with this question.
Level of Cognitive Ability: Application
Client Needs: Physiological Integrity
Integrated Concept/Process: Nursing Process/Implementation
Content Area: Adult Health/Neurological
Reference: Black J, Hawks J, Keene A: *Medical-surgical nursing: clinical management for positive outcomes*, ed 6, Philadelphia, 2001, WB Saunders, p. 1417.

45. *Answer:* 2
Rationale: Typically, seizure assessment includes the time the seizure began, part(s) of the body affected, type of movements and progression of the seizure, changes in pupil size, eye deviation or nystagmus, client condition during the seizure, and postictal status.
Test-Taking Strategy: Use the process of elimination. Option 2 identifies concern about vomiting and subsequent aspiration. The nurse is concerned about aspiration, not from vomiting, but from inhalation of the client's own saliva. Because all other options are standard assessments, option 2 is the answer to the question. Review nursing assessment during a seizure if you had difficulty answering this question.
Level of Cognitive Ability: Comprehension
Client Needs: Physiological Integrity
Integrated Concept/Process: Nursing Process/Data Collection
Content Area: Adult Health/Neurological
Reference: Black J, Hawks J, Keene A: *Medical-surgical nursing: clinical management for positive outcomes*, ed 6, Philadelphia, 2001, WB Saunders, p. 2277.

46. *Answer:* 3
Rationale: Seizure precautions may vary somewhat from agency to agency, but they generally have some commonalities. Usually an airway, oxygen, and suctioning equipment are kept available at the bedside. The side rails of the bed are padded, and the bed is kept in the lowest position. The client has an IV access in place to have a readily accessible route if IV anticonvulsant medications must be administered. The use of padded tongue blades is highly controversial, and they should not be kept at the bedside. Forcing a tongue blade into the mouth during a seizure will more likely harm the client who bites down during seizure activity. Risks include blocking the airway from improper placement, chipping the client's teeth, and subsequent risk of aspirating tooth fragments. If the client has an aura before the seizure, it may give the nurse enough time to place an oral airway before seizure activity begins.
Test-Taking Strategy: This question must be evaluated from the perspective of causing possible harm. No harm can come to the client from any of the options except for the tongue blade. Review seizure precautions if you had difficulty with this question.
Level of Cognitive Ability: Application
Client Needs: Safe, Effective Care Environment
Integrated Concept/Process: Nursing Process/Planning
Content Area: Adult Health/Neurological
Reference: Black J, Hawks J, Keene A: *Medical-surgical nursing: clinical management for positive outcomes*, ed 6, Philadelphia, 2001, WB Saunders, p. 2277.

47. *Answer:* 3
Rationale: Nursing actions during a seizure include providing for privacy, loosening restrictive clothing, removing pillow and raising side rails in bed, and placing the client on one side with the head flexed forward, if possible, to allow the tongue to fall forward and facilitate drainage. The limbs are never restrained, because the strong muscle contractions could cause the client harm. If the client is not in bed when seizure activity begins, the nurse lowers the client to the floor if possible, protects the head with a pad against injury, and moves furniture that may injure the client. Other aspects of care are as described for the client who is in bed.
Test-Taking Strategy: This question must be evaluated from the perspective of causing possible harm. No harm can come to the client from any of the options except for restraining the limbs. Avoid restraints. Review care to a client during a seizure if you had difficulty with this question.
Level of Cognitive Ability: Application
Client Needs: Physiological Integrity
Integrated Concept/Process: Nursing Process/Implementation
Content Area: Adult Health/Neurological
Reference: Black J, Hawks J, Keene A: *Medical-surgical nursing: clinical management for positive outcomes*, ed 6, Philadelphia, 2001, WB Saunders, p. 2277.

48. *Answer:* 3
Rationale: Typical anticonvulsant medication instructions include taking the dose daily to keep the blood level of the drug constant; having a serum drug level drawn before taking the morning dose, avoiding abruptly stopping the medication; avoiding alcohol, checking with the physician before taking over-the-counter medications, avoiding activities where alertness and coordination are required until medication effects are known, providing good oral hygiene and getting regular dental care, and carrying a Medic-Alert bracelet or tag.
Test-Taking Strategy: Use the process of elimination. Options 1 and 2 can be eliminated fairly easily after reading this question, as they are the least likely choices for being correct. Of the two remaining options, medications are not generally taken just before drawing therapeutic serum levels, because the results would be artificially high. This leaves oral hygiene as the correct answer, because of the risk of gingival hyperplasia. Review client education related to phenytoin (Dilantin) if you had difficulty with this question.
Level of Cognitive Ability: Analysis
Client Needs: Health Promotion and Maintenance
Integrated Concept/Process: Nursing Process/Evaluation
Content Area: Adult Health/Neurological
Reference: Black J, Hawks J, Keene A: *Medical-surgical nursing: clinical management for positive outcomes*, ed 6, Philadelphia, 2001, WB Saunders, p. 1927.

49. *Answer:* 2
Rationale: Hemiparesis is a weakness of the face, arm, and leg on one side. The client with one-sided hemiparesis benefits from having objects placed on the unaffected side and within reach. Other helpful activities with hemiparesis include ROM exercises to the affected side and muscle strengthening exercises to the unaffected side.
Test-Taking Strategy: Use the process of elimination. Begin to answer this question by eliminating options 3 and 4 as potentially hazardous to the client. Next distinguish between hemiparesis and unilateral neglect. The client with hemiparesis has weakness on one side; therefore objects should be place on the stronger side. With unilateral neglect, objects are placed on the affected side to train the client to attend to that part of the environment. Knowing this allows you to select option 2 over option 1. Review care to the client with hemiparesis if you had difficulty with this question.
Level of Cognitive Ability: Application
Client Needs: Safe, Effective Care Environment
Integrated Concept/Process: Nursing Process/Planning
Content Area: Adult Health/Neurological
Reference: Black J, Hawks J, Keene A: *Medical-surgical nursing: clinical management for positive outcomes,* ed 6, Philadelphia, 2001, WB Saunders, p. 1957.

50. *Answer:* 1
Rationale: Before the client with dysphagia is started on a diet, the gag and swallow reflexes must have returned. The client is assisted with meals as needed and is given ample time to chew and swallow. Food is placed on the unaffected side of the mouth. Liquids are thickened to avoid aspiration.
Test-Taking Strategy: Use the process of elimination. This question asks you to identify an incorrect item. Option 4 is generally a good action for all clients. Option 3 is correct because the client has better sensation and motion on the unaffected side of the mouth. This narrows your options to two opposing concepts: thin vs. thick liquids. Thickened liquids are easier for the client with impaired facial motion and swallowing ability to manage. Knowing this enables you to choose option 1 as the action to avoid. Review care to the client with residual dysphagia if you had difficulty with this question.
Level of Cognitive Ability: Application
Client Needs: Physiological Integrity
Integrated Concept/Process: Nursing Process/Implementation
Content Area: Adult Health/Neurological
Reference: Black J, Hawks J, Keene A: *Medical-surgical nursing: clinical management for positive outcomes,* ed 6, Philadelphia, 2001, WB Saunders, p. 652.

51. *Answer:* 3
Rationale: Homonymous hemianopsia is loss of half of the visual field. The client with homonymous hemianopsia should have objects placed in the intact field of vision, and the nurse should also approach the client from the intact side. The nurse instructs the client to scan the environment to overcome the visual deficit and does client teaching from within the intact field of vision. The nurse encourages the use of personal eyeglasses if they are available.
Test-Taking Strategy: Use the process of elimination. To answer this question accurately, you must be able to distinguish between homonymous hemianopsia and unilateral neglect. Clients are approached differently with these two deficits. The similarity is that the client must be taught to scan the environment, which is also the answer to this question. Review the concept of homonymous hemianopsia if you are unfamiliar with it.
Level of Cognitive Ability: Analysis
Client Needs: Health Promotion and Maintenance
Integrated Concept/Process: Nursing Process/Evaluation
Content Area: Adult Health/Neurological
Reference: Black J, Hawks J, Keene A: *Medical-surgical nursing: clinical management for positive outcomes,* ed 6, Philadelphia, 2001, WB Saunders, p. 1959.

52. *Answer:* 2
Rationale: Clients with aphasia after CVA often fatigue easily and have a short attention span. General guidelines when trying to communicate with the aphasic client include speaking more slowly and allowing adequate response time, listening to and watching attempts to communicate, and trying to put the client at ease with a caring and understanding manner. Avoid shouting (because the client is not deaf), appearing rushed for a response, and letting family members give all the responses for the client.
Test-Taking Strategy: This question tests a fundamental concept in communicating with the aphasic client. If this question was difficult, review these communication strategies.
Level of Cognitive Ability: Application
Client Needs: Psychosocial Integrity
Integrated Concept/Process: Communication and Documentation
Content Area: Adult Health/Neurological
Reference: Black J, Hawks J, Keene A: *Medical-surgical nursing: clinical management for positive outcomes,* ed 6, Philadelphia, 2001, WB Saunders, p. 1957.

53. *Answer:* 3
Rationale: Placing an eye patch over one eye in the client with diplopia removes the second image and restores more normal vision. The patch is alternated on a daily basis to maintain the strength of the extraocular muscles of the eyes.
Test-Taking Strategy: Use the process of elimination. Knowing that an eye patch will help diplopia only while it is worn, you first eliminate options 1 and 2. If you know that the extraocular muscles weaken with eye patch use, you will select option 3 over 4, as these are small muscles that would lose strength fairly rapidly. Review care to the client with diplopia if you had difficulty with this question.
Level of Cognitive Ability: Comprehension
Client Needs: Physiological Integrity
Integrated Concept/Process: Teaching/Learning
Content Area: Adult Health/Neurological
Reference: Black J, Hawks J, Keene A: *Medical-surgical nursing: clinical management for positive outcomes,* ed 6, Philadelphia, 2001, WB Saunders, p. 1885.

54. *Answer:* 3
Rationale: Myasthenia gravis can often be diagnosed based on clinical signs and symptoms. The diagnosis can be confirmed by injecting the client with a dose of Tensilon. This medication

inhibits the breakdown of an enzyme in the neuromuscular junction, so more acetylcholine binds onto receptors. Muscle strengthening for 3 to 5 minutes after this injection confirms a diagnosis of myasthenia gravis. Another medication, neostigmine (Prostigmin), may also be used because the effect lasts for 1 to 2 hours, allowing for better analysis. For either medication, atropine should be available as the antidote.
Test-Taking Strategy: Knowledge of the purpose and expected findings of the Tensilon test is required to answer this question successfully. Review this test if you had difficulty with this question.
Level of Cognitive Ability: Analysis
Client Needs: Physiological Integrity
Integrated Concept/Process: Nursing Process/Data Collection
Content Area: Pharmacology
Reference: Black J, Hawks J, Keene A: *Medical-surgical nursing: clinical management for positive outcomes,* ed 6, Philadelphia, 2001, WB Saunders, p. 2021.

55. *Answer:* 2
Rationale: The client has speech that is nasal in tone and dysarthritic because of cranial nerve involvement of the muscles governing speech. The nurse listens attentively and verbally, verifies what the client has said, asks questions requiring a yes or no response, and develops alternative communication methods (letter board, picture board, pen and paper, flash cards). Encouraging the client to speak quickly is unsuccessful and counterproductive.
Test-Taking Strategy: Some techniques are useful in communicating with clients with speech impairment, regardless of the specific cause of the difficulty. Options 3 and 4 are classic examples of alternative communication methods that are useful, so you would eliminate them. Because option 1 is also helpful, this leaves option 2 as the correct answer. Speaking quickly is difficult for a client with a speech impairment. Review these communication techniques if you had difficulty with this question.
Level of Cognitive Ability: Application
Client Needs: Psychosocial Integrity
Integrated Concept/Process: Communication and Documentation
Content Area: Adult Health/Neurological
Reference: Black J, Hawks J, Keene A: *Medical-surgical nursing: clinical management for positive outcomes,* ed 6, Philadelphia, 2001, WB Saunders, p. 2021.

56. *Answer:* 3
Rationale: Myasthenic crisis is often caused by undermedication and responds to administration of cholinergic medications such as neostigmine (Prostigmin) and pyridostigmine (Mestinon). Cholinergic crisis (the opposite problem) is caused by excess medication and responds to withholding of medications. Too little exercise and fatty food intake are incorrect. Overexertion and overeating could possibly trigger myasthenic crisis.
Test-Taking Strategy: To answer this question most easily, it is necessary to know that undermedication is a common cause of myasthenic crisis. Review the causes of this type of crisis if you are unfamiliar with them.
Level of Cognitive Ability: Comprehension
Client Needs: Physiological Integrity
Integrated Concept/Process: Nursing Process/Data Collection
Content Area: Adult Health/Neurological
Reference: Black J, Hawks J, Keene A: *Medical-surgical nursing: clinical management for positive outcomes,* ed 6, Philadelphia, 2001, WB Saunders, p. 2022.

57. *Answer:* 2
Rationale: Clients with myasthenia gravis are taught to space out activities over the day to conserve energy and restore muscle strength. It is important to take medications correctly to maintain optimal blood levels. Muscle strengthening exercises are not helpful and can fatigue the client. Overeating, heat, crowds, erratic sleep habits, and emotional stress cause symptoms to exacerbate.
Test-Taking Strategy: Use the process of elimination. If you know that common causes of myasthenic and cholinergic crises are undermedication and overmedication, respectively, you should be able to easily eliminate each of the incorrect options to this question. No other option would prevent both of those complications. It is extremely important that these clients take medications on time to maintain therapeutic blood levels. Review measures to prevent myasthenic and cholinergic crises if you are unfamiliar with them.
Level of Cognitive Ability: Application
Client Needs: Health Promotion and Maintenance
Integrated Concept/Process: Nursing Process/Implementation
Content Area: Adult Health/Neurological
Reference: Black J, Hawks J, Keene A: *Medical-surgical nursing: clinical management for positive outcomes,* ed 6, Philadelphia, 2001, WB Saunders, p. 2022.

58. *Answer:* 3
Rationale: Most ongoing treatment for myasthenia gravis is done in outpatient settings, and the client needs to be aware of the lifestyle changes needed to maintain independence. Taking medications an hour before mealtime gives greater muscle strength for chewing. The client should have portable suction equipment and a portable resuscitation bag available in case of respiratory distress. The client should carry medical identification about the condition. The client should avoid activities that could worsen the symptoms, including stress, infection, heat, surgery, and alcohol.
Test-Taking Strategy: Use the process of elimination. Options 2 and 4 are reasonable courses of action and can be eliminated. To discriminate between the remaining two options, you need to know that premedication an hour before meals gives strength to the muscles (for chewing and swallowing) and that heat and infection (crowds at the beach) trigger myasthenic crisis. Review client education points with myasthenia gravis if you had difficulty with this question.
Level of Cognitive Ability: Comprehension
Client Needs: Health Promotion and Maintenance
Integrated Concept/Process: Teaching/Learning
Content Area: Adult Health/Neurological
Reference: Black J, Hawks J, Keene A: *Medical-surgical nursing: clinical management for positive outcomes,* ed 6, Philadelphia, 2001, WB Saunders, p. 2020.

59. *Answer:* 3
Rationale: The client with Parkinson's disease tends to become withdrawn and depressed, and should become an active participant in own care to prevent this. There should be planned activities throughout the day to inhibit daytime sleeping and boredom. The nurse gives the client encouragement and praises the client for perseverance. Exercise helps prevent progression of the disease and self-care improves self-esteem.
Test-Taking Strategy: Use the process of elimination. Options 1 and 4 are the least plausible of all available answers and may be eliminated first. Option 2 is well intentioned, but is not therapeutic in helping the client to cope with the disease. Option 3 is the best choice. Review care to the client with Parkinson's disease if you had difficulty with this question.
Level of Cognitive Ability: Application
Client Needs: Psychosocial Integrity
Integrated Concept/Process: Nursing Process/Planning
Content Area: Adult Health/Neurological
Reference: Black J, Hawks J, Keene A: *Medical-surgical nursing: clinical management for positive outcomes*, ed 6, Philadelphia, 2001, WB Saunders, p. 2017.

60. *Answer:* 1
Rationale: Parkinsonian crisis can occur with emotional trauma or sudden withdrawal of medications. The client exhibits severe tremors, rigidity, and bradykinesia. The client also displays anxiety, is diaphoretic, and has tachycardia and hyperpnea. The client should be placed in a quiet, dim room and respiratory and cardiac support should be available.
Test-Taking Strategy: Use the process of elimination. Option 4 is not indicated and is eliminated first. Option 3 is not an immediate concern and is eliminated next. Of the remaining two options, there is nothing about parkinsonian crisis that warrants placement of an nasogastric tube. This leaves the correct option, which is to put the client in a dim, quiet room and provide for support of cardiac and respiratory symptoms. Review nursing care for parkinsonian crisis if you had difficulty with this question.
Level of Cognitive Ability: Application
Client Needs: Safe, Effective Care Environment
Integrated Concept/Process: Nursing Process/Implementation
Content Area: Adult Health/Neurological
Reference: Black J, Hawks J, Keene A: *Medical-surgical nursing: clinical management for positive outcomes*, ed 6, Philadelphia, 2001, WB Saunders, p. 2020.

61. *Answer:* 2
Rationale: The client with Parkinson's disease should exercise in the morning when energy levels are highest. The client should avoid sitting in soft, deep chairs, because they are difficult to arise from. The client can rock back and forth to initiate movement. The client should buy clothes with Velcro fasteners and slide locking buckles to support the ability to dress self.
Test-Taking Strategy: Use the process of elimination. Option 1 is not useful to clients with fatigue from any disorder, so this option may be eliminated first. Knowing that the client with Parkinson's disease has difficulty with movement and dexterity helps to eliminate options 3 and 4. Review client teaching points with Parkinson's disease if you had difficulty with this question.
Level of Cognitive Ability: Comprehension
Client Needs: Health Promotion and Maintenance
Integrated Concept/Process: Teaching/Learning
Content Area: Adult Health/Neurological
Reference: Black J, Hawks J, Keene A: *Medical-surgical nursing: clinical management for positive outcomes*, ed 6, Philadelphia, 2001, WB Saunders, p. 2018.

62. *Answer:* 4
Rationale: Facial pain can be minimized by using cotton pads to wash the face, and by using water at room temperature. The client should chew on the unaffected side of the mouth, eat a soft diet, and take in foods and beverages at room temperature. If tooth brushing triggers pain, an oral rinse after meals is sometimes helpful instead.
Test-Taking Strategy: Use the process of elimination. To answer this question most easily, you should know that the pain of trigeminal neuralgia is triggered by mechanical or thermal stimuli. This will help you systematically eliminate each of the incorrect options. Very hot or cold foods are likely to trigger the pain, not relieve it. Review these client education points if you had difficulty with this question.
Level of Cognitive Ability: Comprehension
Client Needs: Health Promotion and Maintenance
Integrated Concept/Process: Teaching/Learning
Content Area: Adult Health/Neurological
Reference: Black J, Hawks J, Keene A: *Medical-surgical nursing: clinical management for positive outcomes*, ed 6, Philadelphia, 2001, WB Saunders, p. 1995.

REFERENCES

Black J, Hawks J, Keene A: *Medical-surgical nursing: clinical management for positive outcomes*, ed 6, Philadelphia, 2001, WB Saunders.

Chernecky C, Berger B: *Laboratory tests and diagnostic procedures*, ed 3, Philadelphia, 2001, WB Saunders.

Clark J, Queener S, Karb V: *Pharmacologic basis of nursing practice*, ed 6, St Louis, 2000, Mosby.

DeWit S: *Fundamental concepts and skills for nursing*, Philadelphia, 2001, WB Saunders.

Hodgson B, Kizior R: *Saunders nursing drug handbook 2002*, Philadelphia, 2002, WB Saunders.

Ignatavicius D, Workman M: *Medical-surgical nursing: critical thinking for collaborative care*, ed 4, Philadelphia, 2002, WB Saunders.

Lehne R: *Pharmacology for nursing care*, ed 4, Philadelphia, 2001, WB Saunders.

Potter P, Perry A: *Fundamentals of nursing*, ed 5, St Louis, 2001, Mosby.

Perry A, Potter P: *Clinical nursing skills and techniques*, ed 5, St Louis, 2002, Mosby

Neurological Medications

I. ANTIMYASTHENIC MEDICATIONS

A. Description
1. Relieve muscle weakness associated with myasthenia gravis by blocking acetycholine breakdown at the neuromuscular junction
2. Used to treat or diagnose myasthenia gravis or to distinguish cholinergic crisis from myasthenic crisis
3. Neostigmine bromide (Prostigmin), pyridostigmine bromide (Mestinon), ambenonium (Mytelase) are used to control myasthenic symptoms
4. Edrophonium chloride (Tensilon) is used to diagnose myasthenia gravis and to distinguish cholinergic crisis from myasthenic crisis

B. Medications (Box 55-1)

C. Side effects: cholinergic crisis (Box 55-2)

D. Implementation
1. Assess neuromuscular status, including reflexes, muscle strength, and gait
2. Monitor the client for signs and symptoms of medication overdose (cholinergic crisis) and underdose (myasthenic crisis)
3. Instruct the client to take medications on time to prevent weakness, because weakness can impair the client's ability to breathe and swallow

BOX 55-1

Antimyasthenic Medications

Edrophonium chloride (Tensilon, Enlon)
Neostigmine bromide (Prostigmin bromide)
Pyridostigmine bromide (Mestinon)
Ambenonium chloride (Mytelase)

BOX 55-2

Signs of Cholinergic Crisis

GI disturbances
Abdominal cramps
Nausea, vomiting, diarrhea
Increased salivation and tearing
Increased bronchial secretions
Sweating
Miosis
Hypertension

4. Instruct the client to take the medication before meals for best absorption
5. Instruct the client to wear a Medic-Alert bracelet
6. Note that antimyasthenic therapy is lifelong
7. Evaluate for medication effectiveness, which is based on the improvement of neuromuscular symptoms or strength without cholinergic signs and symptoms
8. When administering edrophonium (Tensilon), have emergency resuscitation equipment on hand and atropine sulfate available for cholinergic crisis

E. **Tensilon test**
1. Tensilon is injected intravenously (IV)
2. The **Tensilon test** can cause ventricular fibrillation and cardiac arrest
3. Atropine sulfate is the antidote for overdose
4. Diagnosis of myasthenia gravis: most myasthenic clients will show a marked improvement in muscle tone within 30 to 60 seconds after injection, and the muscle improvement lasts 4 to 5 minutes
5. Diagnosis of cholinergic crisis (overdose with anticholinesterase) or myasthenic crisis (undermedication)

a. In cholinergic crisis, muscle tone does not improve after the administration of Tensilon, and muscle twitching may be noted around the eyes and face
b. A Tensilon injection makes the client in cholinergic crisis temporarily worse (negative **Tensilon test**)
c. A Tensilon injection temporarily improves the condition when the client is in myasthenic crisis (positive **Tensilon test**)

II. ANTIPARKINSONIAN MEDICATIONS

A. Description
1. Restore the balance of the neurotransmitters acetylcholine and dopamine in the central nervous system (CNS), decreasing the signs and symptoms of Parkinson's disease
2. These medications include the dopaminergics, which stimulate the dopamine receptors, and the anticholinergics, which block the cholinergic receptors
3. Used for drug-induced parkinsonism, in which neuroleptic agents block dopamine receptors in the CNS, leading to functional loss of dopamine activity
4. Used for Parkinson's disease, in which dopamine-containing neurons in the basal ganglia are destroyed or deficient, which causes loss of fine motor control

B. Dopaminergic medications
1. Description
a. Stimulate the dopamine receptors
b. Increase the amount of dopamine available in the CNS or enhance neurotransmission of dopamine
c. Contraindicated in cardiac, renal, or psychiatric disorders
d. Levodopa taken with a monoamine oxidase inhibitor antidepressant can cause a hypertensive crisis
2. Medications (Box 55-3)
3. Side effects
a. Dyskinesia
b. Involuntary body movements
c. Tachycardia
d. Nausea and vomiting
e. Urinary retention
f. Constipation
g. Dizziness
h. Orthostatic hypotension
i. Confusion
j. Mood changes
k. Hallucinations
4. Implementation
a. Assess vital signs
b. Assess for risk of injury
c. Instruct the client to take the medication with food if nausea and vomiting occur
d. Assess for signs and symptoms of parkinsonism, such as rigidity, tremors, akinesia and bradykinesia, and a stooped-forward posture, shuffling gait, and masked facies
e. Monitor for signs of dyskinesia
f. Instruct the client taking carbidopa-levodopa (Sinemet) to eat low-protein foods, because high-protein diets interfere with medication transport to the CNS
g. Instruct the client to change positions slowly to minimize orthostatic hypotension
h. Instruct the client not to discontinue the medication abruptly
i. Instruct the client to report side effects and symptoms of dyskinesia
j. Instruct the client to avoid alcohol
k. Monitor the client for improvement in signs and symptoms of parkinsonism without the development of severe side effects from the medications
l. Inform the client that urine or perspiration may be discolored and that this is harmless, but it may stain the clothing
m. Advise the client with diabetes mellitus that glucose testing should not be done through urine testing because the results will not be reliable
n. When administering levodopa, instruct the client to avoid excessive vitamin B_6 intake to prevent medication reactions

BOX 55-3

Medications to treat Parkinson's Disease

MEDICATIONS AFFECTING THE AMOUNT OF DOPAMINE
Amantadine (Symmetrel)
Bromocriptine (Parlodel)
Carbidopa-levodopa (Sinemet)
Levodopa (Larodopa, Dopar)
Pergolide mesylate (Permax)
Pramipexole (Mirapex)
Ropinirole (Requip)
Selegiline HCl (Carbex, Eldepryl)
Tolcapone (Tasmar)

ANTICHOLINERGICS
Benztropine mesylate (Cogentin)
Biperiden HCl (Akineton)
Ethopropazine HCl (Parsidol)
Procyclidine HCl (Kemadrin)
Trihexyphenidyl HCl (Artane)

ANTIHISTAMINE
Diphenhydramine HCl (Benadryl)

C. Anticholinergic medications
 1. Description
  a. Block the cholinergic receptors in the CNS, thereby suppressing acetylcholine activity
  b. Reduce the rigidity and some of the tremors but have a minimal effect on the bradykinesia
  c. Contraindicated in clients with glaucoma
  d. The client with chronic obstructive lung disease can develop dry, thick mucus secretions
 2. Medications (Box 55-3)
 3. Side effects
  a. Blurred vision
  b. Dry mouth and dry secretions
  c. Increased pulse rate
  d. Constipation
  e. Urinary retention
  f. Restlessness and confusion
  g. Photophobia
 4. Implementation
  a. Monitor vital signs
  b. Assess for risk of injury
  c. Assess for signs and symptoms of parkinsonism such as rigidity, tremors, akinesia, and bradykinesia; a stooped-forward posture, shuffling gait, and masked facies
  d. Monitor the client for improvement in signs and symptoms
  e. Assess the client's bowel and urinary function and monitor for urinary retention and constipation
  f. Monitor for involuntary movements
  g. Encourage the client to avoid alcohol, smoking, caffeine, and aspirin to decrease gastric acidity
  h. Instruct the client to consult with the physician before taking any nonprescription medications
  i. Instruct the client to minimize dry mouth by increasing fluid intake and by using ice chips, hard candy, or gum
  j. Instruct the client to prevent constipation by increasing fluid and fiber in the diet
  k. Instruct the client to use sunglasses in direct sun because of possible photophobia
  l. Instruct the client to have routine eye examinations to assess for intraocular pressure

III. ANTICONVULSANT MEDICATIONS (Table 55-1)

A. Description
 1. Used to depress abnormal neuronal discharges and prevent the spread of seizures
 2. Used with caution in clients on anticoagulants, aspirin, sulfonamides, cimetidine (Tagamet), and antipsychotics
 3. Absorption is decreased with the use of antacids, calcium preparations, and antineoplastic medications

TABLE 55-1

Anticonvulsant Medications

Medication	Therapeutic Serum Range
Phenytoin (Dilantin)	10-20 μg/mL
Carbamazepine (Tegretol)	3-14 μg/mL
Mephenytoin (Mesantoin)	25-40 μg/mL
Ethotoin (Peganone)	10-50 μg/mL
Phenobarbital (Luminal)	15-40 μg/mL
Primidone (Mysoline)	5-10 μg/mL
Amobarbital (Amytal)	1-5 μg/mL
Mephobarbital (Mebaral)	15-40 μg/mL
Clonazepam (Klonopin)	20-80 ng/mL
Lorazepam (Ativan)	50-240 ng/mL
Ethosuximide (Zarontin)	40-100 μg/mL
Valproic acid (Depakene)	40-100 μg/mL

B. Implementation for clients on anticonvulsants
 1. Initiate seizure precautions
 2. Monitor urinary output
 3. Monitor liver and renal function tests
 4. Monitor for signs of medication toxicity, which would include CNS depression, ataxia, nausea, vomiting, drowsiness, dizziness, restlessness, and visual disturbances
 5. If a seizure occurs, assess seizure activity, including location and duration
 6. Protect client from hazards in the environment during a seizure
C. Client education (Box 55-4)
D. Hydantoins (Box 55-5)
 1. Used to treat seizures
 2. Phenytoin (Dilantin) is also used to treat dysrhythmias
 3. Side effects
  a. Gingival hyperplasia
  b. Reddened gums that bleed easily
  c. Slurred speech
  d. Confusion
  e. Depression
  f. Nausea and vomiting
  g. Constipation
  h. Headaches
  i. Blood dyscrasias: decreased platelet count and decreased white blood cell (WBC) count
  j. Elevated blood glucose
  k. Alopecia
  l. Hirsutism
 4. Implementation
  a. Oral tube feedings may interfere with the absorption of oral phenytoin and diminish the medication's effectiveness; therefore

BOX 55-4

Client Education: Anticonvulsants

Take anticonvulsant with food to decrease GI irritation, but avoid milk and antacids, which impair absorption
If taking liquid medication, shake well before ingesting
Do not discontinue medication
Avoid alcohol
Avoid over-the-counter medications
Wear a Medic-Alert bracelet
Use caution when driving or performing activities that require alertness
Maintain good oral hygiene and use a soft toothbrush
Stress importance of preventive dental-checkups
Stress importance of follow-up care with periodic blood studies related to determining toxicity
Monitor serum glucose levels (diabetes mellitus)
Stress that urine may be a harmless pink-red or red-brown color
Report symptoms of sore throat, bruising, and nosebleeds, which may indicate a blood dyscrasia
Inform the physician if adverse reactions occur, such as gingivitis, nystagmus, slurred speech, rash, or dizziness

BOX 55-5

Hydantoins

Phenytoin (Dilantin)
Mephenytoin (Mesantoin)
Ethotoin (Peganone)
Fosphenytoin (Cerebyx)

feedings should be scheduled as far as possible from the phenytoin administration
b. Monitor therapeutic serum levels to assess for toxicity
c. Monitor for signs of toxicity
d. Instruct the client about the importance of good oral hygiene and regular dental examinations
e. Instruct the client to consult with the physician before taking other medications to ensure compatibility with anticonvulsants

E. Barbiturates (Box 55-6)
1. Used for tonic-clonic seizures and acute episodes of seizures resulting from status epilepticus

BOX 55-6

Barbiturates

Phenobarbital
Primidone (Mysoline)
Amobarbital (Amytal)
Mephobarbital (Mebaral)

2. May also be used as adjuncts to anesthesia
3. Side effects
   a. Drowsiness
   b. Dizziness
   c. Hypotension
   d. Respiratory depression
   e. Tolerance to the medication

F. Benzodiazepines (Box 55-7)
1. To treat absence seizures
2. Diazepam (Valium) is used to treat status epilepticus, anxiety, and skeletal muscle spasms
3. Clorazepate (Tranxene) is used as adjunctive therapy for partial seizures
4. Side effects
   a. Ataxia
   b. Respiratory and cardiac depression
   c. Medication tolerance and drug dependency

G. Succinimides (Box 55-8)
1. Used to treat absence seizures
2. Side effects
   a. Anorexia, nausea, vomiting
   b. Blood dyscrasias

H. Oxazolidinediones (Box 55-9)
1. Used for absence seizures
2. Side effects
   a. Sedation
   b. Photophobia

I. Valproates (Box 55-10)

BOX 55-7

Benzodiazepines

Clonazepam (Klonopin)
Clorazepate (Tranxene)
Diazepam (Valium)
Lorazepam (Ativan)

BOX 55-8

Succinimides

Ethosuximide (Zarontin)
Methsuximide (Celontin)
Phensuximide (Milontin)

BOX 55-9

Oxazolidinediones

Paramethadione (Paradione)
Trimethadione (Tridione)

BOX 55-10

Valproates

Valproic acid (Depakene)
Divalproex sodium (Depakote)

1. Used to treat tonic-clonic, partial, myoclonic, and psychomotor seizures
2. Side effects
   a. Nausea
   b. Vomiting
   c. Abdominal cramps
   d. Diarrhea
   e. Constipation
   f. Hepatotoxicity

J. Iminostilbenes (Box 55-11)
1. Used to treat seizure disorders that have not responded to other anticonvulsants
2. Used to treat trigeminal neuralgia
3. Side effects
   a. Drowsiness
   b. Dizziness
   c. Nausea
   d. Vomiting
   e. Constipation or diarrhea
   f. Visual abnormalities
   g. Dry mouth
   h. Headache

IV. CENTRAL NERVOUS SYSTEM STIMULANTS

A. Description
1. Amphetamines and caffeine stimulate the cerebral cortex of the brain (Box 55-12)
2. Analeptics and caffeine act on the brainstem and medulla to stimulate respiration
3. Anorexiants act on the cerebral cortex and hypothalamus to suppress appetite (Box 55-13)
4. Used to treat narcolepsy and attention deficit hyperactivity disorders
5. Used to treat respiratory depression (Box 55-14)
6. Used as adjunctive therapy for exogenous obesity

B. Side effects
1. Irritability
2. Restlessness
3. Tremors
4. Insomnia
5. Heart palpitations
6. Tachycardia
7. Hypertension
8. Dry mouth
9. Anorexia
10. Weight loss
11. Diarrhea or constipation
12. Impotence
13. Dependence and tolerance

C. Implementation
1. Monitor vital signs
2. Assess mental status
3. Assess height, weight, and growth of the child
4. Monitor complete blood count, WBC, and platelet counts before and during therapy
5. Monitor for side effects
6. Monitor sleep patterns
7. Monitor for withdrawal symptoms such as nausea, vomiting, weakness, and headache
8. Instruct the client to take the medication before meals
9. Instruct the client to avoid foods and beverages containing caffeine to prevent additional stimulation
10. Instruct the client to read labels on over-the-counter products because many contain caffeine

BOX 55-11
Other Anticonvulsants

Carbamazepine (Tegretol)
Felbamate (Felbatol)
Gabapentin (Neurontin)
Lamotrigine (Lamictal)
Tiagabine (Gabitril)
Topiramate (Topamax)

BOX 55-12
Amphetamines

Amphetamine sulfate
Dextroamphetamine sulfate (Dexedrine)
Methamphetamine HCl (Desoxyn)
Methylphenidate HCl (Ritalin)
Pemoline (Cylert)

BOX 55-13
Anorexiants

Diethylpropion HCl (Tenuate, Tepanil)
Mazindol (Sanorex, Mazanor)
Phendimetrazine (Anorex, Bontril, Melfiat, Obalan)
Phentermine HCl (Fastin, Apidex, Zantryl)
Benzphetamine HCl (Didrex)
Phenylpropanolamine (Acutrim, Dexatrim, Phenyldrine)
Sibutramine (Meridia)

BOX 55-14
Treating Respiratory Depression

Aminophylline
Caffeine
Doxapram (Dopram)
Theophylline

11. Instruct the client to avoid alcohol
12. Instruct the client not to discontinue the medication abruptly
13. Instruct the client to take the last daily dose of the CNS stimulant at least 6 hours before bedtime to prevent insomnia
14. Monitor for drug dependence and abuse with amphetamines
15. If a child is taking a CNS stimulant, instruct the parents to notify the school nurse
16. Monitor for calming effects of CNS stimulants within 3 to 4 weeks on children with attention deficit hyperactivity disorder
17. Monitor growth in the child on long-term therapy with methylphenidate HCl (Ritalin)

V. NONNARCOTIC ANALGESICS

A. Nonsteroidal antiinflammatory drugs (NSAIDs) (Box 55-15)
1. Description
a. NSAIDs are aspirin and aspirin-like medications that inhibit the synthesis of prostaglandins
b. They act as an analgesic to relieve pain, as an antipyretic to reduce body temperature, and as an anticoagulant to inhibit platelet aggregation
c. Used to relieve inflammation and pain and in the treatment of rheumatoid arthritis, bursitis, tendinitis, osteoarthritis, and acute gout
d. Contraindicated in hypersensitivity or liver or renal disease
e. Aspirin should not be taken by children with flu symptoms because of the risk of Reye's syndrome
f. Aspirin should not be taken if the client is on an anticoagulant
g. Aspirin and an NSAID should not be taken together because aspirin decreases the blood level and the effectiveness of the NSAID
h. NSAIDs can increase the effects of warfarin (Coumadin), sulfonamides, cephalosporins, and phenytoin (Dilantin)
i. Hypoglycemia can result if ibuprofen (Motrin) is taken with insulin or an oral hypoglycemic medication
j. A high risk of toxicity exists if ibuprofen is taken concurrently with calcium blockers
2. Side effects (Table 55-2)
3. Implementation
a. Assess client for allergies
b. Obtain a medication history and medical history on the client
c. Assess for history of gastric upset or bleeding or liver disease
d. Assess the client for GI upset during medication administration
e. Monitor for edema
f. Monitor serum salicylate (aspirin) level when the client is taking high doses
g. Monitor for signs of bleeding such as tarry stools, bleeding gums, petechiae, ecchymosis, and purpura
h. Instruct the client to take the medication with water, milk, or food

BOX 55-15

Nonsteroidal Antiinflammatory Drugs (NSAIDs)

ACETAMINOPHEN
Acetaminophen (Tylenol)

ASPIRIN AND OTHER SALICYLATES
Aspirin (acetylsalicylic acid) (A.S.A., Aspergum, Bayer, Ecotrin)
Aspirin (acetylsalicylic acid), buffered (Alka-Seltzer, Bufferin)
Choline salicylate (Arthropan)
Diflunisal (Dolobid)
Magnesium salicylate (Doan's, Magan)
Olsalazine (Dipentum)
Salsalate (Amigesic, Disalcid)
Sulfasalazine (Azulfidine)

PROPIONIC ACID DERIVATIVES
Fenoprofen (Nalfon)
Flurbipofen (Ansaid)
Ibuprofen (Motrin, Advil, Nuprin, Medipren)
Ketoprofen (Orudis)
Naproxen (Anaprox, Naprosyn)
Oxaprozin (Daypro)

OTHER NSAIDs
Diclofenac (Voltaren)
Etodolac (Lodine)
Indomethacin (Indocin)
Ketorolac tromethamine (Toradol)
Meclofenamate (Meclomen)
Mefenamic acid (Ponstel)
Nabumetone (Relafen)
Phenylbutazone (Butazolidin, Butazone)
Piroxicam (Feldene)
Sulindac (Clinoril)
Tolmetin (Tolectin)

TABLE 55-2

Side Effects of Aspirin and NSAIDs

Aspirin	NSAIDs
Drowsiness	Hypotension
Tinnitus	Sodium and water retention
Headaches	Gastric irritation
Flushing	Blood dyscrasias
Dizziness	Dizziness
GI symptoms	Tinnitus
Visual changes	Pruritus

i. Enteric-coated form or buffered form of aspirin can be taken to decrease gastric distress
j. Instruct the client that enteric-coated tablets cannot be crushed or broken
k. Advise the client to inform other health care professionals if they are taking high doses of aspirin
l. Note that aspirin should be discontinued 3 to 7 days before surgery to reduce the risk of bleeding
m. Instruct the client to avoid alcoholic beverages

B. Acetaminophen (Tylenol)
1. Description
a. Inhibits prostaglandin synthesis
b. Used to decrease pain and fever
c. Contraindicated in hepatic or renal disease, alcoholism, and hypersensitivity
2. Side effects
a. Anorexia, nausea, vomiting
b. Rash
c. Hypoglycemia
d. Oliguria
e. Hepatotoxicity
3. Implementation
a. Monitor vital signs
b. Assess the client for history of liver dysfunction
c. Monitor for hepatic damage, which includes nausea, vomiting, diarrhea, and abdominal pain
d. Monitor liver enzyme tests
e. Instruct the client that self-medication should not be used longer than 10 days for an adult and 5 days for a child
f. Note that the antidote for Tylenol is acetylcysteine (Mucomyst)
g. Evaluate for the effectiveness of the medication

VI. NARCOTIC ANALGESICS

A. Description
1. Suppress pain impulses but can suppress respiration and coughing by acting on the respiratory and cough center in the medulla of the brainstem
2. Can produce euphoria and sedation
3. Can cause physical dependence
4. Used for relief of mild, moderate, or severe pain

B. Medications (Box 55-16)
1. Codeine sulfate
a. Effective cough suppressant at low doses
b. Can cause constipation
2. Hydromorphone HCl (Dilaudid)
a. Can decrease respiration
b. Can cause constipation
3. Meperidine HCl (Demerol)
a. Can cause hypotension and dizziness
b. Used for acute pain and as a preoperative medication
c. Can **increase intracranial pressure** in head injuries
d. Contraindicated in head injuries and **increased intracranial pressure**, respiratory disorders, hypotension, shock, severe hepatic and renal disease, and in clients taking monoamine oxidase inhibitors
e. Should not be taken with alcohol or sedative hypnotics because it may increase the CNS depression
4. Morphine sulfate
a. Can cause respiratory depression, orthostatic hypotension, and constipation
b. May cause nausea and vomiting because of increased vestibular sensitivity

BOX 55-16

Narcotic Analgesics

Codeine sulfate; Codeine phosphate
Hydromorphone HCl (Dilaudid, HydroStat IR, PMS-Hydromorphone)
Meperidine HCl (Demerol)
Morphine sulfate
Oxycodone HCl with acetaminophen (Percocet)
Oxycodone with aspirin (Percodan)
Propoxyphene napsylate (Darvon-N)
Buprenorphine HCl (Buprenex)
Butorphanol tartrate (Stadol, Stadol NS)
Dezocine (Dalgan)
Nalbuphine HCl (Nubain)
Methadone HCl (Dolophine, Methadose)
Pentazocine HCl (Talwin)
Hydrocodone bitartrate (Hycodan)
Levorphanol tartrate (Levo-Dromoran)
Fentanyl (Duragesic, Sublimaze)
Sufentanil citrate (Sufenta)
Oxycodone (Roxicodone)
Oxymorphone HCl (Numorphan)
Tramadol HCl (Ultram)

   c. Used for acute pain caused by myocardial infarction (MI) or cancer, for dyspnea caused by pulmonary edema, and as a preoperative medication
   d. Contraindicated in severe respiratory disorders, head injuries, **increased intracranial pressure,** severe renal disease, or seizure activity
   e. Used with caution in clients with shock or blood loss
5. Oxycodone with aspirin (Percodan)
   a. Should not be taken by a client allergic to aspirin
   b. Can cause gastric irritation and should be taken with food or plenty of liquids
6. Propoxyphene HCl (Darvon) and propoxyphene napsylate (Darvon-N)
   a. Darvon compound contains aspirin and should not be taken by a client allergic to aspirin
   b. Darvocet-N contains acetaminophen
7. Nalbuphine HCl (Nubain): preferable for treating the pain of an MI because it reduces the oxygen needs of the heart without reducing blood pressure
8. Methadone HCl (Dolophine)
   a. Dilute doses of oral concentrate with at least 90 mL of water
   b. Dilute dispersible tablets in at least 120 mL of water, orange juice, or acidic fruit beverage
   c. Used as a replacement medication for opiate dependence or to facilitate withdrawal
9. Hydrocodone (Hycodan): frequently used for cough suppression

C. Implementation for narcotic analgesics
1. Monitor vital signs
2. Assess the client thoroughly before administering pain medication
3. Initiate nursing measures such as massage, distraction, deep breathing and relaxation exercises, the application of heat or cold as prescribed, and providing care and comfort before administering the narcotic analgesic
4. Administer medications 30 to 60 minutes before painful activities
5. Monitor respiratory rate, and if the rate is less than 12 breaths per minute in an adult, withhold the medication unless ventilatory support is being provided
6. Monitor pulse, and if bradycardia develops, hold the dose and notify the physician
7. Monitor blood pressure for hypotension
8. Auscultate breath sounds because narcotic analgesics suppress the cough reflex
9. Encourage activities such as turning, deep breathing, and incentive spirometry to prevent atelectasis and pneumonia
10. Monitor level of consciousness (LOC)
11. Initiate safety precautions such as side rails, a night light, and supervised ambulation
12. Monitor input and output
13. Assess for urinary retention
14. Instruct the client to take oral doses with milk or a snack to reduce gastric irritation
15. Instruct the client to avoid alcohol
16. Instruct the client to avoid activities that require alertness
17. Note effectiveness of medication
18. Have the narcotic antagonist, oxygen, and resuscitation equipment available

D. Morphine sulfate
1. Side effects
   a. Respiratory depression
   b. Orthostatic hypotension
   c. Urinary retention
   d. Nausea
   e. Vomiting
   f. Constipation
   g. Cough suppression
   h. Reduction in pupillary size
   i. Miosis
2. Implementation
   a. Have naxolone (Narcan) available for overdose
   b. Assess vital signs
   c. Note rate and depth of respirations
   d. Withhold the medication if the respiratory rate is less than 12 breaths per minute; respirations of less than 10 breaths per minute can indicate respiratory distress
   e. Monitor urinary output, which should be at least 600 mL per day
   f. Monitor bowel sounds for decreased peristalsis because constipation can occur
   g. Monitor for pupil changes because pinpoint pupils can indicate morphine overdose
   h. Avoid alcohol or CNS depressants because they can cause respiratory depression
   i. Instruct the client to report dizziness or difficulty breathing

E. Meperidine HCl (Demerol)
1. Side effects
   a. Respiratory depression
   b. Hypotension
   c. Tachycardia
   d. Drowsiness
   e. Constipation
   f. Urinary retention

g. Nausea
h. Vomiting
i. Tremors
2. Implementation
a. Monitor vital signs
b. Monitor for respiratory dysfunction and hypotension
c. Have naloxone (Narcan) available for overdose
d. Monitor for urinary retention
e. Monitor bowel sounds and for constipation

VII. NARCOTIC ANTAGONISTS (Box 55-17)

A. Used to treat respiratory depression from narcotic overdose
B. Implementation
1. Monitor blood pressure, pulse, and respiratory rate every 5 minutes initially, tapering to every 15 minutes, then every 30 minutes until stable
2. Place the client on a cardiac monitor and monitor cardiac rhythm
3. Auscultate breath sounds
4. Have resuscitation equipment available
5. Do not leave the client unattended
6. Monitor the client closely for several hours because when the effects of the antagonist wear off, the client may again display signs of narcotic overdose

VIII. OSMOTIC DIURETICS (Box 55-18)

A. Description
1. Increase osmotic pressure of the glomerular filtrate, inhibiting reabsorption of water and electrolytes
2. Used for oliguria and to prevent renal failure
3. Used to decrease intracranial pressure
4. Used to decrease intraocular pressure in narrow-angle glaucoma

BOX 55-17

Narcotic Antagonists

Nalmefene (Revex)
Naloxone HCl (Narcan)
Naltrexone HCl (ReVia)

BOX 55-18

Osmotic Diuretics

Mannitol (Osmitrol)
Urea (Ureaphil)

5. Mannitol is used with chemotherapy to induce diuresis
B. Side effects
1. Fluid and electrolyte imbalances
2. Pulmonary edema from the rapid shifts of fluid
3. Nausea and vomiting
4. Tachycardia from the rapid fluid loss
5. Hyponatremia and dehydration
C. Implementation
1. Monitor vital signs
2. Monitor weight
3. Monitor urine output
4. Monitor electrolyte levels
5. Monitor lungs and heart sounds for signs of pulmonary edema
6. Monitor for signs of dehydration
7. Monitor neurological status
8. Assess for signs of decreasing intracranial pressure if appropriate
9. Change the client's position slowly to prevent orthostatic hypotension

PRACTICE QUESTIONS

1. A nurse is caring for a client diagnosed with Bell's palsy. The client has been taking acetaminophen (Tylenol) and a Tylenol overdose is suspected. The nurse anticipates that the antidote to be prepared is:
1. Auranofin (Ridaura)
2. Fludarabine (Fludara)
3. Acetylcysteine (Mucomyst)
4. Pentostatin (Nipent)

2. A client with trigeminal neuralgia tells the nurse that acetaminophen (Tylenol) is taken on a frequent daily basis for relief of generalized discomfort. Which of the following would indicate toxicity associated with the medication?
1. Platelet count of 400,000 cells/μL
2. A direct bilirubin level of 2 mg/dL
3. Prothrombin time of 11 seconds
4. Sodium of 140 mEq/L

3. A nurse is assisting in preparing to administer acetylcysteine (Mucomyst) to the client with an overdose of acetaminophen (Tylenol). Which of the following are appropriate actions when administering this antidote?
1. Mixing the medication in a flavored ice drink and allowing the client to drink the medication through a straw
2. Administering the medication by intramuscular injection, mixed in 10 mL of normal saline
3. Administering the medication by intramuscular injection in the gluteal muscle
4. Administering the medication subcutaneously in the deltoid muscle

4. A client is receiving baclofen (Lioresal) for muscle spasms resulting from a spinal cord injury. The nurse monitors the client knowing that which of the following indicates a side effect related to this medication?
   1. Photosensitivity
   2. Slurred speech
   3. Hypertension
   4. Muscle pain
5. A client is suspected of having myasthenia gravis. The physician administers edrophonium (Tensilon) by IV injection to determine the diagnosis. The nurse understands that which of the following would indicate the diagnosis of myasthenia gravis after administration of this medication?
   1. An increase in muscle strength
   2. A decrease in muscle strength
   3. Joint pain
   4. Feelings of faintness, dizziness, hypotension, and signs of flushing in the client
6. A client with myasthenia gravis is suspected of having cholinergic crisis. Which of the following symptoms would indicate that this crisis exists?
   1. Hypotension
   2. Hypertension
   3. Mouth sores
   4. Ataxia
7. A client with myasthenia gravis is receiving pyridostigmine (Mestinon). The nurse monitors for signs and symptoms of cholinergic crisis resulting from overdose of the medication. The nurse checks the medication supply to ensure that which medication is available for administration if a cholinergic crisis occurs?
   1. Vitamin K
   2. Protamine sulfate
   3. Acetylcysteine (Mucomyst)
   4. Atropine sulfate
8. A client with myasthenia gravis becomes increasingly weaker. The physician prepares to identify whether the client is reacting to an overdose of the medication (cholinergic crisis) or an increasing severity of the disease (myasthenic crisis). An injection of edrophonium (Tensilon) is administered. Which of the following would indicate that the client is in cholinergic crisis?
   1. An improvement of the weakness
   2. A temporary worsening of the condition
   3. No change in the condition
   4. Complaints of muscle spasms
9. A client with myasthenia gravis verbalizes complaints of feeling much weaker than normal. The physician plans to implement a diagnostic test to determine if the client is experiencing a myasthenic crisis. The physician administers edrophonium (Tensilon). Which of the following would indicate that the client is experiencing a myasthenic crisis?
   1. Increasing weakness
   2. No change in the condition
   3. A temporary improvement in the condition
   4. An increase in muscle spasms
10. Levodopa (Carbidopa) is prescribed for the client with Parkinson's disease. The nurse monitors the client for adverse reactions to the medication. Which of the following would indicate that the client is experiencing an adverse reaction?
    1. Pruritus
    2. Hypertension
    3. Tachycardia
    4. Impaired voluntary movements
11. Phenytoin (Dilantin), 100 mg orally three times a day, has been prescribed for the client for seizure control. The nurse reinforces instructions regarding the medication to the client. Which of the following statements, if made by the client, would indicate effective teaching?
    1. "It's OK to break the capsules to make it easier for me to swallow them."
    2. "I will use a soft toothbrush to brush my teeth."
    3. "If I forget to take my medication, I can wait until the next dose and eliminate that dose."
    4. "If my throat becomes sore, it's a normal effect of the medication and it's nothing to be concerned about."
12. A client is taking phenytoin (Dilantin) for seizure control. A serum drug level is drawn. Which of the following would indicate a therapeutic serum drug range?
    1. 5 to 10 μg/mL
    2. 10 to 20 μg/mL
    3. 20 to 30 μg/mL
    4. 30 to 40 μg/mL
13. A nonsteroidal antiinflammatory drug (NSAID) is prescribed for the client. To promote the best absorption of the medication, the nurse instructs the client to take the medication:
    1. 60 minutes before meals
    2. After meals
    3. With 8 oz of milk
    4. With an antacid
14. A nurse is caring for a client who is taking phenytoin (Dilantin) for control of seizures. During data collection, the nurse notes that the client is taking birth control pills. Which of the following information should the nurse provide to the client?
    1. The increased risk of thrombophlebitis exists while taking phenytoin (Dilantin) and birth control pills together
    2. The potential decreased effectiveness of the birth control pills exists while taking phenytoin (Dilantin)
    3. The client may stop the medication if it is causing severe gastrointestinal effects

4. Pregnancy should be avoided while taking phenytoin (Dilantin)

15. A client with trigeminal neuralgia is being treated with carbamazepine (Tegretol). Which of the following laboratory results would indicate that the client is experiencing an adverse reaction to the medication?
    1. White blood cell count of 3000/μL
    2. Blood urea nitrogen (BUN) 15 mg/dL
    3. Sodium 140 mEq/L
    4. Uric acid 5.0 ng/dL

16. A client with multiple sclerosis is receiving diazepam (Valium), a centrally acting skeletal muscle relaxant. Which of the following would indicate that the client is experiencing a side effect related to this medication?
    1. Headache
    2. Increased salivation
    3. Urinary retention
    4. Drowsiness

17. A nurse is caring for a client receiving morphine sulfate subcutaneously for pain. Because morphine has been prescribed for this client, which of the following nursing actions would be included in the plan of care?
    1. Monitor the client's temperature
    2. Encourage fluids
    3. Maintain the client in a supine position
    4. Encourage the client to cough and deep breathe

18. Meperidine (Demerol) is prescribed for the client with pain. Which of the following would the nurse monitor for as a side effect of this medication?
    1. Hypertension
    2. Bradycardia
    3. Diarrhea
    4. Urinary retention

19. A nurse is caring for a client with severe back pain. Codeine sulfate has been prescribed for the client. Which of the following would the nurse include in the plan of care while the client is taking this medication?
    1. Monitor for hypertension
    2. Restrict fluid intake
    3. Monitor the bowel activity
    4. Monitor peripheral pulses

20. Dantrolene (Dantrium) is prescribed for a client with spinal cord injury for discomfort resulting from spasticity. The nurse tells the client about the importance of follow-up care and the need for which of the following blood studies?
    1. Sedimentation rate
    2. White blood cell count
    3. Liver function studies
    4. Creatinine

21. A client with epilepsy is taking the prescribed dose of phenytoin (Dilantin) to control seizures. A Dilantin blood level is drawn and the results reveal a level of 35 μg/mL. Which of the following symptoms would be expected as a result of this laboratory result?
    1. No symptoms because this is a normal therapeutic level
    2. Slurred speech
    3. Tachycardia
    4. Nystagmus

22. A physician initiates levodopa therapy for the client with Parkinson's disease. A few days after the client starts the medication, the client complains of nausea and vomiting. The nurse's best instruction to the client is that:
    1. This is an expected side effect of the medication
    2. Taking the medication with food will help to prevent the nausea
    3. Taking an antiemetic is the best measure to prevent the nausea
    4. The nausea and vomiting will decrease when the dose of levodopa is stabilized

23. Mannitol (Osmitrol) is being administered to a client with increased intracranial pressure after a head injury. The nurse assisting in caring for the client knows that which of the following indicates the therapeutic action of this medication?
    1. Induces diuresis by raising the osmotic pressure of glomerular filtrate, thereby inhibiting tubular reabsorption of water and solutes
    2. Induces diuresis by promoting the reabsorption of sodium and water in the loop of Henle
    3. Prevents the filtration of sodium and water through the kidneys
    4. Prevents the filtration of sodium and potassium through the kidneys

24. Carbamazepine (Tegretol) is prescribed for a client with a diagnosis of psychomotor seizures. The nurse reviews the client's health history knowing that this medication is contraindicated if which of the following disorders were present?
    1. Liver disease
    2. Headaches
    3. Hypothyroidism
    4. Diabetes mellitus

25. A client is admitted to the hospital with complaints of back spasms. The client states "I have been taking two to three aspirin every 4 hours for the last week and it hasn't helped my back." Aspirin intoxication is suspected. Which of the following symptoms would indicate aspirin intoxication?
    1. Diarrhea
    2. Constipation
    3. Tinnitus
    4. Photosensitivity

ANSWERS

1. *Answer:* 3
Rationale: The antidote for acetaminophen (Tylenol) is acetylcysteine (Mucomyst). Auranofin (Ridaura) is a gold preparation used in rheumatoid arthritis. Fludarabine (Fludara) and Pentostatin (Nipent) are antineoplastic agents.
Test-Taking Strategy: Knowledge regarding the antidote for acetaminophen (Tylenol), and the medication classifications noted in the options, will assist you in answering this question. It is important to know the antidote for various medications. If you had difficulty with this question, review antidotes.
Level of Cognitive Ability: Comprehension
Client Needs: Physiological Integrity
Integrated Concept/Process: Nursing Process/Planning
Content Area: Pharmacology
Reference: Hodgson B, Kizior R: *Saunders nursing drug handbook 2002*, Philadelphia, 2002, WB Saunders, p. 8.

2. *Answer:* 2
Rationale: In adults, overdose of acetaminophen (Tylenol) causes liver damage. Option 2 is an indicator of liver function, and is the only option that indicates an abnormal laboratory value. The normal direct bilirubin is 0 to 0.3 mg/dL. The normal platelet count is 150,000 to 400,000 cells/μL. The normal prothrombin time is 9.5 to 11.3 seconds. The normal sodium is 135 to 145 mEq/L.
Test-Taking Strategy: Knowledge that acetaminophen (Tylenol) causes liver damage and knowledge of the normal laboratory results will be helpful in answering this question. Reviewing the laboratory values in the options will direct you to option 2, the abnormal value. Also, of all of the options, the bilirubin is the most directly related laboratory value to liver function. Review these signs of toxicity if you had difficulty with this question.
Level of Cognitive Ability: Analysis
Client Needs: Physiological Integrity
Integrated Concept/Process: Nursing Process/Data Collection
Content Area: Pharmacology
Reference: Hodgson B, Kizior R: *Saunders nursing drug handbook 2002*, Philadelphia, 2002, WB Saunders, p. 8.

3. *Answer:* 1
Rationale: Because acetylcysteine (Mucomyst) has a pervasive flavor of rotten eggs, it must be disguised in a flavored ice drink, and is preferably drunk through a straw to minimize contact with the mouth. It is not administered by intramuscular or subcutaneous route.
Test-Taking Strategy: Use the process of elimination. Knowing that the medication is a solution that is also used for nebulization treatments will assist you to selecting the option that indicates an oral route. Note that options 2, 3, and 4 indicate parenteral administration and option 1, the correct option, indicates oral administration. Review this medication if you had difficulty with this question.
Level of Cognitive Ability: Application
Client Needs: Physiological Integrity
Integrated Concept/Process: Nursing Process/Implementation
Content Area: Pharmacology
Reference: Hodgson B, Kizior R: *Saunders nursing drug handbook 2002*, Philadelphia, 2002, WB Saunders, p. 11.

4. *Answer:* 2
Rationale: Side effects of baclofen (Lioresal) include drowsiness, dizziness, weakness, and nausea. Occasional side effects include headache, paresthesia of the hands and feet, constipation or diarrhea, anorexia, hypotension, confusion, and nasal congestion. Paradoxical central nervous system excitement and restlessness can occur along with slurred speech, tremor, dry mouth, nocturia, and impotence.
Test-Taking Strategy: Knowledge regarding the medication is required to answer the question. Option 2 is the option that is most closely associated with a neurological disorder. If you had difficulty with this question, review the side effects related to baclofen (Lioresal).
Level of Cognitive Ability: Application
Client Needs: Physiological Integrity
Integrated Concept/Process: Nursing Process/Data Collection
Content Area: Pharmacology
Reference: Hodgson B, Kizior R: *Saunders nursing drug handbook 2002*, Philadelphia, 2002, WB Saunders, p. 102.

5. *Answer:* 1
Rationale: Edrophonium (Tensilon) is a short-acting acetylcholinesterase inhibitor used as a diagnostic agent. When a new client with suspected myasthenia gravis is given the medication intravenously, an increase in muscle strength should be seen in 1 to 3 minutes. If no response occurs, another dose of edrophonium (Tensilon) is given over the next 2 minutes and muscle strength is again tested. If no increase in muscle strength occurs with this higher dose, the muscle weakness is not caused by myasthenia gravis. Clients receiving injections of this medication commonly demonstrate a drop of blood pressure, feel faint, and dizzy and are flushed.
Test-Taking Strategy: Knowledge regarding this medication as a diagnostic tool for myasthenia gravis is required to answer this question. Review this medication as a diagnostic tool for suspected myasthenia gravis you had difficulty with this question.
Level of Cognitive Ability: Analysis
Client Needs: Physiological Integrity
Integrated Concept/Process: Nursing Process/Evaluation
Content Area: Pharmacology
Reference: Lehne R: *Pharmacology for nursing care*, ed 4, Philadelphia, 2001, WB Saunders, p. 126.

6. *Answer:* 2
Rationale: Cholinergic crisis occurs with an overdose of medication. Indications of cholinergic crisis includes gastrointestinal disturbances, nausea, vomiting, diarrhea, abdominal cramps, increased salivation and tearing, miosis, hypertension, sweating, and increased bronchial secretions.
Test-Taking Strategy: Knowledge regarding both cholinergic and myasthenic crisis is required to answer this question. Review both cholinergic and myasthenic crisis if you had difficulty with this question.
Level of Cognitive Ability: Comprehension
Client Needs: Physiological Integrity
Integrated Concept/Process: Nursing Process/Data Collection
Content Area: Pharmacology
Reference: Black J, Hawks J, Keene A: *Medical-surgical nursing: clinical management for positive outcomes*, ed 6, Philadelphia, 2001, WB Saunders, p. 2022.

7. *Answer:* 4
Rationale: The antidote for cholinergic crisis is atropine sulfate. Vitamin K is the antidote for warfarin sodium (Coumadin). Protamine sulfate is the antidote for heparin, and acetylcysteine (Mucomyst) is the antidote for acetaminophen (Tylenol).
Test-Taking Strategy: Knowledge regarding antidotes for the various medications is required to answer this question. Review antidotes if you had difficulty with this question.
Level of Cognitive Ability: Application
Client Needs: Physiological Integrity
Integrated Concept/Process: Nursing Process/Implementation
Content Area: Pharmacology
Reference: Black J, Hawks J, Keene A: *Medical-surgical nursing: clinical management for positive outcomes,* ed 6, Philadelphia, 2001, WB Saunders, p. 2022.

8. *Answer:* 2
Rationale: An edrophonium (Tensilon) injection makes the client in cholinergic crisis temporarily worse. This is known as a negative Tensilon test.
Test-Taking Strategy: Knowledge regarding the use of this medication as a diagnostic tool to differentiate between cholinergic and myasthenic crisis is required to answer this question. Review this diagnostic test and the differences between cholinergic and myasthenic crisis if you had difficulty with this question.
Level of Cognitive Ability: Analysis
Client Needs: Physiological Integrity
Integrated Concept/Process: Nursing Process/Evaluation
Content Area: Pharmacology
Reference: Black J, Hawks J, Keene A: *Medical-surgical nursing: clinical management for positive outcomes,* ed 6, Philadelphia, 2001, WB Saunders, p. 2022.

9. *Answer:* 3
Rationale: Edrophonium (Tensilon) is administered to determine whether the client is reacting to an overdose of a medication (cholinergic crisis) or an increasing severity of the disease (myasthenic crisis). When the edrophonium (Tensilon) injection is given and the condition improves temporarily, the client is in myasthenic crisis. This is known as a positive Tensilon test.
Test-Taking Strategy: Knowledge regarding the use of this medication as a diagnostic tool to differentiate between cholinergic and myasthenic crisis is required to answer this question. Review this diagnostic test and the differences between cholinergic and myasthenic crisis if you had difficulty with this question.
Level of Cognitive Ability: Analysis
Client Needs: Physiological Integrity
Integrated Concept/Process: Nursing Process/Evaluation
Content Area: Pharmacology
Reference: Black J, Hawks J, Keene A: *Medical-surgical nursing: clinical management for positive outcomes,* ed 6, Philadelphia, 2001, WB Saunders, p. 2022.

10. *Answer:* 4
Rationale: Dyskinesia and impaired voluntary movement may occur with high levodopa dosages. Nausea, anorexia, dizziness, orthostatic hypotension, bradycardia, akinesia (the temporary muscle weakness that lasts 1 minute to 1 hour, also known as "on-off phenomenon"), are frequent side effects of the medication.
Test-Taking Strategy: Use the process of elimination. Knowledge regarding the adverse effects of levodopa (Carbidopa) is required to answer this question. Options 2 and 3 are cardiac-related options, so these options can be eliminated first. Note that the question asks for an adverse reaction; therefore select option 4 over option 1 as the correct answer. Review the adverse effects of carbidopa (Levodopa) if you had difficulty with this question.
Level of Cognitive Ability: Comprehension
Client Needs: Physiological Integrity
Integrated Concept/Process: Nursing Process/Data Collection
Content Area: Pharmacology
Reference: Hodgson B, Kizior R: *Saunders nursing drug handbook 2002,* Philadelphia, 2002, WB Saunders, p. 165.

11. *Answer:* 2
Rationale: Phenytoin (Dilantin) it an anticonvulsant. Gingival hyperplasia, bleeding, swelling, and tenderness of the gums can occur with the use of this medication. The client needs to be taught good oral hygiene, gum massage, and the need for regular dentist visits. The client should not skip medication doses as this could precipitate a seizure. Capsules should not be chewed or broken and they must be swallowed. The client needs to be instructed to report a sore throat, fever, glandular swelling, or any skin reaction, as this indicates hematological toxicity.
Test-Taking Strategy: Use the process of elimination. Note the key words "indicate effective teaching." Eliminate option 3, as the client needs to be encouraged to take medications on time. Also, eliminate option 4 because the client needs to report these symptoms to the physician. Remember, Dilantin capsules should not be broken. Review the side effects related to phenytoin (Dilantin) if you had difficulty with this question.
Level of Cognitive Ability: Comprehension
Client Needs: Health Promotion and Maintenance
Integrated Concept/Process: Teaching/Learning
Content Area: Pharmacology
Reference: Hodgson B, Kizior R: *Saunders nursing drug handbook 2002,* Philadelphia, 2002, WB Saunders, p. 880.

12. *Answer:* 2
Rationale: The therapeutic serum drug level range for phenytoin (Dilantin) is 10 to 20 μg/mL.
Test-Taking Strategy: Knowledge regarding the therapeutic serum range of this medication is required to answer the question. A helpful hint may be to remember that the theophylline therapeutic range and the acetaminophen (Tylenol) therapeutic range are the same as the Dilantin therapeutic range. Remembering this may assist you when answering questions related to any of these three medications. Review this therapeutic level if you had difficulty with this question.
Level of Cognitive Ability: Comprehension
Client Needs: Physiological Integrity
Integrated Concept/Process: Nursing Process/Data Collection
Content Area: Pharmacology
Reference: Hodgson B, Kizior R: *Saunders nursing drug handbook 2002,* Philadelphia, 2002, WB Saunders, p. 880.

13. *Answer:* 1
Rationale: NSAIDs should be given 30 to 60 minutes before or 2 hours after meals to promote the best absorption. Administering the medication with meals, milk, or an antacid will slow the absorption of the medication.
Test-Taking Strategy: Use the process of elimination. Note the similarity between options 2, 3, and 4. Each of these options indicate administering the medication with a food, fluid, or an antacid. Also, note the key words "best absorption." Review this medication if you had difficulty with this question.
Level of Cognitive Ability: Application
Client Needs: Health Promotion and Maintenance
Integrated Concept/Process: Teaching/Learning
Content Area: Pharmacology
Reference: Lehne R: *Pharmacology for nursing care,* ed 4, Philadelphia, 2001, WB Saunders, p. 766.

14. *Answer:* 2
Rationale: Phenytoin (Dilantin) enhances the rate of estrogen metabolism, which can decrease the effectiveness of some birth control pills. Options 1, 3, are 4 are not accurate.
Test-Taking Strategy: Use the process of elimination. Knowledge regarding medication interactions while taking phenytoin (Dilantin) is required to answer the question. Option 1 would cause anxiety in the client. A client should not be instructed to stop anticonvulsant medication. Pregnancy does not need to be "avoided." Review medication interactions related to phenytoin (Dilantin) if you had difficulty with this question.
Level of Cognitive Ability: Application
Client Needs: Health Promotion and Maintenance
Integrated Concept/Process: Nursing Process/Implementation
Content Area: Pharmacology
Reference: Hodgson B, Kizior R: *Saunders nursing drug handbook 2002,* Philadelphia, 2002, WB Saunders, p. 800.

15. *Answer:* 1
Rationale: Adverse effects of carbamazepine (Tegretol) appear as blood dyscrasias, including aplastic anemia, agranulocytosis, thrombocytopenia, leukopenia, cardiovascular disturbances, thrombophlebitis, dysrhythmias, and dermatological effects.
Test-Taking Strategy: Knowledge regarding the adverse effects related to this medication is required to answer the question. If you are familiar with normal laboratory values, you will note that the only option that indicates an abnormal value is option 1. Review the signs of adverse reactions related to this medication if you had difficulty with this question.
Level of Cognitive Ability: Analysis
Client Needs: Physiological Integrity
Integrated Concept/Process: Nursing Process/Data Collection
Content Area: Pharmacology
Reference: Hodgson B, Kizior R: *Saunders nursing drug handbook 2002,* Philadelphia, 2002, WB Saunders, p. 163.

16. *Answer:* 4
Rationale: Incoordination and drowsiness are common side effects resulting from this medication. Options 1, 2, and 3 are incorrect.
Test-Taking Strategy: Note that the question addresses a centrally acting skeletal muscle relaxant. This may assist you in the process of elimination and direct you to the correct option of drowsiness. If you had difficulty with this question, review the side effects associated with diazepam (Valium).
Level of Cognitive Ability: Comprehension
Client Needs: Physiological Integrity
Integrated Concept/Process: Nursing Process/Data Collection
Content Area: Pharmacology
Reference: Hodgson B, Kizior R: *Saunders nursing drug handbook 2002,* Philadelphia, 2002, WB Saunders, p. 330.

17. *Answer:* 4
Rationale: Morphine suppresses the cough reflex. Clients need to be encouraged to cough and deep breathe to prevent pneumonia. Options 1, 2, and 3 are not specifically associated with this medication.
Test-Taking Strategy: Use the process of elimination. Knowledge that morphine suppresses the cough reflex and the respiratory reflex would lead you to the correct option. Additionally, use the ABCs—airway, breathing, and circulation—when selecting the correct option. Review this medication if you had difficulty with this question.
Level of Cognitive Ability: Application
Client Needs: Physiological Integrity
Integrated Concept/Process: Nursing Process/Planning
Content Area: Pharmacology
Reference: Hodgson B, Kizior R: *Saunders nursing drug handbook 2002,* Philadelphia, 2002, WB Saunders, p. 752.

18. *Answer:* 4
Rationale: Side effects of this medication include respiratory depression, orthostatic hypotension, tachycardia, drowsiness and mental clouding, constipation, and urinary retention.
Test-Taking Strategy: Knowledge regarding side effects associated with narcotic analgesics will assist you in answering the question. If you had difficulty with this question review this medication.
Level of Cognitive Ability: Application
Client Needs: Physiological Integrity
Integrated Concept/Process: Nursing Process/Data Collection
Content Area: Pharmacology
Reference: Hodgson B, Kizior R: *Saunders nursing drug handbook 2002,* Philadelphia, 2002, WB Saunders, p. 692.

19. *Answer:* 3
Rationale: While the client is taking codeine sulfate, the nurse would monitor vital signs and for hypotension. The nurse should also increase fluid intake, palpate the bladder for urinary retention, auscultate bowel sounds, and monitor the pattern of daily bowel activity and stool consistency. The nurse should monitor respiratory status and initiate breathing and coughing exercises. Additionally, the nurse monitors the effectiveness of the pain medication.
Test-Taking Strategy: Use the process of elimination recalling that codeine can cause constipation. If you had difficulty with this question, review nursing measures related to the administration of codeine sulfate.
Level of Cognitive Ability: Application
Client Needs: Physiological Integrity

Integrated Concept/Process: Nursing Process/Planning
Content Area: Pharmacology
Reference: Hodgson B, Kizior R: *Saunders nursing drug handbook 2002*, Philadelphia, 2002, WB Saunders, p. 269.

20. *Answer:* 3
Rationale: Dantrolene can cause liver damage and the nurse should monitor the liver function studies. Baseline liver function studies are done before therapy starts, and regular liver function studies are performed throughout therapy. Dantrolene is discontinued if no relief of spasticity is achieved in 6 weeks.
Test-Taking Strategy: Knowledge that this medication is hepatotoxic will direct you to the correct option. If you had difficulty with this question, review this medication.
Level of Cognitive Ability: Application
Client Needs: Physiological Integrity
Integrated Concept/Process: Nursing Process/Implementation
Content Area: Pharmacology
Reference: Hodgson B, Kizior R: *Saunders nursing drug handbook 2002*, Philadelphia, 2002, WB Saunders, p. 306.

21. *Answer:* 2
Rationale: The therapeutic Dilantin level is 10 to 20 μg/mL. At greater than 20 μg/mL, involuntary movements of the eyeballs (nystagmus) appears. At greater than 30 μg/mL, ataxia and slurred speech arise.
Test-Taking Strategy: Knowledge regarding the therapeutic Dilantin level is required to answer this question. Review therapeutic levels and associated signs, if you had difficulty with this question.
Level of Cognitive Ability: Analysis
Client Needs: Physiological Integrity
Integrated Concept/Process: Nursing Process/Evaluation
Content Area: Pharmacology
Reference: Hodgson B, Kizior R: *Saunders nursing drug handbook 2002*, Philadelphia, 2002, WB Saunders, p. 880.

22. *Answer:* 2
Rationale: The best instruction by the nurse is that food will prevent the nausea. Antiemetics from the phenothiazine class should not be used because they block the therapeutic action of dopamine. The other options are incorrect.
Test-Taking Strategy: Use the process of elimination. Note the key word "best" and focus on the issue of the question. It is best to use nonpharmacological approaches first to alleviate the nausea. Additionally, the nurse cannot prescribe medications. Review this medication if you had difficulty with this question.
Level of Cognitive Ability: Application
Client Needs: Physiological Integrity
Integrated Concept/Process: Nursing Process/Implementation
Content Area: Pharmacology
Reference: Hodgson B, Kizior R: *Saunders nursing drug handbook 2002*, Philadelphia, 2002, WB Saunders, p. 165.

23. *Answer:* 1
Rationale: Mannitol (Osmitrol) is an osmotic diuretic that induces diuresis by raising the osmotic pressure of glomerular filtrate, thereby inhibiting tubular reabsorption of water and solutes. It is used to reduce intracranial pressure in the client with head trauma.
Test-Taking Strategy: Use the process of elimination. Read the question carefully noting that it presents a client with increased intracranial pressure. The only option that suggests an action that will produce diuresis and reduce intracranial pressure is option 1. If you had difficulty with this question, review the action of mannitol (Osmitrol).
Level of Cognitive Ability: Comprehension
Client Needs: Physiological Integrity
Integrated Concept/Process: Nursing Process/Evaluation
Content Area: Pharmacology
Reference: Hodgson B, Kizior R: *Saunders nursing drug handbook 2002*, Philadelphia, 2002, WB Saunders, p. 677.

24. *Answer:* 1
Rationale: Tegretol is contraindicated in liver disease, and liver function tests are routinely prescribed for baseline purposes and are monitored during therapy. It is also contraindicated if the client has a history of blood dyscrasias.
Test-Taking Strategy: Knowledge regarding the contraindications associated with Tegretol is required to answer this question. Review this medication if you are unfamiliar with it.
Level of Cognitive Ability: Analysis
Client Needs: Physiological Integrity
Integrated Concept/Process: Nursing Process/Data Collection
Content Area: Pharmacology
Reference: Hodgson B, Kizior R: *Saunders nursing drug handbook 2002*, Philadelphia, 2002, WB Saunders, p. 163.

25. *Answer:* 3
Rationale: Mild intoxication with acetylsalicylic acid (aspirin) is called salicylism and is commonly experienced when the daily dosage is more than 4 grams. Tinnitus (ringing in the ears) is the most frequent effect noted with intoxication. Hyperventilation may occur because salicylate stimulates the respiratory center. Fever may result because salicylate interferes with the metabolic pathways coupling oxygen consumption and heat production. Options 1, 2, and 4 are incorrect.
Test-Taking Strategy: Use the process of elimination. Focus on the issue of the question, aspirin intoxication. Options 1 and 2 relate to gastrointestinal symptoms and can be eliminated. From the remaining options, it is necessary to know that tinnitus is an indication of toxicity. If you had difficulty with this question, review aspirin intoxication.
Level of Cognitive Ability: Comprehension
Client Needs: Physiological Integrity
Integrated Concept/Process: Nursing Process/Data Collection
Content Area: Pharmacology
Reference: Hodgson B, Kizior R: *Saunders nursing drug handbook 2002*, Philadelphia, 2002, WB Saunders, p. 82.

REFERENCES

Black J, Hawks J, Keene A: *Medical-surgical nursing: clinical management for positive outcomes*, ed 6, Philadelphia, 2001, WB Saunders.

Chernecky C, Berger B: *Laboratory tests and diagnostic procedures*, ed 3, Philadelphia, 2001, WB Saunders.

Clark J, Queener S, Karb V: *Pharmacologic basis of nursing practice*, ed 6, St Louis, 2000, Mosby.

DeWit S: *Fundamental concepts and skills for nursing*, Philadelphia, 2001, WB Saunders.

Hodgson B, Kizior R: *Saunders nursing drug handbook 2002*, Philadelphia, 2002, WB Saunders.

Ignatavicius D, Workman M: *Medical-surgical nursing: critical thinking for collaborative care*, ed 4, Philadelphia, 2002, WB Saunders.

Lehne R: *Pharmacology for nursing care*, ed 4, Philadelphia, 2001, WB Saunders.

Potter P, Perry A: *Fundamentals of nursing*, ed 5, St Louis, 2001, Mosby.

Smeltzer S, Bare B: *Brunner and Suddarth's textbook of medical-surgical nursing*, ed 9, Philadelphia, 2000, Lippincott Williams & Wilkins.

UNIT XVII

The Adult Client with a Musculoskeletal Disorder

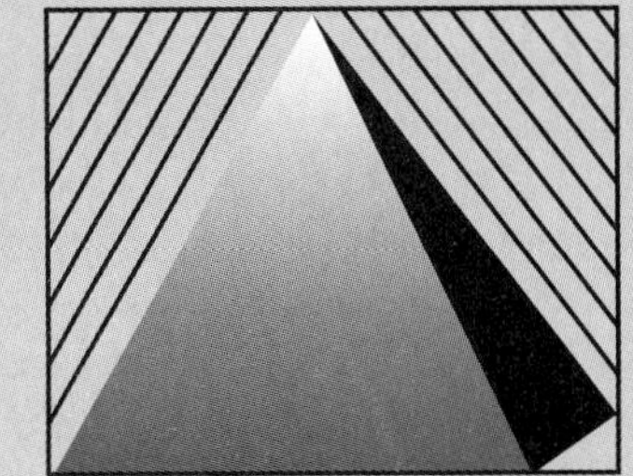

PYRAMID TERMS

Casts Made of plaster or fiberglass to provide immobilization of bone and joints after a fracture or injury.

Compartment Syndrome Increased pressure within one or more compartments causing massive compromise of circulation to an area and causing irreversible neuromuscular damage within 4 to 6 hours of its onset if not treated.

External Fixation Stabilization of a fracture by the use of an external frame, with multiple pins applied through the bone.

Fat Embolism An embolism that can occur 24 to 48 hours after a fracture or within the first 72 hours.

Internal Fixation Stabilization of a fracture that involves the application of screws, plates, pins, or nails to hold the fragments in alignment.

Reduction The procedure that restores the bone to proper alignment.

Traction Force applied in two directions to reduce and immobilize a fracture.

PYRAMID TO SUCCESS

The Pyramid to Success focuses on the emergency care to a client who sustains a fracture or other musculoskeletal injury, monitoring for complications related to fractures, and interventions if complications occur. Nursing care related to casts and traction is emphasized. Skill related to instructing the client in the use of an assistive device such as a cane, walker, or crutches is a pyramid point. Pyramid points also include postoperative care after hip surgery or amputation, and care to the client with rheumatoid arthritis or osteoporosis. Focus on the points related to the psychosocial effects as a result of the musculoskeletal disorder such as unexpected body image changes, and the appropriate and available support services needed for the client. The Integrated Concepts and Processes addressed in this unit include the Clinical Problem-Solving Process (Nursing Process), Caring, Communication and Documentation, Cultural Awareness, Self-Care, and Teaching/Learning.

CLIENT NEEDS

Safe, Effective Care Environment

Asepsis related to wounds
Client rights
Confidentiality regarding disorder and plan of care
Dietary consultation
Establishing priorities
Informed consent for diagnostic treatments and surgical procedures
Physical therapy and occupational therapy referrals
Preventing injury from accidents
Standard (universal) precautions

Health Promotion and Maintenance

Health promotion related to diet and activity
Home care instructions regarding care related to musculoskeletal disorder
Reinforcement regarding the importance of prescribed therapy
Techniques related to data collection of the musculoskeletal system
The aging process and disease prevention

Psychosocial Integrity

Available support systems and utilization of community resources
Cultural, religious, and spiritual influences
Grief and loss related to mobility limitations and restrictions
Sensory and perceptual alterations

Situational role changes as a result of musculoskeletal disorder
The ability to cope with feelings of isolation and loss of independence
Unexpected body image changes as a result of injury or disease

Physiological Integrity

Care related to casts and traction
Complications of a fracture
Complications related to procedures or injuries
Emergency care for a fracture or other injury
Measures to promote comfort
Osteoporosis
Pharmacological medications, actions, agents, side effects, and adverse effects
Postoperative interventions
Promoting normal elimination patterns
Promoting self-care measures
Rheumatoid arthritis
Use of assistive devices for mobility such as canes, walkers, and crutches

REFERENCES

Black J, Hawks J, Keene A: *Medical-surgical nursing: clinical management for positive outcomes*, ed 6, Philadelphia, 2001, WB Saunders.

Chernecky C, Berger B: *Laboratory tests and diagnostic procedures*, ed 3, Philadelphia, 2001, WB Saunders.

Clark J, Queener S, Karb V: *Pharmacologic basis of nursing practice*, ed 6, St Louis, 2000, Mosby.

DeWit S: *Fundamental concepts and skills for nursing*, Philadelphia, 2001, WB Saunders.

Hill S, Howlett H: *Success in practical nursing: personal and vocational issues*, ed 4, Philadelphia, 2001, WB Saunders.

National Council of State Boards of Nursing: *Test plan for the National Council Licensure Examination for Practical/Vocational Nurses*, Chicago, 2001, Author.

Potter P, Perry A: *Fundamentals of nursing*, ed 5, St Louis, 2001, Mosby.

Perry A, Potter P: *Clinical nursing skills and techniques*, ed 5, St Louis, 2002, Mosby.

Wilson J: *Infection control in clinical practice*, ed 2, St Louis, 2002, Balliere Tindall.

56 Musculoskeletal System

I. ANATOMY AND PHYSIOLOGY

A. Skeleton
  1. Axial portion
    a. Cranium
    b. Vertebrae
    c. Ribs
  2. Appendicular portion
    a. Limbs
    b. Shoulders
    c. Hips

B. Types of bones (Box 56-1)
  1. Spongy bone
    a. Located in the ends of long bones and the center of flat and irregular bones
    b. Can withstand forces applied in many directions
  2. Dense (compact) bones
    a. Covers spongy bone
    b. Cylinder around a central marrow cavity
    c. Can withstand force predominantly in one direction
  3. Characteristics of the bones
    a. Support and protect structures of the body
    b. Provide attachments for muscles, tendons, and ligaments
    c. Contain tissue in the central cavities, which aids in formation of blood cells
    d. Assists in regulating calcium and phosphate concentrations
  4. Bone growth
    a. The length of bone growth is a result of the ossification of the epiphyseal cartilage at the ends of bones, and bone growth stops between the ages of 18 and 25 years
    b. The width of bone growth is a result of the activity of osteoblasts and occurs throughout life but does slow down with the aging process
    c. Bone absorption around the bone marrow continues throughout life; therefore bones become weaker with aging

C. Types of joints (Table 56-1)
  1. Characteristics of the joints
    a. Allow movement between bones
    b. Formed where two bones join
    c. Surfaces are covered with cartilage
    d. Enclosed in a capsule
    e. Contain a cavity filled with synovial fluid

BOX 56-1

Types of Bones

Long
Short
Flat
Irregular

TABLE 56-1

Types of Joints

Type	Description
Synarthrosis	Fibrous or fixed joints No movement associated with these joints
Amphiarthrosis	Cartilaginous joints Slightly movable joints
Diarthrosis	Synovial joints Ball-and-socket joints
Condyloid	Freely movable joints Allow frictionless, painless movement

f. Ligaments hold the bone and joint in the correct position
g. Articulation is the meeting point of two or more joints

2. Synovial fluid
a. Found in joint capsule
b. Formed by synovial membrane, which lines joint capsule
c. Lubricates the cartilage
d. Cushion for shocks

D. Muscles
1. Characteristics of muscles
a. Made up of bundles of muscle fibers
b. Provide the force to move bones
c. Assist in maintaining posture
d. Assist with heat production

2. The process of contraction and relaxation
a. Muscle contraction and relaxation require large amounts of adenosine triphosphate (ATP)
b. Contraction also requires calcium, which functions as a catalyst
c. Acetylcholine released by the motor end plate of the motor neuron initiates an action potential
d. Acetylcholine is then destroyed by acetylcholinesterase
e. Calcium is required to contract muscle fibers and acts as a catalyst for the enzyme needed for the sliding together action of actin and myosin
f. After contraction, ATP transports calcium out to allow actin and myosin to slide apart and allow the muscle to relax

3. Skeletal muscles
a. Are attached to two bones and cross at least one joint
b. The point of origin is the point of attachment on the bone closest to trunk
c. The point of insertion is the point of attachment on the bone farthest from the trunk
d. Skeletal muscles act in groups
e. Prime movers contract to produce movement
f. Antagonists relax
g. Synergists contract to stabilize
h. Nerves activate and control the muscles

II. RISK FACTORS ASSOCIATED WITH MUSCULOSKELETAL DISORDERS (Box 56-2)

BOX 56-2

Risk Factors Associated with Musculoskeletal Disorders

Trauma and injury
Falls
Autoimmune disorders
Infection
Degenerative conditions
Obesity
Calcium deficiency
Postmenopausal states
Metabolic disorders
Neoplastic disorders
Hyperuricemia
Medications

III. DIAGNOSTIC TESTS

A. X-ray studies
1. Description: a commonly used procedure to diagnose disorders of the musculoskeletal system
2. Implementation
a. Handle injured area carefully
b. Administer analgesics as prescribed before the procedure particularly if the client is in pain
c. Remove any radiopaque objects such as jewelry
d. Shield the client's testes, ovaries, or pregnant abdomen
e. Client must lie still during an x-ray study
f. Inform the client that exposure to radiation is minimal and not dangerous
g. Health care provider is to wear a lead apron if staying in the room with the client

B. Arthrocentesis
1. Description
a. Involves aspirating synovial fluid, blood, or pus via a needle inserted into a joint cavity
b. Medication may be instilled into the joint if necessary to alleviate inflammation
2. Implementation
a. Obtain an informed consent
b. Apply a compress bandage postprocedure as prescribed
c. Instruct the client to rest the joint for 8 to 24 hours postprocedure
d. Instruct the client to notify the physician if a fever or swelling of the joint occurs

C. Arthrogram
1. Description
a. A radiographic examination of the soft tissues of the joint structures used to diagnose trauma to the joint capsule or ligaments
b. A local anesthetic is used for the procedure and a contrast medium or air is injected

into the joint cavity, and the joint is moved through range of motion (ROM) as a series of x-ray films is taken
2. Implementation
a. Inform the client to fast from food and fluids for 8 hours before the procedure
b. Assess for client allergies to iodine or seafood before the procedure
c. Obtain an informed consent
d. Inform the client that they will need to remain as still as possible except when asked to reposition
e. Minimize the use of the joint for 12 hours after the procedure
f. Instruct the client that the joint may be edematous and tender for 1 to 2 days after the procedure and may be treated with ice packs and analgesics as prescribed
g. Inform the client that if edema and tenderness last longer than 2 days to notify the physician
h. If knee arthrography was performed, an Ace wrap over the knee may be prescribed for 3 to 4 days
i. If air was used for injection, crepitus may be felt in the joint for up to 2 days

D. Arthroscopy
1. Description
a. Provides an endoscopic examination of various joints
b. Articular cartilage abnormalities can be assessed, loose bodies can be removed, and the cartilage trimmed
c. A biopsy may be performed during the procedure
2. Implementation
a. Instruct the client to fast for 8 to 12 hours before procedure
b. Obtain an informed consent
c. Administer pain medication as prescribed postprocedure
d. An elastic wrap should be worn for 2 to 4 days as prescribed
e. Instruct the client that walking without weight bearing is usually permitted after sensation returns but to limit activity for 1 to 4 days as prescribed
f. Instruct the client to elevate extremity as often as possible for 2 days and to place ice on the site to minimize swelling
g. Reinforce instructions regarding the use of crutches, which may be used for 5 to 7 days postprocedure when walking
h. Advise the client to notify the physician if fever, increased knee pain, or edema continues for more than 3 days

E. Bone scan
1. Description
a. Radioisotope is injected intravenously (IV) and will collect in areas that indicate abnormal bone metabolism and some fractures, if they exist
b. The isotope is excreted in urine and feces within 48 hours and is not harmful to others
2. Implementation
a. Hold fluids for 4 hours before the procedure
b. Obtain an informed consent
c. Remove all jewelry and metal objects
d. After injection of the radioisotope, the client must drink 32 ounces of water (if not contraindicated) to promote renal filtering of excess isotope
e. From 1 to 3 hours after injection, have the client void, and then the scanning procedure is performed
f. Inform the client of the need to lie supine during the procedure and that the procedure is not painful
g. No special precautions are required after the procedure because a minimal amount of radioactivity exists in the isotope
h. Monitor the injection site for redness and swelling
i. Encourage oral fluid intake after the procedure

F. Bone or muscle biopsy
1. Description: may be done during surgery or through aspiration, or punch or needle biopsy
2. Implementation
a. Obtain an informed consent
b. Monitor for bleeding, swelling, and hematoma, or severe pain
c. Elevate the site for 24 hours after the procedure to reduce edema
d. Apply ice packs as prescribed to prevent development of a hematoma
e. Monitor for signs of infection after the procedure
f. Inform the client that mild to moderate discomfort is normal after the procedure

G. Electromyography (EMG)
1. Description
a. Measures electrical potential associated with skeletal muscle contractions
b. Needles are inserted into the muscle and recordings of muscular electrical activity are traced on recording paper through an oscilloscope
2. Implementation
a. Obtain an informed consent

b. Instruct the client that the needle insertion is uncomfortable
c. Instruct the client not to take any stimulants or sedatives 24 hours before the procedure
d. Inform the client that slight bruising may occur at needle insertion sites

H. Myelogram
1. Description: injection of dye or air into subarachnoid space to detect abnormalities of the spinal cord and vertebrae
2. Implementation preprocedure
a. Obtain an informed consent
b. Provide hydration for at least 12 hours before the test
c. Assess for allergies to iodine
d. Premedicate for sedation as prescribed
3. Implementation postprocedure
a. Perform vital signs and neurological assessment frequently as prescribed
b. If a water-based dye is used, elevate the head 15 to 30 degrees for 8 hours as prescribed
c. If an oil-based dye is used, keep client flat 6 to 8 hours as prescribed
d. If air is used, keep the head lower than the trunk
e. Force fluids and monitor intake and output

IV. FRACTURES

A. Description: a break in the continuity of the bone caused by trauma, twisting as a result of muscle spasm or indirect loss of leverage, or bone decalcification and disease that results in osteopenia
B. Types of fractures (Box 56-3)
C. Data collection in a fracture of an extremity
1. Pain or tenderness over the involved area
2. Loss of function
3. Obvious deformity
4. Crepitation
5. Erythema, edema, ecchymosis
6. Muscle spasm and impaired sensation
D. Initial care of a fracture of an extremity (Box 56-4)
1. Immobilize affected extremity
2. If a compound fracture exists, splint the extremity and cover the wound with a sterile dressing
E. **Reduction:** restoring the bone to proper alignment
1. Closed **reduction**
a. Performed by manual manipulation
b. May be performed with patient under local or general anesthesia
c. A **cast** may be applied after **reduction**

BOX 56-3

Types of Fractures

Closed or simple: Skin over the fractured area remains intact
Greenstick: One side of the bone is broken and the other is bent; most commonly seen in children
Transverse: The bone is fractured straight across
Oblique: The break extends in an oblique direction
Spiral: The break partially encircles bone
Comminuted: The bone is splintered or crushed, with three or more fragments
Complete: The bone is completely separated by a break into two parts
Incomplete: A partial break in the bone
Open-Compound: The bone is exposed to air through a break in the skin, and soft tissue injury and infection are common
Impacted: A part of fractured bone is driven into another bone
Depressed: Bone fragments are driven inward
Compression: A fractured bone compressed by other bone
Pathological: A fracture due to weakening of the bone structure by pathological processes such as neoplasia or osteomalacia; also called spontaneous fracture

BOX 56-4

Interventions for a Fracture

Reduction
Fixation
Traction
Casts

2. Open **reduction**
a. Involves a surgical intervention
b. May be treated with **internal fixation** devices
c. The client may be placed in **traction** or a **cast** after the procedure

F. Fixation
1. Internal **fixation**
a. Follows open **reduction**
b. Involves the application of screws, plates, pins, or nails to hold the fragments in alignment
c. May involve removal of damaged bone and replacement with a prosthesis
d. Provides immediate bone strength
e. Risk of infection is associated with the procedure
2. External **fixation**
a. An external frame is used with multiple pins applied through the bone
b. Provides more freedom of movement than with **traction**

G. **Traction** (Figure 56-1)
1. Description
   a. The exertion of a pulling force applied in two directions to reduce and immobilize a fracture
   b. Provides proper bone alignment and reduces muscle spasms
2. Implementation
   a. Maintain proper body alignment
   b. Ensure that the weights hang freely and do not touch floor
   c. Do not remove or lift weights without a physician's order
   d. Ensure that pulleys are not obstructed and that ropes in pulleys move freely
   e. Place knots in ropes to prevent slipping
   f. Check ropes for fraying

H. Skeletal **traction** (Figure 56-2)
1. Description: mechanically applied to bone using pins, wires, or tongs
2. Implementation
   a. Monitor color, motion, and sensation (CMS) of the affected extremity
   b. Monitor the insertion sites for redness, swelling, or drainage
   c. Provide insertion site care as prescribed
3. Cervical tongs and halo fixation device (Refer to Chapter 54 regarding care to the client with these types of devices)

I. Skin **traction** (Box 56-5)
1. Description: **traction** applied by the use of elastic bandages or adhesive
2. Cervical skin **traction**
   a. Relieves muscle spasms and compression in upper extremities and neck
   b. Uses a head halter and a chin pad to attach the **traction**

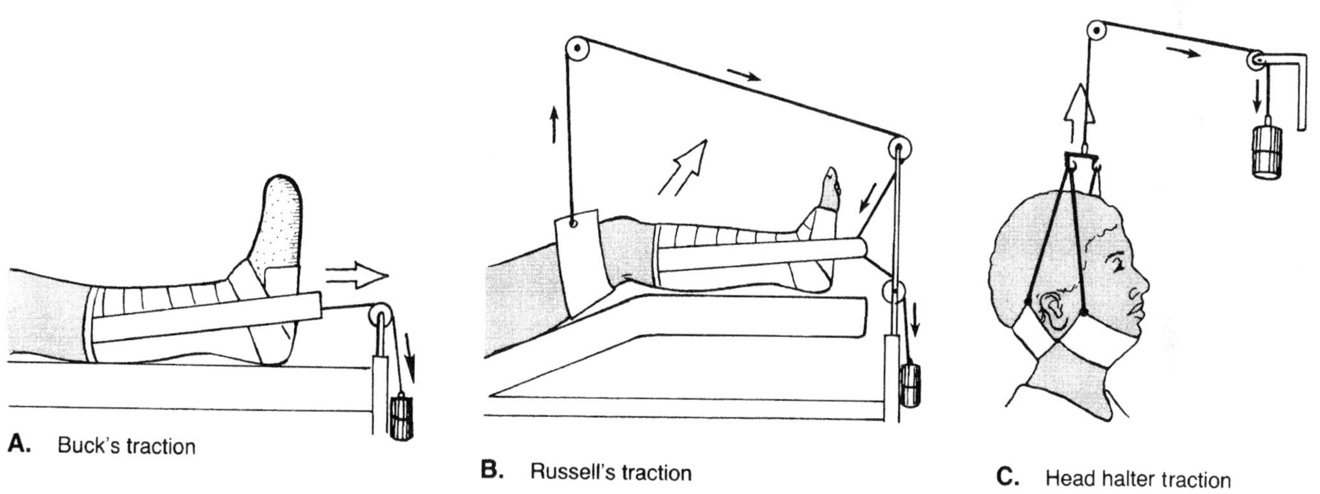

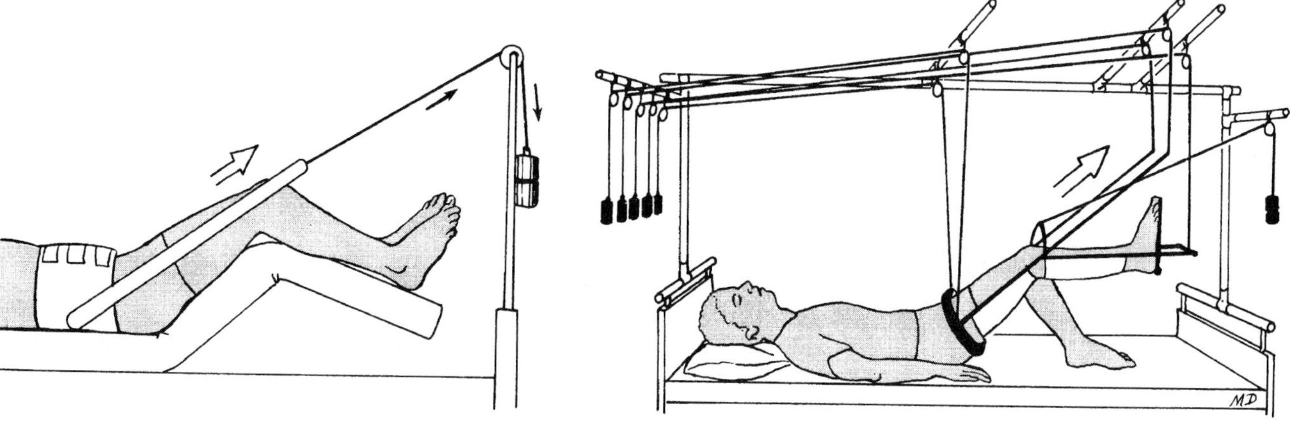

FIG. 56-1 Examples of common types of traction A, B, C, D, E. (From DeWit S: *Essentials of medical surgical nursing*, ed 4, Philadelphia, 1998, WB Saunders.)

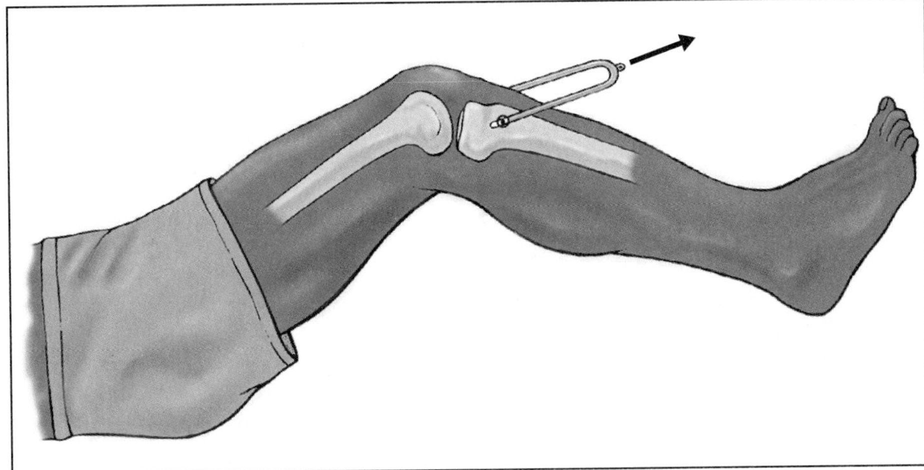

FIG. 56-2 Skeletal traction. (From Monahan, Neighbors: *Medical surgical nursing*, ed 2, Philadelphia, 1998, WB Saunders.)

BOX 56-5

Types: Skin Traction

Cervical traction
Buck's traction
Russell's traction
Pelvic traction

c. Use powder to protect the ears from friction rub
d. Position the client with the head of the bed elevated 30 to 40 degrees and attach the weights to a pulley system over the head of the bed

3. Buck's skin traction
   a. Used to alleviate muscle spasms; immobilizes a lower limb by maintaining a straight pull on the limb with the use of weights
   b. A boot appliance is applied to attach to the **traction**
   c. Weight is attached to a pulley and allow weights to hang freely over edge of bed
   d. Not more than 8 to 10 pounds of weight should be applied
   e. Elevate the foot of the bed to provide the **traction**
4. Russell's skin **traction** (Refer to Chapter 34 regarding information related to this type of traction)
5. Pelvic skin **traction**
   a. Used to relieve low back, hip, or leg pain and to reduce muscle spasm
   b. Apply the **traction** snugly over the pelvis and iliac crest and attach to weights
   c. Use measures as prescribed to prevent the client from slipping down in bed

J. Balanced suspension (Box 56-6)
   1. Description
      a. Used with skin or skeletal **traction**
      b. Used to approximate fractures of femur, tibia, or fibula
      c. Produced by a counterforce other than client
   2. Implementation
      a. Place the client in low-Fowler's position, either on the side or back
      b. Maintain a 20-degree angle from the thigh to the bed
      c. Protect the skin from breakdown
      d. Provide pin care if pins are used with the skeletal **traction**
      e. Clean pin site with sterile normal saline and hydrogen peroxide or Betadine as prescribed or per agency procedure

K. Dunlop's traction
   1. Description: horizontal traction to align fractures of the humerus; vertical traction maintains the forearm in proper alignment
   2. Implementation: nursing care is similar to Buck's traction

L. **Casts**
   1. Description: made of plaster or fiberglass to provide immobilization of bone and joints after a fracture or injury

BOX 56-6

Balanced Suspension

Thomas splint with Pearson attachment
Steinmann pin
Kirschner wires

2. Implementation
   a. Keep **cast** and extremity elevated
   b. Allow a wet **cast** 24 to 48 hours to dry (synthetic casts dry in 20 minutes)
   c. Handle a wet **cast** with the palms of the hand until dry
   d. Turn the extremity unless contraindicated, so that all sides of the wet **cast** will dry
   e. Heat can be used to dry the **cast**
   f. The **cast** will change from a dull to a shiny substance when dry
   g. Examine the skin and **cast** for pressure areas
   h. Monitor the extremity for circulatory impairment such as pain, swelling, discoloration, tingling, numbness, coolness, or diminished pulse
   i. Notify the physician immediately if circulatory compromise occurs
   j. Prepare for bivalving or cutting the **cast** if circulatory impairment occurs
   k. Petal the **cast**; maintain smooth edges around the **cast** to prevent crumbling of the **cast** material
   l. Monitor the client's temperature
   m. Monitor for the presence of a foul odor, which may indicate infection
   n. Monitor drainage by circling the area of drainage on the **cast**
   o. Monitor for warmth on the **cast**
   p. Monitor for wet spots, which may indicate a need for drying, or the presence of drainage under the **cast**
   q. If an open draining area exists on the affected extremity, a cut-out portion of the **cast** or a window will be made by the physician
   r. Instruct the client not to stick objects inside the **cast**
   s. Teach the client to keep the **cast** clean and dry
   t. Instruct the client on isometric exercises to prevent muscle atrophy

V. CRUTCH WALKING

A. Description
   1. An accurate measurement of the client for crutches is important because an incorrect measurement could damage the brachial plexus
   2. The distance between the axilla and arm pieces on the crutches should be two fingers-width in the axilla space
   3. The elbows should be slightly flexed 20 to 30 degrees when walking
   4. When ambulating with the client, stand on the affected side
   5. Instruct the client never to rest the axilla on the axillary bars
   6. Instruct the client to look up and outward when ambulating
   7. Instruct the client to stop ambulation if numbness or tingling in the hands or arms occur

B. Crutch gaits

C. Assisting the client with crutches to sit and stand
   1. Place the unaffected leg against the front of the chair
   2. Move the crutches to affected side and grasp the chair's arm with the hand on the unaffected side
   3. Flex the knee of unaffected leg to lower self into the chair while placing the affected leg straight out in front
   4. Reverse steps to move from a sitting to a standing position

D. Going up and down stairs
   1. Up the stairs
      a. The client moves the unaffected leg up first
      b. The client moves the affected leg and the crutches up
   2. Down the stairs
      a. The client moves the crutches and the affected leg down
      b. The client moves unaffected leg down

VI. CANES AND WALKERS

A. Description: made of a lightweight material with a rubber suction tip at the bottom

B. Implementation
   1. Stand at the affected side of the client when ambulating
   2. The handle should be at the level of the client's greater trochanter
   3. The client's elbow should be flexed at a 25- to 30-degree angle
   4. Instruct the client to hold cane close to the body
   5. Instruct the client to hold cane in the hand on the unaffected side so that cane and weaker leg can work together with each step
   6. Instruct the client to move the cane at the same time as the affected leg
   7. Instruct the client to inspect the rubber tips regularly for worn places

C. Hemicanes or quadripod canes
   1. Used for clients who have the use of only one upper extremity
   2. Hemicanes provide more security than a quadripod cane; however, both types provide more security than a single-tipped cane

3. Position the cane at the client's unaffected side with the straight nonangled side adjacent to the body
4. Position the cane 6 inches from client's side with the hand grips level with the greater trochanter

D. Walker
1. Stand adjacent to the client on the affected side
2. Instruct the client to put all four points of the walker flat on the floor before putting weight on the hand pieces
3. Instruct the client to move the walker forward and to walk into it

VII. COMPLICATIONS OF FRACTURES (Box 56-7)

A. Fat embolism
1. Description
   a. An embolism originating in the bone marrow that occurs after a fracture
   b. Clients with long bone fractures are at the greatest risk for development of **fat embolism**
   c. Usually occurs within 48 hours after the injury
2. Data collection
   a. Restlessness
   b. Mental status changes
   c. Tachycardia, tachypnea, hypotension
   d. Dyspnea
   e. Petechial rash over upper chest and neck
3. Implementation: notify the physician immediately

B. **Compartment syndrome**
1. Description
   a. Increased pressure within one or more compartments causing massive compromise of circulation to an area
   b. Leads to decreased perfusion and tissue anoxia
   c. Within 4 to 6 hours after the onset of **compartment syndrome**, neuromuscular damage is irreversible
2. Data collection
   a. Increased pain and swelling
   b. Pain with passive motion
   c. Inability to move joints
   d. Loss of sensation (paresthesia)
   e. Pulselessness
3. Implementation: notify the physician immediately

C. Infection
1. Description: can be caused by the interruption of the integrity of the skin
2. Data collection
   a. Fever
   b. Pain
   c. Erythema in the area surrounding the fracture
   d. Tachycardia
   e. Elevated white blood cell (WBC) count
3. Implementation: notify the physician

D. Avascular necrosis
1. Description: an interruption in the blood supply to the bony tissue, which results in the death of the bone
2. Data collection
   a. Pain
   b. Decreased sensation
3. Implementation
   a. Notify the physician if pain or decreased sensation occurs
   b. Prepare the client for removal of necrotic tissue because it serves as a focus for infection

E. Pulmonary embolism
1. Description: caused by immobility precipitated by a fracture
2. Data collection
   a. Restlessness and apprehension
   b. Dyspnea
   c. Diaphoresis
3. Implementation
   a. Notify the physician if signs of emboli are present
   b. Anticoagulant therapy may be prescribed

BOX 56-7

Complications of Fractures

Compartment syndrome
Fat emboli
Infection
Avascular necrosis
Pulmonary emboli

VIII. FRACTURED HIP

A. Types
1. Intracapsular
   a. Bone is broken inside the joint
   b. Skin **traction** is applied preoperatively to immobilize and prevent pain
   c. Treatment includes a total hip replacement or **internal fixation** with replacement of the femoral head with a prosthesis
   d. Avoid hip flexion to prevent displacement
2. Extracapsular
   a. Fracture can occur at the greater trochanter or can be an intertrochanteric fracture

b. Trochanteric fracture is outside the joint
c. Preoperative treatment includes balanced suspension **traction**
d. Avoid hip flexion to prevent displacement
e. Surgical treatment includes **internal fixation** with nail-plate, screws, or wires

B. Postoperative implementation
1. Maintain leg and hip in proper alignment
2. Prevent flexion or external or internal rotation
3. Turn the client from back to unaffected side
4. Do not position to affected side unless prescribed by the physician
5. Maintain leg abduction to prevent internal or external rotation
6. Use a trochanter roll to prevent external rotation
7. Ensure that hip flexion angle does not exceed 60 to 80 degrees
8. Elevate the head of the bed 30 to 45 degrees for meals only
9. Ambulate as prescribed by the physician
10. Avoid weight bearing on affected leg as prescribed; instruct client on the use of a walker to avoid weight bearing
11. Keep the operative leg extended, supported, and elevated when getting client out of bed
12. Avoid hip flexion greater than 90 degrees and avoid low chairs when out of bed
13. Monitor the wound for infection or hemorrhage
14. Monitor circulation and sensation of the affected side
15. Maintain Hemovac or Jackson-Pratt drain if in place; maintain compression to facilitate drainage and monitor and record output
16. Drainage should continuously decrease in amount, and by 48 hours postoperatively, drainage should be approximately 30 mL in an 8-hour period
17. Maintain the use of antiembolism stockings and encourage the client to flex and extend feet and ankles
18. Provide continuous passive motion (CPM) as prescribed
19. Instruct the client to avoid crossing legs and bending over activities
20. Physical therapy will begin postoperatively as prescribed by the physician

IX. TOTAL KNEE REPLACEMENT

A. Description: implantation of a device to substitute for the femoral condyles and the tibial joint surfaces

B. Postoperative implementation
1. Monitor the incision for drainage and infection
2. Maintain Hemovac or Jackson-Pratt drain if in place
3. Begin CPM 24 to 48 hours as prescribed to exercise knee and provide moderate flexion and extension
4. Administer analgesics before CPM to decrease pain
5. Leg should not be dangled to prevent dislocation
6. Maintain Ace wrap or antiembolism stockings if prescribed
7. Prepare the client for out of bed activities
8. Avoid weight bearing and instruct the client in crutch walking

X. HERNIATION: INTERVERTEBRAL DISK

A. Description: nucleus of disk protrudes into the annulus causing nerve compression

B. Cervical disk
1. Occurs at C5 to C6 and C6 to C7 interspaces
2. Diagnosis is determined by cervical myelography
3. Causes pain and stiffness in the neck, top of the shoulders, scapula, upper extremities, and head
4. Produces paresthesia and numbness of the upper extremities
5. Implementation
   a. Provide bed rest to relieve pressure, and reduce inflammation and edema
   b. Provide immobilization as prescribed via cervical collar, **traction**, or brace
   c. Apply hot, moist compresses as prescribed to increase the blood flow and relax spasms
   d. Instruct the client to avoid flexing, extending, or rotating the neck
   e. Instruct the client that while sleeping to avoid the prone position and keep the head, spine, and hip in alignment
   f. Instruct the client to avoid long automobile rides
   g. Instruct the client in the use of analgesics, sedatives, antiinflammatory agents, and corticosteroids as prescribed
   h. Prepare the client for a corticosteroid injection into the epidural space if prescribed
   i. Assist the client with the application of a cervical collar or cervical traction as prescribed
6. Cervical collar
   a. Used for cervical disk herniation
   b. Holds head in a neutral or slightly flexed position

c. Client may have to wear a cervical collar 24 hours a day
d. Inspect the skin under the collar for irritation
e. When pain subsides, the client is taught cervical isometric exercises to strengthen the muscles

C. Lumbar disk
1. Occurs at L4 to L5 or L5 to S1 interspaces
2. Diagnosis is determined by lumbar myelography
3. Postural deformity occurs
4. Produces muscle weakness, sensory loss, and the tendon reflexes are altered
5. The client experiences low back pain and muscle spasms with radiation of the pain into one hip and down the leg (sciatica)
6. Pain is aggravated by bending, lifting, straining, sneezing, coughing and is relieved by bed rest
7. Implementation
a. Bed rest on a firm mattress in semi-Fowler's position with moderate hip and knee flexion
b. Apply moist heat and massage as prescribed
c. Instruct the client to sleep on side with knees and hips in a position of flexion with a pillow between the legs
d. Apply pelvic **traction** as prescribed to relieve muscle spasms
e. Begin ambulation gradually as the inflammation and edema subside
f. Instruct the client in the use of muscle relaxants, antiinflammatory medications, and corticosteroids as prescribed
g. Instruct the client in the use of a corset or brace as prescribed
h. Instruct the client regarding correct posture while sitting, standing, walking, and working
i. Instruct the client to lift objects by bending the knees and keeping the back straight, avoiding lifting anything above the elbows
j. Instruct the client regarding a weight control program as prescribed
k. Instruct the client in an exercise program as prescribed to strengthen abdominal and back muscles

D. Disk surgery (Box 56-8)
1. Preoperative implementation
a. Reassure client that surgery will not weaken the back
b. Instruct the client regarding coughing and deep breathing exercises
c. Instruct the client about logrolling and ROM exercises

BOX 56-8

Types of Disk Surgery

Diskectomy: removal of herniated disk tissue and related matter
Laminectomy: removal of the lamina
Laminotomy: division of the lamina of a vertebrae
Diskectomy with fusion: fusion of vertebrae with bone graft
Chemolysis: injections to dissolve affected disk

2. Postoperative implementation: cervical disk
a. Monitor for respiratory difficulty
b. Encourage coughing and deep breathing
c. Monitor for hoarseness and inability to cough effectively because this may indicate laryngeal nerve damage
d. Use throat sprays or lozenges for sore throat and do not use those that may numb the throat, to avoid choking
e. Monitor wound for drainage
f. Provide a soft diet if the client complains of dysphagia
g. Monitor for sudden return of radicular pain, which may indicate that the cervical spine has become unstable
3. Postoperative implementation: lumbar disk
a. Monitor for wound hemorrhage
b. Monitor sensation and motor ability of lower extremities as well as color, temperature, and sensation of toes
c. Monitor for urinary retention, paralytic ileus, and constipation
d. Initiate measures to prevent constipation such as a high-fiber diet, increased fluids, and stool softeners as prescribed
e. When turning and repositioning client, place bed in a flat position and a pillow between the legs; turn the client as a unit (logroll) without twisting the client's back
f. When positioning the client, a pillow is placed under the head with the knees slightly flexed
g. Avoid extreme knee flexion when the client is lying on the side
h. To assist the client out of bed, raise the head of the bed while the client lies on the side; the client's head and shoulders are supported by the first nurse, the client pushes self to a sitting position, while the second nurse eases the legs over side of bed
i. Instruct the client to avoid sitting, as it places a strain on the surgical site
j. Administer narcotics and sedatives as prescribed to relieve pain and anxiety

k. Encourage early ambulation
l. Assist the client with the use of a back brace or corset if prescribed

XI. AMPUTATION (Figure 56-3)

A. Description: the surgical removal of a limb or part of a limb

B. Postoperative implementation
1. Monitor vital signs
2. Monitor for infection and hemorrhage
3. Mark bleeding and drainage on the dressing if it occurs
4. Keep a tourniquet at the bedside
5. Monitor for pulmonary emboli
6. Observe and prevent contractures
7. Monitor for signs of necrosis and neuroma
8. Evaluate for phantom limb pain, explain sensation to the client, and medicate client as prescribed
9. During the first 24 hours, elevate the foot of the bed to reduce edema, then keep the bed flat to prevent hip flexion contractures as prescribed
10. Do not elevate the stump itself, because elevation can cause flexion contracture of the hip joint
11. After 24 and 48 hours postoperatively, position client prone as prescribed to stretch the muscles and prevent flexion contractures of hip
12. In the prone position, place a pillow under the abdomen and stump and keep the legs close together to prevent abduction
13. Maintain application of an Ace wrap or elastic stump shrinker as prescribed to provide stump shrinkage
14. Remove and rewrap the Ace bandage or elastic stump shrinker three to four times a day as prescribed
15. Wash stump with mild soap or water and apply lanolin to skin if dry
16. Massage skin toward the suture line to increase circulation
17. Prepare for a **cast** application if prescribed to prepare the stump for prosthesis
18. Encourage the client to look at the stump
19. Encourage verbalization regarding loss of a body part and assist client to identify coping mechanisms to deal with the loss

C. Implementation for below-the-knee amputation
1. Prevent edema
2. Do not allow the stump to hang over the edge of the bed
3. Do not allow the client to sit for long periods

D. Implementation for above-the-knee amputation
1. Prevent internal or external rotation of the limb
2. Place a sandbag or rolled towel along the outside of the thigh to prevent rotation

E. Rehabilitation
1. Instruct the client in crutch walking
2. Prepare the stump for prosthesis
3. Prepare the client for the fitting of the stump for prosthesis
4. Instruct the client in exercises to maintain ROM
5. Provide psychosocial support to the client

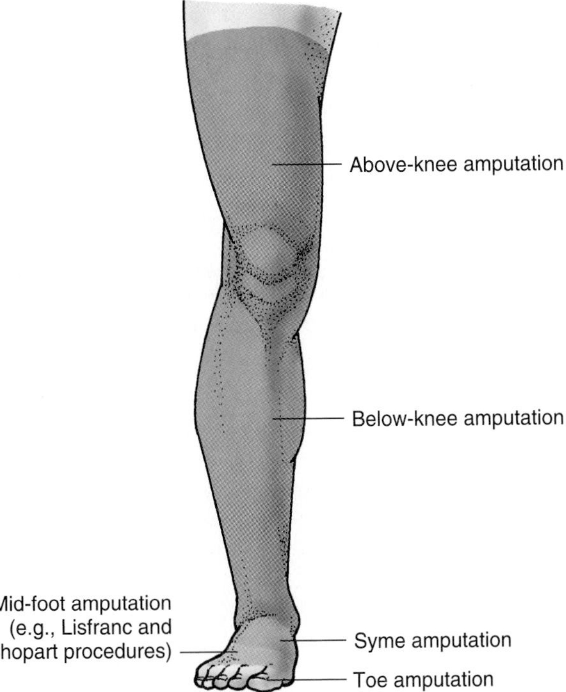

FIG. 56-3 Common levels of lower extremity amputations. (From Ignatavicius D, Workman M: *Medical surgical nursing*, ed 4, Philadelphia, 2002, WB Saunders.)

XII. RHEUMATOID ARTHRITIS (RA)

A. Description
1. Chronic systemic inflammatory disease; the cause is unknown
2. Leads to destruction of connective tissue and synovial membrane within joints
3. Weakens and leads to dislocation of the joint and permanent deformity
4. Formation of pannus occurs at the junction of synovial tissue and articular cartilage projecting into the joint cavity and causing necrosis
5. Exacerbations are increased by physical or emotional stress

6. Risk factors include exposure to infectious agents; fatigue and emotional stress can exacerbate the condition
7. Vasculitis can cause malfunction and eventual failure of an organ or system

B. Data collection
1. Inflammation, tenderness, and stiffness of the joints
2. Moderate to severe pain and morning stiffness lasting longer than 30 minutes
3. Joint deformities, muscle atrophy, and decreased ROM
4. Spongy, soft feeling in joints
5. Low-grade temperature, fatigue, and weakness
6. Anorexia, weight loss, and anemia
7. Elevated sedimentation rate and positive rheumatoid factor
8. X-ray film showing joint deterioration
9. Synovial tissue biopsy presents inflammation

C. Rheumatoid (RA) factor
1. A blood test used to diagnose rheumatoid arthritis
2. Values
   a. Nonreactive: 0 to 39 IU/mL
   b. Weakly reactive: 40 to 79 IU/mL
   c. Reactive: greater than 80 IU/mL

D. Pain
1. Salicylates
   a. Monitor for side effects including tinnitus, gastrointestinal (GI) upset, or prolonged bleeding time
   b. Administer with meals or a snack
   c. Monitor for abnormal bleeding or bruising
2. Nonsteroidal antiinflammatory drugs (NSAIDs)
   a. Administer in combination with salicylates as prescribed if pain and inflammation are not decreased within 6 to 12 weeks after salicylate therapy
   b. Monitor for side effects such as GI upset, central nervous system (CNS) manifestations, skin rash, hypertension, fluid retention, and changes in renal function
3. Corticosteroids: administer as prescribed during exacerbations or severe involvement when commonly used agents are ineffective
4. Antineoplastic medications: administer as prescribed in clients with life-threatening RA
5. Gold salts: administer as prescribed in combination with salicylates and NSAIDs to induce remission and decrease pain and inflammation

E. Physical mobility
1. Preserve joint function
2. Provide ROM exercises to maintain joint motion and muscle strengthening
3. Balance rest and activity
4. Splints during acute inflammation to prevent deformity
5. Prevent flexion contractures
6. Apply heat or cold therapy as prescribed to joints
7. Apply paraffin baths and massage as prescribed
8. Encourage consistency with exercise program
9. Instruct the client to stop exercise if pain increases
10. Exercise only to the point of pain
11. Avoid weight bearing on inflamed joints

F. Self-care (Box 56-9)
1. Assess the need for assistive devices such as higher level toilet seats, chairs, and wheelchairs to facilitate mobility
2. Collaborate with occupational therapy to obtain assistive adaptive devices
3. Instruct the client in alternative strategies for providing activities of daily living

G. Fatigue
1. Identify factors that may contribute to fatigue
2. Monitor for signs of anemia
3. Administer iron, folic acid, and vitamin supplements as prescribed
4. Monitor for drug-related blood loss by testing the stool for occult blood
5. Instruct the client in measures to conserve energy such as pacing activities and obtaining assistance when possible

H. Body image disturbance
1. Assess the client's reaction to body change
2. Encourage the client to verbalize feeling

BOX 56-9

Client Education for RA and Degenerative Joint Disease

Assist the client to identify and correct hazards in the home
Instruct the client in the correct use of assistive adaptive devices
Instruct the client in energy conservation measures
Review prescribed exercise program
Instruct the client to sit in a chair with a high, straight back
Instruct the client to use a small pillow only when lying down
Instruct the client in measures to protect the joints
Instruct the client regarding the prescribed medications
Stress the importance of follow-up visits with the physician

3. Assist the client with self-care activities and grooming
4. Encourage the client to wear street clothes
5. Provide patience and understanding and be aware that the client may be manipulative and demanding

I. Surgical implementation
1. Synovectomy: surgical removal of the synovia to help maintain joint function
2. Arthrodesis: bony fusion of a joint to regain some mobility
3. Joint replacement (arthroplasty): surgical replacement of diseased joints with artificial joints to restore motion to a joint and function to the muscles, ligaments, and other soft tissue structures that control a joint

XIII. OSTEOARTHRITIS (DEGENERATIVE JOINT DISEASE, DJD)

A. Description
1. Progressive degeneration of the joints caused by wear and tear
2. Causes the formation of bony buildup and the loss of articular cartilage in peripheral and axial joints
3. Affects the weight-bearing joints and joints that receive the greatest stress such as the knees, toes, and lower spine
4. The cause is unknown but may be trauma, fractures, infections, obesity

B. Data collection
1. Joint pain that early in the disease process diminishes after rest and intensifies after activity
2. As the disease progresses, pain occurs with slight motion or even at rest
3. Symptoms are aggravated by temperature change and humidity
4. Crepitus
5. Joint enlargement
6. Presence of Heberden's nodes or Bouchard's nodes
7. Limited ROM
8. Difficulty getting up after prolonged sitting
9. Skeletal muscle atrophy
10. Inability to perform activities of daily living
11. Compression of the spine as manifested by radiating pain, stiffness, and muscle spasms in one or both extremities

C. Pain
1. Administer NSAIDs, salicylates, and muscle relaxants as prescribed
2. Prepare the client for corticosteroid injections into joints as prescribed
3. Place affected joint in functional position
4. Immobilize affected joint with a splint or brace
5. Avoid large pillows under the head or knees
6. Provide a bed or foot cradle
7. Position the client prone twice a day
8. Instruct the client on the importance of moist heat, hot packs or compresses, and paraffin dips as prescribed
9. Apply cold applications as prescribed when joint is acutely inflamed
10. Encourage adequate rest, recommending 10 hours of sleep at night and a 1- to- 2 hour nap in the afternoon

D. Nutrition
1. Encourage a well-balanced diet
2. Encourage weight loss if necessary

E. Physical mobility (Box 56-9)
1. Reinforce the exercise program and the importance of participating in the program
2. Instruct the client that exercises should be active rather than passive and to exercise only to the point of pain
3. Instruct the client to stop exercise if pain is increased with exercising
4. Instruct the client to decrease the number of repetitions in an exercise when the inflammation is severe

F. Surgical management
1. Osteotomy: the bone is cut to correct the joint deformity and promote realignment
2. Total joint replacement (TJR)
   a. Performed when all measures of pain relief have failed
   b. Hips and knees are most commonly replaced
   c. Contraindicated in the presence of infection, advanced osteoporosis, and severe inflammation

XIV. OSTEOPOROSIS

A. Description
1. An age-related metabolic disease
2. Bone demineralization results in the loss of bone mass, leading to fragile and porous bones and subsequent fractures
3. Greater bone resorption than bone formation occurs
4. Occurs most commonly in the wrist, hip, and vertebral column
5. Can occur postmenopausal or as a result of a metabolic disorder or calcium deficiency

B. Data collection
1. Back pain after lifting, bending, or stooping
2. Back pain that increases with palpation

3. Pelvic or hip pain, especially with weight bearing
4. Problems with balance
5. Decline in height from vertebrae compression
6. Kyphosis of the dorsal spine
7. Constipation, abdominal distention, and respiratory impairment as a result of movement restriction and spinal deformity
8. Pathological fractures
9. Appearance of thin porous bone on x-ray film

C. Implementation
1. Assess risk for injury
2. Provide a safe and hazard-free environment and assist client to identify hazards in the home environment
3. Use side rails to prevent falls
4. Move the client gently when turning and repositioning
5. Encourage ambulation; assist with ambulation if client is unsteady
6. Instruct the client in the use of assistive devices such as a cane or walker
7. Provide ROM exercises
8. Instruct the client in the use of good body mechanics
9. Instruct the client in exercises to strengthen abdominal and back muscles to improve posture and provide support for the spine
10. Instruct the client to avoid activities that can cause vertebral compression
11. Apply a back brace as prescribed during an acute phase to immobilize the spine and provide spinal column support
12. Encourage the use of a firm mattress
13. Provide a diet high in protein, calcium, vitamins C and D, and iron
14. Encourage adequate fluid intake to prevent renal calculi
15. Instruct the client to avoid alcohol and coffee
16. Administer estrogen or androgens to decrease the rate of bone resorption as prescribed
17. Administer calcium and vitamin D as prescribed for bone metabolism
18. Administer calcitonin as prescribed to inhibit bone loss
19. Administer analgesics, muscle relaxants, and antiinflammatory medications as prescribed

XV. GOUT

A. Description
1. A systemic disease in which urate crystals deposit in joints and other body tissues
2. Leads to abnormal amounts of uric acid in the body
3. Primary gout results from a disorder of purine metabolism
4. Secondary gout involves excessive uric acid in the blood that is caused by another disease

B. Phases
1. Asymptomatic
   a. No symptoms
   b. Serum uric acid is elevated
2. Acute: excruciating pain and inflammation of one or more small joints, especially the great toe
3. Intermittent: Asymptomatic period between acute attacks
4. Chronic
   a. Results from repeated episodes of acute gout
   b. Results in deposits of urate crystals under the skin and within the major organs, especially the renal system

C. Data collection
1. Excruciating pain in the involved joints
2. Swelling and inflammation of joints
3. Tophi (hard, fairly large and irregular shaped deposits in the skin) that may break open and discharge a yellow gritty substance
4. Low-grade fever
5. Malaise and headache
6. Pruritis
7. Presence of renal stones
8. Elevated uric acid levels

D. Implementation
1. Provide a low-purine diet as prescribed
2. Instruct the client to avoid foods as organ meats, wines, aged cheese
3. Encourage a high fluid intake of 2000 mL to prevent stone formation
4. Encourage weight reduction diet if required
5. Instruct the client to avoid alcohol and fat-starvation diets, as they may precipitate a gout attack
6. Increase urinary pH (above 6) by eating alkaline ash foods such as citrus fruits and juices, milk, and other dairy products
7. Provide bed rest during acute attacks
8. Monitor joint ROM ability and appearance of joints
9. Position the joint in mild flexion position during acute attack
10. Elevate affected extremity
11. Protect affected joint from excessive movement or direct contact with sheets
12. Provide heat or cold for local treatments to affected joint as prescribed
13. Administer NSAIDs and antigout medications as prescribed

PRACTICE QUESTIONS

1. A client is complaining of knee pain. The knee is swollen, reddened, and warm to the touch. The nurse interprets that the client's signs and symptoms are not compatible with:
   1. Inflammation
   2. Degenerative disease
   3. Infection
   4. Recent injury
2. A client is treated in the physician's office after a fall, which sprained the ankle. X-ray film has ruled out fracture. Before sending the client home, the nurse would plan to teach the client about which of the following items that is to be avoided in the next 24 hours?
   1. Application of a heating pad
   2. Application of an Ace wrap
   3. Resting the foot
   4. Elevating the ankle on a pillow while sitting or lying down
3. A nurse is collecting physical data of the musculoskeletal system on an assigned client. The nurse would document the presence of which of the following as a normal finding?
   1. Presence of fasciculations
   2. Atrophy on the client's dominant side
   3. Hypertrophy on the client's dominant side
   4. Atrophy on the client's nondominant side
4. A nurse has given dietary instructions to a client to minimize the risk of osteoporosis. The nurse would evaluate that the client understands the recommended changes if the client verbalized to increase intake of which of these foods?
   1. Potatoes
   2. Cheese
   3. Fish
   4. Chicken
5. A nurse is providing care to a client after a bone biopsy. Which of the following actions by the nurse is not needed in the care of this client?
   1. Monitoring site for swelling, bleeding, hematoma
   2. Administering intramuscular narcotic analgesics
   3. Elevating the limb for 24 hours
   4. Monitoring vital signs every 4 hours
6. A nurse has reinforced instructions to the client returning home after arthroscopy of the knee. The nurse would evaluate that the client understands the instructions if the client states to:
   1. Stay off the leg entirely for the rest of the day
   2. Resume regular exercise the following day
   3. Refrain from eating food for the remainder of the day
   4. Report fever or site inflammation to the physician
7. A nurse is caring for the client who is going to have an arthrogram using a contrast medium. Which of the following data collected by the nurse would be of highest priority?
   1. Allergy to iodine or shellfish
   2. Ability of the client to remain still during the procedure
   3. Whether the client has any remaining questions about the procedure
   4. Whether the client wishes to void before the procedure
8. A client with a bone infection is to undergo indium imaging. The client asks the nurse to explain how the procedure is done. The nurse plans the response on the understanding that:
   1. Indium is injected into the bloodstream and collects in normal bone, but not in infected areas
   2. Indium is injected into the bloodstream and highlights the vascular supply to the bone
   3. A sample of the client's leukocytes is tagged with indium and will subsequently accumulate in infected bone
   4. A sample of the client's RBCs is tagged with indium, and will highlight normal bone
9. A client with possible rib fracture has never had a chest x-ray study. The nurse would plan to tell the client which of the following items about the procedure?
   1. The x-rays stimulate a small amount of pain
   2. It is necessary to remove jewelry and any other metal objects
   3. The client will be asked to breathe in and out during the x-ray study
   4. The x-ray technologist will stand next to the client during the x-ray study
10. A nurse is teaching the client who is to have a gallium scan about the procedure. The nurse would include which of the following items as part of the instructions?
    1. The gallium will be injected intravenously 2 to 3 hours before the procedure
    2. The procedure takes about 15 minutes to perform
    3. The client must stand erect during the filming
    4. The client should remain on bed rest for the remainder of the day after the scan
11. A client has had a bone scan. The nurse would evaluate that the client understands the elements of follow-up care if the client states to:
    1. Report any feelings of nausea or flushing
    2. Ambulate at least three times before the end of the day
    3. Eat only small meals for the remainder of the day
    4. Drink plenty of water for a day or two after the procedure
12. A client seeks treatment in the emergency room for a lower leg injury. There is visible deformity to the lower aspect of the leg, and the injured leg appears shorter than the other. The area is painful, swollen,

and beginning to become ecchymotic. The nurse interprets that this client has experienced a:
1. Contusion
2. Fracture
3. Sprain
4. Strain

13. A nurse is one of several people who witness a vehicle hit a pedestrian at fairly low speed on a small street. The individual is dazed and tries to get up. The leg appears fractured. The nurse would:
1. Stay with the person and coax the person to remain still
2. Assist the person to get up and walk to the sidewalk
3. Leave the person for a few moments to call an ambulance
4. Try to manually reduce the fracture

14. A nurse witnesses a client sustain a fall and suspects the leg may be fractured. Which of the following actions is the highest priority of the nurse?
1. Take a set of vital signs
2. Call the radiology department
3. Reassure the client that everything will be fine
4. Immobilize the leg before moving the client

15. A nurse in the emergency room is caring for a client with a fractured arm. The nurse would evaluate that which of the following items is not necessary before reduction of the fracture in the casting room?
1. Explanation of the procedure to the client
2. Administration of an analgesic
3. Anesthesia consent
4. Consent for the procedure

16. A nurse plans to reduce the anxiety of a client who is going to have a plaster cast applied by teaching the client about the procedure. The nurse would not include which of the following items in the discussion?
1. A stockinette will be placed over the leg area to be casted
2. The cast edges may be trimmed with a cast knife
3. The cast will give off heat as it dries
4. The client may bear weight on the cast in one-half hour

17. A nurse is planning to teach the client with a left arm cast about measures to keep the left shoulder from becoming stiff and "frozen." Which of the following suggestions would the nurse include in the teaching plan?
1. Lift the left arm up over the head
2. Lift the right arm up over the head
3. Make a fist with the hand of the casted arm
4. Use a sling on the left arm

18. A client has a fiberglass (nonplaster) cast applied to the lower leg. The client asks the nurse when the client will be able to walk on the cast. The nurse replies that the client will be able to bear weight on the cast:
1. Within 20 to 30 minutes of application
2. In approximately 8 hours
3. In 24 hours
4. In 48 hours

19. A nurse has reinforced instructions with the client with a nonplaster (fiberglass) leg cast about on cast care at home. The nurse would evaluate that the client needs further instructions if the client makes which of the following statements?
1. "I should avoid walking on wet, slippery floors."
2. "It's OK to wipe dirt off the top of the cast with a damp cloth."
3. "I'm not supposed to scratch the skin underneath the cast."
4. "If the cast gets wet, I can dry it with a hair dryer turned to the warmest setting."

20. A client with a hip fracture asks the nurse why Buck's extension traction is being applied before surgery. The nurse's response is based on the understanding that Buck's extension traction primarily:
1. Provides rigid immobilization of the fracture site
2. Provides comfort by reducing muscle spasms, and provides fracture immobilization
3. Lengthens the fractured leg to prevent severing of blood vessels
4. Allows bony healing to begin before surgery

21. A client in skeletal leg traction with an overbed frame and trapeze is not allowed to turn from side to side. Which of the following actions by the nurse would be most useful in trying to provide good skin care to the client?
1. Ask the client to lift up by digging into the mattress with the unaffected leg
2. Push down on the mattress of the bed while administering care
3. Have another nurse tilt the client anyway
4. Ask the client to pull up on a trapeze to lift the hips off the bed

22. A nurse is evaluating the pin sites of a client in skeletal traction. The nurse would be least concerned with which of the following findings?
1. Purulent drainage
2. Serous drainage
3. Pain at a pin site
4. Inflammation

23. A client has Buck's extension traction applied to the right leg. The nurse would plan which of the following interventions to prevent complications of the device?
1. Massage the skin of the right leg with lotion every 8 hours
2. Give pin care once a shift
3. Inspect the skin on the right leg at least once every 8 hours
4. Release the weights on the right leg for ROM exercises daily

24. A nurse is caring for the client who had skeletal traction applied to the left leg. The client is complaining of severe left leg pain. Which of the following actions should the nurse take first?
 1. Medicate the client with an analgesic
 2. Provide pin care
 3. Call the physician immediately
 4. Check the client's alignment in bed
25. A nurse has reinforced instructions regarding specific leg exercises for the client immobilized in right skeletal lower leg traction. The nurse evaluates that the client needs further instruction if the nurse observes the client:
 1. Pulling up on the trapeze
 2. Flexing and extending the feet
 3. Performing active ROM to the right ankle and knee
 4. Doing quadriceps-setting and gluteal-setting exercises
26. A nurse is assessing the casted extremity of a client. The nurse would check for which of the following signs and symptoms indicative of infection?
 1. Coolness and pallor of the extremity
 2. Presence of a "hot spot" on the cast
 3. Diminished distal pulse
 4. Dependent edema
27. A client has sustained a closed fracture and has just had a cast applied to the affected arm. The client is complaining of intense pain. The nurse has elevated the limb, applied an ice bag, and administered an analgesic that was ineffective in relieving the pain. The nurse interprets that this pain may be due to:
 1. Impaired tissue perfusion
 2. The newness of the fracture
 3. The anxiety of the client
 4. Infection under the cast
28. A nurse is assigned to care for a client with multiple trauma admitted to the hospital. The client has a leg fracture and a plaster cast has been applied. In positioning the casted leg, the nurse should:
 1. Keep the leg in a level position
 2. Keep the leg level for 3 hours, and elevate it for 1 hour
 3. Elevate the leg on pillows continuously for 24 to 48 hours
 4. Elevate the leg for 3 hours, and put it flat for 1 hour
29. A client is complaining of skin irritation from the edges of a cast applied the previous day. The nurse should plan for which of the following actions?
 1. Massaging the skin at the rim of the cast
 2. Applying lotion to the skin at the rim of the cast
 3. Using a rough file to smooth the cast edges
 4. Petaling the cast edges with adhesive tape
30. A client is being discharged to home after application of a plaster leg cast. The nurse would evaluate that the client understands proper care of the cast if the client states to:
 1. Avoid getting the cast wet
 2. Use the fingertips to lift and move the leg
 3. Cover the casted leg with warm blankets
 4. Use a padded coat hanger end to scratch under the cast
31. A client being measured for crutches asks the nurse why the crutches cannot rest up underneath the arm for extra support. The nurse's response is based on the understanding that this could result in:
 1. Impaired range of motion while the client ambulates
 2. Skin breakdown in the area of the axilla
 3. Injury to the brachial plexus nerves
 4. A fall and further injury
32. A nurse is planning to reinforce instructions to the client about how to stand on crutches. The nurse plans to incorporate into written instructions to tell the client to place the crutches:
 1. 8 inches to the front and side of the client's toes
 2. 3 inches to the front and side of the client's toes
 3. 20 inches to the front and side of the client's toes
 4. 15 inches to the front and side of the client's toes
33. A nurse is giving the client with a left leg cast crutch-walking instructions using the three-point gait. The client is allowed touch-down of the affected leg. The nurse tells the client to advance the:
 1. Left leg and right crutch, then right leg and left crutch
 2. Crutches and then both legs simultaneously
 3. Crutches and the right leg, then advance the left leg
 4. Crutches and the left leg, then advance the right leg
34. A nurse has given the client instructions regarding crutch safety. The nurse evaluates that the client needs reinforcement of information if the client states:
 1. The need to have spare crutches and tips available
 2. That crutch tips will not slip even when wet
 3. Not to use someone else's crutches
 4. That crutch tips should be inspected periodically for wear
35. A client has slight weakness in the right leg. Based on this data, the nurse determines that the client would benefit most from the use of a:
 1. Walker
 2. Wooden crutch
 3. Lofstrand crutch
 4. Straight leg cane
36. A client who has experienced a cerebrovascular accident (CVA) has partial hemiplegia of the left leg.

The straight leg cane formerly used by the client is not quite sufficient now. The nurse interprets that the client could benefit from the somewhat greater support and stability provided by a:
1. Quad-cane
2. Wooden crutch
3. Lofstrand crutch
4. Wheelchair

37. A client with right-sided weakness needs to learn how to use a cane. The nurse plans to teach the client to position the cane by holding it with the:
1. Left hand, and placing the cane in front of the left foot
2. Right hand, and placing the cane in front of the right foot
3. Left hand, and 6 inches lateral to the left foot
4. Right hand, and 6 inches lateral to the right foot

38. A client who is learning to use a cane is afraid it will slip with ambulation, causing a fall. The nurse provides the client with the greatest reassurance by telling the client that:
1. Canes prevent falls, not cause them
2. The cane has a flared tip with concentric rings to give stability
3. The physical therapist will determine if the cane is inadequate
4. The cane would help to break a fall, even if the client does slip

39. A nurse is evaluating the client's use of a cane for left-sided weakness. The nurse would intervene and correct the client if the nurse observed that the client:
1. Holds the cane on the right side
2. Keeps the cane 6 inches out to the side of the right foot
3. Moves the cane when the right leg is moved
4. Leans on the cane when the right leg swings through

40. A nurse is caring for the client who develops compartment syndrome from a severely fractured arm. The client asks the nurse how this can happen. The nurse's response is based on the understanding that:
1. An injured artery causes impaired arterial perfusion through the compartment
2. The fascia expands with injury, causing pressure on underlying nerves and muscles
3. A bone fragment has injured the nerve supply in the area
4. Bleeding and swelling cause increased pressure in an area that cannot expand

41. A nurse is caring for a client with fresh application of a plaster leg cast. The nurse would plan to prevent development of compartment syndrome by:
1. Elevating the limb and applying ice to the affected leg
2. Elevating the limb and covering the limb with bath blankets
3. Placing the leg in a slightly dependent position and applying ice
4. Keeping the leg horizontal and applying ice to the affected leg

42. A nurse is monitoring a confused elderly client admitted with a hip fracture. Which of the following data obtained by the nurse would not place the client at more risk for altered thought processes?
1. Stress induced by the fracture
2. Hearing aid available and in working order
3. Unfamiliar hospital setting
4. Eyeglasses left at home

43. A nurse is caring for an elderly client who had a hip pinned after being fractured. In planning nursing care, which of the following would the nurse avoid to minimize the chance for further injury?
1. Side rails in the "up" position
2. Use of nightlight in hospital room and bathroom
3. Call bell placed within reach
4. Delays in responding to call light

44. A nurse is repositioning the client who has returned to the nursing unit after internal fixation of a fractured right hip. The nurse should use a:
1. Pillow to keep the right leg abducted during turning
2. Pillow to keep the right leg adducted during turning
3. Trochanter roll to prevent external rotation while turning
4. Trochanter roll to prevent abduction while turning

45. A client who has had a right total knee replacement asks the nurse how long the right leg must be kept in the continuous passive motion (CPM) machine. The nurse's response is based on the understanding that the device should be used:
1. For 30 minutes out of every hour
2. Every other hour for 60 minutes
3. For 3 hours at a time, followed by 1 hour of rest
4. As much as the client can tolerate

46. A nurse has an order to get the client out of bed to a chair on the first postoperative day after total knee replacement. The nurse would plan to do which of the following to protect the knee joint?
1. Apply a knee immobilizer before getting the client up, and elevate the client's surgical leg while sitting
2. Apply an Ace wrap around the dressing and put ice on the knee while sitting
3. Lift the client to the bedside chair leaving the CPM machine in place
4. Obtain a walker to minimize weight bearing by the client on the affected leg

47. A client with diabetes mellitus has had a right below the knee amputation. The nurse would be especially vigilant in monitoring for which of the following signs and symptoms due to the history of diabetes?
   1. Edema of the stump
   2. Hemorrhage
   3. Separation of wound edges
   4. Slight redness of incision
48. A client is admitted to the nursing unit after a left below-the-knee amputation after a crush injury to the foot and lower leg. The client tells the nurse "I think I'm going crazy. I can feel my left foot itching." The nurse interprets the client's statement to be:
   1. A normal response, and indicates the presence of phantom limb sensation
   2. A normal response, and indicates the presence of phantom limb pain
   3. An abnormal response, and indicates the client needs more psychological support
   4. An abnormal response, and indicates the client is in denial about the limb loss
49. A client is complaining of low back pain with radiation down the left posterior thigh. The nurse continues to collect data from the client to see if the pain is worsened or aggravated by:
   1. Bed rest
   2. Application of heat
   3. Bending or lifting
   4. Ibuprofen (Motrin)
50. A client has just undergone spinal fusion after experiencing a herniated lumbar disk. The nurse would avoid which of the following to maintain client safety after this procedure?
   1. Logrolling technique for repositioning
   2. Pillows under the length of the legs
   3. Head of bed flat
   4. Overhead trapeze
51. A nurse has reinforced instructions with a client with herniated lumbar disk about proper body mechanics and other items pertinent to low back care. The nurse evaluates that the client needs further instruction if the client verbalizes to:
   1. Get out of bed by sitting straight up and swinging legs over the side of the bed
   2. Increase fiber and fluids in the diet
   3. Strengthen the back muscles by swimming or walking
   4. Bend at the knees to pick up objects
52. A client who has had spinal fusion and insertion of hardware is extremely concerned with the perceived lengthy rehabilitation period. The client expresses concerns about finances and ability to return to prior employment. The nurse understands that the client's needs could best be addressed by referral to the:
   1. Surgeon
   2. Clinical nurse specialist
   3. Social worker
   4. Physical therapist
53. A nurse is planning to reinforce instructions to the client about proper use of a thoracolumbosacral orthosis after spinal fusion with instrumentation. The nurse would plan to include which of the following teaching points in discussion with the client?
   1. Areas of skin redness at the edges of the brace indicates a good, snug fit
   2. The device is applied before getting out of bed in the morning
   3. The brace should be applied directly next to the skin
   4. The Velcro closures should be fairly loose to avoid constriction
54. A client is being transferred to the nursing unit from the postanesthesia care unit after spinal fusion with Harrington rod insertion. The nurse would prepare to transfer the client from the stretcher to the bed by using:
   1. A bath blanket and the assistance of 3 people
   2. A bath blanket and the assistance of 4 people
   3. A slider board and the assistance of 2 people
   4. A slider board and the assistance of 4 people
55. A client is being discharged to home after spinal fusion with insertion of Harrington rods. The nurse would suggest a consultation with the continuing care nurse regarding the need for follow-up modification of the home environment if the client stated that:
   1. The bedroom and bath are on the second floor of the home
   2. The bathroom has hand railings in the shower
   3. The family has rented a commode for use by the client
   4. There are three steps to get up to the front door
56. A client with a left arm fracture exhibits loss of sensation in the left fingers, pallor, poor capillary refill, and diminished left radial pulse. The nurse should take which of the following actions?
   1. Administer an analgesic
   2. Check the circulation again in 30 minutes
   3. Provide range of motion to the fingers of the left hand
   4. Contact the physician
57. A client is complaining of pain underneath a cast in the area of a bony prominence. The nurse interprets that this client may need to have:
   1. The cast replaced with an air splint
   2. Extra padding put over this area of the cast
   3. The cast bivalved
   4. A window cut in the cast
58. A client is fearful about having an arm cast removed. Which of the following actions by the nurse would be the most helpful?

1. Telling the client that the saw makes a frightening noise
2. Reassuring the client that no one has yet had an arm lacerated
3. Stating that the hot cutting blades cause burns only very rarely
4. Showing the client the cast cutter and explaining how it works

59. A nurse is obtaining a health history from a client and is assessing for risk factors associated with osteoporosis. Which of the following findings is not an associated risk factor?
1. High calcium diet consumption
2. Postmenopausal age
3. Long-term use of corticosteroids
4. Family history of osteoporosis

60. A nurse is providing instructions to a client with osteoporosis regarding appropriate food items to include in the diet. Which of the following food items would provide the least amount calcium?
1. Plain yogurt
2. Seafood
3. Sardines
4. Pork

61. A nurse is caring for a client who is having an acute attack of gout. Which of the following would not be a component of the plan of care for this client?
1. Restricting fluids
2. A low purine diet
3. Bed rest
4. Administration of nonsteroidal antiinflammatory drugs (NSAIDs)

62. A nurse is collecting data on a client with a diagnosis of rheumatoid arthritis (RA). Which of the following would the nurse not expect to note in the client?
1. Complaints of pain that is more severe after exercise
2. Complaints of pain that is more severe on arising in the morning
3. Swollen, shiny joints
4. Skin nodules near bony prominences

ANSWERS

1. *Answer:* 2
Rationale: Redness and heat are associated with musculoskeletal inflammation, infection, or a recent injury. Degenerative disease is accompanied by pain, but there is no redness. Swelling may or may not occur.
Test-Taking Strategy: Use the process of elimination recalling the signs of inflammation. This will easily direct you to option 2. Review the signs of musculoskeletal inflammation if you had difficulty with this question.
Level of Cognitive Ability: Comprehension
Client Needs: Physiological Integrity
Integrated Concept/Process: Nursing Process/Data Collection
Content Area: Adult Health/Musculoskeletal
Reference: DeWit S: *Fundamental concepts and skills for nursing,* Philadelphia, 2001, WB Saunders, p. 205.

2. *Answer:* 1
Rationale: Soft tissue injuries such as sprains are treated by RICE (rest, ice, compression, elevation) for the first 24 hours after the injury. Ice is applied intermittently for 20 to 30 minutes at a time. Heat is not used in the first 24 hours because it could increase venous congestion, which would increase edema and pain.
Test-Taking Strategy: Use the process of elimination. Note the key word "avoided." It is likely that sprains should be rested and elevated, so these options are eliminated. Use of an Ace wrap is also helpful in reducing the pain and swelling, so this cannot be the answer either. By the process of elimination, heat must be the item to avoid in the first 24 hours. Review the measures to treat a sprain if you had difficulty with this question.
Level of Cognitive Ability: Application
Client Needs: Physiological Integrity
Integrated Concept/Process: Nursing Process/Planning
Content Area: Adult Health/Musculoskeletal
Reference: DeWit S: *Fundamental concepts and skills for nursing,* Philadelphia, 2001, WB Saunders, p. 780.

3. *Answer:* 3
Rationale: Hypertrophy, or increased muscle size, on the client's dominant side of up to 1 cm, is considered normal. Atrophy on either side is considered an abnormal finding. Fasciculations are fine muscle twitches that are not normally present.
Test-Taking Strategy: Use the process of elimination noting the key word "normal." Options 2 and 4 are eliminated first because atrophy is not a normal finding. Knowing that fasciculations are not normal helps you to select option 3 over option 1. Review normal musculoskeletal findings if you had difficulty with this question.
Level of Cognitive Ability: Comprehension
Client Needs: Health Promotion and Maintenance
Integrated Concept/Process: Nursing Process/Data Collection
Content Area: Adult Health/Musculoskeletal
Reference: Black J, Hawks J, Keene A: *Medical-surgical nursing: clinical management for positive outcomes,* ed 6, Philadelphia, 2001, WB Saunders, p. 211.

4. *Answer:* 2
Rationale: The major dietary source of calcium is from dairy foods, including milk, yogurt, and a variety of cheeses. Calcium may also be added to certain products, such as orange juice, which are then advertised as being "fortified" with calcium. Calcium supplements are available and recommended for those with typically low calcium intake.

Test-Taking Strategy: Use the process of elimination. Knowing that calcium is required for the client with osteoporosis and which foods are high in calcium are required to answer this question. Review this content if you had difficulty with this question.
Level of Cognitive Ability: Comprehension
Client Needs: Health Promotion and Maintenance
Integrated Concept/Process: Teaching/Learning
Content Area: Adult Health/Musculoskeletal
Reference: DeWit S: *Fundamental concepts and skills for nursing,* Philadelphia, 2001, WB Saunders, p. 474.

5. *Answer:* 2
Rationale: Nursing care after bone biopsy includes monitoring the site for swelling, bleeding, and hematoma formation. The biopsy site is elevated for 24 hours to reduce edema. The vital signs are monitored every 4 hours for 24 hours. The client usually requires mild analgesics; more severe pain usually indicates that complications are arising.
Test-Taking Strategy: Use the process of elimination. Note the key word "not." One way to approach this question is to look at the method of anesthesia used for this procedure. If you know that this procedure is done with the patient under local anesthesia, it makes sense that monitoring vital signs every 4 hours is probably sufficient (option 4). The nurse would routinely monitor for complications (option 1). This narrows the choices to site elevation or narcotic analgesics. Of these two, site elevation makes sense to reduce edema, while narcotic administration by the intramuscular route seems excessive for a local procedure. Thus, option 2 is the answer to the question as stated. Review care to the client after a bone biopsy if you had difficulty with this question.
Level of Cognitive Ability: Application
Client Needs: Physiological Integrity
Integrated Concept/Process: Nursing Process/Implementation
Content Area: Adult Health/Musculoskeletal
Reference: Black J, Hawks J, Keene A: *Medical-surgical nursing: clinical management for positive outcomes,* ed 6, Philadelphia, 2001, WB Saunders, p. 2098.

6. *Answer:* 4
Rationale: After arthroscopy, the client can usually walk carefully on the leg once sensation has returned. The client is instructed to avoid strenuous exercise for at least a few days. The client may resume the usual diet. Signs and symptoms of infection should be reported to the physician.
Test-Taking Strategy: Use the process of elimination. Note the key words "understands the instructions." Options 2 and 3 are the least plausible and may be eliminated first. To differentiate between the last two options, you would need to know that the client can walk on the affected leg once sensation has returned. The client is always taught signs and symptoms of infection to report to the physician. Review home care instructions after arthroscopy if you had difficulty with this question.
Level of Cognitive Ability: Comprehension
Client Needs: Health Promotion and Maintenance
Integrated Concept/Process: Teaching/Learning
Content Area: Adult Health/Musculoskeletal
Reference: Black J, Hawks J, Keene A: *Medical-surgical nursing: clinical management for positive outcomes,* ed 6, Philadelphia, 2001, WB Saunders, pp. 200, 548.

7. *Answer:* 1
Rationale: Because of the risk of allergy to contrast dye, the nurse places highest priority on identifying whether the client has an allergy to iodine or shellfish. The nurse also reinforces information about the test, tells the client about the need to remain still during the procedure, and encourages the client to void before the procedure for comfort.
Test-Taking Strategy: Use the process of elimination. Note the key words "highest priority." This tells you that more than one or all of the options are correct (in fact, they all are). While options 2, 3, and 4 all compete for your priority, only option 1 (allergy to iodine or shellfish) takes obvious first preference. The consequence of possible anaphylactic shock (physiological risk) makes this the correct option. Review care to the client scheduled for an arthrogram if you had difficulty with this question.
Level of Cognitive Ability: Application
Client Needs: Safe, Effective Care Environment
Integrated Concept/Process: Nursing Process/Data Collection
Content Area: Adult Health/Musculoskeletal
Reference: Black J, Hawks J, Keene A: *Medical-surgical nursing: clinical management for positive outcomes,* ed 6, Philadelphia, 2001, WB Saunders, p. 546.

8. *Answer:* 3
Rationale: A sample of the client's blood is collected, and the leukocytes are tagged with indium. The leukocytes are then reinjected into the client. They accumulate in infected areas of bone and can be detected with scanning. No special preparation or aftercare is necessary.
Test-Taking Strategy: Use the process of elimination. This question is difficult if you are not familiar with the procedure. Look at the information. The client has a bone infection. With any type of infection, leukocytes migrate to the area (and bone is not a highly vascular area). This should suggest option 3 as the correct choice in answering this question. Review this diagnostic test if you had difficulty with this question.
Level of Cognitive Ability: Application
Client Needs: Physiological Integrity
Integrated Concept/Process: Nursing Process/Implementation
Content Area: Adult Health/Musculoskeletal
Reference: Black J, Hawks J, Keene A: *Medical-surgical nursing: clinical management for positive outcomes,* ed 6, Philadelphia, 2001, WB Saunders, p. 548.

9. *Answer:* 2
Rationale: An x-ray is a photographic image of a part of the body on a special film, which is used to diagnose a wide variety of conditions. The x-ray itself is painless; any discomfort would arise from repositioning a painful part for filming. The nurse may want to premedicate a client who is at risk for pain. Any radiopaque objects such as jewelry or other metal must be removed. The client is asked to breathe in deeply, and then hold the breath while the chest x-ray study is done. To minimize risk of radiation exposure, the x-ray technologist stands in a separate area protected by a lead wall. The client also wears a lead shield over the gonads.
Test-Taking Strategy: Use the process of elimination. Options 1 and 4 are obviously incorrect and are eliminated first. Of the two remaining options, eliminate option 3 because the client

needs to be still during the x-ray study. Review this diagnostic procedure if you had difficulty with this question.
Level of Cognitive Ability: Application
Client Needs: Safe, Effective Care Environment
Integrated Concept/Process: Nursing Process/Implementation
Content Area: Adult Health/Musculoskeletal
Reference: DeWit S: *Fundamental concepts and skills for nursing,* Philadelphia, 2001, WB Saunders, p. 423.

10. *Answer:* 1
Rationale: A gallium scan is similar to a bone scan, but with injection of gallium isotope instead of technetium Tc 99m. Gallium is injected 2 to 3 hours before the procedure. The procedure takes 30 to 60 minutes to perform. The client must lie still during the procedure. There is no special aftercare.
Test-Taking Strategy: Use the process of elimination. If you know that a gallium scan is similar to a bone scan, then you could begin by eliminating options 3 and 4. The timeframe in option 2 is rather brief, which allows you to choose option 1 as the correct option. Review this test if you had difficulty with this question.
Level of Cognitive Ability: Application
Client Needs: Physiological Integrity
Integrated Concept/Process: Nursing Process/Implementation
Content Area: Adult Health/Musculoskeletal
Reference: Black J, Hawks J, Keene A: *Medical-surgical nursing: clinical management for positive outcomes,* ed 6, Philadelphia, 2001, WB Saunders, p. 548.

11. *Answer:* 4
Rationale: There are no special restrictions after a bone scan. The client is encouraged to drink large amounts of water for 24 to 48 hours to flush the radioisotope from the system. There are no hazards to the client or staff from the minimal amount of radioactivity of the isotope.
Test-Taking Strategy: Use the process of elimination. There is no purpose for options 2 or 3, which allows you to eliminate them first. Nausea and flushing could accompany dye injection during a procedure, but this procedure uses radioisotopes and the question relates to care after the procedure. Thus this option is also eliminated. The only option left is drinking fluids, which will hasten elimination of the isotope from the client's system. Review this diagnostic procedure if you had difficulty with this question.
Level of Cognitive Ability: Comprehension
Client Needs: Physiological Integrity
Integrated Concept/Process: Nursing Process/Evaluation
Content Area: Adult Health/Musculoskeletal
Reference: Black J, Hawks J, Keene A: *Medical-surgical nursing: clinical management for positive outcomes,* ed 6, Philadelphia, 2001, WB Saunders, p. 547.

12. *Answer:* 2
Rationale: Typical signs and symptoms of fracture include pain, loss of function in the area, deformity, shortening of the extremity, crepitus, swelling, and ecchymosis. Not all fractures lead to the development of every sign. A contusion results from a blow to soft tissue and causes pain, swelling, and ecchymosis. A sprain is an injury to a ligament caused by a wrenching or twisting motion. Symptoms include pain, swelling, and inability to use the joint or bear weight normally. A strain results from a pulling force on the muscle. Symptoms include soreness and pain with muscle use.
Test-Taking Strategy: Use the process of elimination. Within the list of signs and symptoms in the question, note the one that states one leg is shorter than another. Only a fractured bone (which shortens with displacement) could cause this sign. This makes it easy to eliminate each of the other incorrect options. Review the signs of a fracture if you had difficulty with this question.
Level of Cognitive Ability: Comprehension
Client Needs: Physiological Integrity
Integrated Concept/Process: Nursing Process/Data Collection
Content Area: Adult Health/Musculoskeletal
Reference: Black J, Hawks J, Keene A: *Medical-surgical nursing: clinical management for positive outcomes,* ed 6, Philadelphia, 2001, WB Saunders, p. 590.

13. *Answer:* 1
Rationale: With a suspected fracture, the client is not moved unless it is dangerous to remain in that spot. The nurse should remain with the client and have someone else call for emergency help. A fracture is not reduced at the scene. Before moving the client, the site of the fracture is immobilized to prevent further injury.
Test-Taking Strategy: Use the process of elimination. Options 2 and 4 are the worst choices and should be eliminated first. Either of these options could result in further injury to the client. Of the two remaining options, the most prudent action would be for the nurse to remain with the client and have someone else call for emergency assistance. Review immediate care to the client with a fracture if you had difficulty with this question.
Level of Cognitive Ability: Application
Client Needs: Physiological Integrity
Integrated Concept/Process: Nursing Process/Implementation
Content Area: Adult Health/Musculoskeletal
Reference: Black J, Hawks J, Keene A: *Medical-surgical nursing: clinical management for positive outcomes,* ed 6, Philadelphia, 2001, WB Saunders, p. 590.

14. *Answer:* 4
Rationale: When a fracture is suspected, it is imperative that the area is splinted before the client is moved. Emergency help should be called for if the client is not hospitalized, and a physician is called for the hospitalized client. The nurse should remain with the client and provide realistic reassurance. The nurse does not prescribe radiology tests.
Test-Taking Strategy: Use the process of elimination. Note the key words "highest priority." Eliminate option 2 because the nurse does not order x-ray studies. Option 3 is eliminated next because the nurse never tells a client that "everything will be fine." Of the last two choices, immobilizing the limb is imperative for the client's safety, which makes it a better choice than taking vital signs. Review care to the client when a fracture is suspected if you had difficulty with this question.
Level of Cognitive Ability: Application
Client Needs: Physiological Integrity
Integrated Concept/Process: Nursing Process/Implementation
Content Area: Adult Health/Musculoskeletal

Reference: Black J, Hawks J, Keene A: *Medical-surgical nursing: clinical management for positive outcomes,* ed 6, Philadelphia, 2001, WB Saunders, p. 590.

15. *Answer:* 3
Rationale: Before a fracture is reduced, the client is informed about the procedure, and consent is obtained. An analgesic is given as prescribed, because the procedure is painful. Administration of anesthesia may or may not be done, depending on severity. Closed reductions may be done in the emergency room without anesthesia. If anesthesia is used, the procedure is done in the operating room.
Test-Taking Strategy: Use the process of elimination. Note the key words "not necessary" and "casting room." Options 1 and 4 are obviously needed, so these options are eliminated first. The question specifically states that the procedure is going to be done in the cast room, which helps you to choose option 3 (anesthesia consent) as the unnecessary item. Review the procedure for reduction of a fracture if you had difficulty with this question.
Level of Cognitive Ability: Comprehension
Client Needs: Physiological Integrity
Integrated Concept/Process: Nursing Process/Evaluation
Content Area: Adult Health/Musculoskeletal
Reference: Black J, Hawks J, Keene A: *Medical-surgical nursing: clinical management for positive outcomes,* ed 6, Philadelphia, 2001, WB Saunders, p. 590.

16. *Answer:* 4
Rationale: The procedure for casting involves washing and drying the skin and placing a stockinette material over the area to be casted. A roll of padding is then applied smoothly and evenly. The plaster is rolled onto the padding, and the edges are trimmed or smoothed as needed. A plaster cast gives off heat as it dries. A plaster cast can tolerate weight bearing once it is dry, which varies from 24 to 72 hours depending on the nature and thickness of the cast.
Test-Taking Strategy: Use the process of elimination. Note the key word "not." Familiarity with the different types of casting materials and their differences helps you to answer this question. Options 1, 2, and 3 are all true for plaster casts. Option 4 is true for nonplaster casts. Review the procedure for applying a cast if you had difficulty with this question.
Level of Cognitive Ability: Application
Client Needs: Psychosocial Integrity
Integrated Concept/Process: Nursing Process/Implementation
Content Area: Adult Health/Musculoskeletal
Reference: Black J, Hawks J, Keene A: *Medical-surgical nursing: clinical management for positive outcomes,* ed 6, Philadelphia, 2001, WB Saunders, p. 602.

17. *Answer:* 1
Rationale: Immobility and the weight of a casted arm may cause the shoulder above an arm fracture to become stiff. The shoulder of a casted arm should be lifted over the head periodically as a preventive measure. The use of slings further immobilizes the shoulder and may be contraindicated. Making fists with the left hand provides isometric exercise to maintain muscle strength. Range of motion of the affected fingers is also a useful general measure. Lifting the right arm is of no particular value.
Test-Taking Strategy: Use the process of elimination. Visualize each of the movements and think about the muscle groups that are moved with each. Options 2 and 4 provide for no movement of the left arm and are eliminated first. Making a fist with hand on the casted arm provides good isometric exercise to the muscles surrounding the fracture but, again, does nothing for the shoulder. The only viable option is raising the arm over the head, which provides some range of motion for the shoulder joint. Review these measures if you had difficulty with this question.
Level of Cognitive Ability: Application
Client Needs: Health Promotion and Maintenance
Integrated Concept/Process: Teaching/Learning
Content Area: Adult Health/Musculoskeletal
Reference: Black J, Hawks J, Keene A: *Medical-surgical nursing: clinical management for positive outcomes,* ed 6, Philadelphia, 2001, WB Saunders, p. 606.

18. *Answer:* 1
Rationale: A fiberglass cast is made of water-activated polyurethane materials, which are dry to the touch within minutes and reach full rigid strength in about 20 minutes. Because of this, the client can bear weight on the cast within 20 to 30 minutes.
Test-Taking Strategy: Use the process of elimination. Familiarity with nonplaster casts is needed to answer this question precisely. Options 3 and 4 should be eliminated first, because these timeframes are similar to the drying times for plaster casts. Knowing that the nonplaster type of cast is lighter and dries extremely quickly may help you to choose the 20 to 30 minute timeframe as correct. Review client teaching points related to casts if you had difficulty with this question.
Level of Cognitive Ability: Application
Client Needs: Health Promotion and Maintenance
Integrated Concept/Process: Nursing Process/Implementation
Content Area: Adult Health/Musculoskeletal
Reference: Black J, Hawks J, Keene A: *Medical-surgical nursing: clinical management for positive outcomes,* ed 6, Philadelphia, 2001, WB Saunders, p. 602.

19. *Answer:* 4
Rationale: Client instructions should include to avoid walking on wet, slippery floors to prevent falls. Surface soil on a cast may be removed with a damp cloth. If the cast gets wet, it can be dried with a hair dryer set to a cool setting to prevent skin breakdown. If the skin under the cast itches, cool air from a hair dryer may be used to relieve it. The client should never scratch under a cast because of risk of skin breakdown and ulcer formation.
Test-Taking Strategy: Use the process of elimination. Note the key words "needs further instructions." Options 1 and 3 are certainly true and are therefore eliminated. Knowledge of nonplaster cast material is needed to discriminate between the last two. A fiberglass cast may be wiped with a damp cloth, as it is water resistant. It may be helpful to remember never to use a hair dryer on a cast, or on the skin under any cast, with the dryer set at the warmest setting; only cool settings are used

to prevent burns. Review client teaching points related to casts if you had difficulty with this question.
Level of Cognitive Ability: Comprehension
Client Needs: Health Promotion and Maintenance
Integrated Concept/Process: Nursing Process/Evaluation
Content Area: Adult Health/Musculoskeletal
Reference: Black J, Hawks J, Keene A: *Medical-surgical nursing: clinical management for positive outcomes,* ed 6, Philadelphia, 2001, WB Saunders, p. 602.

20. *Answer:* 2
Rationale: Buck's extension traction is a type of skin traction often applied after hip fracture before the fracture is reduced in surgery. It reduces muscle spasms and helps to immobilize the fracture. It does not lengthen the leg for the purpose of preventing blood vessel severance. It also does not allow for bony healing to begin.
Test-Taking Strategy: Use the process of elimination. Options 3 and 4 are the least plausible of all the choices and should be eliminated first. To discriminate between the last two, note the words "rigid immobilization" in option 1. Since skin traction uses lighter weights than skeletal traction, this type of traction cannot be said to provide rigid immobilization. Review this type of traction if you had difficulty with this question.
Level of Cognitive Ability: Application
Client Needs: Physiological Integrity
Integrated Concept/Process: Nursing Process/Implementation
Content Area: Adult Health/Musculoskeletal
Reference: Black J, Hawks J, Keene A: *Medical-surgical nursing: clinical management for positive outcomes,* ed 6, Philadelphia, 2001, WB Saunders, p. 599.

21. *Answer:* 4
Rationale: If the client in skeletal traction may not turn from side to side, the nurse should have the client pull up on a trapeze and try to lift the hips off the bed for skin care, bed pan use, and linen changes. If the client is unable to pull up on a trapeze, the nurse can push down on the mattress with one hand while administering care with the other.
Test-Taking Strategy: Use the process of elimination. Option 3 is contraindicated because it ignores a medical order. Option 1 is not feasible as stated. The client cannot lift up from the bed using one foot only. Options 2 and 4 are both acceptable alternatives. Since the question asks which would be "most useful," the answer is option 4. Providing care to the client who can lift the hips off the bed using a trapeze is easier and more efficient than providing care to one who cannot. Review care to the client in traction if you had difficulty with this question.
Level of Cognitive Ability: Application
Client Needs: Physiological Integrity
Integrated Concept/Process: Nursing Process/Implementation
Content Area: Adult Health/Musculoskeletal
Reference: Black J, Hawks J, Keene A: *Medical-surgical nursing: clinical management for positive outcomes,* ed 6, Philadelphia, 2001, WB Saunders, p. 611.

22. *Answer:* 2
Rationale: A small amount of serous oozing is expected at pin insertion sites. Signs of infection such as inflammation, purulent drainage, and pain at the pin site are not expected findings, and should be reported.
Test-Taking Strategy: Use the process of elimination. Options 1 and 4 seem to indicate an infectious problem, and are eliminated. Note the key words "least concerned with." To discriminate between options 2 and 3, look at them carefully. The complaint of pain is at "a pin site" only. It gives no indication that the pain is related to the fracture or muscle spasm. Because serous drainage is an expected finding, you would choose this over the complaint of pain as the answer to the question. Review care to the client in skeletal traction if you had difficulty with this question.
Level of Cognitive Ability: Comprehension
Client Needs: Physiological Integrity
Integrated Concept/Process: Nursing Process/Evaluation
Content Area: Adult Health/Musculoskeletal
Reference: Black J, Hawks J, Keene A: *Medical-surgical nursing: clinical management for positive outcomes,* ed 6, Philadelphia, 2001, WB Saunders, p. 599.

23. *Answer:* 3
Rationale: Buck's extension traction is a type of skin traction. The nurse inspects the skin of the limb in traction at least once every 8 hours for irritation or inflammation. Massaging the skin with lotion is not indicated. The nurse never releases the weights of traction unless specifically ordered by the physician. There are no pins to care for with skin traction.
Test-Taking Strategy: Use the process of elimination. A baseline knowledge of Buck's extension traction allows you to eliminate options 2 and 4 easily. There are no pins, and the nurse never removes weights without a specific order to do so. Because the apparatus would have to be removed to apply lotion, which is unnecessary, the correct option is to inspect the skin. Review care to the client with Buck's extension traction if you had difficulty with this question.
Level of Cognitive Ability: Application
Client Needs: Safe, Effective Care Environment
Integrated Concept/Process: Nursing Process/Planning
Content Area: Adult Health/Musculoskeletal
Reference: Black J, Hawks J, Keene A: *Medical-surgical nursing: clinical management for positive outcomes,* ed 6, Philadelphia, 2001, WB Saunders, p. 599.

24. *Answer:* 4
Rationale: A client who complains of severe pain may need realignment or may have traction weights ordered that are too heavy. The nurse realigns the client and, if ineffective, then calls the physician. After traction has been established, severe leg pain indicates a problem. The client should be medicated after trying to determine and treat the cause. Providing pin care is unrelated to the problem as described.
Test-Taking Strategy: Use the process of elimination. Note the key word "first." Use the steps of the nursing process. Option 4 is the only option that addresses data collection. Review care to the client in skeletal traction if you had difficulty with this question.
Level of Cognitive Ability: Application
Client Needs: Physiological Integrity
Integrated Concept/Process: Nursing Process/Implementation
Content Area: Adult Health/Musculoskeletal

Reference: Black J, Hawks J, Keene A: *Medical-surgical nursing: clinical management for positive outcomes*, ed 6, Philadelphia, 2001, WB Saunders, p. 599.

25. *Answer:* 3
Rationale: Exercise is indicated within therapeutic limits for the client in skeletal traction to maintain muscle strength and range of motion. The client may pull up on the trapeze, perform active ROM with uninvolved joints, and do isometric muscle setting exercises (such as quadriceps- and gluteal-setting exercises). The client may also flex and extend the feet.
Test-Taking Strategy: Use the process of elimination. Note the key words "needs further instruction." Options 1 and 4 are most easily identified as correct actions, and are therefore eliminated as possible answers to this question. To discriminate between options 2 and 3, imagine the lines of pull on the fracture site with the movements described. While flexing and extending the feet does not disrupt the line of pull from the traction, performing active ROM to the affected knee and ankle does. Review care to the client in traction if you had difficulty with this question.
Level of Cognitive Ability: Comprehension
Client Needs: Physiological Integrity
Integrated Concept/Process: Nursing Process/Evaluation
Content Area: Adult Health/Musculoskeletal
Reference: Black J, Hawks J, Keene A: *Medical-surgical nursing: clinical management for positive outcomes*, ed 6, Philadelphia, 2001, WB Saunders, p. 607.

26. *Answer:* 2
Rationale: Signs and symptoms of infection under a casted area include odor or purulent drainage from the cast, or the presence of "hot spots," which are areas of the cast that are warmer than others. The physician should be notified if any of these occur. Signs of impaired circulation in the distal limb include coolness and pallor of the skin, diminished arterial pulse, and edema.
Test-Taking Strategy: Use the process of elimination. Begin to answer this question by thinking of what you would expect to find with infection: redness, swelling, heat, and purulent drainage. With these in mind, options 1 and 3 can be eliminated easily. To discriminate between options 2 and 4, "dependent edema" is not necessarily indicative of infection. Swelling would be continuous. The "hot spot" on the cast could signify infection underneath that area. Review the complications of a cast if you had difficulty with this question.
Level of Cognitive Ability: Application
Client Needs: Physiological Integrity
Integrated Concept/Process: Nursing Process/Data Collection
Content Area: Adult Health/Musculoskeletal
Reference: Black J, Hawks J, Keene A: *Medical-surgical nursing: clinical management for positive outcomes*, ed 6, Philadelphia, 2001, WB Saunders, p. 605.

27. *Answer:* 1
Rationale: Most pain associated with fractures can be minimized with rest, elevation, application of cold, and administration of analgesics. Pain that is not relieved from these measures should be reported to the physician, as it may be due to impaired tissue perfusion, tissue breakdown, or necrosis. Because this is a new closed fracture and cast, infection would not have had time to set in.
Test-Taking Strategy: Use the process of elimination. Options 2 and 3 are the least plausible given the description in the question and are eliminated first. Because the fracture and cast are so new, it is extremely unlikely that infection could have possibly set in. The most likely option is impaired tissue perfusion, as pain from ischemia is not relieved by comfort measures and analgesics. Review the complications of a cast if you had difficulty with this question.
Level of Cognitive Ability: Analysis
Client Needs: Physiological Integrity
Integrated Concept/Process: Nursing Process/Data Collection
Content Area: Adult Health/Musculoskeletal
Reference: Black J, Hawks J, Keene A: *Medical-surgical nursing: clinical management for positive outcomes*, ed 6, Philadelphia, 2001, WB Saunders, p. 601.

28. *Answer:* 3
Rationale: A casted extremity is elevated continuously for the first 24 to 48 hours to minimize swelling and to promote venous drainage.
Test-Taking Strategy: Use the process of elimination. Recall that edema sets in after fracture, and can be augmented by casting. For this reason, options 1 and 2 are the least helpful, and can be eliminated first. There is no useful purpose for the timing in option 4. Review care to the client with a cast, if you had difficulty with this question.
Level of Cognitive Ability: Application
Client Needs: Physiological Integrity
Integrated Concept/Process: Nursing Process/Implementation
Content Area: Adult Health/Musculoskeletal
Reference: Black J, Hawks J, Keene A: *Medical-surgical nursing: clinical management for positive outcomes*, ed 6, Philadelphia, 2001, WB Saunders, p. 602.

29. *Answer:* 4
Rationale: The edges of the cast can be petaled with tape to minimize skin irritation. If a client has a cast applied and returns home, the client can be taught to do the same.
Test-Taking Strategy: Use the process of elimination. Options 1 and 2 are similar, and neither helps to get rid of the cause of the irritation, so they are eliminated first. Imagine the use of a "rough file"; it would create plaster chips and dust that could go underneath the cast. Review cast petaling if you had difficulty with this question.
Level of Cognitive Ability: Application
Client Needs: Physiological Integrity
Integrated Concept/Process: Nursing Process/Planning
Content Area: Adult Health/Musculoskeletal
Reference: Black J, Hawks J, Keene A: *Medical-surgical nursing: clinical management for positive outcomes*, ed 6, Philadelphia, 2001, WB Saunders, p. 603.

30. *Answer:* 1
Rationale: A plaster cast must remain dry to keep its strength. The cast should be handled using the palms of the hands, not the fingertips, until fully dry. Air should circulate freely around the cast to help it dry; the cast also gives off heat as it

dries. The client should never scratch under the cast; a cool hair dryer may be used to eliminate an itch.
Test-Taking Strategy: Knowledge of cast care is needed to answer this question. Knowing that a wet cast can be dented with the fingertips, causing pressure underneath, helps you to eliminate option 2 first. Knowing that the cast needs to dry helps you eliminate option 3 next. Option 4 is dangerous to skin integrity and is immediately eliminated. Plaster casts, once they have dried after application, should not become wet. Review home care instructions for a client with a cast if you had difficulty with this question.
Level of Cognitive Ability: Comprehension
Client Needs: Health Promotion and Maintenance
Integrated Concept/Process: Nursing Process/Evaluation
Content Area: Adult Health/Musculoskeletal
Reference: Black J, Hawks J, Keene A: *Medical-surgical nursing: clinical management for positive outcomes,* ed 6, Philadelphia, 2001, WB Saunders, p. 602.

31. *Answer:* 3
Rationale: Crutches are measured so that the tops are 3 to 4 fingerbreadths or 1 to 2 inches from the axilla. This ensures that the client's axilla are not resting on the crutch, or bearing the weight of the crutch. This could result in injury to the nerves of the brachial plexus.
Test-Taking Strategy: Use the process of elimination recalling the anatomy of the arm and axillary area. Review measures for crutch walking if you had difficulty with this question.
Level of Cognitive Ability: Comprehension
Client Needs: Physiological Integrity
Integrated Concept/Process: Nursing Process/Implementation
Content Area: Adult Health/Musculoskeletal
Reference: Potter P, Perry A: *Fundamentals of nursing,* ed 5, St Louis, 2001, Mosby, p. 1008.

32. *Answer:* 1
Rationale: The classic tripod position is taught to the client before giving instructions on gait. The crutches are placed anywhere from 6 to 10 inches in front and to the side of the client, depending on the client's body size. This provides a wide enough base of support to the client and improves balance.
Test-Taking Strategy: Use the process of elimination: 3 inches and 20 inches seem excessively short and long, respectively. These two options should be eliminated first. Of the two remaining options, 8 inches seems more in keeping with the normal length of a stride for someone wearing a cast than does 15 inches, and is the correct answer. Review crutch walking if you had difficulty with this question.
Level of Cognitive Ability: Application
Client Needs: Health Promotion and Maintenance
Integrated Concept/Process: Nursing Process/Planning
Content Area: Adult Health/Musculoskeletal
Reference: Potter P, Perry A: *Fundamentals of nursing,* ed 5, St Louis, 2001, Mosby, p. 1009.

33. *Answer:* 4
Rationale: A three-point gait requires good balance and arm strength. The crutches are advanced with the affected leg, and then the unaffected leg is moved forward. Option 1 describes a two-point gait. Option 2 describes a swing-to gait. Option 3 describes the three-point gait used for a right leg problem.
Test-Taking Strategy: Option 1 does not provide the support needed for the casted extremity described in the question and should be eliminated. Option 2 is not necessary if the client is allowed to let the extremity touch the floor. Of the two remaining options, option 4 describes support to the left leg. Review crutch walking if you had difficulty with this question.
Level of Cognitive Ability: Application
Client Needs: Health Promotion and Maintenance
Integrated Concept/Process: Nursing Process/Implementation
Content Area: Adult Health/Musculoskeletal
Reference: Potter P, Perry A: *Fundamentals of nursing,* ed 5, St Louis, 2001, Mosby, p. 1008.

34. *Answer:* 2
Rationale: Crutch tips should remain dry. Water could cause slipping by decreasing the surface friction of the rubber tip on the floor. If crutch tips get wet, the client should dry them with a cloth or paper towel. The client should use only crutches measured for the client. The tips should be inspected for wear, and spare crutches and tips should be available if needed.
Test-Taking Strategy: Note the key words "needs reinforcement." Use the process of elimination. Option 3 is certainly a correct statement and is therefore eliminated. Options 1 and 4 are also true. Remember, crutch tips can slip when they get wet, posing a possible threat to the unsuspecting client. Review crutch safety if you had difficulty with this question.
Level of Cognitive Ability: Comprehension
Client Needs: Health Promotion and Maintenance
Integrated Concept/Process: Nursing Process/Evaluation
Content Area: Adult Health/Musculoskeletal
Reference: Potter P, Perry A: *Fundamentals of nursing,* ed 5, St Louis, 2001, Mosby, p. 1008.

35. *Answer:* 4
Rationale: A straight leg cane is useful for the client with slight weakness in one leg. A walker is beneficial to the client with greater or bilateral weakness, or is at risk for falls. Wooden crutches are often used by clients with a leg cast. Lofstrand crutches aid clients who need crutches, but have limited arm strength.
Test-Taking Strategy: Use the process of elimination. Giving a walker to a client with a slight leg weakness is excessive and is eliminated first. Because there is no evidence that the client has weight-bearing difficulty, crutches are also not indicated. This leaves the straight leg cane as the correct choice. Review the purpose of these various assistive devices if you had difficulty with this question.
Level of Cognitive Ability: Comprehension
Client Needs: Physiological Integrity
Integrated Concept/Process: Nursing Process/Evaluation
Content Area: Adult Health/Musculoskeletal
Reference: Potter P, Perry A: *Fundamentals of nursing,* ed 5, St Louis, 2001, Mosby, p. 828.

36. *Answer:* 1
Rationale: A quad-cane may be used by the client requiring greater support and stability than is provided by a straight leg cane. The quad-cane provides a four point base of support and

is indicated for use by clients with partial or complete hemiplegia. Neither crutches nor a wheelchair is indicated for use with a client such as described in the question.
Test-Taking Strategy: Use the process of elimination. Giving a wheelchair to a client with partial hemiplegia is excessive, and this option is eliminated first. Wooden crutches are not indicated, as there is no restriction in weight bearing. A Lofstrand crutch is useful for clients with limited arm strength. This leaves the quad-cane as the correct choice. Review these various assistive devices if you had difficulty with this question.
Level of Cognitive Ability: Comprehension
Client Needs: Physiological Integrity
Integrated Concept/Process: Nursing Process/Evaluation
Content Area: Adult Health/Musculoskeletal
Reference: DeWit S: *Fundamental concepts and skills for nursing,* Philadelphia, 2001, WB Saunders, p. 828.

37. *Answer:* 3
Rationale: The client is taught to hold the cane on the opposite side of the weakness. This is because, with normal walking, the opposite arm and leg move together (called reciprocal motion). The cane is placed 6 inches lateral to the fifth toe.
Test-Taking Strategy: Knowing that the cane is held at the client's side, not in front, helps you to eliminate options 1 and 2 first. Knowing that the preferred method is to have the cane positioned on the stronger side helps you to choose option 3 over option 4. Review client instructions for the use of a cane if you had difficulty with this question.
Level of Cognitive Ability: Application
Client Needs: Health Promotion and Maintenance
Integrated Concept/Process: Self-Care
Content Area: Adult Health/Musculoskeletal
Reference: DeWit S: *Fundamental concepts and skills for nursing,* Philadelphia, 2001, WB Saunders, p. 828.

38. *Answer:* 2
Rationale: A cane should have a slightly flared tip with flexible concentric rings. This tip acts as a shock absorber and provides optimal stability. Options 1, 3, and 4 are not appropriate.
Test-Taking Strategy: Options 1 and 4 are the least plausible of all the choices and may be eliminated first. Neither statement provides any reassurance for the client. Option 3 also provides no information to relieve the client's anxiety. Option 2 is the best answer. It is a true statement and addresses the client's concerns about safety. Review client instructions for the use of a cane if you had difficulty with this question.
Level of Cognitive Ability: Application
Client Needs: Psychosocial Integrity
Integrated Concept/Process: Teaching/Learning
Content Area: Adult Health/Musculoskeletal
Reference: DeWit S: *Fundamental concepts and skills for nursing,* Philadelphia, 2001, WB Saunders, p. 829.

39. *Answer:* 3
Rationale: The cane is held on the stronger side to minimize stress on the affected extremity and to provide a wide base of support. The cane is held 6 inches lateral to the fifth great toe. The cane is moved forward with the affected leg. The client leans on the cane for added support while the stronger side swings through.
Test-Taking Strategy: The wording of this question guides you to look for an incorrect action. Knowing that the cane is held on the stronger side helps you eliminate options 1 and 2 first. To discriminate between the two remaining choices, recall that the client moves the cane with the weaker leg, and leans on it for support when the stronger leg swings through. Review client instructions for cane walking if you had difficulty with this question.
Level of Cognitive Ability: Comprehension
Client Needs: Health Promotion and Maintenance
Integrated Concept/Process: Nursing Process/Evaluation
Content Area: Adult Health/Musculoskeletal
Reference: DeWit S: *Fundamental concepts and skills for nursing,* Philadelphia, 2001, WB Saunders, p. 829.

40. *Answer:* 4
Rationale: Compartment syndrome is caused by bleeding and swelling within a compartment, which is lined by fascia, and does not expand. The bleeding and swelling place pressure on the nerves, muscles, and blood vessels in the compartment, triggering the symptoms.
Test-Taking Strategy: A basic understanding of the concept of a compartment is needed to answer this question. Option 1 should be eliminated first because it is not due to an arterial injury. Knowing that the fascia itself cannot expand eliminates option 2. To discriminate between the last two options, it is necessary to know that bleeding and swelling cause the symptoms, not a nerve injury. Review the cause of compartment syndrome if you had difficulty with this question.
Level of Cognitive Ability: Application
Client Needs: Physiological Integrity
Integrated Concept/Process: Nursing Process/Implementation
Content Area: Adult Health/Musculoskeletal
Reference: Black J, Hawks J, Keene A: *Medical-surgical nursing: clinical management for positive outcomes,* ed 6, Philadelphia, 2001, WB Saunders, p. 605.

41. *Answer:* 1
Rationale: Compartment syndrome is prevented by controlling edema. This is achieved most optimally with the use of elevation and application of ice.
Test-Taking Strategy: Knowing that edema is controlled or prevented with limb elevation helps you to eliminate options 3 and 4 as possible options. To discriminate between the last two options, look at the effects of ice versus bath blankets. Ice will further control edema, whereas bath blankets will produce heat and prevent air circulation needed for the cast to dry. Review measures to prevent compartment syndrome if you had difficulty with this question.
Level of Cognitive Ability: Application
Client Needs: Physiological Integrity
Integrated Concept/Process: Nursing Process/Planning
Content Area: Adult Health/Musculoskeletal
Reference: Black J, Hawks J, Keene A: *Medical-surgical nursing: clinical management for positive outcomes,* ed 6, Philadelphia, 2001, WB Saunders, p. 605.

42. *Answer:* 2
Rationale: Confusion in the elderly client with hip fracture could result from the unfamiliar hospital setting, stress result-

ing from the fracture, concurrent systemic diseases, cerebral ischemia, or side effects of medications. Use of eyeglasses and hearing aids enhance the client's interaction with the environment and can reduce disorientation.
Test-Taking Strategy: Note the key word "not." Stress from the fracture (option 1) and unfamiliar setting (option 3) are not likely to help the client's functional level and are eliminated as possible options. Eyeglasses and hearing aids are both useful adjuncts in communicating with a client. Because the eyeglasses were left at home, they are of no use at the current time. The working hearing aid is the answer to the question. Review the psychosocial aspects of care for the client with a hip fracture if you had difficulty with this question.
Level of Cognitive Ability: Comprehension
Client Needs: Psychosocial Integrity
Integrated Concept/Process: Nursing Process/Data Collection
Content Area: Adult Health/Musculoskeletal
Reference: Black J, Hawks J, Keene A: *Medical-surgical nursing: clinical management for positive outcomes,* ed 6, Philadelphia, 2001, WB Saunders, p. 608.

43. *Answer:* 4
Rationale: Safe nursing actions intended to prevent injury to the client include keeping side rails up, keeping the bed in a low position, and providing a call bell that is within the client's reach. Responding promptly to the client's use of the call light minimizes the chance that the client will try to get up alone, which could result in a fall.
Test-Taking Strategy: Note the key word "avoid." Because options 1 and 3 (side rails up and call bell in reach) are standard nursing actions, they are eliminated. Use of a nightlight would help prevent falls, which is also helpful. This leaves the delay in answering the call light as the correct option. Delays will give the client reason to try to get up unattended and risk another fall and possible injury. Review safety measures for a client after hip surgery if you had difficulty with this question.
Level of Cognitive Ability: Application
Client Needs: Safe, Effective Care Environment
Integrated Concept/Process: Nursing Process/Implementation
Content Area: Adult Health/Musculoskeletal
Reference: DeWit S: *Fundamental concepts and skills for nursing,* Philadelphia, 2001, WB Saunders, p. 838.

44. *Answer:* 1
Rationale: After internal fixation of a hip fracture, the client is turned to the affected side or the unaffected side as prescribed by the surgeon. Before moving the client, the nurse places a pillow between the client's legs to keep the affected leg in abduction. The client is then repositioned while proper alignment and abduction are maintained.
Test-Taking Strategy: A trochanter roll is useful in preventing external rotation, but it is used once the client has been repositioned. It is not used while turning the client. Thus, options 3 and 4 may be readily eliminated. To discriminate between options 1 and 2, use of a pillow would keep the legs abducted, not adducted. Thus option 1 is the correct answer. Review care to the client after hip surgery if you had difficulty with this question.
Level of Cognitive Ability: Application
Client Needs: Physiological Integrity
Integrated Concept/Process: Nursing Process/Implementation
Content Area: Adult Health/Musculoskeletal
Reference: Black J, Hawks J, Keene A: *Medical-surgical nursing: clinical management for positive outcomes,* ed 6, Philadelphia, 2001, WB Saunders, p. 612.

45. *Answer:* 4
Rationale: The client who has received a total knee replacement often has the leg put into a CPM machine while in the postanesthesia care unit. The device increases circulation and movement of the knee joint. It should be used as much as possible.
Test-Taking Strategy: Knowledge of the purpose and effects of a CPM machine is needed to answer this question correctly. Review these concepts if you had difficulty with this question.
Level of Cognitive Ability: Application
Client Needs: Physiological Integrity
Integrated Concept/Process: Nursing Process/Implementation
Content Area: Adult Health/Musculoskeletal
Reference: Black J, Hawks J, Keene A: *Medical-surgical nursing: clinical management for positive outcomes,* ed 6, Philadelphia, 2001, WB Saunders, p. 565.

46. *Answer:* 1
Rationale: The nurse assists the client to get out of bed on the first postoperative day after putting a knee immobilizer on the affected joint for stability. The surgeon orders the weight-bearing limits on the affected leg. The leg is elevated while the client is sitting in the chair to minimize edema.
Test-Taking Strategy: Use the process of elimination. A compression dressing should already be in place on the wound, so option 2 should be eliminated first. Because the CPM machine is used only while the client is in bed, option 3 is incorrect and is also eliminated. To discriminate between the last two options, knowing that ambulation is not started until the second postoperative day would help you choose correctly. The knee immobilizer should be a natural choice when answering a question about protecting a knee joint. Review care to the client after total knee replacement if you had difficulty with this question.
Level of Cognitive Ability: Application
Client Needs: Physiological Integrity
Integrated Concept/Process: Nursing Process/Planning
Content Area: Adult Health/Musculoskeletal
Reference: Black J, Hawks J, Keene A: *Medical-surgical nursing: clinical management for positive outcomes,* ed 6, Philadelphia, 2001, WB Saunders, p. 565.

47. *Answer:* 3
Rationale: Clients with diabetes mellitus are more prone to wound infection and delayed wound healing as a result of disease. Stump edema and hemorrhage are complications in the immediate postoperative period that apply to any client with an amputation. Slight redness of the incision is considered normal, as long it is dry and intact.
Test-Taking Strategy: The question guides you to look for complications that are primarily due to the coexisting condition of diabetes mellitus. Knowing that diabetes increases the client's chances of developing infection and delayed wound healing helps you to eliminate options 1 and 2 first. You would choose

option 3 over option 4 because separation of wound edges is a more serious problem than a slight redness to the incision line, which is considered normal. Review the complications of an amputation if you had difficulty with this question.
Level of Cognitive Ability: Comprehension
Client Needs: Physiological Integrity
Integrated Concept/Process: Nursing Process/Data Collection
Content Area: Adult Health/Musculoskeletal
Reference: Black J, Hawks J, Keene A: *Medical-surgical nursing: clinical management for positive outcomes*, ed 6, Philadelphia, 2001, WB Saunders, p. 1150.

48. ***Answer:*** 1
Rationale: Phantom limb sensations are felt in the area of the amputated limb. These can include itching, warmth, and cold. The sensations are due to intact peripheral nerves in the area amputated. Whenever possible, clients should be prepared for these sensations. The client may also feel painful sensations in the amputated limb, called phantom limb pain. The origin of the pain is less well understood, but the client should be prepared for this, too, whenever possible.
Test-Taking Strategy: Use the process of elimination. By knowing that sensation and pain may be felt in the residual limb helps you to eliminate options 3 and 4 first, because the sensations are not abnormal responses. You would select option 1 over option 2 because the client has described an itching sensation, but has not complained of pain in the residual limb. Review the expected findings after amputation if you had difficulty with this question.
Level of Cognitive Ability: Analysis
Client Needs: Psychosocial Integrity
Integrated Concept/Process: Nursing Process/Evaluation
Content Area: Adult Health/Musculoskeletal
Reference: Black J, Hawks J, Keene A: *Medical-surgical nursing: clinical management for positive outcomes*, ed 6, Philadelphia, 2001, WB Saunders, p. 1410.

49. ***Answer:*** 3
Rationale: Low back pain with radiation into one leg (sciatica) is consistent with herniated lumbar disk. The nurse continues to collect data from the client to see if the pain is aggravated by events that increase intraspinal pressure such as bending, lifting, sneezing, or coughing, or with lifting the leg straight up while supine (straight leg raising test). Options 1, 2, and 4 assist in alleviating pain.
Test-Taking Strategy: To answer this question, recall the basic causes of back pain and the factors that alleviate or aggravate it. With this knowledge, recall that bed rest, heat (or sometimes ice), and nonsteroidal antiinflammatory agents usually relieve back pain, whereas bending, lifting, and straining aggravate it. If this question was difficult, review these concepts.
Level of Cognitive Ability: Application
Client Needs: Physiological Integrity
Integrated Concept/Process: Nursing Process/Data Collection
Content Area: Adult Health/Musculoskeletal
Reference: Black J, Hawks J, Keene A: *Medical-surgical nursing: clinical management for positive outcomes*, ed 6, Philadelphia, 2001, WB Saunders, p. 1984.

50. ***Answer:*** 4
Rationale: After spinal fusion, the head of bed is generally kept in a flat position. The client is logrolled from side to side as ordered. Pillows may be placed under the entire length of the legs by surgeon preference to relieve tension on the lower back. The use of an overhead trapeze is contraindicated because its use could promote twisting of the spine after surgery.
Test-Taking Strategy: Note the key word "avoid." After spinal surgery, the nurse uses positioning techniques and aids that will keep the spine in good alignment. Thus, options 1 and 3 are obviously indicated and are therefore eliminated as items to avoid as this question asks. To discriminate between the last two items, using pillows under the length of the legs promotes slight flexion of the spine while avoiding pressure on the popliteal space (which predisposes to thrombophlebitis). Using an overbed trapeze could allow the client to twist the spine, which is directly contraindicated. Review postoperative care after spinal fusion if you had difficulty with this question.
Level of Cognitive Ability: Application
Client Needs: Physiological Integrity
Integrated Concept/Process: Nursing Process/Implementation
Content Area: Adult Health/Musculoskeletal
Reference: Black J, Hawks J, Keene A: *Medical-surgical nursing: clinical management for positive outcomes*, ed 6, Philadelphia, 2001, WB Saunders, p. 1988.

51. ***Answer:*** 1
Rationale: Clients are taught to get out of bed by sliding near to the edge of the mattress. The client then rolls onto one side and pushes up from the bed using one or both arms. The back is kept straight and the legs are swung over the side. Increasing fluids and dietary fiber helps prevent straining at stool, thereby preventing increases in intraspinal pressure. Walking and swimming are excellent exercises for strengthening lower back muscles. Proper body mechanics includes bending at the knees, not the waist, to lift objects.
Test-Taking Strategy: Note the key words "needs further instruction." Options 3 and 4 are examples of classic interventions that are indicated, and so they are eliminated first. Clients with low back pain should avoid events that increase intraspinal pressure. Option 2 prevents increases in intraspinal pressure. Option 1 causes an increase in intraspinal pressure if you think of the body mechanics involved in getting out of bed this way. Review the principles of proper body mechanics if you had difficulty with this question.
Level of Cognitive Ability: Comprehension
Client Needs: Health Promotion and Maintenance
Integrated Concept/Process: Nursing Process/Evaluation
Content Area: Adult Health/Musculoskeletal
Reference: Black J, Hawks J, Keene A: *Medical-surgical nursing: clinical management for positive outcomes*, ed 6, Philadelphia, 2001, WB Saunders, p. 1991.

52. ***Answer:*** 3
Rationale: After spinal surgery, concerns about finances and employment are best handled by referral to a social worker. This individual will provide information about resources available to the client.

Test-Taking Strategy: An understanding of the roles of the various members of the health care team helps you to answer this question. The physical therapist has the best knowledge of techniques for increasing mobility and endurance. An occupational therapist would have knowledge of techniques for activities of daily living and items related to occupation, but this is not one of the options. The clinical nurse specialist and surgeon do not have information related to financial resources. Review health care professional roles if you had difficulty with this question.
Level of Cognitive Ability: Comprehension
Client Needs: Safe, Effective Care Environment
Integrated Concept/Process: Nursing Process/Evaluation
Content Area: Adult Health/Musculoskeletal
Reference: Black J, Hawks J, Keene A: *Medical-surgical nursing: clinical management for positive outcomes,* ed 6, Philadelphia, 2001, WB Saunders, p. 1987.

53. *Answer:* 2
Rationale: A back brace or thoracolumbosacral orthosis is individually fitted to the client. The brace should not irritate the skin with proper fitting. The brace is applied in the morning before getting out of bed. The closures should be secure, but not overly loose or tight. A layer of clothing is worn between the orthosis and the skin.
Test-Taking Strategy: Skin irritation is not likely to be a good sign and should be eliminated first. Loose connections are also not likely to indicate proper fit, so option 4 should be eliminated next. Of the two remaining options, you would not choose option 3 because the orthosis is likely to become soiled with perspiration or cause skin irritation. Review care to the client with a brace if you had difficulty with this question.
Level of Cognitive Ability: Application
Client Needs: Physiological Integrity
Integrated Concept/Process: Self-Care
Content Area: Adult Health/Musculoskeletal
Reference: DeWit S: *Fundamental concepts and skills for nursing,* Philadelphia, 2001, WB Saunders, p. 830.

54. *Answer:* 4
Rationale: After spinal fusion, with or without instrumentation, the client is transferred from stretcher to bed using a slider board and the assistance of four people. This permits optimal stabilization and support of the spine, while allowing the client to be moved smoothly and gently.
Test-Taking Strategy: Use the process of elimination. This question can be answered by analyzing the level of comfort and stability provided to the client's spine with the amounts of assistance given in each option. Using this approach, you can systematically eliminate each of the incorrect options. Review care to the client after Harrington rod insertion if you had difficulty with this question.
Level of Cognitive Ability: Application
Client Needs: Safe, Effective Care Environment
Integrated Concept/Process: Nursing Process/Implementation
Content Area: Adult Health/Musculoskeletal
Reference: Black J, Hawks J, Keene A: *Medical-surgical nursing: clinical management for positive outcomes,* ed 6, Philadelphia, 2001, WB Saunders, p. 1987.

55. *Answer:* 1
Rationale: Stair climbing may be restricted or limited for several weeks after spinal fusion with instrumentation. The nurse ensures that resources are in place before discharge so that the client may sleep and perform all activities of daily living on a single living level.
Test-Taking Strategy: Use the process of elimination. Options 2 and 3 are obviously useful to the client and can be eliminated. To discriminate between options 1 and 4 (both of which involve stairs), option 4 is the least problematic, whereas option 1 poses a significant problem to the client who is restricted from stair climbing. Review the home care needs of the client after Harrington rod insertion if you had difficulty with this question.
Level of Cognitive Ability: Comprehension
Client Needs: Safe, Effective Care Environment
Integrated Concept/Process: Nursing Process/Planning
Content Area: Adult Health/Musculoskeletal
Reference: Black J, Hawks J, Keene A: *Medical-surgical nursing: clinical management for positive outcomes,* ed 6, Philadelphia, 2001, WB Saunders, p. 1988.

56. *Answer:* 4
Rationale: The client with pallor, slow capillary refill, weakened or lost pulse, and absence of sensation or motion to the distal limb may have arterial damage from a lacerated, contused, thrombosed, or severed artery. These signs can occur with constriction from a tight cast as well. Regardless of the cause, the nurse notifies the physician immediately. Emergency intervention is needed, which could include removal of the constricting bandage, fracture reduction, or surgery to repair the area.
Test-Taking Strategy: Knowing that these signs indicate insufficient arterial circulation, you know that this can lead to irreversible ischemia and damage. Because of this, you eliminate options 1 and 3 first as not being helpful. Rechecking the circulation in 30 minutes loses valuable time for action to restore the impaired circulation and is a poor choice. The physician should be notified immediately. Review the complications of a fracture if you had difficulty with this question.
Level of Cognitive Ability: Application
Client Needs: Physiological Integrity
Integrated Concept/Process: Nursing Process/Implementation
Content Area: Adult Health/Musculoskeletal
Reference: Black J, Hawks J, Keene A: *Medical-surgical nursing: clinical management for positive outcomes,* ed 6, Philadelphia, 2001, WB Saunders, p. 604.

57. *Answer:* 4
Rationale: A window may be cut in a dried cast to relieve pressure, monitor pulses, relieve discomfort, or remove drains. Bivalving the cast involves splitting the cast along both sides to allow space for swelling, facilitate taking x-ray films, or to make a half-cast for use as an intermittent splint. Padding is not placed on top of a cast. The use of an air splint is not indicated.
Test-Taking Strategy: Note the key words "bony prominence." Wherever there is a bony prominence, there is a risk of pressure and skin breakdown. If the pressure area is under a cast, the cast must be removed in that area to relieve the pressure.

Therefore, options 1 and 3 can be readily eliminated. Because extra padding over the area of the cast is not helpful, that option can be eliminated next. This leaves putting a window in the cast as the correct answer. This will relieve the pressure in that one area without disrupting the cast. Review the complications of a cast and the treatments for complications if you had difficulty with this question.
Level of Cognitive Ability: Analysis
Client Needs: Physiological Integrity
Integrated Concept/Process: Nursing Process/Evaluation
Content Area: Adult Health/Musculoskeletal
Reference: Black J, Hawks J, Keene A: *Medical-surgical nursing: clinical management for positive outcomes*, ed 6, Philadelphia, 2001, WB Saunders, p. 604.

58. ***Answer:*** 4
Rationale: Clients may fear having a cast removed because of misconceptions about the cast cutting blade. The nurse should show the cast cutter to the client before it is used and explain that the client may feel heat, vibration, and pressure. The cast cutter resembles a small electric saw with a circular blade. The nurse should reassure the client that the blade does not cut like a saw, but instead cuts the cast by vibrating side to side.
Test-Taking Strategy: Note the key words "most helpful." Option 2 gives no information, although it may be well intentioned, and is eliminated first. Options 1 and 3 give accurate information, but are not reassuring. Option 4 gives the client the most reassurance because it best prepares the client for what will occur when the cast is removed. Review this procedure if you had difficulty with this question.
Level of Cognitive Ability: Application
Client Needs: Psychosocial Integrity
Integrated Concept/Process: Nursing Process/Implementation
Content Area: Adult Health/Musculoskeletal
Reference: DeWit S: *Fundamental concepts and skills for nursing*, Philadelphia, 2001, WB Saunders, p. 811.

59. ***Answer:*** 1
Rationale: Risk factors associated with osteoporosis include a diet that is deficient in calcium. Options 2, 3, and 4 include risk factors associated with osteoporosis. Additional risk factors include sedentary lifestyle, cigarette smoking, excessive alcohol consumption, chronic illness, and long-term use of anticonvulsants and furosemide (Lasix).
Test-Taking Strategy: Knowledge regarding the risk factors associated with osteoporosis is required to answer this question. Review these risk factors if you are not familiar with them.
Level of Cognitive Ability: Comprehension
Client Needs: Health Promotion and Maintenance
Integrated Concept/Process: Nursing Process/Data Collection
Content Area: Adult Health/Musculoskeletal
Reference: Black J, Hawks J, Keene A: *Medical-surgical nursing: clinical management for positive outcomes*, ed 6, Philadelphia, 2001, WB Saunders, p. 566.

60. ***Answer:*** 4
Rationale: Foods high in calcium include plain yogurt, dairy products, seafood, sardines, green vegetables, calcium-fortified orange juice, and cereal. Of the items listed in the options, option 4 would contain the least amount of calcium.
Test-Taking Strategy: Note the key word "least." By the process of elimination, you should easily be directed to option 4. Review foods high in calcium if you had difficulty with this question.
Level of Cognitive Ability: Comprehension
Client Needs: Health Promotion and Maintenance
Integrated Concept/Process: Teaching/Learning
Content Area: Adult Health/Musculoskeletal
Reference: Black J, Hawks J, Keene A: *Medical-surgical nursing: clinical management for positive outcomes*, ed 6, Philadelphia, 2001, WB Saunders, p. 641.

61. ***Answer:*** 1
Rationale: Ample fluid intake is encouraged to promote excretion of uric acid. The client is placed on bed rest until the pain subsides. A diet low in purine is normally prescribed, which includes a decrease in red and organ meat. NSAIDs are used to reduce pain and inflammation.
Test-Taking Strategy: Noting the key words "not" and "acute" will assist in eliminating options 3 and 4. Knowledge that a low purine diet may be recommended for the client with gout will easily direct you to option 1. Review care to the client with gout if you had difficulty with this question.
Level of Cognitive Ability: Comprehension
Client Needs: Health Promotion and Maintenance
Integrated Concept/Process: Nursing Process/Planning
Content Area: Adult Health/Musculoskeletal
Reference: Black J, Hawks J, Keene A: *Medical-surgical nursing: clinical management for positive outcomes*, ed 6, Philadelphia, 2001, WB Saunders, p. 854.

62. ***Answer:*** 1
Rationale: Rheumatoid arthritis is characterized by chronic joint pain of varying intensity that is more severe on arising in the morning. The nurse would note that joint involvement is symmetrical and the joints are swollen, shiny, reddened, and painful. Rheumatoid nodules, which are painless subcutaneous movable skin nodules near bony prominences, may occur anywhere on the body.
Test-Taking Strategy: Note the key word "not." Note that options 1 and 2 are similar in that both address the component of pain and its occurrence. This should lead you to suspect that one of these options is correct. Review the characteristics associated with RA if you had difficulty with this question.
Level of Cognitive Ability: Comprehension
Client Needs: Physiological Integrity
Integrated Concept/Process: Nursing Process/Data Collection
Content Area: Adult Health/Musculoskeletal
Reference: DeWit S: *Fundamental concepts and skills for nursing*, Philadelphia, 2001, WB Saunders, p. 870.

REFERENCES

Black J, Hawks J, Keene A: *Medical-surgical nursing: clinical management for positive outcomes*, ed 6, Philadelphia, 2001, WB Saunders.

Chernecky C, Berger B: *Laboratory tests and diagnostic procedures*, ed 3, Philadelphia, 2001, WB Saunders.

Clark J, Queener S, Karb V: *Pharmacologic basis of nursing practice*, ed 6, St Louis, 2000, Mosby.

DeWit S: *Fundamental concepts and skills for nursing*, Philadelphia, 2001, WB Saunders.

Hodgson B, Kizior R: *Saunders nursing drug handbook 2002*, Philadelphia, 2002, WB Saunders.

Ignatavicius D, Workman M: *Medical-surgical: critical thinking for collaborative care*, ed 4, Philadelphia, 2002, WB Saunders.

Lehne R: *Pharmacology for nursing care*, ed 4, Philadelphia, 2001, WB Saunders.

Potter P, Perry A: *Fundamentals of nursing*, ed 5, St Louis, 2001, Mosby.

Perry A, Potter P: *Clinical nursing skills and techniques*, ed 5, St Louis, 2002, Mosby.

Musculoskeletal Medications

I. SKELETAL MUSCLE RELAXANTS (Box 57-1)

A. Description
1. Act directly on the neuromuscular junction or indirectly on the central nervous system (CNS)
2. Centrally acting muscle relaxants depress neuron activity in the spinal cord or brain
3. Peripheral-acting muscle relaxants act directly on the skeletal muscles
4. Used to prevent or relieve muscle spasms, to treat spasticity associated with spinal cord disease or lesions, for painful musculoskeletal conditions, and for chronic debilitating disorders such as multiple sclerosis, cerebrovascular accident (CVA), or cerebral palsy
5. Contraindicated in severe liver, renal, or heart disease
6. Should not be taken with CNS depressants such as barbiturates, narcotics, and alcohol; sedatives; hypnotics; or tricyclic antidepressants

BOX 57-1

Skeletal Muscle Relaxants

Baclofen (Lioresal)
Carisoprodol (Soma, Vanadom)
Cyclobenzaprine (Flexeril, Cycoflex)
Dantrolene (Dantrium)
Diazepam (Valium)
Metaxalone (Skelaxin)
Methocarbamol (Robaxin, Carbacot, Skelex)
Orphenadrine (Norflex, Flexoject)
Chlorzoxazone (Paraflex, Parafon Forte, Relaxone)
Chlorphenesin (Maolate)
Tizanidine (Zanaflex)

B. Side effects
1. Dizziness and hypotension
2. Drowsiness
3. Dry mouth
4. Gastrointestinal (GI) upset
5. Photosensitivity
6. Liver toxicity

C. Implementation
1. Obtain a medical history
2. Monitor vital signs
3. Monitor for CNS side effects
4. Assess for risk of injury
5. Assess involved joints and muscles for pain and mobility
6. Monitor liver function tests because hepatotoxicity can occur
7. Monitor renal function studies
8. Instruct the client to take the medication with food to decrease GI upset
9. Instruct the client to report side effects
10. Instruct the client to avoid alcohol and CNS depressants
11. Instruct the client to avoid activities requiring alertness

D. Nursing considerations
1. Baclofen (Lioresal)
   a. Causes CNS effects such as drowsiness, dizziness, weakness, and fatigue
   b. Frequently causes nausea, constipation, and urinary retention
   c. Can be administered by the physician by intrathecal infusion using an implantable pump
2. Dantrolene (Dantrium)
   a. Acts directly on skeletal muscles to relieve spasticity
   b. Liver damage is the most serious adverse effect

c. Liver function tests should be monitored before the initiation of treatment and during treatment
d. Can cause GI bleeding, urinary frequency, impotence, photosensitivity, and rash
e. Instruct the client to wear protective clothing when in the sun
f. Instruct the client to notify physician if rash, bloody or tarry stool, or yellow discoloration of the skin or eyes occurs

3. Cyclobenzaprine (Flexeril, Cycoflex)
   a. Contraindicated in clients who have received monoamine oxidase inhibitors (MAOIs) within 14 days of initiation of cyclobenzaprine therapy, and in clients with cardiac disorders
   b. Used with caution in clients with a history of urinary retention, angle-closure glaucoma, and increased intraocular pressure
   c. Should be used only for short term (2 to 3 weeks of therapy)
4. Methocarbamol (Robaxin, Carbocot, Skelex)
   a. Parenteral form is contraindicated in clients with renal impairment
   b. Parenteral form can cause hypotension, bradycardia, anaphylaxis, and seizures
   c. May cause urine to turn brown, black, or green
   d. Inform the client to notify the physician if blurred vision, nasal congestion, urticaria, or rash occurs
5. Chlorzoxazone (Paraflex, Parafon Forte, Relaxone)
   a. Monitor for hypersensitivity reactions such as urticaria, redness or itching, and possibly angioedema
   b. May cause malaise and urine discoloration
6. Carisoprodol (Soma, Vanadom)
   a. Advise the client to take the medication with food to prevent GI upset
   b. Instruct the client to report any rash or hypersensitivity to the physician

II. ANTIGOUT MEDICATIONS (Box 57-2)

A. Description
   1. Decrease inflammation
   2. Reduce uric acid production and increase uric acid excretion to prevent or relieve gout or to manage hyperuricemia
   3. Used cautiously in clients with GI, renal, cardiac, and hepatic disease
   4. Allopurinol (Lopurin, Zyloprim) can increase the effect of warfarin sodium and oral hypoglycemic agents

B. Side effects
   1. Headaches
   2. Nausea, vomiting, and diarrhea
   3. Blood dyscrasias such as bone marrow depression
   4. Flushed skin and skin rash
   5. Uric acid kidney stones
   6. Sore gums
   7. Metallic taste

C. Implementation
   1. Monitor serum uric acid levels
   2. Monitor intake and output
   3. Maintain a fluid intake of at least 2000 to 3000 mL a day to avoid kidney stones
   4. Monitor complete blood cell count (CBC) and renal and liver function studies
   5. Instruct the client to avoid alcohol and caffeine because these products can increase uric acid levels
   6. Instruct the client not to take large doses of vitamin C while taking allopurinol (Zyloprim) because kidney stones may occur
   7. Encourage the client to comply with therapy to prevent elevated uric acid levels, which can trigger a gout attack
   8. Instruct the client to avoid foods high in purine such as wine, alcohol, organ meats, sardines, salmon, and gravy
   9. Instruct the client to take the medication with food
   10. Instruct the client to report side effects to the physician
   11. Advise the client to have a yearly eye examination because visual changes can occur from prolonged use of allopurinol
   12. Caution the client not to take aspirin with these medications because this could trigger a gout attack
   13. Concurrent use of aspirin causes elevated uric acid levels; the client should be instructed to take acetaminophen (Tylenol)

BOX 57-2

Antigout Medications

Allopurinol (Lopurin, Zyloprim)
Colchicine
Probenecid (Benemid)
Sulfinpyrazone (Anturane)

III. ANTIARTHRITIC MEDICATIONS (Box 57-3)

A. Nonsteroidal antiinflammatory medications (NSAIDs) (refer to Chapter 55)
B. Gold therapy
   1. Description

BOX 57-3

Antiarthritic Medications

Auranofin (Ridaura)
Aurothioglucose (Solganal)
Azathioprine (Imuran)
Gold sodium thiomalate (Myochrysine)
Hydroxychloroquine sulfate (Plaquenil)
Methotrexate sodium (Rheumatrex)
Penicillamine (Cuprimine)
Sulfasalazine (Azulfidine)

BOX 57-4

Contraindications for Gold Therapy

Eczema
Urticaria
Colitis
Hemorrhagic conditions
Systemic lupus erythematosus
Renal or hepatic dysfunction
Uncontrolled diabetes mellitus
Congestive heart failure
Recent radiation therapy

a. Referred to as chrysotherapy or heavy-metal therapy
b. Depresses migration of leukocytes and suppresses prostaglandin activity
c. Reduces inflammation by decreasing enzyme release and altering the immune response
d. Primarily used for palliative relief of symptoms in rheumatoid arthritis
e. Contraindications are listed in Box 57-4

2. Side effects
   a. Dizziness
   b. Urticaria and rash
   c. Erythema and dermatitis
   d. Alopecia
   e. Stomatitis
   f. Diarrhea
   g. Hepatitis
   h. Metallic taste in the mouth
   i. Blood dyscrasias such as bone marrow suppression
   j. Photosensitivity reactions
   k. Gold toxicity
3. Implementation
   a. Obtain the client's medical history
   b. Monitor for blood dyscrasias before and during therapy
   c. Monitor for proteinuria and hematuria before and during therapy
   d. When administering the gold injection, monitor the client for 30 minutes after injection for possible allergic reaction
   e. Instruct the client to maintain good oral hygiene
   f. Instruct the client to use sunscreen and protective clothing to prevent photosensitivity reactions
   g. Teach the client about the signs and symptoms of gold toxicity, which include pruritis, skin rash, metallic taste, stomatitis, and diarrhea
   h. If toxicity occurs, dimercaprol (BAL in oil) may be prescribed to enhance gold excretion

PRACTICE QUESTIONS

1. Allopurinol (Zyloprim) has been prescribed for the client. The client asks the nurse about the action of the medication. The nurse responds knowing that it:
   1. Is used for the lysis of thrombi obstructing coronary arteries
   2. Prevents calcium ion entry across cell membranes of the cardiac smooth muscle
   3. Decreases sympathetic outflow from the central nervous system (CNS)
   4. Decreases uric acid production and reduces uric acid concentrations in both the serum and urine
2. A nurse is caring for a client who is taking allopurinol (Zyloprim). Which of the following medications, if prescribed for the client, would the nurse question?
   1. Mebendazole (Vermox)
   2. Ergonovine maleate (Ergotrate)
   3. Warfarin sodium (Coumadin)
   4. Pentazocine (Talwin)
3. A nurse prepares to reinforce instructions to a client who is taking allopurinol (Zyloprim). The nurse plans to include which of the following in the instructions?
   1. Inform the client that the effect of the medication will occur immediately
   2. Instruct the client to drink 3000 mL of fluid per day
   3. Instruct the client to take the medication on an empty stomach
   4. Inform the client that if swelling of the lips occurs, this is a normal expected response
4. A nurse is caring for a client with unstable angina. The client is taking acetylsalicylic acid (aspirin) on a daily basis to reduce the risk of myocardial infarction (MI). Which of the following medication doses would the nurse expect the client to be taking?
   1. 3 grams daily
   2. 325 mg daily

3. 1.3 grams daily
4. 700 mg daily

5. Colchicine is prescribed for a client with a diagnosis of gout. The nurse reviews the client's medical history in the health record knowing that the medication would be contraindicated in which of the following disorders?
   1. Renal failure
   2. Hypothyroidism
   3. Diabetes mellitus
   4. Myxedema
6. A nurse is caring for a client who is taking probenecid (Benemid). The client has been instructed to restrict the diet to low-purine foods. Which of the following foods would the nurse instruct the client to avoid?
   1. Potatoes
   2. Ice cream
   3. Spinach
   4. Scallops
7. A physician prescribes auranofin (Ridaura) for the client with rheumatoid arthritis. Which of the following would indicate to the nurse that the client is experiencing toxicity related to the medication?
   1. Constipation
   2. Complaints of a metallic taste in the mouth
   3. Ringing in the ears
   4. Joint pain
8. A film-coated form of diflunisal (Dolobid) has been prescribed for a client for the treatment of chronic rheumatoid arthritis. The client calls the clinic nurse because of difficulty swallowing the tablets. Which of the following instructions would the nurse provide to the client?
   1. Crush the tablet and mix it with food
   2. Open the tablet and mix the contents with food
   3. Swallow the tablets with large amounts of water or milk
   4. Notify the physician for a medication change
9. A physician instructs an elderly client with rheumatoid arthritis to take ibuprofen (Motrin). The nurse reinforces the instructions knowing that the normal adult dose for this client is which of the following?
   1. 100 mg PO BID
   2. 200 mg PO BID
   3. 300 mg PO TID
   4. 1000 mg PO QID
10. Baclofen (Lioresal) is prescribed for the client with multiple sclerosis. The nurse assists in planning care knowing that the primary therapeutic effect of this medication is which of the following?
   1. Increased muscle tone
   2. Decreased muscle spasms
   3. Decreased local pain and tenderness
   4. Increased range of motion
11. A nurse is monitoring a client receiving baclofen (Lioresal) for side effects related to the medication. Which of the following would indicate that the client is experiencing a side effect?
   1. Drowsiness
   2. Diarrhea
   3. Polyuria
   4. Muscular excitability
12. A nurse is reinforcing discharge instructions to a client receiving baclofen (Lioresal). Which of the following would the nurse plan to include in the instructions?
   1. Restrict fluid intake
   2. Avoid the use of alcohol
   3. Stop the medication if diarrhea occurs
   4. Notify the physician if fatigue occurs
13. An adult client with muscle spasms is taking an oral maintenance dose of baclofen (Lioresal). The nurse reviews the medication record expecting that which of the following doses would be prescribed?
   1. 15 mg QID
   2. 25 mg QID
   3. 30 mg QID
   4. 40 mg QID
14. A client with acute muscle spasms has been taking baclofen (Lioresal). The client calls the clinic nurse because of continuous feelings of weakness and fatigue and asks the nurse about discontinuing the medication. Which of the following responses to the client would be most appropriate?
   1. "It is best that you taper the dose if you intend to stop the medication."
   2. "Weakness and fatigue commonly occur and will diminish with continued medication use."
   3. "It is all right to stop the medication if you think that you can tolerate the muscle spasms."
   4. "You should never stop the medication."
15. Dantrolene sodium (Dantrium) is prescribed for the client experiencing flexor spasms. The client asks the nurse about the action of the medication. The nurse responds knowing that the therapeutic action of this medication is which of the following?
   1. Acts within the spinal cord to suppress hyperactive reflexes
   2. Acts on the central nervous system (CNS) to suppress spasms
   3. Acts directly on the skeletal muscle to relieve spasticity
   4. Depresses spinal reflexes
16. A nurse is reviewing the laboratory studies on a client receiving dantrolene sodium (Dantrium). Which of the following laboratory tests would identify an adverse effect associated with the administration of this medication?
   1. Blood urea nitrogen (BUN)
   2. Creatinine

3. Liver function tests
4. Hematological function tests

17. A nurse is reviewing the record of a client who has been prescribed baclofen (Lioresal). Which of the following disorders, if noted in the client's history, would alert the nurse to contact the physician?
    1. Coronary artery disease
    2. Diabetes mellitus
    3. Seizure disorders
    4. Hyperthyroidism

18. Cyclobenzaprine HCl (Flexeril) is prescribed for the client for muscle spasms. The nurse is reviewing the client's record. Which of the following disorders, if noted in the client's record, would indicate a need to contact the physician regarding the administration of this medication?
    1. Glaucoma
    2. Hyperthyroidism
    3. Emphysema
    4. Diabetes mellitus

19. The client is to receive a prescription for methocarbamol (Robaxin). The nurse reinforces instructions to the client regarding the medication. Which of the following client statements would indicate a need for further education?
    1. "My urine may turn brown or green."
    2. "If my vision becomes blurred I don't need to be concerned about it."
    3. "I might get some nasal congestion from this medication."
    4. "This medication is prescribed to help relieve my muscle spasms."

20. The nurse is reviewing the physician's orders for an adult client who has been admitted to the hospital after sustaining a back injury. Carisoprodol (Soma) is prescribed for the client to relieve muscle spasms. The physician has prescribed 350 mg to be administered QID. When preparing to give this medication, the nurse determines that this dosage is:
    1. The normal adult dosage
    2. A lower than normal dosage
    3. A higher than normal dosage
    4. A dosage requiring further clarification

ANSWERS

1. *Answer:* 4
Rationale: Allopurinol is an antigout medication. It decreases uric acid production by inhibiting the enzyme xanthine oxidase and reduces uric acid concentrations in both serum and urine.
Test-Taking Strategy: Use the process of elimination. Note that options 1 and 2 are similar in that they both address a cardiac situation; this leaves options 3 and 4. Knowledge that this medication is in the antigout classification will assist in directing you to the correct option from those remaining. If you had difficulty with this question, review the action of allopurinol.
Level of Cognitive Ability: Application
Client Needs: Physiological Integrity
Integrated Concept/Process: Nursing Process/Implementation
Content Area: Pharmacology
Reference: Hodgson B, Kizior R: *Saunders nursing drug handbook 2002*, Philadelphia, 2002, WB Saunders, p. 26.

2. *Answer:* 3
Rationale: Allopurinol is an antigout medication that may increase the effect of oral anticoagulants. Warfarin sodium (Coumadin) is an anticoagulant, and if this medication was prescribed for the client, the nurse would question the order. Ergotrate is an antimigraine medication. Talwin is an opioid analgesic. Vermox is an antihelminthic.
Test-Taking Strategy: Knowledge regarding the medication interactions related to allopurinol is required to answer this question. If you had difficulty with this question, review the interactions associated with this medication.
Level of Cognitive Ability: Application
Client Needs: Safe, Effective Care Environment
Integrated Concept/Process: Nursing Process/Implementation
Content Area: Pharmacology
Reference: Hodgson B, Kizior R: *Saunders nursing drug handbook 2002*, Philadelphia, 2002, WB Saunders, p. 26.

3. *Answer:* 2
Rationale: Clients taking allopurinol are encouraged to drink 3000 mL of fluid a day. A full therapeutic effect may take 1 or more weeks. Allopurinol is to be given with or immediately after meals or milk. If the client develops a rash, irritation of the eyes, or swelling of the lips or mouth, he or she should contact the physician, as this may indicate hypersensitivity.
Test-Taking Strategy: Knowledge regarding client instructions related to this medication will assist in answering the question. Option 4 can be easily eliminated because it indicates a hypersensitivity, which is not a normal expected response. From this point, use the process of elimination and nursing knowledge. If you had difficulty with this question, review client instructions related to allopurinol.
Level of Cognitive Ability: Application
Client Needs: Health Promotion and Maintenance
Integrated Concept/Process: Nursing Process/Planning
Content Area: Pharmacology
Reference: Hodgson B, Kizior R: *Saunders nursing drug handbook 2002*, Philadelphia, 2002, WB Saunders, p. 26.

4. *Answer:* 2
Rationale: Aspirin may be used to reduce the risk of recurrent transient ischemic attack (TIA) or stroke, or reduce the risk of myocardial infarction (MI) in clients with unstable angina or

with a history of a previous MI. The normal dose for clients being treated with aspirin to decrease thrombosis and MI is 300 to 325 mg daily. Clients being treated to prevent TIAs are usually prescribed 1.3 grams daily in two to four divided doses. Clients with rheumatoid arthritis are treated with 3.2 to 6 grams daily in divided doses.
Test-Taking Strategy: Use the process of elimination. Note the key words "reduce the risk of MI." This should indicate to you that the client is receiving the medication as a preventive measure, directing you to the lowest dose of medication in the options. If you had difficulty with this question, review aspirin dosages.
Level of Cognitive Ability: Analysis
Client Needs: Physiological Integrity
Integrated Concept/Process: Nursing Process/Data Collection
Content Area: Pharmacology
Reference: Hodgson B, Kizior R: *Saunders nursing drug handbook 2002*, Philadelphia, 2002, WB Saunders, p. 82.

5. *Answer:* 1
Rationale: Colchicine is contraindicated in severe gastrointestinal, renal, hepatic or cardiac disorders, and in clients with blood dyscrasias. Clients with impaired renal function may exhibit myopathy and neuropathy manifested as generalized weakness. This medication should be used with caution in clients with impaired hepatic function, older adults, and debilitated individuals.
Test-Taking Strategy: Use the process of elimination. Note that options 2, 3, and 4 are all endocrine-related disorders. Option 1, the correct option, is different from the others. Review this medication if you had difficulty with this question.
Level of Cognitive Ability: Analysis
Client Needs: Physiological Integrity
Integrated Concept/Process: Nursing Process/Data Collection
Content Area: Pharmacology
Reference: Hodgson B, Kizior R: *Saunders nursing drug handbook 2002*, Philadelphia, 2002, WB Saunders, p. 270.

6. *Answer:* 4
Rationale: Benemid is a medication used for clients with gout to inhibit the reabsorption of uric acid by the kidney and promote excretion of uric acid in the urine. Uric acid is produced when purine is catabolized. Clients are instructed to modify their diets and limit excessive purine intake. High-purine foods to avoid or limit include organ meats, roe, sardines, scallops, anchovies, broth, mincemeat, herring, shrimp, mackerel, gravy, and yeast.
Test-Taking Strategy: Use the process of elimination. Note the key word "avoid." Options 1 and 3 are high-nutrient foods, so eliminate these options first. From this point, use knowledge regarding purpose of the medication, treatment for gout, and food sources high in purine to select the correct option. If you had difficulty with this question, review foods that are high in purine.
Level of Cognitive Ability: Application
Client Needs: Health Promotion and Maintenance
Integrated Concept/Process: Nursing Process/Implementation
Content Area: Pharmacology
Reference: Hodgson B, Kizior R: *Saunders nursing drug handbook 2002*, Philadelphia, 2002, WB Saunders, p. 917.

7. *Answer:* 2
Rationale: Ridaura is the one gold preparation that is given orally rather than by injection. Gastrointestinal reactions including diarrhea, abdominal pain, nausea, and loss of appetite are common early in therapy, but usually subside in the first 3 months. Early symptoms of toxic reactions include a rash, purple blotches, pruritis, mouth lesions, and a metallic taste in the mouth.
Test-Taking Strategy: Use the process of elimination. Option 4, joint pain, can be eliminated because the medication is administered to reduce the joint pain. Note that the question is asking for a toxic effect; therefore from the options remaining, you should be directed to the correct option, metallic taste. Remember, gold is a metal. If you had difficulty with this question, review toxicity related to gold compounds.
Level of Cognitive Ability: Analysis
Client Needs: Physiological Integrity
Integrated Concept/Process: Nursing Process/Data Collection
Content Area: Pharmacology
Reference: Hodgson B, Kizior R: *Saunders nursing drug handbook 2002*, Philadelphia, 2002, WB Saunders, p. 92.

8. *Answer:* 3
Rationale: Dolobid may be given with water, milk, or meals. The tablets should not be crushed or broken open.
Test-Taking Strategy: Use the process of elimination. Eliminate option 4 first as the least likely option. Next, noting the words "film-coated" will assist in eliminating options 1 and 2. Additionally, these options are similar in that they both suggest breaking the tablets. If you had difficulty with this question, review the procedure for administration.
Level of Cognitive Ability: Application
Client Needs: Health Promotion and Maintenance
Integrated Concept/Process: Nursing Process/Implementation
Content Area: Pharmacology
Reference: Hodgson B, Kizior R: *Saunders nursing drug handbook 2002*, Philadelphia, 2002, WB Saunders, p. 342.

9. *Answer:* 3
Rationale: For acute or chronic rheumatoid arthritis or osteoarthritis, the normal PO adult dose for an elderly client is 300 to 800 mg three to four times daily.
Test-Taking Strategy: Use the process of elimination. Noting the word "elderly" in the question will assist in eliminating option 4. From the remaining options, it is necessary to be familiar with normal dosages. Review the normal dosage for this medication if you had difficulty with this question.
Level of Cognitive Ability: Application
Client Needs: Physiological Integrity
Integrated Concept/Process: Teaching/Learning
Content Area: Pharmacology
Reference: Hodgson B, Kizior R: *Saunders nursing drug handbook 2002*, Philadelphia, 2002, WB Saunders, p. 552.

10. *Answer:* 2
Rationale: Baclofen is a skeletal muscle relaxant and acts at the spinal cord level to decrease the frequency and amplitude of muscle spasms in clients with spinal cord injuries or diseases, and in clients with multiple sclerosis.

Test-Taking Strategy: Knowledge that this medication is a skeletal muscle relaxant is required to answer this question. If you knew the action of this medication, you would easily be directed to option 2. Review this medication if you had difficulty with this question.
Level of Cognitive Ability: Comprehension
Client Needs: Physiological Integrity
Integrated Concept/Process: Nursing Process/Planning
Content Area: Pharmacology
Reference: Hodgson B, Kizior R: *Saunders nursing drug handbook 2002*, Philadelphia, 2002, WB Saunders, p. 102.

11. *Answer:* 1
Rationale: Baclofen is a central nervous system (CNS) depressant that frequently causes drowsiness, dizziness, weakness, and fatigue. It can also cause nausea, constipation, and urinary retention. Clients should be warned about the possible reactions.
Test-Taking Strategy: Knowledge that baclofen is a CNS depressant used to treat muscle spasticity will easily direct you to option 1. If you had difficulty with this question, review the side effects of this medication.
Level of Cognitive Ability: Analysis
Client Needs: Physiological Integrity
Integrated Concept/Process: Nursing Process/Data Collection
Content Area: Pharmacology
Reference: Hodgson B, Kizior R: *Saunders nursing drug handbook 2002*, Philadelphia, 2002, WB Saunders, p. 102.

12. *Answer:* 2
Rationale: Baclofen is a central nervous system (CNS) depressant. The client should be cautioned against the use of alcohol and other CNS depressants because baclofen potentiates the depressant activity of these agents. Constipation rather than diarrhea is a adverse effect of baclofen. It is not necessary to restrict fluids, but the client should be warned that urinary retention can occur. Fatigue is related to a CNS effect that is most intense during the early phase of therapy and diminishes with continued medication use. It is not necessary that the client notify the physician.
Test-Taking Strategy: Knowledge that baclofen is a CNS depressant will easily direct you to option 2. If you were unsure of the correct option, use general principles related to medication administration. Alcohol should be avoided with the use of many medications. Review this medication if you had difficulty with this question
Level of Cognitive Ability: Application
Client Needs: Health Promotion and Maintenance
Integrated Concept/Process: Nursing Process/Planning
Content Area: Pharmacology
Reference: Hodgson B, Kizior R: *Saunders nursing drug handbook 2002*, Philadelphia, 2002, WB Saunders, p. 102.

13. *Answer:* 1
Rationale: Baclofen is dispensed in tablets of 10 and 20 mg for oral use. Dosages are low initially and then gradually increased. Maintenance doses range from 15 to 20 mg administered three to four times a day.
Test-Taking Strategy: Knowledge regarding the normal adult maintenance dosage is required to answer this question. Review this maintenance dosage if you had difficulty with this question
Level of Cognitive Ability: Analysis
Client Needs: Physiological Integrity
Integrated Concept/Process: Nursing Process/Data Collection
Content Area: Pharmacology
Reference: Hodgson B, Kizior R: *Saunders nursing drug handbook 2002*, Philadelphia, 2002, WB Saunders, p. 102.

14. *Answer:* 2
Rationale: The client should be instructed that symptoms such as drowsiness, weakness, and fatigue are more intense in the early phase of therapy and diminish with continued medication use. The client should be instructed never to abruptly withdraw or stop the medication because abrupt withdrawal can cause visual hallucinations, paranoid ideation, and seizures. It is best for the nurse to inform the client that these symptoms will subside and encourage the client to continue the use of the medication.
Test-Taking Strategy: Use the process of elimination. Note the key words "most appropriate." Eliminate option 4 first because it is a rather extreme nursing response. Next, eliminate options 1 and 3 because these responses do not represent the scope of nursing practice. Review this medication if you had difficulty with this question
Level of Cognitive Ability: Application
Client Needs: Health Promotion and Maintenance
Integrated Concept/Process: Communication and Documentation
Content Area: Pharmacology
Reference: Hodgson B, Kizior R: *Saunders nursing drug handbook 2002*, Philadelphia, 2002, WB Saunders, p. 102.

15. *Answer:* 3
Rationale: Dantrium acts directly on skeletal muscle to relieve muscle spasticity. The primary action is the suppression of calcium release from the sarcoplasmic reticulum. This in turn decreases the ability of the skeletal muscle to contract.
Test-Taking Strategy: Use the process of elimination. Options 1, 2, and 4 are all similar in that they address central nervous system (CNS) depression (spinal cord, CNS, spinal) and the depression of reflexes. Therefore, eliminate these options. Review this medication if you had difficulty with this question.
Level of Cognitive Ability: Application
Client Needs: Physiological Integrity
Integrated Concept/Process: Nursing Process/Implementation
Content Area: Pharmacology
Reference: Hodgson B, Kizior R: *Saunders nursing drug handbook 2002*, Philadelphia, 2002, WB Saunders, p. 306.

16. *Answer:* 3
Rationale: Dose-related liver damage is the most serious adverse effect of dantrolene. To reduce the risk of liver damage, tests of liver function should be performed before treatment and throughout the treatment interval. It is administered in the lowest effective dosage for the shortest time necessary.
Test-Taking Strategy: Use the process of elimination. Eliminate options 1 and 2 because these tests both assess kidney function.

From the remaining options, it is necessary to recall that this medication affects liver function. Review this medication if you had difficulty with this question.
Level of Cognitive Ability: Analysis
Client Needs: Physiological Integrity
Integrated Concept/Process: Nursing Process/Data Collection
Content Area: Pharmacology
Reference: Hodgson B, Kizior R: *Saunders nursing drug handbook 2002*, Philadelphia, 2002, WB Saunders, p. 306.

17. *Answer:* 3
Rationale: Clients with seizure disorders may have a lowered seizure threshold when baclofen is administered. Concurrent therapy may require an increase in the anticonvulsive medication.
Test-Taking Strategy: Knowledge regarding the contraindications and the cautions associated with the administration of baclofen is required to answer this question. If you are unfamiliar with these contraindications and cautions, review this content.
Level of Cognitive Ability: Analysis
Client Needs: Safe, Effective Care Environment
Integrated Concept/Process: Nursing Process/Data Collection
Content Area: Pharmacology
Reference: Hodgson B, Kizior R: *Saunders nursing drug handbook 2002*, Philadelphia, 2002, WB Saunders, p. 102.

18. *Answer:* 1
Rationale: Because this medication has anticholinergic effects, it should be used with caution with clients who have a history of urinary retention, angle-closure glaucoma, and increased intraocular pressure. Cyclobenzaprine HCl should be used only for short-term 2- to 3-week therapy.
Test-Taking Strategy: Knowledge that this medication has anticholinergic effects will assist in directing you to option 1. If you are unfamiliar with this medication and the contraindications associated with its administration, review this content.
Level of Cognitive Ability: Analysis
Client Needs: Safe, Effective Care Environment
Integrated Concept/Process: Nursing Process/Data Collection
Content Area: Pharmacology
Reference: Hodgson B, Kizior R: *Saunders nursing drug handbook 2002*, Philadelphia, 2002, WB Saunders, p. 287.

19. *Answer:* 2
Rationale: The client needs to be told that the urine may turn brown, black, or green. Other adverse effects include blurred vision, nasal congestion, urticaria, and rash. The client needs to be instructed that, if these adverse effects occur, the physician needs to be notified.
Test-Taking Strategy: Note the key words "need for further education." Use knowledge regarding this medication to direct you to option 2. If you had difficulty with this question, review this medication.
Level of Cognitive Ability: Analysis
Client Needs: Health Promotion and Maintenance
Integrated Concept/Process: Nursing Process/Evaluation
Content Area: Pharmacology
Reference: Hodgson B, Kizior R: *Saunders nursing drug handbook 2002*, Philadelphia, 2002, WB Saunders, p. 707.

20. *Answer:* 1
Rationale: The normal adult dosage for Soma is 350 mg PO three to four times daily.
Test-Taking Strategy: This question may be difficult if you are not familiar with the normal medication dosage. Review this medication if you had difficulty with this question.
Level of Cognitive Ability: Analysis
Client Needs: Physiological Integrity
Integrated Concept/Process: Nursing Process/Evaluation
Content Area: Pharmacology
Reference: Hodgson B, Kizior R: *Saunders nursing drug handbook 2002*, Philadelphia, 2002, WB Saunders, p. 170.

REFERENCES

Black J, Hawks J, Keene A: *Medical-surgical nursing: clinical management for positive outcomes*, ed 6, Philadelphia, 2001, WB Saunders.
Chernecky C, Berger B: *Laboratory tests and diagnostic procedures*, ed 3, Philadelphia, 2001, WB Saunders.
Clark J, Queener S, Karb V: *Pharmacologic basis of nursing practice*, ed 6, St Louis, 2000, Mosby.
DeWit S: *Fundamental concepts and skills for nursing*, Philadelphia, 2001, WB Saunders.
Hodgson B, Kizior R: *Saunders nursing drug handbook 2002*, Philadelphia, 2002, WB Saunders.
Ignatavicius D, Workman M: *Medical-surgical: critical thinking for collaborative care*, ed 4, Philadelphia, 2002, WB Saunders.
Lehne R: *Pharmacology for nursing care*, ed 4, Philadelphia, 2001, WB Saunders.
Potter P, Perry A: *Fundamentals of nursing*, ed 5, St Louis, 2001, Mosby.
Smeltzer S, Bare B: *Brunner and Suddarth's textbook of medical-surgical nursing*, ed 9, Philadelphia, 2000, Lippincott Williams & Wilkins.

UNIT XVIII

The Adult Client with an Immune Disorder

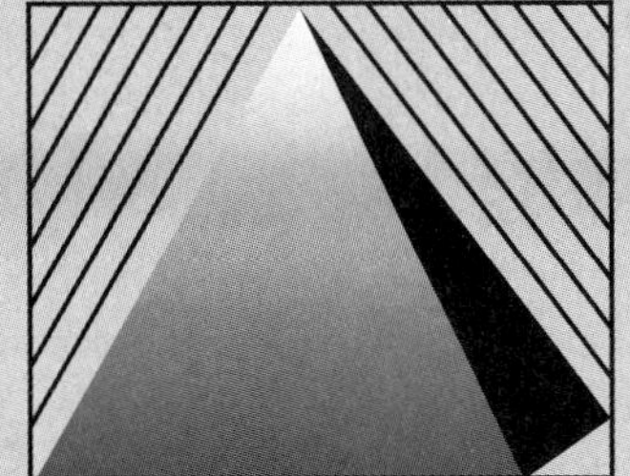

PYRAMID TERMS

Acquired Immunity Received passively from the mother's antibodies, animal serum, or from the production of antibodies in response to a disease. Immunization produces active acquired immunity.

Allergy An abnormal, individual response to certain substances that normally do not trigger such an exaggerated reaction.

Cellular Response A delayed response; also called delayed hypersensitivity. Active against slowly developing bacterial infections.

Humoral Response An immediate response that provides protection against acute, rapidly developing bacterial and viral infections.

Immune Deficiency The absence or inadequate production of immune bodies.

Natural Immunity Also called innate immunity. Is present at birth.

PYRAMID TO SUCCESS

Pyramid points focus on the effects of and complications associated with an immune deficiency. Specific focus relates to the nursing care related to the disorder, the impact of the treatment or disorder, and to client adaptation. Acquired immunodeficiency syndrome is a pyramid focus, along with protecting the client from infection, and preventing the transmission of infection to other individuals. Psychosocial issues relate to social isolation and the body image disturbances that can occur as a result of the immune disorder. The Integrated Concepts and Processes addressed in this unit include the Clinical Problem-Solving Process (Nursing Process), Caring, Communication and Documentation, Cultural Awareness, Self-Care, and Teaching/Learning.

CLIENT NEEDS

Safe, Effective Care Environment

Advance directives
Advocacy related to client's decisions
Asepsis
Client rights
Confidentiality regarding diagnosis
Consultations and referrals
Establishing priorities
Handling hazardous and infectious materials
Informed consent for treatments and procedures
Standard (universal) and protective precautions

Health Promotion and Maintenance

Client lifestyle choices
Expected body image changes
Health promotion programs
Health screening measures
Prevention of disease related to infection

Psychosocial Integrity

Assisting in mobilizing appropriate support and resource systems
Assisting the client and family to cope
Ability to cope, adapt, and/or problem solve during illness or stressful events
Grief and loss related to death and the dying process
Promoting a positive environment to maintain optimal quality of life
Religious, spiritual, and cultural preferences

Physiological Integrity

Diagnostic tests and laboratory values
Managing pain
Monitoring for the expected and unexpected responses to treatments
Promoting nutrition
Protecting the client from the infection
Providing basic care and comfort

REFERENCES

Black J, Hawks J, Keene A: *Medical-surgical nursing: clinical management for positive outcomes*, ed 6, Philadelphia, 2001, WB Saunders.

Chernecky C, Berger B: *Laboratory tests and diagnostic procedures*, ed 3, Philadelphia, 2001, WB Saunders.

Clark J, Queener S, Karb V: *Pharmacologic basis of nursing practice*, ed 6, St Louis, 2000, Mosby.

DeWit S: *Fundamental concepts and skills for nursing*, Philadelphia, 2001, WB Saunders.

Hill S, Howlett H: *Success in practical nursing: personal and vocational issues*, ed 4, Philadelphia, 2001, WB Saunders.

National Council of State Boards of Nursing: *Test plan for the National Council Licensure Examination for Practical/Vocational Nurses*, Chicago, 2001, Author.

Potter P, Perry A: *Fundamentals of nursing*, ed 5, St Louis, 2001, Mosby.

Perry A, Potter P: *Clinical nursing skills and techniques*, ed 5, St Louis, 2002, Mosby.

Wilson J: *Infection control in clinical practice*, ed 2, St Louis, 2002, Balliere Tindall.

Immune Disorders

I. FUNCTIONS OF THE IMMUNE SYSTEM

A. Provides protection against invasion from outside the body, such as microorganisms
B. Protects the body from internal threats
C. Maintains the internal environment by removing dead or damaged cells

II. IMMUNE RESPONSE

A. T and B lymphocytes
1. Migrate to lymphoid tissue where they wait to form either sensitized lymphocytes for **cellular** immunity or antibodies for **humoral** immunity
2. Some B lymphocytes lie dormant until a specific antigen enters the body at which time they greatly increase in number and are available for defense
3. T lymphocytes are responsible for rejection of transplanted tissue
4. Both T and B lymphocytes are necessary for a normal immune response

B. **Humoral response**
1. An immediate response
2. Provides protection against acute, rapidly developing bacterial and viral infections

C. **Cellular response**
1. A delayed response; also called delayed hypersensitivity
2. Active against slowly developing bacterial infections
3. Also involved in autoimmune response, some allergic reactions, and rejection of foreign cells

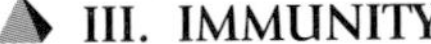

III. IMMUNITY

A. **Natural immunity**
1. Also called innate
2. Present at birth

B. **Acquired immunity**
1. Received passively from the mother's antibodies, animal serum, or from the production of antibodies in response to a disease
2. Immunization produces active **acquired immunity**

IV. IMMUNIZATIONS

(Refer to Chapter 36 regarding immunizations.)

V. LABORATORY STUDIES

A. Antinuclear antibody (ANA)
1. A blood test used in the differential diagnosis of rheumatic diseases, and to detect antinucleoprotein factors and patterns associated with certain autoimmune diseases
2. Positive at a titer of 1:20 or 1:40 depending on the laboratory
3. A positive result does not necessarily confirm a disease

B. Anti-dsDNA antibody test
1. A blood test done specifically to identify or differentiate DNA antibodies found in systemic lupus erythematosus (SLE) or other rheumatic diseases
2. Supports a diagnosis, monitors disease activity and response to therapy, and establishes a prognosis for SLE
3. Values
   a. Negative: less than 70 units by enzyme-linked immunosorbent assay (ELISA)
   b. Borderline: 70 to 200 units
   c. Positive: greater than 200 units

C. Refer to Chapter 10 for testing related to acquired immunodeficiency syndrome (AIDS)

VI. IMMUNE DEFICIENCY

A. Description
1. Absence or inadequate production of immune bodies
2. Can be congenital (primary) or acquired (secondary)
3. Treatment depends on the inadequacy of immune bodies and its primary cause

B. Data collection
1. Factors that decrease immune function
2. Frequent infections
3. Nutritional status
4. Medication history such as corticosteroids
5. History of alcohol or drug abuse

C. Implementation
1. Protect from infection
2. Promote balanced, adequate nutrition
3. Use strict aseptic technique for all procedures
4. Provide psychosocial care regarding lifestyle changes and role changes
5. Instruct the client in measures to prevent infection

VII. HYPERSENSITIVITY AND ALLERGY

A. Description
1. An **allergy** is an abnormal, individual response to certain substances that normally do not trigger such an exaggerated reaction
2. In most types of allergies, a reaction occurs only on second and subsequent contacts with the allergen
3. Skin testing may be done to determine the allergen

B. Data collection
1. History of exposure to allergens
2. Itching, tearing, and burning of eyes
3. Itching and burning of the skin
4. Rashes
5. Nose twitching, nasal stuffiness

C. Implementation
1. Identification of the specific allergen
2. Managing the symptoms with the use of antihistamines, antiinflammatory agents, or corticosteroids
3. Salves, wet compresses, and soothing baths for local reactions
4. Desensitization programs

VIII. ANAPHYLAXIS

A. Description
1. A serious and dramatic allergic reaction with the release of histamine from the damaged cells
2. Can cause shock and death if not treated immediately

B. Data collection
1. Identification of allergies
2. Difficulty breathing
3. Difficulty swallowing
4. Complaints of a swollen tongue
5. Facial edema and swelling of the lips
6. Skin redness
7. Presence of a rash

C. Implementation
1. Establish a patent airway
2. Prepare for the administration of epinephrine (Adrenalin), diphenhydramine HCl (Benadryl), or corticosteroids
3. Provide measures to control shock
4. Provide emotional support
5. Instruct the client to wear a Medic-Alert bracelet
6. Instruct the client in the use of prescribed medication for immediate treatment of a reaction

IX. LATEX ALLERGY

A. Description
1. A hypersensitivity to latex
2. The source of the allergic reaction is thought to be due to the proteins in the natural rubber latex or the various chemicals used in the manufacturing process of the latex from a liquid substance into the finished product
3. Symptoms of the **allergy** can range from mild contact dermatitis to moderately severe symptoms of rhinitis, conjunctivitis, urticaria, and bronchospasm, to severe life-threatening anaphylaxis

B. Common routes of exposure (Box 58-1)
1. Cutaneous: wearing natural latex gloves
2. Percutaneous and parenteral: intravenous (IV) lines and catheters; hemodialysis equipment
3. Mucosal: use of latex condoms, catheters, airways, and nipples
4. Aerosol: aerosolization of powder from latex gloves can occur when gloves are dispensed from the box or when gloves are removed from the hands

C. At-risk individuals
1. Health care workers
2. Individuals who work with manufacturing latex products
3. Females
4. Individuals with spina bifida

BOX 58-1

Common Products that Contain Natural Rubber Latex

Ace bandages (brown)
Adhesive bandages
Ambu bag
Balloons
Band-Aid dressings
Blood pressure cuff (tubing and bladder)
Catheters
Catheter leg bag straps
Condoms
Diaphragms
Elastic pressure stockings
Electrocardiogram pads
Feminine hygiene pads
Gloves
IV catheters, tubing, and rubber injection ports
Levine tubes
Pads for crutches
Prepackaged enema kits
Rubber stoppers on medication vials
Stethoscopes
Syringes

5. Individuals who wear gloves frequently such as food handlers, hairdressers, and auto mechanics
6. Individuals allergic to kiwis, bananas, pineapples, tropical fruits, avocados, potatoes, and chestnuts

D. Data collection
1. Anaphylactic hypersensitivity
   a. Rapid onset
   b. Urticaria, wheezing, dyspnea, laryngeal edema, bronchospasm, tachycardia, angioedema, hypotension, and cardiac arrest
2. Delayed-type hypersensitivity: includes symptoms of contact dermatitis such as pruritus, edema, erythema, vesicles, papules, and crusting and thickening of the skin

E. Implementation
1. Ask the client about a known **allergy** to latex when performing the initial data collection
2. Identify risk factors to a latex **allergy** in the client
3. Individuals with an **allergy**
   a. Avoid latex products
   b. Obtain an emergency medical kit that contains antihistamines and epinephrine
   c. Wear a Medic-Alert bracelet
   d. Inform health care providers and local and paramedic ambulance companies about the **allergy**
   e. Advise the individual to place a warning label in the car window to alert police and paramedics of the **allergy**, in case of a car accident
   f. Provide information about local support groups and resources of alternative products

X. AUTOIMMUNE DISEASE

A. Description
1. Body is unable to recognize its own cells as a part of itself
2. Can affect collagenous tissue

B. Systemic lupus erythematosus
1. Description
   a. A chronic, progressive, systemic inflammatory disease that can cause major organs and systems to fail
   b. Connective tissue and fibrin deposits in blood vessels on collagen fibers and on organs
   c. Leads to necrosis and/or inflammation in blood vessels, lymph nodes, gastrointestinal (GI) tract, pleura
   d. There is no cure for the disease
2. Causes
   a. The cause is unknown and it is thought to be due to a defect in the immunological mechanisms or from genetic origin
   b. Precipitating factors include medications, stress, genetic factors, sunlight or ultraviolet light, and pregnancy
3. Data collection
   a. Precipitating factors such as sunlight, stress, and medications
   b. Dry scaly raised rash on the face or upper body
   c. Fever
   d. Weakness, malaise, and fatigue
   e. Anorexia
   f. Weight loss
   g. Photosensitivity
   h. Joint pain
   i. Erythema of the palms
   j. Butterfly erythema of the face
   k. Anemia
   l. Positive ANA and LE prep
   m. Elevated sedimentation rate
4. Implementation
   a. Monitor skin integrity and provide frequent oral care
   b. Instruct the client to clean skin with a mild soap avoiding harsh and perfume substances
   c. Assist with the use of ointments and creams for rash as prescribed

d. Identify factors contributing to fatigue
e. Administer iron, folic acid, or vitamin supplements as prescribed if anemia occurs
f. Provide a high vitamin and high iron diet
g. Provide a high-protein diet if there is no evidence of kidney disease
h. Instruct the client in measures to conserve energy, such as pacing activities and balancing rest with exercise
i. Administer topical or systemic corticosteroids, salicylates, and nonsteroidal anti-inflammatory drugs (NSAIDs) as prescribed for pain and inflammation
j. Administer hydroxychloroquine (Plaquenil) as prescribed to decrease the inflammatory response
k. Instruct the client to avoid exposure to sunlight and ultraviolet light
l. Monitor for proteinuria and red cell casts in the urine
m. Monitor for bruising, bleeding, and injury
n. Assist with plasmapheresis as prescribed to remove autoantibodies and immune complexes from the blood before organ damage occurs
o. Monitor for signs of organ involvement such as pleuritis, nephritis, pericarditis, neuritis, anemia, and peritonitis
p. Note that lupus nephritis occurs early in the disease process
q. Provide supportive therapy as major organs become affected
r. Provide emotional support and encourage the client to verbalize feelings
s. Provide information regarding support groups and encourage use of community resources

C. Scleroderma (progressive systemic sclerosis)
1. Description
a. A chronic connective tissue disease, similar to SLE, characterized by inflammation, fibrosis, and sclerosis
b. Affects the connective tissue throughout the body
c. Causes fibrotic changes involving the skin, synovial membranes, esophagus, heart, lungs, kidneys, and GI tract
d. Treatment is directed toward forcing the disease into remission and slowing its progress
2. Data collection
a. Pain
b. Stiffness and muscle weakness
c. Pitting edema of the hands and fingers which progresses to the rest of the body
d. Taut and shiny skin that is free from wrinkles
e. Skin tissue is tight, hard and thick, and loses its elasticity
f. Masklike hard skin that adheres to underlying structures
g. Dysphagia
h. Decreased range of motion
i. Joint contractures
j. Inability to perform activities of daily living
3. Implementation
a. Encourage activity as tolerated
b. Maintain a constant room temperature
c. Provide small frequent meals eliminating foods that stimulate gastric secretions such as spicy foods, caffeine, and alcohol
d. Advise the client to sit up for 1 to 2 hours after meals if esophageal involvement exists
e. Provide supportive therapy as the major organs become affected
f. Administer corticosteroids as prescribed for inflammation
g. Provide emotional support and encourage the use of resources as necessary

D. Polyarteritis nodosa
1. Description
a. A collagen disease that causes inflammation of the arteries and thickening and impairment of the circulation
b. Treatment is similar to treatment for SLE
c. Affects middle-aged men and involves every body system
d. The cause is unknown and the prognosis is poor
e. Renal disorders and cardiac involvement are the most frequent causes of death
2. Data collection
a. Malaise and weakness
b. Low-grade fever
c. Severe abdominal pain
d. Bloody diarrhea
e. Weight loss
f. Elevated sedimentation rate
3. Implementation
a. Provide supportive care as required
b. Provide a well-balanced diet
c. Administer corticosteroids and analgesics to control pain and inflammation
d. Provide emotional support and encourage the client to verbalize feelings
e. Initiate support services for the client

E. Pemphigus vulgaris
1. Description
a. A rare disease that occurs predominately between middle and old age
b. The cause is unknown and the disorder is potentially fatal

c. Initial lesions occur on the oral mucosa and then progress to a generalized distribution
d. Treatment is aimed at suppressing the immune response that causes blister formation
2. Data collection
a. Lesions appear as fragile flaccid bullae
b. Partial-thickness wounds that bleed, weep, and form crusts when bullae are disrupted
c. Debilitation, malaise, and pain
d. Chewing and swallowing difficulties
e. Nikolsky's sign: separation of the epidermis caused by rubbing the skin
f. Leukocytosis, eosinophilia, foul-smelling discharge from skin
3. Implementation
a. Provide supportive care
b. Provide oral hygiene and increase fluid intake
c. Soothe oral lesions
d. Assist with oatmeal or potassium permanganate baths as prescribed for relief of symptoms
e. Administer topical or systemic antibiotics as prescribed for secondary infections
f. Administer corticosteroids and cytotoxic agents as prescribed to bring about remission

XI. ACQUIRED IMMUNODEFICIENCY SYNDROME

A. Description
1. An infectious disease characterized by severe deficits in cellular function
2. Manifested clinically by opportunistic infection and/or unusual neoplasms
3. Etiology: human immunodeficiency virus (HIV)
4. The disease has a long incubation period, sometimes up to 10 years or more
5. Manifestations may not appear until late in the infection

B. AIDS-related complex
1. Similar to AIDS
2. Two or more symptoms or two or more laboratory findings characteristic of immunodeficiency
3. Client is not as ill as the AIDS client
4. May lead to AIDS

C. High-risk groups
1. Male homosexuals or bisexuals
2. Intravenous drug abusers
3. Persons receiving blood transfusions (hemophiliacs, surgical clients)
4. Those individuals with frequent exposure to blood and body fluids
5. Heterosexual contact with high-risk individuals
6. Babies born to infected mothers

D. Data collection
1. Malaise, weight loss
2. Lymphadenopathy of at least 3 months
3. Leukopenia
4. Diarrhea
5. Fatigue
6. Night sweats
7. Presence of opportunistic infections
8. *Pneumocystic carinii* pneumonia (major source of mortality)
9. Kaposi's sarcoma: purplish/red lesions of internal organs and skin
10. Candidiasis
11. Fungal infections
12. Cytomegalovirus

E. Implementation
1. Provide respiratory support
2. Administer respiratory treatments as prescribed
3. Administer oxygen as prescribed
4. Maintain fluid and electrolyte balance
5. Monitor for signs of infection
6. Prevent the spread of infection
7. Initiate standard (universal) precautions
8. Provide comfort as necessary
9. Provide meticulous skin care
10. Provide adequate nutritional support as prescribed
11. Refer to Chapters 22 and 36 for additional information on AIDS

PRACTICE QUESTIONS

1. A client is suspected of having systemic lupus erythematous (SLE). The nurse monitors the client knowing that which of the following is a characteristic sign of SLE?
   1. Rash on the face across the bridge of the nose and on the cheeks
   2. Fatigue
   3. Fever
   4. Elevated red blood cell count
2. The nurse is caring for a client with systemic lupus erythematous (SLE). Which of the following would not be a component of the teaching plan for the client to manage fatigue?
   1. To avoid long periods of rest
   2. To sit whenever possible
   3. To take a hot bath in the evening
   4. To engage in moderate low impact exercise when not fatigued
3. A client has requested and undergone testing for human immunodeficiency virus (HIV). The client

now asks what will be done next, as the results of two enzyme-linked immunosorbent assay (ELISA) tests have been positive. The nurse's response is based on the understanding that:

1. The client will probably have a bone marrow biopsy done
2. A Western blot will be done to confirm these findings
3. A CD4 cell count will be done to measure T-helper lymphocytes
4. The client will be definitively diagnosed as HIV positive at this point

4. A nurse is caring for the client with acquired immunodeficiency syndrome (AIDS). The nurse detects early infection with *Pneumocystis carinii* by monitoring the client for which of the following clinical manifestations?
   1. Dyspnea on exertion
   2. Dyspnea at rest
   3. Fever
   4. Cough
5. A client with acquired immunodeficiency syndrome (AIDS) has a concurrent diagnosis of histoplasmosis. The nurse notes during data collection that the client has enlarged lymph nodes. The nurse interprets that:
   1. The client has disseminated histoplasmosis infection
   2. This is a side effect of the medications given to treat AIDS
   3. This indicates that the histoplasmosis is resolving
   4. The client probably has yet another infection that is developing
6. A nurse is caring for the client with acquired immunodeficiency syndrome (AIDS) who is experiencing night fever and night sweats. Which of the following nursing interventions would be the least helpful in managing this symptom?
   1. Keep a change of bed linens nearby in case they are needed
   2. Administer an antipyretic after the client spikes the fever
   3. Make sure the pillow has a plastic cover
   4. Keep liquids at the bedside
7. A client exposed to human immunodeficiency virus (HIV) approximately 3 months ago has seroconverted to HIV-positive status. The nurse anticipates that the client will experience which of the following at this time?
   1. Oral lesions
   2. Purplish skin lesions
   3. Chronic cough
   4. No signs and symptoms
8. A client with acquired immunodeficiency syndrome (AIDS) has raised, dark purplish-colored lesions on the trunk of the body. The nurse anticipates that which of the following procedures will be done to confirm whether these lesions are due to Kaposi's sarcoma?
   1. Enzyme-linked immunosorbent assay (ELISA)
   2. Western blot
   3. Skin biopsy
   4. Lung biopsy
9. A nurse participating in a health fair is setting up a booth on prevention of human immunodeficiency virus (HIV) transmission. A poster is planned that will list sexual behaviors in one of two columns, rated "safe" and "not safe." Which of the following behaviors would the nurse place in the "not safe" column?
   1. Use of latex condoms
   2. Use of "natural skin" condoms
   3. Abstinence
   4. Mutual monogamy
10. A client with acquired immunodeficiency syndrome (AIDS) is experiencing nausea and vomiting. The nurse would make which of the following dietary alterations for this client to enhance nutritional intake?
    1. Avoid dairy products and red meat
    2. Plan large, nutritious meals
    3. Add spices to food for added flavor
    4. Serve foods while they are very warm
11. A client with acquired immunodeficiency syndrome (AIDS) has diarrhea from lactose intolerance and a respiratory infection from *Pneumocystis carinii.* In evaluating the documented plan of care for the nursing diagnosis Impaired Gas Exchange, which of the following would not be considered by the nurse to be a positive outcome criterion for this client?
    1. Is free of complaints of shortness of breath
    2. Expectorates secretions easily
    3. Has clear breath sounds
    4. Limits fluid intake
12. A client with pemphigus vulgaris is being seen in the clinic on a regular basis. The nurse plans care based on which of the following descriptions of this condition?
    1. The presence of skin vesicles found along the nerve caused by a virus
    2. An autoimmune disorder that causes blistering in the epidermis
    3. The presence of red, raised papules and large plaques covered by silvery scales
    4. The presence of tiny red vesicles
13. A nurse is providing dietary instructions to the client with systemic lupus erythematosus (SLE). Which of the following dietary items would the nurse instruct the client to avoid?
    1. Cantaloupe
    2. Broccoli
    3. Turkey
    4. Steak

14. A client is brought to the emergency room and is experiencing an anaphylaxis reaction from eating shellfish. The nurse prepares for which of the following initial actions?
    1. Administration of epinephrine (Adrenalin)
    2. Administration of a corticosteroid
    3. Maintaining a patent airway
    4. Instructing the client on the importance of obtaining a Medic-Alert bracelet
15. A nurse is assisting in planning care for a client with a diagnosis of immune deficiency. The nurse would incorporate which of the following as a priority in the plan of care?
    1. Emotional support to decrease fear
    2. Protecting the client from infection
    3. Encouraging discussion about lifestyle changes
    4. Identifying factors that decreased the immune function
16. A client calls the nurse in the emergency room and tells the nurse that he or she was just stung by a bumble bee while gardening. The client is afraid of a severe reaction because the client's neighbor experienced such a reaction just 1 week ago. The most appropriate nursing action is to:
    1. Ask the client if he or she ever received a bee sting in the past
    2. Tell the client to call an ambulance for transport to the emergency room
    3. Advise the client to soak the site in hydrogen peroxide
    4. Tell the client not to worry about the sting unless difficulty breathing occurs
17. A nurse is assisting in administering immunizations at a health care clinic. The nurse understands that an immunization will provide:
    1. Natural immunity from disease
    2. Acquired immunity from disease
    3. Innate immunity from disease
    4. Protection from all diseases
18. A nurse is assigned to care for a client with systemic lupus erythematosus (SLE). The nurse plans care knowing that this disorder is:
    1. A local rash that occurs as a result of allergy
    2. An inflammatory disease of collagen contained in connective tissue
    3. A disease caused by overexposure to sunlight
    4. A disease caused by the continuous release of histamine in the body
19. A nurse is providing home care instructions to a client who has been diagnosed with a latex allergy. The nurse most appropriately instructs the client to avoid:
    1. Outdoor activities as much as possible
    2. Going to parties
    3. The use of condoms
    4. Sunlight
20. A nurse is collecting data on a client who has been diagnosed with an allergy to latex. In determining the client's risk factors associated with the allergy, the nurse questions the client about an allergy to which food item?
    1. Milk
    2. Bananas
    3. Yogurt
    4. Eggs
21. A nurse is caring for a client who returned to home from the emergency room after treatment for a sprained ankle. The nurse notes that the client was sent home with crutches and needs instructions regarding crutch walking. When collecting data from the client, the nurse discovers that the client has an allergy to latex. Before providing instructions regarding crutch walking, the nurse most appropriately:
    1. Contacts the physician
    2. Covers the crutch pads with cloth
    3. Tells the client that the crutches must be removed from the house immediately
    4. Calls the local medical supply store and asks for a cane to be delivered
22. A nurse is ordering dressing supplies for a client who has an allergy to latex. The nurse asks the medical supply personnel to deliver which of the following?
    1. Adhesive bandages
    2. Band-Aid dressings
    3. Cotton pads and silk tape
    4. Brown Ace bandages

ANSWERS

1. *Answer:* 1

Rationale: Skin lesions or rash on the face across the bridge of the nose and on the cheeks is a characteristic sign of SLE. Fever and fatigue may potentially occur before and during exacerbation. Anemia is most likely to occur in SLE.

Test-Taking Strategy: Note the key words "characteristic sign." Knowledge regarding the manifestations associated with SLE will easily direct you to option 1. If you are unfamiliar with this disorder, review this content.

Level of Cognitive Ability: Application
Client Needs: Physiological Integrity
Integrated Concept/Process: Nursing Process/Data Collection
Content Area: Adult Health/Immune
Reference: Black J, Hawks J, Keene A: *Medical-surgical nursing: clinical management for positive outcomes*, ed 6, Philadelphia, 2001, WB Saunders, p. 2157.

2. *Answer:* 3

Rationale: To help reduce fatigue in the client with SLE, the nurse should instruct the client to sit whenever possible, to avoid hot baths, to schedule moderate low impact exercises when not fatigued, and to maintain a balanced diet. The client is instructed not to rest for long periods because it promotes joint stiffness.

Test-Taking Strategy: Note the key words "not" and "manage fatigue." By using the process of elimination, you should be easily directed to option 3 as being the action that would exacerbate fatigue. If you had difficulty with this question, review measures to prevent fatigue.

Level of Cognitive Ability: Comprehension

Client Needs: Health Promotion and Maintenance

Integrated Concept/Process: Teaching/Learning

Content Area: Adult Health/Immune

Reference: Black J, Hawks J, Keene A: *Medical-surgical nursing: clinical management for positive outcomes*, ed 6, Philadelphia, 2001, WB Saunders, p. 2157.

3. *Answer:* 2

Rationale: If the results of two ELISA tests are positive, the Western blot is done to confirm the findings. If the result of the Western blot is positive, then the client is considered to be positive for HIV, and infected with the HIV virus.

Test-Taking Strategy: Knowledge of the diagnostic tests and procedural steps in diagnosing HIV is needed to answer this question. Review these diagnostic tests if you had difficulty with this question.

Level of Cognitive Ability: Application

Client Needs: Physiological Integrity

Integrated Concept/Process: Nursing Process/Implementation

Content Area: Adult Health/Immune

Reference: Black J, Hawks J, Keene A: *Medical-surgical nursing: clinical management for positive outcomes*, ed 6, Philadelphia, 2001, WB Saunders, p. 2193.

4. *Answer:* 4

Rationale: The client with *Pneumocystis carinii* infection usually has a cough as the first symptom, which begins as nonproductive, then progresses to productive. Later signs include fever, dyspnea on exertion, and finally dyspnea at rest.

Test-Taking Strategy: The key word in the stem of this question is "early." Although all of these symptoms may appear at some point in the client with *Pneumocystis carinii*, knowing that the cough appears first helps you to eliminate each of the other options. Review the early signs of *Pneumocystis carinii* infection if you had difficulty with this question.

Level of Cognitive Ability: Application

Client Needs: Physiological Integrity

Integrated Concept/Process: Nursing Process/Data Collection

Content Area: Adult Health/Immune

Reference: Black J, Hawks J, Keene A: *Medical-surgical nursing: clinical management for positive outcomes*, ed 6, Philadelphia, 2001, WB Saunders, p. 2199.

5. *Answer:* 1

Rationale: Histoplasmosis usually starts as a respiratory infection in the client with AIDS. It then becomes a disseminated infection, with enlargement of lymph nodes, spleen, and liver. Options 2, 3, and 4 are incorrect.

Test-Taking Strategy: Use the process of elimination. Knowing that lymph nodes may enlarge with generalized infection helps you to narrow the choices to options 1 and 4. Because the question contains no information that indicates that option 4 is true, option 1 is the correct choice by elimination. Review disseminated infections in the client with AIDS if you had difficulty with this question.

Level of Cognitive Ability: Analysis

Client Needs: Physiological Integrity

Integrated Concept/Process: Nursing Process/Data Collection

Content Area: Adult Health/Immune

Reference: Black J, Hawks J, Keene A: *Medical-surgical nursing: clinical management for positive outcomes*, ed 6, Philadelphia, 2001, WB Saunders, p. 2204.

6. *Answer:* 2

Rationale: For clients with AIDS who experience night fever and night sweats, it is useful to offer the client an antipyretic of choice before the client goes to sleep. It is also helpful to keep a change of bed linens and night clothes nearby for use. The pillow should have a plastic cover, and a towel may be placed over the pillowcase if there is profuse diaphoresis. The client should have liquids at the bedside to drink.

Test-Taking Strategy: Use the process of elimination. The wording of the question guides you to look for a response that is not the best or most correct action. Options 1 and 3 are helpful from an environmental viewpoint, so they are eliminated first as answers to this question. Knowing that liquids will help prevent dehydration assists you to eliminate this option next. This leaves option 2 as the answer. Because night fever and sweats occur serially, it is most helpful to give the antipyretic before sleep as a prophylactic measure. Review care to the client with AIDS if you had difficulty with this question.

Level of Cognitive Ability: Application

Client Needs: Physiological Integrity

Integrated Concept/Process: Nursing Process/Implementation

Content Area: Adult Health/Immune

Reference: Black J, Hawks J, Keene A: *Medical-surgical nursing: clinical management for positive outcomes*, ed 6, Philadelphia, 2001, WB Saunders, p. 2209.

7. *Answer:* 4

Rationale: The client in stage 1 (seroconversion) acute HIV infection has laboratory documentation of HIV-positive status, but is asymptomatic. After infection and seroconversion in stage 1, the client may remain asymptomatic for 6 months to more than 11 years. The client's T4 cell count is normal during these two stages. The client will begin to show symptoms in stage 3 when the T4 cell count drops below 500/mm^3. At this time, the client experiences opportunistic infections, including oral lesions (thrush) and skin lesions (Kaposi's sarcoma). The client may also experience signs of respiratory infection in stage 3.

Test-Taking Strategy: Use the process of elimination. Read the question carefully noting the 3-month period between exposure and seroconversion. This will direct you to option 4. Review the clinical manifestations associated with HIV if you had difficulty with this question.

Level of Cognitive Ability: Analysis
Client Needs: Physiological Integrity
Integrated Concept/Process: Nursing Process/Data Collection
Content Area: Adult Health/Immune
Reference: Black J, Hawks J, Keene A: *Medical-surgical nursing: clinical management for positive outcomes*, ed 6, Philadelphia, 2001, WB Saunders, p. 2199.

8. *Answer:* 3
Rationale: The skin biopsy is the procedure of choice to diagnose Kaposi's sarcoma, which frequently complicates the clinical picture of the client with AIDS. Lung biopsy would confirm *Pneumocystis carinii* infection. The ELISA and Western blot tests are used to diagnose HIV.
Test-Taking Strategy: Use the process of elimination. Begin to answer this question by eliminating options, 1 and 2, which are used to diagnose whether the client is HIV positive. Knowledge of the meaning of Kaposi's sarcoma, or attention to the words "lesions" and "trunk," will help you to choose correctly between the remaining options. Review the diagnostic testing to confirm Kaposi's sarcoma if you had difficulty with this question.
Level of Cognitive Ability: Analysis
Client Needs: Physiological Integrity
Integrated Concept/Process: Nursing Process/Data Collection
Content Area: Adult Health/Immune
Reference: Black J, Hawks J, Keene A: *Medical-surgical nursing: clinical management for positive outcomes*, ed 6, Philadelphia, 2001, WB Saunders, p. 2205.

9. *Answer:* 2
Rationale: Abstinence is the safest way to avoid HIV infection. The next most reliable method is participation in a mutually monogamous relationship. The use of latex condoms is considered safe, because the latex prevents the transmission of the HIV virus as long as the condom is used properly and remains in place. The use of "natural skin" condoms is not considered safe because the pores in the condom are large enough for the virus to pass through.
Test-Taking Strategy: Use knowledge of transmission of sexually transmitted diseases and universal precautions to answer this question. Note the key words "not safe." The wording of the question tells you that there is one option that is dissimilar from the others, which in this case is the correct answer to the question. Review these preventive measures if you had difficulty with this question.
Level of Cognitive Ability: Application
Client Needs: Health Promotion and Maintenance
Integrated Concept/Process: Teaching/Learning
Content Area: Adult Health/Immune
Reference: Black J, Hawks J, Keene A: *Medical-surgical nursing: clinical management for positive outcomes*, ed 6, Philadelphia, 2001, WB Saunders, p. 2186.

10. *Answer:* 1
Rationale: The AIDS client with nausea and vomiting should avoid fatty products such as diary products and red meat. Meals should be small and frequent to lessen the chance of vomiting. Spices and odorous foods should be avoided, because they aggravate nausea. Foods are best tolerated either cold or at room temperature.
Test-Taking Strategy: Use knowledge of the effects of AIDS on the gastrointestinal tract and general principles for treating nausea and vomiting to answer this question. Doing so will guide you to eliminate systematically each of the incorrect options. Review nutritional support for the client with AIDS if you had difficulty with this question.
Level of Cognitive Ability: Application
Client Needs: Physiological Integrity
Integrated Concept/Process: Nursing Process/Implementation
Content Area: Adult Health/Immune
Reference: Black J, Hawks J, Keene A: *Medical-surgical nursing: clinical management for positive outcomes*, ed 6, Philadelphia, 2001, WB Saunders, p. 2208.

11. *Answer:* 4
Rationale: The status of the client with a diagnosis of Impaired Gas Exchange would be evaluated against the standard outcome criteria for this nursing diagnosis. These would include that the client states that breathing is easier, coughs up secretions effectively, and has clear breath sounds. The client should not limit fluid intake because fluids are needed to decrease the viscosity of secretions for expectoration. The client with diarrhea should also not limit fluid intake because of the risk of dehydration.
Test-Taking Strategy: Use the process of elimination. Note that the stem of the question contains the key word "not." This tells you that the answer to the question is an incorrect goal for the client. Use knowledge related to airway management and fluid balance and the process of elimination to choose correctly. Review care to the client with AIDS if you had difficulty with this question.
Level of Cognitive Ability: Analysis
Client Needs: Physiological Integrity
Integrated Concept/Process: Nursing Process/Evaluation
Content Area: Adult Health/Immune
Reference: Black J, Hawks J, Keene A: *Medical-surgical nursing: clinical management for positive outcomes*, ed 6, Philadelphia, 2001, WB Saunders, p. 2200.

12. *Answer:* 2
Rationale: Pemphigus vulgaris is an autoimmune disease that causes blistering in the epidermis. Clients have large flaccid blisters (bullae). Because the blisters are in the epidermis, they have a very tiny covering of skin and break easily, leaving large denuded areas of skin. On initial examination, clients may have crusting areas instead of intact blisters. Option 1 describes herpes zoster. Option 3 describes psoriasis, and option 4 describes eczema.
Test-Taking Strategy: Use the process of elimination. Knowledge that pemphigus vulgaris is an autoimmune disorder will easily direct you to option 2. If you had difficulty with this question, review the characteristics of this disorder.
Level of Cognitive Ability: Application
Client Needs: Physiological Integrity
Integrated Concept/Process: Nursing Process/Planning
Content Area: Adult Health/Immune
Reference: Black J, Hawks J, Keene A: *Medical-surgical nursing: clinical management for positive outcomes*, ed 6, Philadelphia, 2001, WB Saunders, p. 1310.

13. *Answer:* 4
Rationale: The client with SLE is at risk for cardiovascular disorders such as coronary artery disease and hypertension. The client is advised of lifestyle changes to reduce these risks, which include smoking cessation, prevention of obesity, and hyperlipidemia. The client is advised to reduce salt, fat, and cholesterol intake.
Test-Taking Strategy: Use the process of elimination. Note the key word "avoid" in the question. Use knowledge regarding basic nutritional components of food items to help direct you to option 4. If you had difficulty with this question, review therapeutic management of SLE.
Level of Cognitive Ability: Application
Client Needs: Physiological Integrity
Integrated Concept/Process: Teaching/Learning
Content Area: Adult Health/Immune
Reference: Black J, Hawks J, Keene A: *Medical-surgical nursing: clinical management for positive outcomes*, ed 6, Philadelphia, 2001, WB Saunders, p. 2157.

14. *Answer:* 3
Rationale: The initial action would be to maintain a patent airway. The client would then receive epinephrine. Corticosteroids may also be prescribed. The client will need to be instructed about wearing a Medic-Alert bracelet, but this is not the initial action.
Test-Taking Strategy: Use the ABCs—airway, breathing, and circulation—to answer the question. Airway is always the priority. Review care to the client experiencing an anaphylaxis reaction if you had difficulty with this question.
Level of Cognitive Ability: Application
Client Needs: Physiological Integrity
Integrated Concept/Process: Nursing Process/Planning
Content Area: Adult Health/Immune
Reference: DeWit S: *Fundamental concepts and skills for nursing*, Philadelphia, 2001, WB Saunders, p. 635.

15. *Answer:* 2
Rationale: The client with immune deficiency has inadequate or the absence of immune bodies and is at risk for infection. The priority nursing intervention would be to protect the client from infection. Options 1, 3, and 4 may be components of care but are not the priority.
Test-Taking Strategy: Use Maslow's Hierarchy of Needs theory to answer the question. Remember that physiological needs are the priority. This will easily direct you to option 2. Review the care of a client with immune deficiency if you had difficulty with this question.
Level of Cognitive Ability: Application
Client Needs: Physiological Integrity
Integrated Concept/Process: Nursing Process/Planning
Content Area: Adult Health/Immune
Reference: Black J, Hawks J, Keene A: *Medical-surgical nursing: clinical management for positive outcomes*, ed 6, Philadelphia, 2001, WB Saunders, p. 2136.

16. *Answer:* 1
Rationale: In most types of allergies, a reaction occurs only on second and subsequent contacts with the allergen. The most appropriate action therefore would be to ask the client if he or she ever received a bee sting in the past. Option 2 is unnecessary. Option 3 is not appropriate advice. The client should not be told "not to worry."
Test-Taking Strategy: Use the steps of the nursing process to answer the question. Option 1 is the only option that addresses data collection. Review information related to allergic reactions if you had difficulty with this question.
Level of Cognitive Ability: Application
Client Needs: Physiological Integrity
Integrated Concept/Process: Nursing Process/Implementation
Content Area: Adult Health/Immune
Reference: DeWit S: *Fundamental concepts and skills for nursing*, Philadelphia, 2001, WB Saunders, p. 635.

17. *Answer:* 2
Rationale: Acquired immunity can occur by receiving an immunization that causes antibodies to a specific pathogen to form. Natural (innate) immunity is present at birth. There is no immunization that protects the client from all diseases.
Test-Taking Strategy: Use the process of elimination and knowledge regarding immunity to disease to answer the question. Eliminate option 4 first because of the absolute word "all." Next eliminate options 1 and 3 because they are similar. Review natural and acquired immunity if you had difficulty with this question.
Level of Cognitive Ability: Comprehension
Client Needs: Physiological Integrity
Integrated Concept/Process: Nursing Process/Implementation
Content Area: Adult Health/Immune
Reference: Black J, Hawks J, Keene A: *Medical-surgical nursing: clinical management for positive outcomes*, ed 6, Philadelphia, 2001, WB Saunders, p. 2081.

18. *Answer:* 2
Rationale: SLE is an inflammatory disease of collagen contained in connective tissue. Options 1, 3, and 4 are not associated with this disease.
Test-Taking Strategy: Knowledge regarding the characteristics of SLE is required to answer this question. Review this disorder if you had difficulty with this question.
Level of Cognitive Ability: Comprehension
Client Needs: Physiological Integrity
Integrated Concept/Process: Nursing Process/Planning
Content Area: Adult Health/Immune
Reference: Black J, Hawks J, Keene A: *Medical-surgical nursing: clinical management for positive outcomes*, ed 6, Philadelphia, 2001, WB Saunders, p. 2157.

19. *Answer:* 3
Rationale: Mucosal exposure to latex can occur on contact with latex condoms. The nurse would most appropriately provide instructions to the client about the need to avoid the use of condoms, unless they are latex-free. There is no reason to avoid outdoor activities or sunlight. There is also no reason to avoid parties; however, the client should be informed that certain forms of balloons are made of latex.
Test-Taking Strategy: Use the process of elimination. Note the key word "avoid." Eliminate option 1 and 4 first because they are similar. From the remaining options, focusing on the issue

will direct you to option 3. Review instructions for the client with a latex allergy if you had difficulty with this question.
Level of Cognitive Ability: Application
Client Needs: Health Promotion and Maintenance
Integrated Concept/Process: Teaching/Learning
Content Area: Adult Health/Immune
Reference: Smeltzer S, Bare B: *Brunner and Suddarth's textbook of medical-surgical nursing,* ed 9, Philadelphia, 2000, Lippincott Williams & Wilkins, pp. 1402-1403.

20. *Answer:* 2
Rationale: Individuals who are allergic to bananas, avocados, tropical fruits, kiwis, potatoes, and chestnuts are at risk for developing a latex allergy. This is thought to be due to a possible cross-reaction between the food and the latex allergen. Options 1, 3, and 4 are unrelated to latex allergy.
Test-Taking Strategy: Use the process of elimination and knowledge regarding the food items related to a latex allergy. Eliminate options 1, 3, and 4 because they are similar and all relate to dairy products. Review the food items that are associated with a risk for latex allergy if you had difficulty with this question.
Level of Cognitive Ability: Analysis
Client Needs: Health Promotion and Maintenance
Integrated Concept/Process: Nursing Process/Data Collection
Content Area: Adult Health/Immune
Reference: Phipps W, Sands J, Marek J: *Medical-surgical nursing: concepts and clinical practice,* ed 6, St Louis, 1999, Mosby, p. 511.

21. *Answer:* 2
Rationale: Pads used on crutches contain latex. If the client requires the use of crutches, the nurse can cover the pads with a cloth to prevent cutaneous contact. Option 3 is inappropriate and may alarm the client. The nurse cannot order a cane for a client. Additionally, this type of assistive device may not be appropriate considering this client's injury. There is no reason to contact the physician at this time.
Test-Taking Strategy: Use the process of elimination and knowledge regarding the alternative resources that can be used for a client with an allergy to latex. There are no data in the question that support the need to contact the physician. The nurse should not prescribe assistive devices for the client. Option 3 is not a therapeutic action. Review care to the client with a latex allergy if you had difficulty with this question.
Level of Cognitive Ability: Application
Client Needs: Safe, Effective Care Environment
Integrated Concept/Process: Nursing Process/Implementation
Content Area: Adult Health/Immune
Reference: Smeltzer S, Bare B: *Brunner and Suddarth's textbook of medical-surgical nursing,* ed 9, Philadelphia, 2000, Lippincott Williams & Wilkins, p. 1402.

22. *Answer:* 3
Rationale: Cotton pads and plastic or silk tape are latex-free products. The items identified in options 1, 2, and 4 all contain latex.
Test-Taking Strategy: Use the process of elimination and knowledge regarding the products that contain latex to answer this question. Noting the key words "cotton" and "silk" in option 3 may assist in answering correctly. Review the list of products that contain latex if you had difficulty with this question.
Level of Cognitive Ability: Application
Client Needs: Safe, Effective Care Environment
Integrated Concept/Process: Nursing Process/Implementation
Content Area: Adult Health/Immune
Reference: Smeltzer S, Bare B: *Brunner and Suddarth's textbook of medical-surgical nursing,* ed 9, Philadelphia, 2000, Lippincott Williams & Wilkins, p. 1402.

REFERENCES

Black J, Hawks J, Keene A: *Medical-surgical nursing: clinical management for positive outcomes,* ed 6, Philadelphia, 2001, WB Saunders.

Chernecky C, Berger B: *Laboratory tests and diagnostic procedures,* ed 3, Philadelphia, 2001, WB Saunders.

Clark J, Queener S, Karb V: *Pharmacologic basis of nursing practice,* ed 6, St Louis, 2000, Mosby.

DeWit S: *Fundamental concepts and skills for nursing,* Philadelphia, 2001, WB Saunders.

Hodgson B, Kizior R: *Saunders nursing drug handbook 2002,* Philadelphia, 2002, WB Saunders.

Ignatavicius D, Workman M: *Medical-surgical: critical thinking for collaborative care,* ed 4, Philadelphia, 2002, WB Saunders.

Lehne R: *Pharmacology for nursing care,* ed 4, Philadelphia, 2001, WB Saunders.

Potter P, Perry A: *Fundamentals of nursing,* ed 5, St Louis, 2001, Mosby.

Perry A, Potter P: *Clinical nursing skills and techniques,* ed 5, St. Louis, 2002, Mosby.

Smeltzer S, Bare B: *Brunner and Suddarth's textbook of medical-surgical nursing,* ed 9, Philadelphia, 2000, Lippincott Williams & Wilkins.

Wilson J: *Infection control in clinical practice,* ed 2, St Louis, 2002, Balliere Tindall.

Immunological Medications

I. HUMAN IMMUNODEFICIENCY VIRUS (HIV) AND ACQUIRED IMMUNODEFICIENCY SYNDROME (AIDS) (Box 59-1)

A. Antiinflammatory medications
   1. Sulfasalazine (Azulfidine)
      a. Used to treat toxoplasmosis or nocardiasis
      b. Administered orally
      c. Can cause renal toxicity
      d. Suppresses bone marrow function
      e. Increases photosensitivity
      f. Monitor urine output and complete blood count (CBC)
      g. Monitor the client for sore throat, pallor, purpura, jaundice, and weakness
      h. Encourage fluid intake
      i. Advise the client to avoid exposure to the sun

B. Antiinfective medications
   1. Pentamidine isethionate (Pentam-300)
      a. Used to treat *Pneumocystis carinii* pneumonia
      b. Administered by intramuscular (IM) or intravenous (IV) route
      c. Can cause nephrotoxicity
      d. Monitor blood pressure and heart rate (may cause hypotension)
      e. Monitor for hypoglycemia
      f. Is hepatotoxic and immunosuppressive
      g. Monitor liver function tests and CBC
   2. Metronidazole (Flagyl)
      a. Used to treat cryptosporidiosis and giardiasis
      b. Administered orally or by the IV route
      c. Administer with food or milk
      d. Monitor for dry mouth, dizziness, or fungal infection

BOX 59-1

Medications for HIV and AIDS

ANTIINFLAMMATORY MEDICATIONS
Sulfasalazine (Azulfidine)

ANTIINFECTIVE MEDICATIONS
Pentamidine isethionate (Pentam 300)
Metronidazole (Flagyl)

ANTIFUNGAL MEDICATIONS
Ketonazole (Nizoral)
Fluconazole (Dilfulcan)
Amphotericin B (Fungizone)

ANTIVIRALS
Gancyclovir (Cytovene)
Acyclovir (Zovirax)
Foscarnet (Foscavir)

ANTIRETROVIRALS (NUCLEOSIDE REVERSE TRANSCRIPTASE INHIBITORS)
Zidovudine (Ritrovir, AZT)
Didanosine (Videx)
Lamivudine (Epivir)
Zalcitabine (ddC)

ANTIRETROVIRALS (PROTEASE INHIBITORS)
Saquinavir (Invirase)
Ritonavir (Norvir)
Stavudine (d4T, Zerit)

ANTIFUNGAL, ANTIINFECTIVE, ANTIPROTOZOAL
Dapsone (Avlosulfon, DDS)

ANTIMALARIAL, ANTIPROTOZOAL
Pyrimethamine (Daraprim)

e. Instruct the client to avoid alcohol during treatment

C. Antifungal medications
1. Ketonazole (Nizoral)
a. Used in the treatment of candidiasis, coccidiodomycosis, or histoplasmosis
b. Administered orally
c. Administer with food or milk
d. Instruct the client to avoid antacids for 2 hours after taking the medication because gastric acid is needed to activate the medication
e. Is hepatotoxic
f. Monitor hepatic function
g. Instruct the client to avoid exposure to the sun because the medication increases photosensitivity
h. Instruct the client to avoid alcohol during treatment
2. Fluconazole (Dilfulcan)
a. Used to treat candidiasis
b. Administered orally
c. Is hepatotoxic
d. Monitor for abdominal pain, fever, and diarrhea
e. Monitor hepatic function
3. Amphotericin B (Fungizone)
a. Used to treat candidiasis and other fungal infections
b. Administered by the IV route
c. Is nephrotoxic
d. Can cause thrombophlebitis
e. Suppresses bone marrow function
f. Monitor renal function
g. Monitor infusion site
h. Monitor CBC

D. Antivirals
1. Gancyclovir (Cytovene)
a. Used to treat cytomegalovirus retinitis
b. Administered orally or by the IV route
c. Suppresses bone marrow function
d. Monitor neutrophil and platelet count
e. Administer with food
2. Acyclovir (Zovirax)
a. Used to treat herpes simplex, herpes zoster, or varicella zoster
b. May be administered orally or by the IV route
c. Is nephrotoxic
d. Monitor renal function
e. Encourage fluid intake
f. Is irritating to a blood vessel when administered by the IV route
3. Foscarnet (Foscavir)
a. Used in the treatment of cytomegalovirus retinitis in human immunodeficiency virus (HIV)-infected clients
b. Administered by the IV route
c. Is nephrotoxic
d. Monitor renal function
4. Zidovudine (Ritrovir, AZT)
a. Antiretroviral (nucleoside reverse transcriptase inhibitor)
b. Indicated for clients with HIV seropositivity
c. Administered orally
d. Suppresses bone marrow function
e. Is hepatotoxic and nephrotoxic
f. Monitor CBC, hepatic, and renal function studies
g. Monitor for dizziness because the medication crosses the blood-brain barrier
h. Instruct the client that medication must be administered around the clock
5. Didanosine (Videx)
a. Antiretroviral (nucleoside reverse transcriptase inhibitor)
b. Indicated for clients with HIV seropositivity
c. Administered orally
d. Administer on an empty stomach to enhance absorption
e. Instruct the client to chew tablet or crush
f. Monitor for dizziness, neuropathy, and pancreatitis
6. Lamivudine (Epivir)
a. Antiretroviral (nucleoside reverse transcriptase inhibitor)
b. Indicated for clients with HIV seropositivity
c. Used as prophylaxis for occupational exposure
d. Administered orally
e. Can cause severe pancreatitis
f. Instruct the client to avoid fatty foods
7. Zalcitabine (ddC)
a. Antiretroviral (nucleoside reverse transcriptase inhibitor)
b. Used in the management of HIV infection with other antiretrovirals such as AZT because of the synergistic effect
c. It has also been used as a single agent in clients who are intolerant of other regimens
d. Administered orally (with AZT)
e. Can cause serious liver damage
f. Monitor liver function studies
8. Saquinavir (Invirase)
a. Antiretroviral (protease inhibitor)
b. Used in combination with other antiretroviral medications in the management of HIV infection
c. Administered orally
d. Administered with meals

e. Is best absorbed if the client consumes a high calorie, high-fat meal
f. It can cause photosensitivity and the client is instructed to avoid sun exposure

9. Ritonavir (Norvir)
   a. Antiretroviral (protease inhibitor)
   b. Used in combination with other antiretroviral medications in the management of HIV infection
   c. Administered orally
   d. Administered 1 hour before or two hours after meals because it is best absorbed in a fasting state
   e. Can increase triglyceride levels
   f. Monitor triglyceride levels
10. Stavudine (d4T, Zerit)
   a. Antiretroviral (protease inhibitor)
   b. Used in the management of HIV infection in clients who do not respond to or who cannot tolerate conventional therapy
   c. Administered orally
   d. Can cause peripheral neuropathy
   e. Monitor the client's gait
   f. Ask the client about paresthesias

E. Dapsone (Avlosulfon, DDS)
   1. Antifungal, anti-infective, antiprotozoal
   2. Used for the treatment of toxoplasmosis
   3. Administered orally
   4. Suppresses bone marrow activity
   5. Can cause anemia, peripheral motor weakness, liver damage
   6. Monitor the CBC
   7. Monitor for fever, sore throat, purpura, or jaundice

F. Pyrimethamine (Daraprim)
   1. Antimalarial, antiprotozoal
   2. Used in the treatment of toxoplasmosis or *Pneumocystis carinii* pneumonia
   3. Administered orally
   4. Suppresses bone marrow function
   5. Monitor complete blood count (CBC) and platelet count
   6. Administer with food or milk

II. SYSTEMIC LUPUS ERYTHEMATOSUS (Box 59-2)

BOX 59-2

Systemic Lupus Erythematosus

Azathioprine (Imuran)
Cyclophosphamide (Cytoxan)
Hydroxychloroquine sulfate (Plaquenil)
Prednisone (Deltasone)
Nonsteroidal antiinflammatory drugs

A. Medications: used to control symptoms and to prevent or control serious complications that occur as a result of organ damage by the inflammatory process

B. Azathioprine (Imuran)
   1. Glucocorticoid-sparing effect
   2. Potentiates the immunosuppressive action of glucocorticoids and thereby allows a lower dosage of glucocorticoid to have a greater immunosuppressive action
   3. Monitor CBC and liver function tests

C. Cyclophosphamide (Cytoxan)
   1. Immunosuppressive treatment of diffuse proliferative nephritis and other organ inflammation unresponsive to glucocorticoids
   2. Reserved for use in severe cases because of the adverse side effects

D. Hydroxychloroquine sulfate (Plaquenil)
   1. An antimalarial used to prevent the recurrence of an exacerbation
   2. An eye examination should be performed initially and 6 months after treatment
   3. Administer with meals or a glass of milk

E. Prednisone (Deltasone)
   1. Used at high doses to treat exacerbations and at low doses to control symptoms when other medications do not work
   2. Refer to Chapter 43 for information on glucocorticoids

F. Nonsteroidal antiinflammatory drugs (NSAIDs)
   1. Used to control fever and arthralgia
   2. Refer to Chapter 55 for information on NSAIDs

III. IMMUNIZATIONS

(Refer to Chapter 36.)

PRACTICE QUESTIONS

1. Dapsone (DDS) is prescribed for a client with acquired immunodeficiency syndrome (AIDS) for the treatment of toxoplasmosis. The nurse reinforces medication instructions and tells the client to:
   1. Discontinue the medication if nausea and vomiting develops
   2. Plan to take the medication every 6 hours around the clock
   3. Contact the physician if fever or a sore throat occurs
   4. Report to the clinic weekly for the injections
2. Pyrimethamine (Daraprim) has been added to the medication regimen for the client with acquired immunodeficiency syndrome (AIDS). On review of the client's record, the nurse notes this new prescrip-

tion and plans care knowing that this has been prescribed for the treatment of:

1. Toxoplasmosis
2. Cardiac irregularities
3. Kaposi's sarcoma
4. Nausea and vomiting

3. Saquinavir (Invirase) is prescribed for the client who is human immunodeficiency virus (HIV) seropositive. The nurse reinforces medication instructions and tells the client to:

1. Take the medication on an empty stomach
2. Eat low calorie foods
3. Eat foods that are low in fat
4. Avoid sun exposure

4. The client who is human immunodeficiency virus (HIV) seropositive has been taking Ritonavir (Norvir). The client returns to the clinic for follow-up laboratory tests. The nurse reviews the client's record and expects to note a physician's order for which of the following laboratory tests?

1. Platelet count
2. Triglyceride level
3. Prothrombin time (PT)
4. International normalized ratio (INR)

5. A client who is human immunodeficiency virus (HIV) seropositive has been taking Stavudine (d4T, Zerit). The nurse monitors which of the following most closely while the client is taking this medication?

1. Appetite
2. Gait
3. Gastrointestinal function
4. Level of consciousness (LOC)

6. A client who is human immunodeficiency virus (HIV) seropositive has been taking zalcitabine (ddC) as a component of treatment. The nurse plans to monitor which of the following most closely while the client is taking this medication?

1. Liver function studies
2. Platelet count
3. Red blood cell count
4. Glucose level

7. A nurse is assigned to care for a client with cytomegalovirus retinitis and acquired immunodeficiency syndrome (AIDS) who is receiving foscavir (Foscarnet). The nurse checks the latest results of which of the following laboratory studies while the client is taking this medication?

1. Serum albumin
2. Serum creatinine
3. CD4 cell count
4. Lymphocyte count

8. A client with acquired immunodeficiency syndrome (AIDS) and pneumocystis carinii infection has been receiving pentamidine (Pentam 300). The client develops a fever of 101° F degrees. The nurse does further monitoring of the client, knowing that this sign would most likely indicate:

1. The dose of the medication is too low
2. The client is experiencing toxic effects of the medication
3. The client has developed inadequacy of thermoregulation
4. This is a result of another infection, caused by leukopenic effects of the medication

9. A client with acquired immunodeficiency syndrome (AIDS) has been started on therapy with zidovudine (AZT, Retrovir). The nurse carefully monitors which of the following laboratory results during treatment with this medication?

1. Complete blood count (CBC)
2. Blood urea nitrogen
3. Blood culture
4. Blood glucose level

10. A nurse is reviewing the results of serum laboratory studies drawn on a client with acquired immunodeficiency syndrome (AIDS) who is receiving didanosine (Videx). The nurse interprets that the client may very well have the medication discontinued by the physician because of which of the following significantly elevated results?

1. Serum cholesterol
2. Serum amylase
3. Blood glucose
4. Serum protein

ANSWERS

1. *Answer:* 3

Rationale: Dapsone may be prescribed for the treatment of toxoplasmosis. The medication is taken orally on a daily basis. The medication suppresses bone marrow activity and the complete blood count (CBC) is monitored closely. If the client develops fever, sore throat, purpura, or jaundice, the physician is notified. Medications are available to treat nausea and vomiting and the client should not discontinue the medication if these symptoms occur but should contact the physician.

Test-Taking Strategy: Use the process of elimination. Eliminate option 1 first because the nurse would not tell the client to discontinue the medication. Next, eliminate options 2 and 4 knowing that the medication is administered orally on a daily basis. Review this medication if you had difficulty with this question.

Level of Cognitive Ability: Application

Client Needs: Health Promotion and Maintenance

Integrated Concept/Process: Teaching/Learning

Content Area: Adult Health/Immune

Reference: Lehne R: *Pharmacology for nursing care,* ed 4, Philadelphia, 2001, WB Saunders, p. 898.

2. *Answer:* 1
Rationale: Daraprim is an antimalarial and an antiprotozoal medication. It is used in the treatment of toxoplasmosis or *Pneumocystis carinii* pneumonia. It is not used to treat nausea, vomiting, cardiac irregularities, or Kaposi's sarcoma.
Test-Taking Strategy: Use the process of elimination. Knowledge regarding the action and use of Daraprim is required to answer this question. If you knew that this medication was an antimalarial and an antiprotozoal medication, then you would easily be directed to option 1. Review this medication if you had difficulty with this medication.
Level of Cognitive Ability: Analysis
Client Needs: Physiological Integrity
Integrated Concept/Process: Nursing Process/Planning
Content Area: Adult Health/Immune
Reference: Lehne R: *Pharmacology for nursing care,* ed 4, Philadelphia, 2001, WB Saunders, p. 1088.

3. *Answer:* 4
Rationale: Invirase is an antiretroviral (protease inhibitor) used in combination with other antiretroviral medications in the management of HIV infection. It is administered with meals and is best absorbed if the client consumes a high-calorie, high-fat meals. It can cause photosensitivity and the client is instructed to avoid sun exposure.
Test-Taking Strategy: Use the process of elimination. Knowledge regarding this medication is required to answer this question. Options 2 and 3 can be eliminated first knowing that these dietary measures would not likely be prescribed. From the remaining options, it is necessary to know that this medication can cause photosensitivity. Review this medication if you had difficulty with this question.
Level of Cognitive Ability: Application
Client Needs: Health Promotion and Maintenance
Integrated Concept/Process: Teaching/Learning
Content Area: Adult Health/Immune
Reference: Lehne R: *Pharmacology for nursing care,* ed 4, Philadelphia, 2001, WB Saunders, p. 1041.

4. *Answer:* 2
Rationale: Norvir is an antiretroviral (protease inhibitor) used in combination with other antiretroviral medications in the management of HIV infection. It can increase the triglyceride levels and therefore the client's triglyceride level should be monitored. The platelet count, PT, and INR are not laboratory tests that would specifically be monitored in the client on this medication.
Test-Taking Strategy: Knowledge regarding the side effects of Norvir is required to answer this question. Review this medication if you had difficulty with this question.
Level of Cognitive Ability: Analysis
Client Needs: Physiological Integrity
Integrated Concept/Process: Nursing Process/Planning
Content Area: Adult Health/Immune
Reference: Lehne R: *Pharmacology for nursing care,* ed 4, Philadelphia, 2001, WB Saunders, p. 1032.

5. *Answer:* 2
Rationale: Stavudine is an antiretroviral (protease inhibitor) used in the management of HIV infection in clients who do not respond to or who cannot tolerate conventional therapy. The medication can cause peripheral neuropathy and the nurse should closely monitor the client's gait and ask the client about paresthesia.
Test-Taking Strategy: Knowledge regarding the specific side effects of this medication is required to answer this question. If you are not familiar with this medication and the important data collection measures, review this content.
Level of Cognitive Ability: Application
Client Needs: Physiological Integrity
Integrated Concept/Process: Nursing Process/Data Collection
Content Area: Adult Health/Immune
Reference: Lehne R: *Pharmacology for nursing care,* ed 4, Philadelphia, 2001, WB Saunders, p. 1035.

6. *Answer:* 1
Rationale: Zalcitabine is an antiretroviral (nucleoside reverse transcriptase inhibitor) used in the management of HIV infection with other antiretrovirals. It has also been used as a single agent in clients who are intolerant of other regimens. It can cause serious liver damage and liver function studies should be monitored closely. Options 2, 3, and 4 are not specifically associated with the use of this medication.
Test-Taking Strategy: Knowledge regarding the side effects of zalcitabine is required to answer this question. Review this medication if you had difficulty with this question.
Level of Cognitive Ability: Application
Client Needs: Physiological Integrity
Integrated Concept/Process: Nursing Process/Data Collection
Content Area: Adult Health/Immune
Reference: Lehne R: *Pharmacology for nursing care,* ed 4, Philadelphia, 2001, WB Saunders, p. 1034.

7. *Answer:* 2
Rationale: Foscavir is very toxic to the kidneys. Serum creatinine is monitored prior to therapy, 2 to 3 times per week during induction therapy, and at least weekly during maintenance therapy. It also may cause decreased levels of calcium, magnesium, phosphorus, and potassium in the bloodstream. Thus, these levels are also measured with the same frequency.
Test-Taking Strategy: It is necessary to know the toxicities and important side effects of this medication to discriminate among the various options correctly. Review this medication if you had difficulty with this question.
Level of Cognitive Ability: Application
Client Needs: Physiological Integrity
Integrated Concept/Process: Nursing Process/Data Collection
Content Area: Adult Health/Immune
Reference: Lehne R: *Pharmacology for nursing care,* ed 4, Philadelphia, 2001, WB Saunders, p. 1022.

8. *Answer:* 4
Rationale: Frequent side effects of this medication include leukopenia, thrombocytopenia and anemia. The client should be routinely monitored for signs and symptoms of infection. The client should also have ongoing monitoring of a number

of parameters due to the nature and side effects of the medication, including blood glucose, blood urea nitrogen, serum creatinine, complete blood count, liver function studies, and serum calcium and magnesium levels.
Test-Taking Strategy: Use the process of elimination. Options 2 and 3 are the least plausible given the information in the question, and are eliminated first. To discriminate between the remaining options, you need to know that the medication has leukopenic side effects. Review this medication if you had difficulty with this question.
Level of Cognitive Ability: Analysis
Client Needs: Physiological Integrity
Integrated Concept/Process: Nursing Process/Data Collection
Content Area: Adult Health/Immune
Reference: Lehne R: *Pharmacology for nursing care,* ed 4, Philadelphia, 2001, WB Saunders, p. 1093.

9. ***Answer:*** 1
Rationale: A common side effect of this medication therapy is agranulocytopenia and anemia. The nurse carefully monitors CBC results for these changes. With early HIV infection or in the client who is asymptomatic, CBC levels are monitored monthly for 3 months, then every 3 months thereafter. In clients with advanced disease, they are monitored every 2 weeks for the first 2 months, and then once a month if the medication is tolerated well.
Test-Taking Strategy: It is necessary to know the toxicities and important side effects of this medication to discriminate among the various options correctly. Review this medication if you had difficulty with this question.
Level of Cognitive Ability: Application
Client Needs: Physiological Integrity
Integrated Concept/Process: Nursing Process/Data Collection
Content Area: Adult Health/Immune
Reference: Lehne R: *Pharmacology for nursing care,* ed 4, Philadelphia, 2001, WB Saunders, p. 1031.

10. ***Answer:*** 2
Rationale: A serum amylase level that is increased 1.5 to 2 times normal may signify pancreatitis in the AIDS client, which is potentially fatal. The medication may have to be discontinued. The medication is also hepatotoxic, and can result in liver failure.
Test-Taking Strategy: It is necessary to know the toxicities and important side effects of this medication to discriminate among the various options correctly. Review this medication if you had difficulty with this question.
Level of Cognitive Ability: Comprehension
Client Needs: Physiological Integrity
Integrated Concept/Process: Nursing Process/Evaluation
Content Area: Adult Health/Immune
Reference: Lehne R: *Pharmacology for nursing care,* ed 4, Philadelphia, 2001, WB Saunders, p. 1034.

REFERENCES

Black J, Hawks J, Keene A: *Medical-surgical nursing: clinical management for positive outcomes,* ed 6, Philadelphia, 2001, WB Saunders.

Chernecky C, Berger B: *Laboratory tests and diagnostic procedures,* ed 3, Philadelphia: WB Saunders.

Clark J, Queener S, Karb V: *Pharmacologic basis of nursing practice,* ed 6, St Louis, 2000, Mosby.

DeWit S: *Fundamental concepts and skills for nursing,* Philadelphia, 2001, WB Saunders.

Hodgson B, Kizior R: *Saunders nursing drug handbook 2002,* Philadelphia, 2002, WB Saunders.

Ignatavicius D, Workman M: *Medical-surgical: Critical thinking for collaborative care,* ed 4, Philadelphia, 2002, WB Saunders.

Lehne R: *Pharmacology for nursing care,* ed 4, Philadelphia, 2001, WB Saunders.

Potter P, Perry A: *Fundamentals of nursing,* ed 5, St Louis, 2001, Mosby.

Perry A, Potter P: *Clinical nursing skills and techniques,* ed 5, St Louis, 2002, Mosby.

Smeltzer S, Bare B: *Brunner & Suddarth's Textbook of medical-surgical nursing,* ed 9, Philadelphia, 2000, Lippincott Williams & Wilkins.

Wilson J: *Infection control in clinical practice,* ed 2, St Louis, 2002, Balliere Tindall.

UNIT XIX

The Adult Client with a Mental Health Disorder

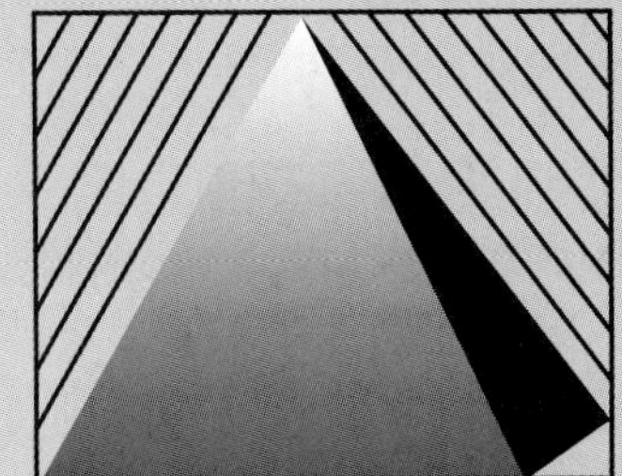

PYRAMID TERMS

Abuse An act of misuse, deceit, or exploitation. The wrong or improper use or action toward another individual that results in injury, damage, maltreatment, or corruption.

Addiction Also known as drug dependence. Incorporates the concepts of loss of control with respect to the use of a drug, taking the drug despite related problems and complications, and a tendency to relapse.

Coping Mechanisms Methods of adjusting to environmental stress without altering one's own goals or purposes. Can include both conscious and unconscious mechanisms.

Crisis A temporary state of disequilibrium in which an individual's usual coping mechanisms or problem-solving methods fail. It can result in personality growth or personality disorganization.

Defense Mechanisms A coping mechanism (protective defense) of the ego that attempts to protect the individual from feelings of inadequacy and worthlessness and prevent awareness of anxiety. When anxiety is too painful, the individual copes by using defense mechanisms to protect the ego and decrease anxiety.

Milieu The physical and social environment in which an individual lives. Milieu therapy focuses on positive physical and social environmental manipulation to produce positive change.

Restraints Physical restraints include any manual method or mechanical device, material, or equipment that inhibits free movement. Chemical restraints includes the administration of medications for the specific purpose of inhibiting a specific behavior or movement.

Seclusion Placing a client alone in a specially designed room for protection and close supervision. It is the last measure in a process to maximize safety to the client and others.

Suicide The ultimate act of self-destruction, in which an individual purposefully ends his or her own life.

Suicide Attempt Any willful, self-inflicted, or life-threatening attempt by an individual that has not lead to death.

PYRAMID TO SUCCESS

The Pyramid to Success focuses on the therapeutic nurse-client relationship, client rights, and the ethical and legal issues related to the care of the client with a mental health disorder. Pyramid points focus on the use of restraints, seclusion, and electroconvulsive therapy (ECT). Focus on care to the client with an addiction, such as an eating disorder, or drug or alcohol disorder. Additional focus areas include anxiety, depression, suicide, abuse and violence, posttraumatic stress disorders, obsessive-compulsive disorders, schizophrenia, and bipolar disorders. Pyramid points address the use of medications prescribed for the client with a mental health disorder, particularly lithium carbonate (Eskalith) and the benzodiazepines. The Integrated Concepts and Processes addressed in this unit include Caring, the Clinical Problem-Solving Process (Nursing Process), Communication and Documentation, Cultural Awareness, Self-Care, and Teaching/Learning.

CLIENT NEEDS

Safe, Effective Care Environment

Client advocacy
Client rights
Confidentiality
Establishing priorities
Ethical practice
Informed consent related to treatments, such as restraints, seclusion, and electroconvulsive therapy (ECT)
Legal responsibilities related to reporting incidence of violence and abuse
Psychiatric consultations and referrals
Providing safety to client and others
Use of restraints and seclusion

Health Promotion and Maintenance

Family interaction patterns
Health promotion programs related to addictions
Individual lifestyle choices

Psychosocial Integrity

Abuse and neglect
Behavioral interventions
Chemical dependency
Coping mechanisms
Crisis intervention
Domestic violence
End of life issues
Grief and loss
Mental health concepts and illness
Religious and spiritual influences on health
Stress management
Suicide
Support systems
Therapeutic environment
Therapeutic nurse-client relationship

Physiological Integrity

Abusive and self-destructive behavior
Alterations in body systems related to addictions
Elimination
Expected effects of medications
Medication administration
Nutrition
Personal hygiene measures
Potential complications related to medications and ECT
Rest and sleep

REFERENCES

Black J, Hawks J, Keene A: *Medical-surgical nursing: clinical management for positive outcomes*, ed 6, Philadelphia, 2001, WB Saunders.

Chernecky C, Berger B: *Laboratory tests and diagnostic procedures*, ed 3, Philadelphia, 2001, WB Saunders.

Clark J, Queener S, Karb V: *Pharmacologic basis of nursing practice*, ed 6, St Louis, 2000, Mosby.

DeWit S: *Fundamental concepts and skills for nursing*, Philadelphia, 2001, WB Saunders.

Hill S, Bauer B: *Mental health nursing*, Philadelphia, 2002, WB Saunders.

Hill S, Howlett H: *Success in practical nursing: personal and vocational issues*, ed 4, Philadelphia, 2001, WB Saunders.

Keltner N, Schwecke L, Bostrom C: *Psychiatric nursing*, ed 3, St Louis, 1999, Mosby.

National Council of State Boards of Nursing: *Test plan for the National Council Licensure Examination for Practical/Vocational Nurses*, Chicago, 2001, Author.

Potter P, Perry A: *Fundamentals of nursing*, ed 5, St Louis, 2001, Mosby.

Perry A, Potter P: *Clinical nursing skills and techniques*, ed 5, St Louis, 2002, Mosby.

Wilson J: *Infection control in clinical practice*, ed 2, St Louis, 2002, Balliere Tindall.

Varcarolis E: *Foundations of psychiatric mental health nursing*, ed 4, Philadelphia, 2002, WB Saunders.

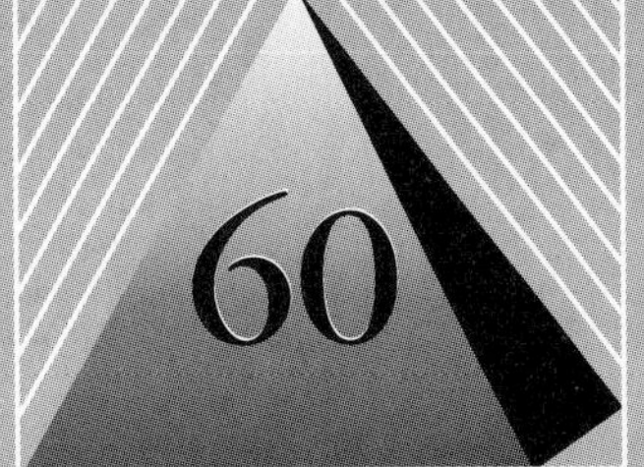

Foundations of Psychiatric Mental Health Nursing

I. MENTAL HEALTH

A. A lifelong process of successful adaptation to a changing internal and external environment

B. The individual is in contact with reality and the environment and possesses the ability to love, work, and resolve conflicts within a framework of reasonability

C. The individual has psychobiological resilience

II. PSYCHIATRIC/MENTAL HEALTH ILLNESS

A. Description
1. Loss of the ability to respond to the environment in ways that is in accord with oneself or society's expectations
2. Characterized by thought or behavior patterns that impair functioning and cause the individual distress

B. Personality characteristics
1. Is unaccepting of self and dislikes self
2. Has an unrealistic perception of strengths and weaknesses
3. Thoughts and perceptions may not be reality based
4. Is unable to find meaning and purpose in life
5. Lacks direction and productivity in life
6. Has difficulty in meeting own needs
7. Depends on others for thought and actions

C. Adaptations to stress
1. Feels out of control with self and with the environment
2. Has a negative perception of the environment
3. Has ineffective **coping mechanisms**

D. Interpersonal relationships
1. Is unable to love and care for others
2. Is unable to feel loved by others or accept feelings from others

III. COPING AND DEFENSE MECHANISMS

A. **Coping mechanisms**
1. Coping involves any effort to decrease the stress response
2. **Coping mechanisms** can be either constructive or destructive in nature; they can be task oriented related to direct problem solving, or can be a defense-oriented regulating response to protect oneself
3. Destructive **coping mechanisms** often cause a mental health disorder because the problem that causes the disorder is avoided
4. Neurotic or psychotic behaviors can typically result when **coping mechanisms** become destructive

B. **Defense mechanisms** (Box 60-1)
1. **Coping mechanism** (protective defenses) of the ego that attempt to protect the individual from feelings of inadequacy and worthlessness and prevent awareness of anxiety
2. When anxiety is too painful, the individual copes by using **defense mechanisms** to protect the ego and decrease anxiety

C. Implementation
1. Assess the client's use of the **defense mechanism**
2. Determine if the use of the **defense mechanism** characterizes unhealthy adjustment
3. Facilitate appropriate use of **defense mechanisms**
4. Avoid criticizing the behavior and the use of **defense mechanisms**
5. Assist the client to identify the source of the anxiety
6. Assist the client to explore methods to reduce the anxiety

BOX 60-1

Types of Defense Mechanisms

Compensation: Putting forth extra effort to achieve in areas in which one has a real or imagined deficiency
Conversion: The expression of emotional conflicts through physical symptoms
Denial: Disowning consciously intolerable thoughts and impulses
Displacement: Feelings toward one person are directed to another who is less threatening, thereby satisfying an impulse with a substitute object
Dissociation: The blocking off of an anxiety-provoking event or period of time from the conscious mind
Fantasy: Gratification by imaginary achievements and wishful thinking
Fixation: Never advancing to the next level of emotional development and organization; the persistence in later life of interests and behavior patterns appropriate to an earlier age
Identification: The unconscious attempt to change oneself to resemble an admired person
Insulation: Withdrawing into passivity and becoming inaccessible to avoid further threatening situations
Intellectualization: Excessive reasoning to avoid feeling; the thinking is disconnected from feelings, and situations are dealt with at a cognitive level
Introjection: A type of identification in which the individual incorporates the traits or values of another into self
Isolation: Response in which a person blocks feelings associated with an unpleasant experience
Projection: Transferring one's internal feelings, thoughts, and unacceptable ideas and traits to someone else
Rationalization: An attempt to make unacceptable feelings and behavior acceptable by justifying the behavior
Reaction formation: Developing conscious attitudes and behaviors and acting out behaviors opposite to what one really feels
Regression: Returning to an earlier developmental stage to express an impulse in order to deal with reality
Repression: An unconscious process in which the client blocks undesirable and unacceptable thoughts from conscious expression
Sublimation: Replacement of an unacceptable need, attitude, or emotion with one more socially acceptable
Substitution: The replacement of a valued unacceptable object with an object that is more acceptable to the ego
Suppression: The conscious, deliberate forgetting of unacceptable or painful thoughts, ideas, and feelings
Symbolization: The conscious use of an idea or object to represent another actual event or object; many times the meaning is not clear because the symbol may be representative of something unconscious
Undoing: Engaging in behavior that is considered to be opposite of a previous unacceptable behavior, thought, or feeling

IV. THE NURSE-CLIENT RELATIONSHIP

A. Principles
1. Respect the client and value the client as an individual
2. Care for the client in a holistic manner
3. Maintain appropriate limits
4. Remember that empathy is therapeutic and sympathy is nontherapeutic
5. Maintain honest and open communication
6. Encourage expression of the client's feelings
7. Assist the client to develop resources

B. Phases of the therapeutic relationship
1. Orientation/initiation phase
   a. Establish boundaries and trust with the client
   b. Identify the expectations of the relationship
   c. Assess the anxiety in the client
   d. Define goals with the client
2. Working/continuation phase
   a. Promote an attitude of acceptance
   b. Assist the client to express feelings
   c. Identify problems
   d. Continue to assess and evaluate problems
   e. Promote insight and the use of constructive **coping mechanisms**
   f. Increase the client's independence
3. Termination/separation phase
   a. Prepare the client for termination and separation on initial contact
   b. Evaluate progress and achievement of goals
   c. Identify and deal with termination and separation issues
   d. Encourage the client to discuss feelings about termination
   e. Transfer the client to other support systems
   f. Do not promise the client that the relationship will be continued

V. THERAPEUTIC COMMUNICATION PROCESS

A. Principles
1. Communication includes both verbal and nonverbal expression
2. Successful communication includes appropriateness, efficiency, flexibility, and feedback
3. Anxiety in either the nurse or the client impedes communication

4. Communication needs to be goal directed within a professional framework

B. Therapeutic communication techniques and blocks to communication (Table 60-1)

VI. DIAGNOSTIC AND STATISTICAL MANUAL OF MENTAL DISORDERS

A. A classification system developed by the American Psychiatric Association used to determine a medical diagnosis

B. Knowledge of the criteria for a particular psychiatric diagnosis will assist the nurse in making a clinical decision about a nursing diagnosis

VII. TYPES OF MENTAL HEALTH ADMISSIONS AND DISCHARGES (Box 60-2)

A. Voluntary admission
1. Any citizen of lawful age may apply in writing (usually on a standard admission form) for admission to the hospital
2. Sought by the client or the client's guardian if the client is too ill but voluntarily seeks assistance
3. Client agrees to accept treatment
4. Civil rights are fully retained by the client
5. Client is free to sign himself or herself out of the hospital

B. Involuntary admission
1. Involuntary admission may be necessary when a person is mentally ill, is a danger to self or others, or is in need of psychiatric treatment or physical care
2. An admission status in which a person who has the legal capacity to consent to mental

BOX 60-2

Client Rights

Right to accessible health care
Right to a coordination and continuity of health care
Right to courteous and individualized health care
Right to information about the qualifications, names, and titles of personnel delivering care
Right to refuse observation by those not directly involved in care
Right to privacy and confidentiality
Right to informed consent
Right to treatment
Right to refuse treatment
Right to treatment in the least restrictive setting
Right not to be subjected to unnecessary restraints
Right to habeas corpus; may request a hearing at any time to be released from the hospital
Right to information about diagnosis, prognosis, and treatment
Right to information on the charges for service
Right to communicate with people outside the hospital through written correspondence, telephone, and personal visits
Right to keep clothing and personal effects
Right to be employed
Right to religious freedom
Right to execute wills
Right to retain licenses, privileges, or permits established by the law, such as a driver's or professional license

TABLE 60-1

Therapeutic Communication Techniques and Blocks to Communication

Therapeutic Techniques	Blocks
Listening	Giving advice
Being silent	Changing the subject
Respecting the client	Giving approval or disapproval
Providing recognition and acknowledgment	Challenging the client
Providing feedback	Making stereotypical comments
Offering to assist	Making value judgments
Focusing and refocusing	Providing false reassurance
Clarifying and validating	Placing the client's feelings on hold
Reflecting	Asking the client "Why?"
Making observations	Being defensive
Giving information	
Presenting reality	
Summarizing	
Using open-ended questions	
Providing nonverbal encouragement	
Maintaining neutral responses	
Encouraging formulation of plan of action	

health treatment refuses to do so and is involuntarily detained for treatment by the state
3. The client who is involuntarily admitted does not lose his or her right of informed consent
4. The length of time for hospitalization is specified by the state and varies from state to state
5. The client is considered legally competent until he or she has been declared incompetent through a legal proceeding
6. If the nurse believes that a client lacks competency, action should be initiated to have a legal guardian appointed from the court
7. Categories
   a. Evaluation and emergency care
   b. Certification for observation and treatment
   c. Extended or indeterminate commitment

C. Release from the hospital
1. Description
   a. Depends on the client's admission status
   b. The client who sought voluntary admission has the right to demand and receive release
   c. Some states provide for conditional release of voluntary clients, which enables the treating physician or administrator to order continued treatment on an outpatient basis if the clinical needs of the client would warrant further care
2. Conditional release
   a. Usually requires outpatient treatment for a specified period to determine the client's compliance with medication protocol, ability to meet basic needs, and ability to reintegrate into the community
   b. A voluntary client who is conditionally released cannot be reinstitutionalized without the client's consent, unless the institution complies with the procedures for involuntary admission
   c. An involuntary client who is conditionally released may be reinstitutionalized while the commitment is still in effect without recommencement of formal admission procedures
3. Discharge
   a. Discharge (unconditional release) is the termination of the client-institution relationship
   b. This release may be ordered by the psychiatrist, court ordered, or administratively ordered
   c. The administration officer of an institution has the discretion to discharge clients
   d. In most states, clients can institute a court proceeding to seek a judicial discharge (writ of habeas corpus)
   e. Discharge planning and follow-up care are important for the continued well-being of the client with a mental health disorder
   f. After-care case managers are needed to facilitate the client's adaptation back into the community and to provide early referral if the treatment plan is not followed

VIII. MILIEU THERAPY

A. Description
1. **Milieu** is the physical and social environment in which an individual lives
2. Provides a safe environment that is adapted to the individual client's needs and also provides greater comfort and freedom of expression than has been experienced in the past by the client
3. Staffed by persons trained to provide support and understanding and individual attention
4. All members contribute to the planning and functioning of the setting
5. The power hierarchy is diminished because all members are viewed as significant and valuable members of the community

B. Focus
1. Positive environmental manipulation, both physical and social, in order to effect a positive change
2. Client's rights through involvement in setting goals, freedom of movement, and informal relationships with staff
3. Group and social interaction
4. Use of community meetings, activity groups, social skills groups, and physical exercise programs

IX. PSYCHOTHERAPY

A. Description
1. Use of a group of techniques to modify feelings, attitudes, and behaviors in clients
2. Therapist uses both verbal and nonverbal means of communication to build a relationship with the client

B. Focus
1. The basic concept involves understanding
2. The focus in on issues of importance to the client, purpose of the interaction, identification of the roles of the therapist and client, and the use of primarily verbal means of communication
3. Nonverbal techniques include silence, body language, facial expressions, and respect for personal space

C. Levels of psychotherapy

1. Supportive therapy: allows the client to express feelings, explore alternatives, and make decisions in a safe, caring environment
2. Reeducative therapy: involves learning new ways of perceiving and behaving
3. Reconstructive therapy: involves deep psychotherapy or psychoanalysis

X. BEHAVIOR AND BEHAVIOR MODIFICATION

A. Behavior therapy
   1. An approach to bring about behavioral change
   2. It includes a group of diversified approaches for dealing with maladaptive behavior
   3. The belief is that most behaviors are learned
   4. Maladaptive behavior is a way of dealing with stress, and the therapy is an approach to bring about a change in the behavior

B. Self-control therapy
   1. Combination of cognitive and behavioral approaches
   2. A basic theme is that talking to oneself can direct and control actions more effectively
   3. Useful to deal with stress

C. Desensitization
   1. The reduction of intense reactions to a stimulus by repeated exposure to the stimulus in a weaker and milder form
   2. Gradually over a period of time, exposure is increased until the fear of the object or situation has ceased

D. Aversion therapy
   1. Negative reinforcement is a technique to change behavior
   2. A stimulus attractive to the client is paired with an unpleasant event in hopes of endowing the stimulus with negative properties

E. Modeling: the therapist provides a role model for specified identified behaviors, and the client learns through imitation

F. Operant conditioning: entails rewarding a client for desired behaviors and is the basis for behavior modification

XI. COGNITIVE THERAPY

A. An active, directive time-limited structured approach used to treat a variety of psychiatric disorders

B. Therapeutic techniques are designed to identify reality testing and correct distorted conceptualization and the dysfunctional belief underlying these cognitions

C. The client learns to master problems in situations that he or she previously considered insuperable, by evaluating and correcting their thinking

D. The cognitive therapist helps the client to think and act more realistically and adaptively about his or her psychological problems so as to reduce symptoms

E. Various cognitive and behavioral strategies are used in cognitive therapy

XII. GROUP AND GROUP THERAPY

A. Stages of group development
   1. Initial stage
      a. Involves superficial rather that open and trusting communication
      b. Members are becoming acquainted with each other and are searching for similarity between themselves and other group members
      c. Members may be unclear about the purpose or goals of the group
      d. A certain amount of structuring of group norms, roles, and responsibilities take place
   2. Working stage
      a. During this stage, the real work of the group is accomplished
      b. Members are familiar with each other, the group leader, and the group roles, and they feel free to approach their problems and to attempt to solve their problems
      c. Conflict and cooperation surface during the group's work
   3. Termination stage
      a. The group evaluates the experience and explores members' feelings about it and the impending separation
      b. Provides an opportunity for members who have difficulty with termination to learn to deal more realistically and comfortably with this normal part of human experience

B. Community support groups
   1. Promote identification, clarification, understanding, role modeling, feelings of togetherness, and group cohesion
   2. Prevent the individual member from feeling lonely and isolated
   3. Help members decrease levels of stress and increase levels of self-acceptance
   4. Members are better able to deal with the problems that they brought to the group
   5. The outcome is rewarding, and the members develop new or more effective patterns of behavior
   6. Some groups evolve into educational models that enhance communication, self-image,

body image, problem solving, decision making, and growth processes

C. Family therapy
   1. Specific intervention mode based on the premise that the members, with the presenting symptoms, signal the presence of pain in the entire family
   2. The therapist works to assist the family to identify and express their thoughts and feelings, define family roles and rules, try new, more productive styles of relating, and restore strength to the family

PRACTICE QUESTIONS

1. A nurse assists in planning care for a client scheduled to be discharged from a mental health clinic. The nurse knows that unresolved feelings related to loss may resurface during which phase of the therapeutic nurse-client relationship?
   1. Orientation phase
   2. Working phase
   3. Termination phase
   4. Trusting phase
2. A client with depression who attempted suicide says to the nurse, "I should have died. I've always been a failure. Nothing ever goes right for me." The most therapeutic response by the nurse is:
   1. "I don't see you as a failure."
   2. "Feeling like this is all part of being ill."
   3. "You've been feeling like a failure for a while?"
   4. "You have everything to live for."
3. A client states to the nurse, "I haven't slept at all the last couple of nights." The most therapeutic response by the nurse is:
   1. "Go on......"
   2. "Sleeping?"
   3. "The last couple of nights?"
   4. "You're having difficulty sleeping?"
4. While the male nurse is gathering psychosocial data from a female client, the client states, "I don't want to discuss this—it's private and personal." Which statement by the male nurse indicates a therapeutic response?
   1. "This often happens to me. Perhaps you would find it easier to speak to a nurse who is female."
   2. "I am a nurse and as such I'll have you know that all information is kept confidential."
   3. "I know that some of these questions are difficult for you, but as a nurse, I must legally respect your confidentiality."
   4. "This is difficult for you to speak about, but I am trying to perform a complete data collection and I am no different from a female nurse, if that's your problem."
5. A nurse is caring for a Native-American client who says, "I don't want you to touch me. I'll take care of myself!" The most therapeutic response by the nurse is:
   1. "I will respect your feelings. I'll just leave this cup for you to collect your urine in. After breakfast, I will take more blood from you."
   2. "If you didn't want our care, why did you come here?"
   3. "Why are you being so difficult? I only want to help you."
   4. "Sounds like you're feeling pretty troubled by all of us. Let's work together so you can do everything for yourself as you request."
6. A nurse is assigned to care for a client who is experiencing altered thought processes. The nurse is told that the client believes that the food is being poisoned. Which communication technique does the nurse plan to use to encourage the client to eat?
   1. Open-ended questions and silence
   2. Offering opinions about the necessity of adequate nutrition
   3. Identifying the reasons that the client may not want to eat
   4. Focusing on self-disclosure regarding food preferences
7. A nurse is assigned to care for a client admitted to the hospital after sustaining an injury from a house fire. The client attempted to save a neighbor involved in the fire but in spite of the client's efforts, the neighbor died. Which action would the nurse be engaged in with the client during the working phase of the nurse-client relationship?
   1. Identifying the client's potential for self-harm
   2. Identifying the client's ability to function
   3. Inquiring about the client's perception of the neighbor's death
   4. Inquiring about the client's feelings that may block coping
8. A client who has just been sexually assaulted is very quiet and calm. The nurse identifies this behavior as indicative of which defense mechanism?
   1. Denial
   2. Projection
   3. Rationalization
   4. Intellectualization
9. A nurse is assisting with the data collection on a client admitted to the psychiatric unit. The nurse reviews the data obtained and identifies which of the following as a priority concern?
   1. The presence of bruises on the client's body
   2. The client's report of not eating or sleeping
   3. The client's report of suicidal thoughts
   4. The significant other disapproving of the treatment

10. Laboratory work is prescribed on a client who has been experiencing delusions. When the laboratory technician approaches the client to obtain a specimen of the client's blood, the client begins to shout "You're all vampires. Let me out of here!" The nurse who is present at the time would respond most appropriately by stating which of the following?
    1. "The technician is not going to hurt you, but is going to help you!"
    2. "What makes you think that the technician is a vampire?"
    3. "The technician will leave and come back later for your blood."
    4. "It must be fearful to think others want to hurt you."
11. An inebriated client is brought to the emergency department by the local police. The client is told that the physician will be in to see the client in about 30 minutes. The client becomes very loud and offensive and wants to be seen by the physician immediately. The nurse assisting to care for the client would plan for which most appropriate nursing intervention?
    1. Attempt to talk with the client to deescalate the behavior
    2. Watch the behavior escalate before intervening
    3. Inform the client that he or she will be asked to leave if the behavior continues
    4. Offer to take the client to an examination room until he or she can be treated
12. A client is admitted to a psychiatric unit for treatment of psychotic behavior. The client is at the locked exit door, and is shouting, "Let me out. There's nothing wrong with me. I don't belong here." The nurse identifies this behavior as:
    1. Projection
    2. Denial
    3. Regression
    4. Rationalization
13. A client says to the nurse, "I'm going to die, and I wish my family would stop hoping for a 'cure'! I get so angry when they carry on like this! After all, I'm the one who's dying." The most therapeutic response by the nurse is:
    1. "You're feeling angry that your family continues to hope for you to be 'cured'?"
    2. "I think we should talk more about your anger with your family."
    3. "Well, it sounds like you're being pretty pessimistic. After all, years ago people died of pneumonia."
    4. "Have you shared your feelings with your family?"
14. A nurse employed in a psychiatric unit is assigned to care for a client admitted to the unit 2 days ago. On review of the client's record, the nurse notes that the admission was an informal voluntary admission. Based on this type of admission, the nurse would expect which of the following?
    1. The client will be very resistant to treatment measures
    2. The client's family will be very resistant to treatment measures
    3. The client will be angry and will refuse care
    4. The client will participate in the treatment plan
15. A licensed practical nurse (LPN) enters a client's room, and the client is demanding release from the hospital. The LPN reviews the client's record and notes that the client was admitted 2 days ago for treatment of an anxiety disorder, and that the admission was a voluntary admission. The LPN reports the findings to the registered nurse (RN) and expects that the RN will take which of the following actions?
    1. Tell the client that discharge is not possible at this time
    2. Call the client's family
    3. Contact the physician
    4. Persuade the client to stay a few more days
16. A client is admitted to the psychiatric nursing unit. When collecting data from the client, the nurse notes that the client is admitted by involuntary status. Based on this type of admission, the nurse most likely expects that the client:
    1. Presents a harm to self
    2. Requested the admission
    3. Consented to the admission
    4. Provided written application to the facility for admission
17. A nurse is caring for a client who is scheduled for electroconvulsive therapy. The nurse notes that an informed consent has not been obtained for the procedure. On review of the record, the nurse notes that the admission was an involuntary hospitalization. Based on this information, the nurse determines that:
    1. An informed consent does not need to be obtained
    2. An informed consent should be obtained from the family
    3. An informed consent needs to be obtained from the client
    4. The physician will obtain the informed consent
18. After a group therapy session, a client approaches the licensed practical nurse (LPN) and verbalizes a need for seclusion because of uncontrollable feelings. The LPN reports the findings to the registered nurse (RN) and expects that the RN will take which of the following actions?
    1. Inform the client that seclusion has not been prescribed
    2. Obtain an informed consent
    3. Call the client's family
    4. Place the client in seclusion immediately

19. A nurse is providing care to a client admitted to the hospital with a diagnosis of anxiety disorder. The nurse is talking with the client. The client says to the nurse, "I have a secret that I want to tell you. You won't tell anyone about it, will you?" The most appropriate nursing response is which of the following?
    1. "No, I won't tell anyone."
    2. "I cannot promise to keep a secret."
    3. "If you tell me the secret, I will tell it to your doctor."
    4. "If you tell me the secret, I will need to document it in your record."
20. A nurse is greeted by a neighbor in a local grocery store. The neighbor says to the nurse, "How is Carol doing? She is my best friend and is seen at your clinic every week." The most appropriate nursing response is which of the following?
    1. "I'm not suppose to discuss this, but since you are my neighbor, I can tell you that she is doing great!"
    2. "I'm not suppose to discuss this, but since you are my neighbor, I can tell you that she really has some problems!"
    3. "If you want to know about Carol, you need to ask her yourself."
    4. "I cannot discuss any client situation with you."
21. A client was involuntarily admitted to the psychiatric unit because of episodes of extremely violent behavior. The client is demanding to be discharged from the hospital. The licensed practical nurse (LPN) reports the information to the registered nurse (RN) and the RN does not allow the client to leave. The LPN understands that which of the following represents the legal ramifications associated with the RN's behavior?
    1. The RN will be charged with imprisonment
    2. The RN will be charged with assault
    3. The RN will be charged with slander
    4. No charge will be made against the RN because the RN's actions are reasonable
22. A nurse is preparing a client for the termination phase of the nurse client relationship. Which of the following nursing tasks would the nurse most appropriately plan for this phase?
    1. Identify expected outcomes
    2. Plan short-term goals
    3. Assist in making appropriate referrals
    4. Assist in developing realistic solutions
23. During the termination phase of the nurse-client relationship, the clinic nurse observes that the client continuously demonstrates bursts of anger. The most appropriate interpretation of the behavior is that the client:
    1. Requires further treatment and is not ready to be discharged
    2. Is displaying typical behaviors that can occur during termination
    3. Needs to be admitted to the hospital
    4. Needs to be referred to the psychiatrist as soon as possible
24. An 18-year-old woman is admitted to an inpatient psychiatric unit with the diagnosis of anorexia nervosa. A behavior therapy approach is used as part of her treatment plan. The nurse understands that the purpose of this approach is to:
    1. Help the client identify and examine dysfunctional thoughts and beliefs
    2. Emphasize social interaction with clients who withdraw
    3. Provide a supportive environment
    4. Examine conflicts and past issues
25. Milieu therapy is prescribed for a client. The nurse understands that this type of therapy can best be described as which of the following?
    1. A form of behavior modification therapy
    2. A cognitive approach to changing behavior
    3. The client is involved in setting goals
    4. A behavioral approach to changing behavior
26. Disulfiram (Antabuse) is prescribed for a client with a problem related to alcohol. The nurse understands that this medication works on the principle of which of the following therapies?
    1. Desensitization
    2. Self-control therapy
    3. Milieu therapy
    4. Aversion therapy
27. A client with an eating disorder is attending group meetings with Overeaters Anonymous. Which of the following is not a characteristic of this form of self-help group?
    1. People who have a similar problem are able to help others
    2. It is designed to serve people who have a common problem
    3. The members provide support to each other
    4. The leader is a nurse or psychiatrist
28. A client is attending a Gambler's Anonymous meeting for the first time. The model used by this group is the 12-step program developed by Alcoholics Anonymous. The nurse understands that the first step in the 12-step program is which of the following?
    1. Stating that the gambling will be stopped
    2. Discontinuing relationships with friends who are gamblers
    3. Substituting gambling for other activities
    4. Admitting to having a problem
29. A nurse is assisting in conducting a group therapy session and a client with a manic disorder is monopolizing the group. The most appropriate nursing action is which of the following?

1. Suggest that the client stop talking and try listening to others
2. Ask the client to leave
3. Tell the client to stop monopolizing the group
4. Refer the client to another group

30. A nurse is assisting in monitoring a group therapy session. During this session, the members are identifying tasks and boundaries. The nurse understands that these activities are characteristic of which stage of group development?
   1. Forming
   2. Storming
   3. Norming
   4. Performing

ANSWERS

1. *Answer:* 3
Rationale: In the termination phase, the relationship comes to a close. Ending treatment may sometimes be traumatic for clients who have come to value the relationship and the help. Because loss is an issue, any unresolved feelings related to loss may resurface during this phase. Options 1, 2, and 4 are incorrect.
Test-Taking Strategy: Note the key words "unresolved" and "loss" in the question. Consider the phases of the therapeutic nurse-client relationship to direct you to option 3. Review these phases and the nursing implications if you had difficulty with this question.
Level of Cognitive Ability: Comprehension
Client Needs: Psychosocial Integrity
Integrated Concept/Process: Caring
Content Area: Mental Health
Reference: Hill S, Bauer B: *Mental health nursing,* Philadelphia, 2002, WB Saunders, p. 248.

2. *Answer:* 3
Rationale: Responding to the feelings expressed by a client is an effective therapeutic communication technique. The correct option is an example of the use of restating. Options 1, 2, and 4 block communication because they minimize the client's experience and do not facilitate exploration of the client's expressed feelings.
Test-Taking Strategy: Use therapeutic communication techniques. Select the option that directly addresses the client feelings and concerns. Option 3 is the only option that is stated in the form of a question and is open-ended; thus it will encourage the verbalization of feelings. Review these techniques if you had difficulty with this question.
Level of Cognitive Ability: Application
Client Needs: Psychosocial Integrity
Integrated Concept/Process: Communication and Documentation
Content Area: Mental Health
Reference: Hill S, Bauer B: *Mental health nursing,* Philadelphia, 2002, WB Saunders, p. 62.

3. *Answer:* 4
Rationale: Option 4 identifies the therapeutic communication technique of restatement. Although it is a technique that has a prompting component to it, it repeats the client's major theme and provides the perception of the problem from the client's perspective. Option 1 allows the client to direct the discussion when it needs to be more focused at this point. Option 2 uses reflection that simply repeats the client's last words to prompt further discussion. Option 3 focuses on the number of nights rather than the specific problem of sleep.
Test-Taking Strategy: Use therapeutic communication techniques. Option 4 identifies restatement and repeats the client's major theme. Review therapeutic communication techniques if you had difficulty with this question.
Level of Cognitive Ability: Application
Client Needs: Psychosocial Integrity
Integrated Concept/Process: Communication and Documentation
Content Area: Mental Health
Reference: Hill S, Bauer B: *Mental health nursing,* Philadelphia, 2002, WB Saunders, p. 62.

4. *Answer:* 3
Rationale: When reading the question, you do not know whether the client is responding to the nurse's gender or is simply uncomfortable sharing personal information. The most therapeutic response for the male nurse is not to bring what may be his own gender issues into the response at this time. Options 1, 2, and 4 are nontherapeutic responses.
Test-Taking Strategy: Use therapeutic communication techniques. Option 1 is not therapeutic because the response clearly ignores the fact that this is not about the nurse, but is about the client and the client's discomfort. In option 2, the nurse becomes somewhat angry, which is not therapeutic. In option 4, the nurse begins responding correctly with an empathic stance but becomes involved in a gender defense and becomes somewhat defensive. Review therapeutic communication techniques if you had difficulty with this question.
Level of Cognitive Ability: Application
Client Needs: Psychosocial Integrity
Integrated Concept/Process: Communication and Documentation
Content Area: Mental Health
Reference: Varcarolis E: *Foundations of psychiatric mental health nursing,* ed 4, Philadelphia, 2002, WB Saunders, p. 254.

5. *Answer:* 4
Rationale: The most therapeutic response is the one that reflects the client's feelings and offers the client control of care. In option 1, the nurse uses avoidance and information giving. Option 2 is an aggressive and nontherapeutic communication technique. Option 3 is social and nontherapeutic because it

labels the client's behavior and is likely to provoke anger from the client.
Test-Taking Strategy: Use therapeutic communication techniques and knowledge regarding cultural issues related to Native-Americans to answer the question. Review these cultural issues if you had difficulty with this question.
Level of Cognitive Ability: Application
Client Needs: Psychosocial Integrity
Integrated Concept/Process: Cultural Awareness
Content Area: Mental Health
Reference: Varcarolis E: *Foundations of psychiatric mental health nursing*, ed 4, Philadelphia, 2002, WB Saunders, p. 254.

6. *Answer:* 1
Rationale: Open-ended questions and silence are strategies used to encourage clients to discuss their problem. Options 2 and 3 do not encourage the client to express feelings. The nurse should not offer opinions and should encourage the client to identify the reasons for the behavior. Option 4 is not a client-centered intervention.
Test-Taking Strategy: Use the process of elimination. Eliminate options 2 and 3 first because they do not support client expression of feelings. Eliminate option 4 next because it is not a client-centered intervention. Focusing on the client's feelings will direct you to option 1. Review therapeutic communication techniques if you had difficulty with this question.
Level of Cognitive Ability: Application
Client Needs: Psychosocial Integrity
Integrated Concept/Process: Caring
Content Area: Mental Health
Reference: Varcarolis E: *Foundations of psychiatric mental health nursing*, ed 4, Philadelphia, 2002, WB Saunders, p. 253.

7. *Answer:* 4
Rationale: The client must first deal with feelings and negative responses before the client is able to work through the meaning of the crisis. Option 4 pertains directly to the client's feelings. Options 1, 2, and 3 do not directly address the client's feelings.
Test-Taking Strategy: Use the process of elimination. Focusing on the feelings of the client will direct you to option 4. Review the phases of the nurse-client relationship if you had difficulty with this question.
Level of Cognitive Ability: Application
Client Needs: Psychosocial Integrity
Integrated Concept/Process: Nursing Process/Implementation
Content Area: Mental Health
Reference: Varcarolis E: *Foundations of psychiatric mental health nursing*, ed 4, Philadelphia, 2002, WB Saunders, p. 222.

8. *Answer:* 1
Rationale: Denial is a response by victims of sexual abuse. It is described as an adaptive and protective reaction. Projection is blaming or "scapegoating." Rationalization is justifying the unacceptable attributes about himself or herself. Intellectualization is the excessive use of abstract thinking or generalizations to decrease painful thinking.
Test-Taking Strategy: Use the process of elimination and knowledge regarding defense mechanisms. Note the key words "calm" and "quiet." These behaviors are indicative of denial in a sexually abused victim. If you had difficulty with this question, review content related to the sexually abused victim and defense mechanisms.
Level of Cognitive Ability: Comprehension
Client Needs: Psychosocial Integrity
Integrated Concept/Process: Nursing Process/Data Collection
Content Area: Mental Health
Reference: Varcarolis E: *Foundations of psychiatric mental health nursing*, ed 4, Philadelphia, 2002, WB Saunders, p. 26.

9. *Answer:* 3
Rationale: The client's thoughts are extremely important when verbalized. Suicidal thoughts are the highest priority. Options 1, 2, and 4 will all affect the treatment of the client but are not of greatest importance at this time.
Test-Taking Strategy: The client is the focus of the question; therefore eliminate option 4. Focus on the key words "priority concern" and use prioritizing skills. Remember, if the client verbalizes suicidal thoughts, it is a priority concern. Review data collection techniques related to the suicidal client if you had difficulty with this question.
Level of Cognitive Ability: Analysis
Client Needs: Psychosocial Integrity
Integrated Concept/Process: Nursing Process/Data Collection
Content Area: Mental Health
Reference: Varcarolis E: *Foundations of psychiatric mental health nursing*, ed 4, Philadelphia, 2002, WB Saunders, p. 641.

10. *Answer:* 4
Rationale: Option 4 is the only option that recognizes the client's need. This response helps the client to focus on the emotion underlying the delusion, but does not argue with it. If the nurse attempts to change the client's mind, the delusion may in fact be even more strongly held.
Test-Taking Strategy: Use therapeutic communication techniques and knowledge regarding the dynamics of delusions and how delusions meet the client's underlying needs. This will direct you to option 4. Additionally, option 4 focuses on the client's feelings. Review therapeutic communication techniques if you had difficulty with this question.
Level of Cognitive Ability: Application
Client Needs: Psychosocial Integrity
Integrated Concept/Process: Communication and Documentation
Content Area: Mental Health
Reference: Varcarolis E: *Foundations of psychiatric mental health nursing*, ed 4, Philadelphia, 2002, WB Saunders, p. 531.

11. *Answer:* 4
Rationale: Safety of the client, other clients, and staff is of prime concern. When dealing with an impaired individual, trying to talk may be out of the question. Waiting to intervene could cause the client to become even more agitated and a threat to others. Option 3 would only further aggravate an already agitated individual. Option 4 is in effect an isolation technique that allows for separation from others and provides a less stimulating environment where the client can maintain dignity.

Test-Taking Strategy: Focus on the issue of the question and use the process of elimination. Noting that the client is inebriated will assist in directing you to option 4. Option 4 most directly addresses the situation and the behavior and feelings of the client. Review nursing interventions for a client who is inebriated if you had difficulty with this question.
Level of Cognitive Ability: Application
Client Needs: Psychosocial Integrity
Integrated Concept/Process: Nursing Process/Planning
Content Area: Mental Health
Reference: Varcarolis E: *Foundations of psychiatric mental health nursing*, ed 4, Philadelphia, 2002, WB Saunders, p. 110.

12. ***Answer:*** 2
Rationale: Denial is refusal to admit to a painful reality, which is treated as if it does not exist. In projection, a person unconsciously rejects emotionally unacceptable features and attributes them to other people, objects, or situations. In regression, the client returns to an earlier, more comforting, although less mature way of behaving. Rationalization is justifying the unacceptable attributes about oneself.
Test-Taking Strategy: Use the process of elimination. Note the key words "There's nothing wrong with me." Select the response that recognizes the client's attempt to avoid looking at the reality of the situation. If you had difficulty with this question, review defense mechanisms.
Level of Cognitive Ability: Comprehension
Client Needs: Psychosocial Integrity
Integrated Concept/Process: Nursing Process/Data Collection
Content Area: Mental Health
Reference: Varcarolis E: *Foundations of psychiatric mental health nursing*, ed 4, Philadelphia, 2002, WB Saunders, p. 292.

13. ***Answer:*** 1
Rationale: Reflection is the therapeutic communication technique that redirects the client's feelings back in order to validate what the client is saying. In option 2, the nurse attempts to use focusing, but the attempt to discuss central issues seems premature. In option 3, the nurse makes a judgment and is nontherapeutic in the one-on-one relationship. In option 4, the nurse is attempting to assess the client's ability to openly discuss feelings with family members. Although this may be appropriate, the timing is somewhat premature and closes off facilitation of the client's feelings.
Test-Taking Strategy: Use therapeutic communication techniques. Note that option 1 uses the therapeutic technique of reflection and also focuses on the client's feelings. Options 2, 3, and 4 are nontherapeutic at this time. Review therapeutic communication techniques if you had difficulty with this question.
Level of Cognitive Ability: Application
Client Needs: Psychosocial Integrity
Integrated Concept/Process: Communication and Documentation
Content Area: Mental Health
Reference: Varcarolis E: *Foundations of psychiatric mental health nursing*, ed 4, Philadelphia, 2002, WB Saunders, p. 253.

14. ***Answer:*** 4
Rationale: Generally, voluntary admission is sought by the client or client's guardian through a written application to the facility. If the client seeks voluntary admission, the most likely expectation is that the client will participate in the treatment program.
Test-Taking Strategy: Use the process of elimination. Note the key words "informal voluntary admission." This will easily direct you to option 4. Additionally, note that options 1, 2, and 3 are similar. Review the various types of hospital admission processes if you had difficulty with this question.
Level of Cognitive Ability: Comprehension
Client Needs: Psychosocial Integrity
Integrated Concept/Process: Nursing Process/Planning
Content Area: Mental Health
Reference: Varcarolis E: *Foundations of psychiatric mental health nursing*, ed 4, Philadelphia, 2002, WB Saunders, p. 171.

15. ***Answer:*** 3
Rationale: Generally, voluntary admission is sought by the client or client's guardian through a written application to the facility. Voluntary clients have the right to demand and obtain release. The best nursing action is to contact the physician.
Test-Taking Strategy: Use the process of elimination. Noting the type of hospital admission will assist in eliminating option 1. It is inappropriate to "persuade" a client to stay in the hospital. Option 2 should be eliminated based simply on the issue of client rights and the issue of confidentiality. Review the various types of hospital admission and discharge processes if you had difficulty with this question.
Level of Cognitive Ability: Application
Client Needs: Safe, Effective Care Environment
Integrated Concept/Process: Nursing Process/Implementation
Content Area: Mental Health
Reference: Varcarolis E: *Foundations of psychiatric mental health nursing*, ed 4, Philadelphia, 2002, WB Saunders, p. 171.

16. ***Answer:*** 1
Rationale: Involuntary admission is made without the client's consent. Involuntary admission is necessary when a person is a danger to self or others or is in need of psychiatric treatment or physical care. Options 2, 3, and 4 describe the process of voluntary admission.
Test-Taking Strategy: Use the process of elimination. Note the key words "involuntary status." This should easily direct you to option 1. Also, note that options 2, 3, and 4 are similar. Review the process of involuntary admission if you had difficulty with this question.
Level of Cognitive Ability: Comprehension
Client Needs: Psychosocial Integrity
Integrated Concept/Process: Nursing Process/Planning
Content Area: Mental Health
Reference: Varcarolis E: *Foundations of psychiatric mental health nursing*, ed 4, Philadelphia, 2002, WB Saunders, p. 171.

17. ***Answer:*** 3
Rationale: Clients who are involuntarily admitted do not lose their right to informed consent. The informed consent needs to be obtained from the client. Options 1, 2, and 4 are incorrect.
Test-Taking Strategy: Use the process of elimination and knowledge regarding the hospital admission processes and client's rights to answer this question. Focusing on the issue of

client's rights will direct you to option 3. Review client's rights if you had difficulty with this question.
Level of Cognitive Ability: Comprehension
Client Needs: Safe, Effective Care Environment
Integrated Concept/Process: Nursing Process/Planning
Content Area: Mental Health
Reference: Varcarolis E: *Foundations of psychiatric mental health nursing,* ed 4, Philadelphia, 2002, WB Saunders, p. 171.

18. *Answer:* 2
Rationale: A client may request to be secluded or restrained. Federal laws require the consent of the client unless an emergency situation exists in which an immediate risk to the client or others can be documented. The use of seclusion and restraint is permitted only on the written order of a physician, which must be reviewed and renewed every 24 hours, and which also must specify the type of restraint to be used.
Test-Taking Strategy: Use the process of elimination. There is no reason to call the family at this time; therefore eliminate option 3. Knowing that a physician's written order is necessary in this situation will assist in eliminating option 4. Option 1 is not the best choice because this information, if given to a client experiencing uncontrollable feelings, may cause escalation of the feelings. Review the procedures for seclusion if you had difficulty with this question.
Level of Cognitive Ability: Application
Client Needs: Safe, Effective Care Environment
Integrated Concept/Process: Nursing Process/Implementation
Content Area: Mental Health
Reference: Varcarolis E: *Foundations of psychiatric mental health nursing,* ed 4, Philadelphia, 2002, WB Saunders, p. 175.

19. *Answer:* 2
Rationale: The nurse should never promise to keep a secret. Secrets are appropriate in a social relationship but not in a therapeutic one. The nurse needs to be honest with the client and tell the client that a promise cannot be made to keep the secret.
Test-Taking Strategy: Use the process of elimination and therapeutic communication techniques. Option 1 can be easily eliminated because it is inappropriate. Also, options 3 and 4 are not only inappropriate, but are to an extent threatening and may even block further communication. Review the principles related to a therapeutic nurse-client relationship if you had difficulty with this question.
Level of Cognitive Ability: Application
Client Needs: Psychosocial Integrity
Integrated Concept/Process: Communication and Documentation
Content Area: Mental Health
Reference: Varcarolis E: *Foundations of psychiatric mental health nursing,* ed 4, Philadelphia, 2002, WB Saunders, p. 254.

20. *Answer:* 4
Rationale: A nurse is required to maintain confidentiality regarding clients and their care. Confidentiality is basic to the therapeutic relationship and is a client's right. Option 3 is correct in a sense; however, it is a rather blunt statement. Both options 1 and 2 identify statements that do not maintain client confidentiality.
Test-Taking Strategy: Use the process of elimination. Focus on the issue of the question, maintaining confidentiality. This should easily assist you in eliminating options 1 and 2. From the remaining options, select option 4 over option 3 because it is most direct and correct. Option 3 is a rather blunt and somewhat rude statement. Review confidentiality issues if you had difficulty with this question.
Level of Cognitive Ability: Application
Client Needs: Safe, Effective Care Environment
Integrated Concept/Process: Communication and Documentation
Content Area: Mental Health
Reference: Varcarolis E: *Foundations of psychiatric mental health nursing,* ed 4, Philadelphia, 2002, WB Saunders, p. 187.

21. *Answer:* 4
Rationale: False imprisonment is an act with the intent to confine a person to a specific area. A nurse can be charged with false imprisonment if the nurse prohibits a client from leaving the hospital if the client was voluntarily admitted and if there are no agency policies or legal reasons for detaining the client. On the other hand, if the client was involuntarily admitted or had agreed to an evaluation before discharge, the nurse's actions are reasonable.
Test-Taking Strategy: Use the process of elimination. Noting the key words "involuntarily admitted" will assist to eliminate option 1 and direct you to option 4. Options 2 and 3 are unrelated to the issue of the question and can be easily eliminated. Review the issues related to false imprisonment and hospital admissions if you had difficulty with this question.
Level of Cognitive Ability: Comprehension
Client Needs: Safe, Effective Care Environment
Integrated Concept/Process: Nursing Process/Implementation
Content Area: Mental Health
Reference: Varcarolis E: *Foundations of psychiatric mental health nursing,* ed 4, Philadelphia, 2002, WB Saunders, p. 178.

22. *Answer:* 3
Rationale: Tasks of the termination phase include evaluating client performance, evaluating achievement of expected outcomes, evaluating future needs, making appropriate referrals, and dealing with the common behaviors associated with termination. Options 1, 2, and 4 identify the tasks of the working phase of the relationship.
Test-Taking Strategy: Noting the key words "termination phase" should direct you to option 3. If you are unfamiliar with the appropriate tasks of the phases of the nurse-client relationship, review this content.
Level of Cognitive Ability: Application
Client Needs: Psychosocial Integrity
Integrated Concept/Process: Nursing Process/Planning
Content Area: Mental Health
Reference: Varcarolis E: *Foundations of psychiatric mental health nursing,* ed 4, Philadelphia, 2002, WB Saunders, p. 945.

23. *Answer:* 2
Rationale: In the termination phase of a relationship, it is normal for a client to demonstrate a number of regressive behaviors. Typical behaviors include return of symptoms, anger, withdrawal, and minimizing the relationship. The anger that

the client is experiencing is a normal behavior during the termination phase and does not necessarily indicate the need for hospitalization or treatment.
Test-Taking Strategy: Use the process of elimination. Note the key words "termination phase." This alone may assist in directing you to option 2. Additionally, note the similarity among options 1, 3, and 4. These options address the need for further supervised treatment. If you are unfamiliar with the client behaviors associated with the termination phase, review this content.
Level of Cognitive Ability: Analysis
Client Needs: Psychosocial Integrity
Integrated Concept/Process: Nursing Process/Evaluation
Content Area: Mental Health
Reference: Varcarolis E: *Foundations of psychiatric mental health nursing*, ed 4, Philadelphia, 2002, WB Saunders, p. 934.

24. *Answer:* 1
Rationale: Behavior therapy is used to help clients identify and examine dysfunctional thoughts as well as identify and examine values and beliefs that maintain these thoughts. Options 2, 3, and 4 are incorrect.
Test-Taking Strategy: Use the process of elimination. Note the key word "behavior." Focusing on this key word should direct you to option 1. If you are unfamiliar with this type of therapy and its purpose, review this content.
Level of Cognitive Ability: Comprehension
Client Needs: Psychosocial Integrity
Integrated Concept/Process: Nursing Process/Implementation
Content Area: Mental Health
Reference: Varcarolis E: *Foundations of psychiatric mental health nursing*, ed 4, Philadelphia, 2002, WB Saunders, p. 941.

25. *Answer:* 3
Rationale: Milieu therapy provides a safe environment that is adapted to the individual client's needs and also provides greater comfort and freedom of expression than has been experienced in the past by the client. All members contribute to the planning and functioning of the setting.
Test-Taking Strategy: Use the process of elimination. Note that options 1, 2, and 4 are similar and that option 3 identifies a global description. Review this model of care if you had difficulty with this question.
Level of Cognitive Ability: Comprehension
Client Needs: Psychosocial Integrity
Integrated Concept/Process: Nursing Process/Implementation
Content Area: Mental Health
Reference: Varcarolis E: *Foundations of psychiatric mental health nursing*, ed 4, Philadelphia, 2002, WB Saunders, p. 43.

26. *Answer:* 4
Rationale: Aversion therapy, also known as aversion conditioning or negative reinforcement, is a technique used to change behavior. In this therapy, a stimulus (alcohol) attractive to the client is paired with an unpleasant event in hopes of instituting the stimulus with negative properties. Desensitization is the reduction of intense reactions to a stimulus by repeated exposure to the stimulus in a weaker and milder form. Milieu therapy provides positive environmental manipulation, both physical and social, to effect a positive change in the client. Self-control therapy combines cognitive and behavioral approaches and is useful to deal with stress.
Test-Taking Strategy: Focus on the information in the question. Recalling that aversion therapy is a form of negative reinforcement will easily direct you to the correct option. If you had difficulty with this question, review this form of therapy.
Level of Cognitive Ability: Comprehension
Client Needs: Psychosocial Integrity
Integrated Concept/Process: Nursing Process/Implementation
Content Area: Mental Health
Reference: Varcarolis E: *Foundations of psychiatric mental health nursing*, ed 4, Philadelphia, 2002, WB Saunders, p. 42.

27. *Answer:* 4
Rationale: The sponsor of a self-help group is an experienced member of the group. A nurse or psychiatrist may be asked by the group to serve as a resource but would not be the leader of the group. Options 1, 2, and 3 are characteristics of a self-help group.
Test-Taking Strategy: Use the process of elimination and note the key word "not" in the stem of the question. Note that options 1, 2, and 3 are similar. This should direct you to option 4. Review the characteristics of a self-help group if you had difficulty with this question.
Level of Cognitive Ability: Comprehension
Client Needs: Psychosocial Integrity
Integrated Concept/Process: Nursing Process/Implementation
Content Area: Mental Health
Reference: Varcarolis E: *Foundations of psychiatric mental health nursing*, ed 4, Philadelphia, 2002, WB Saunders, p. 941.

28. *Answer:* 4
Rationale: The first step in the 12-step program is to admit that a problem exists. Options 1 and 2 are unrealistic as a first step in the process to recovery. Although option 3 may be a strategy, it is not the first step.
Test-Taking Strategy: Note the key words "first step" in the question. This will easily assist in directing you to option 4. If you are unfamiliar with the 12-step program, review this content.
Level of Cognitive Ability: Comprehension
Client Needs: Psychosocial Integrity
Integrated Concept/Process: Nursing Process/Implementation
Content Area: Mental Health
Reference: Varcarolis E: *Foundations of psychiatric mental health nursing*, ed 4, Philadelphia, 2002, WB Saunders, p. 772.

29. *Answer:* 1
Rationale: If a client is monopolizing the group, it is important that the nurse be direct and decisive. The best action is to suggest that the client stop talking and try listening to others. Although option 3 may be a direct response, option 1 is the most therapeutic direct statement. Options 2 and 4 are inappropriate.
Test-Taking Strategy: Use the process of elimination. Eliminate options 2 and 4 first because they are similar. Use therapeutic communication techniques to assist in directing you to option 1. If you had difficulty with this question, review therapeutic communication techniques.
Level of Cognitive Ability: Application
Client Needs: Psychosocial Integrity

Integrated Concept/Process: Nursing Process/Implementation
Content Area: Mental Health
Reference: Varcarolis E: *Foundations of psychiatric mental health nursing,* ed 4, Philadelphia, 2002, WB Saunders, p. 246.

30. *Answer:* 1
Rationale: In the forming or initial stage, the members are identifying tasks and boundaries. Storming involves responding emotionally to tasks. In the norming stage, members express intimate personal opinions and feelings around personal tasks. In the performing stage, members direct group energy toward the completion of tasks.
Test-Taking Strategy: Use the process of elimination. Note the key word "identifying" in the question. This key word should assist in directing you to option 1. If you had difficulty with this question, review the stages of group development.
Level of Cognitive Ability: Comprehension
Client Needs: Psychosocial Integrity
Integrated Concept/Process: Nursing Process/Implementation
Content Area: Mental Health
Reference: Varcarolis E: *Foundations of psychiatric mental health nursing,* ed 4, Philadelphia, 2002, WB Saunders, p. 942.

REFERENCES

Fortinash K, Holoday-Worret P: *Psychiatric mental health nursing,* ed 2, St Louis, 2000, Mosby.

Hill S, Bauer B: *Mental health nursing,* Philadelphia, 2002, WB Saunders.

Keltner N, Schwecke L, Bostrom C: *Psychiatric nursing,* ed 3, St Louis, 1999, Mosby.

Varcarolis E: *Foundations of psychiatric mental health nursing,* ed 4, Philadelphia, 2002, WB Saunders.

61

Mental Health Disorders

I. ANXIETY

A. Description
1. A subjective, individual experience
2. A normal response to stress
3. A feeling of apprehension, uneasiness, uncertainty, or dread
4. Occurs as a result of threats that may be misperceived or misinterpreted
5. May precede new experiences
6. Occurs as a result of a threat to identity or self-esteem
7. May result when values are threatened

B. Types of anxiety
1. Normal: a healthy type of anxiety
2. Acute: precipitated by imminent loss or change that threatens the sense of security
3. Chronic: anxiety that the individual has lived with for a long time

C. Levels of anxiety
1. Mild
   a. Associated with the tension of every day life
   b. The individual is alert
   c. The perceptual field is increased
   d. Can be motivating, produce growth and creativity, and increase learning
2. Moderate
   a. The focus is on immediate concerns
   b. Narrows the perceptual field
   c. Selective inattentiveness occurs
   d. Learning and problem solving still take place
3. Severe
   a. Feeling that something bad is about to happen
   b. A significant reduction in perceptual field occurs
   c. Focus is on specific details or scattered details
   d. All behavior is directed at relieving the anxiety
   e. Learning and problem solving are not possible
   f. The individual needs direction to focus
4. Panic
   a. Associated with dread and terror and a sense of impending doom
   b. The personality is disorganized
   c. The individual is unable to communicate or function effectively
   d. Increased motor activity occurs
   e. Loss of rational thoughts with distorted perception
   f. Inability to concentrate
   g. If prolonged, panic can lead to exhaustion and death

D. Implementation
1. Recognize the anxiety
2. Establish trust
3. Protect the client
4. Do not attack **coping mechanisms**
5. Do not force the client into situations that provoke anxiety
6. Decrease stimulation in the environment
7. Modify the environment by setting limits or limiting interaction with others
8. Provide creative outlets
9. Provide activities that limit the amount of time for destructive behavior
10. Promote relaxation techniques
11. Administer antianxiety medications as prescribed

E. Implementation: mild to moderate levels
1. Help the client identify the anxiety
2. Encourage the client to talk about feelings and concerns

3. Help the client identify thoughts and feelings that occur before the onset of anxiety
4. Encourage problem solving
5. Encourage gross motor exercise

F. Implementation: severe to panic levels
1. Reduce the anxiety quickly
2. Use a calm manner
3. Always remain with the client
4. Minimize environmental stimuli
5. Provide clear, simple statements
6. Use a low-pitched voice
7. Attend to the physical needs of the client
8. Provide gross motor activity
9. Administer antianxiety medications as prescribed

II. GENERALIZED ANXIETY DISORDER

A. Description
1. An unrealistic anxiety in which the cause can usually be identified
2. Physical symptoms occur

B. Data collection
1. Chronic muscular tension
2. Restlessness
3. Episodes of trembling and shakiness
4. Chronic fatigue
5. Dizziness
6. Inability to relax
7. Inability to concentrate
8. Sleep problems
9. Inability to recognize the connection between anxiety and physical symptoms
10. The client is focused on the physical discomfort

C. Panic disorder
1. Description
   a. The cause usually cannot be identified
   b. It produces a sudden onset with feelings of intense apprehension and dread
   c. Severe, recurrent, intermittent anxiety attacks, lasting 5 to 30 minutes occur
2. Data collection
   a. Choking sensation
   b. Labored breathing
   c. Pounding heart
   d. Chest pain
   e. Dizziness
   f. Nausea
   g. Blurred vision
   h. Numbness or tingling of extremities
   i. A sense of unreality and helplessness
   j. A fear of being trapped and going crazy
   k. A fear of dying
3. Implementation
   a. Attend to physical symptoms
   b. Assist the client to identify the thoughts that arouse the anxiety and identify the basis for these thoughts
   c. Assist the client to change unrealistic thoughts to more realistic thoughts
   d. Utilize cognitive restructuring
   e. Administer antianxiety medications as prescribed

III. POSTTRAUMATIC STRESS DISORDER

A. Description: after experiencing a psychologically traumatic event, outside the range of usual experience, the individual reexperiences the event via recurrent and intrusive dreams or flashbacks

B. Stressors
1. A natural disaster
2. Combat
3. Victim of rape
4. Accidents
5. Victim of crime or violence
6. Victim of sexual, physical, and emotional **abuse**
7. Reexperiencing the event as flashbacks

C. Data collection
1. Emotional numbness
2. Detachment
3. Depression
4. Anxiety
5. Sleep disturbances and nightmares
6. Hypervigilance
7. Guilt about surviving
8. Poor concentration and avoidance of activities that trigger the memory of the event

D. Implementation
1. Desensitization through gradual exposure to the event or situations similar to the event
2. Instructing the client in relaxation techniques
3. Providing individual therapy addressing loss of control issues or anger
4. Using support groups
5. Using hypnotherapy

IV. PHOBIAS

A. Description
1. An irrational fear of an object or situation that persists although the person may recognize it as unreasonable
2. Is associated with panic level anxiety and the anxiety is severe if the object, situation, or activity cannot be avoided
3. **Defense mechanisms** commonly used include repression and displacement

B. Types
1. Agoraphobia

a. Fear of being alone in open or public places where escape might be difficult
b. The individual may not leave home
c. The individual experiences fear or a sense of helplessness or embarrassment if the attack occurs
d. The individual avoids situations that may trigger the attack

2. Social phobia
a. Fear of situations in which one might be embarrassed or criticized and the fear of making a fool of oneself
b. Can include the fear of eating in public, public speaking, or performing

3. Specific phobia: a fear of a single object, activity, or situation such as snakes, closed spaces, and flying

C. Implementation
1. Stay with the client when the anxiety is high to promote safety and security
2. Identify the basis of the anxiety
3. Allow the client to verbalize feelings about the anxiety-producing object or situation because frequently talking about the feared object is the first step in the desensitization process
4. Desensitization by gradually introducing the individual to the feared object or situation in small doses
5. Teach relaxation techniques such as breathing exercises, muscle-relaxation exercises, and visualization of pleasant situations
6. Do not force contact with the phobic object or situation

V. OBSESSIVE-COMPULSIVE DISORDER

A. Obsessions: preoccupation with persistent intrusive thoughts and ideas

B. Compulsions
1. Repeated performance of rituals or purposeless behaviors designed to prevent some event, divert unacceptable thoughts, and decrease anxiety
2. Obsessions and compulsions often occur together and can disrupt normal activities
3. Anxiety occurs if obsessions or compulsions are resisted and from being powerless to resist the thoughts or rituals
4. Obsessive thoughts can involve issues of violence, aggression, sexual behavior, orderliness, or religion
5. Intrusive thoughts uncontrollably interrupt conscious thoughts and the ability to function

C. Behavior patterns
1. Decrease the anxiety
2. Are associated with the obsessive thoughts
3. Neutralize the thought
4. During stressful times, the ritualistic behavior increases
5. **Defense mechanisms** include repression, displacement, and undoing

D. Implementation
1. Identify the situations that precipitate the behavior
2. Do not interrupt the compulsive behaviors
3. Allow time for the client to perform rituals
4. Provide for client safety related to the behaviors
5. Implement a schedule for the client that distracts from the behaviors
6. Set limits on rituals that may interfere with the client's physical well-being to protect from physical harm
7. Encourage the client to verbalize concerns
8. Gradually assist the client to decrease the frequency of compulsive behaviors by establishing a written contract

VI. SOMATOFORM DISORDERS

A. Description
1. Characterized by persistent worry or complaints regarding physical illness when there is no supporting physical findings
2. The client focuses on the physical signs and symptoms and is unable to control them
3. The physical signs and symptoms increase with psychosocial stressors
4. The anxiety is redirected into a somatic concern

B. Somatization disorder (Box 61-1)
1. Description
a. Occurs over a period of years and usually presents before age 30
b. The client has multiple physical complaints involving multiple systems
c. The emotional stress can result from anxiety, fear, depression, worry, or repressed anger
d. The client may unconsciously use somatization for secondary gains such as increased attention and decreased responsibilities

BOX 61-1

Types of Somatoform Disorders

Somatization disorder
Hypochondriasis
Conversion disorder

2. Data collection
   a. Physical complaints of abdominal pain, denial of emotional problems, signs of anxiety, fear, and low self-esteem
   b. Psychosexual symptoms
   c. Secondary gain

C. Hypochondriasis
1. Description
   a. The preoccupation with fears of having a serious disease
   b. No evidence of physical illness exists
   c. Causes a significant impaired social and occupational functioning
2. Data collection
   a. Preoccupation with physical functioning
   b. Frequent somatic complaints
   c. Difficulty expressing feelings
   d. Extensive use of home remedies or nonprescription medications
   e. Repeatedly visiting the doctor
   f. Secondary gain
   g. Fatigue and insomnia
   h. Anxiety

D. Conversion disorder
1. Description
   a. A physical symptom or a deficit suggesting loss or altered body function related to psychological conflict or a neurological disorder
   b. An expression of a psychological conflict or need
   c. The most common conversion symptoms are blindness, deafness, paralysis, and the inability to talk
   d. There is no organic cause
   e. Symptoms are not intentionally produced by the client
   f. Symptoms are directly related to the conflict and to decrease the anxiety
2. Data collection
   a. "La Belle Indifference": unconcerned with symptoms
   b. Physical limitation or disability
   c. Feelings of guilt, anxiety, or frustration
   d. Low self-esteem and feelings of inadequacy
   e. Unexpressed anger or conflict
   f. Secondary gain
3. Implementation
   a. Obtain a nursing history and assess for physical problems
   b. Do not reinforce the sick role
   c. Discourage verbalization about physical symptoms by not responding with positive reinforcement
   d. Explore with the client the needs being met by symptoms
   e. Assist the client to identify alternative ways of meeting needs
   f. Assist the client to relate feelings and conflicts to physical symptoms
   g. Allow a specific time period to discuss physical complaints because the client will feel less threatened if this behavior is limited rather than stopped completely
   h. Assure the client that physical illness has been ruled out
   i. Explore the source of anxiety and stimulate verbalization of anxiety
   j. Encourage the use of relaxation techniques as the anxiety increases
   k. Convey an understanding that symptoms are real to the client
   l. Implement pain-reduction measures as required
   m. Report and assess any new physical complaint
   n. Encourage diversional activities to decrease the client's focus on self
   o. Provide positive feedback for accomplishments to increase self-esteem
   p. Assist the client in recognizing his or her feelings and emotions
   q. Contract with the client to engage in relationships with others to redirect interest
   r. Administer antianxiety medications as prescribed

VII. DISSOCIATIVE DISORDER

A. Description
1. A disruption in integrative functions of memory, consciousness, or identity
2. Associated with exposure to a traumatic event

B. Dissociative identity disorder (multiple personality)
1. Description
   a. Two or more fully developed distinct and unique personalities within the person
   b. Personalities may take full control of the client, one at a time
   c. The personalities may or may not be aware of each other
2. Data collection
   a. The inability to recall important information too extensive to be explained by ordinary forgetfulness
   b. Transition from one personality to the other is related to stress and is sudden
   c. Dissociation is used as a method of distancing and defending self from anxiety and traumatizing experiences

C. Dissociative amnesia

1. Description
   a. Inability to recall important personal information because it is anxiety provoking
   b. Memory impairment may be impartial or almost complete
2. Data collection
   a. Localized: the client blocks out all memories about a specific period
   b. Selective: the client recalls some but not all memories about a specific period
   c. Generalized: loss of all memory about past life

D. Dissociative fugue
1. Description
   a. The assumption of a new identity in a new environment
   b. The disorder may occur suddenly
2. Data collection
   a. May drift from place to place
   b. Develops few social relationships
   c. When the fugue lifts the client returns home and is unable to recall the fugue state

E. Depersonalization disorder
1. Description: an altered self-perception in which one's own reality is temporarily lost or changed
2. Data collection
   a. Feelings of detachment
   b. Intact reality testing

F. Implementation
1. Develop a trusting relationship with the client
2. Encourage verbal expression of painful experiences, anxieties, and concerns
3. Explore methods of coping
4. Identify sources of conflict
5. Focus on the client's strengths and skills
6. Orient the client
7. Provide nondemanding simple routines
8. Allow client to progress at own pace
9. Use stress-reduction techniques
10. Use individual, group, and/or family psychotherapy to integrate dissociated aspects of personality or memory and to expand self-awareness

VIII. BIPOLAR DISORDER

A. Description
1. Characterized by episodes of mania and depression with periods of normal mood and activity in between
2. The treatment medication of choice is lithium carbonate (Eskalith), which can be toxic and therefore requires regular monitoring of serum lithium levels

B. Data collection (Box 61-2)

C. Implementation for mania
1. Remove hazardous objects from the environment
2. Monitor the client's sleep patterns
3. Assess the client closely for fatigue
4. Provide frequent rest periods
5. Use comfort measures to promote sleep
6. Provide a private room if possible
7. Administer hypnotic or sedative medication as prescribed
8. Encourage the client to ventilate feelings
9. Use calm, slow interactions
10. Help the client focus on one topic during the conversation
11. Ignore or distract the client from grandiose thinking
12. Present reality to the client

BOX 61-2

Bipolar Disorders

MANIA

Inappropriate affect
Restlessness
Flight of ideas
Inability to eat or sleep because of involvement in more important things
Extroverted personality
Delusional self-confidence
Initiation of activity
High and unstable affect
Becomes angry quickly
Pressure of speech
Grandiose and persecutory delusions
Inappropriate dress
Urgent motor activity
Significant decrease in appetite
Inability to sleep yet still active
Sexually promiscuous
Distracted by environmental stimuli
Unlimited energy

DEPRESSION

Decreased emotion and physical activity
Inability to make quick decisions
Introverted personality
Lack of initiative
Lack of self-confidence
Internalizing hostility
Loss of interest in appearance
Lack of energy
Easily fatigued
Withdrawn from groups
Lack of sexual interest

13. Don't argue with the client
14. Limit group activities and assess the client's tolerance level
15. Provide high-calorie finger foods and fluids
16. Supervise the client's choice of clothing
17. Reduce environmental stimuli
18. Set limits on inappropriate behaviors
19. Provide physical activities and outlets for tension
20. Avoid competitive games
21. Provide gross motor activities such as walking
22. Provide simple and direct explanations for routine procedures
23. Provide structured activities or one-to-one activities with the nurse
24. Supervise the administration of medication

IX. SCHIZOPHRENIA

A. Description
   1. A group of mental disorders characterized by psychotic features, inability to trust others, disordered thought processes, and disrupted interpersonal relationships
   2. Schizophrenia causes disturbances in affect, mood, behavior, and thought processes

B. Data collection
   1. Physical characteristics
      a. Disheveled appearance
      b. Body image distortions
      c. Preoccupied with somatic complaints
      d. Neglects eating, sleeping, and elimination
   2. Motor activity (Box 61-3)
      a. Catatonic posturing: holding bizarre postures for long periods of time
      b. Catatonic excitement: moving excitedly with no environmental stimuli
      c. May be totally immobilized
      d. Unable to respond to commands, or responds only to commands
      e. Waxy flexibility
      f. Movements may be repetitive or stereotyped
      g. Motor activity may be increased as evidenced by agitation, pacing, inability to sleep, loss of appetite and weight, and impulsiveness
      h. May be unable to initiate activity, known as volition or anergia
   3. Emotional characteristics
      a. Mistrust
      b. Views the world as threatening and unsafe
      c. Feelings not easily interpreted
      d. Ambivalence manifested as compulsive rituals, negativism, and overcompliance
      e. May display feelings of helplessness, anxiety, anger, guilt and depression, decreased self-esteem
   4. Compulsive rituals: attempts to solve conflicting feelings by constant, repetitive activity, which may be stereotyped or seem meaningless
   5. Overcompliance: attempts to deny responsibility for any action by doing only what another exactly instructs
   6. Affective disturbances
      a. Flat affect or inappropriate affect
      b. Altered thought processes
   7. Thought processes
      a. Impaired reality testing
      b. Fragmentation of thoughts
      c. Blocking
      d. Loose associations
      e. Autistic thinking
      f. Perceives environment in a totally self-centered way
      g. Neologisms
      h. Magical thinking
      i. Unable to conceptualize meaning in words or thoughts
      j. Unable to organize facts logically
      k. Delusions
   8. Types of delusions (Box 61-4)
      a. Loss of reference in which the client believes that certain events, situations, or interactions are directly related to self
      b. Delusions of persecution in which the client believes that he or she is being harassed, threatened, or persecuted by some powerful force

BOX 61-3

Abnormal Motor Behaviors: Description and Types

Description: abnormal motor behavior or activity, displayed by the mentally ill client, occurring as a result of a psychiatric disorder

Akathisia: displaying motor restlessness and muscular quivering; the client is unable to sit or lie quietly

Echolalia: repeating the speech of another person

Echopraxia: repeating the movements of another person

Parkinson-like symptoms: making masklike faces, drooling, and having shuffling gait, tremors, and muscular rigidity

Waxy flexibility: having one's arms or legs placed in a certain position and holding that same position for hours

Dyskinesia: impairment of the power of voluntary movements

BOX 61-4

Delusions

Description

A false belief held to be true even when there is evidence to the contrary

TYPES

Persecution: the thought that one is being singled out for harm by others

Grandeur: the false belief that one is a very powerful and important person

Jealousy: the false belief that one's partner or mate is going out with other people

c. Delusions of grandeur in which the client attaches special significance to self in relation to others or the universe and has an exaggerated sense of self that has no basis in reality
d. Somatic delusions in which the client believes that his or her body is changing or responding in an unusual way that has no basis in reality

9. Perceptual distortions (Box 61-5)
   a. Illusions that may be brief experiences with a misinterpretation or exaggeration of reality
   b. Hallucinations such as perceiving objects, sensations, or images with no basis in reality (Box 61-6)
10. Language and communication disturbances (Box 61-7)
    a. Related to disorders in the thought process
    b. Unable to organize language
    c. Difficulty communicating clearly
    d. Inappropriate responses to a situation
    e. A single word or phrase may represent the whole meaning of the conversation, and the client may feel that he or she has communicated adequately
    f. May develop private language

C. Types of schizophrenia
1. Paranoid schizophrenia
   a. Suspiciousness
   b. Hostility
   c. Delusions
   d. Auditory hallucinations
   e. Anxiety and anger
   f. Aloofness
   g. Persecutory themes
   h. Violence
2. Disorganized schizophrenia
   a. Extreme social withdrawal
   b. Disorganized speech or behavior
   c. Flat or inappropriate affect

BOX 61-5

Abnormal Thought Processes

Description: abnormal thought processes, displayed by the mentally ill client, occurring as a result of a psychiatric disorder

Neologisms: words that an individual makes up that only have meaning for the individual themselves; is often part of a delusional system

Looseness of association: the individual's thinking is haphazard, illogical, and confused and connections in thought are interrupted; seen mostly in schizophrenic disorders

Flight of ideas: a constant flow of speech in which the individual jumps from one topic to another in rapid succession; there is a connection between topics although it is sometimes difficult to identify; is seen in manic states

Blocking: a sudden cessation of a thought in the middle of a sentence; the client is unable to continue the train of thought; often sudden new thoughts come up unrelated to the topic

Circumstantiality: before getting to the point or answering a question, the individual gets caught up in countless details and explanations

Confabulation: filling a memory gap with detailed fantasy believed by the teller; the purpose of confabulation is to maintain self-esteem; seen in organic conditions such as Korsakoff's psychosis

Word salad: a mixture of words and phrases that have no meaning

BOX 61-6

Preoccupation in Thought Content: Hallucinations

A sense perception for which no external stimuli exists

Can have an organic or functional etiology

TYPES

Visual: seeing things that are not there

Auditory: hearing voices when none are present

Olfactory: smelling smells that do not exist

Tactile: feeling touch sensations in the absence of stimuli

Gustatory: experiencing taste in the absence of stimuli

   d. Silliness unrelated to speech
   e. Stereotyped behaviors
   f. Grimacing mannerisms
   g. Inability to perform activities of daily living (ADL)
3. Catatonic schizophrenia
   a. Marked psychomotor disturbances
   b. Immobility
   c. Stupor
   d. Waxy flexibility
   e. Excessive purposeless motor activity
   f. Echolalia

BOX 61-7

Language and Communication Disturbance

Neologism: a new word devised that has special meaning only to the client
Echolalia: repetition of words or phrases heard from another person
Verbigeration: purposeless repetition of words or phrases
Metonymic speech: mental confusion exhibited by the use of a word that is not the precise term intended but is of similar meaning
Clang association: repetition of words or phrases that are similar in sound but in no other way
Word salad: form of speech in which words or phrases are connected meaninglessly
Stilted language: an inappropriate and overly formal communication pattern usually written and seems artificial and intellectual
Pressured speech: speaks as if the words are being forced out quickly
Mutism: absence of verbal speech

g. Automatic obedience
h. Stereotyped or repetitive behavior

4. Undifferentiated schizophrenia
   a. Does not meet criteria for paranoid, disorganized, or catatonic schizophrenia
   b. Delusions and hallucinations
   c. Disorganized speech
   d. Disorganized or catatonic behavior
   e. Flat affect
   f. Social withdrawal
5. Residual schizophrenia
   a. Diagnosed as schizophrenic in the past
   b. May last for many years
   c. The client exhibits marked social isolation and withdrawal and impaired role functioning

D. Implementation (Box 61-8)

E. Implementation: active hallucinations
1. Monitor for hallucination cues
2. Intervene with a one-to-one contact
3. Decrease stimuli or move the client to another area
4. Avoid conveying to the client that you are also experiencing the hallucination
5. Respond verbally to anything real that the client talks about
6. Avoid touching the client
7. Encourage the client's expression of feelings
8. During the hallucination, attempt to engage the client's attention through a concrete activity
9. Accept behavior and do not joke about or judge the client's behavior
10. Provide easy activities and a structured environment with routine ADL

BOX 61-8

Implementation for Schizophrenia

Assess the client's physical needs
Set limits on the client's behavior when it interferes with others and becomes disruptive
Maintain a safe environment
Initiate one-to-one interactions and progress to small groups as tolerated
Spend time with the client even if the client is unable to respond
Monitor for altered thought processes
Maintain ego boundaries and avoid touching the client
Limit time of interaction with the client
Avoid an overly warm approach
A neutral approach is less threatening
Do not make promises to the client that cannot be kept
Establish daily routines
Assist the client to improve grooming and accept responsibility for personal care
Sit with client in silence if necessary
Provide short, brief, and frequent contact with the client
Tell the client when you are leaving
Tell the client when you don't understand
"Do not go along" with the client's delusions or hallucinations
Provide simple concrete activities such as puzzles or word games
Reorient the client as necessary
Assist the client to establish what is real and unreal
Stay with the client if the client is frightened
Speak to the client in a simple, direct, and concise manner
Reassure the client that the environment is safe
Remove the client from group situations if the client behavior is too bizarre, disturbing, or dangerous to others
Set realistic goals
Initially do not offer choices to the client and gradually assist the client in making own decisions
Assess physical needs
Use containers for food, especially with the paranoid schizophrenic
Provide a radio or tape player at night for insomnia
Explain in detail everything being done
Set limits on the client's behavior if the client is unable to do so
Decrease excessive stimuli in the environment
Monitor for suicide risk
Assist the client to use alternative means to express feelings such as through music, art therapy, or writing

11. Monitor for signs of increasing fear, anxiety, or agitation
12. Provide **seclusion** as necessary
13. Administer medications as prescribed

F. Implementation: delusions
1. Interact on the basis of reality
2. Encourage the client to express feelings
3. Do not dispute with the client or try to convince the client that delusions are false
4. Begin with activities on a one-to-one basis
5. Alter hospital routines as necessary such as using canned or packaged food, food in containers, or food from home
6. Recognize accomplishments and provide positive feedback for successes

X. PARANOID DISORDERS

A. Description
1. The client demonstrates suspiciousness and mistrust of others
2. The client is often viewed by others as hostile, stubborn, and defensive
3. Concrete, pervasive, delusional system characterized by persecutory and grandiose beliefs

B. Behaviors
1. Suspicious and mistrustful
2. Emotionally distant
3. Distorts reality
4. Poor insight
5. Hypervigilance
6. Low self-esteem
7. Highly sensitive, difficulty in admitting own error, and takes pride in being correct
8. Hypercritical and intolerant of others
9. Hostile, aggressive, and quarrelsome
10. Evasive
11. Concrete thinking

C. Delusions
1. Serves purpose in establishing identity and self-esteem
2. Grandiose and persecutory delusions
3. Process of delusion includes denial, projection, and rationalization
4. As trust in others increases, the need for delusions decreases

D. Types
1. Paranoid personality
   a. Suspicious
   b. Nonpsychotic
   c. No hallucinations or delusions
   d. No symptoms of schizophrenia
2. Paranoid state
   a. Onset abrupt in response to stress and subsides when stress decreases
   b. No hallucinations but experiences paranoid delusions
   c. May be sensitive and suspicious before the development of delusions
   d. Psychotic state
   e. No symptoms of schizophrenia
3. Paranoia
   a. Client appears normal except for delusional system
   b. Single highly organized delusional system
   c. Not bizarre
   d. No hallucinations
   e. Reserved and sensitive before onset
   f. Psychotic state
   g. No symptoms of schizophrenia
4. Paranoid schizophrenia
   a. Before onset the client becomes cold, withdrawn, distrustful, resentful, argumentative, sarcastic, and defiant
   b. Bizarre, numerous, and changeable delusions
   c. Delusions become less logical as client becomes more disorganized
   d. Persecutory hallucinations
   e. Psychotic state
   f. All symptoms of schizophrenia present

E. Implementation (Box 61-9)

BOX 61-9

Implementation for Paranoid Disorders

Assess for suicide risk
Diminish suspicious behavior
Establish trusting relationship
Promote increased self-esteem
Remain calm, nonthreatening, and nonjudgmental
Provide continuity of care
Respond honestly to the client
Follow through on commitments made to the client
Acknowledge the client's feelings, but tell the client that you do not share the client's interpretation of an event
Provide a daily schedule of activities
Assist the client to identify diversionary activities
Gradually introduce the client to groups
Refocus conversation to reality-based topics
Use role playing to help the client identify thoughts and feelings
Provide positive reinforcement for successes
Do not argue with client regarding client's delusions
Use concrete, specific words
Do not be secretive with the client
Do not whisper in the client's presence
Assure the client that he or she will be safe
Involve the client in noncompetitive tasks
Provide the client with the opportunity to complete small tasks
Monitor eating, drinking, sleeping, and elimination patterns
Limit physical contact
Monitor for agitation and decrease stimuli as needed

XI. PERSONALITY DISORDERS

A. Description
   1. Includes various inflexible maladaptive behavior patterns or traits that may impair functioning and relationships
   2. The individual usually remains in touch with reality and typically has a lack of insight into his or her behavior
   3. Stress exacerbates manifestations of a personality disorder
   4. In severe cases, the personality disorder may deteriorate to a psychotic state

B. Characteristics
   1. Poor impulse control
      a. Acting out to manage internal pain
      b. Forms of acting out include physical and verbal attacks, manipulation, substance **abuse**, promiscuous sexual behaviors, and **suicide attempts**
   2. Mood characteristics
      a. Experience abandonment and depression
      b. Moods include rage, guilt, fear, and emptiness
   3. Impaired judgment
      a. Have difficulty with problem solving
      b. Unable to perceive consequences of behavior
   4. Impaired reality testing: distort reality and often project their own feelings onto others
   5. Impaired object relations: rigid and inflexible and have difficulty in intimate relationships
   6. Impaired self-perception: distorted self-perception and experience self-hate or self-idealization
   7. Impaired thought processes
      a. Concrete or diffuse thinking
      b. Difficulty concentrating
      c. Impaired memory
   8. Impaired stimulus barrier
      a. Unable to regulate incoming sensory stimuli
      b. Increased excitability
      c. Excessive response to noise and light
      d. Poor attention span
      e. Agitated
      f. Insomnia

C. Schizoid personality disorder
   1. Description: characterized by an inability to form warm, close social relationships
   2. Data collection
      a. Social detachment and lack of close relationships
      b. Interest in solitary activities
      c. Aloof and indifferent
      d. Restricted expression of emotions
      e. Lack of interest in others

D. Schizotypal personality disorder
   1. Description: exhibit abnormal or highly unusual thoughts, perceptions, and speech and behavior patterns
   2. Data collection
      a. Suspicious
      b. Paranoia
      c. Magical thinking
      d. Odd thinking and speech
      e. Relationship deficits

E. Paranoid personality disorder
   1. Description: characterized by suspiciousness and mistrust of others
   2. Data collection
      a. Suspicious and distrusting
      b. Argumentative
      c. Hostile, aloof
      d. Rigid, critical, and controlling of others
      e. Grandiosity

F. Histrionic personality disorder
   1. Description
      a. Characterized by overly dramatic and intensely expressive behavior
      b. The client is lively and dramatic and enjoys being the center of attention
      c. Interpersonal relations may be poor
   2. Data collection
      a. Attention seeking
      b. Needs to be the center of attention
      c. Sexually seductive or provocative
      d. Self-dramatizing and theatrical
      e. Overly concerned with appearance
      f. Has romantic fantasies and controls partners
      g. Bores easily
      h. Displays dependency

G. Narcissistic personality disorder
   1. Description
      a. Characterized by an increased sense of self-importance
      b. The client is preoccupied with fantasies and has a constant need for attention and admiration
   2. Data collection
      a. Grandiosity
      b. Requires admiration and inflated accomplishments
      c. Overestimates abilities and underestimates contributions of others
      d. Lacks empathy and sensitivity to the needs of others

H. Avoidant personality disorder
   1. Description: characterized by social withdrawal and extreme sensitivity to potential rejection
   2. Data collection

a. Feelings of inadequacy
b. Hypersensitive to reactions of others and reacts poorly to criticism
c. Social inhibition
d. Lack of support systems

I. Dependent personality disorder
1. Description
a. The individual lacks self-confidence and the ability to function independently
b. Passively allows others to make decisions and assume responsibility for major areas in his or her life
2. Data collection
a. Difficulty making decisions
b. Lacks autonomy
c. Cannot tolerate being alone and must always have a close relationship
d. Needs others to assume responsibility and make decisions

J. Obsessive-compulsive personality disorder
1. Description: the client has difficulty expressing warm and tender emotions and reflects perfectionism, stubbornness, the need to control others, and a devotion to work
2. Data collection
a. Orderliness and perfectionism
b. Overconscientious
c. Inflexible and preoccupied with details and rules
d. Devoted to work and lacks leisure activities and friendships
e. Miserly and stubborn
f. Hoards worthless objects

K. Antisocial personality disorder
1. Description
a. A pattern of irresponsible and antisocial behavior
b. Characterized by selfishness, inability to maintain lasting relationships, poor sexual adjustment, failure to accept social norms, irritability, and aggressiveness
2. Data collection
a. Perceives the world as hostile
b. Superficial charm and hostility
c. No shame or guilt
d. Self-centered
e. Unreliable
f. Easily bored
g. Poor work history
h. Unable to tolerate frustration
i. Views others as objects to be manipulated
j. Poor judgment
k. Impulsive

▲ L. Borderline personality disorder
1. Description
a. Characterized by instability in interpersonal relationships, mood, and self-image
b. Behavior may be impulsive and unpredictable
2. Data collection
a. Unclear identity
b. Unstable and intense
c. Extreme shifts in mood
d. Easily angered
e. Easily bored
f. Argumentative
g. Depression
h. Self-destructive behavior
i. Manipulation
j. Unable to tolerate anxiety
k. Chronic feelings of emptiness and fear of being alone
l. Splitting

M. Passive aggressive personality disorder
1. Description
a. Characterized by passively expressing covert aggression rather than dealing with it directly
b. The behavior can interfere with both social and work activities
2. Data collection
a. Procrastination
b. Stubbornness
c. Intentional inefficiency
d. Forgetfulness
e. Dependency

N. Implementation ▲
1. Maintain safety against self-destructive behaviors
2. Allow the client to make choices and be as independent as possible
3. Encourage the client to discuss feelings rather than act them out
4. Provide consistency in response to client's acting-out behaviors
5. Discuss expectations and responsibilities with the client
6. Discuss the consequences that will follow certain behaviors
7. Inform the client that harm to self, others, and property is unacceptable
8. Identify splitting behavior
9. Assist the client to deal directly with anger
10. Develop a written contract with the client
11. Encourage the client to keep a journal recording daily feelings
12. Encourage the client to participate in group activities and praise nonmanipulative behavior
13. Set and maintain limits to decrease manipulative behavior

14. Remove the client from group situations in which attention-seeking behaviors occur
15. Provide realistic praise for positive behaviors in social situations

XII. ELECTROCONVULSIVE THERAPY (ECT)

A. Description
1. An effective treatment for depression that consists of inducing a grand mal (tonic-clonic) seizure by passing an electrical current through electrodes that are attached to the temples
2. The administration of a muscle relaxant minimizes seizure activity, preventing damage to long bones and cervical vertebrae
3. The usual course is 6 to 12 treatments given two to three times a week
4. Maintenance ECT once a month may help to decrease the relapse rate for the client with recurrent depression
5. ECT is not a permanent cure
6. Not necessarily effective in the client with depression and personality disorders, those with drug dependence, or those with depression secondary to situational or social difficulties
7. At-risk clients include those with recent myocardial infarction, cerebrovascular accident, or cerebral vascular malformation, or clients with intracranial mass lesions

B. Uses
1. Clients with major depressive and bipolar depressive disorders, especially when psychotic symptoms are present such as delusions of guilt, somatic delusions, and delusions of infidelity
2. Clients who have depression with marked psychomotor retardation and stupor
3. Manic clients whose conditions are resistant to lithium and antipsychotic medications and in clients who are rapid cyclers (a client with a bipolar disorder who has many episodes of mood swings close together)
4. Clients with schizophrenia (especially catatonia), those with schizoaffective syndromes, and psychotic clients

C. Indications for use
1. When antidepressant medications have no effect
2. When there is a need for a rapid definitive response, such as when a client is suicidal or homicidal
3. When the client is in extreme agitation or stupor
4. When the risks of other treatments outweigh the risk of ECT
5. When the client has a history of poor medication response, a history of good ECT response, or both
6. When the client prefers it

D. Preprocedure
1. Explain the procedure to the client
2. Encourage the client to discuss feelings, including myths regarding ECT
3. Teach the client and family what to expect
4. Informed consent must be obtained when voluntary clients are being treated
5. For involuntary clients, when informed consent cannot be obtained, permission may be obtained from the next of kin, although in some states the permission for ECT must be obtained from the court
6. NPO after midnight or at least 4 hours before treatment
7. Baseline vital signs are taken
8. The client is requested to void
9. Hairpins, contact lenses, and dentures are removed
10. Administer preoperative medication if prescribed; glycopyrrolate (Robinul) or atropine sulfate may be prescribed to prevent the potential for aspiration and to minimize bradydysrhythmias in response to electrical stimulants

E. During the procedure
1. Place a blood pressure cuff on one of the client's arms
2. An intravenous line is inserted, and electroencephalographic and electrocardiographic electrodes are attached
3. A pulse oximeter is placed onto the client's finger
4. Blood pressure is monitored throughout the treatment
5. Medications administered may include a short-acting anesthetic such as methohexital sodium (Brevital Sodium) or thiopental sodium (Pentothal), and a muscle relaxant such as succinylcholine (Anectine)
6. 100% oxygen by mask via positive pressure is administered throughout the procedure
7. An airway or bite block is placed to prevent biting the tongue
8. Electrical stimulus is administered and the seizure should last 30 to 60 seconds

F. Postprocedure
1. The client will be transported to a recovery room with the blood pressure cuff and oximeter in place, where oxygen, suction, and other emergency equipment are available

2. Once the client is awake, talk to the client and take vital signs
3. The client may be confused; provide frequent orientation (brief, distinct, and simple) and reassurance
4. Client returns to the nursing unit when a 90% oxygen saturation level is maintained, vital signs are stable, and mental status is satisfactory
5. Assess the gag reflex before giving the client fluids, food, or medication

G. Potential side effects
1. Major side effects with bilateral treatment are confusion, disorientation, and short-term memory loss
2. The client may be confused and disorientated on awakening
3. Memory deficits may occur, but memory usually recovers completely, although some clients have memory loss lasting up to 6 months

XIII. COGNITIVE IMPAIRMENT DISORDERS

A. Autism: refer to Chapter 28
B. Attention deficit hyperactivity disorder (ADHD): refer to Chapter 28
C. Tourette's disorder: refer to Chapter 28
D. Dementia and Alzheimer's disease
1. Dementia
a. Organic syndrome with progressive deterioration in intellectual functioning
b. Long- and short-term memory loss occurs with impairment in judgment, abstract thinking, problem-solving ability, and behavior
c. Results in a self-care deficit
d. The most common type of dementia is Alzheimer's disease
2. Alzheimer's disease (Box 61-10)
a. An irreversible form of senile dementia from nerve cell deterioration
b. Individuals with Alzheimer's disease experience cognitive deterioration and progressive loss of ability to carry out ADLs

BOX 61-10

Alzheimer's Disease

Amnesia: inability to learn new information or to recall previously learned information
Agnosia: failure to recognize or identify objects despite intact sensory function
Aphasia: language disturbance in understanding and expressing the spoken word
Apraxia: inability to perform motor activities despite intact motor function

c. The client experiences a steady decline in physical and mental functioning and usually requires nursing home placement in the final stages of the illness
3. Implementation
a. Identify and reinforce retained skills
b. Provide continuity of care
c. Orient to the environment
d. Furnish environment with familiar possessions
e. Acknowledge the client's feelings
f. Assist the client and family members to manage memory deficits and behavior changes
g. Encourage the family members to express feelings about caregiving
h. Provide the caregiver support, and identify available resources and support groups
i. Monitor ADLs
j. Remind the client how to perform self-care activities
k. Maintain independence
l. Provide consistent routines
m. Provide exercise, such as walking with an escort
n. Avoid activities that tax the memory
o. Allow plenty of time to complete a task
p. Use constant encouragement in a step-by-step approach
q. Provide activities that distract and occupy time, such as listening to music, coloring, and watching TV
r. Provide mental stimulation with simple games or activities
4. Wandering
a. Provide a safe environment
b. Prevent unsafe wandering
c. Provide close supervision
d. Close and secure doors
e. Use identification bracelets and electronic surveillance
5. Communication
a. Adapt to the communication level of the client
b. Use a firm volume and a low-pitched voice to communicate
c. Stand directly in front of the client and maintain eye contact
d. Call the client by name and identify self; wait for a response
e. Use a calm and reassuring voice
f. Use pantomime gestures if the client is unable to understand spoken words
g. Use slow, clear, verbal communication techniques
h. Use short words and simple sentences

i. Ask only one question at a time, and give one direction at a time
j. Repeat questions if necessary, but do not rephrase

6. Impaired judgment
   a. Remove throw rugs, toxic substances, and dangerous electrical appliances from the environment
   b. Reduce hot water heater temperature
7. Altered thought processes
   a. Call the client by name
   b. Orient the client frequently
   c. Use familiar objects in the room
   d. Place a calendar and clock in a visible place
   e. Maintain familiar routines
   f. Allow the client to reminisce
   g. Make tasks simple
   h. Allow time for the client to complete a task
   i. Provide positive reinforcement for positive behaviors
8. Altered sleep patterns
   a. Allow client to wander in a safe place until he or she becomes tired
   b. Prevent shadows in the room
   c. Avoid the use of hypnotics, as they cause confusion
9. Agitation
   a. Assess the precipitant of the agitation
   b. Reassure the client
   c. Remove items that can be hazardous during the time of agitation
   d. Approach the client slowly and calmly from the front; then speak, gesture, and move slowly
   e. Remove the client to a less stressful environment
   f. Use touch gently
   g. Do not argue with the client or restrain the client
   h. Distract the client with questions about the problem, and gradually turn the attention to something else

XIV. PSYCHOSEXUAL ALTERATIONS

A. Sexuality
   1. One's sense of being a sexual individual
   2. Includes how one looks, behaves, and relates to others

B. Sexual expression
   1. Heterosexuality: male-female sexual relationships
   2. Homosexuality: sexual attraction to a member of the same sex
   3. Bisexuality: sexual attraction to and activity with both sexes
   4. Transvestitism: obsession with wearing clothing of the opposite sex

C. Alterations in sexual behavior
   1. Transsexualism: feeling that one's sex is inappropriate and desiring to acquire sexual characteristics of the opposite sex
   2. Exhibitionism: sexual urges and fantasies and exposing genitals to strangers
   3. Fetishism: using nonliving objects for sexual gratification
   4. Pedophilia: desiring sexual activity with a child under age 13
   5. Sexual masochism: sexual gratification that involves receiving pain
   6. Sexual sadism: sexual gratification that involves inflicting pain
   7. Voyeurism: sexual gratification through observing others disrobing or engaging in sexual activity
   8. Zoophilia: intense sexual arousal or desire for sexual contact with animals
   9. Frotteurism: intense sexual arousal or desire when rubbing against a nonconsenting person

D. Implementation
   1. Assessment of sexual history and precipitating event for sexual disorder
   2. Encourage the client to explore personal beliefs
   3. Provide a nonjudgmental attitude
   4. Provide supportive psychotherapy
   5. Initiate psychoanalysis as prescribed

PRACTICE QUESTIONS

1. A nurse collects data on a client with an admitting diagnosis of bipolar affective disorder—mania. The symptom presentation that requires the nurse's immediate intervention is:
   1. The client's outlandish behaviors and inappropriate dress
   2. The client's grandiose delusions of being a royal descendent of King Arthur
   3. The client's nonstop physical activity and poor nutritional intake
   4. The client's constant, incessant talking that includes sexual innuendoes and teasing the staff
2. A client in a manic state emerges from her room. She is topless and is making sexual remarks and gestures toward staff and peers. The best initial nursing action is to:
   1. Quietly approach the client, escort her to her room, and assist her in getting dressed
   2. Approach the client in the hallway and insist that she go to her room

3. Confront the client on the inappropriateness of her behaviors and offer her a time-out
4. Ask the other clients to ignore her behavior; eventually she will return to her room

3. A nurse reviews the activity schedule for the day and determines that the best activity that the manic client could participate in is:
    1. A brown-bag luncheon and a book review
    2. Tetherball
    3. A paint-by-number activity
    4. A deep breathing and progressive relaxation group

4. A client who is delusional says to the nurse "The federal guards were sent to kill me." The nurse's best response will be:
    1. "The guards are not out to kill you."
    2. "I don't believe this is true."
    3. "I don't know anything about the guards. Do you feel afraid that people are trying to hurt you?"
    4. "What makes you think the guards were sent to hurt you?"

5. A woman comes into the emergency room in a severe state of anxiety after a car accident. The most important nursing intervention is to:
    1. Remain with the client
    2. Put the client in a quiet room
    3. Teach the client deep breathing
    4. Encourage the client to talk about her feelings and concerns

6. A male client with delirium becomes agitated and confused in his room at night. The best initial intervention by the nurse is to:
    1. Use a night-light and turn off the television
    2. Keep the television and a soft light on during the night
    3. Move the client next to the nurse's station
    4. Play soft music during the night, and maintain a well-lit room

7. A nurse is collecting data on a client who is actively hallucinating. Which of the following nursing statements would be most therapeutic at this time?
    1. "I talked to the voices you're hearing and they won't hurt you now."
    2. "I can hear the voice and she wants you to come to dinner."
    3. "Sometimes people hear things or voices others can't hear."
    4. "I know you feel 'they are out to get you' but it's not true."

8. A nurse is caring for a client with a diagnosis of depression. The nurse monitors for signs of constipation and urinary retention knowing that these problems are most likely due to:
    1. Inadequate dietary intake and dehydration
    2. Lack of exercise and poor diet
    3. Poor dietary choices
    4. Psychomotor retardation and side effects of medication

9. A client is admitted to the inpatient unit and is being considered for electroconvulsive therapy (ECT). The client appears calm but the family is hypervigilant and anxious. The client's mother begins to cry and states "My son's brain will be destroyed. How can the doctor do this to him?" The nurse's best response to this remark is:
    1. "It sounds as though you need to speak to the psychiatrist."
    2. "Your son has decided to have this treatment. You should support him."
    3. "Perhaps you'd like to see the ECT room and speak to the staff."
    4. "It sounds as though you have some concerns about the ECT procedure. Why don't we all sit down together and discuss any concerns you may have."

10. A nurse is caring for a client who has been treated with long-term antipsychotic medication. As part of the nursing care plan, the nurse monitors for tardive dyskinesia (TD). In the event that TD occurs, the nurse would most likely observe:
    1. Abnormal movements and involuntary movements of the mouth, tongue, and face
    2. Abnormal breathing through the nostrils
    3. Severe headache, flushing, tremor, and ataxia
    4. Severe hypertension, migraine headache, and "marbles in the mouth" syndrome

11. A client who is diagnosed with pedophilia and was recently paroled as a sex offender says, "I'm in treatment and I have served my time, now this group has posters of me all over the neighborhood telling about me with my picture on it." Which of the following is the most appropriate response by the nurse?
    1. "You understand that people fear for their children but you're feeling unfairly treated?"
    2. "When children are hurt as you hurt them, people want you isolated."
    3. "You seem angry but you have committed serious crimes against several children so your neighbors are frightened."
    4. "You're lucky it doesn't escalate into something pretty scary after your crime"

12. A nurse is discharging a client with a history of command hallucinations to harm self or others. The nurse instructs the client about interventions for hallucinations and anxiety and determines that the client understands the interventions when the client states:
    1. "My medications won't make me anxious."
    2. "I can call my therapist when I'm hallucinating so that I can talk about my feelings and plans and not hurt anyone."

3. "I'll go to a support group and talk so that I won't hurt anyone."
4. "I won't get anxious or hear things if I get enough sleep and eat well."

13. A nurse observes that a client is psychotic, pacing, agitated, and presenting aggressive gestures. The client's speech pattern is rapid and the client's affect is belligerent. Based on these observations, the nurse's immediate priority of care is to:
   1. Provide safety for the client and other clients on the unit
   2. Offer the client a less stimulated area to calm down and gain control
   3. Provide the clients on the unit with a sense of comfort and safety
   4. Assist the staff in caring for the client in a controlled environment
14. A nurse is caring for a male client diagnosed with catatonic stupor. The client is lying on the bed with the body pulled into a fetal position. The most appropriate nursing intervention is which of the following?
   1. Leave the client alone and intermittently check on him
   2. Take the client into the dayroom with other clients so they can help watch him
   3. Sit beside the client in silence and verbalize occasional open-ended questions
   4. Ask direct questions to encourage talking
15. A mother of a teenage client with an anxiety disorder is concerned about her daughter's progress on discharge. She states that her daughter "stashes food, eats all the wrong things that make her hyperactive," and "hangs out with the wrong crowd." In helping the mother prepare for her daughter's discharge, the nurse instructs the mother to:
   1. Restrict the daughter's socializing time with her friends
   2. Consider taking time from work to help her daughter readjust to the home environment
   3. Restrict the amount of chocolate and caffeine products in the home
   4. Keep her daughter out of school until she can adjust to the school environment
16. A client is unwilling to go out of the house for fear of "doing something crazy in public." Because of this fear, the client remains homebound except when accompanied outside by the spouse. The nurse determines that the client has:
   1. Social phobia
   2. Agoraphobia
   3. Claustrophobia
   4. Hypochondriasis
17. A client reports that crying spells have been a major problem over the past several weeks, and that the doctor said that depression is probably the reason. The nurse observes that the client is sitting slumped in the chair and the clothes that the client is wearing are not fitting well. The nurse interprets that further data collection should focus on:
   1. Sleep patterns
   2. Onset of the crying spells
   3. Weight loss
   4. Medication compliance
18. A client was admitted to a medical unit with acute blindness. Many tests are performed and there seems to be no organic reason why this client cannot see. The nurse later learns that the client became blind after witnessing a hit and run car accident, when a family of three were killed. The nurse suspects that the client may be experiencing a:
   1. Psychosis
   2. Conversion disorder
   3. Dissociative disorder
   4. Repression
19. A manic client announces to everyone in the dayroom that a stripper is coming to perform this evening. When the psychiatric aide firmly states that this behavior is not appropriate, the manic client becomes verbally abusive and threatens physical violence to the aide. Based on the analysis of this situation, the nurse determines that the most appropriate action would be to:
   1. With assistance, escort the manic client to his or her room and administer PRN haloperidol (Haldol)
   2. Tell the client that smoking privileges are revoked for 24 hours
   3. Orient the client to time, person, and place
   4. Tell the client that the behavior is not appropriate
20. A nurse is preparing a client for electroconvulsive therapy (ECT), which is scheduled for the next morning. Which of the following would not be a component of the plan of care?
   1. Withhold food and fluids for 6 hours before the treatment
   2. Have the client void before the procedure
   3. Remove dentures and contact lenses before the procedure
   4. Administer tap water enemas on the evening before the procedure

ANSWERS

1. *Answer:* 3
Rationale: Mania is a mood characterized by excitement, euphoria, hyperactivity, excessive energy, decreased need for sleep, and impaired ability to concentrate or complete a single train of thought. It is a period when the mood is predominantly elevated, expansive, or irritable. Option 3 identifies a physiological need requiring immediate intervention.
Test-Taking Strategy: Use the process of elimination and note the key words "immediate intervention." Use Maslow's Hierarchy of Needs theory to assist in answering the question. Option 3 indicates a potential disruption in the client's physiological status. Review care to the client with mania if you had difficulty with this question.
Level of Cognitive Ability: Comprehension
Client Needs: Psychosocial Integrity
Integrated Concept/Process: Nursing Process/Data Collection
Content Area: Mental Health
Reference: Hill S, Bauer B: *Mental health nursing,* Philadelphia, 2002, WB Saunders, p. 225.

2. *Answer:* 1
Rationale: A person who is experiencing mania lacks insight and judgment, has poor impulse control, and is highly excitable. The nurse must take control without increasing the client's stress or anxiety. A quiet, firm approach while distracting the client (walking him or her to his or her room and assisting with dressing) achieves the goal of having him or her dressed appropriately and preserving psychosocial integrity. Option 4 is inappropriate. "Insisting" that the client go to his or her room may meet with a great deal of resistance. Confronting the client and offering the client a consequence of "time-out" may be meaningless.
Test-Taking Strategy: Use the process of elimination and focus on the issue of the question. Noting that the issue relates to having the client dress appropriately will direct you to option 1. Review care to the client with mania if you had difficulty with this question.
Level of Cognitive Ability: Application
Client Needs: Psychosocial Integrity
Integrated Concept/Process: Nursing Process/Implementation
Content Area: Mental Health
Reference: Hill S, Bauer B: *Mental health nursing,* Philadelphia, 2002, WB Saunders, p. 225.

3. *Answer:* 2
Rationale: A person who is experiencing mania is overactive, full of energy, lacks concentration, and has poor impulse control. The client needs an activity that will allow him or her to use excess energy, yet not endanger others during the process. Options 1, 3, and 4 are relatively sedate activities that require concentration, a quality that is lacking in the manic state. Such activities may lead to increased frustration and anxiety for the client. Tetherball is an exercise that uses the large muscle groups of the body and is a great way to expend the increased energy this client is experiencing.
Test-Taking Strategy: Use the process of elimination. Note the similarity in options 1, 3, and 4 in that they are relatively sedate activities that require concentration. Review the appropriate interventions for a manic client if you had difficulty with this question.
Level of Cognitive Ability: Application
Client Needs: Psychosocial Integrity
Integrated Concept/Process: Nursing Process/Implementation
Content Area: Mental Health
Reference: Hill S, Bauer B: *Mental health nursing,* Philadelphia, 2002, WB Saunders, p. 225.

4. *Answer:* 3
Rationale: Disagreeing with delusions may make the client more defensive, and the client may cling to the delusions even more. It is most therapeutic for the nurse to empathize with the client's experience. Options 1 and 2 are statements that disagree with the client. Option 4 is encouraging discussion regarding the delusion.
Test-Taking Strategy: Use therapeutic communication techniques for the client experiencing delusions. Eliminate options 1 and 2 because they are similar and are statements that disagree with the client. Option 4 is encouraging discussion regarding the delusion. Review communication techniques for the client experiencing delusions if you had difficulty with this question.
Level of Cognitive Ability: Application
Client Needs: Psychosocial Integrity
Integrated Concept/Process: Communication and Documentation
Content Area: Mental Health
Reference: Hill S, Bauer B: *Mental health nursing,* Philadelphia, 2002, WB Saunders, p. 125.

5. *Answer:* 1
Rationale: If a client is left alone with severe anxiety, he or she may feel abandoned and become overwhelmed. Placing the client in a quiet room is also indicated, but the nurse must stay with the client. It is not possible to teach the client deep breathing until the anxiety decreases. Encouraging the client to discuss concerns and feelings would not take place until the anxiety has decreased.
Test-Taking Strategy: Use the process of elimination. Note the key word "severe." Eliminate options 3 and 4 first knowing that these actions are not possible when the client is in a severe state of anxiety. From the remaining options, the best action is to remain with the client. Review care to the client with severe anxiety if you had difficulty with this question.
Level of Cognitive Ability: Application
Client Needs: Psychosocial Integrity
Integrated Concept/Process: Nursing Process/Implementation
Content Area: Mental Health
Reference: Hill S, Bauer B: *Mental health nursing,* Philadelphia, 2002, WB Saunders, p. 149.

6. *Answer:* 1
Rationale: It is important to provide a consistent daily routine and a low stimulating environment when the client is agitated and confused. Noise levels including a radio and television may add to the confusion and disorientation. Moving the client next to the nurses' station is not the initial action.
Test-Taking Strategy: Use the process of elimination. Note the key word "initial" in the stem of the question. Eliminate

options 2 and 4 first because they are similar. From the remaining options, recalling that a low stimulating environment is best will direct you to option 1. Review measures related to the client with agitation and confusion if you had difficulty with this question.
Level of Cognitive Ability: Application
Client Needs: Psychosocial Integrity
Integrated Concept/Process: Nursing Process/Implementation
Content Area: Mental Health
Reference: Hill S, Bauer B: *Mental health nursing,* Philadelphia, 2002, WB Saunders, p. 125.

7. *Answer:* 3
Rationale: It is important for the nurse to reinforce reality with the client. Options 1, 2, and 4 do not reinforce reality but rather the hallucination that the voices are real.
Test-Taking Strategy: Use the process of elimination. Note that options 1, 2, and 4 all indicate reinforcement to the client that the voices are real. Option 3 is the only statement that indicates reality. Review nursing interventions related to the client who is hallucinating if you had difficulty with this question.
Level of Cognitive Ability: Application
Client Needs: Psychosocial Integrity
Integrated Concept/Process: Communication and Documentation
Content Area: Mental Health
Reference: Hill S, Bauer B: *Mental health nursing,* Philadelphia, 2002, WB Saunders, p. 317.

8. *Answer:* 4
Rationale: Constipation can be related to inadequate food intake, lack of exercise, and poor diet. In this situation, urinary retention is most likely due to medications. Option 4 is the only option that addresses both constipation and urinary retention.
Test-Taking Strategy: Use the process of elimination and focus on the data in the question. Options 1, 2, and 3 are all similar and address diet. Option 4 addresses both concerns, constipation and urinary retention. If you had difficulty with this question, review the interventions for a client with depression and the effects of medications prescribed for this disorder.
Level of Cognitive Ability: Comprehension
Client Needs: Physiological Integrity
Integrated Concept/Process: Nursing Process/Data Collection
Content Area: Mental Health
Reference: Hill S, Bauer B: *Mental health nursing,* Philadelphia, 2002, WB Saunders, p. 137.

9. *Answer:* 4
Rationale: The nurse needs to encourage the family and client to verbalize their fears and concerns. Option 4 is the only option that encourages verbalization. Options 1, 2, and 3 avoid dealing with the client or family concerns.
Test-Taking Strategy: Use therapeutic communication techniques and focus on the client's feelings and concerns. This will direct you to option 4. Review these techniques if you had difficulty with this question.
Level of Cognitive Ability: Application
Client Needs: Psychosocial Integrity
Integrated Concept/Process: Nursing Process/Implementation
Content Area: Mental Health
Reference: Varcarolis E: *Foundations of psychiatric mental health nursing,* ed 4, Philadelphia, 2002, WB Saunders, p. 254.

10. *Answer:* 1
Rationale: Tardive dyskinesia is a severe reaction associated with the long-term use of antipsychotic medication. The clinical manifestations are abnormal movements (dyskinesia) and involuntary movements of the mouth, tongue, and face. In its more severe form, tardive dyskinesia involves the fingers, arms, trunk, and respiratory muscles. When this occurs, the medication is discontinued.
Test-Taking Strategy: Knowledge regarding the clinical manifestations of tardive dyskinesia is required to answer this question. If you had difficulty with this question, review the characteristics associated with this reaction.
Level of Cognitive Ability: Comprehension
Client Needs: Physiological Integrity
Integrated Concept/Process: Nursing Process/Data Collection
Content Area: Mental Health
Reference: Varcarolis E: *Foundations of psychiatric mental health nursing,* ed 4, Philadelphia, 2002, WB Saunders, p. 548.

11. *Answer:* 1
Rationale: Focusing and verbalizing the implied is the most therapeutic communication because it assists the client to clarify thinking and to relook at what the client is really saying. Option 1 is the only option that reflects the use of this therapeutic communication technique. Option 2 is insensitive and anxiety-provoking. Option 3 does not facilitate client expression of feelings. Option 4 gives advice and also does not facilitate the client's expression of feelings.
Test-Taking Strategy: Use therapeutic communication techniques to answer the question. Remembering to focus on the client's feelings and concerns will direct you to option 1. Review these techniques if you had difficulty with this question.
Level of Cognitive Ability: Application
Client Needs: Psychosocial Integrity
Integrated Concept/Process: Communication and Documentation
Content Area: Mental Health
Reference: Varcarolis E: *Foundations of psychiatric mental health nursing,* ed 4, Philadelphia, 2002, WB Saunders, p. 254.

12. *Answer:* 2
Rationale: There may be an increased risk for impulsive and/or aggressive behavior if a client is receiving command hallucinations to harm (self) or others. Talking about the auditory hallucinations can interfere with the subvocal muscular activity associated with a hallucination. Option 2 is a specific agreement to seek help and evidences self-responsible commitment and control over own behavior.
Test-Taking Strategy: Use the process of elimination. Note the relationship between the word "hallucinations" in the question and in the correct option. Review care to the client with command hallucinations if you had difficulty with this question.
Level of Cognitive Ability: Comprehension
Client Needs: Psychosocial Integrity

Integrated Concept/Process: Teaching/Learning
Content Area: Mental Health
Reference: Varcarolis E: *Foundations of psychiatric mental health nursing*, ed 4, Philadelphia, 2002, WB Saunders, p. 533.

13. ***Answer:*** 1
Rationale: Safety to the client and other clients is the priority. Option 1 is the only option that addresses the client and other clients' safety needs. Option 2 addresses the client's needs. Option 3 addresses other clients' needs. Option 4 is not client centered.
Test-Taking Strategy: Use the process of elimination and focus on the issue, safety. Option 1 is the global option and addresses the safety of all. Review care to the psychotic client if you had difficulty with this question.
Level of Cognitive Ability: Application
Client Needs: Safe, Effective Care Environment
Integrated Concept/Process: Nursing Process/Implementation
Content Area: Mental Health
Reference: Varcarolis E: *Foundations of psychiatric mental health nursing*, ed 4, Philadelphia, 2002, WB Saunders, p. 109.

14. ***Answer:*** 3
Rationale: Clients with catatonic stupor may be immobile and mute, and require consistent, repeated approaches. The nurse facilitates communication with the client by sitting in silence, asking open-ended questions, and pausing to provide opportunities for the client to respond. The nurse would not leave the client alone. Option 2 relies on other clients to care for this client, which is an inappropriate expectation. Asking direct questions to this client is not therapeutic. Option 3 is the best action because it provides for client supervision and communication as appropriate.
Test-Taking Strategy: Use the process of elimination. Eliminate option 1 because the nurse would not leave the client alone. Eliminate option 2 next because this action relies on other clients to care for this client. Eliminate option 4 because asking direct questions to this client is not therapeutic. Review care to the client with catatonic stupor if you had difficulty with this question.
Level of Cognitive Ability: Application
Client Needs: Psychosocial Integrity
Integrated Concept/Process: Nursing Process/Implementation
Content Area: Mental Health
Reference: Varcarolis E: *Foundations of psychiatric mental health nursing*, ed 4, Philadelphia, 2002, WB Saunders, p. 558.

15. ***Answer:*** 3
Rationale: Clients with anxiety disorder should abstain from, or limit their intake of, caffeine, chocolate, and alcohol. These products have the potential to increase anxiety. Options 1 and 4 are unreasonable and are an unhealthy approach. It may not be realistic for a family member to take time away from work.
Test-Taking Strategy: Use the process of elimination. Options 1, 2, and 4 are similar and are concerned with monitoring or curtailing the client's physical activities. Option 3 addresses preparation of the client's environment and focuses on the concern or issue expressed in the question. Review discharge planning for the client with anxiety if you had difficulty with this question.
Level of Cognitive Ability: Application
Client Needs: Health Promotion and Maintenance
Integrated Concept/Process: Teaching/Learning
Content Area: Mental Health
Reference: Varcarolis E: *Foundations of psychiatric mental health nursing*, ed 4, Philadelphia, 2002, WB Saunders, p. 283.

16. ***Answer:*** 2
Rationale: Agoraphobia is a fear of being alone in open or public places where escape might be difficult. Agoraphobia includes experiencing fear or a sense of helplessness or embarrassment if a phobic attack occurs. Avoidance of such situations usually results in the reduction of social and professional interactions. Social phobia focuses more on specific situations, such as the fear of speaking, performing, or eating in public. Claustrophobia is a fear of closed-in places. Clients with hypochondriacal symptoms focus their anxiety on physical complaints and are preoccupied with their health.
Test-Taking Strategy: Use the process of elimination and focus on the data in the question. Knowledge regarding the specific types of phobias and associated client behaviors is required to answer this question. If you had difficulty with this question, review phobia types and associated client behaviors.
Level of Cognitive Ability: Comprehension
Client Needs: Psychosocial Integrity
Integrated Concept/Process: Nursing Process/Data Collection
Content Area: Mental Health
Reference: Varcarolis E: *Foundations of psychiatric mental health nursing*, ed 4, Philadelphia, 2002, WB Saunders, p. 313.

17. ***Answer:*** 3
Rationale: All of the options are possible issues to address; however, weight loss is the first item that needs further data collection, because an ill fit of clothing could indicate a problem with nutrition. The client has already told the nurse that the crying spells have been a problem. Medication or sleep patterns are not mentioned or addressed in the question.
Test-Taking Strategy: Use the process of elimination and Maslow's Hierarchy of Needs theory to answer the question. Focusing on the data in the question will assist in eliminating options 1, 2, and 4. Review the priorities of care for a client with depression if you had difficulty with this question.
Level of Cognitive Ability: Analysis
Client Needs: Physiological Integrity
Integrated Concept/Process: Nursing Process/Data Collection
Content Area: Mental Health
Reference: Varcarolis E: *Foundations of psychiatric mental health nursing*, ed 4, Philadelphia, 2002, WB Saunders, p. 465.

18. ***Answer:*** 2
Rationale: A conversion disorder is the alteration or loss of a physical function that cannot be explained by any known pathophysiological mechanism. It is thought to be an expression of a psychological need or conflict. In this situation, the client witnessed an accident that was so psychologically painful that the client became blind. A dissociative disorder is a disturbance or alteration in the normally integrative functions of identity, memory, and consciousness. Psychosis is a state in which a person's mental capacity to recognize reality, communicate, and relate to others is impaired, thus interfering with the person's capacity to deal with life demands.

Repression is a coping mechanism in which unacceptable feelings are kept out of awareness.
Test-Taking Strategy: Use the process of elimination. Noting that the client evidences no organic reason to account for the blindness will direct you to option 2. If you had difficulty with this question, review conversion disorders and defense mechanisms.
Level of Cognitive Ability: Comprehension
Client Needs: Psychosocial Integrity
Integrated Concept/Process: Nursing Process/Data Collection
Content Area: Mental Health
Reference: Varcarolis E: *Foundations of psychiatric mental health nursing*, ed 4, Philadelphia, 2002, WB Saunders, p. 292.

19. ***Answer:*** **1**
Rationale: The client is at risk for injury to self and others and therefore should be escorted out of the dayroom. Hyperactive and agitated behavior usually responds to haloperidol (Haldol). Option 2 may increase the agitation that already exists in this client. Orientation will not halt the behavior. Telling the client that the behavior is not appropriate has already been attempted by the psychiatric aide.
Test-Taking Strategy: Use the process of elimination and therapeutic interventions for the manic client. Options 2, 3, and 4 will not deescalate the client's agitation. If you had difficulty with this question, review the appropriate interventions in dealing with a manic client.
Level of Cognitive Ability: Application
Client Needs: Psychosocial Integrity
Integrated Concept/Process: Nursing Process/Implementation
Content Area: Mental Health
Reference: Varcarolis E: *Foundations of psychiatric mental health nursing*, ed 4, Philadelphia, 2002, WB Saunders, p. 109.

20. ***Answer:*** 4
Rationale: Enemas are not a component of the pretreatment care for a client scheduled for ECT. Options 1, 2, and 3 are a part of the pretreatment plan. Additionally, an informed consent is required and the nurse should teach the client and family what to expect with ECT and allow the client to discuss his or her feelings regarding the procedure.
Test-Taking Strategy: Use the process of elimination and note the key word "not." Knowledge regarding the pretreatment care for the client scheduled for ECT is required to answer this question. If you had difficulty with this question, review this procedure.
Level of Cognitive Ability: Application
Client Needs: Physiological Integrity
Integrated Concept/Process: Nursing Process/Planning
Content Area: Mental Health
Reference: Varcarolis E: *Foundations of psychiatric mental health nursing*, ed 4, Philadelphia, 2002, WB Saunders, p. 477.

REFERENCES

Fortinash K, Holoday-Worret P: *Psychiatric mental health nursing*, ed 2, St Louis, 2000, Mosby.

Hill S, Bauer B: *Mental health nursing*, Philadelphia, 2002, WB Saunders.

Keltner N, Schwecke L, Bostrom C: *Psychiatric nursing*, ed 3, St Louis, 1999, Mosby.

Varcarolis E: *Foundations of psychiatric mental health nursing*, ed 4, Philadelphia, 2002, WB Saunders.

62 Addictions

I. EATING DISORDERS

A. Description: characterized by uncertain self-identification and grossly disturbed eating habits

B. Compulsive overeating
1. Bingelike overeating without purging
2. Food consumption is out of the individual's control and occurs in a stereotyped fashion
3. Client may be repulsed by eating, and the eating relieves tension but does not produce pleasure
4. Is aware that eating patterns are abnormal and feels depressed after eating
5. Eats secretly during a binge and consumes high-calorie and easily digestible food
6. Repeatedly tries to diet but without success
7. Lacks interest in exercise programs and feels helpless and hopeless about weight
8. When experiencing guilt, anger, depression, boredom, loneliness, inadequacy, or ambivalence, responds by eating

C. Anorexia nervosa
1. Description
   a. The onset is often associated with a stressful life event
   b. The client intensely fears obesity
   c. Body image is distorted, and the client has a disturbed self-concept
   d. Preoccupied with foods that prevent weight gain and has a phobia against foods that produce weight gain
   e. The eating disorder can be life-threatening
   f. Death can occur from starvation, **suicide**, or electrolyte imbalance
2. Data collection
   a. Refusal to eat and appetite loss
   b. Appetite denial
   c. Feelings of lack of control
   d. Self-induced vomiting and self-administered enemas
   e. Exercises compulsively
   f. Overachiever and perfectionist
   g. Decreased temperature, pulse, and blood pressure
   h. Weight loss
   i. Gastrointestinal disturbances
   j. Constipation
   k. Electrolyte imbalances
   l. Scaly, dry skin
   m. Sleep disturbances
   n. Hormone deficiencies
   o. Amenorrhea for at least three consecutive menstrual periods
   p. Teeth and gum deterioration
   q. Cyanosis and numbness of extremities
   r. Esophageal varices from vomiting
   s. Bone degeneration

D. Bulimia nervosa
1. Description
   a. The client indulges in eating binges followed by purging behaviors
   b. Most clients remain within a normal weight range but feel that their lives are dominated by the eating-related conflict
2. Data collection
   a. Preoccupied with body shape and weight
   b. Consumes high-calorie food in secret; guilt about secretive eating
   c. Binge, purge syndrome
   d. Attempts to lose weight through diets, vomiting, enemas, cathartics, and amphetamines or diuretics
   e. Needs to control yet experiences feelings of powerlessness or loss of control
   f. Low self-esteem
   g. Poor interpersonal relationships

h. Mood swings
i. Self-mutilating behavior; **suicide** thoughts and attempts at **suicide**
j. Electrolyte imbalances
k. Loss of tooth enamel and dental decay
l. Stomach ulcers and rectal bleeding
m. Esophageal varicose from vomiting
n. Cardiac disease and hypertension

E. Implementation: clients with an eating disorder
1. Assess the client's nutritional status
2. Establish a contract with the client concerning the diet plan for the day
3. Assist the client in identifying precipitators to the eating disorder
4. Encourage the client to state feelings about the eating behavior
5. Be accepting and nonjudgmental, expressing neither approval nor disapproval of the behavior
6. Encourage behavior modification techniques
7. Provide praise and positive reinforcement for accomplishments
8. Supervise the client during mealtimes and for a specified period after meals
9. Set a time limit for each meal
10. Provide a pleasant, relaxed environment for eating
11. Monitor for signs of physical complications related to the eating disorder
12. Record intake and output (I&O)
13. Weigh the client daily at the same time, using the same scale, after the client voids
14. When weighing the client, ensure that the client is wearing the same clothing as when the previous weight was taken
15. Monitor and restore fluid and electrolyte balance
16. Monitor elimination patterns
17. Assess and monitor the client's activity level
18. Encourage the client to participate in diversional activities
19. Assess the client's suicidal potential
20. Administer antidepressant medication as prescribed
21. Encourage psychotherapy as prescribed
22. Refer the client to support groups

II. SUBSTANCE ABUSE DISORDERS

A. Description: behavioral changes associated with regular substance **abuse** that affects the central nervous system (CNS)

B. Substance dependence (Box 62-1)
1. Pattern of repeated use of a substance, which usually results in tolerance, withdrawal, and compulsive drug-taking behavior

BOX 62-1

CAGE Screening Test

C: Have you ever felt the need to cut down on your drinking or drug use?
A: Have you ever been annoyed at criticism of your drinking or drug use?
G: Have you ever felt guilty about something you have done when you have been drinking or taking drugs?
E: Have you ever had an "eye opener," drinking or taking drugs first thing in the morning to get going or to avoid withdrawal symptoms?

2. Client takes substances in larger amounts and over longer periods of time than was intended
3. Client has the desire to cut down but has unsuccessful efforts to decrease or discontinue use
4. Daily activities revolve around the use of a substance

C. Substance tolerance: the need for increased amounts of the substance to achieve the desired effect

D. Substance **abuse**
1. Client recurrently uses substances
2. Client experiences recurrent, significant harmful consequences related to the use of substances
3. Client has legal problems related to substance **abuse**

E. Substance withdrawal
1. Physiological and/or substance-specific cognitive symptoms
2. Occurs when blood levels decrease in an individual with prolonged heavy use of a substance

F. Precipitating factors of substance **abuse**
1. Rebellion and peer group pressure in adolescence
2. Pleasure-seeking experience, because the substance decreases physical and emotional pain
3. Group influence and peer pressure
4. Depression
5. Loss and grieving

G. Dysfunctional behaviors of substance **abuse**
1. Insensitive to self and others
2. Manipulative
3. Impulsiveness
4. Anger, including physical and verbal **abuse**
5. Avoidance of relationships, with physical and emotional distancing
6. Sense of self-importance and requiring special treatment
7. Denial, blaming everything but the substance

8. Codependent and expects others to accept behavior
9. Low self-esteem
10. Depression

III. ALCOHOL ABUSE

A. Description
   1. Alcohol is a CNS depressant affecting all body tissues
   2. Physical dependence is a biological need for alcohol to avoid physical withdrawal symptoms
   3. Psychological dependence is a craving for the subjective effect of alcohol

B. Risk factors
   1. Biological predisposition
   2. Depressed and highly anxious characteristics
   3. Low self-esteem
   4. Poor self-control
   5. History of rebelliousness, poor school performance, delinquency
   6. Poor parental relationships

C. Data collection
   1. Slurred speech
   2. Uncoordinated movements
   3. Unsteady gait
   4. Restlessness
   5. Belligerence
   6. Confusion
   7. Sneaking drinks, drinking in the morning, and experiencing blackouts
   8. Binge drinking
   9. Arguments about drinking
   10. Missing work
   11. Increased tolerance to alcohol
   12. Intoxication, with blood alcohol levels greater than or equal to 0.08% to 0.1% (80 to 100 mg alcohol/dL blood) or higher

D. Psychological symptoms
   1. Depression
   2. Hostility
   3. Suspiciousness
   4. Rationalization
   5. Irritability
   6. Isolation
   7. Decrease in inhibitions
   8. Decrease in self-esteem
   9. Denial that a problem exists

E. Complications associated with chronic alcohol use
   1. Vitamin deficiencies
      a. Vitamin B deficiency causing peripheral neuropathies
      b. Thiamine deficiency causing Korsakoff's syndrome
   2. Alcohol-induced persistent amnesiac disorder causing severe memory problems
   3. Wernicke's encephalopathy, causing confusion, ataxia, and abnormal eye movements
   4. Hepatitis; cirrhosis of the liver
   5. Esophagitis and gastritis
   6. Pancreatitis
   7. Anemias
   8. Immune system dysfunctions
   9. Brain damage
   10. Peripheral neuropathy
   11. Cardiac disorders

IV. ALCOHOL WITHDRAWAL

A. Description
   1. Occurs when an addicted person stops ingesting alcohol
   2. Can occur 6 to 8 hours after drinking has ended or decreased, and symptoms can last 5 days or longer
   3. Alcohol withdrawal is highly individual, and some clients experience mild withdrawal symptoms requiring minimal medical supervision; others experience severe symptoms that can be life-threatening

B. Stages of withdrawal
   1. Stage 1
      a. May begin 6 to 8 hours after last ingestion or a significant decrease in usual consumption of alcohol
      b. Anxiety
      c. Anorexia
      d. Insomnia
      e. Tremors
      f. Hyperalertness
      g. Internal shaking
      h. Nausea and vomiting
      i. Headache
      j. Increased pulse and blood pressure
      k. Depression
   2. Stage 2
      a. May begin 8 to 12 hours after the last ingestion or a significant decrease in usual consumption of alcohol
      b. Profound confusion
      c. Gross tremors
      d. Nervousness
      e. Disorientation
      f. Illusions
      g. Auditory and visual hallucinations
      h. Nightmares
   3. Stage 3
      a. May begin 12 to 48 hours after the last ingestion or a significant decrease in usual consumption of alcohol

b. Severe hallucinations
c. Seizures
4. Stage 4
a. May begin 3 to 5 days after the last ingestion or a significant decrease in usual alcohol consumption
b. Confusion, disorientation, clouding of consciousness, and delirium
c. Hypertension, diaphoresis, tachycardia
d. Visual and tactile hallucinations
e. Fluctuating levels of consciousness
f. Fever (103° F to 104° F)
g. Tremors
h. Uncontrolled tachycardia
i. Severe psychomotor activity
j. Agitation
k. Hallucinations
l. Sleeplessness
m. A medical emergency

C. Implementation
1. Initiate seizure precautions
2. Administer chlordiazepoxide (Librium) as prescribed for withdrawal and anticonvulsive effects
3. Administer diazepam (Valium) or pentobarbital (phenobarbital) as prescribed to produce sedation and control withdrawal
4. Administer phenytoin (Dilantin) to prevent seizures
5. Administer vitamin B_1 (thiamine) as prescribed for malnutrition
6. Administer magnesium sulfate as prescribed to increase the effectiveness of vitamin B_1 and help reduce postwithdrawal seizures
7. Hydrate the client
8. Monitor vital signs frequently
9. Monitor I&O
10. Orient client frequently
11. Maintain minimal stimuli
12. Approach the client in an accepting and nonjudgmental manner
13. Assist the client to use assertive techniques rather than manipulation to meet needs
14. Set limits on manipulative behavior
15. Direct the client to focus on the substance **abuse** problem
16. Limit the client's blame-placing or rationalizing to explain the substance **abuse** problem
17. Encourage the client to participate in group therapy and support groups
18. Encourage the client to attend weekly Alcoholics Anonymous (AA) meetings

D. Disulfiram (Antabuse) therapy
1. Description
a. An alcohol deterrent used for alcoholic dependence
b. The medication sensitizes the client to alcohol, so a disulfiram-alcohol reaction occurs if alcohol is ingested
c. The client must abstain from alcohol for at least 12 hours before the initial dose is administered
d. The client must avoid drinking for 14 days after disulfiram therapy has been discontinued; otherwise the client is at risk for disulfiram-alcohol reaction
2. Negative physiological responses
a. Throbbing headache
b. Flushing
c. Nausea
d. Copious vomiting
e. Diaphoresis
f. Dizziness
g. Blurred vision and confusion
h. Hypotension
i. Dyspnea
j. Palpitations and tachycardia
k. Chest pain
3. Client education
a. Educate as to the effects of the medication
b. Instruct the client that the effects of the medication may occur for several days after discontinuance
c. Ensure that the client agrees to abstain from alcohol and any alcohol-containing substances
d. Instruct the client to avoid the use of substances that contain alcohol, such as cough medicines, rubbing compounds, vinegar, mouthwashes, and aftershave lotions

V. HALLUCINOGENS (Box 62-2)
A. Causes psychosis, with distorted perception, heightened sense of awareness, grandiosity, hallucinations, mystical experiences, and distortions of time and space
B. May harm self when under the influence
C. No withdrawal syndrome when discontinued, but flashbacks may occur for several months after use stops

BOX 62-2

Hallucinogens

Lysergic acid diethylamide (LSD)
Mescaline
Peyote
Phencyclidine (PCP)
Psilocybin (derived from mushrooms)

D. Bad trips may result in panic and unpredictable psychotic behaviors

VI. CANNABIS

A. Can include marijuana, "pot," "hashish"
B. Causes altered state of awareness, relaxation, and mild euphoria
C. Decreases inhibitions
D. Decreased motivation from prolonged use
E. Can cause possible psychosis
F. Physiological effects include slowed reflexes
G. Causes drying of mucous membranes and reddening of the eyes

VII. OPIOIDS (Box 62-3)

A. Description
1. Cause mental and physical deterioration
2. High risk for infection with human immunodeficiency virus (HIV) or hepatitis virus if taken intravenously
3. Cause decreased response to pain, respiratory depression, constriction of pupils, euphoria, apathy, impaired judgment

B. Withdrawal
1. Methadone blocks the action of opioids and may be used to assist with withdrawal
2. Signs of withdrawal include anxiety; yawning; diaphoresis; cramping; rhinorrhea; achiness and muscle twitching; anorexia; insomnia; increased temperature, respiration, and blood pressure; nausea, vomiting, and diarrhea; and restlessness
3. Overdose of opioids can lead to coma, respiratory depression, and death

VIII. CENTRAL NERVOUS SYSTEM DEPRESSANTS (Box 62-4)

A. Description
1. Act as a depressant, sedative, and hypnotic
2. Cause physical and psychological dependence
3. Cause euphoria
4. Can cause depression and hostility
5. Impaired judgment and lack of coordination can occur
6. Slurring of speech and decreased inhibitions can occur
7. Tolerance can develop

B. Withdrawal: causes increased temperature, tachycardia, postural hypotension, insomnia, tremors, agitation, apprehension, weakness, seizures, and psychosis

BOX 62-3

Opiates

Codeine
Heroin ("China white," synthetic heroin)
Meperidine hydrochloride (Demerol)
Methadone
Morphine sulfate
Opium

BOX 62-4

Central Nervous System Depressants

Barbiturates
Benzodiazapines
Methaqualone (Quaaludes, "sopers")

IX. CNS STIMULANTS (Box 62-5)

A. Description
1. Stimulants lead to alertness and extra energy
2. Effects include euphoria, hyperactivity, insomnia, anorexia and weight loss, tachycardia and hypertension, psychotic behavior
3. Psychological dependence and tolerance can occur
4. Sudden death has been associated with cocaine **abuse**

B. Withdrawal
1. Crash
2. Depression
3. Lack of energy

X. IMPLEMENTATION: WITHDRAWAL

A. Initiate seizure precautions
B. Hydrate the client
C. Monitor vital signs every hour
D. Monitor I&O
E. Orient the client frequently
F. Maintain minimal stimuli
G. Approach the client in an accepting and nonjudgmental manner

BOX 62-5

Central Nervous System Stimulants

Amphetamines
Benzedrine inhalers
Caffeine
Cocaine, "crack"
Diet pills
Methylenedioxylmethamphetamine (Ecstasy)

H. Direct the client's focus to the substance **abuse** problem
I. Identify with client situations that precipitate angry feelings
J. Limit the client's blame-placing or rationalizing to explain the substance **abuse** problem
K. Assist the client to use assertive techniques rather than manipulation to meet needs
L. Set limits on manipulative behavior and verbal and physical **abuse**
M. Hold the client firmly to reasonable limits, consistently reinforcing rules, with reasonable consequences for breaking rules
N. Hold the client accountable for all behaviors
O. Assist the client to explore strengths and weaknesses
P. Encourage time-out if the client is losing control
Q. Encourage the client to participate in unit activities
R. Encourage the client to participate in group therapy and support groups
S. See Box 62-6 for a list of therapies
T. Box 62-7 delineates nursing care for clients

BOX 62-6

Therapies for Substance Abuse Clients

Community treatment programs
Family counseling
Psychotherapy
Self-help groups
Transitional living programs

BOX 62-7

Withdrawal: Nursing Care

Obtain information regarding the drug type and amount consumed
Assess vital signs
Remove unnecessary objects from the environment
Provide one-to-one supervision if necessary
Provide a quiet, calm environment with minimal stimuli
Maintain client orientation
Ensure the client's safety by implementing seizure precautions
Use restraints, if necessary and prescribed, to prevent the client from harming self and others
Provide for physical needs
Provide food and fluids as tolerated
Administer medications as prescribed to decrease withdrawal symptoms
Collect blood and urine samples for drug screening

PRACTICE QUESTIONS

1. A nurse is caring for a female client who was recently admitted for anorexia nervosa. The nurse enters the client's room and notes that the client is engaged in rigorous push-ups. Which nursing action is most appropriate?
   1. Allow the client to complete her exercise program
   2. Tell the client that she is not allowed to exercise rigorously
   3. Interrupt the client and offer to take her for a walk
   4. Interrupt the client and weigh immediately
2. A nurse is caring for a client with anorexia nervosa. The nurse monitoring the client's behavior understands that the client with anorexia nervosa manages anxiety by:
   1. Always reinforcing self-approval
   2. Having the need to always make the right decision
   3. Engaging in immoral acts
   4. Observing rigid rules and regulations
3. A nurse is developing a plan of care for the hospitalized client with bulimia nervosa. Which of the following would not be included in the plan of care?
   1. Monitoring intake and output
   2. Monitoring electrolyte levels
   3. Observing for excessive exercise
   4. Checking for the presence of laxatives and diuretics in the client's belongings
4. A nurse is monitoring a client who abuses alcohol for signs of alcohol withdrawal. Which of the following would alert the nurse to the potential for delirium tremors (DTs)?
   1. Hypertension, changes in level of consciousness, hallucinations
   2. Hypotension, ataxia, vomiting
   3. Stupor, agitation, muscular rigidity
   4. Hypotension, coarse hand tremor, agitation
5. A spouse of a client admitted for alcohol withdrawal says to the nurse "I should get out of this bad situation." The most helpful response by the nurse would be:
   1. "I agree with you. You should get out of this situation."
   2. "What do you find difficult about this situation?"
   3. "Why don't you tell your husband about this."
   4. "This is not the best time to make that decision."
6. A nurse is caring for a client who is suspected to be dependent on drugs. Which of the following questions would be most appropriate for the nurse to ask when collecting data from the client regarding drug abuse?
   1. "Why did you get started on these drugs?"
   2. "How long did you think you could take these drugs without someone finding out?"
   3. "How much do you use and what effect does it have on you?"

4. The nurse does not ask any questions in fear that the client is in denial and will throw the nurse out of the room

7. A client who has been drinking alcohol on a regular basis admits to having "a problem." The client is asking for assistance with the problem. The nurse would support the client to attend which of the following community groups?
   1. Al Anon
   2. Alcoholics Anonymous
   3. Families Anonymous
   4. Fresh Start
8. A client with a diagnosis of anorexia nervosa, who is in a state of starvation, is in a two-bed room. A newly admitted client will be assigned to this client's room. Which of the following clients would be an appropriate choice as this client's roommate?
   1. A client with pneumonia
   2. A client receiving diagnostic tests
   3. A client who could benefit from the client's assistance at mealtime
   4. A client who thrives on managing others
9. A client has been hospitalized and has participated in substance abuse therapy group sessions. On discharge, the client has consented to participate in Alcoholics' Anonymous (AA) community groups. Which of the following statements by the client would best indicate to the nurse that the client has well assimilated therapy session topics, coping response styles, and has processed information effectively for self-use?
   1. "I know I'm ready to be discharged; I feel like I can say "no" and leave a group of friends if they are drinking . . ." No Problem."
   2. "This group has really helped a lot. I know it will be different when I go home. But I'm sure that my family and friends will all help me like the people in this group have . . . They'll all help me . . . I know they will . . . They won't let me go back to my old ways."
   3. "I'm looking forward to leaving here; I know that I will miss all of you. So, I'm happy and I'm sad, I'm excited and I'm scared. I know that I have to work hard to be strong and that everyone isn't going to be as helpful as you people."
   4. "I'll keep all my appointments; go to all my AA groups; I'll do everything I'm supposed to . . . Nothing will go wrong that way . . ."
10. A nurse is assigned to care for a client at risk for alcohol withdrawal. The nurse monitors the client knowing that the early signs of withdrawal will develop within how much time after cessation or reduction of alcohol intake?
    1. Within a few hours
    2. After several hours
    3. In 1 week
    4. In 2 to 3 weeks
11. A nurse determines that the wife of an alcoholic client is benefiting from attending an Al Anon group when the nurse hears the wife say:
    1. "My attendance at the meetings has helped me to see that I provoke my husband's violence."
    2. "I no longer feel that I deserve the beatings my husband inflicts on me."
    3. "I can tolerate my husband's destructive behaviors now that I know they are common with alcoholics."
    4. "I enjoy attending the meetings because they get me out of the house and away from my husband."
12. A female client with anorexia nervosa is a member of a support group. The client verbalizes that she would like to buy some new clothes but her finances are limited. Group members brought some used clothes to the client to replace the client's old clothes. The client believed that the new clothes were much too tight, so she reduced her calorie intake to 800 calories daily. The nurse identifies this behavior as:
    1. Normal
    2. Indicative of the client's ambivalence
    3. Evidence of the client's altered/distorted body image
    4. Regression
13. A hospitalized client with a history of alcohol abuse tells the nurse, "I am leaving now. I have to go. I don't want any more treatment. I have things that I have to do right away." The client has not been discharged. In fact, the client is scheduled for an important diagnostic test to be performed in 1 hour. After discussing the client's concerns with the client, the client dresses and begins to walk out of the hospital room. The most appropriate nursing action is to:
    1. Restrain the client until the physician can be reached
    2. Call security to block all exit areas
    3. Tell the client that he or she cannot return to this hospital again if the client leaves now
    4. Call the nursing supervisor
14. A nurse is collecting data from a client with a diagnosis of bulimia nervosa. The nurse understands that which of the following is not a characteristic finding in this disorder?
    1. Enlarged parotid glands
    2. Dental erosion
    3. Electrolyte imbalances
    4. Body weight well below ideal range
15. A nurse is caring for a client who has a history of opioid abuse and is monitoring the client for signs of withdrawal. Which of the following observations, if made by the nurse, are indicative of the clinical manifestations associated with withdrawal from opioids?

1. Increased blood pressure and pulse with low-grade fever, yawning, restlessness, anxiety, craving, diarrhea, and mydriasis
2. Tachycardia, mild hypertension, sweating, nausea, vomiting, and marked tremors
3. Increased appetite, irritability, anxiety, restlessness, and altered concentration
4. Depressed feelings, high drug craving, fatigue with a desire to sleep, agitation, and paranoia

ANSWERS

1. *Answer:* 3
Rationale: Clients with anorexia nervosa are frequently preoccupied with rigorous exercise and push themselves beyond normal limits to work off caloric intake. The nurse must provide for appropriate exercise as well as place limits on rigorous activities. Options 1, 2, and 4 are inappropriate nursing actions.
Test-Taking Strategy: Use the process of elimination. Focus on the key words "most appropriate." Also, focus on the need for the nurse to set firm limits with clients who have this disorder. If you had difficulty with this question, review interventions for the client with anorexia nervosa.
Level of Cognitive Ability: Application
Client Needs: Physiological Integrity
Integrated Concept/Process: Nursing Process/Implementation
Content Area: Mental Health
Reference: Hill S, Bauer B: *Mental health nursing,* Philadelphia, 2002, WB Saunders, p. 174.

2. *Answer:* 4
Rationale: Clients with anorexia nervosa have the desire to please others. Their need to be correct or perfect interferes with rational decision-making processes. These clients are moralistic. Rules and rituals help these clients manage their anxiety.
Test-Taking Strategy: Use the process of elimination and focus on the issue, managing anxiety. Eliminate options 1 and 2 because of the absolute word "always." Option 3 is not characteristic of the client with anorexia. Review the characteristics associated with this disorder if you had difficulty with this question.
Level of Cognitive Ability: Analysis
Client Needs: Psychosocial Integrity
Integrated Concept/Process: Nursing Process/Data Collection
Content Area: Mental Health
Reference: Hill S, Bauer B: *Mental health nursing,* Philadelphia, 2002, WB Saunders, p. 174.

3. *Answer:* 3
Rationale: Excessive exercise is a characteristic of anorexia nervosa, not a characteristic of clients with bulimia. Frequent vomiting, in addition to laxative and diuretic abuse, may lead to dehydration and electrolyte imbalance. Assessing for dehydration and electrolyte imbalance are important nursing actions. Option 3 is the only option that is not a characteristic of bulimia.
Test-Taking Strategy: Use the process of elimination. Note the key word "not" in the stem of the question. Options 1, 2, and 4 are similar and directly or indirectly infer concern about fluid and electrolyte balance. Option 3 is different from the other options. Review the characteristics associated with bulimia nervosa if you had difficulty with this question.
Level of Cognitive Ability: Analysis
Client Needs: Physiological Integrity
Integrated Concept/Process: Nursing Process/Planning
Content Area: Mental Health
Reference: Hill S, Bauer B: *Mental health nursing,* Philadelphia, 2002, WB Saunders, p. 174.

4. *Answer:* 1
Rationale: The symptoms associated with DTs typically are anxiety, insomnia, anorexia, hypertension, disorientation, visual or tactile hallucinations, changes in level of consciousness, agitation, fever, and delusions.
Test-Taking Strategy: Use the process of elimination. Review each option carefully to ensure that all of the symptoms are contained in the correct option. Eliminate options 2 and 4 first knowing that hypertension rather than hypotension occurs. From the remaining options, recalling that the client who is stuporous is not likely to exhibit agitation will direct you to option 1. Review these symptoms if you had difficulty with this question.
Level of Cognitive Ability: Analysis
Client Needs: Physiological Integrity
Integrated Concept/Process: Nursing Process/Data Collection
Content Area: Mental Health
Reference: Hill S, Bauer B: *Mental health nursing,* Philadelphia, 2002, WB Saunders, p. 117.

5. *Answer:* 2
Rationale: The most helpful response is the one that encourages the client to problem-solve. Giving advice implies that the nurse knows what is best and can also foster dependency. The nurse should not agree with the client, nor should the nurse request that the client provide explanations.
Test-Taking Strategy: Use therapeutic communication techniques. Eliminate option 3 because of the word "why," which should be avoided in communication. Eliminate option 1 because the nurse is agreeing with the client. Eliminate option 4 because this option places the client's feelings on hold. Option 2 is the only option that addresses the client's feelings. Review therapeutic communication techniques if you had difficulty with this question.
Level of Cognitive Ability: Application
Client Needs: Psychosocial Integrity
Integrated Concept/Process: Communication and Documentation

Content Area: Mental Health
Reference: Hill S, Bauer B: *Mental health nursing,* Philadelphia, 2002, WB Saunders, p. 58.

6. ***Answer:*** 3
Rationale: Whenever the nurse performs an assessment for a client who is dependent on drugs, it is best for the nurse to attempt to elicit information by being nonjudgmental and direct. Option 1 is incorrect because it is judgmental, off focus, and reflects the nurse's bias. Option 2 is incorrect because it is judgmental, insensitive, and aggressive, which is nontherapeutic. Option 4 is incorrect because it indicates passivity on the nurse's part and uses rationalization to avoid the therapeutic nursing intervention.
Test-Taking Strategy: Use the process of elimination and therapeutic communication techniques to answer the question. Also, focus on the words "most appropriate." Review assessment of a client who is a substance abuser if you had difficulty with this question.
Level of Cognitive Ability: Application
Client Needs: Health Promotion and Maintenance
Integrated Concept/Process: Nursing Process/Data Collection
Content Area: Mental Health
Reference: Hill S, Bauer B: *Mental health nursing,* Philadelphia, 2002, WB Saunders, p. 62.

7. ***Answer:*** 2
Rationale: Alcoholics Anonymous is a major self-help organization for the treatment of alcoholism. Option 1 is a group for families of alcoholics. Option 3 is for parents of children who abuse substances. Option 4 is for nicotine addicts.
Test-Taking Strategy: Use the process of elimination. If you are unfamiliar with these support groups, note the relationship between "drinking" in the question and "Alcoholics" in the correct option. Familiarize yourself with the purpose of specific support groups if you had difficulty with this question.
Level of Cognitive Ability: Application
Client Needs: Health Promotion and Maintenance
Integrated Concept/Process: Self-Care
Content Area: Mental Health
Reference: Hill S, Bauer B: *Mental health nursing,* Philadelphia, 2002, WB Saunders, p. 118.

8. ***Answer:*** 2
Rationale: The client receiving diagnostic tests is an acceptable roommate. The client with anorexia is most likely experiencing hematological complications, such as leukopenia. Having a roommate with pneumonia would place the client with anorexia nervosa at risk for infection. The client with anorexia nervosa should not be put in a situation in which they are able to focus on the nutritional needs of others or being managed by others, because this may contribute to sublimation and suppression of their own hunger.
Test-Taking Strategy: Use the process of elimination and note the key words "in a state of starvation." Recalling the characteristics associated with anorexia nervosa will direct you to option 2. Review care of the client with anorexia nervosa if you have difficulty with this question.
Level of Cognitive Ability: Analysis
Client Needs: Safe, Effective Care Environment
Integrated Concept/Process: Nursing Process/Planning
Content Area: Mental Health
Reference: Hill S, Bauer B: *Mental health nursing,* Philadelphia, 2002, WB Saunders, p. 175.

9. ***Answer:*** 3
Rationale: In option 3, the client is expressing real concern and ambivalence about discharge from the hospital. The client also demonstrates reality in the statement. Option 1 indicates client denial. In option 2, the client is relying heavily on others. In option 4, the client is concrete and procedure-oriented; again, the client states that "nothing will go wrong that way" if the client follows all the directions.
Test-Taking Strategy: Use the process of elimination and select the option that identifies the most realistic client verbalization. This will easily direct you to option 3. Review care to the client with a substance abuse problem if you had difficulty with this question.
Level of Cognitive Ability: Analysis
Client Needs: Psychosocial Integrity
Integrated Concept/Process: Nursing Process/Evaluation
Content Area: Mental Health
Reference: Varcarolis E: *Foundations of psychiatric mental health nursing,* ed 4, Philadelphia, 2002, WB Saunders, p. 772.

10. ***Answer:*** 1
Rationale: Early signs of alcohol withdrawal develop within a few hours after cessation or reduction of alcohol and peaks after 24 to 48 hours.
Test-Taking Strategy: Use the process of elimination. Note the key word "early." This will assist in directing you to option 1. If you are unfamiliar with the manifestations associated with alcohol withdrawal, review this content.
Level of Cognitive Ability: Comprehension
Client Needs: Physiological Integrity
Integrated Concept/Process: Mental Health
Reference: Varcarolis E: *Foundations of psychiatric mental health nursing,* ed 4, Philadelphia, 2002, WB Saunders, p. 757.

11. ***Answer:*** 2
Rationale: Al Anon support groups are a protected, supportive opportunity for spouses and significant others to learn what to expect and to obtain suggestions about successful behavioral changes. Option 2 is the most healthy response because it exemplifies an understanding that the alcoholic partner is responsible for his behavior and cannot be allowed to blame family members for loss of control. In option 1, the nonalcoholic partner indicates responsibility when the spouse loses control. Option 3 indicates that the wife remains codependent. Option 4 indicates that the group is being seen as an escape, not a place to work on issues.
Test-Taking Strategy: Use the process of elimination. Identify the client of the question and identify the option that most directly addresses the issue of the question, that is, benefiting from attending an Al Anon group. Review the purpose of this type of support group if you had difficulty with this question.
Level of Cognitive Ability: Analysis
Client Needs: Psychosocial Integrity

Integrated Concept/Process: Nursing Process/Evaluation
Content Area: Mental Health
Reference: Varcarolis E: *Foundations of psychiatric mental health nursing,* ed 4, Philadelphia, 2002, WB Saunders, p. 772.

12. *Answer:* 3
Rationale: Altered/distorted body image is a concern of clients with anorexia nervosa. Although the client may struggle with ambivalence and present with regressed behavior, the client's coping pattern relates to the basic issue of distorted body image. The nurse should address this need in the support group.
Test-Taking Strategy: Use the process of elimination. Focus on the information provided in the question to determine that the issue relates to a distorted body image. This will easily direct you to option 3. If you had difficulty with this question, review the characteristics associated with the client with anorexia nervosa.
Level of Cognitive Ability: Comprehension
Client Needs: Psychosocial Integrity
Integrated Concept/Process: Nursing Process/Data Collection
Content Area: Mental Health
Reference: Varcarolis E: *Foundations of psychiatric mental health nursing,* ed 4, Philadelphia, 2002, WB Saunders, p. 415.

13. *Answer:* 4
Rationale: A nurse can be charged with false imprisonment if a client is made to wrongfully believe that he or she cannot leave the hospital. Most health care facilities have documents, which the client is asked to sign, that relate to the client's responsibilities when the client leaves against medical advice. The client should be asked to sign this document before leaving. The nurse should request that the client wait to speak to the physician before leaving, but if the client refuses to do so, the nurse cannot hold the client against their will. Restraining the client and calling security to block exits constitute false imprisonment. Any client has a right to health care and cannot be told otherwise.
Test-Taking Strategy: Use the process of elimination. Keeping the concept of false imprisonment in mind, eliminate options 1 and 2 because they are similar. Eliminate option 3 knowing that any client has a right to health care. Review the points related to false imprisonment if you had difficulty with this question.
Level of Cognitive Ability: Application
Client Needs: Safe, Effective Care Environment
Integrated Concept/Process: Nursing Process/Implementation
Content Area: Mental Health
Reference: Varcarolis E: *Foundations of psychiatric mental health nursing,* ed 4, Philadelphia, 2002, WB Saunders, p. 178.

14. *Answer:* 4
Rationale: Clients with bulimia nervosa may not initially appear to be physically or emotionally ill. They are often at or slightly below ideal body weight. On further inspection, the client demonstrates enlargement of the parotid glands with dental erosion and caries if the client has been inducing vomiting. Electrolyte imbalances are present.
Test-Taking Strategy: Use the process of elimination and note the key word "not." Knowledge regarding the characteristics noted in bulimia nervosa will assist in answering this question. Option 4 is a characteristic sign of anorexia nervosa, not bulimia nervosa. Review the characteristics of these disorders if you had difficulty with this question.
Level of Cognitive Ability: Comprehension
Client Needs: Physiological Integrity
Integrated Concept/Process: Nursing Process/Data Collection
Content Area: Mental Health
Reference: Varcarolis E: *Foundations of psychiatric mental health nursing,* ed 4, Philadelphia, 2002, WB Saunders, p. 425.

15. *Answer:* 1
Rationale: Opioids are central nervous system depressants. They generally cause drowsiness and the feeling of being out of touch with the world. Option 1 identifies the clinical manifestations associated with withdrawal from opioids. Option 2 describes withdrawal from alcohol. Option 3 describes withdrawal from nicotine. Option 4 describes withdrawal from cocaine.
Test-Taking Strategy: Use the process of elimination. Focus on the issue of the question, the clinical manifestations associated with withdrawal from opioids. If you had difficulty with this question, review the manifestations associated with opioid withdrawal.
Level of Cognitive Ability: Analysis
Client Needs: Physiological Integrity
Integrated Concept/Process: Nursing Process/Data Collection
Content Area: Mental Health
Reference: Hill S, Bauer B: *Mental health nursing,* Philadelphia, 2002, WB Saunders, p. 114.

REFERENCES

Fortinash K, Holoday-Worret P: *Psychiatric mental health nursing,* ed 2, St Louis, 2000, Mosby.

Hill S, Bauer B: *Mental health nursing,* Philadelphia, 2002, WB Saunders.

Keltner N, Schwecke L, Bostrom C: *Psychiatric nursing,* ed 3, St Louis, 1999, Mosby.

Varcarolis E: *Foundations of psychiatric mental health nursing,* ed 4, Philadelphia, 2002, WB Saunders.

Crisis Theory and Intervention

I. CRISIS INTERVENTION

A. Description
1. **Crisis** is a temporary state of severe emotional disorganization resulting from failure of **coping mechanisms** and/or lack of support
2. Decision making and problem solving are inadequate
3. Treatment is immediate, supportive, and directly responsive to the immediate **crisis** to assist the client and/or the family through the stressful situation

B. Phases of a **crisis**
1. Phase 1: external precipitating event
2. Phase 2
   a. Perception of threat
   b. Increase in anxiety
   c. Client may cope or resolve **crisis**
3. Phase 3
   a. Failure of coping
   b. Increasing disorganization
   c. Physical symptoms emerge
   d. Relationship problems
4. Phase 4
   a. Mobilization of internal and external resources
   b. Resolutions related to precrisis functioning include functioning at a higher level, at the same level, or at a lower level

C. **Crisis** intervention
1. Treatment is immediate, supportive, and directly responsive to the immediate **crisis**
2. Goal-directed intervention
3. Feelings of the client are acknowledged
4. Provides opportunities for expression and validation of feelings
5. Connections are made between the meaning of the event and the **crisis**
6. Explores alternative **coping mechanisms** and tries out new behaviors

II. GRIEVING

A. Description
1. A normal human process that occurs in response to a loss
2. Progresses through various stages, and the entire process may take up to 3 years

B. Data collection
1. Crying
2. Guilt and anger
3. Fatigue and lethargy
4. Insomnia
5. Depression
6. Agitation
7. Anorexia
8. Ambivalence
9. Somatic complaints
10. Sense of detachment and unreality
11. Denial

C. Implementation
1. Assess the client's progress through the grieving process
2. Encourage the client to express feelings about the loss and its significance on life
3. Encourage expression of angry feelings
4. Explain the normal stages of the grieving process to the client
5. Assist the client to make appropriate future plans related to changes caused by the loss
6. Encourage the client to work through the feelings associated with the loss

III. DEPRESSION

A. Description

1. Affects feelings, thoughts, and behaviors
2. Can occur after a loss, including loss of self-esteem, the end of a significant relationship, the death of a loved one, or a traumatic event
3. The loss is followed by grief and mourning, and if this process does not resolve, depression results
4. Depression may be mild, moderate, or severe
5. Treatment includes counseling, antidepressant medication, and electroconvulsive therapy (ECT)

B. Mild depression
1. Triggered by an external event, and the experience follows the normal grief reaction
2. Lasts less than 2 weeks
3. Feeling sad
4. Feeling let down or disappointed
5. Mild alterations in sleep patterns
6. Feeling less alert
7. Irritability
8. Not interested in spending time with others
9. Increased use of alcohol or drugs

C. Moderate depression
1. Persists over time
2. The person experiences a sense of change and often seeks help
3. Despondent and gloomy
4. Feels dejected
5. Low self-esteem
6. Helplessness and powerlessness
7. May experience intense anxiety and anger
8. Diurnal variation: may feel better at a certain time of the day, such as in the morning
9. Slow thought processes and difficulty in concentrating
10. Rumination: persistent thinking about and discussion of a particular subject
11. Negative thinking and suicidal thoughts
12. Sleep disturbances
13. Social withdrawal
14. Anorexia, weight loss, and fatigue
15. Somatic complaints
16. Menstrual changes
17. Increased use of alcohol or drugs

D. Severe depression
1. Intense and pervasive
2. Despair and hopelessness
3. Guilt and worthlessness
4. Flat affect
5. May show agitation and pace about
6. Poor posture and unkempt appearance
7. Decreased speech
8. Self-destructive thoughts; however, the client may lack energy to act on the thought
9. Social withdrawal
10. Poor concentration and overwhelmed by simple tasks
11. Severe psychomotor retardation
12. Anorexia and marked weight loss
13. Constipation and urinary retention
14. Lack of sexual interest
15. Terminal insomnia
16. Diurnal variation: the person feels worse in the morning and better as the day goes on
17. Delusions and hallucinations

E. Implementation
1. Altered thought processes
   a. Encourage the client to discuss losses or changes in life situation
   b. Encourage the client to express sadness or anger, and allow adequate time for verbal responses
   c. Assist in developing short-term goals
   d. Encourage the use of problem solving and positive thinking
   e. Limit decision making
   f. Spend short periods of time throughout the day with the client
   g. Be on time when a schedule is planned with the client
   h. Sit in silence with the client who is not verbalizing
   i. Use simple, concrete words when communicating
   j. Avoid a cheerful attitude
2. Risk for self-harm
   a. Assess for **suicide** clues, and intervene to provide safety precautions as necessary
   b. Ask the client directly, "Have you thought of hurting yourself?"
   c. Assess lethality of plans
   d. Do not leave the client alone for extended periods
   e. If the client has a suicidal plan, place on a one-to-one supervision
   f. Form a suicidal contract with the client
3. Activity intolerance
   a. Encourage daily exercise
   b. Assist with activities of daily living (ADLs) if the client is unable to perform them
   c. Begin with one-to-one activities
   d. Provide activities for easy mastery to increase self-esteem and assist in alleviating guilt feelings
   e. Provide activities that require little orientation (card games, drawing)
   f. Engage in gross motor activities (walking)
   g. Eventually bring the client into small group activities, and then large groups
4. Altered nutrition
   a. Ensure adequate nutrition

b. Offer small, high-calorie, high-protein snacks and fluids throughout the day
c. Stay with the client during meals
d. Weigh the client weekly
e. Assess bowel patterns for constipation

5. Assess for sleep pattern disturbance
a. Ensure adequate sleep
b. Provide rest periods after activities
c. Encourage the client to dress and stay out of bed during the day
d. Provide relaxation measures at bedtime
e. Decrease environmental stimuli at bedtime
f. Spend time with the client before bedtime

IV. SUICIDAL BEHAVIOR

A. Description
1. Suicidal clients characteristically have feelings of worthlessness, guilt, and hopelessness that are so overwhelming that they feel unable to go on with life and unfit to live
2. The nurse caring for a depressed client always considers the possibility of **suicide**

B. High-risk groups
1. Those with a history of previous **suicide attempts**
2. Family history of **suicide attempts**
3. Adolescents
4. Elderly clients
5. Disabled or terminally ill adults
6. Clients with personality disorders
7. Clients with organic brain syndrome or dementia
8. Depressed or psychotic clients
9. Substance **abusers**

C. Clues
1. Giving away personal, special, and prized possessions
2. Canceling social engagements
3. Making out or changing a will
4. Taking out or changing insurance policies
5. Positive or negative changes in behavior
6. Poor appetite
7. Sleeping difficulties
8. Feelings of hopelessness
9. Difficulty in concentrating
10. Loss of interest in activities
11. Client statements that indicate an intent to attempt **suicide**
12. Sudden calmness or improvement in a depressed client
13. Client questions about poisons, guns, or other lethal objects

D. Data collection
1. The plan
a. Does the client have a plan?
b. What is the plan, how lethal is the plan, and how likely is death to occur?
c. Does the client have the means to carry out the plan?
2. Client history of attempts
a. Were there **suicide attempts** in the past? What were the outcomes?
b. Was the client accidentally rescued?
c. Have the past attempts and methods been the same, or have methods increased in lethality?
3. Psychosocial
a. Is the client alone or alienated from others?
b. Is hostility or depression present?
c. Do hallucinations exist?
d. Is substance **abuse** present?
e. Any recent losses or physical illness?
f. Any environmental or lifestyle changes?

E. Implementation
1. Initiate **suicide** precautions
2. Remove harmful objects
3. Do not leave the client alone
4. Provide a one-to-one supervision at all times
5. Provide a nonjudgmental, caring attitude
6. Develop a contract that is written, dated, and signed and indicates alternative behavior at times of suicidal thoughts
7. Encourage the client to talk about feelings and to identify positive aspects about self
8. Encourage active participation in own care
9. Keep the client active by assigning simple tasks
10. Check that visitors do not leave harmful objects in the client's room
11. Identify support systems
12. Do not allow the client to leave the unit unless accompanied by a staff member
13. Continue to assess the client's **suicide** potential

V. ABUSIVE BEHAVIORS

A. Anger
1. A feeling of annoyance that may be displaced onto an object or person
2. Is used to avoid anxiety and gives a feeling of power in situations in which the person feels out of control

B. Violence: the physical force that is threatening to the safety of self and others

C. Aggression: can be harmful and destructive when not controlled

D. Data collection
1. History of violence or self-harm

2. Poor impulse control and low tolerance of frustration
3. Defiant and argumentative
4. Verbal threats
5. Increased pacing and agitation
6. Muscle rigidity
7. Flushed face
8. Glaring
9. Loud voice

E. Implementation
1. Acknowledge anger
2. Set limits on behavior
3. Listen actively and assist the client to deal with the consequences of anger
4. Provide safety for expressing anger and safety to others

F. **Restraints** and **seclusion**
1. Description
a. Physical **restraints**: any manual method or mechanical device, material, or equipment that inhibits free movement
b. **Seclusion**: the last step in a process to maximize safety of a client and others in which a client is placed alone in a specially designed room for protection and close supervision
c. Chemical **restraints**: medications given for a very specific purpose of inhibiting a specific behavior or movement; has an impact on the client's ability to relate to the environment
2. Use of **restraints** and **seclusion**
a. Should never be used as punishment or for the convenience of the health care staff
b. The least restrictive means of **restraint** for the shortest duration should be used
c. Used when behavior is physically harmful to the client or others
d. Used when the disruptive behavior presents a danger to the facility
e. Used when alternative or less restrictive measures are insufficient in protecting the client or others from harm
f. Used when the client anticipates that a controlled environment would be helpful and requests **seclusion**
g. Requires a written order of a physician that must be reviewed and renewed every 24 hours and that also must specify the type of **restraint** to be used
h. In an emergency, the charge nurse may place a client in **restraint** or **seclusion** and obtain a written or verbal order as soon as possible thereafter
i. Laws require the consent of the client unless an emergency situation exists and can be documented
j. The client must be removed from **restraint** or **seclusion** when safer and quieter behavior is observed
k. While in **restraint** or **seclusion**, the client must be protected from all sources of harm
l. The nurse must document the behavior leading to **restraint** or **seclusion** and the time the client is placed in and released from **restraint** or **seclusion**
m. The client in **restraint** or **seclusion** must be assessed every 15 to 30 minutes for physical needs, safety, and comfort; these observations are also documented

VI. FAMILY VIOLENCE

A. Description
1. The violence begins with threats or verbal or physical minor assaults, and the victim attempts to comply with the requests of the **abuser**
2. The **abuser** loses control and becomes destructive and harmful while the victim attempts to protect himself or herself; the **abuser** then becomes loving and attempts to make peace
3. The behavior of the **abuser** may be an attempt for closeness and companionship
4. The **abuser** believes that violence is normal and that the victim is responsible for the **abuse**
5. Outsiders are not aware of what is happening in the family, and when outsiders try to enter the family, the family feels assaulted
6. Family members are socially isolated and lack of autonomy and trust among each other exists
7. Caring and intimacy in the family are absent
8. Family members expect other members in the family to meet their needs, but none are able to do so
9. The **abuser** threatens to abandon the family

B. Characteristics of **abusers**
1. Impaired self-esteem
2. Strong dependency needs
3. Narcissistic and suspicious
4. History of sexual **abuse** during childhood
5. Perceive victims as their property and believe that they are entitled to **abuse** them

C. Characteristics of victims
1. Feel trapped, dependent, helpless, and powerless
2. Depressed
3. Low self-esteem and blame themselves for the problems

D. Implementation
1. Report cases of suspected **abuse**

2. Assess situations associated with family violence
3. Assess for evidence of physical injuries
4. Ensure privacy and confidentiality during assessment, and provide a nonjudgmental and empathetic approach to foster trust
5. Assist in resolving family dysfunction with prescribed therapies
6. Encourage psychotherapy, counseling, group therapy, and support groups to assist family members to develop coping strategies
7. Encourage individual therapy for victims that promotes coping with the trauma and prevents further psychological conflict
8. Provide individual therapy for **abusers** that focuses on preventing violent behavior and repairing relationships
9. Ensure that the victim is not left alone with **abuser**
10. Assist the victim to understand his or her participation in the **abuse**
11. Assist the victim to develop self-protective abilities and other problem-solving abilities
12. Provide support and assistance in coping with contacting the legal system
13. Assist the family to identify an access to community and personal resources

VII. CHILD ABUSE (SEE CHAPTER 28)

A. Description: involves emotional or physical **abuse** or neglect, as well as sexual exploitation or molestation by caretakers or other individuals

B. Data collection
1. Physical **abuse**
   a. Unexplained bruises, burns, or fractures
   b. Bald spots on scalp
   c. Apprehensive child
   d. Extreme aggressiveness or withdrawal
   e. Fear of parents
   f. Lack of crying when approached by a stranger
2. Physical neglect
   a. Inadequate weight gain
   b. Poor hygiene
   c. Consistent hunger
   d. Inconsistent school attendance
   e. Constant fatigue
   f. Reports of lack of child supervision
   g. Delinquency
3. Emotional **abuse**
   a. Speech disorders
   b. Habit disorders, such as sucking, biting, rocking
   c. Psychoneurotic reactions
   d. Learning disorders
   e. **Suicide attempts**
4. Sexual **abuse**
   a. Difficulty walking or sitting
   b. Torn, stained, or bloody underclothing
   c. Pain, swelling, or itching of the genitals
   d. Bruises, bleeding, or lacerations in the genital or anal area
   e. Unwillingness to change clothes or unwillingness to participate in gym activities
   f. Poor peer relations
   g. Delinquency
   h. Changes in sleep patterns
   i. Self-disruptive behavior

C. Implementation 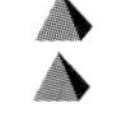
1. Report cases of suspected **abuse**
2. Support the child during a thorough physical assessment
3. Assess injuries
4. Place the child in an environment that is safe, thereby preventing further injury
5. Move slowly around the child
6. Avoid loud noises around the child
7. Communicate with the child at the child's eye level
8. Reassure the child that he or she is not a bad person, that the child is loved and not responsible for the **abuser's** behavior
9. Do not rescue the child from the parents
10. Document in an objective manner information related to the suspected **abuse**
11. Assess parents' strengths and weaknesses, normal **coping mechanisms,** and presence or absence of support systems
12. Assist the family in identifying stressors and alternative ways to express feelings
13. Provide education to the parents and refer the parents to **crisis** hotlines and community support systems

VIII. ELDER ABUSE

A. Description
1. **Abuse** can be physical, sexual, psychological, or financial
2. Neglect can include unintentional failure to care for the elder person's needs or an intentional neglect, such as abandonment
3. Victims may attempt to dismiss injuries as accidental, and **abusers** may prevent victims from receiving proper medical care to avoid discovery
4. Victims are often socially isolated
5. Victims may be care providers for the **abusers**

B. Data collection
1. Physical **abuse**

a. Fractures
b. Lacerations
c. Punctures
d. Bruises
e. Burns
2. Sexual **abuse**
a. Torn or stained underclothing
b. Discomfort or bleeding in the genital area
c. Difficulty in walking or sitting
d. Unexplained genital infections or disease
3. Psychological **abuse**
a. Confusion
b. Fearful and agitated
c. Changes in appetite and weight
d. Withdrawn and loss of interest in self and social activities
4. Financial **abuse**
a. Fearful when discussing finances
b. Confused, inaccurate, or no knowledge of finances
c. Inability to pay bills
5. Neglect
a. Disheveled appearance
b. Dehydration and malnutrition
c. Dressed inadequately or inappropriately
d. Lacking physical needs, such as glasses, hearing aids, and dentures
e. Skin breaks
f. Signs of medication overdose

C. Implementation
1. Report cases of suspected **abuse**
2. Assess for physical injuries
3. Assist with providing care to treat physical injuries
4. Assist with legal procedures, such as police reports, order of protection, and court-ordered counseling
5. Explore alternative living arrangements that are least restrictive and disruptive to the victim
6. Assist with financial management protection
7. Encourage counseling and provide referrals to emergency community resources
8. Refer to protective services for adults
9. Arrange counseling and treatment for the **abuser**

IX. RAPE AND SEXUAL ASSAULT

A. Description
1. Engaging another person in a sexual act and/or sexual intercourse through the use of force and without the consent of the sexual partner
2. The victim is not required by law to report the rape or assault
3. The victim is often blamed by others and often receives no support from significant others
4. Acquaintance rapes involve someone known to the victim
5. Statutory rape is the act of sexual intercourse with someone under the age of legal consent even if there is consent from the minor

B. Data collection
1. Female client
a. Obtain the date of the last menstrual period
b. Determine the form of birth control used and the last act of intercourse before the rape
c. Determine duration of intercourse, orifices violated, and penile penetration
d. Determine whether a condom was used by perpetrator
2. Discuss shame, embarrassment, and humiliation
3. Discuss anger and revenge
4. Discuss fear of telling others for fear of not being believed

C. Rape trauma syndrome
1. Sleep disturbances, nightmares
2. Loss of appetite
3. Fears, anxiety, phobias, suspicion
4. Decrease in activities and motivation
5. Disruptions in relationships with partner, family, friends
6. Self-blame, guilt, shame
7. Lowered self-esteem, feelings of worthlessness
8. Somatic complaints

D. Implementation
1. Encourage the client not to shower, bathe, douche (female), or change clothing
2. Assist with the female pelvic examination and obtaining specimens to detect for semen
3. Preserve any evidence
4. Treat physical injuries
5. Provide client safety
6. Assist the client to refrain from self-blame
7. Reinforce to the client that survival of the assault is most important; if the victim survived the rape, then he or she did exactly what was necessary to stay alive
8. Refer to **crisis** intervention and support groups

PRACTICE QUESTIONS

1. A nurse is reviewing the health care record of a client admitted to the psychiatric unit. The nurse notes that the admission nurse has documented that the client is experiencing anxiety as a result of a situational

crisis. The nurse would determine that this type of crisis could be caused by:
1. A fire that destroyed the client's home
2. A recent rape episode experienced by the client
3. The death of a loved one
4. Witnessing a murder

2. A nurse is gathering data from a client in crisis. When determining the client's perception of the precipitating event that led to the crisis, the most appropriate question to ask is:
   1. "What leads you to seek help now?"
   2. "Who is available to help you?"
   3. "What do you usually do to feel better?"
   4. "With whom do you live?"
3. A nurse is assisting in developing a plan of care for the client in a crisis state. When developing the plan, the nurse will consider which of the following?
   1. Presenting symptoms in a crisis situation are similar for all individuals experiencing a crisis
   2. A crisis state indicates that the individual is suffering from an emotional illness
   3. A crisis state indicates that the individual is suffering from a mental illness
   4. A client's response to a crisis is individualized and what constitutes a crisis for one person may not constitute a crisis for another person
4. A nurse observes that a client with a potential for violence is agitated, pacing up and down the hallway, and is making aggressive and belligerent gestures at other clients. Which of the following statements would be most appropriate to make to this client?
   1. "What is causing you to become agitated?"
   2. "You need to stop that behavior now!"
   3. "You will need to be restrained if you do not change your behavior."
   4. "You will need to be placed in seclusion!"
5. During a conversation with a depressed client on a psychiatric unit, the client says to the nurse "My family would be better off without me." The nurse's best response is:
   1. "Everyone feels this way when they are depressed."
   2. "Have you talked to your family about this?"
   3. "You sound very upset. Are you thinking of hurting yourself?"
   4. "You will feel better once your medication begins to work."
6. A nurse is caring for an older adult client who has recently lost her husband. The client says, "No one cares about me anymore. All the people I loved are dead." Which of the following responses by the nurse is most therapeutic?
   1. "That seems rather unlikely to me."
   2. "You must be feeling all alone at this point?"
   3. "I don't believe that and neither do you."
   4. "Right! Why not just `pack it in'?"
7. A nurse is planning care for a client who is being hospitalized because the client has been displaying violent behavior and is at risk for potential harm to others. Which of the following would not be a component of the plan of care?
   1. Keep the door to the client's room open when with the client
   2. Assign the client to a room at the end of the hall to avoid disturbing the other clients
   3. Face the client when providing care
   4. Ensure that a security officer is within the immediate area
8. Which behaviors observed by the nurse might lead to the suspicion that a depressed female adolescent client may be suicidal?
   1. The client becomes angry while speaking on the telephone and slams the receiver down on the hook
   2. The client runs out of the therapy group swearing at the group leader and runs to her room
   3. The client gets angry with her roommate when the roommate borrows the client's clothes without asking
   4. The client gives away a prized CD and a cherished autograph picture of the performer
9. A client is admitted to the psychiatric unit after a serious suicidal attempt by hanging. The nurse's most important aspect of care is to maintain client safety. This is accomplished best by:
   1. Assigning a staff member to the client who will remain with the client at all times
   2. Admitting the client to a seclusion room where all potentially dangerous articles are removed
   3. Removing the client's clothing and placing the client in a hospital gown
   4. Requesting that a peer remain with the client at all times
10. The police arrive at the emergency room with a client who has seriously lacerated both wrists. The initial nursing action is to:
    1. Examine and treat the wound sites
    2. Secure and record a detailed history
    3. Encourage and assist the client to ventilate feelings
    4. Administer an antianxiety agent
11. A nurse receives a telephone call from a male client who states that he wants to kill himself and has a bottle of sleeping pills in front of him. The best nursing action is to:
    1. Insist that the client give you his name and address so that you can get the police there immediately
    2. Keep the client talking and allow the client to ventilate feelings
    3. Use therapeutic communications, especially the reflection of feelings

4. Keep the client talking, signal to another staff member to trace the call so that appropriate help can be sent

12. A nurse is caring for a client with severe depression. Which of the following activities would be most appropriate for this client?
   1. Paint by number
   2. A puzzle
   3. Drawing
   4. Checkers

13. A client in a severe major depressive episode is unable to address activities of daily living. The most appropriate nursing intervention is to:
   1. Feed, bathe, and dress the client as needed until the client can perform these activities independently
   2. Structure the client's day so that adequate time can be devoted to the client's assuming responsibility for the activities of daily living
   3. Offer the client choices and consequences to the failure to comply with the expectation of maintaining activities of daily living
   4. Have the client's peers confront the client about how the noncompliance in addressing activities of daily living affects the milieu

14. An elderly male client who is a victim of elder abuse and the family have been attending weekly counseling sessions. Which of the following statements, if made by the abusive family member, would indicate that he or she has learned positive coping skills?
   1. "I will be more careful to make sure that my father's needs are met."
   2. "I am so sorry and embarrassed that the abusive event occurred. It won't happen again."
   3. "I feel better able to care for my father now that I know where to obtain assistance."
   4. "Now that my father is moving into my home, I will need to change my ways."

15. A nurse is assisting in planning care for a client being admitted to the nursing unit who attempted suicide. Which of the following priority nursing interventions will the nurse include in the plan of care?
   1. Check the whereabouts of the client every 15 minutes
   2. Suicide precautions with 30 minute checks
   3. One-to-one suicide precautions
   4. Ask that the client report suicidal thoughts immediately

ANSWERS

1. *Answer:* 3

Rationale: A situational crisis arises from external rather than internal sources. External situations that could precipitate crisis include loss of or change of a job, the death of a loved one, abortion, a change in financial status, divorce, the addition of new family members, pregnancy, and severe illness. Options 1, 2, and 4 identify adventitious crisis. An adventitious crisis is not a part of every day life, is unplanned, and accidental.

Test-Taking Strategy: Use the process of elimination and focus on the key words "situational crisis." This will assist in eliminating options 1, 2, and 4 because of the nature of their similarity. If you had difficulty with this question, review the types of crisis.

Level of Cognitive Ability: Comprehension

Client Needs: Psychosocial Integrity

Integrated Concept/Process: Nursing Process/Data Collection

Content Area: Mental Health

Reference: Varcarolis E: *Foundations of psychiatric mental health nursing*, ed 4, Philadelphia, 2002, WB Saunders, p. 617.

2. *Answer:* 1

Rationale: A nurse's initial task when gathering data from a client in crisis is to assess the individual or family and the problem. The more clearly the problem can be defined, the better the chance a solution can be found. Option 1 will assist in determining data related to the precipitating event that led to the crisis. Options 2 and 4 identify situational supports. Option 3 identifies personal coping skills.

Test-Taking Strategy: Use the process of elimination. Note the key words "precipitating event." Focus on these key words when selecting the correct option. Eliminate options 2 and 4 because this information will determine support systems. Eliminate option 3 because this question would be asked when determining coping skills. Review data collection methods for a client in crisis if you had difficulty with this question.

Level of Cognitive Ability: Application

Client Needs: Psychosocial Integrity

Integrated Concept/Process: Nursing Process/Data Collection

Content Area: Mental Health

Reference: Varcarolis E: *Foundations of psychiatric mental health nursing*, ed 4, Philadelphia, 2002, WB Saunders, p. 616.

3. *Answer:* 4

Rationale: Although each crisis response can be described in similar terms as far as presenting symptoms are concerned, what constitutes a crisis for one person may not constitute a crisis for another person because each is a unique individual. Being in a crisis state does not mean that the client is suffering from an emotional or mental illness.

Test-Taking Strategy: Use the process of elimination. Eliminate option 1 because of the word "all." Next eliminate options 2 and 3 because a crisis does not indicate "illness." Review the

characteristics of a crisis state if you had difficulty with this question.
Level of Cognitive Ability: Comprehension
Client Needs: Psychosocial Integrity
Integrated Concept/Process: Nursing Process/Data Collection
Content Area: Mental Health
Reference: Varcarolis E: *Foundations of psychiatric mental health nursing*, ed 4, Philadelphia, 2002, WB Saunders, p. 616.

4. *Answer:* 1
Rationale: The best statement is to ask the client what is causing the agitation. This will assist the client to become aware of the behavior and will assist the nurse in planning appropriate interventions for the client. Option 2 is demanding behavior, which could cause increased agitation in the client. Options 3 and 4 are threats to the client and are inappropriate.
Test-Taking Strategy: Use the process of elimination. Eliminate option 2 because of the demand that it places on the client. Eliminate options 3 and 4 because they indicate threats to the client. Review appropriate nursing interventions for the agitated client if you had difficulty with this question.
Level of Cognitive Ability: Application
Client Needs: Psychosocial Integrity
Integrated Concept/Process: Communication and Documentation
Content Area: Mental Health
Reference: Varcarolis E: *Foundations of psychiatric mental health nursing*, ed 4, Philadelphia, 2002, WB Saunders, p. 666.

5. *Answer:* 3
Rationale: Clients who are depressed may be at risk for suicide. It is critical for the nurse to assess suicidal ideation and plan. The client should be directly asked if a plan for self-harm exists. Options 1, 2, and 4 are not therapeutic responses.
Test-Taking Strategy: Use therapeutic communication techniques. Option 3 is the only option that deals directly with the client's feelings. Additionally, clients at risk for suicide need to be directly assessed regarding the potential for self-harm. Review data collection techniques for the depressed client if you had difficulty with this question.
Level of Cognitive Ability: Application
Client Needs: Psychosocial Integrity
Integrated Concept/Process: Nursing Process/Data Collection
Content Area: Mental Health
Reference: Varcarolis E: *Foundations of psychiatric mental health nursing*, ed 4, Philadelphia,' 2002, WB Saunders, p. 640.

6. *Answer:* 2
Rationale: The client is experiencing loss and is feeling hopeless. The most therapeutic response by the nurse is the one that attempts to translate words into feelings. In option 1, the nurse is voicing doubt, which is often used when a client verbalizes delusional ideas. In option 3, the nurse is disagreeing with the client, which implies that the nurse has passed judgment on the client's ideas or opinions. In option 4, the nurse uses sarcasm, which gives advice and is nontherapeutic as a nursing response.
Test-Taking Strategy: Use therapeutic communication techniques. Option 2 is the only option that focuses on the client's feelings. Review therapeutic communication techniques if you had difficulty with this question.
Level of Cognitive Ability: Application
Client Needs: Psychosocial Integrity
Integrated Concept/Process: Communication and Documentation
Content Area: Mental Health
Reference: Varcarolis E: *Foundations of psychiatric mental health nursing*, ed 4, Philadelphia, 2002, WB Saunders, p. 254.

7. *Answer:* 2
Rationale: The client should be placed in a room near the nurses' station and not at the end of a long, relatively unprotected corridor. The nurse should not isolate self with a potentially violent client. The door to the client's room should be kept open, and the nurse should never turn away from the client. A security officer or male aide should be within immediate call if there is a suspicion that an act of violence is imminent.
Test-Taking Strategy: Use the process of elimination. Note the key word "not" in the stem of the question. Keeping in mind that safety is the issue, you should easily be able to select the correct option. If you had difficulty with this question, review guidelines in caring for the violent client.
Level of Cognitive Ability: Application
Client Needs: Safe, Effective Care Environment
Integrated Concept/Process: Nursing Process/Implementation
Content Area: Mental Health
Reference: Varcarolis E: *Foundations of psychiatric mental health nursing*, ed 4, Philadelphia, 2002, WB Saunders, p. 679.

8. *Answer:* 4
Rationale: A depressed, suicidal client often "gives" away that which is of value as a way of saying "good-bye" and wanting to be remembered. Options 1, 2, and 3 identify acting-out behaviors.
Test-Taking Strategy: Use the process of elimination. Options 1, 2, and 3 are similar in that they deal with anger and "acting out behaviors," which are often typical of any adolescent. Option 4 is different in nature and an action that could indicate that the client may be "saying good-bye." Review the clues that indicate suicide if you had difficulty with this question.
Level of Cognitive Ability: Analysis
Client Needs: Psychosocial Integrity
Integrated Concept/Process: Nursing Process/Data Collection
Content Area: Mental Health
Reference: Varcarolis E: *Foundations of psychiatric mental health nursing*, ed 4, Philadelphia, 2002, WB Saunders, p. 641.

9. *Answer:* 1
Rationale: Hanging is a serious suicide attempt. The plan of care must reflect action that will promote the client's safety. Constant observation status (one-on-one) with a staff member who is never less than an arm's length away is the best intervention.
Test-Taking Strategy: Use the process of elimination. Eliminate option 2 because seclusion should not be the initial intervention. Eliminate option 4 next because the responsibility to safeguard a client is not the peer's responsibility. Eliminate option 3 because removing one's clothing will not maximize

all possible safety strategies. Review nursing interventions for the client at risk for suicide if you had difficulty with this question.
Level of Cognitive Ability: Application
Client Needs: Safe, Effective Care Environment
Integrated Concept/Process: Nursing Process/Implementation
Content Area: Mental Health
Reference: Varcarolis E: *Foundations of psychiatric mental health nursing,* ed 4, Philadelphia, 2002, WB Saunders, p. 643.

10. *Answer:* 1
Rationale: The initial nursing action is to examine and treat the self-inflicted injuries. Injuries from lacerated wrists can lead to a life-threatening situation. Other interventions may follow after the client has been treated medically.
Test-Taking Strategy: Use Maslow's Hierarchy of Needs theory to prioritize. Physiological needs come first. Option 1 addresses the physiological need. Review care to the client who attempted suicide if you had difficulty with this question.
Level of Cognitive Ability: Application
Client Needs: Physiological Integrity
Integrated Concept/Process: Nursing Process/Implementation
Content Area: Mental Health
Reference: Varcarolis E: *Foundations of psychiatric mental health nursing,* ed 4, Philadelphia, 2002, WB Saunders, p. 385.

11. *Answer:* 4
Rationale: In a crisis, the nurse must take an authoritative, active role to promote the client's safety. A bottle of sleeping pills in front of a client who verbalizes he wants to kill himself is a "crisis." The client's safety is of prime concern. Keeping the client on the phone and getting help to the client is the best intervention. The word "insist" may anger the client and he might hang up. Option 2 lacks the authoritative action stance of securing the client's safety. Using therapeutic communication is important, but overuse of "reflection" may sound uncaring or superficial and is lacking direction/solutions to the immediate problem of the client's safety.
Test-Taking Strategy: Use the process of elimination and focus on the client's safety. Although each of the options may seem appropriate, the best option is option 4. It is the most global option and encompasses every necessary action. Review interventions for the client who is suicidal if you had difficulty with this question.
Level of Cognitive Ability: Application
Client Needs: Safe, Effective Care Environment
Integrated Concept/Process: Nursing Process/Implementation
Content Area: Mental Health
Reference: Varcarolis E: *Foundations of psychiatric mental health nursing,* ed 4, Philadelphia, 2002, WB Saunders, p. 616.

12. *Answer:* 3
Rationale: Concentration and memory are poor in a client with severe depression. When a client has a diagnosis of severe depression, the nurse needs to provide activities that require little concentration. Activities that have no right or wrong choices or decisions minimize opportunities for the client to put themselves down.
Test-Taking Strategy: Use the process of elimination. Note the similarities in options 1, 2, and 4 in that they all require concentration. It is important to remember that clients with depression have difficulty concentrating and need activities that require little concentration. Review care to the client with severe depression if you had difficulty with this question.
Level of Cognitive Ability: Application
Client Needs: Psychosocial Integrity
Integrated Concept/Process: Nursing Process/Implementation
Content Area: Mental Health
Reference: Varcarolis E: *Foundations of psychiatric mental health nursing,* ed 4, Philadelphia, 2002, WB Saunders, p. 460.

13. *Answer:* 1
Rationale: The client with depression may not have the energy or interest to complete activities of daily living. Often, severely depressed clients are unable to perform even the simplest of activities of daily living. The nurse assumes this role and completes these tasks with the client. Options 2 and 3 are incorrect because the client lacks the energy and motivation to perform these tasks independently. Option 4 will increase the client's feelings of poor self-esteem and unworthiness.
Test-Taking Strategy: Use the process of elimination. Note the key words "severe major depressive episode." Eliminate options 2 and 3 because the client lacks the energy and motivation to do these independently. In addition, option 3 may lead to increased feelings of worthlessness as the client fails to meet expectations. Option 4 will increase the client's feelings of poor self-esteem and unworthiness. Review care to the client with severe depression if you had difficulty with this question.
Level of Cognitive Ability: Application
Client Needs: Physiological Integrity
Integrated Concept/Process: Nursing Process/Implementation
Content Area: Mental Health
Reference: Varcarolis E: *Foundations of psychiatric mental health nursing,* ed 4, Philadelphia, 2002, WB Saunders, p. 467.

14. *Answer:* 3
Rationale: Elder abuse is sometimes the result of family members who are being expected to care for their aging parents. This care can cause the family to become overextended, frustrated, or financially depleted. Knowing where to turn in the community for assistance in caring for aging family members can bring the much needed relief. Using these alternatives is a positive alternative coping strategy that many families use.
Test-Taking Strategy: Use the process of elimination and focus on the issue, a coping strategy. Only option 3 identifies a means of coping with the issues. The other options are statements of good faith or promises, which may or may not be kept in the future. Option 3 outlines a definitive plan for how to handle the pressure associated with the father's care. Review effective coping strategies if you had difficulty with this question.
Level of Cognitive Ability: Analysis
Client Needs: Health Promotion and Maintenance
Integrated Concept/Process: Nursing Process/Evaluation
Content Area: Mental Health
Reference: Varcarolis E: *Foundations of psychiatric mental health nursing,* ed 4, Philadelphia, 2002, WB Saunders, p. 710.

15. *Answer:* 3
Rationale: One-to-one suicide precautions are required for the client who has attempted suicide. Options 1 and 2 may be

appropriate but not at the present time considering the situation. Option 4 may also be an appropriate nursing intervention, but the priority is stated in option 3. The best option is constant supervision so that the nurse may intervene as needed if the client attempts to cause harm to self.

Test-Taking Strategy: Use the process of elimination. Note the key word "priority" in the stem of the question. Recalling that one-to-one suicide precaution is the priority in caring for a suicidal client will direct you to option 3. Review interventions for the suicidal client if you had difficulty with this question.

Level of Cognitive Ability: Application

Client Needs: Safe, Effective Care Environment

Integrated Concept/Process: Nursing Process/Implementation

Content Area: Mental Health

Reference: Varcarolis E: *Foundations of psychiatric mental health nursing,* ed 4, Philadelphia, 2002, WB Saunders, p. 639.

REFERENCES

Fortinash K, Holoday-Worret P: *Psychiatric mental health nursing,* ed 2, St Louis, 2000, Mosby.

Hill S, Bauer B: *Mental health nursing,* Philadelphia, 2002, WB Saunders.

Keltner N, Schwecke L, Bostrom C: *Psychiatric nursing,* ed 3, St Louis, 1999, Mosby.

Varcarolis E: *Foundations of psychiatric mental health nursing,* ed 4, Philadelphia, 2002, WB Saunders.

64 Psychiatric Medications

I. SELECTIVE SEROTONIN REUPTAKE INHIBITORS (SSRI) (Box 64-1)

A. Description
1. Inhibit serotonin uptake
2. Produce an antidepressant response

B. Side effects
1. Nausea and diarrhea
2. Dry mouth
3. Central nervous system (CNS) stimulation
4. Photosensitivity
5. Insomnia
6. Nervousness
7. Headache
8. Dizziness
9. Weight loss

C. Implementation
1. Monitor vital signs
2. Monitor weight
3. Initiate safety precautions, particularly if dizziness occurs
4. Instruct the client to take a single dose in the morning to prevent insomnia
5. Administer with a snack or with meals to reduce the risk of dizziness and light-headedness
6. Monitor the suicidal client, especially during improved mood and increased energy levels
7. Instruct client that fluoxetine (Prozac) should be taken early in the day to avoid interference with sleep
8. For the client on long-term therapy, monitor liver and renal function tests
9. Monitor the white blood cell (WBC) and neutrophil counts and discontinue the medication, as prescribed, if levels fall below normal
10. If priapism (painful, prolonged penile erection) occurs, notify the physician immediately
11. Instruct the client to change positions slowly to avoid a hypotensive effect
12. Instruct the client to avoid alcohol
13. Instruct the client to report any visual changes to the physician

BOX 64-1

Selective Serotonin Reuptake Inhibitors (SSRI)

Citalopram (Celexa)
Fluoxetine (Prozac)
Fluvoxamine (Luvox)
Paroxetine HCl (Paxil)
Sertraline HCl (Zoloft)
Venlafaxine (Effexor)

II. TRICYCLIC ANTIDEPRESSANTS (Box 64-2)

A. Description
1. Block the reuptake of norepinephrine and serotonin at the presynaptic neuron
2. Used to treat depression
3. May reduce seizure threshold
4. May reduce effectiveness of antihypertensive agents
5. Concurrent use with alcohol or antihistamines can cause CNS depression
6. Concurrent use with monoamine oxidase inhibitors (MAOIs) can cause hypertensive crisis

B. Side effects
1. Anticholinergic effects
2. Dry mouth

BOX 64-2

Tricyclic Antidepressants

Amitriptyline HCl (Elavil)
Amoxapine (Asendin)
Bupropion (Wellbutrin, Zyban)
Clomipramine (Anafranil)
Desipramine HCl (Norpramin)
Doxepin HCl (Sinequan)
Fluoxetine HCl (Prozac)
Imipramine HCl (Tofranil)
Maprotiline (Ludiomil)
Mirtazapine (Remeron)
Nefazodone HCl (Serzone)
Nortriptyline HCl (Aventyl)
Protriptyline HCl (Vivactil)
Trazodone HCl (Desyrel)
Trimipramine maleate (Surmontil)

3. Decreased gastrointestinal (GI) motility and constipation
4. Difficulty voiding
5. Dilated pupils and blurred vision
6. Photosensitivity
7. Cardiovascular disturbances
8. Tachycardia, dysrhythmias
9. Orthostatic hypotension
10. Sedation
11. Weight gain
12. Anxiety, restlessness, and irritability
13. Decreased or increased libido, with ejaculatory and erection disturbances

C. Implementation
1. Instruct the client that the medication may take several weeks to produce the desired effect (client response may not occur until 2 to 4 weeks after the first dose)
2. Monitor the suicidal client, especially during improved mood and increased energy levels
3. Instruct the client to change positions slowly to avoid a hypotensive effect
4. Monitor pattern of daily bowel activity
5. Assess for urinary retention
6. For the client on long-term therapy, monitor liver and renal function tests
7. Administer with food or milk if GI distress occurs
8. Administer the entire daily oral dose at one time, preferably at bedtime
9. Instruct the client to avoid alcohol and nonprescription medications to prevent adverse medication interactions
10. Instruct the client to avoid driving and other activities requiring alertness
11. When the medication is discontinued, it should be tapered gradually

III. MONOAMINE OXIDASE INHIBITORS (Box 64-3)

A. Description
1. Inhibit MAO enzyme, which is present in the brain, blood platelets, liver, spleen, and kidneys
2. Inhibition of the MAO enzyme metabolizes amines, norepinephrine, and serotonin, and the concentration of these amines increases
3. Used for depression in the client who has not responded to other antidepressant therapies, including electroconvulsive therapy
4. Concurrent use with amphetamines, antidepressants, dopamine, epinephrine, guanethidine, levodopa, methyldopa, nasal decongestants, norepinephrine, reserpine, tyramine-containing foods, and vasoconstrictors may cause hypertensive crisis
5. Concurrent use with narcotic analgesics may cause hypertension, hypotension, coma, or seizures

B. Side effects
1. Orthostatic hypotension
2. Restlessness
3. Insomnia
4. Dizziness
5. Weakness, lethargy
6. GI upset
7. Dry mouth
8. Weight gain
9. Peripheral edema
10. Anticholinergic effects
11. CNS stimulation, including anxiety, agitation, and mania
12. Delay in ejaculation

C. Hypertensive crisis
1. Hypertension
2. Occipital headache radiating frontally
3. Neck stiffness and soreness
4. Nausea and vomiting
5. Sweating
6. Fever and chills
7. Clammy skin
8. Dilated pupils
9. Palpitations, tachycardia, or bradycardia
10. Constricting chest pain

BOX 64-3

Monoamine Oxidase Inhibitors (MAOIs)

Isocarboxazid (Marplan)
Phenelzine sulfate (Nardil)
Tranylcypromine sulfate (Parnate)

11. Antidote for hypertensive crisis: 5 to 10 mg phentolamine (Regitine) intravenous (IV) injection

D. Implementation
1. Monitor blood pressure frequently for hypertension
2. Monitor for signs of hypertensive crisis
3. If palpitations or frequent headaches occur, notify the physician and discontinue the medication as prescribed
4. Administer with food if GI distress occurs
5. Instruct the client that the medication effect may be noted during the first week of therapy, but maximum benefit may take up to 3 weeks
6. Instruct the client to report headache, neck stiffness, or neck soreness immediately
7. Instruct the client to change positions slowly to prevent orthostatic hypotension
8. Instruct the client to avoid caffeine or over-the-counter preparations such as weight-reducing pills or medications for hay fever and colds
9. Monitor for client compliance with medication administration
10. Instruct the client to carry a Medic-Alert card indicating that a MAOI medication is prescribed
11. Avoid administering the medication in the evening because insomnia may result
12. MAOIs should be tapered and discontinued 7 to 14 days before surgery
13. When the medication is discontinued, it should be discontinued gradually
14. Instruct the client to avoid foods that require bacteria or molds for their preparation or preservation or those that contain tyramine (Box 64-4)

IV. ANTIMANIC MEDICATIONS (Box 64-5)

A. Description
1. Affect cellular transport mechanism and alter both the presynaptic and postsynaptic events affecting serotonin, thus enhancing serotonin function
2. Concurrent use with diuretics, fluoxetine, methyldopa, or nonsteroidal antiinflammatory medications increases lithium reabsorption by the kidney, or inhibits lithium excretion, either of which increases the risk of lithium toxicity
3. Acetazolamide, aminophylline, phenothiazines, or sodium bicarbonate may increase renal excretion of lithium, reducing its effectiveness
4. The therapeutic dose is only slightly less than the amount producing toxicity
5. The therapeutic drug serum level of lithium is 0.6 to 1.2 mEq/L
6. The causes of an increase in lithium level include decreased sodium intake, fluid and electrolyte loss associated with severe sweating, dehydration, diarrhea, or diuretic therapy, illness, or overdose
7. Serum lithium levels should be checked every 1 to 2 months or whenever any behavioral change suggests an altered serum level
8. Blood samples to check serum lithium levels should be drawn in the morning, 12 hours after the last dose was taken

B. Side effects
1. Polyuria
2. Polydipsia
3. Anorexia, nausea
4. Dry mouth
5. Mild thirst
6. Weight gain
7. Abdominal bloating
8. Soft stools or diarrhea
9. Fine hand tremors
10. Inability to concentrate
11. Muscle weakness

BOX 64-4

Tyramine Foods to Avoid

Cheese, especially aged, except cottage cheese
Sour cream
Pickled herring
Avocados
Bananas
Papaya
Broad beans
Figs
Overripe fruit
Brewer's yeast
Meat extracts and tenderizers
Yogurt
Sausage, bologna, pepperoni, salami
Soy sauce
Raisins
Red wine, beer, sherry
Beef or chicken liver
Caffeine as coffee, tea, or chocolate

BOX 64-5

Antimanic Medications

Lithium carbonate (Eskalith, Lithane, Lithobid)
Lithium citrate (Cibalith-S)

12. Lethargy
13. Fatigue
14. Headache
15. Hair loss

C. Implementation
1. Monitor the suicidal client, especially during improved mood and increased energy levels
2. Administer the medication with food to minimize GI irritation
3. Instruct the client to maintain a fluid intake of 6 to 8 glasses of water a day
4. Instruct the client to avoid excessive amounts of coffee, tea, or cola, which have a diuretic effect
5. Instruct the client to maintain an adequate salt intake
6. Do not administer diuretics while the client is taking lithium
7. Instruct the client to avoid alcohol
8. Instruct the client to avoid over-the-counter medications
9. Instruct the client that he or she may take a missed dose within 2 hours of scheduled time; otherwise the client should skip the missed dose and take the next dose at the scheduled time
10. Instruct the client not to adjust the dosage without consulting the physician, because lithium should be tapered off and not discontinued abruptly
11. Instruct the client in the signs and symptoms of lithium toxicity
12. Instruct the client to notify the physician if polyuria, prolonged vomiting, diarrhea, or fever occurs
13. Instruct the client that the therapeutic response to the medication will be noted in 1 to 3 weeks
14. Monitor electrocardiogram, renal function tests, and thyroid tests

D. Lithium toxicity
1. Description
   a. Occurs when ingested lithium cannot be detoxified and excreted by the kidneys
   b. Symptoms of toxicity begin to appear when the serum lithium level is 1.5 to 2.0 mEq/L
2. Mild toxicity
   a. Serum lithium level at 1.5 mEq/L
   b. Apathy
   c. Lethargy
   d. Diminished concentration
   e. Mild ataxia
   f. Coarse hand tremors
   g. Slight muscle weakness
3. Moderate toxicity
   a. Serum lithium level of 1.5 to 2.5 mEq/L
   b. Nausea, vomiting
   c. Severe diarrhea
   d. Mild to moderate ataxia and incoordination
   e. Slurred speech
   f. Tinnitus
   g. Blurred vision
   h. Muscle twitching
   i. Irregular tremors
4. Severe toxicity
   a. Serum lithium level above 2.5 mEq/L
   b. Nystagmus
   c. Muscle fasciculations
   d. Deep tendon hyperreflexia
   e. Visual or tactile hallucinations
   f. Oliguria or anuria
   g. Impaired level of consciousness (LOC)
   h. Tonic-clonic seizures or coma leading to death
5. Implementation for lithium toxicity
   a. Hold lithium and notify the physician
   b. Monitor vital signs and LOC
   c. Monitor cardiac status
   d. Prepare to obtain lithium level; electrolyte, blood urea nitrogen, and creatinine counts; and complete blood cell count
   e. Monitor for suicidal tendencies and institute **suicide** precautions

V. ANTIANXIETY OR ANXIOLYTIC MEDICATIONS

A. Description
1. Depress the CNS, thereby increasing the effects of gamma-aminobutyric acid (GABA), which produces relaxation and may depress the limbic system
2. Benzodiazepines have anxiety reducing (anxiolytic), sedative-hypnotic, muscle relaxing, and anticonvulsant actions (Box 64-6)

BOX 64-6

BENZODIAZEPINES

Alprazolam (Xanax)
Chlordiazepoxide HCl (Librium)
Clonazepam (Klonopin)
Clorazepate (Tranxene)
Diazepam (Valium)
Estazolam (ProSom)
Flurazepam (Dalmane)
Halazepam (Paxipam)
Lorazepam (Ativan)
Oxazepam (Serax)
Prazepam (Centrax)
Quazepam (Doral)
Temazepam (Restoril)
Triazolam (Halcion)

B. Side effects
  1. Daytime sedation
  2. Ataxia
  3. Dizziness
  4. Headaches
  5. Blurred or double vision
  6. Hypotension
  7. Tremor
  8. Amnesia
  9. Slurred speech
  10. Urinary incontinence
  11. Constipation
  12. Paradoxical CNS excitement

C. Acute toxicity
  1. Somnolence
  2. Confusion
  3. Diminished reflexes and coma
  4. Flumazenil (Romazicon), a benzodiazepine antagonist, administered IV, will reverse benzodiazepine intoxication in 5 minutes
  5. The client being treated for an overdose of a benzodiazepine may experience agitation, restlessness, discomfort, and anxiety

D. Implementation
  1. Monitor for motor responses such as agitation, trembling, and tension
  2. Monitor for autonomic responses such as cold clammy hands and sweating
  3. Monitor for paradoxical CNS excitement during early therapy, particularly in older and debilitated individuals
  4. Monitor for visual disturbances, as the medications can worsen glaucoma
  5. Monitor liver and renal function tests and blood counts
  6. Reduce the medication dose, as prescribed, for the older adult client and for the client with impaired liver function
  7. Initiate safety precautions because the older adult client is at risk for falling when taking the medication for sleep or anxiety
  8. Assist with ambulation if drowsiness or light-headedness occurs
  9. Instruct the client that drowsiness usually disappears during continued therapy
  10. Instruct the client to avoid tasks that require alertness until the response to the medication is established
  11. Instruct the client to avoid alcohol
  12. Instruct the client not to take other medications without consulting the physician
  13. Instruct the client not to withdraw the medication abruptly

E. Withdrawal
  1. To lessen withdrawal symptoms, the dosage of a benzodiazepine should be tapered gradually over 2 to 6 weeks
  2. Abrupt or too rapid withdrawal results in:
    a. Restlessness
    b. Irritability
    c. Insomnia
    d. Hand tremors
    e. Abdominal or muscle cramps
    f. Sweating
    g. Vomiting
    h. Seizures

VI. MEDICATIONS FOR INSOMNIA AND ANXIETY (Box 64-7)

A. Description
  1. Depress the reticular activating system by promoting the inhibitory synaptic action of the neurotransmitter GABA
  2. Used for short-term treatment of insomnia or for sedation to relieve anxiety, tension, and apprehension

B. Side effects
  1. Confusion
  2. Irritability
  3. Allergic reactions
  4. Agranulocytosis
  5. Thrombocytopenia purpura
  6. Megaloblastic anemia

C. Overdose
  1. Tachycardia
  2. Hypotension
  3. Cold and clammy skin
  4. Dilated pupils
  5. Weak and rapid pulse
  6. Signs of shock
  7. Depressed respirations
  8. Absent reflexes
  9. Coma and death may result from respiratory and cardiovascular collapse

BOX 64-7

Barbiturates and Sedative-Hypnotic Anxiolytics

BARBITURATES

Amobarbital sodium (Amytal Sodium)
Aprobarbital sodium (Alurate Sodium)
Butabarbital sodium (Butisol Sodium)
Pentobarbital sodium (Nembutal Sodium)
Phenobarbital sodium (Luminal Sodium)
Secobarbital sodium (Seconal Sodium)

SEDATIVE-HYPNOTIC ANXIOLYTICS

Buspirone (BuSpar)
Chloral hydrate (Noctec)
Ethchlorvynol (Placidyl)
Hydroxyzine HCl (Atarax)
Meprobamate (Equanil)
Zolpidem tartrate (Ambien)

D. Withdrawal
   1. Severe withdrawal symptoms begin within 24 hours after the medication is discontinued in an individual with severe drug dependence
   2. Gradual withdrawal is used to detoxify a dependent person
   3. Anxiety
   4. Insomnia
   5. Nightmares
   6. Daytime agitation
   7. Tremors
   8. Delirium
   9. Seizures

E. Implementation
   1. Administer lower doses as prescribed for the elderly client
   2. Medications should be used with caution in the client who has suicidal tendencies or a history of drug **addiction**
   3. Maintain safety by supervising ambulation and using side rails at night
   4. Instruct the client to take the medication as directed
   5. Instruct the client to avoid driving or operating hazardous equipment if drowsiness, dizziness, or unsteadiness occurs
   6. Instruct the client to avoid alcohol
   7. For insomnia, instruct the client to take the medication 30 minutes before bedtime
   8. Instruct the client that a hangover effect may occur in the morning
   9. Instruct the client not to discontinue the medication abruptly
   10. Instruct the client taking chloral hydrate to take the medication with food, a full glass of water, fruit juice, or ginger ale to improve the taste and to prevent gastric irritation

VII. ANTIPSYCHOTIC MEDICATIONS (Box 64-8)

A. Description
   1. Improve the thought processes and the behavior of the client with psychotic symptoms, especially the client with schizophrenia
   2. Block dopamine receptors in the brain, thereby reducing the psychotic symptoms
   3. Block the chemoreceptor trigger zone and vomiting center in the brain, producing an antiemetic effect
   4. Phenothiazines lower the seizure threshold
   5. Antipsychotics should not be given with other antipsychotic or antidepressant medications

B. Side effects
   1. Anticholinergic effects
   2. Dry mouth
   3. Increased heart rate
   4. Urinary retention
   5. Constipation
   6. Hypotension
   7. Drowsiness
   8. Blood dyscrasias
   9. Pruritis
   10. Photosensitivity

C. Extrapyramidal syndrome
   1. Parkinsonism
      a. Tremors
      b. Masklike facies
      c. Rigidity
      d. Shuffling gait
   2. Dystonia
      a. Facial grimacing
      b. Abnormal or involuntary eye movements
   3. Akathisia
      a. Restlessness
      b. Constant moving about
   4. Tardive dyskinesia
      a. Protrusion of the tongue
      b. Chewing motion
      c. Involuntary movement of the body and extremities

D. Implementation
   1. Monitor vital signs
   2. Monitor for extrapyramidal syndrome
   3. Monitor for symptoms of neuroleptic malignant syndrome
   4. Monitor urine output
   5. Monitor serum glucose

BOX 64-8

Antipsychotic Medications

PHENOTHIAZINES
Acetophenazine maleate (Tindal)
Chlorpromazine HCl (Thorazine)
Fluphenazine HCl (Prolixin)
Perphenazine (Trilafon)
Prochlorperazine (Compazine)
Promazine HCl (Sparine)
Thioridazine HCl (Mellaril)
Trifluoperazine (Stelazine)
Triflupromazine HCl (Vesprin)

OTHER ANTIPSYCHOTICS
Clozapine (Clozaril)
Haloperidol (Haldol)
Loxapine HCl (Loxitane)
Molindone HCl (Moban)
Olanzapine (Zyprexa)
Risperidone (Risperdal)
Thiothixene HCl (Navane)

6. Note that the client taking an antipsychotic medication may require long-term medication for parkinsonian symptoms
7. Administer the medication with food or milk to decrease gastric irritation
8. For oral use, the liquid form might be preferred because some clients hide tablets in the mouth to avoid taking them
9. Note that the absorption rate is faster with the liquid form
10. Avoid skin contact with the liquid concentrate to prevent contact dermatitis
11. Protect the liquid concentrate from light
12. Dilute the liquid concentrate with fruit juice
13. Inform the client that a full therapeutic effect of the medication may not be evident for 3 to 6 weeks after initiation of therapy; however, an observable therapeutic response may be apparent after 7 to 10 days
14. Inform the client that phenothiazines may cause a harmless pinkish to red-brown urine color
15. Instruct the client to use sunscreen, hats, and protective clothing when outdoors
16. Instruct the client to avoid alcohol or other CNS depressants
17. Instruct the client to change positions slowly to avoid orthostatic hypotension
18. Instruct the client to report signs of agranulocytosis, including sore throat, fever, and malaise
19. Instruct the client to report signs of liver dysfunction including jaundice, malaise, fever, and right upper abdominal pain
20. When antipsychotics are discontinued, the medication dosage should be reduced gradually to avoid sudden recurrence of psychotic symptoms

VIII. NEUROLEPTIC MALIGNANT SYNDROME

A. Description
   1. A potentially fatal syndrome that may occur at any time during therapy with neuroleptic medications (antipsychotic or antischizophrenic medications)
   2. Although it is rare, it is more commonly seen at the initiation of therapy, after the client is changed from one medication to another, after a dosage increase, or when a combination of medications are used

B. Data collection
   1. Dyspnea or tachypnea
   2. Tachycardia or irregular pulse rate
   3. Fever
   4. High or low blood pressure
   5. Increased sweating
   6. Loss of bladder control
   7. Skeletal muscle rigidity
   8. Pale skin
   9. Excessive weakness or fatigue
   10. Altered LOC
   11. Seizures
   12. Severe extrapyramidal side effects
   13. Difficulty swallowing
   14. Excessive salivation
   15. Oculogyric crisis
   16. Dyskinesia
   17. Elevated WBC count
   18. Elevated liver function tests
   19. Elevated creatinine phosphokinase level

C. Implementation
   1. Notify the physician
   2. Monitor vital signs
   3. Initiate safety and seizure precautions
   4. The neuroleptic medication is discontinued
   5. Monitor LOC
   6. Administer antipyretics as prescribed
   7. Use a cooling blanket to lower the body temperature
   8. Monitor electrolytes and IV fluids as prescribed

IX. MEDICATIONS TO TREAT ATTENTION DEFICIT HYPERACTIVITY DISORDER (ADHD) (Box 64-9)

A. Children with ADHD may require medication to reduce hyperactive behavior and lengthen attention span

B. Medications that are most effective in controlling this disorder are CNS stimulants

C. CNS stimulants, which increase agitation and activity in adults, have a calming effect on children with ADHD and increase alertness and sensitivity to stimuli

D. Implementation
   1. Monitor for CNS side effects
   2. Instruct the client and parents that over-the-counter medications need to be avoided
   3. Instruct the client and parents that the last dose of the day should be taken at least 6

BOX 64-9

Medications to Treat Attention Deficit Hyperactivity Disorder (ADHD)

Amphetamine
Dextroamphetamine sulfate (Dexedrine)
Methamphetamine HCl (Desoxyn)
Methylphenidate HCl (Ritalin)
Pemoline (Cylert)

hours before bedtime (14 hours for extended-release forms) to prevent insomnia
4. Monitor height and weight (particularly in children)
5. Reinforce that several weeks of therapy may be necessary before the therapeutic effect can be evaluated
6. Instruct the client and parents that a drug-free period may be prescribed to allow growth of the child if the medication has caused growth retardation
7. Methylphenidate (Ritalin) should be taken on an empty stomach, 30 to 45 minutes before a meal or snack

X. MEDICATIONS TO TREAT ALZHEIMER'S DISEASE

A. Acetylcholinesterase inhibitors may be used to treat Alzheimer's disease to improve cognitive functions in the early stages

B. Donepezil (Aricept)
1. A reversible inhibitor of acetylcholinesterase
2. Used to treat mild to moderate dementia of Alzheimer's disease
3. Common side effects include nausea and diarrhea
4. Can slow the heart rate through its vagotonic effect

C. Tacrine (Cognex)
1. A centrally acting acetylcholinesterase inhibitor
2. Used to treat mild to moderate dementia of Alzheimer's disease
3. Side effects include ataxia, loss of appetite, nausea, vomiting, and diarrhea
4. An adverse effect is hepatotoxicity; liver function studies need to be monitored

PRACTICE QUESTIONS

1. A nurse has administered a dose of diazepam (Valium) to the client. The nurse would take which of the following most important actions before leaving the client's room?
   1. Drawing the shades closed
   2. Putting up the side rails on the bed
   3. Giving the client a bedpan
   4. Turning the volume on the television set down
2. A nurse is assisting in preparing a teaching plan for a client who is taking lithium carbonate (Eskalith). Which of the following would not be a component of the teaching plan?
   1. Lithium blood levels must be monitored very closely
   2. Contact the physician if excessive diarrhea, vomiting, or diaphoresis occurs
   3. Take the lithium with meals
   4. Decrease fluid intake while taking the lithium
3. A client with a psychotic disorder is being treated with haloperidol (Haldol). Which of the following would indicate the presence of a toxic effect of this medication?
   1. Hypotension
   2. Nausea
   3. Excessive salivation
   4. Blurred vision
4. Buspirone HCl (BuSpar) is prescribed for a client with an anxiety disorder. The nurse instructs the client regarding the medication and informs the client that which of the following are characteristics of this medication?
   1. The medication can produce a sedating effect
   2. Tolerance can occur with the medication
   3. The medication is addicting
   4. Dizziness and nervousness may occur
5. Neuroleptic malignant syndrome is suspected in a client who is taking chlorpromazine (Thorazine). Which of the following medications would the nurse prepare in anticipation of being prescribed to treat this adverse reaction related to the use of chlorpromazine?
   1. Phytonadione (vitamin K)
   2. Bromocriptine (Parlodel)
   3. Enalapril maleate (Vasotec)
   4. Protamine sulfate
6. A nurse is caring for a hospitalized client who has been taking clozapine (Clozaril) for the treatment of a schizophrenic disorder. The nurse evaluates the laboratory studies that have been prescribed for the client. Which of the following laboratory studies will the nurse specifically review to monitor for an adverse reaction associated with the use of this medication?
   1. White blood cell (WBC) count
   2. Platelet count
   3. Cholesterol level
   4. Blood urea nitrogen
7. Disulfiram (Antabuse) is prescribed for a client who is seen in the psychiatric health care clinic. The nurse is collecting data on the client and is providing instructions regarding the use of this medication. Which of the following data are most important for the nurse to obtain before administration of this medication?
   1. When the last alcoholic drink was consumed
   2. A history of diabetes insipidus
   3. A history of hyperthyroidism
   4. When the last full meal was consumed
8. A nurse is collecting data on a client and the client's spouse reports that the client is taking donepezil HCl (Aricept). Which of the following disorders would the nurse suspect that this client may have based on the use of this medication?

1. Dementia
2. Obsessive compulsive disorder
3. Seizure disorder
4. History of schizophrenia

9. Fluoxetine HCl (Prozac) is prescribed for the client. The nurse provides instructions to the client regarding the administration of the medication. Which of the following statements if made by the client indicates an understanding regarding the administration of the medication:
   1. "I should take the medication right before bedtime."
   2. "I should take the medication with my evening meal."
   3. "I should take the medication at noon time with an antacid."
   4. "I should take the medication in the morning when I first arise."

10. A nursing student is assigned to care for a client with a diagnosis of schizophrenia. Haloperidol (Haldol) is prescribed for the client. The nursing instructor asks the student to describe the action of the medication. Which of the following statements if made by the nursing student indicates an understanding of the action of this medication?
    1. It blocks the uptake of norepinephrine and serotonin
    2. It blocks the binding of dopamine to the postsynaptic dopamine receptors in the brain
    3. It is a serotonin reuptake blocker
    4. It inhibits the breakdown of released acetylcholine

11. A client receiving lithium carbonate (Eskalith) complains of loose, watery stools and difficulty walking. The nurse would expect the serum lithium level to be which of the following?
    1. 0.7 mEq/L
    2. 1.0 mEq/L
    3. 1.2 mEq/L
    4. 1.7 mEq/L

12. When teaching a client who is being started on imipramine HCl (Tofranil), the nurse would inform the client that the desired effects of the medication may:
    1. Start during the first week of administration
    2. Start during the second week of administration
    3. Not occur for 2 to 3 weeks of administration
    4. Not occur until after a month of administration

13. A client receiving thioridazine (Mellaril) complains that they feel very "faint" when he or she tries to get out of bed in the morning, The nurse recognizes this complaint as a symptom of:
    1. Psychosomatic symptoms
    2. Cardiac dysrhythmias
    3. Respiratory insufficiency
    4. Postural hypotension

14. A client who is on lithium carbonate (Eskalith) therapy is scheduled for surgery. The nurse informs the client that:
    1. The medication will be discontinued several days before surgery and resumed by injection in the immediate postoperative period
    2. The medication is to be taken until the day of surgery and resumed by injection in the immediate postoperative period
    3. The medication will be discontinued 1 to 2 days before the surgery and resumed as soon as full oral intake is allowed
    4. The medication will be discontinued a week before the surgery and resumed a week after surgery

15. A client receiving a tricyclic antidepressant arrives at the mental health clinic. Which observation would indicate that the client is correctly following the medication plan?
    1. Reports sleeping 12 hours per night and 3 to 4 hours during the day
    2. Arrives at the clinic neat and appropriate in appearance
    3. Reports not going to work for this past week
    4. Complains of not being able to "do anything" anymore

16. A nurse is performing a follow-up teaching session with a client discharged 1 month ago. The client is taking fluoxetine (Prozac). What information would be important for the nurse to gather regarding the adverse effects related to the medication?
    1. Problems with excessive sweating
    2. Gastrointestinal dysfunctions
    3. Cardiovascular symptoms
    4. Problems with mouth dryness

17. A client taking buspirone HCl (BuSpar) for 1 month returns to the clinic for a follow-up visit. Which of the following manifestations would indicate medication effectiveness?
    1. No reports of alcohol withdrawal symptoms
    2. No paranoid thought processes
    3. No rapid heartbeats or anxiety
    4. No thought broadcasting or delusions

18. A client taking lithium carbonate (Eskalith) reports vomiting, abdominal pain, diarrhea, blurred vision, tinnitus, and tremors. The lithium level is checked as a part of the routine follow-up evaluation and the level is 3.0 mEq/L. The nurse knows this level is:
    1. Normal
    2. Slightly above normal
    3. Excessively below normal
    4. Toxic

19. A client is placed on chloral hydrate (Noctec) for short-term treatment. What nursing action would

best indicate a clear understanding of the major side effect of this medication?
1. Monitoring neurological signs every 2 hours
2. Monitoring the blood pressure every 4 hours
3. Instructing the client to call for ambulation assistance
4. Lowering the bed and clearing a path to the bathroom at bedtime

20. A client admitted to the hospital gives the nurse a bottle of clomipramine (Anafranil). The nurse notes that the medication has not been taken by the client in 2 months. What behaviors observed in the client would validate noncompliance with this medication?
    1. Frequent hand washing with hot soapy water
    2. Complaints of hunger
    3. A pulse rate below 60 beats per minute
    4. Complaints of insomnia
21. An adult client is administered haloperidol (Haldol) intramuscularly twice a day. After 3 days of therapy, which of the following should be implemented first at the beginning of the nursing shift?
    1. Check vital signs, compare the data with the client's record
    2. Assess the physical safety of other unit clients
    3. Monitor the client's nutritional intake
    4. Assess the client's orientation and delusional status
22. Diphenhydramine HCl (Benadryl) is used in the treatment of allergic rhinitis for a hospitalized client with a chronic psychotic disorder. This medication will not be continued at home because the nurse is aware that:
    1. Allergic symptoms are short term
    2. Poor compliance causes this medication to fail to reach its therapeutic blood level
    3. Addictive properties are enhanced in the presence of psychotropic medications
    4. This medication promotes long-term extrapyramidal symptoms
23. A client arrives at the health care clinic and tells the nurse that they have been doubling the daily dosage of bupropion (Wellbutrin) to aid them in getting better faster. Which ongoing data collection is required based on this information?
    1. Monitor for orthostatic hypotension
    2. Monitor for seizure activity
    3. Monitor for weight gain
    4. Monitor for insomnia
24. Immediately after taking a routine evening dose of alprazolam (Xanax), a client says "I'm not sure I should have taken that stuff." The best response by the nurse would be:
    1. "You are afraid of the media claims about this medication."
    2. "Your depression will fade once the medication begins to work."
    3. "Anxiety is expected with any new experience."
    4. "Lets talk about how you feel about Xanax for a while."
25. A physician orders phenobarbital sodium (Luminal Sodium) 10 mg by mouth daily. The medication bottle is labeled 15 mg per 5 mL. What will the nurse administer?
    1. 2.5 mL
    2. 3.3 mL
    3. 5 mL
    4. 10 mL
26. A client is discharged on phenobarbital sodium (Luminal Sodium) 200 mg by mouth twice day. Which of the following statements, if made by the client, reflects an accurate understanding of safety precautions with this medication?
    1. "I can take my medication at any time during the day."
    2. "Using a daily dosing system container is critical to the prevention of an overdose."
    3. "Drinking one beer may change the way my medication works."
    4. "I can take my medication with food."
27. Fluphenazine (Prolixin) is administered to a client daily. The nurse plans to monitor for the common side effects of the medication. Which of the following would the nurse include in the plan of care?
    1. Monitor the blood pressure every 2 hours
    2. Review the white blood cell (WBC) results daily
    3. Offer a nutritious snack between meals
    4. Offer hard candy or gum periodically
28. A depressed client who is on tranylcypromine sulfate (Parnate) has been instructed on diet. The nurse feels confident that the client understands the diet when given a choice of restaurant foods if the client selects:
    1. Pepperoni pizza, salad, and cola
    2. Roasted chicken, roasted potatoes, and beer
    3. Pickled herring, french fries, and milk
    4. Fried haddock, baked potato, and cola
29. A client is being treated for depression with amitriptyline HCl (Elavil). During the initial phases of treatment, the most important nursing intervention is:
    1. Ordering the client a tyramine-free diet
    2. Recognizing that frequent blood levels are necessary because there is a narrow range between therapeutic and toxic blood levels of this medication
    3. Getting baseline postural blood pressures on the client before administering the medication and each time the medication is dispensed to the client, especially during the initial days of treatment
    4. Checking the client for anticholinergic effects

30. A client who is on lithium carbonate (Eskalith) will be discharged at the end of the week. In formulating a discharge teaching plan, the nurse will instruct the client that it is most important to:
    1. Avoid soy sauce, wine, and aged cheese
    2. Take medication only as prescribed because it can become addicting
    3. Check with the psychiatrist before using any over-the-counter medications or prescription medications
    4. Have the lithium level checked every 2 weeks

ANSWERS

1. *Answer:* 2
Rationale: Diazepam is a sedative/hypnotic with anticonvulsant and skeletal muscle relaxant properties. The nurse should institute safety measures before leaving the client's room to ensure that the client does not injure self. The most frequent side effects of this medication are dizziness, drowsiness, and lethargy. For this reason, the nurse puts the side rails up on the bed before leaving the room to prevent falls. Options 1, 3, and 4 may be helpful measures that provide a comfortable, restful environment. However, option 2 is the one that provides for the client's safety needs.
Test-Taking Strategy: Use the process of elimination. Note that the stem of the question contains the key words "most important." This tells you that more than one or all of the options may be partly or totally correct. Use Maslow's Hierarchy of Needs theory to prioritize remembering that physiological and safety needs are a priority. Review nursing care for a client taking diazepam if you had difficulty with this question.
Level of Cognitive Ability: Application
Client Needs: Safe, Effective Care Environment
Integrated Concept/Process: Nursing Process/Implementation
Content Area: Pharmacology
Reference: Hodgson B, Kizior R: *Saunders nursing drug handbook 2002*, Philadelphia, 2002, WB Saunders, p. 330.

2. *Answer:* 4
Rationale: Because therapeutic and toxic dosage ranges are so close, lithium blood levels must be monitored very closely, more frequently at first and then once every several months. The client should be instructed to contact the physician if excessive diarrhea, vomiting or diaphoresis occurs. Lithium is irritating to the gastric mucosa; therefore lithium should be taken with meals. A normal diet and normal salt and fluid intake (1500 to 3000 mL per day) should be maintained because lithium decreases sodium reabsorption by the renal tubules, which could cause sodium depletion. A low-sodium intake causes lithium retention and could lead to toxicity.
Test-Taking Strategy: Use the process of elimination and note the key word "not" in the stem of the question. Remember that generally, it is important that clients be taught to maintain an adequate fluid intake. This principle will easily direct you to option 4. Review the client teaching points related to the administration of this medication if you had difficulty with this question.
Level of Cognitive Ability: Application
Client Needs: Health Promotion and Maintenance
Integrated Concept/Process: Nursing Process/Planning
Content Area: Pharmacology
Reference: Hodgson B, Kizior R: *Saunders nursing drug handbook 2002*, Philadelphia, 2002, WB Saunders, p. 654.

3. *Answer:* 3
Rationale: Toxic effect include extrapyramidal symptoms noted as marked drowsiness and lethargy, excessive salivation, and a fixed stare. Akathisia, acute dystonias, and tardive dyskinesia are also toxic effects. Hypotension, nausea, and blurred vision are occasional side effects.
Test-Taking Strategy: Use the process of elimination and note the key words "toxic effect." Select option 3 because "excessive" salivation indicates a toxic effect. Review the toxic effects of this medication if you had difficulty with this question.
Level of Cognitive Ability: Analysis
Client Needs: Physiological Integrity
Integrated Concept/Process: Nursing Process/Data Collection
Content Area: Pharmacology
Reference: Hodgson B, Kizior R: *Saunders nursing drug handbook 2002*, Philadelphia, 2002, WB Saunders, p. 525.

4. *Answer:* 4
Rationale: Buspirone HCl is used in the management of anxiety disorders. The advantages of this medication is that it is not sedating, tolerance does not develop, and it is not addicting. Dizziness, nausea, headaches, nervousness, light-headedness, and excitement, which generally are not major problems, are side effects of the medication.
Test-Taking Strategy: Knowledge regarding the side effects and advantages of buspirone HCl is required to answer this question. Review this medication and its use if you had difficulty with this question.
Level of Cognitive Ability: Application
Client Needs: Physiological Integrity
Integrated Concept/Process: Nursing Process/Implementation
Content Area: Pharmacology
Reference: Hodgson B, Kizior R: *Saunders nursing drug handbook 2002*, Philadelphia, 2002, WB Saunders, p. 143.

5. *Answer:* 2
Rationale: Bromocriptine is an antiparkinsonian prolactin inhibitor used in the treatment of neuroleptic malignant syndrome. Vitamin K is the antidote for warfarin (Coumadin) overdose. Protamine sulfate is the antidote for heparin overdose.

Enalapril maleate is an antihypertensive that is used in the treatment of hypertension.
Test-Taking Strategy: Knowledge regarding the treatment for neuroleptic malignant syndrome is required to answer this question. If you are unfamiliar with the various medications used as antidotes or treatments for various syndromes, review this content.
Level of Cognitive Ability: Application
Client Needs: Physiological Integrity
Integrated Concept/Process: Nursing Process/Planning
Content Area: Pharmacology
Reference: Hodgson B, Kizior R: *Saunders nursing drug handbook 2002*, Philadelphia, 2002, WB Saunders, p. 135.

6. *Answer:* 1
Rationale: Hematological reactions can occur in the client taking clozapine and include agranulocytosis and mild leukopenia. The WBC count should be assessed before initiating treatment and should be monitored closely during the use of this medication. The client should also be monitored for signs indicating agranulocytosis, which may include sore throat, malaise, and fever. Options 2, 3, and 4 are unrelated to this medication.
Test-Taking Strategy: Knowledge regarding the adverse effects that can occur in association with the use of clozapine is required to answer this question. If you are unfamiliar with these adverse reactions and the laboratory studies that need to be monitored, review this content.
Level of Cognitive Ability: Application
Client Needs: Physiological Integrity
Integrated Concept/Process: Nursing Process/Data Collection
Content Area: Pharmacology
Reference: Hodgson B, Kizior R: *Saunders nursing drug handbook 2002*, Philadelphia, 2002, WB Saunders, p. 266.

7. *Answer:* 1
Rationale: Disulfiram is used as an adjunct treatment for selective clients with chronic alcoholism who want to remain in a state of enforced sobriety. Clients must abstain from alcohol intake for at least 12 hours before the initial dose of the medication is administered. The most important assessment is to determine when the last alcoholic intake was consumed. The medication is used with caution in clients with diabetes mellitus, hypothyroidism, epilepsy, cerebral damage, nephritis, and hepatic disease. It is also contraindicated in severe heart disease, psychosis, or hypersensitivity related to the medication.
Test-Taking Strategy: Use the process of elimination. Recalling that the medication is used as an adjunct treatment for selective clients with chronic alcoholism will assist in directing you to option 1. Review this medication if you had difficulty with this question.
Level of Cognitive Ability: Analysis
Client Needs: Physiological Integrity
Integrated Concept/Process: Nursing Process/Data Collection
Content Area: Pharmacology
Reference: Varcarolis E: *Foundations of psychiatric mental health nursing*, ed 4, Philadelphia, 2002, WB Saunders, p. 776.

8. *Answer:* 1
Rationale: Donepezil HCl is a cholinergic agent that is used in the treatment of mild to moderate dementia of the Alzheimer's type. It enhances cholinergic functions by increasing the concentration of acetylcholine. It slows the progression of Alzheimer's disease. Options 2, 3, and 4 are incorrect.
Test-Taking Strategy: Knowledge regarding the use of donepezil HCl is required to answer this question. Review this medication if you had difficulty with this question.
Level of Cognitive Ability: Analysis
Client Needs: Physiological Integrity
Integrated Concept/Process: Nursing Process/Data Collection
Content Area: Pharmacology
Reference: Hodgson B, Kizior R: *Saunders nursing drug handbook 2002*, Philadelphia, 2002, WB Saunders, p. 369.

9. *Answer:* 4
Rationale: Fluoxetine HCl is administered in the early morning without consideration to meals. Options 1, 2, and 3 are incorrect.
Test-Taking Strategy: Knowledge regarding client instructions related to the use of fluoxetine HCl is required to answer this question. If you are unfamiliar with the use of this medication and the client teaching points, review this content.
Level of Cognitive Ability: Analysis
Client Needs: Health Promotion and Maintenance
Integrated Concept/Process: Teaching/Learning
Content Area: Pharmacology
Reference: Hodgson B, Kizior R: *Saunders nursing drug handbook 2002*, Philadelphia, 2002, WB Saunders, p. 464.

10. *Answer:* 2
Rationale: Haloperidol acts by blocking the binding of dopamine to the postsynaptic dopamine receptors in the brain. Imipramine HCl (Tofranil) blocks the reuptake of norepinephrine and serotonin. Donepezil HCl (Aricept) inhibits the breakdown of released acetylcholine. Fluoxetine HCl (Prozac) is a potent serotonin reuptake blocker.
Test-Taking Strategy: Knowledge regarding the action of haloperidol is required to answer this question. Review this medication if you had difficulty with this question.
Level of Cognitive Ability: Comprehension
Client Needs: Physiological Integrity
Integrated Concept/Process: Teaching/Learning
Content Area: Pharmacology
Reference: Hodgson B, Kizior R: *Saunders nursing drug handbook 2002*, Philadelphia, 2002, WB Saunders, p. 525.

11. *Answer:* 4
Rationale: The therapeutic serum level of lithium is 0.6 to 1.2 mEq/L. Serum lithium levels above the therapeutic level will produce signs of toxicity.
Test-Taking Strategy: Focus on the data in the question, noting that the client is experiencing loose, watery stools and difficulty waking. Recalling the therapeutic serum level of lithium will direct you to option 4. Review this therapeutic level and the signs of toxicity if you had difficulty with this question.
Level of Cognitive Ability: Analysis
Client Needs: Physiological Integrity
Integrated Concept/Process: Nursing Process/Data Collection
Content Area: Pharmacology
Reference: Hodgson B, Kizior R: *Saunders nursing drug handbook 2002*, Philadelphia, 2002, WB Saunders, p. 654.

12. *Answer:* 3
Rationale: The therapeutic effects of administration of imipramine HCl (Tofranil) may not occur for 2 to 3 weeks after the antidepressant therapy has been initiated.
Test-Taking Strategy: Knowledge regarding the therapeutic effect of imipramine HCl (Tofranil) is required to answer this question. Review this medication if you had difficulty with this question.
Level of Cognitive Ability: Application
Client Needs: Physiological Integrity
Integrated Concept/Process: Nursing Process/Implementation
Content Area: Pharmacology
Reference: Hodgson B, Kizior R: *Saunders nursing drug handbook 2002*, Philadelphia, 2002, WB Saunders, p. 562.

13. *Answer:* 4
Rationale: Thioridazine can cause postural hypotension. The client needs to be taught to get out of bed slowly and to rise from a sitting position slowly because of this untoward effect related to the medication. Options 1, 2, and 3 are unrelated to the use of this medication.
Test-Taking Strategy: Use the process of elimination. Noting the key word "faint" in the question will direct you to option 4. Review the effects of this medication if you had difficulty with this question.
Level of Cognitive Ability: Analysis
Client Needs: Psychosocial Integrity
Integrated Concept/Process: Nursing Process/Data Collection
Content Area: Pharmacology
Reference: Hodgson B, Kizior R: *Saunders nursing drug handbook 2002*, Philadelphia, 2002, WB Saunders, p. 1069.

14. *Answer:* 3
Rationale: The client who is on lithium carbonate must be off the medication for 1 to 2 days before a scheduled surgical procedure and can resume the medication when full oral intake is ordered after the surgery. Options 1, 2, and 4 are incorrect.
Test-Taking Strategy: Use the process of elimination. Recalling that lithium carbonate is an oral medication and is not given as an injection will assist in eliminating options 1 and 2. Option 4 identifies a period of time that is unreasonable and therefore eliminate this option. Review this medication if you had difficulty with this question.
Level of Cognitive Ability: Application
Client Needs: Physiological Integrity
Integrated Concept/Process: Nursing Process/Implementation
Content Area: Pharmacology
Reference: Hodgson B, Kizior R: *Saunders nursing drug handbook 2002*, Philadelphia, 2002, WB Saunders, p. 654.

15. *Answer:* 2
Rationale: Depressed individuals will sleep for long periods, are not able to go to work, and feel as if they cannot "do anything." Once they have had some therapeutic effect from their medication, they will report resolution of many of these complaints as well as demonstrate an improvement in their appearance.
Test-Taking Strategy: Use the process of elimination. The observations identified in options 1, 3, and 4 are all symptoms of depression. The improvement in appearance indicates a therapeutic response to the medication and thus compliance with the medication regimen. Review the expected effects of tricyclic antidepressants if you had difficulty with this question.
Level of Cognitive Ability: Analysis
Client Needs: Physiological Integrity
Integrated Concept/Process: Nursing Process/Evaluation
Content Area: Pharmacology
Reference: Varcarolis E: *Foundations of psychiatric mental health nursing*, ed 4, Philadelphia, 2002, WB Saunders, p. 474.

16. *Answer:* 2
Rationale: The most common adverse reactions related to fluoxetine include central nervous system and gastrointestinal (GI) system dysfunction. This medication affects the GI system by causing nausea and vomiting, cramping, and diarrhea. Options 1, 3, and 4 are not associated side effects of this medication.
Test-Taking Strategy: Knowledge regarding the side effects and adverse reactions related to fluoxetine is required to answer this question. Review these side effects and adverse reactions if you had difficulty with this question.
Level of Cognitive Ability: Application
Client Needs: Physiological Integrity
Integrated Concept/Process: Nursing Process/Data Collection
Content Area: Pharmacology
Reference: Hodgson B, Kizior R: *Saunders nursing drug handbook 2002*, Philadelphia, 2002, WB Saunders, p. 464.

17. *Answer:* 3
Rationale: Buspirone HCl is not recommended for the treatment of drug or alcohol withdrawal, paranoid thought disorders, or schizophrenia (thought broadcasting or delusions). Buspirone HCl is most often indicated for the treatment of anxiety and aggression.
Test-Taking Strategy: Knowledge regarding the use of buspirone HCl will direct you to the correct option. Review this medication if you had difficulty with this question.
Level of Cognitive Ability: Analysis
Client Needs: Physiological Integrity
Integrated Concept/Process: Nursing Process/Evaluation
Content Area: Pharmacology
Reference: Hodgson B, Kizior R: *Saunders nursing drug handbook 2002*, Philadelphia, 2002, WB Saunders, p. 143.

18. *Answer:* 4
Rationale: The therapeutic serum level of lithium is 0.6 to 1.2 mEq/L. A level of 3 mEq/L indicates toxicity.
Test-Taking Strategy: Knowledge regarding the therapeutic serum level of lithium will direct you to option 4. Review this level if you had difficulty with this question.
Level of Cognitive Ability: Comprehension
Client Needs: Physiological Integrity
Integrated Concept/Process: Nursing Process/Data Collection
Content Area: Pharmacology
Reference: Hodgson B, Kizior R: *Saunders nursing drug handbook 2002*, Philadelphia, 2002, WB Saunders, p. 654.

19. *Answer:* 3
Rationale: Chloral hydrate causes sedation and impairment of motor coordination; therefore safety measures need to be implemented. The client is instructed to call for assistance

with ambulation. Options 1 and 2 are not specifically associated with the use of this medication. Although option 4 is an appropriate nursing intervention, it is most important to instruct the client to call for assistance with ambulation.
Test-Taking Strategy: Use the process of elimination and note the key word "best." Recalling the action and effects of the medication will assist in eliminating options 1 and 2. From the remaining options, focus on the issue, client safety. Option 3 is the client-oriented action, whereas option 4 allows the client to ambulate independently, placing the client at risk for injury. Review the nursing interventions related to this medication if you had difficulty with this question.
Level of Cognitive Ability: Application
Client Needs: Safe, Effective Care Environment
Integrated Concept/Process: Nursing Process/Implementation
Content Area: Pharmacology
Reference: Hodgson B, Kizior R: *Saunders nursing drug handbook 2002*, Philadelphia, 2002, WB Saunders, p. 220.

20. *Answer:* 1
Rationale: Clomipramine is commonly used in the treatment of obsessive-compulsive disorder. Handwashing is a common obsessive-compulsive behavior. Weight gain is a common side effect of this medication. Tachycardia and sedation are side effects. Insomnia may occur as a seldom side effect.
Test-Taking Strategy: Recalling that clomipramine is commonly used to treat obsessive-compulsive disorder will direct you to option 1. Review the purpose of this medication if you had difficulty with this question.
Level of Cognitive Ability: Analysis
Client Needs: Physiological Integrity
Integrated Concept/Process: Nursing Process/Evaluation
Content Area: Pharmacology
Reference: Hodgson B, Kizior R: *Saunders nursing drug handbook 2002*, Philadelphia, 2002, WB Saunders, p. 256.

21. *Answer:* 4
Rationale: Haloperidol is used to treat clients exhibiting psychotic features. Hallucinations, delusions, and altered thought processes may cause a client to be a danger to themselves and others. Vital signs are routine and not specific to this situation. The physical safety of other clients is not a direct assessment of this client. Monitoring nutritional intake has no specific value as outlined in this situation.
Test-Taking Strategy: Use the process of elimination and note the key word "first." Identify the client of the question and eliminate option 2. From the remaining options, focus on the action and use of the medication to direct you to option 4. Review the nursing interventions related to this medication if you had difficulty with this question.
Level of Cognitive Ability: Application
Client Needs: Physiological Integrity
Integrated Concept/Process: Nursing Process/Implementation
Content Area: Pharmacology
Reference: Hodgson B, Kizior R: *Saunders nursing drug handbook 2002*, Philadelphia, 2002, WB Saunders, p. 525.

22. *Answer:* 3
Rationale: The addictive properties of diphenhydramine HCl are enhanced when used with psychotropic medications. Allergic symptoms may not be short term and will occur if allergens are present in the environment. Poor compliance may be a problem with psychotic clients, but this issue is not the priority in this situation. Diphenhydramine HCl may be used as a primary management tool for extrapyramidal symptoms and mild medication-induced movement disorders.
Test-Taking Strategy: Knowledge regarding the properties of diphenhydramine HCl (Benadryl) is required to answer this question. Review this medication if you had difficulty with this question.
Level of Cognitive Ability: Comprehension
Client Needs: Physiological Integrity
Integrated Concept/Process: Nursing Process/Planning
Content Area: Pharmacology
Reference: Hodgson B, Kizior R: *Saunders nursing drug handbook 2002*, Philadelphia, 2002, WB Saunders, p. 352.

23. *Answer:* 2
Rationale: Bupropion does not cause significant orthostatic blood pressure changes. Seizure activity is common in dosages greater than 450 mg a day. Bupropion frequently causes a drop in body weight. Insomnia is a side effect, but seizure activity causes a greater client risk.
Test-Taking Strategy: Use the process of elimination and note that the question asks for the assessment data that are required. Noting that the client has been doubling the medication dose and recalling that seizure activity can occur with higher than recommended doses will direct you to option 2. Review this medication if you had difficulty with this question.
Level of Cognitive Ability: Application
Client Needs: Health Promotion and Maintenance
Integrated Concept/Process: Nursing Process/Data Collection
Content Area: Pharmacology
Reference: Hodgson B, Kizior R: *Saunders nursing drug handbook 2002*, Philadelphia, 2002, WB Saunders, p. 141.

24. *Answer:* 4
Rationale: The nurse should focus on assessing the reason for the client's concern. The nurse would add anxiety to the client by mentioning media concerns. Alprazolam is used to treat anxiety, not depression. Cliche responses (option 3) do not express genuine concern.
Test-Taking Strategy: Use therapeutic communication techniques. Remembering to always address the client's feelings first will direct you to option 4. Review these techniques if you had difficulty with this question.
Level of Cognitive Ability: Application
Client Needs: Psychosocial Integrity
Integrated Concept/Process: Communication and Documentation
Content Area: Pharmacology
Reference: Hodgson B, Kizior R: *Saunders nursing drug handbook 2002*, Philadelphia, 2002, WB Saunders, p. 30.

25. *Answer:* 2
Rationale: Follow the formula for the calculation of the medication dose. The physician orders 10 mg.

$$\frac{\text{Desired}}{\text{Available}} \times \text{volume} = \text{dose} \qquad \frac{10 \text{ mg}}{15 \text{ mg}} \times 5 \text{ mL} = 3.33 \text{ ml}$$

Test-Taking Strategy: Use the formula for medication calculations to answer the question. Note that a conversion is not necessary with this calculation problem. Review medication calculations if you had difficulty with this question.
Level of Cognitive Ability: Application
Client Needs: Physiological Integrity
Integrated Concept/Process: Nursing Process/Implementation
Content Area: Pharmacology
Reference: DeWit S: *Fundamental concepts and skills for nursing,* Philadelphia, 2001, WB Saunders, p. 642.

26. *Answer:* 3
Rationale: Phenobarbital sodium should not be taken with other central nerves system agents such as alcohol. The medication should be taken at the same time every day. Dose containers are helpful to prevent dose omissions but will not prevent an overdose. The medication may be taken without regard to meals.
Test-Taking Strategy: Use the process of elimination and note the key words "accurate understanding." Recalling that alcohol should not be consumed when the client is taking a prescription medication will direct you to the correct option. Review the teaching points related to this medication if you had difficulty with this question.
Level of Cognitive Ability: Analysis
Client Needs: Health Promotion and Maintenance
Integrated Concept/Process: Nursing Process/Evaluation
Content Area: Pharmacology
Reference: Hodgson B, Kizior R: *Saunders nursing drug handbook 2002,* Philadelphia, 2002, WB Saunders, p. 872.

27. *Answer:* 4
Rationale: Dry mouth is a common side effect of this medication. Frequent mouth rinsing with water, sucking on hard candy, and chewing gum will alleviate this common side effect. Hypotension and hypertension are rare side effects of fluphenazine. Leukopenia is common but not viewed as a serious health threat, and the WBC would not be obtained on a daily basis. Weight gain is a common side effect and frequent snacks will enhance this problem.
Test-Taking Strategy: Use the process of elimination. Eliminate options 1 and 2 first. It is unlikely that the client would need blood pressure monitoring every 2 hours or that a WBC count will be drawn daily. From the remaining options, recalling the side effects of this medication will direct you to option 4. Review the common side effects related to this medication if you had difficulty with this question.
Level of Cognitive Ability: Application
Client Needs: Physiological Integrity
Integrated Concept/Process: Nursing Process/Planning
Content Area: Pharmacology
Reference: Hodgson B, Kizior R: *Saunders nursing drug handbook 2002,* Philadelphia, 2002, WB Saunders, p. 467.

28. *Answer:* 4
Rationale: Tranylcypromine sulfate is a monoamine oxidase inhibitor (MAOI) used to treat depression. A tyramine-restricted diet is required while on this medication to avoid hypertensive crisis, a life-threatening side effect of the medication. Foods to be avoided are meats prepared with tenderizer, smoked or pickled fish, beef or chicken liver, and dry sausage (salami, pepperoni, bologna). In addition, figs, bananas, aged cheese, yogurt, sour cream, beer, red wine, alcoholic beverages, soy sauce, yeast extract, chocolate, caffeine, and aged, pickled, fermented or smoked foods need to be avoided. Many over-the-counter medications also contain tyramine and must be avoided as well.
Test-Taking Strategy: Knowledge that tranylcypromine sulfate is an MAOI medication and knowledge of which foods need to be avoided with these medications is necessary to answer this question. Review these foods if you had difficulty with this question.
Level of Cognitive Ability: Analysis
Client Needs: Health Promotion and Maintenance
Integrated Concept/Process: Nursing Process/Evaluation
Content Area: Pharmacology
Reference: Hodgson B, Kizior R: *Saunders nursing drug handbook 2002,* Philadelphia, 2002, WB Saunders, p. 1108.

29. *Answer:* 3
Rationale: Amitriptyline HCl is a tricyclic antidepressant often used to treat depression. It causes orthostatic changes and can produce hypotension and tachycardia. This can be frightening to the client and dangerous because it may result in dizziness and client falls. The client must be instructed to move slowly from a lying to a sitting to a standing position to avoid injury if these effects are experienced. The client may also experience sedation, dry mouth, constipation, blurred vision, and other anticholinergic effects, but these are transient and will diminish with time.
Test-Taking Strategy: Use the process of elimination. Recalling the adverse effects of the tricyclic antidepressants will direct you to option 3. Review this medication if you had difficulty with this question.
Level of Cognitive Ability: Application
Client Needs: Physiological Integrity
Integrated Concept/Process: Nursing Process/Implementation
Content Area: Pharmacology
Reference: Hodgson B, Kizior R: *Saunders nursing drug handbook 2002,* Philadelphia, 2002, WB Saunders, p. 52.

30. *Answer:* 3
Rationale: Lithium is the medication of choice to treat manic-depressive illness. Many over-the-counter (OTC) medications interact with lithium, and the client is instructed to avoid OTC medications while taking lithium. Lithium is not addicting and although serum lithium levels need to be monitored, it is not necessary to check these levels every 2 weeks. A tyramine-free diet is associated with monoamine oxidase inhibitors.
Test-Taking Strategy: Use the process of elimination. General principles related to medication administration will direct you to option 3. Review this medication if you had difficulty with this question.
Level of Cognitive Ability: Application
Client Needs: Health Promotion and Maintenance
Integrated Concept/Process: Teaching/Learning
Content Area: Pharmacology
Reference: Hodgson B, Kizior R: *Saunders nursing drug handbook 2002,* Philadelphia, 2002, WB Saunders, p. 654.

REFERENCES

DeWit S: *Fundamental concepts and skills for nursing,* Philadelphia, 2001, WB Saunders.

Fortinash K, Holoday-Worret P: *Psychiatric mental health nursing,* ed 2, St Louis, 2000, Mosby.

Hill S, Bauer B: *Mental health nursing,* Philadelphia, 2002, WB Saunders.

Hodgson B, Kizior R: *Saunders nursing drug handbook 2002,* Philadelphia, 2002, WB Saunders.

Keltner N, Schwecke L, Bostrom C: *Psychiatric nursing,* ed 3, St Louis, 1999, Mosby.

Varcarolis E: *Foundations of psychiatric mental health nursing,* ed 4, Philadelphia, 2002, WB Saunders.

UNIT XX

The Gerontological Client

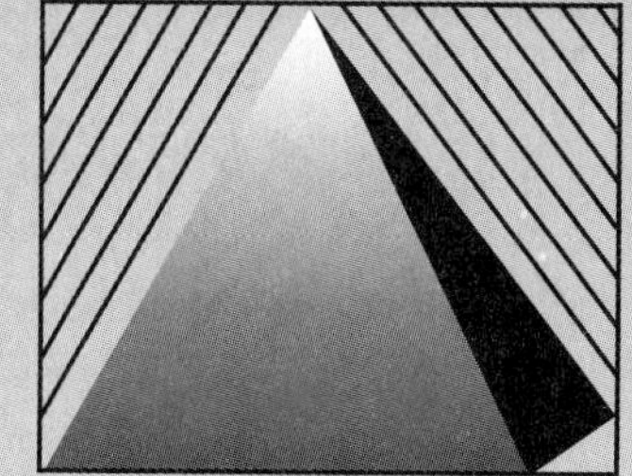

PYRAMID TERMS

Abuse The willful infliction of pain, injury, or mental anguish. Unreasonable confinement or willful deprivation of services, including medical care. Abuse can include failure to prevent injury, verbal assaults, the demand to perform demeaning tasks, theft, or mismanagement of personal belongings.

Aging The biopsychosocial process of change occurring between birth and death.

Alzheimer's Disease An irreversible form of dementia. Individuals with Alzheimer's disease experience cognitive deterioration and progressive loss of ability to carry out the activities of daily living. The client experiences a steady decline in physical and mental functioning that frequently requires caregivers to seek outside resources for assistance.

Dementia Organic syndrome identified by gradual and progressive deterioration in intellectual functioning. Long- and short-term memory loss occurs, with impairment in judgment, abstract thinking, problem-solving ability, and behavior. Results in a self-care deficit. The most common type of dementia is Alzheimer's disease.

Depression A functional disorder of mood that is not linked with aging. The depression may be precipitated by losses related to aging. Depression can be manifested by cognitive impairment or may be the cause of a decline in mental status. Depression can be identified by feelings of sadness, hopelessness, and worthlessness and a decreased interest in activities.

Exploitation Illegal or improper use of the individual's resources.

Gerontology The study of the process of aging.

Neglect The lack of providing services necessary for physical or mental health.

Self-Neglect The person chooses to avoid medical care or other services that could improve optimal function. Unless declared legally incompetent, an individual has the right to refuse care.

PYRAMID TO SUCCESS

The Pyramid to Success focuses on safety issues, the prevention of injury, restraints, abuse and neglect, depression, dementia, and Alzheimer's disease. Pyramid points also focus on methods of communication, particularly when deficits exist. When a question is presented on NCLEX-PN, if an age is identified in the case of the question, note the age. If the age represents an elderly client, use gerontological nursing concepts when answering the question. The Integrated Concepts and Processes addressed in this unit include Clinical Problem-Solving Process (Nursing Process), Caring, Communication and Documentation, Cultural Awareness, Self-Care, and Teaching/Learning.

CLIENT NEEDS

Safe, Effective Care Environment

Accident prevention
Advance directives
Appropriate procedures for safety
Client rights and advocacy
Confidentiality
Continuity of care
Informed consent
Use of restraints

Health Promotion and Maintenance

Aging process
Expected body image changes
Family systems
Lifestyle choices
The prevention and early detection of disorders associated with aging

The importance of follow-up visits to the physician
The importance of safety, exercise, and nutrition
The safe use of medications

Psychosocial Integrity

Abuse and neglect
Adjustment to potential deterioration in physical and mental health and well-being
Changes and adjustment in role function
Coping mechanisms
Grief and loss
Loss of the quantity and quality of relationships
Religious and spiritual resources
Sensory/perceptual alterations
Situational role changes
The threat to independent functioning
The use of resources for the client and family

Physiological Integrity

Alterations in body systems and the related risks resulting from the aging process
Assistive devices
Elimination
Mobility and immobility
Nutrition and oral hydration
Personal hygiene
Rest and sleep
Safe medication administration

REFERENCES

Black J, Hawks J, Keene A: *Medical-surgical nursing: clinical management for positive outcomes*, ed 6, Philadelphia, 2001, WB Saunders.
DeWit S: *Fundamental concepts and skills for nursing*, Philadelphia, 2001, WB Saunders.
Hodgson B, Kizior R: *Saunders nursing drug handbook 2002*, Philadelphia, 2002, WB Saunders.
Lueckenotte A: *Gerontologic nursing*, ed 2, St Louis, 2000, Mosby.
National Council of State Boards of Nursing: *Test plan for the National Council Licensure Examination for Practical/Vocational Nurses*, Chicago, 2001, Author.
Potter P, Perry A: *Fundamentals of nursing*, ed 5, St Louis, 2001, Mosby.

Care of the Gerontological Client

I. PHYSIOLOGICAL CHANGES OF AGING

A. Integumentary system
1. Loss of pigment in hair and skin
2. Increased nail thickness and decreased nail growth
3. Thinning of the epidermis
4. Easy bruising and tearing of the skin
5. Reduction in blood flow to the skin
6. Decreased skin turgor
7. Loss of elasticity and subcutaneous fat
8. Wrinkling of the skin
9. Dry, itchy, cracked skin
10. Inadequate sweating
11. Seborrheic dermatitis and keratosis formation

B. Neurological system
1. Changes in mental status
2. Slowed reflexes
3. Loss of balance
4. Dizziness and syncope
5. Slight tremors
6. Difficulty with fine motor movement
7. Changes in sleep patterns such as decreased total sleep with earlier risings
8. Increased susceptibility to hypothermia and hyperthermia

C. Musculoskeletal system
1. Posture and stature changes causing a decrease in height
2. Kyphosis of the dorsal spine
3. Muscle mass decreases and muscles atrophy
4. Joint capsule components deteriorate
5. Decreased mobility, range of motion, flexibility, and stability
6. Increased stiffness
7. Decrease in physical strength
8. Decrease in muscular coordination
9. Change of gait, with shortened step and wider base
10. Increased brittleness of the bones
11. Decrease in deep tendon reflexes

D. Cardiopulmonary system
1. Energy and endurance diminish
2. Lowered tolerance to exercise
3. Decreased stretch and compliance of the chest wall
4. Decreased rib mobility and lung tone
5. Decreased strength and function of respiratory muscles
6. Decreased depth of respirations and oxygen intake
7. Decreased ability to cough and expectorate sputum
8. Decreased size and number of alveoli
9. Decreased compliance of the heart muscle
10. Heart valves become thicker and more rigid
11. Decreased efficiency of blood return to the heart and decreased cardiac output
12. Decreased resting heart rate
13. Increased blood pressure
14. Susceptible to postural hypotension

E. Hematological and immune systems
1. Hemoglobin and hematocrit levels remain within normal range but average toward the low end of normal
2. Lymphocyte counts tend to be low
3. Decreased resistance to infection and disease
4. Prone to increased blood clotting

F. Gastrointestinal system
1. Decreased appetite, thirst, and oral intake
2. Decreased need for calories
3. Digestive disturbances
4. Decreased stomach-emptying time
5. Increased tendency toward constipation
6. Tooth loss

7. Difficulty in chewing and swallowing food
8. Decreased absorption of carbohydrates, proteins, fats, and vitamins
9. Decreased lean body weight

G. Endocrine system
1. Decreased secretion of hormones, with specific changes related to each hormone function
2. Decreased metabolic rate
3. Decreased glucose tolerance
4. Resistance to insulin in peripheral tissues

H. Renal system
1. Decreased kidney size, function, and ability to concentrate urine
2. Decreased glomerular filtration rate
3. Decreased capacity of the bladder
4. Increased residual urine and increased incidence of infection and incontinence
5. Impaired medication excretion

I. Reproductive system
1. Decreased testosterone production and decreased size of testes
2. Changes in the prostate leading to urinary problems
3. Decreased secretion of hormones with the cessation of menses
4. Vaginal changes, including decreased muscle tone and lubrication

J. Special senses
1. Decreased visual acuity
2. Decreased accommodation in eyes
3. Decreased peripheral vision and increased sensitivity to glare
4. Increased adjustment time to changes in light
5. Presbyopia and cataract formation
6. Possible loss of hearing ability
7. Inability to discern taste of food
8. Decreased smell acuity
9. Changes in touch
10. Decreased pain awareness

II. PSYCHOSOCIAL ASPECTS OF AGING (Box 65-1)

A. Adjustments to retirement and loss of income
B. Changes in role function

BOX 65-1

Concerns of the Older Population

Adequate income
Functional limitations from chronic illness and disability
Ability to maintain independence
Becoming a burden to loved ones
Isolation
Dependence on governmental and social systems
Access to social support systems

C. Coping with change and new life situations
D. Changes in social life
E. Diminished quantity and quality of relationships
F. Coping with loss
G. Adjustment to potential deterioration in physical and mental health and well-being
H. Threat to independent functioning
I. Loss of skills and competencies developed early in life

III. ELDER ABUSE AND NEGLECT

A. Description
1. Involves physical, psychological, financial, and social **abuse**
2. Can involve a violation of the client's rights
3. Individuals at most risk include those who are dependent because of immobility or altered mental status
4. Factors that contribute to **abuse** and **neglect** include long-standing family violence, caregiver stress, and the individual's increasing dependence

B. Types
1. **Abuse**
   a. The willful infliction of pain, injury, or mental anguish
   b. Unreasonable confinement or willful deprivation of services, including medical care
   c. Can include failure to prevent injury, verbal assaults, the demand to perform demeaning tasks, theft, or mismanagement of personal belongings
2. **Neglect:** the lack of provision of services necessary for physical or mental health
3. **Self-neglect**
   a. The person chooses to avoid medical care or other services that would improve optimal functioning
   b. Unless declared legally incompetent, an individual has the right to refuse care
4. **Exploitation:** illegal or improper use of the individual's resources
5. Data collection: **abuse** and **neglect**
   a. Abrasions, lacerations, and bruises
   b. Burns
   c. Sprains, fractures, or dislocations
   d. Pressure sores
   e. Injuries inconsistent with history
   f. Frequent falls
   g. Untreated medical problems
   h. Inappropriate dress and poor hygiene
   i. Excessive drowsiness
   j. Overmedication or undermedication
   k. Malnutrition
   l. Dehydration

m. Expression of fear in response to touch
6. Implementation
a. Assess for signs of **abuse** and **neglect**
b. Report cases of **abuse** and **neglect**, as mandated by all states
c. Initiate protective services
d. Assess for dysfunctional family systems
e. Promote family functioning and initiate appropriate contact with resources

IV. USE OF RESTRAINTS

A. Physical restraints used to prevent injury are to be avoided, and alternative methods to provide safety must be assessed before the use of physical restraints
B. A physician's order must be obtained for the use of restraints
C. Discuss the use of restraints with the client and family
D. Obtain client and family consent for the use of restraints
E. Use the least restrictive device for restraint
F. Use only restraints that have been manufactured as a safety restraint
G. Observe the client frequently, and monitor for alterations in skin integrity and circulation as a result of the restraints
H. Restraints need to be removed at frequent intervals (per agency policy) to assess for complications and to allow for mobility and range of motion
I. Always follow the institutional policy regarding the use of restraints

V. MEDICATIONS

A. Major problems with prescription medications include adverse affects, medication interactions, medication errors, noncompliance, and the cost
B. Determine the use of over-the-counter medications
C. Keep the use of medications to a minimum
D. Medication dosages are normally prescribed at one third to one half of the normal adult doses
E. Closely monitor for adverse effects and response to therapy because of the increased risk for medication toxicity
F. Note that a common sign of an adverse reaction in older adults is an acute change in mental status
G. Assess for medication interactions in the client taking multiple medications
H. Advise the client to use one pharmacy and to notify the consulting physicians of the medications taken
I. Administration of medications
1. Place the client in a sitting position when administering medication
2. Check for mouth dryness because medication may stick and dissolve in mouth
3. Administer liquid preparations if the client has difficulty swallowing tablets
4. Crush tablets if necessary and give with textured food (nectar, applesauce) if not contraindicated
5. Do not crush enteric-coated tablets and do not open capsules
6. If administering a suppository, do not insert suppository immediately after removing from the refrigerator
7. A suppository may take longer to dissolve because of decreased body core temperature
8. When administering parenteral medication, monitor the site because it may ooze medication or bleed because of decreased tissue elasticity
9. Do not use an immobile limb for administering parenteral medication
10. Monitor client compliance with taking prescribed medications
11. Monitor for safety in correctly taking medications
12. Use a medication cassette to facilitate proper administration of medication

VI. DEMENTIA

A. Description
1. Organic syndrome with progressive deterioration in intellectual functioning
2. Long- and short-term memory loss occurs, with impairment in judgment, abstract thinking, problem-solving ability, and behavior
3. Results in a self-care deficit
4. The most common type of **dementia** is **Alzheimer's disease**

B. **Alzheimer's disease**
1. An irreversible form of senile **dementia**
2. Individuals with **Alzheimer's disease** experience cognitive deterioration and progressive loss of ability to carry out the activities of daily living
3. The client experiences a steady decline in physical and mental functioning that frequently requires caregivers to seek outside resources for assistance

C. Data collection
1. Begins with mild memory impairment
2. The client has difficulty remembering names, appointments, and where things are

3. The client is indifferent and occasionally irritable
4. As the disease progresses, moderate memory impairment, particularly of recent events, occurs
5. The client develops a decrease in orientation, is restless, and paces about
6. As the progression of the disease continues, the client develops severely impaired cognitive function, disorientation, delusions, and agitation
7. Limb rigidity and flexion posture
8. Urinary and fecal incontinence

D. Implementation
1. Identify and reinforce retained skills
2. Assist the client and family members to manage memory deficits and behavior changes
3. Encourage the family members to express feelings about caregiving
4. Provide caregiver support and identify the resources and support groups available
5. Provide continuity of care
6. Orient the client to the environment
7. Furnish the environment with familiar possessions
8. Acknowledge the client's feelings
9. Monitor activities of daily living
10. Remind how to perform self-care activities
11. Maintain independence as much as possible
12. Provide consistent routines
13. Provide exercise with supervision, such as walking with an escort
14. Avoid activities that tax the memory
15. Allow plenty of time to complete a task
16. Use constant encouragement in a step-by-step approach
17. Provide mental stimulation with simple games or activities
18. Provide activities that distract and occupy time, such as listening to music, coloring, and watching TV

E. Implementation for Specific Behaviors
1. Wandering
   a. Provide a safe environment
   b. Prevent unsafe wandering
   c. Provide close supervision
   d. Close and secure doors
   e. Use identification bracelets and electronic surveillance devices
2. Communication
   a. Adapt to the communication level of the client
   b. Use a calm and reassuring voice
   c. Use pantomime gestures if the client is unable to understand spoken words
   d. Use slow, clear, verbal communication techniques
   e. Use short words and simple sentences
   f. Call the client by name, identify self, and wait for a response
   g. Ask only one question at a time and give one direction at a time
   h. Repeat questions if necessary, but do not rephrase because this may cause confusion in the client
   i. Stand directly in front of the client and maintain eye contact
   j. Listen and observe the emotion expressed by the client
3. Impaired judgment
   a. Eliminate throw rugs, toxic substances, dangerous electrical appliances, or any other objects that can present a risk of injury
   b. Reduce hot water heater temperature
4. Altered thought processes
   a. Orient the client frequently
   b. Place a calendar and clock in a visible place
   c. Call the client by name
   d. Place familiar objects in the room
   e. Maintain familiar routines
   f. Make tasks simple and allow time for the client to complete a task
   g. Allow the client to reminisce
5. Altered sleep patterns
   a. Allow the client to wander in a safe place until he or she becomes tired
   b. Prevent shadows in the room
   c. Avoid the use of hypnotics and sedatives because they cause confusion and aggravate the sundown effect
6. Agitation
   a. Assess the precipitant of the agitation
   b. Reassure the client
   c. Remove items that can be hazardous during the time of agitation
   d. Approach the client slowly and calmly from the front; then speak, gesture, and move slowly
   e. Use touch gently
   f. Take the client to a less stressful environment
   g. Distract the client with questions about the problem, and gradually turn the attention to something else
   h. Do not argue with the client or restrain the client

VII. DEPRESSION

A. Description

1. A functional disorder of mood that is not linked with **aging**
2. The **depression** may be manifested by cognitive impairment or may be the cause of a decline in mental status
3. **Depression** can be identified by feelings of sadness, hopelessness, worthlessness, and a decreased interest in activities

B. Data collection
1. Difficulty concentrating
2. Feelings of inadequacy and sadness
3. Difficulty sleeping or excessive sleeping
4. Weight gain or loss
5. Vegetative symptoms
6. Constipation
7. Loss of interest in activities
8. Decreased endurance and energy
9. Preoccupation with physical health
10. Thoughts of death or suicide

C. Implementation
1. Assess for signs associated with **depression**
2. Monitor for the risk of suicide and notify the physician
3. Implement safety precautions for suicide risk
4. Provide and reinforce positive experiences
5. Provide a variation in the daily schedule, but limit changes because change is anxiety-producing for the older client
6. Allow the client to talk and reminisce
7. Maintain reality
8. Initiate counseling as appropriate
9. Refer to Chapter 64 for information about the prescribed medications for depression

VIII. PAIN

A. Description
1. Pain can occur from numerous causes and most often occurs as a result of degenerative changes in the musculoskeletal system
2. The failure to alleviate pain in the older client can lead to functional limitations affecting the ability to function independently

B. Data collection
1. Agitation
2. Moaning
3. Crying
4. Restlessness
5. Verbal reporting of pain

C. Implementation
1. Monitor the client for signs of pain
2. Identify the pattern of pain
3. Identify the precipitating factor(s) for the pain
4. Monitor the impact of the pain on activities of daily living
5. Provide pain relief through measures such as distraction, relaxation, massage, and biofeedback
6. Administer pain medication as prescribed and instruct the client in their use
7. Evaluate the effects of pain-reducing measures

IX. IMPAIRED VISION AND HEARING

A. Description
1. Because of the physiological changes that occur with the **aging** process, clients develop decreased visual and hearing acuity
2. Such conditions as loss of sight and hearing, cataracts, glaucoma, and presbyopia can develop

B. Data collection and implementation: refer to Chapter 52

X. ALTERED SKIN INTEGRITY

A. Description
1. Physiological changes include thinning of the epidermis, easy bruising and tearing of the skin, and the reduction in blood flow to the skin
2. Altered skin integrity often occurs in the bedridden or immobile client

B. Data collection and implementation: refer to Chapter 38 regarding information on decubitus

XI. IMPAIRED MOBILITY

A. Description
1. Usually occurs as a result of multiple types of problems and diseases
2. Impaired mobility can occur as a result of decreased physical function related to cardiovascular, pulmonary, musculoskeletal, or neurological disease, or accidents

B. Data collection
1. Existing disease processes
2. Ambulation ability
3. Ability to care for self

C. Implementation
1. Assess risk of injury
2. Determine cause of mobility restriction
3. Assess mobility restrictions related to disease processes
4. Monitor limitations related to all self-care activities
5. Maintain activity through exercise and guided activities
6. Provide rest periods between activities and in the afternoon

7. Break activities up to last no longer than 20 minutes
8. Perform activities that require a high level of energy in the morning
9. Determine the best assistive aid or adaptive device for the client
10. Demonstrate and monitor the safe use of the assistive device
11. Monitor skin for integrity
12. Provide range of motion to prevent deformities and contractures
13. Monitor respiratory status and encourage deep breathing to promote lung expansion

D. Assistive devices: refer to Chapter 56 for information on canes and walkers

XII. FRACTURED HIP

A. Description
1. The most disabling type of fracture for the older adult
2. Usually caused by falls with direct trauma to the hip

B. Data collection and implementation: refer to Chapter 56

XIII. PNEUMONIA

A. Description: causes of pneumonia in the older client include the effects of the **aging** process on the respiratory system, weakness and the inability to cough, malnutrition, and the use of medications

B. Data collection
1. Acute change in mental status
2. Confusion
3. Cough
4. Fever
5. Increased respiratory rate
6. Chest pain
7. Dyspnea
8. Chest radiograph confirmation

C. Implementation
1. Monitor vital signs
2. Assess lung sounds
3. Administer oxygen as prescribed
4. Administer respiratory therapy as prescribed
5. Administer antibiotics as prescribed
6. Provide adequate rest with some progressive activity
7. Mobilize the bed rest client as soon as possible
8. Provide adequate nutrition and hydration
9. Encourage the client to receive immunization against influenza and pneumococcal pneumonia to prevent the infection

XIV. NUTRITIONAL INTAKE

A. Description
1. Physiological requirements decrease with age
2. The older client is at risk for inadequate nutritional and fluid intake as a result of the inability to prepare food, loss of dentition, loss of appetite, lack of exercise, loss of taste and smell sensation, loss of interest in eating, **depression**, or lack of financial resources

B. Data collection
1. Appetite
2. Hydration status
3. Body weight
4. Ability to feed self
5. Ability to chew and swallow
6. Fluid and calorie intake
7. Ability to prepare food and mobilize the resources to shop

C. Implementation
1. Assess appetite
2. Monitor for signs of dehydration and malnutrition
3. Monitor body weight
4. Assess ability to chew and swallow
5. Monitor intake of food and fluids
6. Assess food likes and dislikes
7. Provide small, frequent, nutritious meals
8. Offer nutritious between-meal drinks and snacks
9. Assess ability to prepare food and to shop for food
10. Provide resources necessary to supply the client with adequate food

XV. CONSTIPATION

A. Description
1. Normal elimination does not occur because of a structural problem or disease state
2. Constipation is a frequent complaint regarding bowel function of older people

B. Data collection
1. Frequency of defecation
2. Usual time for defecation
3. Dietary habits
4. Use of laxatives or enemas

C. Implementation
1. Determine the cause of constipation
2. Reestablish typical bowel habits
3. Maintain regular defecation
4. Promote comfort and privacy during defecation
5. Increase fluid intake

6. Add fiber to the diet
7. Provide anal lubricant
8. Administer stool softeners as prescribed
9. Use suppositories sparingly, limiting the type to glycerin or Dulcolax as prescribed
10. Use enemas sparingly, limiting the use to small cleansing enemas such as Fleet as prescribed
11. Avoid the use of mineral oil as a laxative because of problems associated with the absorption of fat-soluble vitamins and the risk of aspiration

XVI. DIARRHEA

A. Description
   1. Frequent defecation of loose or liquid stools
   2. Infections may cause diarrhea
   3. Fecal impaction may cause overflow diarrhea, with stool oozing around the impaction
   4. Antibiotic-associated diarrhea, such as that caused by *Clostridium difficile,* is a problem for older individuals, particularly if they are hospitalized

B. Data collection
   1. Frequency of defecation
   2. Usual time for defecation
   3. Dietary habits
   4. Use of laxatives or enemas
   5. Stool oozing
   6. Signs of dehydration
   7. Electrolyte values

C. Implementation
   1. Assess causative factor
   2. Initiate interventions, as prescribed based on causative factor
   3. Assess for fluid deficit and dehydration
   4. Monitor intake and output (I&O) and electrolyte levels
   5. Increase dietary bulk and fiber
   6. Monitor skin around anal area

XVII. URINARY INCONTINENCE

A. Description
   1. The involuntary release or leakage of urine
   2. The physiological changes that occur in the kidney and bladder as a result of the **aging** process may lead to the urinary incontinence problems experienced by some older clients

B. Data collection
   1. Contributing factors
   2. I&O
   3. Urinary incontinence patterns
   4. Urinary retention

BOX 65-2

Kegel exercises

Contract pubococcygeus muscle
Hold contraction for 10 seconds
Relax for 10 seconds
Work up to 25 repetitions three times a day

   5. Signs of urinary infection, such as burning, frequency, foul odor, or confusion
   6. Urinalysis results

C. Implementation
   1. Monitor I&O
   2. Monitor urinary patterns
   3. Assess contributing factors such as a bladder infection; distance to the bathroom; difficulty ambulating or removing clothing; or coughing, sneezing, or laughing
   4. Establish a toileting schedule such as every 2 hours, or before and after activities, meals, sleep, and rest periods
   5. Provide easy access to bathroom
   6. Ensure adequate fluid intake
   7. Provide a protection plan for accidents to avoid embarrassment
   8. Instruct the client about the use of incontinence aids such as pads or briefs
   9. Provide skin care and monitor for skin breakdown
   10. Teach Kegel exercises to control stress and urge incontinence (Box 65-2)

PRACTICE QUESTIONS

1. A nurse is assigned to care for an older client with hearing loss. The nurse plans care knowing that older clients:
   1. Are often distracted
   2. Respond to low-pitched tones
   3. Have middle ear changes
   4. Develop moist cerumen production
2. An older client is admitted to the hospital with a diagnosis of malnutrition. The nurse is told that blood will be drawn to determine if the client has a protein deficiency. The nurse understands that which of the following blood tests will be done?
   1. Creatinine
   2. Transferrin
   3. Calcium
   4. Sodium
3. A nurse is assigned to care for an older client. To reduce the risk of aspiration during meals, the nurse positions the client:
   1. Upright in a chair
   2. On the left side in bed

3. In low-Fowler's position with the legs elevated
4. On the right side in bed

4. A nurse is assigned to care for an older client who is receiving nutrition via a nasogastric tube. Before administering the tube feeding, the priority nursing action is:
   1. Check the placement of the tube
   2. Check the last time medications were given
   3. Check the time of the last feeding
   4. Warm the feeding to 103° F
5. An older hypertensive client is taking lisinopril (Prinivil, Zestril) 10 mg PO daily. The nurse reinforces instructions to the client regarding the medication. Which statement, if made by the client, indicates that further teaching is necessary?
   1. "I take the pill after breakfast each day."
   2. "I need to change my position slowly."
   3. "If I get a bad headache, I should call my doctor immediately."
   4. "I can skip a dose once a week."
6. Which of the following clients would most likely be a victim of elder abuse?
   1. A 90-year-old woman with advanced Parkinson's disease
   2. A 68-year-old man with newly diagnosed cataracts
   3. A 70-year-old woman with early-diagnosed Lyme disease
   4. A 75-year-old man with moderate hypertension
7. An older female client tells the nurse that she is afraid that she will fall while going to the bathroom at night. Which suggestion, if made by the nurse, indicates that the nurse understands the visual changes affecting older clients?
   1. "Use a bell to call your daughter if you need to get up."
   2. "Keep a night-light on in the bedroom and bathroom."
   3. "Use a commode in your bedroom at night."
   4. "Limit your fluid intake during the day."
8. A nurse is assisting in planning group activities for older clients. Which of the following activities would best promote health and maintenance among older adults?
   1. Gardening every day for an hour
   2. Cycling three times a week for 20 minutes
   3. Sculpting once a week for 40 minutes
   4. Walking three to five times a week for 30 minutes
9. A nurse is assigned to care for an older client. Which of the following activities performed by the nurse fosters reminiscence in the client?
   1. Displaying calendars and clocks
   2. Encouraging client participation in a pottery class
   3. Setting up a pet therapy session
   4. Having story-telling time
10. A nurse is caring for an immobile older client who is on bed rest. The nurse plans care knowing that which of the following problems has the highest priority for the client?
    1. Oral mucous membrane irritation
    2. Respiratory congestion
    3. Impaired memory
    4. Loneliness
11. A nurse is caring for an older client at home. Which situation in the home noted by the nurse requires immediate attention?
    1. An operable smoke detector
    2. A prefilled medication tray
    3. Unsecured scatter rugs
    4. Clear exit passageways
12. Which statement, if made by an older client, indicates to the nurse that teaching about bowel elimination is necessary?
    1. "I drink 6 to 8 glasses of water per day."
    2. "I walk 1 to 2 miles per day."
    3. "I need to decrease fiber in my diet."
    4. "I have a bowel movement every other day."
13. Which of the following situations, if practiced by a nurse, is an example of ageism?
    1. Accepting differences among older adults
    2. Allowing older adults to make decisions
    3. Informing the older adult of his or her rights
    4. Advising older adults to forego aggressive treatment
14. The nurse plans to monitor an older client for medication toxicity knowing that which of the following age-related body changes may cause medication toxicity?
    1. Decreased cough efficiency and decreased vital capacity
    2. Decreased lean body mass and decreased glomerular filtration rate
    3. Decreased salivation and decreased gastrointestinal motility
    4. Decreased muscle strength and loss of bone density
15. A nurse is caring for an older male client who resides in a nursing home. The nurse plans which of the following to encourage autonomy in the client?
    1. Scheduling his barber appointments
    2. Allowing him to choose social activities
    3. Decorating his room
    4. Planning his meals
16. A nurse plans care for an older client knowing that the client is less able to regulate hot and cold bodily changes because of alterations in the activity of the:
    1. Parotid glands
    2. Thymus gland
    3. Pineal gland
    4. Sweat glands

17. A nurse is caring for an older client who is a widow. Which behavior, if engaged in by the client, indicates ineffective coping?
    1. Requesting to visit her husband's grave once a month
    2. Participating in a senior citizen's program
    3. Looking at old snapshots of her family
    4. Neglecting her personal grooming
18. When communicating with an older client who is hearing impaired, the nurse initially:
    1. Stands in front of the client
    2. Exaggerates lip movements
    3. Obtains a sign language interpreter
    4. Pantomimes and writes the client notes
19. A nurse is providing instructions to an older client regarding measures to improve sleep. Which statement, if made by the client, indicates that further teaching is necessary?
    1. "I will drink hot chocolate before bedtime."
    2. "I have stopped smoking cigars."
    3. "I swim three times a week."
    4. "I read for 40 minutes before bedtime."
20. A nurse is caring for an older male client at home. The nurse observes that the client is confined to his room by his daughter-in-law. When the nurse suggests he walk to the den and join the family, he says, "I'm in everyone's way. My son needs for me to stay here." The most important action for the nurse to take is to:
    1. Suggest to the client and family that they consider a nursing home for the client
    2. Identify support systems to the client and family such as respite care and senior citizens
    3. Say nothing as it is best for the nurse to remain neutral and wait to be asked for help
    4. Say to the daughter-in-law, "Confining your father to his room is inhumane."
21. A nurse is caring for an older male client at home. The nurse notes that the client has several bruises on his back, hips, and chest. The medication count and the client's mental status indicate that he is receiving too much sedation. The client says, "My son gets tired having to tend to me at night. I'm always wet and it's all my fault. My son can't help being a little rough." Which of the following responses by the nurse would be most appropriate?
    1. "You're saying that when you're incontinent at night, you feel at fault and that you feel your son can't help being rough?"
    2. "Oh, he can't, can he? I intend to report this abusive behavior to the police."
    3. "Well, I know you feel that you're a bother but you pay your way and then some. I'll talk with your son and clear this right up."
    4. "Let's not dwell on this. After all, you are doing quite well and maybe we can arrange for you to go to a nursing home on the weekends."
22. A nurse has reviewed the record of an assigned older client. Which of the following data would indicate a potential complication associated with the skin of an aging client?
    1. Wrinkling, baldness, and gray hair
    2. Thinning and loss of elasticity in the skin
    3. Deepening of expression lines and wrinkling
    4. Crusting of the skin
23. A nurse has reviewed the record of an assigned older adult client. Which of the following data would indicate a potential complication associated with the eyes of an older adult client?
    1. Vision is 20/20
    2. Irregular lens or cornea
    3. Vision is 20/30
    4. Lens opacity
24. A nurse is assigned to care for a client with a diagnosis of Alzheimer's disease. Which of the following will the nurse most likely expect to note when collecting data about the client?
    1. Inability to talk
    2. One-sided paralysis
    3. Disorientation
    4. Urinary and fecal incontinence
25. A nurse is caring for an older immobilized client. Which nursing intervention will prevent respiratory complications in the client?
    1. Monitoring vital signs every shift
    2. Decreasing oral fluid intake
    3. Changing the client's position every 2 hours
    4. Instructing the client to bear down every hour and hold the breath

ANSWERS

1. *Answer:* 2

Rationale: Presbycusis refers to the age-related irreversible degenerative changes of the inner ear leading to decreased hearing acuity. These changes cause a decreased response to high-frequency sounds. Low-pitched tones of the voice are more easily heard and interpreted by older clients. Options 1, 3, and 4 are incorrect.

Test-Taking Strategy: Knowledge regarding the physiological changes that occur with hearing among older individuals is required to answer this question. If you had difficulty with this question, review these changes and the characteristics of presbycusis.

Level of Cognitive Ability: Comprehension

Client Needs: Physiological Integrity

Integrated Concept/Process: Nursing Process/Planning

Content Area: Adult Health/Ear
Reference: Lueckenotte A: *Gerontologic nursing,* ed 2, St Louis, 2000, Mosby, p. 711.

2. *Answer:* 2
Rationale: Serum transferrin is an iron-transport protein that can be measured directly or calculated as an indirect measurement of the total iron-binding capacity. The blood creatinine, calcium, or sodium levels do not measure protein.
Test-Taking Strategy: Use the process of elimination and note the key words "protein deficiency." The only option that refers to the analysis of protein is option 2. Review the purpose of these laboratory tests if you had difficulty with this question.
Level of Cognitive Ability: Comprehension
Client Needs: Physiological Integrity
Integrated Concept/Process: Nursing Process/Implementation
Content Area: Fundamental Skills
Reference: Lueckenotte A: *Gerontologic nursing,* ed 2, St Louis, 2000, Mosby, p. 189.

3. *Answer:* 1
Rationale: It is preferable to get clients out of bed and sitting in a chair for meals. This position facilitates chewing and swallowing and prevents the reflux of stomach contents and aspiration. Options 2, 3, and 4 do not identify positions that will reduce the risk of aspiration.
Test-Taking Strategy: Use the process of elimination. Focus on the issue of the question "reduce the risk of aspiration." This should easily direct you to option 1. Review the measures that will prevent aspiration if you had difficulty with this question.
Level of Cognitive Ability: Application
Clients Needs: Physiological Integrity
Integrated Concept/Process: Nursing Process/Implementation
Content Area: Fundamental Skills
Reference: Lueckenotte A: *Gerontologic nursing,* ed 2, St Louis, 2000, Mosby, p. 509.

4. *Answer:* 1
Rationale: Before administering a feeding, the nurse checks the placement of the tube by aspirating gastric contents and measuring the pH. Formulas are administered at room temperature. Options 2 and 3, although useful data, are not priority actions.
Test-Taking Strategy: Use the process of elimination and focus on the issue of the question. Use the ABCs—airway, breathing, and circulation—to answer the question. To prevent the complication of aspiration, the priority would be to verify accurate placement of the tube. Review the principles related to nasogastric tube feedings, if you had difficulty with this question.
Level of Cognitive Ability: Application
Clients Needs: Physiological Integrity
Integrated Concept/Process: Nursing Process/Implementation
Content Area: Fundamental Skills
Reference: DeWit S: *Fundamental concepts and skills for nursing,* Philadelphia, 2001, WB Saunders, p. 503.

5. *Answer:* 4
Rationale: Lisinopril is an antihypertensive, angiotensin-converting enzyme inhibitor. Adverse effects include headache, dizziness, fatigue, orthostatic hypotension, tachycardia, and angioedema. Specific client education points include taking one pill a day, not skipping or stopping the medication without consulting the physician, and monitoring for side effects and adverse reactions. The client should notify the physician if side effects occur.
Test-Taking Strategy: Use the process of elimination. Note the key words "further teaching is necessary." Remembering that clients should never skip doses of medication will easily direct you to option 4. If you had difficulty with this question review this medication.
Level of Cognitive Ability: Comprehension
Clients Needs: Health Promotion and Maintenance
Integrated Concept/Process: Teaching/Learning
Content Area: Pharmacology
Reference: Hodgson B, Kizior R: *Saunders nursing drug handbook 2002,* Philadelphia, 2002, WB Saunders, p. 652.

6. *Answer:* 1
Rationale: The typical abuse victim is a woman of advanced age with few social contacts and at least one physical or mental impairment that limits the ability to perform activities of daily living. In addition, the client most likely lives alone or with the abuser and depends on the abuser for care.
Test-Taking Strategy: Note the key words "most likely." Use the process of elimination and identify the client that is most defenseless as the result of the disease process. This will direct you to option 1. If you had difficulty with this question, review content related to elder abuse.
Level of Cognitive Ability: Comprehension
Clients Needs: Psychosocial Integrity
Integrated Concept/Process: Nursing Process/Data Collection
Content Area: Mental Health
Reference: Lueckenotte A: *Gerontologic nursing,* ed 2, St Louis, 2000, Mosby, p. 252.

7. *Answer:* 2
Rationale: Because it takes longer to adapt to changes from dark to light and vice versa, older people are at a greater risk of falls and injuries. Clients should be instructed to keep a night-light on in the bedroom and bathroom to prevent an unsafe environment. Any place where there is a sudden change from dark to light or from light to dark can be dangerous. Options 1 and 3 do not promote independence. Limiting fluid intake can cause dehydration in older adults.
Test-Taking Strategy: Focus on the issue of the question, the physiological eye changes that occur in the older adults. Using the process of elimination will easily direct you to option 2. Review the physiological changes that occur in the older adults if you had difficulty with this question.
Level of Cognitive Ability: Application
Clients Needs: Safe, Effective Care Environment
Integrated Concept/Process: Nursing Process/Implementation
Content Area: Fundamental Skills
Reference: Lueckenotte A: *Gerontologic nursing,* ed 2, St Louis, 2000, Mosby, p. 234.

8. *Answer:* 4
Rationale: Exercise and activity are essential for health promotion and maintenance in the older adult and to achieve an

optimal level of functioning. One of the best exercises for an older adult is walking, progressing to 30 minute sessions three to five times each week. Swimming and dancing are also beneficial. Options 1, 2, and 3 may be appropriate activities for some older adults but are not the best activities.
Test-Taking Strategy: Use the process of elimination. Focus on the key words "best promote." Option 4 is the best exercise for an older adult. Review health promotion in the older adult if you had difficulty with this question.
Level of Cognitive Ability: Application
Clients Needs: Health Promotion and Maintenance
Integrated Concept/Process: Nursing Process/Planning
Content Area: Fundamental Skills
Reference: Lueckenotte A: *Gerontologic nursing,* ed 2, St Louis, 2000, Mosby, p. 212.

9. *Answer:* 4
Rationale: Older adults who like to retell stories or past events need to be provided the opportunity to do so. This is called life review or reminiscence. Option 1 indicates reality orientation techniques. Options 2 and 3 indicate socialization and physical activity.
Test-Taking Strategy: Use the process of elimination. Note the relationship between "fosters reminiscence" in the question and "story-telling time" in the correct option. If you had difficulty with this question, review reminiscence therapy.
Level of Cognitive Ability: Application
Clients Needs: Psychosocial Integrity
Integrated Concept/Process: Nursing Process/Implementation
Content Area: Mental Health
Reference: Lueckenotte A: *Gerontologic nursing,* ed 2, St Louis, 2000, Mosby, p. 133.

10. *Answer:* 2
Rationale: A client who is immobile is at risk for the development of pneumonia and skin break down. Although options 1, 3, and 4 may be important problems to address, option 2 identifies airway, the highest priority.
Test-Taking Strategy: Use Maslow's Hierarchy of Needs theory and the ABCs—airway, breathing, and circulation—to answer the question. This will direct you to option 2. Airway is the priority. Review priority needs of the immobile client on bed rest if you had difficulty with this question.
Level of Cognitive Ability: Application
Clients Needs: Physiological Integrity
Integrated Concept/Process: Nursing Process/Planning
Content Area: Fundamental Skills
Reference: Lueckenotte A: *Gerontologic nursing,* ed 2, St Louis, 2000, Mosby, p. 212.

11. *Answer:* 3
Rationale: Some of the causes of trauma in an older client include an unsteady gait, the presence of unsecured scatter rugs, cluttered passageways, inoperable smoke detectors, and medication administration errors.
Test-Taking Strategy: Use the process of elimination. Note the key words "requires immediate attention." There is one unsafe situation among the options, the presence of unsecured scatter rugs. To prevent falls, rugs need to be secured. The other options presented all ensure safety for the client. Review safety measures for the older client if you had difficulty with this question.
Level of Cognitive Ability: Comprehension
Clients Needs: Safe, Effective Care Environment
Integrated Concept/Process: Nursing Process/Data Collection
Content Area: Fundamental Skills
Reference: Lueckenotte A: *Gerontologic nursing,* ed 2, St Louis, 2000, Mosby, p. 237.

12. *Answer:* 3
Rationale: Adequate dietary fiber is one of the most important factors in aiding bowel function. The retention of water by the fiber has the ability to soften stools and promote regularity. Fluids and exercise facilitate bowel elimination. Also remember that the client's elimination pattern is individual.
Test-Taking Strategy: Use the process of elimination. Note the key words "teaching about bowel elimination is necessary." General knowledge regarding measures to promote bowel elimination will direct you to option 3. Review these measures if you had difficulty with this question.
Level of Cognitive Ability: Comprehension
Clients Needs: Health Promotion and Maintenance
Integrated Concept/Process: Nursing Process/Evaluation
Content Area: Fundamental Skills
Reference: Lueckenotte A: *Gerontologic nursing,* ed 2, St Louis, 2000, Mosby, p. 544.

13. *Answer:* 4
Rationale: Ageism is a form of prejudice, in which older adults are stereotyped by characteristics found in only a few members of their group. Options 1, 2, and 3 are supportive roles that the nurse engages in when dealing with older adults. Option 4 suggests that the nurse does not think that older adults are worthy of aggressive treatment and demonstrates ageism.
Test-Taking Strategy: Use the process of elimination and focus on the issue of the question. Understanding the definition of ageism will easily direct you to option 4. Review the meaning of this term if you had difficulty with this question.
Level of Cognitive Ability: Comprehension
Clients Needs: Psychosocial Integrity
Integrated Concept/Process: Nursing Process/Implementation
Content Area: Fundamental Skills
Reference: Lueckenotte A: *Gerontologic nursing,* ed 2, St Louis, 2000, Mosby, p. 14.

14. *Answer:* 2
Rationale: The older client is at risk for developing medication toxicity because of decreased lean body mass and age-associated decreased glomerular filtration rate. Options 1, 3, and 4 do not contribute to medication toxicity.
Test-Taking Strategy: Use the process of elimination and knowledge regarding the physiological changes associated with aging. Note that option 2 is the only option that addresses renal excretion. If you had difficulty with this question, review the physiological changes associated with aging.
Level of Cognitive Ability: Comprehension
Clients Needs: Physiological Integrity
Integrated Concept/Process: Nursing Process/Planning
Content Area: Fundamental Skills

Reference: Lueckenotte A: *Gerontologic nursing,* ed 2, St Louis, 2000, Mosby, p. 430.

15. *Answer:* 2
Rationale: Autonomy is the personal freedom to direct one's own life as long as it does not impinge on the rights of others. Loss of autonomy, and therefore independence, is a fear among older adults. To promote independence in clients, it is essential to provide them choices. Option 2 is the only option that allows the client to be a decision maker.
Test-Taking Strategy: Use the process of elimination. Note the similarity between options 1, 3, and 4 in that the nurse is the decision maker for the client. If you had difficulty with this question, review the definition of autonomy.
Level of Cognitive Ability: Application
Clients Needs: Safe, Effective Care Environment
Integrated Concept/Process: Nursing Process/Planning
Content Area: Fundamental Skills
Reference: Potter P, Perry A: *Fundamentals of nursing,* ed 5, St Louis, 2001, Mosby, p. 348.

16. *Answer:* 4
Rationale: Sweat glands control temperature regulation. As aging progresses, alterations in sweat gland activity make the glands less effective in temperature regulation, so the aging person is less able to regulate hot and cold bodily changes. The parotid glands are responsible for the drainage of saliva, which plays an important role in digestion. The pineal gland is a major site of melatonin biosynthesis. The thymus gland plays an immunological role throughout life.
Test-Taking Strategy: Use the process of elimination. Note the relationship between "hot and cold bodily changes" in the question and "sweat glands" in the correct option. If you had difficulty with this question, review the functions of the glands identified in each option.
Level of Cognitive Ability: Comprehension
Clients Needs: Physiological Integrity
Integrated Concept/Process: Nursing Process/Planning
Content Area: Fundamental Skills
Reference: Lueckenotte A: *Gerontologic nursing,* ed 2, St Louis, 2000, Mosby, p. 202.

17. *Answer:* 4
Rationale: Coping mechanisms are behaviors used to decrease stress and anxiety. In response to a death, ineffective coping is manifested by an extreme behavior that in some instances may be harmful to the individual either physically or psychologically. Options 1, 2, and 3 are positive activities that the individual is engaging in to get on with her life. Option 4 is indicative of a behavior that identifies an ineffective coping behavior in the grieving process.
Test-Taking Strategy: Use the process of elimination and note the key words "ineffective coping." Note the similarity in options 1, 2, and 3 in that they are positive responses. Review effective and ineffective coping mechanisms if you had difficulty with this question.
Level of Cognitive Ability: Comprehension
Clients Needs: Psychosocial Integrity
Integrated Concept/Process: Nursing Process/Data Collection
Content Area: Fundamental Skills
Reference: Potter P, Perry A: *Fundamentals of nursing,* ed 5, St Louis, 2001, Mosby, p. 618.

18. *Answer:* 1
Rationale: The nurse would ensure that the hearing-impaired client can see the nurse when speaking by providing adequate lighting and by standing in front of the client. The nurse should enunciate words clearly but not exaggerate lip movements. If the client is profoundly hearing impaired and uses signing, a sign language interpreter should be obtained. If a client cannot understand by reading lips, the nurse would try using gestures, pantomiming, or writing notes.
Test-Taking Strategy: Use the process of elimination. Note the key word "initially." To communicate effectively with a hearing-impaired client, the nurse first makes sure that the client can see her or him. There are no data in the question to indicate that options 2, 3, or 4 are necessary interventions. If you had difficulty with this question, review interventions for the hearing impaired.
Level of Cognitive Ability: Application
Clients Needs: Physiological Integrity
Integrated Concept/Process: Communication and Documentation
Content Area: Fundamental Skills
Reference: Potter P, Perry A: *Fundamentals of nursing,* ed 5, St Louis, 2001, Mosby, p. 464.

19. *Answer:* 1
Rationale: The client should avoid caffeinated beverages and stimulants such as tea, cola, and chocolate before bedtime. The client should exercise regularly because exercise enhances sleep. Smoking is avoided. Reading before bedtime can assist in inducing sleep.
Test-Taking Strategy: Use the process of elimination. Focus on the key words "further teaching is necessary." Options 2, 3, and 4 are positive responses indicating that the client has learned the methods of improving sleep. Review the measures to improve sleep if you had difficulty with this question.
Level of Cognitive Ability: Comprehension
Clients Needs: Physiological Integrity
Integrated Concept/Process: Teaching/Learning
Content Area: Fundamental Skills
Reference: Lueckenotte A: *Gerontologic nursing,* ed 2, St Louis, 2000, Mosby, p. 203.

20. *Answer:* 2
Rationale: Assisting clients and families to become knowledgeable regarding available community support systems is a role of the nurse. The suggestion to commit the client to a nursing home is premature. While the data provided tells you that this elder requires nursing care, the extent of nursing care is unknown. Observing that the client has begun to be confined to his room makes it necessary for the nurse to intervene legally and ethically, so option 3 is not appropriate and is passive in terms of advocacy. Option 4 is incorrect and judgmental.
Test-Taking Strategy: Note the key words "most appropriate." Use therapeutic communication techniques and principles related to ethical and legal issues to answer the question. If you had difficulty with this question, review the role of the nurse in providing support to the family.

Level of Cognitive Ability: Application
Client Needs: Safe, Effective Care Environment
Integrated Concept/Process: Nursing Process/Implementation
Content Area: Fundamental Skills
Reference: Lueckenotte A: *Gerontologic nursing,* ed 2, St Louis, 2000, Mosby, p. 166.

21. *Answer:* 1
Rationale: The elder who is abused classically excuses the abuser. Option 1 summarizes and focuses on the content of the client's message and restates so that the client can hear himself making excuses about his son's physical abuse. In option 2, the nurse is sarcastic and without further investigation moves to report the incident. In option 3, the nurse confirms the client's fear that he is a "bother," begins to insinuate that his son is using his money and that this situation will be cleared up just by the nurse's talking with the client's son. Option 4 is incorrect because it advocates avoiding the issue.
Test-Taking Strategy: Use therapeutic communication techniques to answer the question. Option 1 is the only statement that reflects these techniques. If you had difficulty with this question, review therapeutic communication techniques and the blocks to communication.
Level of Cognitive Ability: Application
Client Needs: Psychosocial Integrity
Integrated Concept/Process: Communication and Documentation
Content Area: Mental Health
Reference: Lueckenotte A: *Gerontologic nursing,* ed 2, St Louis, 2000, Mosby, p. 37.

22. *Answer:* 4
Rationale: The normal physiological changes that occur in the skin of the older adult includes thinning of the skin, loss of elasticity, deepening of expression lines, and wrinkling. Baldness and graying of the hair occur. Crusting of the skin would indicate a potential complication.
Test-Taking Strategy: Note the key words "potential complication." Use the process of elimination and knowledge regarding normal expected findings to assist in directing you to the correct option. Review these normal findings and those that indicate a complication if you had difficulty with this question.
Level of Cognitive Ability: Comprehension
Client Needs: Physiological Integrity
Integrated Concept/Process: Nursing Process/Data Collection
Content Area: Adult Health/Integumentary
Reference: Lueckenotte A: *Gerontologic nursing,* ed 2, St Louis, 2000, Mosby, p. 304.

23. *Answer:* 4
Rationale: One of the eye conditions that occurs in the older adult is cataracts. Cataracts result in a loss of opacity of the crystalline lens, causing visual disturbances. Option 1 describes normal vision. Option 2 describes an astigmatism. Option 3 describes near-normal vision.
Test-Taking Strategy: Note the key words "older adult client" and "potential complication." Recalling that cataracts is a condition associated with the older adult client will easily direct you to option 4. Review age-related changes of the eye if you had difficulty with this question.
Level of Cognitive Ability: Comprehension
Client Needs: Physiological Integrity
Integrated Concept/Process: Nursing Process/Data Collection
Content Area: Adult Health/Eye
Reference: Lueckenotte A: *Gerontologic nursing,* ed 2, St Louis, 2000, Mosby, p. 699.

24. *Answer:* 3
Rationale: In Alzheimer's disease, memory impairment and disorientation occur. Options 1, 2, and 4 are not findings associated with this disease.
Test-Taking Strategy: Use the process of elimination. Recalling that Alzheimer's disease is a form of dementia will easily direct you to option 3. If you had difficulty with this question, review the findings associated with the disorder.
Level of Cognitive Ability: Comprehension
Client Needs: Physiological Integrity
Integrated Concept/Process: Nursing Process/Data Collection
Content Area: Fundamental Skills
Reference: Lueckenotte A: *Gerontologic nursing,* ed 2, St Louis, 2000, Mosby, p. 638.

25. *Answer:* 3
Rationale: The nurse should check the immobilized client's vital signs every 4 hours to identify an elevated temperature that suggests infection. The nurse would encourage fluid intake to loosen secretions and thus enable the client to expectorate more easily. Frequent position change helps to mobilize lung secretions and prevent pooling. It is important to encourage coughing and deep breathing to mobilize lung secretions. Clients should be instructed to avoid the Valsalva maneuver or any activity involving holding the breath.
Test-Taking Strategy: Note the key words "prevent respiratory complications." Use the process of elimination. Changing the position of the immobilized client will help prevent pooling of lung secretions. Options 1, 2, and 4 do not assist the client to improve ventilatory efforts. Review these measures if you had difficulty with this question.
Level of Cognitive Ability: Application
Clients Needs: Physiological Integrity
Integrated Concept/Process: Nursing Process/Implementation
Content Area: Fundamental Skills
Reference: Lueckenotte A: *Gerontologic nursing,* ed 2, St Louis, 2000, Mosby, p. 212.

REFERENCES

Black J, Hawks J, Keene A: *Medical-surgical nursing: clinical management for positive outcomes,* ed 6, Philadelphia, 2001, WB Saunders.

DeWit S: *Fundamental concepts and skills for nursing,* Philadelphia, 2001, WB Saunders.

Hodgson B, Kizior R: *Saunders nursing drug handbook 2002,* Philadelphia, 2002, WB Saunders.

Jarvis C: *Physical examination and health assessment,* ed 3, Philadelphia, 2000, WB Saunders.

Lueckenotte A: *Gerontologic nursing,* ed 2, St Louis, 2000, Mosby.

Potter P, Perry A: *Fundamentals of nursing,* ed 5, St Louis, 2001, Mosby.

UNIT XXI

Comprehensive Test

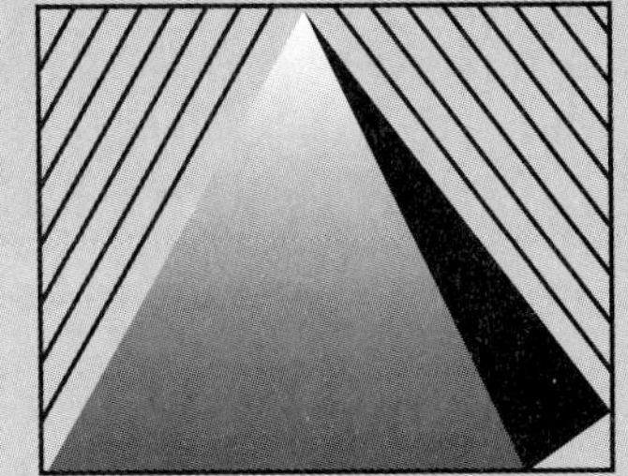

QUESTIONS

1. Before administering an intermittent tube feeding through a nasogastric tube, the nurse checks for gastric residual. The nurse understands that the rationale for checking gastric residual before administering the tube feeding is to:
   1. Confirm proper nasogastric tube placement
   2. Observe the digestion of formula
   3. Check fluid and electrolyte status
   4. Evaluate absorption of the last feeding
2. A client is complaining of gas pains after surgery and requests medication. The nurse selects which of the following medications from the PRN medication list to give to the client?
   1. Magnesium hydroxide (Milk of Magnesia, MOM)
   2. Droperidol (Inapsine)
   3. Acetaminophen (Tylenol)
   4. Simethicone (Mylicon)
3. A client is admitted to the hospital with a diagnosis of major depression. The nurse collects data on the client and identifies that a major concern is the client's altered nutrition related to poor nutritional intake. The most appropriate nursing intervention related to this concern is:
   1. Explain to the client the importance of a good nutritional intake
   2. Weigh the client three times a week, before breakfast
   3. Report the nutritional concern to the psychiatrist and obtain a nutritional consult as soon as possible
   4. Consult with the nutritionist, offer the client several small frequent meals a day, and schedule brief nursing interactions with the client during these times
4. A client received 20 units of NPH insulin subcutaneously at 8:00 AM. The nurse should check the client for a hypoglycemic reaction at:
   1. 10:00 AM
   2. 11:00 AM
   3. 5:00 PM
   4. 11:00 PM
5. A nurse assists in developing a plan of care for a client with hyperparathyroidism receiving calcitonin (Calcimar). Which outcome has the highest priority regarding this medication?
   1. Absence of side effects
   2. Achievement of normal serum calcium levels
   3. Relief of pain
   4. Verbalization of appropriate medication knowledge
6. DuoDerm is prescribed for a client with a leg ulcer. The nurse is assisting in preparing a plan of care for the client and most appropriately includes which of the following in the plan?
   1. Change the DuoDerm daily
   2. Apply the DuoDerm over a dry, sterile dressing
   3. Change the DuoDerm weekly
   4. Apply the DuoDerm over a normal saline-soaked dressing
7. A nursing instructor asks a nursing student about the etiology of hemophilia. The student responds correctly by telling the instructor that:
   1. Hemophilia is a Y-linked hereditary disorder
   2. Males inherit hemophilia from their fathers
   3. Females inherit hemophilia from their mothers
   4. Hemophilia A results from deficiency of factor VIII
8. A 4-year-old child is admitted to the hospital for abdominal pain. The mother reports that the child has been pale, excessively tired, and is bruising very easily. On physical examination lymphadenopathy and hepatosplenomegaly are noted, and diagnostic studies are ordered because acute lymphocytic leukemia (ALL) is suspected. The nurse understands that which of the following tests will confirm this diagnosis?

1. White blood cell (WBC) count
2. A lumbar puncture
3. Bone marrow biopsy
4. A platelet count

9. A child with leukemia is complaining of nausea. The nurse suspects that the nausea is related to the medication therapy. The nurse, concerned about the child's nutritional status, would most appropriately offer which of the following during this episode of nausea?
   1. The child's favorite foods
   2. Cool, clear liquids
   3. Low-protein foods
   4. Low-calorie foods
10. A child with a brain tumor is admitted to the hospital for "debulking" of the tumor. To ensure a safe environment for this child, the nurse suggests to include which of the following in the plan of care?
    1. Assisting the child with ambulation at all times
    2. Avoiding contact with other children on the nursing unit
    3. Initiating seizure precautions
    4. Using a wheelchair for out of bed activities
11. A client is diagnosed with stage I of Lyme disease. The nurse reviews the client's health record knowing that which of the following is a characteristic of this stage?
    1. Signs of neurological disorders
    2. Enlarged and inflamed joints
    3. Arthralgias
    4. Flulike symptoms
12. A nurse is assisting in caring for a client who has a placenta previa. The nurse understands that a cervical examination will not be performed on the client primarily because it could:
    1. Increase the chance of infection
    2. Initiate premature labor
    3. Cause profound hemorrhage
    4. Rupture the fetal membranes
13. A mother is breastfeeding her newborn infant. The mother complains to the nurse that she is experiencing nipple soreness. The nurse provides which of the following suggestions to the client?
    1. Avoid rotating breastfeeding positions so that the nipple will toughen
    2. Stop nursing during the period of nipple soreness to allow the nipples to heal
    3. Nurse the newborn infant less frequently and substitute a bottle feeding until the nipples become less sore
    4. Position the newborn infant with the ear, shoulder, and hip in straight alignment and with the baby's stomach against the mother's
14. A nurse is caring for a client with a diagnosis of agoraphobia. Which of the following behaviors would the nurse expect the client to describe when communicating with the client about the disorder?
    1. A need to wash hands several times before eating a meal
    2. A fear of leaving the house
    3. A fear of speaking in public
    4. A fear of riding in elevators
15. A nurse is preparing to deliver a food tray to a client whose religion is Jewish. The nurse checks the food on the tray and notes that the client has received a roast beef dinner with whole milk as a beverage. Which action will the nurse take?
    1. Deliver the food tray to the client
    2. Call the dietary department and ask for a new meal tray
    3. Replace the whole milk with fat-free milk
    4. Ask the dietary department to replace the roast beef with pork
16. A client is brought to the emergency room by the ambulance team after collapsing at home. Cardiopulmonary resuscitation is attempted but is unsuccessful. The wife of the client tells the nurse that the client is an organ donor and that the eyes are to be donated. Which of the following is the most appropriate nursing action?
    1. Elevate the head of the bed of the deceased and place dry sterile dressings over the eyes
    2. Call the National Donor Association to confirm that the client is a donor
    3. Close the deceased client's eyes and place wet saline gauze pads and an ice pack on the eyes
    4. Ask the wife to obtain the legal documents regarding organ donation from the lawyer
17. A nurse is caring for a client with Alzheimer's disease who is agitated. The nurse implements which intervention to calm this agitated client?
    1. Plays a radio
    2. Turns the lights out
    3. Puts an arm around the client's waist
    4. Encourages group participation
18. A nurse administers a dose of scopolamine to a preoperative client. The nurse tells the client to expect which of the following side effects of the medication?
    1. Excessive urination
    2. Diaphoresis
    3. Dry mouth
    4. Pupillary constriction
19. A nurse is reinforcing instructions regarding methods to prevent Lyme disease. Which of the following would not be part of these instructions?
    1. Avoid the use of insect repellents because it will attract the ticks
    2. Wear long-sleeved tops and long pants in wooded areas
    3. Wear a hat in wooded areas
    4. Wear closed shoes and socks that can be pulled up over the pants when walking in the woods

20. A nurse is caring for a child diagnosed with Down syndrome. In describing the disorder to the parents, the nurse bases the explanation on the fact that Down syndrome is a:
   1. Condition characterized by above average intellectual functioning with deficits in adaptive behavior
   2. Condition characterized by average intellectual functioning and the absence of deficits in adaptive behavior
   3. Congenital condition that results in moderate to severe retardation and has been linked to an extra group G chromosome
   4. Condition characterized by subaverage intellectual functioning with the absence of deficits in adaptive behavior
21. A client with the diagnosis of major depression becomes more anxious on the unit, reports sleeping poorly, and seems be more irritable with staff and family. The nurse interprets the client's behavior as:
   1. The client is at increased risk for suicide
   2. A normal response to hospitalization
   3. The client is dealing with pertinent issues
   4. The client may need some time off the unit
22. A client is admitted with a venous stasis leg ulcer. The nurse assesses the ulcer expecting to note that it:
   1. Has a pale-colored base
   2. Is deep, with even edges
   3. Has little granulation tissue
   4. Has brown pigmentation surrounding it
23. A nurse is told that a client's potassium level is 3.2 mEq/L. Which of the following would the nurse note on the cardiac monitor as a result of the laboratory value?
   1. Elevated T waves
   2. Absent P waves
   3. Elevated ST segment
   4. U waves
24. An adult client with hepatic encephalopathy has a serum ammonia level of 95 μg/dL and receives treatment with lactulose syrup. The nurse would evaluate that the client had the best and most realistic response if the level changed to which of the following after medication administration?
   1. 80 μg/dL
   2. 40 μg/dL
   3. 10 μg/dL
   4. 5 μg/dL
25. A nurse assists in developing a plan of care for the child with meningitis. Which of the following would be the priority problem for this child?
   1. Ineffective cerebral tissue perfusion
   2. Parental knowledge deficit
   3. Dysfunctional family process
   4. Acute pain
26. A nurse is caring for a postoperative client. The physician has prescribed a clear liquid diet. In planning to initiate this diet, which of the following priority items would the nurse place at the bedside?
   1. Code cart
   2. A straw
   3. Cardiac monitor
   4. Suction equipment
27. A client is diagnosed as having irritable bowel syndrome. The nurse avoids telling the client to:
   1. Maintain a low-residue diet
   2. Provide fiber and bulk in the diet
   3. Eat regular meals
   4. Drink 8 to10 cups of liquid each day
28. A depressed client is ready for discharge. The nurse feels comfortable that the client has a good understanding of the disease process when the client states:
   1. "I'll never let this happen to me again. I won't let my boss or my job or my family get to me!"
   2. "It's important for me to eat well, exercise, and to take my medication. If I begin to lose my appetite or not sleep well, I've got to get in to see my doctor."
   3. "I've learned I am a good person and that I am worthy of giving and receiving love. I don't need anyone, I have myself to rely on!"
   4. "I don't know what happened to me. I've always been able to make decisions for myself and for my business. I don't ever want to feel so weak or vulnerable again!"
29. A nurse has given the client taking ethambutol (Myambutol) information about the medication. The nurse evaluates that the client understands the instructions if the client states to immediately report:
   1. Distressing gastrointestinal (GI) side effects
   2. Impaired sense of hearing
   3. Orange-red discoloration of body secretions
   4. Difficulty discriminating the color red from green
30. A nurse is caring for an elderly client with a diagnosis of myasthenia gravis and has reinforced self-care instructions. Which statement by the client indicates that further teaching is necessary?
   1. "I can change the time of my medication on the mornings that I feel strong."
   2. "I rest each afternoon after my walk."
   3. "If I get abdominal cramps and diarrhea, I should call my doctor."
   4. "I cough and deep breathe many times during the day."
31. A nurse is preparing to provide instructions to a client with Addison's disease regarding diet therapy. The nurse understands that which of the following diets would most likely be prescribed for this client?

1. Low sodium
2. High sodium
3. Low protein
4. Low carbohydrate

32. A client with diabetes mellitus who has been controlled with daily insulin has been placed on atenolol (Tenormin) for the control of angina pectoris. Because of the effects of the medication, the nurse checks which of the following signs or symptoms as the most reliable indicator of hypoglycemia?
    1. Tachycardia
    2. Sweating
    3. Blood glucose level
    4. Nervousness

33. A nurse is asked to regulate the flow rate of an IV solution being administered to a client. The IV bag contains 50 mL of solution and the solution is to be administered over 30 minutes. The administration set has a drop factor of 10 drops (gtts) per mL. The nurse would regulate the roller clamp on the infusion set to deliver how many drops per minute?
    1. 9
    2. 17
    3. 30
    4. 50

34. A nurse has reviewed the record of an assigned elderly client. Which of the following data would indicate a potential complication associated with age-related changes in the musculoskeletal system?
    1. Decrease in height
    2. Decrease in lean body mass
    3. Overall sclerotic lesions
    4. Changes in structural bone tissue

35. A nurse reinforces home care instructions to the mother of a child with Reye's syndrome. Which of the following statements by the mother indicates a need for further instruction?
    1. "I need to decrease the stimuli at home to prevent intracranial pressure."
    2. "I need to give frequent, small, nutritious meals to decrease the amount of vomiting."
    3. "I need to have the child nap during the day to provide rest."
    4. "I need to check for jaundiced skin and eyes every day."

36. A physician orders potassium chloride (KCl) elixir 20 mEq PO BID. The medication label states KCl, 30 mEq per 15 mL. The nurse prepares to administer the morning dose. How many milliliters will the nurse administer to the client?
    1. 10 mL
    2. 15 mL
    3. 32 mL
    4. 40 mL

37. A nurse is caring for a client who has bipolar disorder with aggressive social behavior. Which of the following activities would be most appropriate for this client?
    1. Ping pong
    2. Writing
    3. Chess
    4. Basketball

38. A client who chronically uses nonsteroidal antiinflammatory drugs (NSAIDs) has been taking misoprostol (Cytotec). The nurse understands that misoprostol was prescribed to:
    1. Decrease the platelet count
    2. Decrease the white blood cell count
    3. Relieve epigastric pain
    4. Relieve diarrhea

39. The nurse reads the chart of a client that was seen by the physician and notes that the physician has documented that the client has Lyme disease stage III. Which of the following clinical manifestations would the nurse expect to note in the client?
    1. Generalized skin rash
    2. Cardiac irregularity
    3. Enlarged and inflamed joints
    4. Paralysis in the extremity where the tick bite occurred

40. A physician orders 500 mL of 0.9% NS to run over 5 hours. The drop factor is 10 drops per 1 mL. The nurse plans to adjust the flow rate at how many drops per minute?
    1. 15 drops
    2. 17 drops
    3. 20 drops
    4. 22 drops

41. Which of the following data would the nurse determine as indicating that the client is experiencing a major depressive episode?
    1. The client is a male
    2. The client states, "Since my wife died last week, I've been waking up hours before I should and I'm tired all day."
    3. The client uses marijuana
    4. The client states, "The last three weeks, I'm doing all the things I used to do but I'm not enjoying them."

42. A nurse is assisting in planning discharge instructions for a postoperative client. Which of the following instructions would be least appropriate to include in the postoperative discharge plan of care?
    1. Wound care
    2. Activity restrictions
    3. Personal hygiene
    4. Turn and deep breathe

43. A nursing student is asked to discuss juvenile rheumatoid arthritis (JRA) at a clinical conference scheduled at the end of the clinical day. Which of

the following would not be included in the discussion?
1. It most often occurs before the age of 16 years
2. It is twice as likely to occur in boys than girls
3. The cause is unknown
4. Clinical manifestations include morning stiffness and painful, stiff, swollen joints

44. A nurse is caring for a child with spina bifida who has a neurogenic bladder. As part of the nursing care plan, the nurse would monitor for urinary tract infections. The nurse would anticipate that the most likely medication to be prescribed prophylactically would be:
1. Prednisone (Deltasone)
2. Furosemide (Lasix)
3. Sulfisoxazole (Gantrisin)
4. Immune globulin IV

45. A nurse provides medication instructions to a client with peptic ulcer disease. Which statement by the client indicates the best understanding of the medication therapy?
1. "The cimetidine (Tagamet) will cause me to produce less stomach acid."
2. "Sucralfate (Carafate) will change the fluid in my stomach."
3. "Antacids will coat my stomach."
4. "Omeprazole (Prilosec) will coat the ulcer and help it heal."

46. In planning activities for the depressed client, especially during the early stages of hospitalization, which of the following is best?
1. Provide an activity that is quiet and solitary in nature to avoid increased fatigue, such as working on a puzzle or reading a book
2. Plan nothing until the client asks to participate in milieu
3. Offer the client a menu of daily activities and insist that the client participate in all of them
4. Provide a structured daily program of activities and encourage the client to participate

47. A nurse is assisting in preparing a plan of care for a 4-year-old child hospitalized with nephrotic syndrome. The nurse suggests which intervention regarding diet therapy as most appropriate for this child?
1. Provide a high-protein diet
2. Discourage visitors at mealtimes
3. Encourage the child to eat in the playroom with others
4. Provide a high-sodium diet

48. A nursing instructor asks a student to describe the pathophysiology that occurs in Cushing's disease. Which statement by the student indicates an accurate understanding of this disorder?
1. "It is characterized by an oversecretion of glucocorticoid hormones."
2. "It is characterized by an undersecretion of glucocorticoid hormones."
3. "It is characterized by an oversecretion of insulin."
4. "It is characterized by an undersecretion of corticotropic hormones."

49. The nursing instructor asks the nursing student about the physiology related to the cessation of ovulation that occurs during pregnancy. Which of the following responses, if made by the student, indicates an understanding of this physiological process?
1. "Ovulation ceases during pregnancy because the circulating levels of estrogen and progesterone are high."
2. "Ovulation ceases during pregnancy because the circulating levels of estrogen and progesterone are low."
3. "The low levels of estrogen and progesterone increase the release of the follicle-stimulating hormone and the luteinizing hormone."
4. "The high levels of estrogen and progesterone promote the release of the follicle-stimulating hormone and luteinizing hormone."

50. A nurse is assisting in collecting data on a child with seizures. The nurse is interviewing the child's parents to establish their adjustment to caring for their child with a chronic illness. Which of the following statements by a parent would indicate a need for further teaching?
1. "Our child is involved in a swim program with neighbors and friends."
2. "Our child sleeps in our bedroom at night."
3. "Our babysitter just completed cardiopulmonary resuscitation (CPR) training."
4. "We worry about injuries when our child has a seizure."

51. A client is taking lansoprazole (Prevacid) for the chronic management of Zollinger-Ellison syndrome. The nurse advises the client to take which of the following products if needed for a headache?
1. Acetaminophen (Tylenol)
2. Ibuprofen (Motrin)
3. Naprosyn (Aleve)
4. Acetylsalicylic acid (aspirin)

52. A depressed client verbalizes feelings of low self-esteem and self-worth typified by statements such as "I'm such a failure. . . I can't do anything right!" The best nursing action would be to:
1. Tell the client that this is not true; that we all have a purpose in life
2. Remain with the client and sit in silence; this will encourage the client to verbalize feelings
3. Reassure the client that you know how the client is feeling and that things will get better
4. Identify recent behaviors or accomplishments that demonstrate skill ability

53. A nurse is assigned to care for an infant with cryptorchidism. The nurse anticipates that the most likely diagnostic studies to be prescribed would be those that check:
    1. Kidney function
    2. Babinski reflex
    3. DNA synthesis
    4. Chromosomal analysis
54. A nurse is caring for a client with a diagnosis of pemphigus. The nurse understands that a hallmark sign characteristic of this condition is:
    1. Homan's sign
    2. Chvostek's sign
    3. Trousseau's sign
    4. Nikolsky's sign
55. A client asks the nurse about the causes of acne. The nurse most appropriately responds by telling the client:
    1. "It is caused by eating chocolate, nuts, and fatty foods."
    2. "It is caused by oily skin."
    3. "The exact cause is not known."
    4. "It is caused as a result of exposure to heat and humidity."
56. The nurse is reviewing the health record of a pregnant client at 16 weeks of gestation. The nurse would expect to note documentation that the fundus of the uterus is located at which of the following areas?
    1. Midway between the symphysis pubis and the umbilicus
    2. At the umbilicus
    3. Just above the symphysis pubis
    4. At the level of the xiphoid process
57. After diagnosis of Lyme disease stage I, the nurse would anticipate that which of the following will be part of the treatment plan for the client?
    1. No treatment unless symptoms develop
    2. A 3-week course of oral antibiotic therapy
    3. Treatment with intravenous (IV) penicillin G
    4. Daily oatmeal baths for 2 weeks
58. A nurse is assigned to care for a child with a compound fracture of the arm that occurred as a result of a fall. The nurse plans care knowing that this type of fracture involves which of the following?
    1. The bone is broken but the skin over the area of the break is not
    2. The risk of infection is greater than the risk in a simple fracture
    3. One side of the bone is broken and the other side is bent
    4. The entire bone is broken across its width
59. A nursing student is asked to discuss the topic of clubfoot at a clinical conference. The student plans to tell the group that clubfoot:
    1. Is a rare deformity of the skeletal system
    2. Always occurs bilaterally
    3. Affects girls more often than boys
    4. Is a congenital anomaly
60. A client with type 1 diabetes mellitus is to begin an exercise program and the nurse is reinforcing instructions to the client regarding the program. Which of the following should the nurse include in the teaching plan?
    1. Perform exercise during peak times of insulin
    2. Administer insulin after exercising
    3. Take a blood glucose test before exercising
    4. Try to exercise before mealtime
61. A nurse is caring for an older client who is terminally ill. Which of the following signs indicates to the nurse that death may be imminent?
    1. Cold clammy skin and irregular noisy breathing
    2. Eupnea and normal body temperature
    3. Presence of swallowing reflex and active bowel sounds
    4. Rubor and hyperactive reflexes
62. A nurse has given the client with tuberculosis instructions for proper handling and disposal of respiratory secretions. The nurse evaluates that the client understands the instructions if the client verbalizes to:
    1. Wash hands at least four times a day
    2. Turn the head to the side if coughing or sneezing
    3. Discard used tissues in a plastic bag
    4. Brush the teeth and rinse the mouth once a day
63. A client has been taking isoniazid (INH) for a month and a half. The client complains to the nurse about numbness, paresthesias, and tingling in the extremities. The nurse interprets that the client is experiencing:
    1. Small blood vessel spasm
    2. Impaired peripheral circulation
    3. Hypercalcemia
    4. Peripheral neuritis
64. A nurse is preparing a 2-year-old child with suspected nephrotic syndrome for a renal biopsy to confirm the diagnosis. The mother asks the nurse "Will my child ever look thin again?" The nurse most appropriately responds by saying:
    1. "Wearing loose-fitting clothing should help conceal the extra weight."
    2. "In most cases, medication and diet will control fluid retention."
    3. "Do you feel guilty because you didn't notice the weight gain?"
    4. "When children are little, it's expected they'll look a little chubby."
65. A nurse is caring for a client hospitalized with acute exacerbation of chronic obstructive pulmonary disease (COPD). Which of the following would the nurse expect to note in this client?

1. Increased oxygen saturation with exercise
2. A shortened expiratory phase of respiration
3. Dyspnea on exertion
4. Hypocapnia

66. A nurse is caring for a client with a nasogastric tube connected to continuous gastric suction. The nurse observes that the client is mouth breathing, has dry mucous membranes, and a foul breath odor. In planning care, which nursing intervention would be most appropriate to maintain the integrity of this client's oral mucosa?
    1. Offer small sips of water frequently
    2. Encourage the client to suck on sour, hard candy
    3. Brush the teeth frequently; use mouthwash and water
    4. Use lemon-glycerin swabs to provide oral hygiene

67. A client is admitted to the hospital with possible rheumatic endocarditis. The nurse would check the client for signs and symptoms of concurrent:
    1. Viral infection
    2. Yeast infection
    3. Staphylococcal infection
    4. Streptococcal infection

68. A client taking hydrochlorothiazide (HydroDIURIL, HCTZ) has been started on triamterene (Dyrenium) as well. The client asks the nurse why both medications are required. The nurse formulates a response based on the understanding that:
    1. Triamterene is a potassium-sparing diuretic, whereas hydrochlorothiazide is a potassium-losing diuretic
    2. Hydrochlorothiazide is a potassium-sparing diuretic, whereas triamterene is a potassium-losing diuretic
    3. Both are weak potassium-losing diuretics
    4. Both are weak potassium-sparing diuretics

69. A Vigilon burn dressing is prescribed for the client with a partial-thickness burn to the arm. The nurse assisting in developing a plan of care for the client understands that the dressing will need to be changed:
    1. Daily
    2. Every 2 days
    3. Weekly
    4. Twice a week

70. A client who has begun taking fosinopril (Monopril) is very distressed, telling the nurse that he or she cannot taste food normally since beginning the medication 2 weeks ago. The nurse provides the best support to the client by:
    1. Requesting that the physician change the order to another brand of angiotensin-converting enzyme (ACE) inhibitor
    2. Reassuring the client that this is expected and generally disappears in 2 to 3 months
    3. Telling the client not to take the medication with food
    4. Suggesting that the client taper the dose until taste returns to normal

71. A nurse is planning to administer amlodipine (Norvasc) to a client. The nurse plans to check which of the following before giving the medication?
    1. Check blood pressure and pulse
    2. Check respiratory rate
    3. Check heart rate and respiratory rate
    4. Check level of consciousness and blood pressure

72. A client had an aortic valve replacement 2 days ago. This morning the client says to the nurse, "I don't feel any better than I did before surgery." The most appropriate response by the nurse is:
    1. "It's only the second day post-op. Cheer up."
    2. "This is a normal frustration, it'll get better."
    3. "You are concerned that you don't feel any better after surgery."
    4. "You will feel better in a week or two."

73. A nurse is assigned to care for a client admitted to the hospital with a diagnosis of systemic lupus erythematosus (SLE). The nurse reviews the physician's orders expecting to note that which of the following medications are prescribed?
    1. Antibiotic
    2. Narcotic analgesic
    3. Antidiarrheal
    4. Corticosteroid

74. A nurse administers an injection to a client with a diagnosis of acquired immunodeficiency syndrome (AIDS). After administering the medication, the nurse disposes the used needle by:
    1. Placing it in a puncture-resistant container
    2. Laying the needle and syringe on the bedside table and carefully recapping the needle
    3. Asking the client to recap the needle
    4. Recapping the needle before placing it in a puncture-resistant container

75. A nurse is assisting in conducting a research study and is identifying clients in the community at risk for latex allergy. Which client population is at most risk for developing this type of allergy?
    1. The homeless
    2. Individuals living in a group home
    3. Children in daycare centers
    4. Hairdressers

76. A client has just had a cast removed, and the underlying skin is yellow-brown and crusted. The nurse gives the client instructions for skin care. The nurse evaluates that the client has misunderstood the directions if the client states to:
    1. Soak the skin and wash it gently
    2. Scrub the skin vigorously with soap and water

3. Apply an emollient lotion to enhance softening
4. Use a sunscreen on the skin if exposed for a period of time

77. A client has skeletal traction applied to the right leg, and has an overhead trapeze available for use. The nurse would monitor which of the following as a high-risk area for pressure and breakdown?
    1. Scapulae
    2. Back of the head
    3. Right heel
    4. Left heel
78. A client has been placed in Buck's extension traction. The nurse can provide for countertraction to reduce shear and friction by:
    1. Slightly elevating the head of the bed
    2. Slightly elevating the foot of the bed
    3. Providing an overhead trapeze
    4. Using a footboard
79. A nurse has given the client with Bell's palsy instructions on preserving muscle tone in the face and preventing denervation. The nurse decides that the client needs additional information if the client stated to:
    1. Expose the face to cold and drafts
    2. Massage the face with a gentle upward motion
    3. Wrinkle the forehead, blow out the cheeks, and whistle
    4. Use a device for electrical stimulation of the face
80. A nurse is admitting a client with Guillain-Barré syndrome to the nursing unit. The client has an ascending paralysis to the level of the waist. Knowing the complications of the disorder, the nurse brings which of the following items into the client's room?
    1. Nebulizer and pulse oximeter
    2. Flashlight and incentive spirometer
    3. ECG monitoring electrodes and intubation tray
    4. Blood pressure cuff and flashlight
81. A client is admitted with an exacerbation of multiple sclerosis (MS). The nurse is assessing the client for possible precipitating risk factors. Which of the following factors, if stated by the client, would the nurse note as being unrelated to the exacerbation?
    1. A stressful week at work
    2. Ingestion of more fruits and vegetables
    3. A recent bout of the flu
    4. Inability to sleep well
82. A most common side effect associated with the administration of aluminum hydroxide gel (Amphojel) is:
    1. Diarrhea
    2. Constipation
    3. Muscle weakness
    4. Headache
83. A client with hyperphosphatemia is receiving aluminum hydroxide gel (Amphojel). The nurse understands that the usual adult dosage for this medication is:
    1. 10 mL BID
    2. 15 mL TID
    3. 30 mL QD
    4. 30 mL TID
84. A client with chronic renal failure is receiving ferrous sulfate (Feosol). Which of the following is a common side effect associated with this medication?
    1. Diarrhea
    2. Constipation
    3. Headache
    4. Weakness
85. A nurse is trying to communicate with a hearing-impaired client. Which of the following strategies by the nurse would be least helpful when talking to this client?
    1. Not showing frustration through facial expression
    2. Smiling continuously during conversation
    3. Facing the client directly while speaking
    4. Facing the client so that light falls on own face
86. A nurse is preparing to administer digoxin (Lanoxin) 0.125 mg orally to a client with congestive heart failure. The nurse checks which most important vital sign before administering the medication?

    Answer: ________________
87. A postoperative client has an order to receive an intravenous (IV) infusion of 1000 mL of normal saline solution over a period of 10 hours. The drop (gtt) factor for the intravenous infusion set is 15gtt/mL. The nurse sets the flow rate at how many drops per minute?

    Answer: ________________
88. A hospitalized child is diagnosed with respiratory syncytial virus (RSV). The nurse assisting in caring for the child obtains the necessary supplies to implement which type of precautions that will prevent transmission of the virus?

    Answer: ________________
89. A nurse is preparing to administer a prescribed intramuscular (IM) dose of meperidine hydrochloride (Demerol) 35 mg to a client. The medication label reads meperidine hydrochloride 50 mg per mL. How many mL will the nurse administer to the client?

    Answer: ________________
90. A nurse is calculating a client's 24-hour fluid intake. The client consumed coffee (8 oz), water (8 oz), and orange juice (6 oz) for breakfast; soup (4 oz) and iced tea (8 oz) for lunch; and a glass of milk (10 oz), a cup of tea (8 oz), and a glass of water (8 oz) for dinner. Additionally, the client consumed

24 oz of water during the day. How many mL did the client consume in the 24-hour period?
Answer: ________________

91. A nurse is preparing to suction a client through the client's tracheostomy tube. Select all interventions that the nurse would perform for this procedure.
_____Set the wall suction unit pressure at 160 mmHg
_____Don clean gloves before the procedure
_____Oxygenate the client before suctioning
_____Moisten the suction catheter tip in sterile saline solution before insertion
_____Apply suction while inserting the catheter
_____Advance the catheter until resistance is met and then pull the catheter back 1 cm
_____Apply suction while rotating and withdrawing the catheter
_____Allow no more than 10 seconds to suction

92. A nurse is preparing to administer an enema to an adult client. Select all interventions that the nurse would perform for this procedure.
_____Don gloves
_____Place the client in the right Sims' position
_____Ensure that the temperature of the solution is between 100 degrees F (37.8 degrees C) and 105 degrees F (40.5 degrees C)
_____Hang the container containing the enema solution 24 inches above the client's anus
_____Lubricate the enema tube and insert it approximately 4 inches
_____Clamp the tubing if the client expresses discomfort during the procedure

93. A nurse is assigned to care for an adult client who had a cerebrovascular accident and is aphasic. Select all appropriate interventions for communicating with the client.
_____Face the client when talking
_____Give the client directions using short phrases and simple terms
_____Avoid the use of body language when talking to the client
_____Use pantomime when talking to enhance words
_____Phrase what was said differently the second time, if there is a need to repeat something
_____Speak slowly and maintain eye contact

94. A nurse is preparing to set up a sterile field using the principles of aseptic technique to perform a dressing change. Select all appropriate interventions.
_____Use a dry table that is below waist level
_____Place the sterile field 1 foot behind the working area and out of view of the client
_____Open the distal flap of a sterile package first
_____Avoid placing items within 1 inch of any area surrounding the outer edge of the sterile field
_____Don clean gloves before touching items on the sterile field

95. A nurse is preparing to take an axillary temperature using a glass thermometer. Select all interventions that apply.
_____Shake down the mercury in the thermometer to 96 degrees F or below
_____Ensure that the client's axilla is moist before placing the thermometer
_____Place the thermometer in the center of the axilla
_____Place the client's arm at his or her side after putting the thermometer in place
_____Leave the thermometer in place for 8 to 10 minutes

ANSWERS

1. *Answer:* 4
Rationale: All the stomach contents are aspirated and measured before administering a tube feeding. This procedure measures the gastric residual. The gastric residual is assessed to confirm whether undigested formula from a previous feeding remains and thereby evaluates the absorption of the last feeding. It is important to assess gastric residual because administration of a tube feeding to a full stomach could result in over-distention, thus predispose the client to regurgitation and possible aspiration.
Test-Taking Strategy: Note that the issue of the question is the purpose of assessing residual. Focusing on this issue should direct you to option 4. Review this procedure if you had difficulty with this question.
Level of Cognitive Ability: Comprehension
Client Needs: Physiological Integrity
Integrated Concept/Process: Nursing Process/Data Collection
Content Area: Adult Health/Gastrointestinal
Reference: DeWit S: *Fundamental concepts and skills for nursing.* Philadelphia, 2001, WB Saunders, p. 503.

2. *Answer:* 4
Rationale: Simethicone is an antiflatulent used in the relief of pain resulting from excessive gas in the gastrointestinal tract. MOM is an antacid and laxative. Droperidol is used to treat postoperative nausea and vomiting. Acetaminophen is a non-narcotic analgesic.
Test-Taking Strategy: Use the process of elimination and note the key words "gas pains." Knowledge of the classifications to the medications in the options will direct you to option 4. If this question was difficult, review this medication.
Level of Cognitive Ability: Application
Client Needs: Physiological Integrity

Integrated Concept/Process: Nursing Process/Implementation
Content Area: Pharmacology
Reference: Hodgson B, Kizior R: *Saunders nursing drug handbook 2002*, Philadelphia, 2002, WB Saunders, p. 1007.

3. *Answer:* 4
Rationale: Change in appetite is one of the major symptoms of depression. Offering the client several small frequent meals and the nurse's presence at that time to support, encourage, or perhaps even feed the client are the most appropriate interventions. The client is experiencing poor concentration and will not understand the importance of an adequate nutritional intake. Weighing the client does not address how to increase nutritional intake. Reporting the nutritional problems to the psychiatrist is to some degree correct, but does not suggest how one might increase food intake.
Test-Taking Strategy: Use the process of elimination and focus on the issue, poor nutritional intake. Option 4 is the only option that addresses the altered nutrition concretely and designs a method in which the client will feasibly increase the nutritional intake. Review care to the client with depression if you had difficulty with this question.
Level of Cognitive Ability: Application
Client Needs: Physiological Integrity
Integrated Concept/Process: Nursing Process/Implementation
Content Area: Mental Health
Reference: Hill S, Bauer B: *Mental health nursing*, Philadelphia, 2002, WB Saunders, p. 133.

4. *Answer:* 3
Rationale: NPH is an intermediate-acting insulin. The onset of action is 3 to 4 hours, it peaks in 4 to 12 hours, and its duration of action is 16 to 20 hours. Hypoglycemic reactions most likely occur during peak time.
Test-Taking Strategy: Knowledge regarding the onset, peak, and duration of action for NPH insulin is required to answer this question. Recalling that peak action is between 4 to 12 hours will direct you to option 3. Review the characteristics of NPH insulin if you had difficulty with this question.
Level of Cognitive Ability: Application
Client Needs: Physiological Integrity
Integrated Concept/Process: Nursing Process/Implementation
Content Area: Pharmacology
Reference: Ignatavicius D, Workman M: *Medical-surgical: critical thinking for collaborative care*, ed 4, Philadelphia, 2002, WB Saunders, p. 1458.

5. *Answer:* 2
Rationale: Calcitonin can lower plasma calcium levels in clients with hypercalcemia secondary to hyperparathyroidism. The highest priority outcome in this client situation would be a reduction in serum calcium levels.
Test-Taking Strategy: Use the process of elimination. Noting the client diagnosis will assist in directing you to option 2. Additionally, note the relationship between the name of the medication and the word "calcium" in option 2. Review this medication if you had difficulty with this question.
Level of Cognitive Ability: Analysis
Client Needs: Physiological Integrity
Integrated Concept/Process: Nursing Process/Evaluation
Content Area: Adult Health/Endocrine
Reference: Lehne R: *Pharmacology for nursing care*, ed 4, Philadelphia, 2001, WB Saunders, p. 809.

6. *Answer:* 3
Rationale: DuoDerm contains hydroactive particles embedded in a polymer base, which are softened by wound moisture and act as a protective gel over healing tissue. It is applied directly to the wound and can be left in place up to 7 days.
Test-Taking Strategy: Knowledge regarding the use of DuoDerm is required to answer this question. Review this type of protective dressing if you had difficulty with this question.
Level of Cognitive Ability: Application
Client Needs: Physiological Integrity
Integrated Concept/Process: Nursing Process/Planning
Content Area: Pharmacology
Reference: Lewis S, Heitkemper M, Dirksen S: *Medical-surgical nursing: assessment and management of clinical problems*, ed 5, St Louis, 2000, Mosby. p. 205.

7. *Answer:* 4
Rationale: Males inherit hemophilia from their mothers and females inherit the carrier status from their fathers. Some females who are carriers have an increased tendency to bleed and, although it is rare, females can have hemophilia if their fathers have the disorder and their mothers are carriers of the genetic disorder. Hemophilia is inherited in a recessive manner via a genetic defect on the X chromosome. Hemophilia A results from a deficiency of factor VIII. Hemophilia B (Christmas disease) is a deficiency of factor IX.
Test-Taking Strategy: Knowledge regarding hemophilia and related etiology is required to answer the question. Review this disorder if you had difficulty with this question.
Level of Cognitive Ability: Comprehension
Client Needs: Physiological Integrity
Integrated Concept/Process: Teaching/Learning
Content Area: Child Health
Reference: Schulte E, Price D, Gwin J: *Thompson's pediatric nursing*, ed, 8, Philadelphia, 2001, WB Saunders, p. 235.

8. *Answer:* 3
Rationale: The confirmatory test for leukemia is microscopic examination of bone marrow obtained by bone marrow aspirate and biopsy. A lumbar puncture may be done to look for blast cells in the spinal fluid that are indicative of central nervous system disease. The WBC count may be high or low in leukemia. An altered platelet count occurs as a result of chemotherapy.
Test-Taking Strategy: Use the process of elimination. Note the key word "confirm." This key word and recalling that the bone marrow is affected in leukemia will direct you to option 3. Review diagnostic studies related to leukemia if you had difficulty with this question.
Level of Cognitive Ability: Comprehension
Client Needs: Physiological Integrity
Integrated Concept/Process: Nursing Process/Data Collection
Content Area: Child Health
Reference: Schulte E, Price D, Gwin J: *Thompson's pediatric nursing*, ed 8, Philadelphia, 2001, WB Saunders, p. 232.

9. *Answer:* 2
Rationale: When the child is nauseated, it is best to offer cool, clear liquids because they are soothing and better tolerated. It is best not to offer favorite foods when the child is nauseated because foods eaten during times of nausea will be associated with being sick. It is best to offer small frequent meals of high-protein and high-calorie content.
Test-Taking Strategy: Use the process of elimination. The issue of the question relates to nutritional status in a child with nausea. You should easily be able to eliminate options 3 and 4. From the remaining options, you may be tempted to select option 1. Recalling the issue related to nausea will assist in directing you to option 2. Review interventions related to these issues if you had difficulty with this question.
Level of Cognitive Ability: Application
Client Needs: Physiological Integrity
Integrated Concept/Process: Nursing Process/Implementation
Content Area: Child Health
Reference: Schulte E, Price D, Gwin J: *Thompson's pediatric nursing,* ed 8, Philadelphia, 2001, WB Saunders, p. 339.

10. *Answer:* 3
Rationale: Both preoperative and postoperative seizure precautions should be considered for any child with a brain tumor. A thorough neurological assessment should be performed on the child and the child's safety should be assessed before allowing the child to get out of bed without help. Options 1 and 4 are not required unless functional deficits exist. Option 2 is not necessary.
Test-Taking Strategy: Use the process of elimination. Note the key words "safe environment." Eliminate options 1 and 4 first because they are similar. Additionally, note the words "all times" in option 1. Eliminate option 2 because it is unnecessary. Review care to the child with a brain tumor if you had difficulty with this question.
Level of Cognitive Ability: Application
Client Needs: Safe, Effective Care Environment
Integrated Concept/Process: Nursing Process/Planning
Content Area: Child Health
Reference: Wong D, Hockenberry-Eaton M: *Wong's essentials of pediatric nursing,* ed 6, St Louis, 2001, Mosby, 1087.

11. *Answer:* 4
Rationale: The hallmark of stage I is the development of a skin rash at the site of the tick bite. The rash develops into a concentric ring, giving it a bull's eye appearance. The lesion enlarges up to 50 to 60 cm, and smaller lesions develop farther away from the original tick bite. In stage I, most infected persons develop flulike symptoms that last 7 to 10 days and these symptoms may recur later.
Test-Taking Strategy: Use the process of elimination and eliminate options 2 and 3 first because they are similar. Next, note that the question asks for the characteristic of stage I. From the remaining options, select the least serious, as the issue of the question relates to stage I. If you had difficulty with this question, review the stages of Lyme disease.
Level of Cognitive Ability: Comprehension
Client Needs: Physiological Integrity
Integrated Concept/Process: Nursing Process/Data Collection
Content Area: Adult Health/Integumentary
Reference: Black J, Hawks J, Keene A: *Medical-surgical nursing: clinical management for positive outcomes,* ed 6, Philadelphia, 2001, WB Saunders, 1829.

12. *Answer:* 3
Rationale: Because the placenta is implanted low in the uterus, cervical examination could cause disruption of the placenta and initiate profound hemorrhage. The other options are also correct, but the profound hemorrhage is of the greatest concern in this instance.
Test-Taking Strategy: Use the process of elimination. Note the key word "primarily." Recalling that bleeding is a primary concern will direct you to option 3. Review the care of the client with placenta previa if you had difficulty with this question.
Level of Cognitive Ability: Comprehension
Client Needs: Physiological Integrity
Integrated concept/Process: Nursing Process/Implementation
Content Area: Maternity
Reference: Burroughs A, Leifer G: *Maternity nursing,* ed 8, Philadelphia, 2002, WB Saunders, p. 226.

13. *Answer:* 4
Rationale: Comfort measures for nipple soreness include positioning the newborn with the ear, shoulder, and hip in straight alignment and with the baby's stomach against the mother's. Options 1, 2, and 3 do not identify measures that will alleviate the nipple soreness.
Test-Taking Strategy: Use the process of elimination to answer the question. Knowledge regarding the self-care measures to promote comfort to the mother with nipple soreness is required to answer the question. Review these measures if you had difficulty with this question.
Level of Cognitive Ability: Application
Client Needs: Health Promotion and Maintenance
Integrated Concept/Process: Self-Care
Content Area: Maternity
Reference: Murray S, McKinney E, Gorrie T: *Foundations of maternal-newborn nursing,* ed 3, Philadelphia, 2002, WB Saunders, p. 594.

14. *Answer:* 2
Rationale: Agoraphobia is a fear of leaving the house and experiencing panic attacks when doing so. Option 1 describes an obsessive-compulsive behavior. Option 3 describes a social phobia. Option 4 describes claustrophobia.
Test-Taking Strategy: Use the process of elimination. Focus on the key word "agoraphobia." This focus will assist in directing you to option 2. If you had difficulty with this question, review the various types of phobias.
Level of Cognitive Ability: Comprehension
Client Needs: Psychosocial Integrity
Integrated Concept/Process: Nursing Process/Data Collection
Content Area: Mental Health
Reference: Varcarolis E: *Foundations of psychiatric mental health nursing,* ed 4, Philadelphia, 2002, WB Saunders, p. 313.

15. *Answer:* 2
Rationale: In the Jewish religion, the dairy-meat combination is not acceptable. Pork and pork products are not allowed in the traditional Jewish religion. The nurse would not deliver

the food tray to the client and would ask the dietary department to deliver a new meal tray.
Test-Taking Strategy: Use the process of elimination recalling that the dairy-meat combination is not acceptable in the Jewish religion. Review the dietary rules of this religious group if you had difficulty with this question.
Level of Cognitive Ability: Application
Client Needs: Physiological Integrity
Integrated Concept/Process: Cultural Awareness
Content Area: Fundamental Skills
Reference: Hill S, Howlett H: *Success in practical/vocational nursing: from student to leader*, ed 4, Philadelphia, 2001, WB Saunders, p. 161.

16. *Answer:* 3
Rationale: When a corneal donor dies, the eyes are closed and gauze pads wet with saline are placed over them with a small ice pack. Within 2 to 4 hours the eyes are enucleated. The cornea is usually transplanted within 24 to 48 hours. The head of the bed should also be elevated.
Test-Taking Strategy: Use the process of elimination. Note that the issue relates to donation of the eyes. This should assist in eliminating options 2 and 4. From the remaining options, knowledge regarding care to the eyes of the deceased who is a donor will direct you to option 3. Review this procedure if you had difficulty with the question.
Level of Cognitive Ability: Application
Client Needs: Safe, Effective Care Environment
Integrated Concept/Process: Nursing Process/Implementation
Content Area: Fundamental Skills
Reference: Potter P, Perry A: *Fundamentals of nursing*, ed 5, St Louis, 2001, Mosby, p. 636.

17. *Answer:* 3
Rationale: Nursing interventions for the Alzheimer client who is angry, frustrated, or agitated include decreasing environmental stimuli, approaching the client calmly and with assurance, not demanding anything from the client, and distracting the client. It is important that the nurse reach out, touch, hold a hand, put an arm around the waist, or in some way maintain physical contact. Playing a radio may increase stimuli and turning the lights out may produce more agitation. The client with Alzheimer's disease would not be a candidate for group work if he or she is agitated.
Test-Taking Strategy: Use the process of elimination. Remember, calmly touching the client or putting an arm around his or her waist tends to distract the client and decrease the fear, frustration, or agitation being experienced by the client. Review care to the client with Alzheimer's disease if you had difficulty with this question.
Level of Cognitive Ability: Application
Clients Needs: Psychosocial Integrity
Integrated Concept/Process: Nursing Process/Implementation
Content Area: Fundamental Skills
Reference: Lueckenotte A: *Gerontologic nursing*, ed 2, St Louis, 2000, Mosby, p. 214.

18. *Answer:* 3
Rationale: Scopolamine is an anticholinergic medication that causes the frequent side effects of dry mouth, urinary retention, decreased sweating, and dilation of the pupils. The other options are incorrect.
Test-Taking Strategy: Use the process of elimination. Recalling that this medication is an anticholinergic will easily direct you to option 3. If this medication is unfamiliar to you, review the side effects associated with anticholinergics.
Level of Cognitive Ability: Application
Client Needs: Physiological Integrity
Integrated Concept/Process: Nursing Process/Implementation
Content Area: Pharmacology
Reference: Hodgson B, Kizior R: *Saunders nursing drug handbook 2002*, Philadelphia, 2002, WB Saunders, p. 998.

19. *Answer:* 1
Rationale: In the prevention of Lyme disease, individuals need to be instructed to use an insect repellent on the skin and clothes when in an area where ticks are likely to be found. Long-sleeved tops and long pants, closed shoes, and a hat or cap should be worn. If possible, heavily wooded areas or areas with thick underbrush should be avoided. Socks can be pulled up and over pant legs to prevent ticks from entering under clothing.
Test-Taking Strategy: Note the key word "not." Use the process of elimination noting that option 1 uses the word "avoid." If you had difficulty with this question, review measures to prevent contact with ticks.
Level of Cognitive Ability: Application
Client Needs: Safe, Effective Care Environment
Integrated Concept/Process: Self-Care
Content Area: Adult Health/Integumentary
Reference: Ignatavicius D, Workman M: *Medical-surgical: critical thinking for collaborative care*, ed 4, Philadelphia, 2002, WB Saunders, p. 361.

20. *Answer:* 3
Rationale: Down syndrome is a form of mental retardation. It is a congenital condition that results in moderate to severe mental retardation. The syndrome has been linked to an extra group G chromosome, chromosome 21 (trisomy 21).
Test-Taking Strategy: Use the process of elimination. Eliminate options 1 and 2 first because average and above average intelligence are not associated with this disorder. Eliminate option 4 because deficits in adaptive behavior do occur with Down syndrome. Knowing that Down syndrome is associated with an extra chromosome will assist in directing you to the correct option. Review the characteristics of this syndrome if you had difficulty with this question.
Level of Cognitive Ability: Comprehension
Client Needs: Physiological Integrity
Integrated Concept/Process: Nursing Process/Implementation
Content Area: Child Health Schulte E, Price D, Gwin J: *Thompson's pediatric nursing*, ed 8, Philadelphia, 2001, WB Saunders, p. 247.

21. *Answer:* 1
Rationale: The behaviors identified in the question may be manifested by the client who is contemplating suicide. Many of these symptoms are symptoms of the depressed client; however, with this client these behaviors have increased. Hospitalization may actually lessen these symptoms in the depressed client, as a feeling of hope or relief may occur once

treatment begins. Dealing with pertinent issues may be traumatic, but this is not the best option for the question. Time off the unit for this client could put the client at risk for injury.
Test-Taking Strategy: Use the process of elimination and focus on the client behaviors addressed in the question. Of the options presented, option 1 is the priority. If you had difficulty with this question, review the characteristics and client behaviors related to suicide.
Level of Cognitive Ability: Analysis
Client Needs: Psychosocial Integrity
Integrated Concept/Process: Nursing Process/Data Collection
Content Area: Mental Health
Reference: Varcarolis E: *Foundations of psychiatric mental health nursing*, ed 4, Philadelphia, 2002, WB Saunders, p. 641.

22. ***Answer:*** 4
Rationale: Venous leg ulcers, also called stasis ulcers, tend to be more superficial than arterial ulcers, and the ulcer bed is pink. The edges of the ulcer are uneven, and there is evidence of granulation tissue. There is a brown pigmentation to the skin from the accumulation of metabolic waste products resulting from venous stasis. The client also exhibits peripheral edema.
Test-Taking Strategy: Use the process of elimination. This question is asking you to discriminate between signs and symptoms of arterial and venous leg ulcers. Knowing that the information in options 1, 2, and 3 is due to tissue malnutrition (and thus an arterial problem) will assist in answering the question. Review the characteristics of a venous stasis ulcer if you had difficulty with this question.
Level of Cognitive Ability: Comprehension
Client Needs: Physiological Integrity
Integrated Concept/Process: Nursing Process/Data Collection
Content Area: Adult Health/Cardiovascular
Reference: Ignatavicius D, Workman M: *Medical-surgical: critical thinking for collaborative care*, ed 4, Philadelphia, 2002, WB Saunders, p. 745.

23. ***Answer:*** 4
Rationale: A serum potassium level below 3.5 mEq/L is indicative of hypokalemia. Potassium deficit is the most common electrolyte imbalance and is potentially life threatening. Cardiac changes include peaked P waves, flat T waves, depressed ST segment, and prominent U waves.
Test-Taking Strategy: Use the process of elimination. From the information in the question, you need to determine that this is a hypokalemic condition. From this point, it is necessary to know the cardiac changes that are expected when hypokalemia exists. Review these cardiac effects if you had difficulty with this question.
Level of Cognitive Ability: Analysis
Client Needs: Physiological Integrity
Integrated Concept/Process: Nursing Process/Data Collection
Content Area: Fundamental Skills
Reference: DeWit S: *Fundamental concepts and skills for nursing.* Philadelphia, 2001, WB Saunders, p. 447.

24. ***Answer:*** 2
Rationale: The normal serum ammonia level is 35 to 65 μg/dL. In the client with hepatic encephalopathy, the serum level is not likely to drop below normal. The most optimal yet realistic change would be to 40 μg/dL, which falls in the normal range. A level of 80 μg/dL represents insufficient effect of the medication.
Test-Taking Strategy: Familiarity with the normal serum ammonia level is needed to answer this question. It is also necessary to understand the association between hepatic encephalopathy and this laboratory value. Review this test and the desirable effects of this medication if you had difficulty with this question.
Level of Cognitive Ability: Analysis
Client Needs: Physiological Integrity
Integrated Concept/Process: Nursing Process/Data Collection
Content Area: Adult Health/Gastrointestinal
Reference: Chernecky C, Berger B: *Laboratory tests and diagnostic procedures*, ed 3, Philadelphia, 2001, WB Saunders, p. 150.

25. ***Answer:*** 1
Rationale: Ineffective cerebral tissue perfusion is the priority nursing diagnosis for the child with meningitis. Pain related to meningeal irritation may also be an appropriate problem, but is not the priority. There are no data in the question to indicate that options 2 and 3 are a problem.
Test-Taking Strategy: Use Maslow's Hierarchy of Needs theory to assist in eliminating options 2 and 3. Next, use the ABCs—airway, breathing and circulation—to direct you to option 1. Tissue perfusion relates to circulation. Review care to the child with meningitis if you had difficulty with this question.
Level of Cognitive Ability: Application
Client Needs: Physiological Integrity
Integrated Concept/Process: Nursing Process/Planning
Content Area: Child Health
Reference: Schulte E, Price D, Gwin J: *Thompson's pediatric nursing*, ed 8, Philadelphia, 2001, WB Saunders, p. 148.

26. ***Answer:*** 4
Rationale: In a postoperative client, a concern related to initiating a diet is aspiration. Suction equipment must be available. A cardiac monitor and a code cart are unnecessary. A straw may help the client sip fluids, but is not necessary.
Test-Taking Strategy: Note the key words "postoperative" and "priority." Use the ABCs—airway, breathing, and circulation—to answer this question. Option 4 will maintain airway clearance. If you had difficulty with this question, review care to the postoperative client.
Level of Cognitive Ability: Application
Client Needs: Physiological Integrity
Integrated Concept/Process: Nursing Process/Planning
Content Area: Fundamental Skills
Reference: DeWit S: *Fundamental concepts and skills for nursing,* Philadelphia, 2001, WB Saunders, p. 489.

27. ***Answer:*** 1
Rationale: The client with irritable bowel syndrome should be encouraged to include fiber and bulk in the diet to help produce bulky soft stools and establish regular bowel habits. Eating regular meals, drinking 8 to10 cups of liquids each day, and chewing food slowly promote normal bowel function.
Test-Taking Strategy: Use the process of elimination. Note the key word "avoids" in the stem of the question. Also note that options 1 and 2 are opposite client instructions. This should indicate that one of these options is the correct one. Recalling

that the goal is to establish regular bowel habits will assist in directing you to option 1. Review dietary measures for the client with irritable bowel syndrome if you had difficulty with this question.
Level of Cognitive Ability: Application
Client Needs: Health Promotion and Maintenance
Integrated Concept/Process: Nursing Process/Implementation
Content Area: Adult Health/Gastrointestinal
Reference: Ignatavicius D, Workman M: *Medical-surgical: critical thinking for collaborative care,* ed 4, Philadelphia, 2002, WB Saunders, p. 1242.

28. *Answer:* 2
Rationale: The exact causes of depression are not known but it is believed to be related to a biochemical disruption of neurotransmitters in the brain. Diet, exercise, and medication are recognized treatment of the disease process. Option 2 is the only option that incorporates a holistic treatment approach, including good nutrition, exercise, and medication.
Test-Taking Strategy: Use the process of elimination. Options 1, 3, and 4 offer no insight on the part of the client regarding the disease process. Also, note that option 2 is the global option. Review care to the client with depression if you had difficulty with this question.
Level of Cognitive Ability: Analysis
Client Needs: Psychosocial Integrity
Integrated Concept/Process: Nursing Process/Evaluation
Content Area: Mental Health
Reference: Hill S, Bauer B: *Mental health nursing,* Philadelphia, 2002, WB Saunders, p. 225.

29. *Answer:* 4
Rationale: Ethambutol causes optic neuritis, which decreases visual acuity and the ability to discriminate between the colors red and green. This poses a potential safety hazard when driving a motor vehicle. The client is taught to immediately report this symptom. The client is also taught to take the medication with food if GI upset occurs. Impaired hearing results from antitubercular therapy with streptomycin. Orange-red discoloration of secretions occurs with rifampin (Rifadin).
Test-Taking Strategy: Use the process of elimination. Option 1 is the least likely symptom to report; rather, it should be managed by taking the medication with food. Thus this option may be eliminated first. From the remaining options, it is necessary to know that this medication causes optic neuritis and difficulty with red-green discrimination. If this question was difficult, review the side effects of this medication.
Level of Cognitive Ability: Comprehension
Client Needs: Health Promotion and Maintenance
Integrated Concept/Process: Nursing Process/Evaluation
Content Area: Adult Health/Respiratory
Reference: Hodgson B, Kizior R: *Saunders nursing drug handbook 2002,* Philadelphia, 2002, WB Saunders, p. 421.

30. *Answer:* 1
Rationale: The client with myasthenia gravis should be taught that timing of anticholinesterase medication is critical. It is important to instruct the client to administer the medication on time to maintain a chemical balance at the neuromuscular junction. If the medication is not given on time, the client may become too weak to swallow. Options 2, 3, and 4 include the necessary information that the client needs to understand to maintain health with this neurological degenerative disease.
Test-Taking Strategy: Use the process of elimination and note the key words "further teaching is necessary." Basic principles related to medication administration will easily direct you to option 1. Remember, clients should not adjust dosage and medication times. If you had difficulty with this question, review the guidelines related to medication administration.
Level of Cognitive Ability: Comprehension
Clients Needs: Health Promotion and Maintenance
Integrated Concept/Process: Teaching/Learning
Content Area: Adult Health/Neurological
Reference: DeWit S: *Fundamental concepts and skills for nursing,* Philadelphia, 2001, WB Saunders, p. 651.

31. *Answer:* 2
Rationale: A high sodium, high complex carbohydrate, and high protein diet will be prescribed for the client with Addison's disease. To prevent excess fluid and sodium loss, the client is instructed to maintain an adequate salt intake of up to 8 grams of sodium daily and to increase salt intake during hot weather, before strenuous exercise, and in response to fever, vomiting, or diarrhea.
Test-Taking Strategy: Knowledge regarding the pathophysiology associated with Addison's disease will assist in answering this question. If you were unfamiliar with this disorder, review this content.
Level of Cognitive Ability: Comprehension
Client Needs: Physiological Integrity
Integrated Concept/Process: Nursing Process/Planning
Content Area: Adult Health/Endocrine
Reference: Black J, Hawks J, Keene A: *Medical-surgical nursing: clinical management for positive outcomes,* ed 6, Philadelphia, 2001, WB Saunders, p. 403.

32. *Answer:* 3
Rationale: Beta-adrenergic blocking agents, such as atenolol, inhibit the appearance of signs and symptoms of acute hypoglycemia, which would include nervousness, increased heart rate, and sweating. Therefore the client receiving this medication should adhere to the therapeutic regimen, and monitor blood glucose levels carefully. Option 3 is the most reliable indicator of hypoglycemia.
Test-Taking Strategy: Use the process of elimination. Note the use of the word "most reliable" in the stem. This indicates that more than one option could be partially or completely correct. Each of these options is, in fact, a sign or symptom of hypoglycemia. Knowledge of the masking effects of beta-adrenergic blocking agents helps you to choose the blood glucose level as the most reliable indicator. Review this medication if you had difficulty with this question.
Level of Cognitive Ability: Application
Client Needs: Physiological Integrity
Integrated Concept/Process: Nursing Process/Data Collection
Content Area: Pharmacology
Reference: Hodgson B, Kizior R: *Saunders nursing drug handbook 2002,* Philadelphia, 2002, WB Saunders, p. 85.

33. *Answer:* 2
Rationale: The formula for calculating IV drip rates is:

$$\text{gtts/minute} = \frac{\text{Volume (mL)} \times \text{drop factor (gtts/mL)}}{\text{time (in minutes)}}$$

$$= \frac{50 \text{ mL} \times 10 \text{ gtts/mL}}{30 \text{ minutes}} = \frac{500}{30}$$

$$= 16.66 \text{ or } 17\text{gtts/min}$$

Test-Taking Strategy: To calculate the answer to this question correctly, you must be familiar with the standard formula for calculating IV flow rates. Review this formula if you had difficulty with this question.
Level of Cognitive Ability: Application
Client Needs: Physiological Integrity
Integrated Concept/Process: Nursing Process/Implementation
Content Area: Fundamental Skills
Reference: DeWit S: *Fundamental concepts and skills for nursing,* Philadelphia, 2001, WB Saunders, p. 723.

34. *Answer:* 3
Rationale: Sclerotic lesions occur as bone resorption increases and results in replacement of original bone with fibrous material. This condition occurs in Paget's disease, an age-related disorder. Options 1, 2, and 4 identify normal age-related changes in the musculoskeletal system.
Test-Taking Strategy: Use the process of elimination. Note the key words "potential complication." Recalling the normal age-related musculoskeletal findings will assist in directing you to the correct option. Review these normal findings and those that indicate a complication if you had difficulty with this question.
Level of Cognitive Ability: Comprehension
Client Needs: Physiological Integrity
Integrated Concept/Process: Nursing Process/Data Collection
Content Area: Adult Health/Musculoskeletal
Reference: Lueckenotte A: *Gerontologic nursing,* ed 2, St Louis, 2000, Mosby, p. 744.

35. *Answer:* 2
Rationale: The vomiting that occurs in Reye's syndrome is caused by cerebral edema and is a symptom of intracranial pressure. Small frequent meals will not affect the amount of vomiting. Options 1, 3, and 4 are all correct statements. Decreasing stimuli and providing rest decrease stress on the brain tissue. Checking for jaundice will assist in identifying the presence of liver complications, which are characteristic of Reye's syndrome.
Test-Taking Strategy: Note the key words "need for further instruction." Recalling the causes of vomiting with Reye's syndrome will direct you to option 2. Review the pathophysiology associated with Reye's syndrome if you had difficulty with this question.
Level of Cognitive Ability: Comprehension
Client Needs: Health Promotion and Maintenance
Integrated Concept/Process: Teaching/Learning
Content Area: Child Health
Reference: Schulte E, Price D, Gwin J: *Thompson's pediatric nursing,* ed 8, Philadelphia, 2001, WB Saunders, p. 279.

36. *Answer:* 1
Rationale: Follow the formula for dosage calculation.

Formula:

$$\frac{\text{Desired}}{\text{Available}} \times \text{mL} = \text{mL per dose}$$

$$\frac{20 \text{ mEq}}{30 \text{ mEq}} \times 15 \text{ mL} = 10 \text{ mL}$$

Test-Taking Strategy: Follow the formula for the calculation of the correct dose. Label each figure including the answer. Focus on the key information: 30 mEq per 15 mL. Recheck your work and make sure that the answer makes sense. Review medication calculations if you had difficulty with this question.
Level of Cognitive Ability: Application
Client Needs: Physiological Integrity
Integrated Concept/Process: Nursing Process/Planning
Content Area: Fundamental Skills
Reference: DeWit S: *Fundamental concepts and skills for nursing,* Philadelphia, 2001, WB Saunders, p. 642.

37. *Answer:* 2
Rationale: Solitary activities that require a short attention span with mild physical exertion are the most appropriate activities initially for a client who is aggressive. Writing (journaling), walks with staff, and finger painting are activities that minimize stimuli and provide a constructive release for tension. Competitive games should be avoided because they can stimulate aggression and increase psychomotor activity.
Test-Taking Strategy: Use the process of elimination. Options 1, 3, and 4 are similar in that they are activities that the client cannot do alone. Review care to the client with aggressive behavior if you had difficulty with this question.
Level of Cognitive Ability: Application
Client Needs: Psychosocial Integrity
Integrated Concept/Process: Nursing Process/Implementation
Content Area: Mental Health
Reference: Hill S, Bauer B: *Mental health nursing,* Philadelphia, 2002, WB Saunders, p. 137.

38. *Answer:* 3
Rationale: The client who chronically uses NSAIDs is prone to gastric mucosal injury. Misoprostol is specifically given to prevent this occurrence. Diarrhea can be a side effect of the medication, but is not an intended effect. Options 1 and 2 are incorrect.
Test-Taking Strategy: Use the process of elimination and focus on the data in the question. Recalling the effects of NSAIDs will direct you to option 3. Review the action of this medication if you had difficulty with this question.
Level of Cognitive Ability: Analysis
Client Needs: Physiological Integrity
Integrated Concept/Process: Nursing Process/Implementation
Content Area: Pharmacology
Reference: Hodgson B, Kizior R: *Saunders nursing drug handbook 2002,* Philadelphia, 2002, WB Saunders, p. 742.

39. *Answer:* 3
Rationale: Stage III develops within a month to several months after initial infection. It is characterized by arthritic symptoms, such as arthralgias and enlarged or inflamed

joints, which can persist for several years after the initial infection. Cardiac and neurological dysfunctions occur in stage II. A rash occurs in stage I. Paralysis of the extremity where the tick bite occurred is not a directly related characteristic of Lyme disease.
Test-Taking Strategy: Use the process of elimination. Remember that a rash occurs in stage I, cardiac and neurological disorders in stage II, and joint involvement in stage III. If you had difficulty with this question, review the clinical manifestations associated with Lyme disease.
Level of Cognitive Ability: Comprehension
Client Needs: Physiological Integrity
Integrated Concept/Process: Nursing Process/Data Collection
Content Area: Adult Health/Integumentary
Reference: Black J, Hawks J, Keene A: *Medical-surgical nursing: clinical management for positive outcomes*, ed 6, Philadelphia, 2001, WB Saunders, p. 1829.

40. *Answer:* 2
Rationale: The prescribed 500 mL is to be infused over 5 hours. Follow the formula and multiply 500 mL by 10 (gtt factor). Then, divide the result by 300 minutes (5 hours × 60 minutes). The infusion is to run at 16.6 or 17 drops per minute.
Formula:

$$\frac{\text{Total volume in mL} \times \text{drop factor}}{\text{Time in minutes}}$$
$$= \text{Flow rate in drops per minute}$$
$$\frac{500 \text{ mL} \times 10 \text{ drops}}{300 \text{ minutes}} = \frac{5000}{300}$$
$$= 16.6 \text{ or } 17 \text{ drops per minute}$$

Test-Taking Strategy: Follow the formula for calculating the infusion rate for an IV infusion. Label the problem and the answer. Make sure that the answer makes sense. Be sure to change 5 hours to minutes. Review the formula for calculating infusion rates if you had difficulty with this question.
Level of Cognitive Ability: Application
Client Needs: Physiological Integrity
Integrated Concept/Process: Nursing Process/Planning
Content Area: Fundamental Skills
Reference: DeWit S: *Fundamental concepts and skills for nursing*, Philadelphia, 2001, WB Saunders, p. 723.

41. *Answer:* 4
Rationale: Major depression occurs twice as frequently in females as in males. Reacting to loss by experiencing altered sleep for 1 week is a normal grief response. Although depression is often associated with substance abuse, it alone would not indicate a major depression. Option 4 describes anhedonia (loss of pleasure in activities previously enjoyed).
Test-Taking Strategy: Focus on the issue, a major depressive episode. Use the process of elimination and knowledge of the epidemiology of and criteria for major depression to answer the question. Review the manifestations related to depression if you had difficulty with this question.
Level of Cognitive Ability: Analysis
Client Needs: Psychosocial Integrity
Integrated Concept/Process: Nursing Process/Data Collection
Content Area: Mental Health
Reference: Varcarolis E: *Foundations of psychiatric mental health nursing*, ed 4, Philadelphia, 2002, WB Saunders, p. 463.

42. *Answer:* 4
Rationale: The type of planning and instruction required varies with each individual and type of surgery. Specific instructions that the client needs to receive before discharge should include wound care, activity restrictions, dietary instructions, postoperative medication instructions, personal hygiene, and follow-up appointments. Turning and deep breathing are taught in the preoperative period.
Test-Taking Strategy: Use the process of elimination and note the key words "least appropriate." Options 1, 2, and 3 refer to information that needs to be taught in the postoperative period. Option 4 refers to information that should be taught in the preoperative period. Review instructions related to the preoperative and postoperative period if you had difficulty with this question.
Level of Cognitive Ability: Application
Client Needs: Health Promotion and Maintenance
Integrated Concept/Process: Nursing Process/Planning
Content Area: Fundamental Skills
Reference: DeWit S: *Fundamental concepts and skills for nursing*, Philadelphia, 2001, WB Saunders, p. 756.

43. *Answer:* 2
Rationale: JRA is twice as likely to occur in girls as boys. Options 1, 3, and 4 are accurate regarding this disorder.
Test-Taking Strategy: Note the key word "not." Knowledge regarding the etiology and clinical manifestations associated with JRA will direct you to option 2. Review this disorder if you are unfamiliar with JRA.
Level of Cognitive Ability: Comprehension
Client Needs: Physiological Integrity
Integrated Concept/Process: Nursing Process/Planning
Content Area: Child Health
Reference: Schulte E, Price D, Gwin J: *Thompson's pediatric nursing*, ed 8, Philadelphia, 2001, WB Saunders, p. 282.

44. *Answer:* 3
Rationale: The most likely medication to be prescribed to prevent urinary tract infection would be an antibiotic. A common prescribed medication is sulfisoxazole (Gantrisin). The neurogenic bladder prevents the bladder from completely emptying because of the decrease in muscle tone. Prednisone relieves allergic reactions and inflammation rather than preventing infection. Furosemide promotes diuresis and decreases edema caused by congestive heart failure. Immune globulin IV assists with antibody production with immune-compromised clients.
Test-Taking Strategy: Knowledge of the actions and uses of these medications is required to answer this question. Focusing on the data in the question will assist in directing you to option 3. Review these medications if you had difficulty with this question.
Level of Cognitive Ability: Comprehension
Client Needs: Physiological Integrity
Integrated Concept/Process: Nursing Process/Planning
Content Area: Pharmacology
Reference: Lehne R: *Pharmacology for nursing care*, ed 4, Philadelphia, 2001, WB Saunders, p. 965.

45. ***Answer:*** 1
Rationale: Cimetidine, a histamine H_2-receptor antagonist, will decrease the secretion of gastric acid. Sucralfate promotes healing by coating the ulcer. Antacids neutralize acid in the stomach. Omeprazole inhibits gastric acid secretion.
Test-Taking Strategy: Knowledge regarding the actions of the medications used to treat peptic ulcers is required to answer this question. If you are unfamiliar with these medications or their actions, review this content.
Level of Cognitive Ability: Comprehension
Client Needs: Health Promotion and Maintenance
Integrated Concept/Process: Teaching/Learning
Content Area: Adult Health/Gastrointestinal
Reference: Ignatavicius D, Workman M: *Medical-surgical: critical thinking for collaborative care,* ed 4, Philadelphia, 2002, WB Saunders, p. 1226.

46. ***Answer:*** 4
Rationale: A depressed person often suffers with depressed mood and is often withdrawn. Also, the person experiences difficulty concentrating, loss of interest or pleasure, low energy, fatigue, and feelings of worthlessness and poor self-esteem. The plan of care needs to provide successful experiences in a stimulating yet structured environment.
Test-Taking Strategy: Use the process of elimination. Options 1 and 2 are eliminated first because they are too restrictive and offer little or no structure and stimulation. Option 3 is eliminated next because of the absolute word "all" in this option. Review care to the client with depression if you had difficulty with this question.
Level of Cognitive Ability: Application
Client Needs: Psychosocial Integrity
Integrated Concept/Process: Nursing Process/Planning
Content Area: Mental Health
Reference: Hill S, Bauer B: *Mental health nursing,* Philadelphia, 2002, WB Saunders, p.133.

47. ***Answer:*** 3
Rationale: Mealtimes should center on pleasurable socialization. Encourage the child to eat meals with other children on the unit. A diet that is normal in protein with a sodium restriction is usually prescribed.
Test-Taking Strategy: Use the process of elimination. Eliminate options 1 and 4 first. A diet that is normal in protein with a sodium restriction is usually prescribed. Option 2 diminishes the importance of socialization at mealtime. This leaves option 3 as the correct option. Review dietary recommendations for the child with nephrotic syndrome if you had difficulty with this question.
Level of Cognitive Ability: Application
Client Needs: Physiological Integrity
Integrated Concept/Process: Nursing Process/Planning
Content Area: Child Health
Reference: Schulte E, Price D, Gwin J: *Thompson's pediatric nursing,* ed 8, Philadelphia, 2001, WB Saunders, p. 167.

48. ***Answer:*** 1
Rationale: Cushing's syndrome is characterized by an oversecretion of glucocorticoid hormones. Addison's disease is characterized by the failure of the adrenal cortex to produce and secrete adrenocorticol hormones. Options 3 and 4 are inaccurate in regard to Cushing's syndrome.
Test-Taking Strategy: Use the process of elimination. Option 3 can be eliminated first. Remembering that in C"u"shing's (up) syndrome, there is an oversecretion and in A"dd"ison's (down), there is an undersecretion will direct you to option 1. Review this disorder if you had difficulty with this question.
Level of Cognitive Ability: Comprehension
Client Needs: Physiological Integrity
Integrated Concept/Process: Teaching/Learning
Content Area: Adult Health/Endocrine
Reference: Black J, Hawks J, Keene A: *Medical-surgical nursing: clinical management for positive outcomes,* ed 6, Philadelphia, 2001, WB Saunders, p. 1416.

49. ***Answer:*** 1
Rationale: Ovulation ceases during pregnancy because the circulating levels of estrogen and progesterone are high, inhibiting the release of follicle-stimulating hormones and luteinizing hormones, which are necessary for ovulation. Options 2, 3, and 4 are incorrect.
Test-Taking Strategy: Knowledge regarding the hormonal changes that occur during the menstrual cycle and during pregnancy is required to answer this question. Review these hormonal changes if you had difficulty with this question.
Level of Cognitive Ability: Comprehension
Client Needs: Physiological Integrity
Integrated Concept/Process: Teaching/Learning
Content Area: Maternity
Reference: Murray S, McKinney E, Gorrie T: *Foundations of maternal-newborn nursing,* ed 3, Philadelphia, 2002, WB Saunders, p. 122.

50. ***Answer:*** 2
Rationale: Parents are especially concerned about seizures that might go undetected at nighttime. The nurse should suggest a baby monitor. Reassurance by the nurse should ensure parental confidence and decrease parental overprotection. Options 1 and 3 demonstrate parents' ability to choose respite care and activities appropriately. Option 4 is a common concern. Parents need to be reminded that, as the child grows, they can not always observe their child, but that their knowledge of seizure activity and care are appropriate to minimize complications.
Test-Taking Strategy: Use the process of elimination and note the key words "need for further teaching." Option 2 identifies a need to provide parents with an alternate manner to monitor for night seizures. Review parent teaching regarding seizures if you had difficulty with this question.
Level of Cognitive Ability: Comprehension
Client Needs: Psychosocial Integrity
Integrated Concept/Process: Nursing Process/Evaluation
Content Area: Child Health
Reference: Schulte E, Price D, Gwin J: *Thompson's pediatric nursing,* ed 8, Philadelphia, 2001, WB Saunders, p. 223.

51. ***Answer:*** 1
Rationale: Zollinger-Ellison syndrome is a hypersecretory condition of the stomach. The client should avoid taking medications that are irritating to the stomach lining. Irritants would

include aspirin and nonsteroidal antiinflammatory drugs (options 2 and 3). The client should be advised to take acetaminophen for headache.
Test-Taking Strategy: Use the process of elimination. Remember that similar options are not likely to be correct. With this in mind, eliminate options 2 and 3 first. Choose Tylenol over aspirin because it is least irritating to the stomach. Review this medication and this disorder if you had difficulty with this question.
Level of Cognitive Ability: Application
Client Needs: Physiological Integrity
Integrated Concept/Process: Nursing Process/Implementation
Content Area: Pharmacology
Reference: Hodgson B, Kizior R: *Saunders nursing drug handbook 2002*, Philadelphia, 2002, WB Saunders, p. 8.

52. *Answer:* 4
Rationale: Feelings of low self-esteem and worthlessness are common symptoms of the depressed client. An effective plan of care is to provide successful experiences for the client that are challenging but will not be met with failure to enhance the client's personal self-esteem. Reminders of the client's past accomplishments or personal successes are ways to interrupt the client's negative self-talk and distorted cognitive view of themselves.
Test-Taking Strategy: Use the process of elimination and therapeutic communication techniques. Eliminate options 1 and 3 because the nurse is offering an opinion and devaluing the client's feelings. Eliminate option 2 because in this situation, silence can be interpreted as agreeing with the client's feelings. Review care to the client with depression if you had difficulty with this question.
Level of Cognitive Level: Application
Client Needs: Psychosocial Integrity
Integrated Concept/Process: Nursing Process/Implementation
Content Area: Mental Health
Reference: Hill S, Bauer B: *Mental health nursing*, Philadelphia, 2002, WB Saunders, p. 134.

53. *Answer:* 1
Rationale: Cryptorchidism may be the result of hormone deficiency, intrinsic abnormality of a testis, or a structural problem. Diagnostic tests would assess kidney function, as the kidneys and testes arise from the same germ tissue. Babinski's reflex tests neurological function. DNA synthesis and a chromosomal analysis are unrelated to this diagnosis.
Test-Taking Strategy: Use the process of elimination and knowledge regarding the anatomical occurrence of cryptorchidism. Cryptorchidism, undescended or hidden testicles, relates to the genitourinary system. Option 2 relates to neurological function. Options 3 and 4 relate to the structure of cells. Option 1 is the only option that relates to the genitourinary system. Review this disorder if you had difficulty with this question.
Level of Cognitive Ability: Comprehension
Client Needs: Physiological Integrity
Integrated Concept/Process: Nursing Process/Planning
Content Area: Child Health
Reference: Schulte E, Price D, Gwin J: *Thompson's pediatric nursing*, ed 8, Philadelphia, 2001, WB Saunders, p. 149.

54. *Answer:* 4
Rationale: A hallmark sign of pemphigus is Nikolsky's sign. Nikolsky's sign is the ability to rub off the epidermis by slight friction or injury. Trousseau's sign is a sign for tetany in which carpal spasm can be elicited by compressing the upper arm and causing ischemia to the nerves distally. Chvostek's sign seen in tetany is a spasm of the facial muscles elicited by tapping the facial nerve in the region of the parotid gland. Homan's sign, a sign of thrombosis in the leg, is discomfort behind the knee on forced dorsiflexion of the foot.
Test-Taking Strategy: Use the process of elimination. If you knew that Homan's sign was related to thrombophlebitis and that Chvostek's sign and Trousseau's sign were related to tetany, then by the process of elimination, you would select option 4. If you had difficulty with this question, review these various signs.
Level of Cognitive Ability: Comprehension
Client Needs: Physiological Integrity
Integrated Concept/Process: Nursing Process/Data Collection
Content Area: Adult Health/Integumentary
Reference: Black J, Hawks J, Keene A: *Medical-surgical nursing: clinical management for positive outcomes*, ed 6, Philadelphia, 2001, WB Saunders, p. 1422.

55. *Answer:* 3
Rationale: The exact cause of acne is unknown. There is no evidence that consumption of foods such as chocolate, nuts, or fatty foods causes acne. Exacerbations that coincide with the menstrual cycle result from hormonal activity. Heat, humidity, and excessive perspiration also play a role in increased acne.
Test-Taking Strategy: Use the process of elimination. Note the key words "most appropriate" and focus on the issue, the causes of acne. Options 1, 2, and 4 relate specifically to factors that exacerbate acne. Review this disorder and its causes if you had difficulty with this question.
Level of Cognitive Ability: Application
Client Needs: Physiological Integrity
Integrated Concept/Process: Nursing Process/Implementation
Content Area: Adult Health/Integumentary
Reference: Schulte E, Price D, Gwin J: *Thompson's pediatric nursing*, ed 8, Philadelphia, 2001, WB Saunders, p. 340.

56. *Answer:* 1
Rationale: At 12 weeks' gestation, the uterus extends out of the maternal pelvis and can be palpated above the symphysis pubis. At 16 weeks, the fundus reaches midway between the symphysis pubis and the umbilicus. At 20 weeks, the fundus is located at the umbilicus. By 36 weeks, the fundus reaches its highest level at the xiphoid process.
Test-Taking Strategy: Knowledge regarding the patterns of uterine growth is required to answer this question. Focus on the weeks of gestation identified in the question to assist in directing you to the correct option. Review this uterine growth pattern if you had difficulty with this question.
Level of Cognitive Ability: Comprehension
Client Needs: Physiological Integrity
Integrated Concept/Process: Nursing Process/Data Collection
Content Area: Maternity
Reference: Murray S, McKinney E, Gorrie T: *Foundations of maternal-newborn nursing*, ed 3, Philadelphia, 2002, WB Saunders, p. 120.

57. *Answer:* 2
Rationale: Prevention, public education, and early diagnosis are vital to the control and treatment of Lyme disease. A 3-week course of oral antibiotic therapy is recommended during stage I. Later stages of Lyme disease may require therapy with intravenous antibiotics, such as penicillin G. Oatmeal baths will not help a systemic disorder.
Test-Taking Strategy: Use the process of elimination. Note the key words "stage I." Eliminate option 3 because IV antibiotics will not be administered in this stage. Eliminate option 4 because although oatmeal baths may be helpful for pruritis, they would not be helpful to treat a systemic disorder. Waiting for symptoms to develop is an incorrect option. Review the treatment associated with Lyme disease if you had difficulty with this question.
Level of Cognitive Ability: Comprehension
Client Needs: Physiological Integrity
Integrated Concept/Process: Nursing Process/Planning
Content Area: Adult Health/Integumentary
Reference: Ignatavicius D, Workman M: *Medical-surgical: critical thinking for collaborative care*, ed 4, Philadelphia, 2002, WB Saunders, p. 361.

58. *Answer:* 2
Rationale: In a compound fracture, a wound in the skin leads to the broken bone, and there is an added danger of infection. Option 1 describes a simple fracture. Option 3 describes a greenstick fracture. Option 4 describes a complete fracture.
Test-Taking Strategy: Use the process of elimination. Noting the key word "compound" will assist in directing you to option 2. Review the various types of fractures if you had difficulty with this question.
Level of Cognitive Ability: Comprehension
Client Needs: Physiological Integrity
Integrated Concept/Process: Nursing Process/Planning
Content Area: Child Health
Reference: Schulte E, Price D, Gwin J: *Thompson's pediatric nursing*, ed 8, Philadelphia, 2001, WB Saunders, p. 190.

59. *Answer:* 4
Rationale: Clubfoot, one of the most common deformities of the skeletal system, is a congenital anomaly characterized by a foot that has been twisted inward or outward. The condition generally affects both feet and boys are affected twice as often as girls.
Test-Taking Strategy: Use the process of elimination. Eliminate option 1 because of the word "rare" and option 2 because of the word "always." From the remaining options, it is necessary to know that this disorder is a congenital anomaly. Review this disorder if you had difficulty with this question.
Level of Cognitive Ability: Comprehension
Client Needs: Physiological Integrity
Integrated Concept/Process: Nursing Process/Planning
Content Area: Child Health
Reference: Wong D, Hockenberry-Eaton M: *Wong's essentials of pediatric nursing*, ed 6, St Louis, 2001, Mosby, p.1225.

60. *Answer:* 3
Rationale: A blood glucose test performed before exercising provides information to the client regarding the need to eat a snack first. Exercising during the peak times of insulin or before mealtime places the client at risk for hypoglycemia. Insulin should be administered as prescribed.
Test-Taking Strategy: The issue of the question relates to the occurrence of a hypoglycemic reaction. Use the process of elimination keeping in mind this issue and the action of insulin and exercise on the blood glucose level. You should easily be able to eliminate options 1, 2, and 4. Review the effects of exercise if you had difficulty with this question.
Level of Cognitive Ability: Application
Client Needs: Health Promotion and Maintenance
Integrated Concept/Process: Self-Care
Content Area: Adult Health/Endocrine
Reference: DeWit S: *Fundamental concepts and skills for nursing*, Philadelphia, 2001, WB Saunders, p. 447.

61. *Answer:* 1
Rationale: The clinical signs of impending or approaching death include inability to swallow; pitting edema; decreased gastrointestinal and urinary tract activity; bowel and bladder incontinence; loss of motion, sensation, and reflexes; cold or clammy skin; cyanosis; lowered blood pressure; noisy or irregular respiration; and Cheyne-Stokes respirations.
Test-Taking Strategy: Use the process of elimination and eliminate options 2 and 3 because these identify normal findings. Option 4 does not identify signs of approaching death. If you had difficulty with this question, review the signs associated with impending or approaching death.
Level of Cognitive Ability: Comprehension
Clients Needs: Physiological Integrity
Integrated Concept/Process: Nursing Process/Data Collection
Content Area: Fundamental Skills
Reference: Lueckenotte A: *Gerontologic nursing*, ed 2, St Louis, 2000, Mosby, p. 378.

62. *Answer:* 3
Rationale: The client with tuberculosis should wash the hands carefully after each contact with respiratory secretions. The client should cover the mouth and nose when laughing, sneezing, or coughing. Used tissues are discarded in a plastic bag. Oral care should be performed more than once a day.
Test-Taking Strategy: Use the process of elimination. Note that the question specifically relates to information about handling and disposal of secretions. The only options that address this topic directly are options 2 and 3. Because turning the head to the side for coughing and sneezing does not specifically address the handling of secretions, eliminate option 2. Disposal of tissues in a plastic bag is correct. Review home care instructions related to TB if you had difficulty with this question.
Level of Cognitive Ability: Comprehension
Client Needs: Health Promotion and Maintenance
Integrated Concept/Process: Teaching/Learning
Content Area: Adult Health/Respiratory
Reference: Ignatavicius D, Workman M: *Medical-surgical: critical thinking for collaborative care*, ed 4, Philadelphia, 2002, WB Saunders, p. 588.

63. *Answer:* 4
Rationale: A common side effect of isoniazid (INH) is peripheral neuritis. This is manifested by numbness, tingling, and

paresthesias in the extremities. This side effect can be minimized with pyridoxine (vitamin B_6) intake.
Test-Taking Strategy: Use the process of elimination. Options 1 and 2 would not cause the signs and symptoms presented in the question but instead would be manifested by pallor and coolness. Thus options 1 and 2 can be eliminated first. From the remaining options, it is necessary to know either that peripheral neuritis is a side effect of the medication, or that these signs and symptoms do not correlate with hypercalcemia. Review the side effects associated with isoniazid if you had difficulty with this question.
Level of Cognitive Ability: Comprehension
Client Needs: Physiological Integrity
Integrated Concept/Process: Nursing Process/Data Collection
Content Area: Adult Health/Respiratory
Reference: Hodgson B, Kizior R: *Saunders nursing drug handbook 2002*, Philadelphia, 2002, WB Saunders, p. 599.

64. *Answer:* 2
Rationale: It is important to give the mother information that addresses her concern. Most children experience remission with treatment. Options 1 and 3 are nontherapeutic and may add to the mother's guilt. Option 4 does not acknowledge the concern and is a stereotypical response.
Test-Taking Strategy: Use therapeutic communication techniques and focus on the mother's concern. Options 1, 3, and 4 do not address the mother's concern and are inappropriate and nontherapeutic responses. Remember, always address the mother's feelings and concerns. Review this disorder and therapeutic communication techniques if you had difficulty with this question.
Level of Cognitive Ability: Application
Client Needs: Physiological Integrity
Integrated Concept/Process: Communication and Documentation
Content Area: Child Health
Reference: *Potter P, Perry A:* Fundamentals of nursing, *ed 5, St Louis, 2001, Mosby,* p. 459.

65. *Answer:* 3
Rationale: Clinical manifestations of COPD include hypoxemia, hypercapnia, dyspnea on exertion and at rest, oxygen desaturation with exercise, use of accessory muscles of respirations, and a prolonged expiratory phase of respiration. The chest x-ray film will reveal a hyperinflated chest and a flattened diaphragm if the disease is advanced.
Test-Taking Strategy: Use the process of elimination. Eliminate option 1 because oxygen desaturation rather than saturation would occur. Next eliminate option 2 because in the client with COPD, a prolonged expiratory phase of respiration would be noted. From the remaining options, reading carefully will assist in directing you to option 3 as the correct option. If you are unfamiliar with the manifestations associated with COPD, review this content.
Level of Cognitive Ability: Comprehension
Client Needs: Physiological Integrity
Integrated Concept/Process: Nursing Process/Data Collection
Content Area: Adult Health/Respiratory
Reference: Ignatavicius D, Workman M: *Medical-surgical: critical thinking for collaborative care*, ed 4, Philadelphia, 2002, WB Saunders, p. 541.

66. *Answer:* 3
Rationale: After the nasogastric tube is in place, mouth care is extremely important. With one nares occluded, the client tends to mouth breathe, drying the mucous membranes. Frequent small sips of water would be contraindicated when the client is on gastric suction. The hard candy would increase the salivation, but would not be useful in cleaning the oral cavity. Lemon-glycerin swabs have a drying or irritating effect on the mucous membranes.
Test-Taking Strategy: Use the process of elimination and focus on the issue, maintaining the integrity of the oral mucosa. Recalling that a client on gastric suction will be NPO and swallowing water or other liquids would be prohibited will assist in eliminating options 1 and 2. From the remaining options, eliminate option 4 because lemon-glycerin swabs are drying to the mucosa. Review care to the client with a nasogastric tube if you had difficulty with this question.
Level of Cognitive Ability: Application
Client Needs: Physiological Integrity
Integrated Concept/Process: Nursing Process/Implementation
Content Area: Adult Health/Gastrointestinal
Reference: DeWit S: *Fundamental concepts and skills for nursing*, Philadelphia, 2001, WB Saunders, p. 495.

67. *Answer:* 4
Rationale: Rheumatic endocarditis is a major indicator of rheumatic fever, which is a complication of infection with group A beta-hemolytic streptococcal infections. It is frequently triggered by streptococcal pharyngitis. Options 1, 2, and 3 are incorrect.
Test-Taking Strategy: Use the process of elimination. Recalling that streptococcal infections are largely responsible for rheumatic heart disease will direct you to option 4. Review the causes of endocarditis if you had difficulty with this question.
Level of Cognitive Ability: Application
Client Needs: Physiological Integrity
Integrated Concept/Process: Nursing Process/Data Collection
Content Area: Adult Health/Cardiovascular
Reference: Ignatavicius D, Workman M: *Medical-surgical: critical thinking for collaborative care*, ed 4, Philadelphia, 2002, WB Saunders, p. 718.

68. *Answer:* 1
Rationale: Potassium-sparing diuretics include amiloride (Midamor), spironolactone (Aldactone), and triamterene (Dyrenium). They are weak diuretics that are of particular use when combined with potassium-losing diuretics. This is especially useful when medication and dietary supplement of potassium are not appropriate.
Test-Taking Strategy: From the construct of this question, the options are visually divided into two sets: options 1 and 2, and options 3 and 4. Neither 3 nor 4 makes sense, so eliminate these first. From the remaining options, it is especially helpful to remember that hydrochlorothiazide is potassium-losing. This will help you answer correctly by using the process of elimination. Review this medication if you had difficulty with this question.
Level of Cognitive Ability: Application
Client Needs: Physiological Integrity
Integrated Concept/Process: Nursing Process/Implementation

Content Area: Pharmacology
Reference: Hodgson B, Kizior R: *Saunders nursing drug handbook 2002*, Philadelphia, 2002, WB Saunders, p. 535.

69. *Answer:* 1
Rationale: A Vigilon dressing is used to clean small partial-thickness burns. It is a colloidal suspension on a polyethylene mesh support, is permeable to gases and water vapor, and provides a moist environment. It is changed daily.
Test-Taking Strategy: Use the process of elimination. Eliminate options 2 and 4 first because they are similar time frames. From the remaining options, recalling the use of this type of burn covering will assist in directing you to option 1. Review this type of burn covering if you had difficulty with this question.
Level of Cognitive Ability: Comprehension
Client Needs: Physiological Integrity
Integrated Concept/Process: Nursing Process/Planning
Content Area: Pharmacology
Reference: Ignatavicius D, Workman M: *Medical-surgical: critical thinking for collaborative care*, ed 4, Philadelphia, 2002, WB Saunders, p. 1564.

70. *Answer:* 2
Rationale: ACE inhibitors, such as fosinopril, cause temporary impairment of taste (dysgeusia). The nurse can tell the client that this effect usually disappears in 2 to 3 months even with continued therapy, and can provide nutritional counseling if appropriate to avoid weight loss. Options 1, 3, and 4 are inappropriate actions.
Test-Taking Strategy: Use the process of elimination. Eliminate option 4 first because it is an inappropriate nursing action. The nurse does not encourage dosage changes on any prescribed medication. Taking the medication with food is not going to change the taste of the food, so option 3 can be eliminated next. From the remaining options, you need to know that this effect occurs with all medications in the ACE inhibitor group. Thus you are left with the correct option, which is supporting the client through teaching. Review the effects of ACE inhibitors if you had difficulty with this question.
Level of Cognitive Ability: Application
Client Needs: Psychosocial Integrity
Integrated Concept/Process: Nursing Process/Implementation
Content Area: Pharmacology
Reference: Hodgson B, Kizior R: *Saunders nursing drug handbook 2002*, Philadelphia, 2002, WB Saunders, p. 484.

71. *Answer:* 1
Rationale: Before administering a calcium channel blocking agent, the nurse should check the blood pressure and heart rate, which could both decrease in response to the action of this medication.
Test-Taking Strategy: To answer this question, you must know that amlodipine is a calcium channel blocker, and that this group of medications decrease the rate and force of cardiac contraction. This in turn lowers the pulse rate and blood pressure. Option 2 can be eliminated first because it is unrelated to the medication. With options 3 and 4, note that only half of the option is correct. When answering questions such as these, with two items per option, both of the items must be correct for that option to be correct. Review this medication if you had difficulty with this question.
Level of Cognitive Ability: Application
Client Needs: Physiological Integrity
Integrated Concept/Process: Nursing Process/Planning
Content Area: Pharmacology
Reference: Hodgson B, Kizior R: *Saunders nursing drug handbook 2002*, Philadelphia, 2002, WB Saunders, p. 54.

72. *Answer:* 3
Rationale: Paraphrasing is restating the client's message in the nurse's own words. Option 3 uses the therapeutic communication technique of paraphrasing. The client is frustrated and is searching for understanding. Options 1, 2, and 4 are inappropriate communication techniques. Option 1 belittles the client's concerns. Option 2 and 4 offer false reassurance by the nurse.
Test-Taking Strategy: Use therapeutic communication techniques to answer the question. Option 3 focuses on the client's feelings. Review therapeutic communication techniques if you had difficulty with this question.
Level of Cognitive Ability: Application
Client Needs: Psychosocial Integrity
Integrated Concept/Process: Communication and Documentation
Content Area: Adult Health/Cardiovascular
Reference: Potter P, Perry A: *Fundamentals of nursing*, ed 5, St Louis, 2001, Mosby, p. 460.

73. *Answer:* 4
Rationale: Treatment of SLE is based on the systems involved and symptoms. Treatment normally consists of antiinflammatories, corticosteroids, and immunosuppressants. Options 1, 2, and 3 are not a standard component of medication therapy.
Test-Taking Strategy: Knowledge regarding the treatment for SLE is required to answer the question. If you are unfamiliar with the treatments normally prescribed in this disease, review this content.
Level of Cognitive Ability: Analysis
Client Needs: Physiological Integrity
Integrated Concept/Process: Nursing Process/Planning
Content Area: Adult Health/Immune
Reference: Black J, Hawks J, Keene A: *Medical-surgical nursing: clinical management for positive outcomes*, ed 6, Philadelphia, 2001, WB Saunders, p. 2157.

74. *Answer:* 1
Rationale: The correct procedure for needle disposal is to dispose of uncapped needles and sharps in a hard-wall, puncture-resistant container, immediately after use. Needles are not recapped.
Test-Taking Strategy: Use the process of elimination and principles related to the safe disposal of needles and syringes to answer the question. Note that options 2, 3, and 4 are similar in that they all address recapping the needle. Review these principles if you had difficulty with this question.
Level of Cognitive Ability: Application
Client Needs: Safe, Effective Care Environment
Integrated Concept/Process: Nursing Process/Implementation

Content Area: Adult Health/Immune
Reference: DeWit S: *Fundamental concepts and skills for nursing,* Philadelphia, 2001, WB Saunders, p. 863.

75. *Answer:* 4
Rationale: Individuals at risk for developing a latex allergy include health care workers; individuals who work with manufacturing latex products; females; individuals with spina bifida; individuals who wear gloves frequently such as food handlers, hairdressers, and auto mechanics; individuals allergic to kiwis, bananas, pineapples, passion fruits, avocados, and chestnuts.
Test-Taking Strategy: Focus on the issue, a latex allergy. Recalling the cause and the source of the allergic reaction will easily direct you to option 4. Review the cause of this type of allergy and the individuals at risk if you had difficulty with this question.
Level of Cognitive Ability: Analysis
Client Needs: Health Promotion and Maintenance
Integrated Concept/Process: Nursing Process/Data Collection
Content Area: Adult Health/Immune
Reference: Smeltzer S, Bare B: *Brunner and Suddarth's textbook of medical-surgical nursing,* ed 9, Philadelphia, 2000, Lippincott Williams & Wilkins, p. 1401.

76. *Answer:* 2
Rationale: The skin under a casted area may be discolored and crusted with dead skin layers. The client should gently soak and wash the skin for the first few days. The skin should be patted dry, and a lubricating lotion should be applied. Clients often want to scrub the dead skin away, which irritates the skin. The client should avoid overexposing the skin to the sunlight.
Test-Taking Strategy: Note the key word "misunderstood." Option 3 is obviously helpful and therefore cannot be the answer to the question as stated. Option 4 is good advice if the skin has been covered and is eliminated next. Options 1 and 2 seem to oppose each other, making it likely that one of them is correct. Because vigorous scrubbing is more likely to be irritating than providing gentle soaking, it is the most likely choice as the answer to the question. Review skin care measures after cast removal if you had difficulty with this question.
Level of Cognitive Ability: Comprehension
Client Needs: Health Promotion and Maintenance
Integrated Concept/Process: Nursing Process/Evaluation
Content Area: Adult Health/Musculoskeletal
Reference: DeWit S: *Fundamental concepts and skills for nursing,* Philadelphia, 2001, WB Saunders, p. 811.

77. *Answer:* 4
Rationale: Common areas that are under pressure and are at risk for breakdown include the elbows (if they are used for repositioning instead of a trapeze) and the heel of the good leg (which is used as a brace when pushing up in bed). Other pressure points caused by the traction include the ischial tuberosity, popliteal space, and Achilles tendon.
Test-Taking Strategy: Note the key words "high-risk area." Thus you would compare each of the options in terms of their relative risk and choose the one that is greatest. The right heel is eliminated first because it is off the bed in the traction setup. The overhead trapeze would diminish the likelihood that the scapulae and back of the head would be immobile. This leaves the left heel as the answer to the question. This makes sense, given that the client would use the unaffected heel to push into the mattress during repositioning. With repeated use, this could cause the left heel to become reddened and break down. Review the complications of skeletal traction if you had difficulty with this question.
Level of Cognitive Ability: Application
Client Needs: Physiological Integrity
Integrated Concept/Process: Nursing Process/Data Collection
Content Area: Adult Health/Musculoskeletal
Reference: Black J, Hawks J, Keene A: *Medical-surgical nursing: clinical management for positive outcomes,* ed 6, Philadelphia, 2001, WB Saunders, p. 599.

78. *Answer:* 2
Rationale: The part of the bed under an area in traction is usually elevated to aid in countertraction. For the client in Buck's extension traction (which is applied to a leg), the foot of the bed is elevated.
Test-Taking Strategy: To answer this question accurately, you need to understand the principles of traction and countertraction, and be familiar with Buck's extension traction. Option 3 is not used for the purpose of countertraction and is eliminated first. Knowing that Buck's extension traction is applied to the leg helps you eliminate option 1. Of the two remaining choices, option 4 places undue pressure on the client's unaffected foot. Furthermore, a footboard is not used for the purpose of providing countertraction. Option 2 provides a force that opposes the traction force effectively without harming the client. Review care to the client in Buck's extension traction if you had difficulty with this question.
Level of Cognitive Ability: Application
Client Needs: Physiological Integrity
Integrated Concept/Process: Nursing Process/Implementation
Content Area: Adult Health/Musculoskeletal
Reference: Black J, Hawks J, Keene A: *Medical-surgical nursing: clinical management for positive outcomes,* ed 6, Philadelphia, 2001, WB Saunders, p. 599.

79. *Answer:* 1
Rationale: Prevention of muscle atrophy with Bell's palsy is accomplished with the use of facial massage, facial exercises, and electrical stimulation of the nerves. Exposure to cold or drafts is avoided. Local application of heat to the face may improve blood flow and provide comfort.
Test-Taking Strategy: Use the process of elimination. Evaluate each of the options with regard to their effect on preserving muscle tone in the face. Options 2, 3, and 4 are plausible choices. Option 1 is unrelated to muscle tone and is also contraindicated in clients with this condition. Because of this, option 1 is the answer to this question as stated. Review this disorder if you had difficulty with this question.
Level of Cognitive Ability: Comprehension
Client Needs: Health Promotion and Maintenance
Integrated Concept/Process: Teaching/Learning
Content Area: Adult Health/Neurological
Reference: Black J, Hawks J, Keene A: *Medical-surgical nursing: clinical management for positive outcomes,* ed 6, Philadelphia, 2001, WB Saunders, p. 1996.

80. *Answer:* 3
Rationale: The client with Guillain-Barré syndrome is at risk for respiratory failure because of ascending paralysis. An intubation tray should be available for use. Another complication of this syndrome is cardiac dysrhythmias, which necessitates the use of ECG monitoring. Because the client is immobilized, the nurse should routinely assess for deep vein thrombosis and pulmonary embolism.
Test-Taking Strategy: Use the process of elimination. With an ascending paralysis, the client is at risk for involvement of respiratory muscles and subsequent respiratory failure. This knowledge makes you look for an option that coincides with this line of thought. Option 3 is the only option that includes an intubation tray, which would be needed if the client status deteriorated to needing intubation and mechanical ventilation. This option most directly addresses airway. Review care to the client with Guillain-Barré syndrome if you had difficulty with this question.
Level of Cognitive Ability: Application
Client Needs: Physiological Integrity
Integrated Concept/Process: Nursing Process/Implementation
Content Area: Adult Health/Neurological
Reference: Black J, Hawks J, Keene A: *Medical-surgical nursing: clinical management for positive outcomes,* ed 6, Philadelphia, 2001, WB Saunders, p. 2016.

81. *Answer:* 2
Rationale: The onset or exacerbation of MS is preceded by a number of different factors. These include emotional stress, fatigue, infection, physical injury, and pregnancy. There are no known methods of primary prevention. Intake of fruit and vegetables is an unrelated item.
Test-Taking Strategy: Use the process of elimination. If you examine each of the options, all but the fruit and vegetables option involves physiological or psychological stress. Because this option differs from the others, it is the likely correct answer. Review the precipitating risk factors associated with MS if you had difficulty with this question.
Level of Cognitive Ability: Comprehension
Client Needs: Physiological Integrity
Integrated Concept/Process: Nursing Process/Data Collection
Content Area: Adult Health/Neurological
Reference: Black J, Hawks J, Keene A: *Medical-surgical nursing: clinical management for positive outcomes,* ed 6, Philadelphia, 2001, WB Saunders, p. 2014.

82. *Answer:* 2
Rationale: Aluminum-containing antacids are constipating and the client should be instructed to take a stool softener or additional bulk-type laxatives to relieve this uncomfortable side effect. Options 1, 3, and 4 are not side effects of this medication.
Test-Taking Strategy: Knowledge regarding the purpose and side effects associated with administration of this important medication is required to answer this question. If you are unfamiliar with this medication, review this information.
Level of Cognitive Ability: Comprehension
Client Needs: Physiological Integrity
Integrated Concept/Process: Nursing Process/Data Collection
Content Area: Pharmacology
Reference: Lehne R: *Pharmacology for nursing care,* ed 4, Philadelphia, 2001, WB Saunders, p. 856.

83. *Answer:* 4
Rationale: The usual adult dose of aluminum hydroxide gel is 30 to 60 mL or 1 to 3 capsules before each meal or three times a day.
Test-Taking Strategy: Knowledge regarding the usual adult dosage for aluminum hydroxide gel is required to answer this question. If you are unfamiliar with this medication, review this information.
Level of Cognitive Ability: Comprehension
Client Needs: Physiological Integrity
Integrated Concept/Process: Nursing Process/Implementation
Content Area: Pharmacology
Reference: Lehne R: *Pharmacology for nursing care,* ed 4, Philadelphia, 2001, WB Saunders, p. 856.

84. *Answer:* 2
Rationale: Feosol is an iron supplement used to treat anemia. Constipation is a frequent and uncomfortable side effect associated with the administration of oral iron supplements. Stool softeners are often prescribed to prevent constipation.
Test-Taking Strategy: Recalling that oral iron can cause constipation will easily direct you to option 2. If you had difficulty with this question, review the side effects of Feosol.
Level of Cognitive Ability: Comprehension
Client Needs: Physiological Integrity
Integrated Concept/Process: Nursing Process/Data Collection
Content Area: Pharmacology
Reference: Lehne R: *Pharmacology for nursing care,* ed 4, Philadelphia, 2001, WB Saunders, p. 592.

85. *Answer:* 2
Rationale: Clients who are hearing impaired rely on visual cues to assist them to comprehend the conversation of others. Smiling continuously is the least helpful strategy because the smile distorts the appearance of the mouth if the client is trying to read lips. Facing the client and standing so there is light on the nurse's face are helpful because they assist the client to lip read. Taking care not to show frustration or annoyance with the client's impairment is also helpful to preserve the client's self-esteem.
Test-Taking Strategy: Note the key words "least helpful." To answer this question carefully, you must be familiar with general communication strategies as well as those that are helpful for the hearing impaired. If this question was difficult, review these communication strategies.
Level of Cognitive Ability: Application
Client Needs: Psychosocial Integrity
Integrated Concept/Process: Communication and Documentation
Content Area: Adult Health/Ear
Reference: DeWit S: *Fundamental concepts and skills for nursing,* Philadelphia, 2001, WB Saunders, p. 93.

86. ***Answer***: Apical heart rate
Rationale: Digoxin is a cardiac glycoside that is used to treat congestive heart failure and acts by increasing the force of myocardial contraction. Since bradycardia may be a clinical

sign of toxicity, the nurse counts the apical heart rate for 1 full minute before administering the medication. If the pulse rate is below 60 beats per minute in an adult client, the nurse would withhold the medication, report the pulse rate to the registered nurse who would then contact the physician.
Test-Taking Strategy: Noting that the client has congestive heart failure and recalling the action and nursing interventions related to administering this medication will assist in answering this question. Review nursing interventions related to the administration of digoxin if you had difficulty with this question.
Level of Cognitive Ability: Application
Client Needs: Physiological Integrity
Integrated Process: Nursing Process/Implementation
Content Area: Pharmacology
Reference: Hodgson, B., & Kizior, R. (2004). *Saunders nursing drug handbook 2004*. Philadelphia: W.B. Saunders, p. 310.

87. ***Answer***: 25gtt/minute
Rationale: Use the formula for calculating IV flow rates.
Formula:

$$\frac{\text{Total volume to infuse} \times \text{gtt factor}}{\text{Time in minutes}} = \text{gtt/minute}$$

$$\frac{1000 \text{ mL} \times 15 \text{ gtt/mL}}{10 \text{ hours} \times 60 \text{ minutes}} = \frac{15{,}000}{600} = 25 \text{ gtt/min}$$

Test-Taking Strategy: Follow the formula for calculating an IV flow rate and remember to change hours to minutes. Once you have done the calculation, recheck your work and make sure that the answer makes sense. If you had difficulty with this question, review IV flow rates.
Level of Cognitive Ability: Application
Client Needs: Physiological Integrity
Integrated Process: Nursing Process/Implementation
Content Area: Fundamental Skills
Reference: deWit, S. (2001) *Fundamental concepts and skills for nursing*. Philadelphia: W.B. Saunders, p. 723.

88. ***Answer***: Contact precautions
Rationale: RSV is a common causative agent of bronchiolitis, is easily communicable, and is acquired mainly through contact with contaminated surfaces. RSV can live on skin or paper for up to 1 hour and on cribs and other nonporous surfaces up to 6 hours. Although it is not airborne, it is highly communicable. Contact precautions are necessary. Meticulous handwashing decreases the spread of organisms.
Test-Taking Strategy: Recalling that RSV is acquired through contact with contaminated surfaces will assist in answering this question. Review care of the hospitalized child with RSV if you had difficulty with this question.
Level of Cognitive Ability: Application
Client Needs: Safe, Effective Care Environment
Integrated Process: Nursing Process/Planning
Content Area: Child Health
Reference: James, S., Ashwill, J., & Droske, S. (2002). *Nursing care of children: Principles & practice* (2nd ed.). Philadelphia; W.B. Saunders, p. 646.

89. ***Answer***: 0.7 mL
Rationale: Use the medication calculation formula and note the prescribed dose (35 mg) and the available dose (50 mg per mL).
Formula:

$$\frac{\text{Desired}}{\text{Available}} \times 1 \text{ mL} = \text{mL per dose}$$

$$\frac{35 \text{ mg}}{50 \text{ mg}} \times 1 \text{ mL} = 0.7 \text{ mL}$$

Test-Taking Strategy: Follow the formula for the calculation of the correct dose noting the prescribed dose and the available dose. Note that the prescribed dose is a smaller amount than the dose available. This indicates that the amount to be given will be less than 1 mL. Once you have done the calculation, recheck your work, and make sure that the answer makes sense. If you had difficulty with this question, review medication calculation problems.
Level of Cognitive Ability: Application
Client Needs: Physiological Integrity
Integrated Process: Nursing Process/Implementation
Content Area: Fundamental Skills
Reference: deWit, S. (2001) *Fundamental concepts and skills for nursing*. Philadelphia: W.B. Saunders, pp. 642-643.

90. ***Answer***: 2520 (or 2520 mL)
Rationale: The client consumed a total of 84 oz of fluid. Since 1 oz is equal to 30 mL, multiply 84 oz by 30 mL. This yields 2520 mL.
Test-Taking Strategy: Focus on the issue, the total mL that the client consumed in a 24-hour period. Recalling that 1 oz equals 30 mL will assist in answering the question. Review the procedure for changing ounces to mL if you had difficulty with this question.
Level of Cognitive Ability: Comprehension
Client Needs: Physiological Integrity
Integrated Process: Nursing Process/Data Collection
Content Area: Fundamental Skills
Reference: deWit, S. (2001) *Fundamental concepts and skills for nursing*. Philadelphia: W.B. Saunders, p. 455.

91. ***Answer***:
-Oxygenate the client before suctioning
-Moisten the suction catheter tip in sterile saline solution before insertion
-Advance the catheter until resistance is met and then pull the catheter back 1 cm
-Apply suction while rotating and withdrawing the catheter
-Allow no more than 10 seconds to suction
Rationale: Wall suction unit pressure is set between 80 and 120 mmHg maximum. Pressure set at a higher level can cause trauma to respiratory tract tissues. Strict asepsis needs to be maintained and the nurse would wear sterile gloves to perform this procedure. The client should be preoxygenated using a resuscitator bag to prevent hypoxia during suctioning. Moistening the suction catheter tip in sterile saline solution before insertion lubricates the catheter and makes it easier to introduce. Suction is not applied on insertion of the catheter

because it will deplete oxygen and can traumatize tissues. When inserting the catheter, resistance will occur when the catheter reaches the carina (junction of the main bronchi). At this point the nurse pulls the catheter back 1 cm. The nurse applies suction while rotating and withdrawing the catheter to remove secretions around the circumference of the trachea. Suctioning for more than 10 seconds depletes the client's oxygen.
Test-Taking Strategy: Focus on the issue, suctioning procedure through a tracheostomy. The priority issues to think about when answering this question include maintaining oxygenation, maintaining asepsis, and preventing tissue trauma. This will assist in selecting the correct interventions. Review suctioning procedure if you had difficulty with this question.
Level of Cognitive Ability: Application
Client Needs: Physiological Integrity
Integrated Process: Nursing Process/Implementation
Content Area: Adult Health/Respiratory
Reference: deWit, S. (2001) *Fundamental concepts and skills for nursing*. Philadelphia: W.B. Saunders, pp. 537-538.

92. ***Answer***:
-Don gloves
-Ensure that the temperature of the solution is between 100 degrees F (37.8 degrees C) and 105 degrees F (40.5 degrees C)
-Lubricate the enema tube and insert it approximately 4 inches
-Clamp the tubing if the client expresses discomfort during the procedure
Rationale: The nurse wears gloves when administering an enema to prevent the transfer of microorganisms. To administer an enema, the nurse places the client in the left Sims' position because the enema solution will travel up the colon more easily in this position. The temperature of the solution should be between 100 degrees F (37.8 degrees C) and 105 degrees F (40.5 degrees C). Solution that is too hot will burn the client and solution that is too cool will cause cramping. The container containing the enema solution is hung about 12 to 18 inches above the client's anus. A flow of solution that is too forceful can damage the bowel. The tube is lubricated for easy insertion and is inserted approximately 4 inches in an adult. If the client complains of cramping or discomfort during the procedure, the nurse clamps the tubing until the discomfort subsides.
Test-Taking Strategy: Visualize the procedure for administering an enema. Thinking about the anatomy of the bowel and the precautions that need to be taken to prevent trauma to rectal tissue will assist in identifying the correct interventions. Review the procedure for administering an enema if you had difficulty with this question.
Level of Cognitive Ability: Application
Client Needs: Physiological Integrity
Integrated Process: Nursing Process/Implementation
Content Area: Fundamental Skills
Reference: deWit, S. (2001) *Fundamental concepts and skills for nursing*. Philadelphia: W.B. Saunders, pp. 593-594.

93. ***Answer***:
-Face the client when talking
-Give the client directions using short phrases and simple terms
-Use pantomime when talking to enhance words
-Speak slowly and maintain eye contact
Rationale: A client who is aphasic has difficulty expressing or understanding language. The nurse would face the client when talking, establish and maintain eye contact, and speak slowly and distinctly. The nurse should use pantomime when talking to enhance words and body language to enhance the message. The nurse would give the client directions using short phrases and simple terms and phrase questions so that they can be answered with a yes or no. If there is a need to repeat something, the nurse should use the same words a second time.
Test-Taking Strategy: Recall that a client who is aphasic has difficulty expressing or understanding language. Using the principles related to communicating to a client who is hearing-impaired will assist in identifying the correct interventions. Review the guidelines for communicating with an aphasic client if you had difficulty with this question.
Level of Cognitive Ability: Application
Client Needs: Physiological Integrity
Integrated Process: Communication and Documentation
Content Area: Fundamental Skills
Reference: deWit, S. (2001) *Fundamental concepts and skills for nursing*. Philadelphia: W.B. Saunders, p. 93.

94. ***Answer***:
-Open the distal flap of a sterile package first
-Avoid placing items within 1 inch of any area surrounding the outer edge of the sterile field
Rationale: A dry table that is above waist level is used to set up a sterile field. Moisture will contaminate the sterile field and anything below waist level is considered contaminated according to the principles of surgical asepsis. The sterile field must be kept in sight at all times and the nurse should not turn away from it. If this happens, the nurse cannot be sure that it is still sterile. Sterile packages are opened away from the nurse's body and the distal flap of a sterile package is opened first. This prevents contaminating the pack by reaching over the exposed sterile contents after the other flaps are opened. An area of 1 inch surrounding the outer edge of the sterile field must be considered unsterile and sterile items are not placed in this 1 inch area. Sterile not clean gloves are used. An unsterile item touching a sterile item contaminates the sterile item.
Test-Taking Strategy: Focus on the issue, the principles of aseptic technique. Thinking about these principles and visualizing each intervention will assist in identifying those that are appropriate. Review the principles of aseptic technique if you had difficulty with this question.
Level of Cognitive Ability: Application
Client Needs: Safe, Effective Care Environment
Integrated Process: Nursing Process/Implementation
Content Area: Fundamental Skills
Reference: deWit, S. (2001) *Fundamental concepts and skills for nursing*. Philadelphia: W.B. Saunders, pp. 236; 241-242.

95. ***Answer***:
-Shake down the mercury in the thermometer to 96 degrees F or below
-Place the thermometer in the center of the axilla
-Leave the thermometer in place for 8 to 10 minutes

Rationale: If the mercury in the thermometer is above 96 degrees F, the nurse would shake down the mercury with a flick action of the wrist. The nurse places the thermometer in the client's dry axilla because a wet axilla will give a false reading of body temperature. The nurse asks the client to hold the arm tightly against the chest (not at his or her side), resting the arm on the chest. When taking an axillary temperature, longer contact is needed than with an oral temperature to obtain an accurate reading and the thermometer is left in place for 8 to 10 minutes.

Test-Taking Strategy: Focus on the issue, taking an axillary temperature using a glass thermometer. Visualize each of the interventions to assist in identifying the correct actions. Review the procedure for taking an axillary temperature if you had difficulty with this question.
Level of Cognitive Ability: Application
Client Needs: Physiological Integrity
Integrated Process: Nursing Process/Implementation
Content Area: Fundamental Skills
Reference: deWit, S. (2001) *Fundamental concepts and skills for nursing*. Philadelphia: W.B. Saunders, pp. 344-345.

REFERENCES

Black J, Hawks J, Keene A: *Medical-surgical nursing: clinical management for positive outcomes*, ed 6, Philadelphia, 2001, WB Saunders.

Burroughs A, Leifer G: *Maternity nursing*, ed 8, Philadelphia, 2002, WB Saunders.

Chernecky C, Berger B: *Laboratory tests and diagnostic procedures*, ed 3, Philadelphia, 2001, WB Saunders.

DeWit S: *Fundamental concepts and skills for nursing*, Philadelphia, 2001, WB Saunders.

Hill S, Bauer B: *Mental health nursing*, Philadelphia, 2000, WB Saunders.

Hodgson B, Kizior R: *Saunders nursing drug handbook 2002*, Philadelphia, 2002, WB Saunders.

Ignatavicius D, Workman M: *Medical-surgical: critical thinking for collaborative care*, ed 4, Philadelphia, 2002, WB Saunders.

Lehne R, *Pharmacology for nursing care*, ed 4, Philadelphia, 2001, WB Saunders.

Lewis S, Heitkemper M, Dirksen S: *Medical-surgical nursing: assessment and management of clinical problems*, ed 5, St Louis, 2000, Mosby.

Lueckenotte A: *Gerontologic nursing*, ed 2, St Louis, 2000, Mosby.

Murray S, McKinney E, Gorrie T: *Foundations of maternal-newborn nursing*, ed 3, Philadelphia, 2002, WB Saunders.

Potter P, Perry A: *Fundamentals of nursing*, ed 5, St Louis, 2001, Mosby.

Schulte E, Price D, Gwin J: *Thompson's pediatric nursing*, ed 8, Philadelphia, 2001, WB Saunders.

Smeltzer S, Bare B: *Brunner and Suddarth's textbook of medical-surgical nursing*, ed 9, Philadelphia, 2000, Lippincott Williams & Wilkins.

Varcarolis E: *Foundations of psychiatric mental health nursing*, ed 4, Philadelphia, 2002, WB Saunders.

Wong D, Hockenberry-Eaton M: *Wong's essentials of pediatric nursing*, ed 6, St Louis, 2001, Mosby.

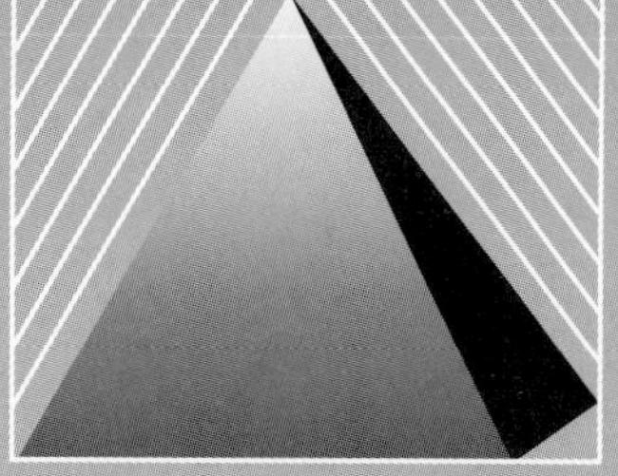

Index

A

Page numbers followed by *f* indicates figures, *t* indicates tables, and *b* indicates boxes.

B

C

E

F

H

I

M

O

T

U

V